MW01600446

Gary R. Lichtenstein
Editor

# Medical Therapy
# of Ulcerative Colitis

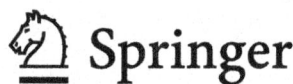 Springer

*Editor*
Gary R. Lichtenstein, MD, FACP, FACG, AGAF
Professor of Medicine
University of Pennsylvania School of Medicine
Director, Center for Inflammatory Bowel Diseases
University of Pennsylvania Health System
Hospital of the University of Pennsylvania
Gastroenterology Division
Philadelphia, PA, USA

ISBN 978-1-4939-4166-7      ISBN 978-1-4939-1677-1 (eBook)
DOI 10.1007/978-1-4939-1677-1
Springer New York Heidelberg Dordrecht London

© Springer Science+Business Media New York 2014
Softcover reprint of the hardcover 1st edition 2014
This work is subject to copyright. All rights are reserved by the Publisher, whether the whole or part of the material is concerned, specifically the rights of translation, reprinting, reuse of illustrations, recitation, broadcasting, reproduction on microfilms or in any other physical way, and transmission or information storage and retrieval, electronic adaptation, computer software, or by similar or dissimilar methodology now known or hereafter developed. Exempted from this legal reservation are brief excerpts in connection with reviews or scholarly analysis or material supplied specifically for the purpose of being entered and executed on a computer system, for exclusive use by the purchaser of the work. Duplication of this publication or parts thereof is permitted only under the provisions of the Copyright Law of the Publisher's location, in its current version, and permission for use must always be obtained from Springer. Permissions for use may be obtained through RightsLink at the Copyright Clearance Center. Violations are liable to prosecution under the respective Copyright Law.
The use of general descriptive names, registered names, trademarks, service marks, etc. in this publication does not imply, even in the absence of a specific statement, that such names are exempt from the relevant protective laws and regulations and therefore free for general use.
While the advice and information in this book are believed to be true and accurate at the date of publication, neither the authors nor the editors nor the publisher can accept any legal responsibility for any errors or omissions that may be made. The publisher makes no warranty, express or implied, with respect to the material contained herein.

Springer is part of Springer Science+Business Media (www.springer.com)

# Preface

Since the landmark description of ulcerative colitis by Dr. Samuel Wilks and Dr. Walter Moxon in 1859, much has been learned about the etiology, pathogenesis, and treatment of these two idiopathic inflammatory bowel disorders. Ulcerative colitis occurs at any age, spares no socioeconomic class, and has the potential to significantly impair patient's quality of life. Substantial progress has been made in the past decade related to ulcerative colitis; however, improvements and expansion of the medical armamentarium used to treat patients with ulcerative colitis have had the greatest impact on patients' lives.

This textbook entitled "Medical Therapy of Ulcerative Colitis" represents the first edition. The authors who were assimilated to contribute to this textbook are the key opinion leaders who are regionally, nationally, and internationally recognized as authorities in inflammatory bowel disease. These authors have made major contributions to the literature that has focused on medical therapy of inflammatory bowel specifically ulcerative colitis. In this book, the authors discuss the current medical therapies and review the clinical trial data that established the foundation for their use. The individual chapters in this book not only review the current medical therapy in use for treatment of patients with Ulcerative Colitis but they also review the basic pathophysiologic principles supporting the use of these and future therapeutics. The utility of mesalamine derivatives, conventional and novel corticosteroids, immunomodulators, AntiTNF therapy, and small adhesion molecules are reviewed in detail. Additionally, novel therapeutics that have potential impact and significance to the practicing physician are highlighted.

I am grateful to my contributors for providing superb, detailed, critical chapters amid their already busy schedules. I am most appreciative and extend thanks to all my colleagues, patients, and those who have supported research in the field, who have helped me uncover and extend the boundaries of my knowledge in inflammatory bowel disease. Lastly, I am most appreciative of my wife Nancy and my children Danielle and Julie for allowing me to spend countless hours doing what I thoroughly enjoy: patient care, research, and education. I feel it is a privilege to do what I do and I thank all for facilitating my enjoyment.

Philadelphia, PA, USA                                Gary R. Lichtenstein, MD, FACP, FACG, AGAF

# Contents

# Contributors

**Faten N. Aberra, M.D., M.S.C.E.** Division of Gastroenterology, Department of Medicine, Hospital of the University of Pennsylvania, Perelman School of Medicine at the University of Pennsylvania, Philadelphia, PA, USA

**Jean-Paul Achkar, M.D., F.A.C.G.** Department of Gastroenterology and Hepatology, Cleveland Clinic, Cleveland, OH, USA

**Anita Afzali, M.D., M.P.H.** Division of Gastroenterology, Department of Internal Medicine, University of Washington, Seattle, WA, USA

**Lindsey Albenberg, D.O.** Department of Gastroenterology, Hepatology, and Nutrition, Children's Hospital of Philadelphia, Philadelphia, PA, USA

**Gert Van Assche, M.D., Ph.D.** Pediatrics, Division of Gastroenterology, Heptaology, and Nutrition, The Children's Hospital of Philadelphia, University of Pennsylvania, Philadelphia, PA, USA

**Robert N. Baldassano, M.D.** Pediatrics, Division of Gastroenterology, Heptaology, and Nutrition, The Children's Hospital of Philadelphia, University of Pennsylvania, Philadelphia, PA, USA

**Daniel C. Baumgart, M.D., Ph.D.** Department of Medicine, Division of Gastroenterology and Hepatology Charité Medical Center - Virchow Hospital, Medical School of the Humboldt, University of Berlin, Germany, Berlin, Germany

**Theodore M. Bayless, M.D.** Department of Gastroenterology, Johns Hopkins Medical Institutions, Baltimore, MD, USA

**Adam M. Berg, M.D.** Department of Gastroenterology, Boston Medical Center, Boston University School of Medicine, Boston, MA, USA

**Wojciech Blonski, M.D., Ph.D.** Department of Internal Medicine, United Health Services, Wilson Memorial Center, Johnson City, NY, USA

**Gregory P. Botta, M.D., Ph.D.** Division of Gastroenterology, University of Pennsylvania Perelman School of Medicine, Philadelphia, PA, USA

**Alan L. Buchman, M.D., M.S.P.H.** Division of Gastroenterology, Feinberg School of Medicine, Northwestern University, Chicago, IL, USA

**Anna M. Buchner, M.D., Ph.D.** Department of Gastroenterology, University of Pennsylvania Hospital, Philadelphia, PA, USA

**Chalermrat Bunchorntavakul, M.D.** Division of Gastroenterology and Hepatology, Department of Medicine, Hospital of the University of Pennsylvania, Philadelphia, PA, USA

**Robert Burakoff, M.D., M.P.H.** Department of Gastroenterology, Brigham and Women's Hospital, Boston, MA, USA

**María Chaparro, M.D., Ph.D.** Gastroenterology, La Princesa University Hospital, Madrid, Spain

**Adam S. Cheifetz, M.D.** Division of Gastroenterology, Center for Inflammatory Bowel Disease, Beth Israel Deaconess Medical Center, Boston, MA, USA

**Russell D. Cohen, M.D.** Section of Gastroenterology, Department of Medicine, Inflammatory Bowel Disease Center, The University of Chicago Medical Center, Chicago, IL, USA

**Raymond K. Cross, M.D., M.S.** Department of Medicine, University of Maryland, Baltimore, MD, USA

**Carmen Cuffari, M.D.** Pediatrics, The Johns Hopkins University, Baltimore, MD, USA

**Sushila Dalal, M.D.** Section of Gastroenterology, Department of Medicine, University of Chicago Medical Center, Chicago, IL, USA

**Themistocles Dassopoulos, M.D.** Department of Medicine, Barnes Jewish Hospital, Washington University, St. Louis, MO, USA

**Francis A. Farraye, M.D., M.Sc.** Section of Gastroenterology, Boston Medical Center, Boston University School of Medicine, Boston, MA, USA

**Marc Ferrante, M.D., Ph.D.** Department of Gastroenterology, University Hospitals Leuven, Leuven, Belgium

**Andreas Fischer, M.D.** Department of Medicine, Division of Gastroenterology and Hepatology Charité Medical Center - Virchow Hospital, Medical School of the Humboldt, University of Berlin, Germany, Berlin, Germany

**Subrata Ghosh, M.D., F.R.C.P.** Department of Medicine, University of Calgary, Calgary, AB, Canada

**Philip M. Ginsburg, M.D., F.A.C.G.** Gastroenterology Center of Connecticut, Yale-New Haven Hospital, Hamden, CT, USA

**Javier P. Gisbert, M.D., Ph.D.** Department of Gastroenterology, La Princesa University Hospital, Madrid, Spain

**Sarah R. Goeppinger, B.A.** Department of Medicine/Gastroenterology, University of Chicago Medicine, Chicago, IL, USA

**Daniel W. Hommes, M.D., Ph.D.** Division of Digestive Diseases, UCLA Center for Inflammatory Bowel Diseases, Los Angeles, CA, USA

**Marietta Iacucci, M.D., Ph.D.** Division of Gastroenterology, Department of Medicine, University of Calgary, Calgary, AB, Canada

**Kim L. Isaacs, M.D., Ph.D.** Department of Gastroenterology and Hepatology, University of North Carolina at Chapel Hill, Chapel Hill, NC, USA

**Pascal Juillerat, M.D., M.Sc.** Gastroenterology Department, Crohn's and Colitis Center, Massachusetts General Hospital, Boston, MA, USA

**Sunanda Kane, M.D., M.S.P.H.** Division of Gastroenterology and Hepatology, Department of Medicine, Mayo Clinic, Rochester, MN, USA

**Seymour Katz, M.D.** New York University School of Medicine, Great Neck, NY, USA

**Judith Kelsen, M.D.** Pediatrics, Division of Gastroenterology, Heptaology, and Nutrition, Children's Hospital of Philadelphia, University of Pennsylvania, Philadelphia, PA, USA

**Caroline Kerner, M.D., M.S.C.E.** Division of Gastroenterology, Department of Medicine, University of Pennsylvania, Pennsylvania Hospital, Philadelphia, PA, USA

**Asher Kornbluth, M.D.** The Henry D. Janowitz Division of Gastroenterology, The Icahn School of Medicine at Mount Sinai, New York, NY, USA

**Joshua R. Korzenik, M.D.** Department of Gastroenterology, BWH Crohn's and Colitis Center, Brigham and Women's Hospital, Chestnut Hill, MA, USA

**Conor Lahiff, M.D.** Gastrointestinal Unit, Division of Gastroenterology, Beth Israel Deaconess Medical Center, Boston, MA, USA

**Brett Lashner, M.D.** Gastroenterology and Hepatology, Cleveland Clinic, Cleveland, OH, USA

**Scott D. Lee, M.D.** Division of Gastroenterology, Department of Inflammatory Bowel Disease Program, University of Washington, Seattle, WA, USA

**Jonathon Levine, M.D.** Gastroenterology, Harvard Medical School, Boston, MA, USA

**James D. Lewis, M.D., M.S.C.E.** Department of Medicine, University of Pennsylvania, Philadelphia, PA, USA

**Yue Li, M.D.** Department of Gastroenterology, Digestive Disease Institute, Cleveland Clinic Foundation, Peking Union Medical College Hospital, Beijing, China

**Gary R. Lichtenstein, M.D., F.A.C.P., F.A.C.G., A.G.A.F.** Professor of Medicine, University of Pennsylvania School of Medicine, Director, Center for Inflammatory Bowel Diseases University of Pennsylvania Health System Hospital of the University of Pennsylvania, Gastroenterology Division, Philadelphia, PA, USA

**Seth Lipka, M.D.** Department of Medicine, Nassau University Medical Center, East Meadow, NY, USA

**Edward V. Loftus Jr., M.D.** Division of Gastroenterology and Hepatology, Mayo Clinic, Rochester, MN, USA

**Randy Longman, M.D., Ph.D.** Division of Gastroenterology and Hepatology, Department of Medicine, The Jill Roberts Center for IBD, New York Presbyterian Hospital/Weill Cornell Medical Center, Weill Cornell Medical College, New York, NY, USA

**Richard P. MacDermott, M.D., M.A.C.G., A.G.A.F.** Department of Gastro-enterology, Inflammatory Bowel Diseases Center, Albany Medical Center, Albany, NY, USA

**Gerassimos J. Mantzaris, M.D., Ph.D., A.G.A.F.** Department of Gastroenterology, Evangelismos Hospital, Athens, Attica, Greece

**Alan C. Moss, M.D.** Center for Inflammatory Bowel Disease, Beth Israel Deaconess Medical Center, Boston, MA, USA

**Prashant R. Mudireddy, M.D.** Department of Gastroenterology, Lennox Hill Hospital, New York, NY, USA

**Seamus J. Murphy, F.R.C.P., Ph.D.** Department of Medicine, Daisy Hill Hospital, Newry, Co. Down, N. Ireland

**Mark T. Osterman, M.D., M.S.C.E.** Division of Gastroenterology, Department of Medicine, Pennsylvania Presbyterian Medical Center, University of Pennsylvania, Philadelphia, PA, USA

**Rebecca Palmer, M.R.C.P.** Transitional Gastroenterology Unit, John Radcliffe Hospital, Oxford, UK

**Keely R. Parisian, M.D.** Digestive Disease Institute, Cleveland Clinic Foundation, Cleveland, OH, USA

**Sandra M. Quezada, M.D., M.S.** Department of Medicine, University of Maryland, Baltimore, MD, USA

**Farzana Rashid, M.D.** Department of Gastroenterology, The University of Pennsylvania School of Medicine, Philadelphia, PA, USA

**K. Rajender Reddy, M.D.** Gastroenterology and Hepatitis Division, Department of Internal Medicine, Hospital of the University of Pennsylvania, Philadelphia, PA, USA

**Miguel Reguiero, M.D.** Department of Gastroenterology, Hepatology, and Nutrition, University of Pittsburgh Medical Center, Pittsburgh, PA, USA

**David T. Rubin, M.D.** Section of Gastroenterology, Department of Medicine, University of Chicago, Chicago, IL, USA

**Paul Rutgeerts, M.D., Ph.D., F.R.C.P.** Department of Gastroenterology, University Hospitals Leuven, Leuven, Belgium

**Atsushi Sakuraba, M.D., Ph.D.** Department of Medicine, University of Chicago, Chicago, IL, USA

**Sunil Samuel, M.B.B.S., Ph.D.** Department of Gastroenterology, Nottingham University Hospitals NHS Trust, Nottingham, Nottinghamshire, UK

**Ellen J. Scherl, M.D., A.G.A.F., F.A.C.G.** Division of Gastroenterology and Hepatology, Department of Medicine, The Jill Roberts Center for IBD, New York Presbyterian Hospital/ Weill Cornell Medical Center, Weill Cornell Medical College, New York, NY, USA

**Frank I. Scott, M.D., M.S.C.E.** Division of Gastroenterology, Department of Medicine, University of Pennsylvania Health System, Perelman School of Medicine, University of Pennsylvania, Philadelphia, PA, USA

**Bo Shen, M.D.** Department of Gastroenterology, Cleveland Clinic Foundation, Cleveland, OH, USA

**Anthony M. Sofia, M.D.** Department of Medicine, University of Chicago Medicine, Chicago, IL, USA

**Jason M. Swoger, M.D., M.P.H.** Department of Gastroenterology, Hepatology, and Nutrition, University of Pittsburgh Medical Center, Pittsburgh, PA, USA

**Simon Travis, D.Phil., F.R.C.P.** Translational Gastroenterology Unit, John Radcliffe Hospital, Oxford, UK

**Fernando Velayos, M.D., M.P.H.** Department of Gastroenterology, University of California, San Francisco, San Francisco, CA, USA

**Séverine Vermeire, M.D., Ph.D.** Department of Gastroenterology, University Hospitals Leuven, Leuwen, Belgium

**Hongha T. Vu, M.D.** Department of Gastroenterology, Barnes Jewish Hospital, Washington University, St. Louis, MO, USA

**Michelle Vu, M.D.** Division of Digestive Diseases, University of California, Los Angeles, CA, USA

**Susan Hongha T. Vu, M.D.** Department of Gastroenterology, Barnes Jewish Hospital, Washington University, St. Louis, MO, USA

**Alissa Walsh, F.R.A.C.P.** Gastroenterology Unit, St. Vincent's Hospital, Sydney, Australia

**Ming-Hsi Wang, M.D., Ph.D.** Department of Gastroenterology and Hepatology, Cleveland Clinic, Cleveland, OH, USA

**Chelle L. Wheat, M.P.H.** Department of Inflammatory Bowel Disease, University of Washington, Seattle, WA, USA

**Xinjun Cindy Zhu, M.D., M.S.** Division of Gastroenterology, Department of Medicine, Inflammatory Bowel Diseases Center, Albany Medical Center, Albany, NY, USA

# The History of Medical Therapy of Ulcerative Colitis

Prashant R. Mudireddy, Wojciech Blonski,
and Gary R. Lichtenstein

**Keywords**
Ulcerative colitis • Medical therapy • History

## Introduction

Ulcerative colitis is a chronic inflammatory bowel disease of unknown etiology that affects the colon. There has been an increased knowledge in the understanding of ulcerative colitis in the last 100 years. But there are several examples in the medical literature to suggest that a diarrheal disease similar to ulcerative colitis had been described many centuries ago.

## Early History

In ancient Chinese medicine, the Yellow Emperor's Canon of Internal Medicine (722 BC) described symptoms (abdominal pain, diarrhea, rectal bleeding) of a disease resembling ulcerative colitis [1]. Many Roman physicians, including Hippocrates (460–377 BC), Aretaeus (80–138 AD), and Soranus (170 AD), reported various forms of chronic diarrhea

P.R. Mudireddy, M.D. (✉)
Department of Gastroenterology, Lenox Hill Hospital,
100 East, 77th St., New York, NY 10075, USA
e-mail: prashantmudireddy@yahoo.com

W. Blonski, M.D., Ph.D.
Department of Internal Medicine, Cyclosporine for Ulcerative
Colitis, United Health Services, Wilson Memorial Center,
Picciano Building 4th Floor, 33-57 Harrison St., Johnson City,
NY 13790, USA
e-mail: blonskiw@gmail.com

G.R. Lichtenstein, M.D., F.A.C.P., F.A.C.G., A.G.A.F. (✉)
Gastroenterology Division, Hospital of the University of
Pennsylvania, University of Pennsylvania School of Medicine,
Philadelphia, PA, USA
e-mail: gary.lichtenstein@uphs.upenn.edu

associated with blood and an ulcerated bowel [2]. Epidemics of dysentery which occurred in colonial America and worldwide and "bloody flux" described by T. Sydenham (in 1669–1670) were definitely infectious in origin, but these illnesses may have included instances of chronic ulcerative colitis [1]. P. J. E. Wilson noted that Prince Charles (1745), the Young Pretender to the Scottish throne, suffered from ulcerative colitis [3]. He also suggested that Prince Charles cured himself by following a milk-free diet [3]. Burch et al. described a case of Sir William Johnson, the Mohawk Baronet, who might have suffered from ulcerative colitis and its extraintestinal manifestations [4]. Sir William Johnson, who was originally from Ireland, first started having health problems (upper respiratory symptoms, sleeplessness, and fatigability) in 1755 [4]. In 1756, he developed bloody flux. This continued over the next 5 years, and by 1761 he developed high fevers, jaundice, and abdominal pain. He tried a number of medications including purgatives and electuaries without relief. Over the next 13 years, in addition to worsening of his bowel symptoms, he developed edema, gum problems, excessive bleeding from razor cuts, sore eyes, and joint pains suggesting extraintestinal manifestations. He succumbed to his illness in 1774. Since it is highly unlikely that single continuous infection can cause these recurring and remitting symptoms, Burch et al. suggested that inflammatory bowel disease may have been responsible for Sir William Johnson's illness [4].

The term ulcerative colitis was first used in medical literature in mid-nineteenth century [5]. Dr. Samuel Wilkes was first to refer the disease by its name [5]. In his testimony to a criminal court in the trial of Dr. Smethurst, which was published as a letter in *The Medical Times and Gazette* in 1859, he used the term ulcerative colitis while describing the postmortem of Miss Isabella Banks. She was a young woman

G.R. Lichtenstein (ed.), *Medical Therapy of Ulcerative Colitis*,
DOI 10.1007/978-1-4939-1677-1_1, © Springer Science+Business Media New York 2014

who had died from acute diarrheal illness [2, 6]. He reported that the mucosa of the entire colon along with the terminal ileum was severely ulcerated end to end. He further stated her ulcerated bowel found on postmortem was caused by arsenic poisoning. This almost led to hanging of Dr. Smethurst (Miss Banks was his mistress), but many wrote letters in his support and he was granted pardon by Home Secretary [2, 6].

Several years later, the Surgeon General of the Union Army during the American Civil War also used the term ulcerative colitis in his publication, *The Medical and Surgical History of the Rebellion, U.S.A* [7]. In this publication, he described the pathological specimens of over 200 cases of ulcerative colitis and even took microphotographs of the specimens, a remarkable achievement for that time. The microphotographs were taken with the help of an improvised microscope with camera lucida and using photolithography [7].

In 1862, Habershon for the first time reported the presence of pseudopolyps in a patient with ulcerative colitis in *Diseases of Abdomen* [1, 2]. He wrote: "In the third stage we find ulceration, sometimes merely as minute circular ulcers, but generally of a more extensive character; the ulcers are often oval in form, placed in the transverse axis of the intestine, their edges are irregular and undermined, and their base is formed by the cellular or muscular coats. These ulcerations gradually extend and coalesce, till nearly the whole of the mucous surface is destroyed, except here and there prominent isolated portions, which become intensely congested, and resemble polypoid growths" (JB Kirsner 2001 chap. 1, p. 16). Similar pseudopolyps of the colon were also described by Woodward (in 1881) of the United States in a 44-year-old male patient who died from prolonged bloody diarrhea [1].

For the first time in 1875, Wilkes and Moxon writing in *Lectures on Pathological Anatomy* distinguished "simple ulcerative colitis" from "febrile epidemic dysentery" [1, 2]. Wilkes wrote: "the term colitis is sometimes used as though synonymous with dysentery. Our usual language has indeed been too indefinite, nay, incorrect, in speaking of all affections of the large intestine as dysenteric......there is quite as much reason to regard febrile epidemic dysentery as a disease distinct from simple ulcerative colitis as there is to regard febrile epidemic diphtheria as a disease distinct from croup" [2, p. 44]. Sir William Allchin in 1885 described extensive denudation with large ulcers in the colonic mucosa of a young woman who died from an acute diarrhea [1, 2]. He further wrote: "it is to be regretted that the term dysentery is not restricted to the true tropical malady and it should not at once be applied in an adjective form to any diarrhea dependent upon ulceration of the colon when factors for the production of the specific disease are, as far as can be recognized, wanting" [2, p. 44].

By 1893, many British physicians attending the Harveian Society of London meeting and physicians from other European countries (Germany, Italy, and France) started to recognize the emergence of a diarrheal illness that was different from epidemic bacillary dysentery prevalent at that time [1]. W. Hale-White, a British physician wrote: "The condition observed is one of intense inflammation of the mucosa progressing to ulceration but the area of distribution and the degree of intensity vary from cecum to anus, occasionally even extending into the ileum, with complete destruction of the mucous membrane over large areas to merely a few discrete ulcers in the lower part of the bowel" [1, p. 17]. I. Boas (Germany) in 1903, for the first time, clinically differentiated ulcerative colitis from bacillary dysentery [1, p. 18].

Around the late nineteenth century, the surgical management of ulcerative colitis started to emerge. In 1893, Mayo Robson of London performed an inguinal colostomy to allow irrigation of the ulcerated bowel with tincture of *Hamamelis* and boracic acid [1]. In 1902, Weir of New York introduced appendicostomy to allow irrigation with methylene blue, silver nitrate, and bismuth [1].

## Twentieth Century

The first cooperative effort to correlate clinical findings found in a number of ulcerative colitis patients was done in 1909 in a London symposium [1]. The clinical features, treatments, and statistics of over 300 cases of ulcerative colitis were reviewed during this symposium [1]. It was also noted that the mortality was very high—over 50 % of cases died in hospital from various complications like perforation, peritonitis, hemorrhage, septic infection, pulmonary embolism, liver disease, and malnutrition [1]. Interestingly, the occurrence of ulcerative colitis among family members was considered a mere coincidence. Since the time of this symposium, ulcerative colitis increased in popularity and started to be recognized as a distinct clinical entity by physicians worldwide. During this early period, physicians implicated bacteria as the etiologic agent of ulcerative colitis [1]. Accordingly, the treatments included "slop diets," Sydenham's remedy (3 pints of milk soured by lactic acid), astringents, opium, tincture of *Hamamelis*, and rectal instillations of boracic acid, silver nitrate, "coli vaccine," or creolin [1].

In 1909, Hawkins reviewed 85 cases of ulcerative colitis. Again, the mortality rate was high in his case series [1]. Forty-one patients had died of various complications. He too suggested bacteria as the possible etiologic agent. He divided patients into five groups—acute, chronic, dysenteric diarrhea, acute or chronic disease, and hemorrhagic disease [1]. At 1913 at the Paris Congress of Medicine, ulcerative colitis was one of the principal subjects, a recognition of increasing awareness of ulcerative colitis [1]. That same year, the first radiological appearance of ulcerative colitis was described independently by Stierlin and Kienbock [1].

The first American case report was published by Bassler of New York in 1913 [8]. Also in 1913, Brown of St. Louis, USA, suggested ileostomy for ulcerative colitis patients [9]. This was based on the principal of bowel rest, i.e., diversion of fecal stream away from the inflamed colon [19 m]. In 1919, Logan of the Mayo Clinic reported 117 cases of ulcerative colitis [10]. Many of the patients in his case series were under the age of 50 years [10]. In 1921, Yeoman of New York published a case series of 65 patients [11].

By the 1920s and 1930s, reports of cases of ulcerative colitis started coming from all over the world. Ulcerative colitis became a well-known disease entity. In 1921, Hurst of London suggested that an organism related to *B. dysenteriae* was the cause of ulcerative colitis [1]. His treatments included daily colonic irrigation of the colon with silver nitrate and injection of large amounts of polyvalent antidysenteric serum [1]. Strauss from Berlin (1923) in his paper on ulcerative colitis recommended treatment with a bland diet and blood transfusions [12]. In 1925, Bargen and his colleagues reported *diplostreptococci* from the rectal ulcerations of patients with ulcerative colitis [13]. They also showed that rabbits injected intravenously with the broth containing *diplostreptococci* developed colonic lesions [13]. The following year, Buie reviewing 473 cases at Mayo Clinic agreed with Bargen's theory [14]. But this theory lost credibility when Paulson and Mones failed to confirm this [15, 16].

During this period, the local and extraintestinal complications of ulcerative colitis were also acknowledged. Lister (1899) reported an association between hepatitis and ulcerative colitis [1]. Wilson (1904) reported a case of ulcerative colitis complicated by perforation and peritonitis [17]. In 1907, Lockhart-Mummery with the help of an electrically illuminated proctosigmoidoscope found carcinoma of the colon in 7 of 36 patients with ulcerative colitis [18]. Later in 1928, Bargen reported 20 cases of malignant disease in ulcerative colitis patients—17 with adenocarcinoma, 2 with lymphosarcoma, and one with lymphatic leukemia [19]. Again in 1929, he reported a total of 268 complications in 693 patients with ulcerative colitis [20]. The complications included polyposis; colonic stricture; perirectal abscess (in retrospect likely due to Crohn's colitis not ulcerative colitis—though Crohn's colitis was not a recognized entity at this time); skin lesions; and arteritis [20]. The association between ulcerative colitis and chronic interstitial nephritis was reported by Hale-White [1]. Crohn in 1925 reported ocular complications in his patients with ulcerative colitis. He proposed that vitamin A deficiency led to keratomalacia and xerophthalmia in these patients [21].

In the 1930s, efforts to find the etiology continued, while more reports of ulcerative colitis cases started to be reported. Hern (1931) reviewed 50 cases of ulcerative colitis and suggested an infectious etiology [1]. He wrote: "the primary factor in ulcerative colitis acted through the blood stream with secondary infection of the mucosal surface by resident colon bacilli and streptococci … causing deep and diffuse involvement of the submucosa and mucous membranes" (JB Kirsner 2001 chap. 1, p. 22). In 1933, Hardy and Bulmer of England reported 95 cases of ulcerative colitis [1]. Ulcerative colitis was a major subject of discussion at the 1935 International Congress of Gastroenterology in Brussels, Belgium [1]. Participants came from many European countries and the United States reflecting the growing interest in the disease among the gastroenterologists [1]. One of the most important issues discussed included familial ulcerative colitis by Hamburger and Bensaude [1].

During the 1930s to 1950s, the awareness of ulcerative colitis increased in the United States [1]. Reports came from many US centers, particularly the Mayo Clinic [22, 23], Philadelphia [24], and the University of Chicago [25–27]. Many new findings were reported during this period like occurrence of ulcerative colitis in patients above 50 years [28, 29], complications like arterial and venous thrombosis [30], hepatic insufficiency [31], clubbed fingers [32], increased frequency of uric acid and calcium oxalate stones [33], iron deficiency anemia, arthritis, dermatological disorder, psychogenic problems [34], acute fulminant ulcerative colitis [35], and pyoderma gangrenosum [36].

Numerous papers highlighting the occurrence of hepatic disease and involvement of joints in ulcerative colitis were also published. In 1958, Brooke and Slaney (of England) suggested portal bacteremia as a factor responsible for development of sclerosing cholangitis [37]. Bywaters and Ansell noticed a high incidence of sacroiliac joint involvement [38]. Fernandez-Herlihy described rheumatoid spondylitis, arthralgias, rheumatoid arthritis, and acute toxic arthritis in their patients [39]. McEwen-Kirsner noticed involvement of peripheral joints and spondylitis in their patients [40].

By the late 1950s, the distribution of the disease extended beyond a few European countries and the United States [1]. Reports of the disease started coming from countries like Greece, Turkey, Iran, Syria, South Africa, Australia, New Zealand, India, and Japan [1]. In fact, at the 1958 World Congress of Gastroenterology Conference in Washington D.C., Matsunaga reported 300 cases of ulcerative colitis in Japan [41].

During the 1950s and 1960s, colon cancer complicating the course of ulcerative colitis received a lot of attention. Dawson and Pryse-Davies (1959) as well as Goldgraber and Kirsner (1964) reported increased colorectal cancer risk in ulcerative colitis patients [42, 43]. Devroede noted that young patients with long-standing disease had a higher risk of cancer [44]. Another group from Mayo Clinic reported colorectal cancer in 98 of 1,564 patients with ulcerative colitis [45].

In 1963–1964, Edwards and Truelove from Oxford, United Kingdom, described the course and prognosis of ulcerative colitis [46, 47]. They analyzed a total of 624 patients with ulcerative colitis. They suggested that the principal factors contributing to mortality were severity of illness, extent of the disease, and age greater than 60 years [46, 47]. They also described several local and systemic complications in their patients like ischiorectal abscesses, fistulas, strictures, inflammatory polyposis, acute dilatation of the colon, perforation, massive bleeding, colon cancer, pyoderma gangrenosum, erythema nodosum, ankylosing spondylitis, pulmonary embolism, anemia, and osteoporosis [46, 47]. Around 14 % of their patients needed radical surgery and another 6 % underwent conservative surgery [46, 47].

Currently, our understanding of ulcerative colitis and its complications has increased greatly, but the etiology still remains obscure.

## History of Ulcerative Colitis in Children

In 1923, Helmholz of the Mayo Clinic was probably the first person to describe clinical features of ulcerative colitis in children in his five case series [48]. Later in 1926, Bourne of England in his review of ten cases of ulcerative colitis described one child with ulcerative colitis [49]. A Mayo Clinic report in 1940 contained a total of 95 children with ulcerative colitis [50]. And the 1955 report by Bargen and Kennedy had 139 cases of ulcerative colitis in children [51]. They concluded that ulcerative colitis in children had a similar course to adults, and it was not as rare as previously thought [51]. The youngest patient ever reported to have ulcerative colitis was a 21-day-old male infant [52]. He ultimately succumbed to his disease following an operation for rapidly deteriorating ulcerative colitis [52]. Other prominent physicians who made significant contribution to IBD literature in children include R. Lagercrantz, Kirsner, Hijmans and Enzer, Durham and Korelitz, and Davidson [1].

The impact of ulcerative colitis on growth and sexual development of children was also recognized during those early years [1]. Davidson of the Bronx Memorial Hospital in 1939 reported impaired growth and development in three children with ulcerative colitis [53]. A group from the University of Chicago (Ricketts, Benditt, and Palmer) reported an association between ulcerative colitis and "infantilism" [54]. They attributed the impaired growth to multiple nutritional deficiencies [54]. Welch et al. in 1937 tried to explain the nutritional deficiencies by demonstrating substantial fecal losses of proteins and electrolytes [55]. This was later confirmed by Sappington and Bockus in 1949 and Kirsner and Sheffner in 1950 [56, 57].

## History of Ulcerative Colitis in Pregnancy

During the 1909 London symposium, for the first time the impact of ulcerative on pregnancy was discussed [1]. But over the next 30 years, very little was done to explore this further [1]. In 1931, Barnes and Hayes of the United States reported three cases of pregnant women with ulcerative colitis [58]. All three patients had a poor outcome—all three died either during pregnancy or in puerperium [58]. One of the patients had a family history of Bright's disease (a form of nephritis), and the other two had chronic nephritis [58]. This led him to conclude that ulcerative colitis in pregnancy is associated with advanced renal insufficiency called azotemic colitis [58]. In 1951, Abramson of Boston reviewed 46 pregnancies in 33 patients with ulcerative colitis [59]. He noticed that four out of five patients who had acute exacerbation of ulcerative colitis during pregnancy and three out of four patients who had acute exacerbation during puerperium died [59]. Given these high mortality rates, therapeutic abortions were recommended in patients with severe ulcerative colitis. In 1955, MacDougall reviewed a total of 100 pregnancies in 64 ulcerative colitis patients [60]. He concluded that ulcerative colitis did not adversely affect the pregnancy [60]. The following year, Crohn studied a total of 150 pregnancies in 110 patients with ulcerative colitis and concluded that the onset or recurrences of ulcerative colitis were most frequent during the first trimester of pregnancy and during puerperium [61].

The first authoritative literature on pregnancy, fertility, and IBD was published in 1985 by Korelitz [62]. He suggested that ulcerative colitis and pregnancy were two independent processes, and therapeutic abortion did not affect the course of ulcerative colitis [70 m]. His recommendation was that one should become pregnant during a quiescent period and continue the medical treatment with steroids and sulfasalazine in addition to increased nutritional intake [62].

## History of Etiology of Ulcerative Colitis

The etiology of ulcerative colitis to date remains obscure. Many theories have been proposed over the years in an effort to explain its etiology.

## Infectious Agents

By the middle of nineteenth century, ulcerative colitis was differentiated from infectious diarrhea by its intermittent and prolonged course, but it was still hard to convince many physicians of its noninfectious nature. In the late nineteenth century and early twentieth century, bacteria were implicated as the possible etiology of ulcerative colitis. *Bacillary dysenteriae* was probably the most common agent thought to cause ulcerative colitis [1]. Some of the other bacterial organisms implicated included *Entamoeba histolytica*, *Salmonella typhi*, *and Shigella dysenteriae* [1].

In 1921, Hurst of London proposed an organism related to *B. dysenteriae* as the possible cause of ulcerative colitis and even advocated giving patients polyvalent antidysenteric serum [1]. In the United States during the 1920s, focal infections such as dental abscesses were thought to be the source of the disease, and removal of the teeth, gall bladder, and appendices were encouraged [63]. Bargen in 1925 found *diplostreptococci* in the cultures of rectal ulcerations and implicated them as the etiologic agents [13]. But his theory soon lost credibility. In 1931, Hern wrote: "the primary factor in ulcerative colitis acted through the blood stream with secondary infection of the mucosal surface by the resident colon bacilli and streptococci...............causing deep and diffuse involvement of the submucosa and the mucous membrane" (JB Kirsner 2001 chap. 1, p. 22). Many such theories have been proposed by various authors, but studies have failed to prove the infectious etiology of ulcerative colitis.

## Psychogenic Factors

In the 1930s, psychogenic factors were implicated as the possible etiology of ulcerative colitis [1]. Murray and Sullivan noticed a chronological association between the onset of bowel symptoms and emotional disturbance [64, 65]. "Typical ulcerative colitis" personality was described in patients with ulcerative colitis and included traits such as immaturity, indecisiveness, overdependence, sensitivity, and inhibited relationships and critical emotional events [66].

Almy et al. proposed that emotional stress effects in the colonic mucosa in patients with ulcerative colitis caused increased hyperemia, vascular engorgement, increased mucous secretions, and increased colonic motor activities [67]. Kern et al. using a balloon technique studied the motility of the distal colon in nonspecific ulcerative colitis patients and found a decrease or absence of phasic activity [68]. It correlated with severe diarrhea, and he attributed this to psychogenic-induced autonomic bombardment of the colon [68]. Later, Meyer found an increased production of lysozyme, mucinase enzyme, in patients with active ulcerative colitis during emotional stress [69]. It was proposed that lysozyme destroyed the colonic mucous lining and increased vulnerability of the colon to invasive pathogens and other cytotoxic agents [69]. But this theory also lost credibility because it was shown in vitro that lysozyme was incapable of dissolving the human mucosa [70]. Since there was no evidence to show that ulcerative colitis patients had a different emotional makeup from the general population, it was concluded that psychogenic factors do not cause ulcerative colitis but contribute to the disease exacerbation, chronicity, and severity [71].

## Genetic Factors

In 1909 at the London symposium, ulcerative colitis cases among family members were mentioned. But at that time, it was considered a mere coincidence [1]. This view was held by physicians until the 1950s when cases of familial IBD were described again. Kirsner and Palmer introduced the concept of "individual vulnerability" in 1954 [1]. This was later revised to describe genetically influenced individual disease susceptibility [1]. In 1958, Schlesinger and Platt noted that a family history of having ulcerative colitis was present in 17 % of 60 children with ulcerative colitis [72]. Additionally, Ashkenazi Jews were found to be at least four times more likely to develop ulcerative colitis than other ethnicities.

## Allergy

In 1925, Andresen suggested that cow's milk might be responsible for the development of ulcerative colitis [5]. Later, Truelove and his colleagues showed that some patients achieved remission of their disease when milk products were excluded from their diet, and they suffered relapse when they were reintroduced. They also showed that the titers of antibodies to milk protein were significantly higher in patients with colitis compared to the normal population [73, 74]. It was suggested that patients who developed colitis usually stopped breastfeeding in their first month of life [75]. This theory also gained credibility when Wright and Truelove in their controlled trial found that milk-free diet was only marginally beneficial to patients with ulcerative colitis [76].

## Immune Mechanisms and Autoimmunity

In the 1940s, various diseases of unknown etiology were attributed to immune and autoimmune mechanisms [66]. Kirsner and Goldgraber described a series of clinical experiences occurring during 1930s and 1940s which suggested possible involvement of immune mechanisms as the etiology of ulcerative colitis [77]. The examples of such events included abrupt onset of ulcerative colitis after food poisoning, association with allergy (asthma, hay fever) or other immune diseases (autoimmune hemolytic anemia), occurrence of IBD among the family members, and response to steroids [77].

The first studies suggesting that ulcerative colitis was an autoimmune disease were done by Broberger and Perlmann [78]. In 1959, they showed the presence of hemagglutinin antibodies to the colonic mucosa in 20 out of 30 children with ulcerative colitis [78]. They further demonstrated that the leukocytes from patients with ulcerative colitis had a cytotoxic effect on colon cells in tissue culture, and this effect was inhibited by pretreatment with colon antigen [78]. But the studies by Harrison (1965) and Wright and Truelove (1966) showed the presence of colon autoantibodies in only 15–20 % of patients with ulcerative colitis [79, 80]. They saw little correlation between the clinical course of ulcerative colitis and the presence of circulating antibodies [79, 80]. So it was unclear whether patients developed antibodies as a cause or as an effect of pathological changes occurring in the colon of patients with ulcerative colitis [5]. By the 1970s, study of immune mechanisms in ulcerative colitis patients became an active area of research [66].

## History of Treatment of Ulcerative Colitis

The treatment of ulcerative colitis has undergone significant changes in the last 70–80 years. This has led to decreased mortality and improved lifestyle of patients with ulcerative colitis.

## Early Treatments

The early treatments included both medical and surgical approaches. In 1893, Mayo Robson performed inguinal colostomy to permit daily irrigation with tincture of *Hamamelis* and boracic acid solution [1]. R. F. Weir in 1902 did an appendicostomy to irrigate the colon with a 5 % methylene blue solution and 1:5,000 silver nitrate or bismuth solution [1]. In the early twentieth century, when an infectious etiology was thought to be the cause of ulcerative colitis, the treatments included "slop diets," "Sydenham's remedy" (three pints of milk soured with lactic acid), astringents, opium, tincture of *Hamamelis* and rectal instillations of boracic acid, silver nitrate, "coli vaccine," or creolin to control infections [1]. During this period, the preferred surgery was appendicostomy, and if the appendix was previously removed, the valvulari cecostomy was done [1].

In 1913, Brown of the United States suggested ileostomy to rest the colon [1]. This procedure gained popularity in 1930s and 1940s [1]. Hurst in 1921, who proposed that an organism closely related to *B. dysenteriae* was the cause of ulcerative colitis, recommended colonic irrigation with silver

nitrate and administration of polyvalent antidysenteric serum [1]. Other popular treatments in 1930s included enemas of tannin, silver nitrate, or bismuth subnitrate, the anti-amebic compound yatren as an anti-inflammatory agent, nutritional supplements, blood transfusions, "elimination diets," and fecal bacterial vaccines [1]. During the 1940s and 1950s when psychogenic factors were implicated as a cause of ulcerative colitis, psychoanalysis was a major approach [81].

With introduction of sulfonamides in the 1930s and adrenocorticotropic hormone (ACTH) in the 1940s, the treatment of ulcerative colitis has changed dramatically.

## Aminosalicylates

Sulfasalazine was first developed by Dr. Nana Svartz, a Swedish physician in the late 1930s, while working at Karolinska Institute in Stockholm [82, 83]. Initially the drug was named salicylazosulfapyridine, which was later abbreviated to salazopyrin and finally changed to azulfidine or sulfasalazine [82, 83]. It contains sulfapyridine (an antibiotic) and 5-aminosalicylic acid (an anti-inflammatory) linked by a diazo bond. Dr. Svartz initially used sulfasalazine to treat patients with rheumatoid arthritis, but the results were not encouraging. But unexpectedly when used in patients with ulcerative colitis, it led to significant improvement in their diarrhea. She published the first case report of use of sulfasalazine in an ulcerative colitis patient in 1942, followed by results of a large uncontrolled study in 1948 [82, 84]. In her uncontrolled study, Dr. Svartz noticed a 75–80 % improvement rates demonstrating its high efficacy in ulcerative colitis patients [84].

Because of World War II, sulfasalazine did not reach the United States until early 1950s and the United Kingdom until late 1950s [85]. By 1960, Dr. Svartz had treated 439 ulcerative colitis patients with sulfasalazine, and about 77 % of them showed improvement in their symptoms [85]. Similarly impressive results were reported by Morrison (1953) and Moertal and Bargen (1959) [85].

In 1962, Baron et al. published the first placebo controlled trial demonstrating the efficacy of oral sulfasalazine in patients with active ulcerative colitis [86]. A dose of 4 g per day for 3 weeks produced remission in 80 % of patients compared to 35 % in the placebo group [86]. In 1965, Mickiewicz reported the efficacy of sulfasalazine in maintaining remission [87]. He found that patients taking sulfasalazine 2 g per day for a 12-month period had a relapse rate of 21 % compared to 73 % in placebo group [87]. Since then, sulfasalazine has been used routinely in management of ulcerative colitis, both to treat active colitis and to maintain remission.

Peppercorn and Goldman of the United States in 1973 described the metabolism of sulfasalazine [88]. They suggested that the colonic bacteria split the diazo bond yielding 5-aminosalicylic acid (5-ASA) and sulfapyridine [88]. After this, research to identify the active moiety providing the therapeutic benefit in ulcerative colitis started. In 1977, Azad Khan and Truelove published their classic article in a non-placebo, controlled design and showed that 5-aminosalicylic acid (ASA) was the active therapeutic moiety of sulfasalazine by comparing the response to sulfasalazine, sulfapyridine, and 5-ASA enemas in patients with active ulcerative colitis [89]. These results were confirmed by Klotz in 1980 [90]. He demonstrated that rectal 5-ASA suppositories were superior to both oral sulfapyridine and sulfasalazine [90]. Van Hees compared the efficacy of suppositories of 5-ASA, sulfapyridine, and placebo in patients with active proctitis. Remission rate in those received 5-ASA was 60 % compared to only 27 % and 13 % in those who received placebo and sulfapyridine, respectively [91].

In 1983, Taffet and Das studied the adverse effects of sulfasalazine and described the options of desensitization in those who are intolerant to sulfasalazine [92]. In the same year, Chan et al. reported on the use of two new sulfasalazine analogs—ipsalazide and balsalazide [93]. In 1985, Selby et al. published results of another new oral 5-ASA formulation, olsalazine, in which two molecules of 5-ASA are connected by an azo bond. The results showed an acceptable efficacy of this new formulation [94].

In 1988, Riley et al. observed superior efficacy of enteric-coated 5-ASA over sulfasalazine in ulcerative colitis patients in their double-blind, double-dummy trial [95]. They also showed that delayed release 5-ASA was an effective treatment for maintaining remission in ulcerative colitis patients and had fewer side effects compared to enteric-coated sulfasalazine [95]. In the same year, McIntyre published the first randomized double blind of balsalazide. In recent years, new and high-strength formulations of 5-ASA using Multi Matrix System® (MMX) have been developed. Clinical trials by Lichtenstein and by Kamm have demonstrated superiority of this new delivery system over placebo in inducing remission in ulcerative colitis patients [96–99]. These trials established the efficacy of once-daily mesalamine formulation. Subsequently, Lichtenstein published data that led to regulatory approval of another once-daily formulation Apriso for maintenance of remission in patients with ulcerative [100] colitis.

## Systemic Corticosteroids

The second major breakthrough in the treatment of ulcerative colitis came with introduction of adrenocorticotropic hormone (ACTH) in late 1940s. In 1948, Kirsner et al. first suggested that the corticosteroids have beneficial effect on the clinical course of ulcerative colitis [26]. In early 1950s, several uncontrolled trials of ACTH, cortisone, and hydrocortisone were published which supported these clinical observations [26, 101–106].

In 1955, the first placebo controlled study demonstrating the effectiveness of corticosteroids in ulcerative colitis patients was published by Truelove and Witts [107]. They included a total of 213 patients of which 109 received cortisone (100 mg per day for 6 weeks) and another 101 received placebo. There was a clear benefit in the favor of cortisone, especially those being treated for their first attack [107]. Again in 1959, Truelove and Witts reported that cortisone and intramuscular ACTH were equally effective in patients having their first attack of ulcerative colitis and that ACTH was more effective than cortisone in those having recurrence. They also noticed that those who received ACTH had more frequent relapses [108].

In 1960, Lennard-Jones et al. showed that oral prednisone (40–60 mg per day) was significantly more effective than placebo in inducing remission in patients with ulcerative colitis [109]. Then in 1962, Baron et al. studied the optimal dose of prednisone in patients with mild-to-moderate disease [110]. Both 40 and 60 mg doses were effective compared to 20 mg dose. But they also noticed more frequent side effects with 60 mg doses [110]. In 1978, Powell-Tuck et al. compared once-daily dose of prednisolone to four times per day doses (same total dose) of prednisolone and at 2 weeks found no difference in clinical or sigmoidoscopic response and side effects in the two groups [111].

Truelove and Jewell in 1974 conducted another landmark study. In an uncontrolled, prospective trial, they studied the use of intravenous steroids in severe ulcerative colitis attacks. A response rate of 60 % was reported within 5 days of IV prednisolone 60 mg/day. They recommended emergent surgery for patients not recovering within 5 days [112]. Subsequent studies found that corticosteroid-naïve patients with severe ulcerative colitis attack responded well to intravenous corticotrophin, and those with prior history of steroid use showed good response to intravenous hydrocortisone [113–115].

The role of steroids in maintaining remission was first studied by Truelove and Witt in 1959. They did not see any reduction in relapse rate in those receiving low cortisone compared to those on placebo [108]. Subsequently, Lennard-Jones et al. found that daily oral prednisolone also did not decrease the relapse rate at 6 months [116].

Recently, budesonide MMX gained regulatory approval for the treatment of patients with active ulcerative colitis [117]. This once-daily formulation has demonstrated fewer steroid-related side effects in this mild to moderately active patient population.

## Topical Corticosteroids

The use of topical steroids in ulcerative colitis patients was first reported by Truelove in 1956–1957 [118, 119]. He found that around 65 % of ulcerative colitis patients with distal disease who received hydrocortisone in the form of a retention enema showed good symptomatic and sigmoidoscopic response [118, 119]. These observations led him to conduct a controlled clinical trial where patients receiving a 120 ml enema containing 100 mg of hydrocortisone were compared to those receiving placebo. At 1 week, 55 % of the patients receiving steroid enemas showed clinical response compared to only 5 % in placebo group [120]. But hydrocortisone enemas were used as a maintenance therapy (nightly on Saturdays and Sundays for 6 months), and the relapse rate was similar to placebo [120]. Truelove also studied the effect of combination therapy with oral and rectal steroids (20 mg of prednisolone and 100 mg hydrocortisone enema) in patients with active colitis [121]. All patients receiving combination therapy showed good response compared to monotherapy with oral steroids or rectal enemas [121]. In 1958, Watkinson confirmed the effect of hydrocortisone enemas in inducing remission in patients with less severe attacks of ulcerative colitis [122]. In 1960, Matts showed the effectiveness of prednisolone-21-phosphate enemas in the treatment of ulcerative colitis compared to placebo [123]. He also found that betamethasone enemas were effective in the treatment of active ulcerative colitis [124].

In addition to enemas, other topical delivery systems of steroids have also been studied in ulcerative patients. In 1962, Lennard-Jones et al. conducted a double-blind controlled trial of prednisolone-21-phosphate suppositories in proctitis and demonstrated superior clinical and sigmoidoscopic improvement compared to placebo [125]. In 1979, Farthing et al, showed that steroid foams instilled through the rectum reached the proximal sigmoid and sometimes even reached the descending colon by using a radionuclide scanning technique [126]. The following year, Ruddell et al. in a randomized study of 30 patients with proctosigmoiditis showed that hydrocortisone in foam base was as effective as hydrocortisone enemas and also noted that patients preferred the convenience of foam [127]. In 1985, Somerville showed that hydrocortisone enemas were as effective as prednisolone enemas and also found that patients tolerated foams better than enemas [128].

Due to the side effects of steroids resulting from systemic absorption, steroids with minimal systemic bioavailability were developed. One such steroid preparation was beclomethasone dipropionate (BDP). In 1982, Kumana et al. showed that BDP enemas were comparable to betamethasone enemas in terms of clinical response in nine patients with distal colitis, but only BDP did not interfere with hypothalamic-pituitary-adrenal axis function [129]. In 1984, Hamilton et al. conducted a single-blind crossover study comparing poorly absorbed prednisolone metasulphobenzoate enemas with low-dose oral prednisone in patients with active distal colitis. Enemas produced a greater clinical and sigmoidoscopic improvement compared to the low oral dose [130]. In another study, McIntyre et al. (1985) compared prednisolone metasulphobenzoate enemas to prednisolone-21-phosphate enemas in patients with distal colitis and found them to be equally effective, but prednisolone metasulphobenzoate had much lower systemic absorption [131].

More recently, new steroids like tixocortol pivalate and budesonide with minimal systemic bioavailability have been developed [132]. In 1986 Hanauer et al. in a large multicenter study showed that tixocortol enemas were as effective as hydrocortisone in patients with left-sided ulcerative colitis [132]. Budesonide is structurally similar to 16-alpha-hydroxyprednisolone. In 1987, Danielson et al. in a randomized controlled study compared the effect of budesonide enemas to prednisolone-21-phosphate enemas in patients with distal colitis [132]. Both enemas were equal in clinical efficacy, though budesonide produced greater sigmoidoscopic and histological improvements [132].

## Antibiotics

Antibiotics have not been shown to be effective in the treatment of ulcerative colitis. In 1972, Davies conducted a double-blind trial comparing metronidazole suppositories (500 mg three times daily) to placebo in 22 patients with proctitis [133]. He did not find any advantage of metronidazole compared to placebo [133]. Chapman in 1986 randomly treated 39 patients with severe ulcerative colitis with intravenous metronidazole and placebo. Patients in both groups also received intravenous steroids and topical steroids [134]. Again, intravenous metronidazole was not superior to placebo [134].

Another antibiotic that has been studied in ulcerative colitis patients was vancomycin. Dickinson et al. in 1985 performed a double-blind trial comparing vancomycin 500 mg orally to placebo given over 7 days [135]. But they did not find any benefit of using vancomycin in patients with active ulcerative colitis [133]. Though antibiotics are not beneficial in treatment of active colitis, they are still indicated in patients with infectious complications and perforation.

## Diet Therapy

Various dietary treatments have been proposed in the treatment of ulcerative colitis. Dickinson et al. in 1980 conducted a prospective controlled trial comparing intravenous hyperalimentation and total bowel rest versus regular diet and no intravenous fluids [136]. Prednisone was continued in both groups. Both groups had similar outcomes [136]. In another controlled trial, McIntyre et al. randomized patients with severe ulcerative colitis to bowel rest and total parenteral nutrition versus oral diet and intravenous fluids and electrolytes [137]. Prednisolone was continued in both groups. The authors noted that 60 % of the patients on bowel rest and TPN needed surgery compared to 42 % of those on regular diet [137].

A high-fiber diet was also considered in the treatment of ulcerative colitis especially for maintaining remission. In a controlled study, Davies and Rhodes randomized patients in remission to either continuing sulfasalazine or stopping sulfasalazine and starting a high-fiber diet [138]. A high relapse rate of 75 % was noticed in high-fiber diet group compared to 20 % in sulfasalazine group [138]. Thus, diet itself only has a role as a supportive therapy.

## Disodium Cromoglycate

This compound was tried as a treatment option in patients with ulcerative colitis based on the premise that allergy played a role in its pathogenesis. In 1976, Heatley et al. in their placebo controlled trial compared clinical response in those treated with 8 weeks of oral and rectal cromoglycate and those treated with placebo [139]. No statistically significant improvement was noticed in the cromoglycate group [139]. In the same year, Mani et al. noticed that 6 months of treatment with cromoglycate led to improvement in sigmoidoscopic findings compared to placebo, but the stool frequency remained unchanged [140]. Cromoglycate was found inferior to placebo to sulfasalazine in the treatment of active colitis by Langman et al. [141].

Studies done to evaluate the efficacy of cromoglycate in maintaining remission also did not yield positive results. Cromoglycate was found to be inferior to sulfasalazine and no better than placebo in maintaining remission by Dronfield et al. [142]. Willoughby showed that use of cromoglycate alone in treatment of ulcerative colitis led to higher relapse rates than those treated with sulfasalazine alone or combination of sulfasalazine and cromoglycate [143].

## Immunosuppressive Drugs

### 6-Mercaptopurine and Azathioprine

Immunosuppressive drugs were first used in ulcerative colitis based on the observations that immune mechanisms may play a role in its pathogenesis. In 1950, Hitchings and Elion initiated the studies of 6-mercaptopurine (6-MP), and in 1958, Schwartz and his colleagues showed its ability to inhibit immune response to a protein antigen [144, 145].

In 1962, Bean of Australia was first to report the use of 6-mercaptopurine in patients with ulcerative colitis [146]. He treated a patient with refractory ulcerative colitis with 6-MP (initial dose of 300 mg/day, then 50 mg on alternate days) and noticed a dramatic response. The patient remained in remission for 2 years [146]. Later, Bean published a case series of seven patients successfully treated with 6-MP [147]. This heralded the era of antimetabolite therapy of ulcerative colitis. Following Bean's report, several uncontrolled trials of 6-MP and azathioprine were published. In 1966, Bowen et al. of the United States reported that eight out of ten patients treated with azathioprine showed improvement [148]. One of the patients was successfully weaned off steroids for the first time in 3 years, while another patient noticed improvement in his arthritis and pyoderma gangrenosum [148]. But significant side effects were also reported by this group. These included leukopenia, thrombocytopenia, and alopecia [148]. Avery Jones et al. reported a case of death from sepsis after few weeks of azathioprine in a 19-year-old girl with ulcerative colitis [149].

In 1968, Mackay et al. of Melbourne, Australia, reported satisfactory response in 9 of the 12 ulcerative colitis patients treated with azathioprine [150]. The patients also received ACTH and prednisolone. This led the authors to conclude that combination of azathioprine and steroids was superior to azathioprine alone [150]. Korelitz (1972) of the United States reported a case series of 14 patients treated with 6-MP and noted clinical improvement in 11 patients [151].

The first controlled clinical trial of azathioprine in ulcerative colitis patients was published in 1972 by Jewell and Truelove [152]. They used azathioprine to prevent relapse. Eleven of 20 patients treated with azathioprine were symptom-free at 1 year compared to only 5 out of 20 in placebo group. But the difference in response between the two groups did not reach a statistical significance [152]. In 1975, two double-blind controlled clinical trials were published [153, 154]. Rosenberg et al. of the University of Chicago, United States, included 30 patients in their study, and the main objective of the study was to see if azathioprine helped reduce steroid dose. They found that though the final steroid dose was lower in azathioprine group compared to placebo, there was no significant clinical or endoscopic improvement [153]. The trial by Caprilli et al. compared clinical response in 20 patients with acute proctocolitis treated with azathioprine versus sulfasalazine. Both drugs produced significant improvement in clinical symptoms and endoscopic findings. So authors concluded that azathioprine was effective in the treatment of acute proctocolitis without concomitant use of steroids [154].

In 1982, the controlled clinical trial by Kirk et al. showed that azathioprine led to statistically significant steroid sparing and improvement in the disease activity of chronic ulcerative colitis [155]. Also no major side effects were described except severe nausea [155]. Authors concluded that azathioprine should be used in patients with chronic ulcerative colitis in whom conventional treatment with steroids and sulfasalazine has failed and in whom surgery is inappropriate [155]. Lobo et al. in 1990 reported an initial remission rate of 46 % (13/28) in ulcerative colitis patients treated with azathioprine, and 11 of these 13 patients maintained remission at 2 years [156]. Also in 1990, Adler and Korelitz presented results of treatment with 6-MP in 87 steroid-refractory patients [157]. They noticed that steroid use was eliminated in 48 % of their patients with good symptom control after a mean treatment period of 2.5 months. The mean steroid-free period was 10.9 months [157]. Hawthorne et al. in 1993 studied the effect of the azathioprine withdrawal in 67 patients in remission [158]. Patients in whom azathioprine was continued were in remission for at least 2 years compared to 59 % relapse rate in placebo group [158]. Currently, azathioprine and 6-MP are increasingly used to maintain long-term remission in ulcerative colitis patients.

## Cyclosporine A

It is an immunosuppressive drug derived from soil fungus *Trichoderma polysporum* [159]. It has a rapid onset of action and was discovered by Borel et al. in 1976 [159]. The first case report of successful treatment of a patient with severe ulcerative colitis with cyclosporine was published in 1984 by Gupta et al. [160]. Following this, many uncontrolled studies have been published showing the efficacy of cyclosporine A in the treatment of patients with severe ulcerative colitis [161–164].

The first randomized placebo controlled trial comparing cyclosporine to placebo in the treatment of patients with severe steroid-refractory ulcerative colitis was published by Lichtiger et al. in 1994 [165]. The clinical response rates which were achieved within a mean time of 7 days was 82 % (9/11 patients) in those patients who received cyclosporine A and 0 % (0/9) in patients who received placebo [165]. Cyclosporine A is now one of the treatments of choice in patients presenting with acute severe steroid-refractory ulcerative colitis.

## Biologics

In the 1990s, studies showed increased concentrations of tumor necrosis factor alpha (TNF-α) in the blood, stool, and colonic tissues of patients with IBD [166–168]. This led to the use of anti-TNF-α agents in the treatment of ulcerative colitis patients.

Infliximab, a chimeric monoclonal antibody directed against TNF-α, was the first biologic approved by FDA for the treatment of ulcerative colitis. It is approved for the treatment of moderate-to-severe disease. Three randomized pilot studies evaluated the efficacy of infliximab in the management of steroid-refractory ulcerative colitis [169–171].

Following these pilot studies, in 2005, the first multicenter randomized placebo controlled trial of infliximab for induction and maintenance of remission in patients with steroid-refractory ulcerative colitis was published (ACT 1 and ACT 2) [172]. In Acute Colitis Trial 1 (ACT 1), a total of 364 patients who did not respond to either steroids alone or in combination with antimetabolites were randomly assigned to placebo, infliximab 5 mg/kg, or infliximab 10 mg/kg [172]. Patients were followed for a total of 54 weeks. The clinical response rates at week 8 were 37.2 %, 69.4 %, and 61.5 % for patients receiving placebo, infliximab 5 mg/kg, and infliximab 10 mg/kg, respectively. At week 54, there was significant difference in the clinical remission rates between infliximab group and placebo group [172]. In ACT 2, the efficacy of infliximab was assessed in patients with moderate-to-severe ulcerative colitis who did not respond to 5-ASA or steroids alone or in combination with antimetabolites [172]. Again, infliximab was found superior to placebo in both inducing remission and maintaining remission at week 30 [172].

Recently, the results of a fully humanized monoclonal antibody adalimumab have been published [173]. Adalimumab has gained regulatory approval for ulcerative colitis. Golimumab is a fully humanized monoclonal immunoglobulin directed against TNF-α which has been shown to be effective in ulcerative colitis. In 2013, golimumab gained approval for the treatment of ulcerative colitis. It has been shown to be effective for induction and maintenance of remission in patients with ulcerative colitis [174, 175].

Additionally, a number of biologics targeting various pro-inflammatory cytokines and chemokines involved in the inflammatory cascade are being studied.

## Conclusion

Ulcerative colitis or a diarrheal illness similar to it has been described in the medical literature many centuries ago. But our knowledge of ulcerative colitis has increased significantly only in the last 50–60 years. The treatment of ulcerative colitis has changed dramatically since the introduction of sulfasalazine and steroids. Medical therapy has improved both the mortality rate and quality of life and lifestyle of patients suffering from this disease. Currently, we are in an era of biologics. It remains to be seen what other new treatments will emerge in the next few years and if we will be able to achieve the cure of ulcerative colitis.

## References

1. Kirsner JB. Ulcerative colitis. In: Kirsner JB, editor. Origins and directions of inflammatory bowel disease. Dordrecht: Kluwer Academic Publishers; 2001. p. 13–54.

2. Alexander-Williams J. Historical review. In: Alan RB, Rhodes JM, Hanauer SB, Keighley MRB, Alexander-Williams J, Fazio VW, editors. Inflammatory bowel diseases. 3rd ed. Edinburgh: Churchill Livingstone; 1983. p. 3–10.
3. Wilson PJE. The young pretender. Br Med J. 1961;2:1226.
4. Burch W, Gump DW, Krawitt EL, Burch W, Gump DW, Krawitt EL. Historical case report of Sir William Johnson, the Mohawk Baronet. Am J Gastroenterol. 1992;87:1023–5.
5. De Dombal FT. Ulcerative colitis: definition, historical background, aetiology, diagnosis, natural history and local complications. Postgrad Med J. 1968;44(515):684–92.
6. Fielding JF. "Inflammatory" bowel disease. Br Med J (Clin Res Ed). 1985;290(6461):47–8.
7. Crohn BB. An historic note on ulcerative colitis. Gastroenterology. 1962;42:366–7.
8. Bassler A. Ulcerative colitis. Interstate Med J. 1913;20:705–6.
9. Brown J. The value of complete physiological rest of the large bowel in the treatment of certain ulcerative and obstructive lesions of this organ. Surg Gynecol Obstet. 1913;16:610–3.
10. Logan A. Chronic ulcerative colitis: a review of one hundred and seventeen cases. Northwest Med. 1919;18:1–9.
11. Yeomans F. Chronic ulcerative colitis. JAMA. 1921;77:2043–8.
12. Strauss H. Ueber colitis-probleme. Dtsch Med Wochschr. 1923;49:1568–70.
13. Bargen JA, LA Logan A. The etiology of chronic ulcerative colitis: experimental studies with suggestions for a more rational form of treatment. Arch Intern Med. 1925;36:818–29.
14. Buie L. Chronic ulcerative colitis. JAMA. 1926;87:1271–4.
15. Paulson M. Chronic ulcerative colitis with reference to a bacterial etiology. Experimental studies. Arch Int Med. 1928;41:75.
16. Mones PG, Sanjuan P. Colitis ulcerosa graves non amibianas:etiologic diagnostico and tratamiento medico. Barcelona: Salvat Editores S.A.; 1935. p. 49.
17. Wilson A. A case of ulcerative colitis with multiple perforations. Lancet. 1904;2:1208–9.
18. Lockhart-Mummery J. The causes of colitis: with special reference to its surgical treatment, with an account of 36 cases. Lancet. 1907;1:1638–43.
19. Bargen JA, Dixon C. Chronic ulcerative colitis associated with carcinoma. Arch Surg. 1928;17:561–76.
20. Bargen J. Complications and sequelae of ulcerative colitis. Ann Intern Med. 1929;3:335–52.
21. Crohn B. Ocular lesions complicating ulcerative colitis. Am J Med Sci. 1925;169:260–7.
22. Sloan Jr WP, Bargen JA, Gage RP. Life histories of patients with chronic ulcerative colitis: a review of 2,000 cases. Gastroenterology. 1950;16:25–38.
23. Bockus HL, Roth JL, Buchman E, Kalser M, Staub WR, Finkelstein A, Valdes-Dapena A. Life history of nonspecific ulcerative colitis: relation of prognosis to anatomical and clinical varieties. Gastroenterologia. 1956;86:549–81.
24. Roth JL, Valdes-Dapena A, Stein GN, Bockus HL. Toxic megacolon in ulcerative colitis. Gastroenterology. 1959;37:239–55.
25. Ricketts WE, Palmer WL. Complications of chronic non-specific ulcerative colitis. Gastroenterology. 1946;7:55–66.
26. Kirsner JB, Palmer WL, et al. Clinical course of chronic nonspecific ulcerative colitis. J Am Med Assoc. 1948;137(11):922–8.
27. Goldgraber MB, Humphreys EM, Kirsner JB, Palmer WL. Carcinoma and ulcerative colitis, a clinical-pathologic study. II. Statistical analysis. Gastroenterology. 1958;34(5):840–6.
28. Brust JCM, Bargen JA. Chronic ulcerative colitis among elderly persons. Minnesota Med. 1935;18:583–5.
29. Banks BM, Klayman MI. Idiopathic ulcerative colitis beginning after the age of fifty. N Engl J Med. 1953;249(3):91–6.
30. Bargen JA, Barker N. Extensive arterial and venous thrombosis complicating ulcerative colitis. Arch Intern Med. 1936;58:17–31.
31. Comfort MW, Bargen J, Morlock CG. The association of chronic ulcerative colitis (colitis gravis) with hepatic insufficiency. Med Clin North Am. 1938;22:1089–97.
32. Schlicke CP, Bargen J. Clubbed fingers and ulcerative colitis. Am J Dig Dis. 1940;7:17–22.
33. Lindahl WW, Bargen J. Nephrolithiasis complicating chronic ulcerative colitis after ileostomy. A report of six cases. J Urol. 1941;46:183–92.
34. Jankelson IR, McClure C, Sweetsir FN. Chronic ulcerative colitis II. Complications outside the digestive tract. Rev Gastroenterol. 1942;9:99–104.
35. Chisholm T. Acute fulminating ulcerative colitis with massive perforation and peritonitis – report of a case. Arch Surg. 1946;53:362–76.
36. Ricketts WE, Kirsner JB, Rothman S. Pyoderma gangrenosum in chronic non-specific ulcerative colitis; a report of three cases. Am J Med. 1948;5:69–75.
37. Brooke BN, Slaney G. Portal bacteraemia in ulcerative colitis. Lancet. 1958;1(7032):1206–7.
38. Bywaters EG, Ansell BM. Arthritis associated with ulcerative colitis; a clinical and pathological study. Ann Rheum Dis. 1958;17(2):169–83.
39. Fernandez-Herhily L. The articular manifestations of chronic ulcerative colitis; an analysis of 555 cases. N Engl J Med. 1959; 261(6):259–63.
40. McEwen C, Lingg C, Kirsner JB, Spencer JA. Arthritis accompanying ulcerative colitis. Am J Med. 1962;33:923–41.
41. Matsunaga F. Clinical studies in ulcerative colitis and its related increase in Japan. Proc World Congress of Gastroenterology, Washington, vol. 2. Baltimore: Williams and Wilkins; 1958. p. 955–60.
42. Dawson IM, Pryse-Davies J. The development of carcinoma of the large intestine in ulcerative colitis. Br J Surg. 1959;47:113–28.
43. Goldgraber MB, Kirsner JB. Carcinoma of the colon in ulcerative colitis. Cancer. 1964;17:657–65.
44. Devroede GJ, Taylor WF, Sauer WG, Jackman RJ, Stickler GB. Cancer risk and life expectancy of children with ulcerative colitis. N Engl J Med. 1971;285(1):17–21.
45. Bargen JA, Sauer WG, Sloan WP, Gage RP. The development of cancer in chronic ulcerative colitis. Gastroenterology. 1954;26(1):32–7.
46. Edwards FC, Truelove SC. The course and prognosis of ulcerative colitis. Gut. 1963;4:299–315.
47. Edwards FC, Truelove SC. The course and prognosis of ulcerative colitis. III. Complications. Gut. 1964;5:1–22.
48. Helmholz H. Chronic ulcerative colitis in childhood. Am J Dis Child. 1923;26:418–30.
49. Bourne G. Chronic ulcerative colitis in children. Arch Dis Child. 1926;1:175–81.
50. Jackman RJ, Bargen JA, Helmholz HF. Life histories of ninety-five children with chronic ulcerative colitis: A statistical study based on comparison with a whole group of eight hundred and seventy-one patients. Am J Dis Child. 1940;59:459–67.
51. Bargen JA, Kennedy RL. Chronic ulcerative colitis in children. Postgrad Med. 1955;17:127–31.
52. Beranbaum SL, Waldron RJ. Chronic ulcerative colitis; case report in a newborn infant. Pediatrics. 1952;9:773–8.
53. Davidson M. Juvenile ulcerative colitis. Arch Intern Med. 1939;64:1187–95.
54. Ricketts WE, Benditt EP, Palmer WL. Chronic ulcerative colitis with infantilism and carcinoma of the colon. Gastroenterology. 1945;5:272–80.
55. Stuart WC, Mildred A, Wakefield EG. Metabolic studies in ulcerative colitis. J Clin Invest. 1937;16:161–8.
56. Sappington TS, Bockus HL. Nitrogen metabolism in chronic idiopathic ulcerative colitis and its therapeutic significance. Ann Intern Med. 1949;31:282–302.

57. Kirsner JB, Sheffner AL. Studies on amino acid excretion in man; effect of various protein supplements in a normal man, two patients with benign gastric ulcer and two patients with chronic ulcerative colitis. J Clin Invest. 1950;29:828.

58. Barnes CS, Hayes H. Ulcerative colitis complicating pregnancy and the puerperium. Am J Obstet Gynecol. 1931;22:907–12.

59. Abramson D, Jankelson IR, Milner LR. Pregnancy in idiopathic ulcerative colitis. Am J Obstet Gynecol. 1951;61:121–9.

60. Macdougall I. Ulcerative colitis and pregnancy. Lancet. 1956;271:641–3.

61. Crohn BB, Yarnis H, Crohn EB, Walter RI, Gabrilove LJ. Ulcerative colitis and pregnancy. Gastroenterology. 1956;30:391–403.

62. Korelitz BI. Pregnancy, fertility, and inflammatory bowel disease. Am J Gastroenterol. 1985;80:365–70.

63. Bargen J. Experimental studies on the etiology of chronic ulcerative colitis (preliminary report). JAMA. 1924;83:332.

64. Murray C. Psychogenic factors in the etiology of ulcerative colitis. Am J Dig Dis. 1930;180:239.

65. Sullivan A. Psychogenic factors and ulcerative colitis. Am J Dig Dis. 1935;2:651.

66. Kirsner JB. Historical origins of current IBD concepts. World J Gastroenterol. 2001;7(2):175–84.

67. Almy TP, Kern Jr F, Tulin M. Alterations in colonic function in man under stress; experimental production of sigmoid spasm in healthy persons. Gastroenterology. 1949;12:425–36.

68. Kern Jr F, Almy TP, Abbot FK, Bogdonoff MD. The motility of the distal colon in nonspecific ulcerative colitis. Gastroenterology. 1951;19:492–503.

69. Meyer K, Gellhorn A, Prudden JF, et al. Lysozyme in chronic ulcerative colitis. Proc Soc Exp Biol (N Y). 1947;65:221–2.

70. Glass GB, Pugh BL, et al. Observations on the treatment of human gastric and colonic mucus with lysozyme. J Clin Invest. 1950;29:12–9.

71. Karush A, Daniels GE, O'Connor JF, Stern LO, Karush A, Daniels GE, O'Connor JF, Stern LO. The response to psychotherapy in chronic ulcerative colitis. I. Pretreatment factors. Psychosom Med. 1968;30:255–76.

72. Schlesinger B, Platt J. Ulcerative colitis in childhood and a follow-up study. Proc R Soc Med. 1958;51:733–5.

73. Truelove SC. Ulcerative colitis provoked by milk. Br Med J. 1961;1(5220):154–60.

74. Taylor KB, Truelove SC. Circulating antibodies to milk proteins in ulcerative colitis. Br Med J. 1961;2(5257):924–9.

75. Acheson ED, Truelove SC. Early weaning in the aetiology of ulcerative colitis. A study of feeding in infancy in cases and controls. Br Med J. 1961;2(5257):929–33.

76. Wright R, Truelove SC. A controlled therapeutic trial of various diets in ulcerative colitis. Br Med J. 1965;2(5454):138–41.

77. Kirsner JB, Goldgraber MB. Hypersensitivity, autoimmunity, and the digestive tract. Gastroenterology. 1960;38:536–62.

78. Broberger O, Perlmann P. Autoantibodies in human ulcerative colitis. J Exp Med. 1959;110:657–74.

79. Harrison WJ, Oxon BM. Autoantibodies against intestinal and gastric mucous cells in ulcerative colitis. Lancet. 1965;285(7400):1346–50.

80. Wright R, Truelove SC. Auto-immune reactions in ulcerative colitis. Gut. 1966;7:32–40.

81. Kirsner JB. Historical origins of medical and surgical therapy of inflammatory bowel disease. Lancet. 1998;352(9136):1303–5.

82. Svartz N. Salazopyrin- a new sulfanilamide preparation. A. Therapeutic results in rheumatoid arthritis. B. Therapeutic results in ulcerative colitis. C. Toxic manifestations on treatment with sulfanilamide preparations. Acta Med Scand. 1942;110:577–90.

83. Svartz N. Sulfasalazine: II. Some notes on the discovery and development of salazopyrin. Am J Gastroenterol. 1988;83:497–503.

84. Svartz N. The treatment of 124 cases of ulcerative colitis with salazopyrine and attempts of desensitization in cases of hypersensitiveness to sulfa. Acta Med Scand. 1948;139 suppl 206:465–72.

85. Watkinson G. Sulphasalazine: a review of 40 years' experience. Drugs. 1986;32 Suppl 1:1–11. Review.

86. Baron JH, Connell AM, Lennard-Jones JE, Jones FA. Sulphasalazine and salicylazosulphadimidine in ulcerative colitis. Lancet. 1962;1:1094–6.

87. Misiewicz JJ, Lennard-Jones JE, Connell AM, Baron JH, Jones FA. Controlled trial of sulphasalazine in maintenance therapy for ulcerative colitis. Lancet. 1965;1:185–8.

88. Peppercorn MA, Goldman P. Distribution studies of salicylazosulfapyridine and its metabolites. Gastroenterology. 1973;64(2):240–5.

89. Azad Khan AK, Piris J, Truelove SC. An experiment to determine the active therapeutic moiety of sulphasalazine. Lancet. 1977;2:892–5.

90. Klotz U, Maier K, Fischer C, Heinkel K. Therapeutic efficacy of sulfasalazine and its metabolites in patients with ulcerative colitis and Crohn's disease. N Engl J Med. 1980;303:1499–502.

91. van Hees PA, Bakker JH, van Tongeren JH. Effect of sulphapyridine, 5-aminosalicylic acid, and placebo in patients with idiopathic proctitis: a study to determine the active therapeutic moiety of sulphasalazine. Gut. 1980;21(7):632–5.

92. Taffet SL, Das KM. Sulfasalazine. Adverse effects and desensitization. Dig Dis Sci. 1983;28(9):833–42. Review.

93. Chan RP, Pope DJ, Gilbert AP, Sacra PJ, Baron JH, Lennard-Jones JE. Studies of two novel sulfasalazine analogs, ipsalazide and balsalazide. Dig Dis Sci. 1983;28:609–15.

94. Selby WS, Barr GD, Ireland A, Mason CH, Jewell DP. Olsalazine in active ulcerative colitis. Br Med J (Clin Res Ed). 1985;291:1373–5.

95. Riley SA, Mani V, Goodman MJ, Herd ME, Dutt S, Turnberg LA. Comparison of delayed release 5 aminosalicylic acid (mesalazine) and sulphasalazine in the treatment of mild to moderate ulcerative colitis relapse. Gut. 1988;29:669–74.

96. D'Haens G, Hommes D, Engels L, Baert F, van der Waaij L, Connor P, Ramage J, Dewit O, Palmen M, Stephenson D, Joseph R. Once daily MMX mesalazine for the treatment of mild-to-moderate ulcerative colitis: a phase II, dose-ranging study. Aliment Pharmacol Ther. 2006;24:1087–97.

97. Sandborn WJ, Kamm MA, Lichtenstein GR, Lyne A, Butler T, Joseph RE. MMX Multi Matrix System mesalazine for the induction of remission in patients with mild-to-moderate ulcerative colitis: a combined analysis of two randomized, double-blind, placebo-controlled trials. Aliment Pharmacol Ther. 2007;26:205–15.

98. Kamm MA, Sandborn WJ, Gassull M, Schreiber S, Jackowski L, Butler T, Lyne A, Stephenson D, Palmen M, Joseph RE. Once-daily, high-concentration MMX mesalamine in active ulcerative colitis. Gastroenterology. 2007;132:66–75. quiz 432–3.

99. Lichtenstein GR, Kamm MA, Boddu P, Gubergrits N, Lyne A, Butler T, Lees K, Joseph RE, Sandborn WJ. Effect of once- or twice-daily MMX mesalamine (SPD476) for the induction of remission of mild to moderately active ulcerative colitis. Clin Gastroenterol Hepatol. 2007;5:95–102.

100. Lichtenstein GR, Gordon GL, Zakko S, Murthy U, Sedghi S, Pruitt R, Merchant K, Shaw A, Bortey E, Forbes W. Once-daily mesalamine capsules for maintenance of remission of ulcerative colitis: a phase III placebo-controlled trial. Aliment Pharmacol Ther. 2010;32(8):990–9. doi:10.1111/j.1365-2036.2010.04438.x. Epub 2010 Aug 18.

101. Gray SJ, Reifenstein RW, Benson Jr JA. ACTH therapy in ulcerative colitis and regional enteritis. N Engl J Med. 1951;245(13):481–7.

102. Elliott JM, Giansiracusa JE. ACTH and cortisone in the treatment of ulcerative colitis; an evaluation of their prolonged administration. N Engl J Med. 1954;250(23):969–76.

103. Maltby EJ, Dickson RC, O'sullivan PM. The use of ACTH and cortisone in idiopathic ulcerative colitis. Can Med Assoc J. 1956;74(1):4–9.

104. Kirsner JB, Sklar M, Palmer WL. The use of ACTH, cortisone, hydrocortisone and related compounds in the management of ulcerative colitis; experience in 180 patients. Am J Med. 1957; 22(2):264–74.

105. Zetzel L, Atin HL. ACTH and adrenalcorticosteroids in the treatment of ulcerative colitis. Am J Dig Dis. 1958;3(12):916–30.

106. Kirsner JB, Palmer WL, Spencer JA, Bicks RO, Johnson CF. Corticotropin (ACTH) and the adrenal steroids in the management of ulcerative colitis: observations in 240 patients. Ann Intern Med. 1959;50(4):891–927.

107. Truelove SC, Witts LJ. Cortisone in ulcerative colitis; final report on a therapeutic trial. Br Med J. 1955;2:1041–8.

108. Truelove SC, Witts LJ. Cortisone and corticotrophin in ulcerative colitis. Br Med J. 1959;1(5119):387–94.

109. Lennard-Jones JE, Longmore AJ, Newell AC, Wilson CW, Jones FA. An assessment of prednisone, salazopyrin, and topical hydrocortisone hemisuccinate used as out-patient treatment for ulcerative colitis. Gut. 1960;1:217–22.

110. Baron JH, Connell AM, Kanaghinis TG, Lennard-Jones JE, Jones AF. Out-patient treatment of ulcerative colitis. Comparison between three doses of oral prednisone. Br Med J. 1962;2(5302): 441–3.

111. Powell-Tuck J, Bown RL, Lennard-Jones JE. A comparison of oral prednisolone given as single or multiple daily doses for active proctocolitis. Scand J Gastroenterol. 1978;13(7):833–7.

112. Truelove SC, Jewell DP. Intensive intravenous regimen for severe attacks of ulcerative colitis. Lancet. 1974;1(7866):1067–70.

113. Kaplan HP, Portnoy B, Binder HJ, Amatruda T, Spiro H. A controlled evaluation of intravenous adrenocorticotropic hormone and hydrocortisone in the treatment of acute colitis. Gastroenterology. 1975;69(1):91–5.

114. Powell-Tuck J, Buckell NA, Lennard-Jones JE. A controlled comparison of corticotropin and hydrocortisone in the treatment of severe proctocolitis. Scand J Gastroenterol. 1977;12(8):971–5.

115. Meyers S, Sachar DB, Goldberg JD, Janowitz HD. Corticotropin versus hydrocortisone in the intravenous treatment of ulcerative colitis. A prospective, randomized, double-blind clinical trial. Gastroenterology. 1983;85(2):351–7.

116. Lennard-Jones JE, Misiewicz JJ, Connell AM, Baron JH, Jones FA. Prednisone as maintenance treatment for ulcerative colitis in remission. Lancet. 1965;1(7378):188–9.

117. Sandborn WJ, Travis S, Moro L, Jones R, Gautille T, Bagin R, et al. Once-daily budesonide MMX® extended-release tablets induce remission in patients with mild to moderate ulcerative colitis: results from the CORE I study. Gastroenterology. 2012;143: 1218–26.

118. Truelove SC. Treatment of ulcerative colitis with local hydrocortisone. Br Med J. 1956;2(5004):1267–72.

119. Truelove SC. Treatment of ulcerative colitis with local hydrocortisone hemisuccinate sodium. Br Med J. 1957;1(5033):1437–43.

120. Truelove SC, Hambling MH. Treatment of ulcerative colitis with local hydrocortisone hemisuccinate sodium; a report on a controlled therapeutic trial. Br Med J. 1958;2(5104):1072–7.

121. Truelove SC. Systemic and local corticosteroid therapy in ulcerative colitis. Br Med J. 1960;1(5171):464–7.

122. Watkinson G. Treatment of ulcerative colitis with topical hydrocortisone hemisuccinate sodium; a controlled trial employing restricted sequential analysis. Br Med J. 1958;2(5104):1077–82.

123. Matts SGF. Local treatment of ulcerative colitis with prednisolone-21-phosphate enemata. Lancet. 1960;1:517–9.

124. Matts SG. Betamethasone enemata in ulcerative colitis. Gut. 1962;3:312–4.

125. Lennard-Jones JE, Baron JH, Connell AM, Jones FA. A double blind controlled trial of prednisolone-21-phosphate suppositories in the treatment of idiopathic proctitis. Gut. 1962;3:207–10.

126. Farthing MJ, Rutland MD, Clark ML. Retrograde spread of hydrocortisone containing foam given intrarectally in ulcerative colitis. Br Med J. 1979;2(6194):822–4.

127. Ruddell WS, Dickinson RJ, Dixon MF, Axon AT. Treatment of distal ulcerative colitis (proctosigmoiditis) in relapse: comparison of hydrocortisone enemas and rectal hydrocortisone foam. Gut. 1980;21(10):885–9.

128. Somerville KW, Langman MJ, Kane SP, MacGilchrist AJ, Watkinson G, Salmon P. Effect of treatment on symptoms and quality of life in patients with ulcerative colitis: comparative trial of hydrocortisone acetate foam and prednisolone 21-phosphate enemas. Br Med J (Clin Res Ed). 1985;291(6499):866.

129. Kumana CR, Seaton T, Meghji M, Castelli M, Benson R, Sivakumaran T. Beclomethasone dipropionate enemas for treating inflammatory bowel disease without producing Cushing's syndrome or hypothalamic pituitary adrenal suppression. Lancet. 1982; 1(8272):579–83.

130. Hamilton I, Pinder IF, Dickinson RJ, Ruddell WS, Dixon MF, Axon AT. A comparison of prednisolone enemas with low-dose oral prednisolone in the treatment of acute distal ulcerative colitis. Dis Colon Rectum. 1984;27(11):701–2.

131. McIntyre PB, Macrae FA, Berghouse L, English J, Lennard-Jones JE. Therapeutic benefits from a poorly absorbed prednisolone enema in distal colitis. Gut. 1985;26(8):822–4.

132. Crotty B, Jewell DP. Drug therapy of ulcerative colitis. Br J Clin Pharmacol. 1992;34(3):189–98. Review.

133. Davies PS, Rhodes J, Heatley RV, Owen E. Metronidazole in the treatment of chronic proctitis: a controlled trial. Gut. 1977;18(8): 680–1.

134. Chapman RW, Selby WS, Jewell DP. Controlled trial of intravenous metronidazole as an adjunct to corticosteroids in severe ulcerative colitis. Gut. 1986;27(10):1210–2.

135. Dickinson RJ, O'Connor HJ, Pinder I, Hamilton I, Johnston D, Axon AT. Double blind controlled trial of oral vancomycin as adjunctive treatment in acute exacerbations of idiopathic colitis. Gut. 1985;26(12):1380–4.

136. Dickinson RJ, Ashton MG, Axon AT, Smith RC, Yeung CK, Hill GL. Controlled trial of intravenous hyperalimentation and total bowel rest as an adjunct to the routine therapy of acute colitis. Gastroenterology. 1980;79(6):1199–204.

137. McIntyre PB, Powell-Tuck J, Wood SR, Lennard-Jones JE, Lerebours E, Hecketsweiler P, Galmiche JP, Colin R. Controlled trial of bowel rest in the treatment of severe acute colitis. Gut. 1986;27(5):481–5.

138. Davies PS, Rhodes J. Maintenance of remission in ulcerative colitis with sulphasalazine or a high-fibre diet: a clinical trial. Br Med J. 1978;1(6126):1524–5.

139. Heatley RV, Calcraft BJ, Rhodes J, Owen E, Evans BK. Disodium cromoglycate in the treatment of chronic proctitis. Gut. 1975; 16(7):559–63.

140. Mani V, Lloyd G, Green FH, Fox H, Turnberg LA. Treatment of ulcerative colitis with oral disodium cromoglycate. A double-blind controlled trial. Lancet. 1976;1(7957):439–41.

141. Langman MJS, Dronfield MW. Disodium cromoglycate maintenance treatment of ulcerative colitis. Acta Allergol. 1977;13:76–81.

142. Dronfield MW, Langman MJ. Comparative trial of sulphasalazine and oral sodium cromoglycate in the maintenance of remission in ulcerative colitis. Gut. 1978;19(12):1136–9.

143. Willoughby CP, Heyworth MF, Piris J, Truelove SC. Comparison of disodium cromoglycate and sulphasalazine as maintenance therapy for ulcerative colitis. Lancet. 1979;1(8108):119–22.

144. Hitchings GH, Elion GB, Falco EA, Russell PB, Vanderwerff H. Studies on analogs of purines and pyrimidines. Ann N Y Acad Sci. 1950;52(8):1318–35.

145. Schwartz R, Stack J, Dameshek W. Effect of 6-mercaptopurine on antibody production. Proc Soc Exp Biol Med. 1958;99(1):164–7.

146. Bean RH. The treatment of chronic ulcerative colitis with 6-mercaptopurine. Med J Aust. 1962;49(2):592–3.

147. Bean RH. Treatment of ulcerative colitis with anti-metabolites. Br Med J. 1966;1.

148. Bowen GE, Irons Jr GV, Rhodes JB, Kirsner JB. Early experiences with azathioprine in ulcerative colitis; a note of caution. JAMA. 1966;195:460–4.

149. Jones FA, Lennard-Jones JE, Hinton JM, Reeves WG. Dangers of immunosuppressive drugs in ulcerative colitis. Br Med J. 1966;1(5500):1418.

150. Present DH. 6-Mercaptopurine and other immunosuppressive agents in the treatment of Crohn's disease and ulcerative colitis. Gastroenterol Clin North Am. 1989;18(1):57–71. Review.

151. Korelitz BI, Wisch N. Long term therapy of ulcerative colitis with 6-mercaptopurine: a personal series. Am J Dig Dis. 1972;17(2):111–8.

152. Jewell DP, Truelove SC. Azathioprine in ulcerative colitis: an interim report on a controlled therapeutic trial. Br Med J. 1972;1(5802):709–12.

153. Rosenberg JL, Wall AJ, Levin B, Binder HJ, Kirsner JB. A controlled trial of azathioprine in the management of chronic ulcerative colitis. Gastroenterology. 1975;69(1):96–9.

154. Caprilli R, Carratù R, Babbini M. Double-blind comparison of the effectiveness of azathioprine and sulfasalazine in idiopathic proctocolitis. Preliminary report. Am J Dig Dis. 1975;20(2):115–20.

155. Kirk AP, Lennard-Jones JE. Controlled trial of azathioprine in chronic ulcerative colitis. Br Med J (Clin Res Ed). 1982;284(6325):1291–2.

156. Lobo AJ, Foster PN, Burke DA, Johnston D, Axon AT. The role of azathioprine in the management of ulcerative colitis. Dis Colon Rectum. 1990;33(5):374–7.

157. Adler DJ, Korelitz BI. The therapeutic efficacy of 6-mercaptopurine in refractory ulcerative colitis. Am J Gastroenterol. 1990;85(6):717–22.

158. Hawthorne AB, Logan RF, Hawkey CJ, Foster PN, Axon AT, Swarbrick ET, Scott BB, Lennard-Jones JE. Randomised controlled trial of azathioprine withdrawal in ulcerative colitis. BMJ. 1992;305(6844):20–2.

159. Hodgson HJ. Cyclosporin in inflammatory bowel disease. Aliment Pharmacol Ther. 1991;5(4):343–50. Review.

160. Gupta S, Keshavarzian A, Hodgson HJ. Cyclosporin in ulcerative colitis. Lancet. 1984;2:1277–8.

161. Kirschner BS, Whitington PF, Black DD, Bostwick D. Cyclosporin-induced remission in severe colitis unresponsive to corticosteroid therapy (abstract). Pediatr Res. 1987;21:271A.

162. Shelley ED, Shelley WB. Cyclosporine therapy for pyoderma gangrenosum associated with sclerosing cholangitis and ulcerative colitis. J Am Acad Dermatol. 1988;18(5 Pt 1):1084–8.

163. Bianchi Porro G, Panza E, Petrillo M. Cyclosporin A in acute ulcerative colitis (letter to editor). Ital J Gastroenterol. 1987;19:40–1.

164. Stange EF, Fleig WE, Rehklau E, Ditschuneit H. Cyclosporin A treatment in inflammatory bowel disease. Dig Dis Sci. 1989;34(9):1387–92.

165. Lichtiger S, Present DH, Kornbluth A, Gelernt I, Bauer J, Galler G, Michelassi F, Hanauer S. Cyclosporine in severe ulcerative colitis refractory to steroid therapy. N Engl J Med. 1994;330(26):1841–5.

166. Braegger CP, Nicholls S, Murch SH, Stephens S, MacDonald TT. Tumour necrosis factor alpha in stool as a marker of intestinal inflammation. Lancet. 1992;339:89–91.

167. Murch SH, Braegger CP, Walker-Smith JA, MacDonald TT. Location of tumour necrosis factor alpha by immunohistochemistry in chronic inflammatory bowel disease. Gut. 1993;34:1705–9.

168. Murch SH, Lamkin VA, Savage MO, Walker-Smith JA, MacDonald TT. Serum concentrations of tumour necrosis factor alpha in childhood chronic inflammatory bowel disease. Gut. 1991;32:913–7.

169. Chey WY. Infliximab for patients with refractory ulcerative colitis. Inflamm Bowel Dis. 2001;7 Suppl 1:S30–3.

170. Chey WY, Hussain A, Ryan C, Potter GD, Shah A. Infliximab for refractory ulcerative colitis. Am J Gastroenterol. 2001;96:2373–81.

171. Sands BE, Tremaine WJ, Sandborn WJ, Rutgeerts PJ, Hanauer SB, Mayer L, Targan SR, Podolsky DK. Infliximab in the treatment of severe, steroid-refractory ulcerative colitis: a pilot study. Inflamm Bowel Dis. 2001;7:83–8.

172. Rutgeerts P, Sandborn WJ, Feagan BG, Reinisch W, Olson A, Johanns J, Travers S, Rachmilewitz D, Hanauer SB, Lichtenstein GR, de Villiers WJ, Present D, Sands BE, Colombel JF. Infliximab for induction and maintenance therapy for ulcerative colitis. N Engl J Med. 2005;353:2462–76.

173. Afif W, Leighton JA, Hanauer SB, Loftus Jr EV, Faubion WA, Pardi DS, Tremaine WJ, Kane SV, Bruining DH, Cohen RD, Rubin DT, Hanson KA, Sandborn WJ. Open-label study of adalimumab in patients with ulcerative colitis including those with prior loss of response or intolerance to infliximab. Inflamm Bowel Dis. 2009;15(9):1302–7.

174. Sandborn WJ, Feagan BG, Marano C, Zhang H, Strauss R, Johanns J, Adedokun OJ, Guzzo C, Colombel JF, Reinisch W, Gibson PR, Collins J, Järnerot G, Rutgeerts P. Subcutaneous golimumab maintains clinical response in patients with moderate-to-severe ulcerative colitis. Gastroenterology. 2013;146(1):96–109.e1. doi:pii: S0016-5085(13)00886-X. 10.1053/j.gastro.2013.06.010.

175. Sandborn WJ, Feagan BG, Marano C, Zhang H, Strauss R, Johanns J, Adedokun OJ, Guzzo C, Colombel JF, Reinisch W, Gibson PR, Collins J, Järnerot G, Hibi T, Rutgeerts P, PURSUIT-SC Study Group. Subcutaneous golimumab induces clinical response and remission in patients with moderate to severe ulcerative colitis. Gastroenterology. 2013;146(1):85–95, quiz e14–5. doi:pii: S0016-5085(13)00846-9. 10.1053/j.gastro.2013.05.048. [Epub ahead of print].

# The Role of the Food and Drug Administration in Medical Therapy for Ulcerative Colitis

**2**

Conor Lahiff, Alan C. Moss, and Adam S. Cheifetz

**Keywords**

Ulcerative colitis • Treatment • Clinical trials • Food and Drug Administration (FDA) • Medication • Biologic agents

## Introduction and Background

Ulcerative colitis (UC) affects approximately 1 in 400 people internationally [1], with a higher prevalence in the Western hemisphere, although more recently incidence and prevalence rates have been rising in the rest of the world, particularly in Asia [2]. The majority of UC patients are prescribed with medication for induction or maintenance of remission [3]. In addition to standard therapies, recent developments in immunology have identified novel therapeutic pathways and biologic agents to treat inflammatory bowel disease (IBD). There are currently 11 drugs and biologic agents (including prednisolone, sulfasalazine, balsalazide, budesonide MMX, infliximab, adalimumab, golimumab, and different preparations of mesalamines) approved by the Food and Drug Administration (FDA) to treat UC (Table 2.1). At present, there are 145 registered clinical trials evaluating therapeutics for managing adult UC, including drugs, biologic agents, and clinical tools for therapeutic monitoring of treatment response and disease activity (www.clinicaltrials.gov, accessed 6/2/2013).

The Food and Drug Administration (FDA) has the responsibility to ensure the safety and efficacy of all prescription drugs used in the United States and is "responsible for protecting the public health by assuring the safety, efficacy and security of human and veterinary drugs, biological products, medical devices, our nation's food supply, cosmetics and products that emit radiation" [4]. In IBD, a major role for the FDA is the assessment of new agents as they navigate the drug development pipeline to approval and increasingly in post-marketing surveillance.

## History of the FDA

The FDA has broad oversight and responsibility for all medical products in the United States. Its legislative basis originated in the Federal Food, Drug, and Cosmetic Act of 1938, which required that new medications be tested for safety before they could be marketed, and these results submitted to the FDA. This act developed after the sulfanilamide elixir disaster of 1937, when over 100 people died from poisoning by diethylene glycol contained in this "medication." The teratogenic effects of thalidomide became known in Europe in the late 1950s, leading to its removal from the market in 1961. This resulted in the FDA garnering more power. In 1962, the Kefauver-Harris Amendment expanded the FDA's responsibility and required drug manufacturers to demonstrate that their products were both safe and effective prior to marketing. These amendments raised the standard of evidence significantly for pharmaceutical companies. Due to the stricter nature of the laws, one-third of marketed drugs were eliminated

C. Lahiff, M.D. (✉)
Gastrointestinal Unit, Mater Hospital,
Whitty Building 4th Floor, Eccles St., Dublin 7, Ireland

Division of Gastroenterology, Center for Inflammatory Bowel Disease, Beth Israel Deaconess Medical Center, 330 Brookline Avenue, Boston, MA 02215, USA
e-mail: conorlahiff@physicians.ie

A.C. Moss, M.D. • A.S. Cheifetz, M.D.
Division of Gastroenterology, Center for Inflammatory Bowel Disease, Beth Israel Deaconess Medical Center, 330 Brookline Avenue, Boston, MA 02215, USA
e-mail: amoss@bidmc.harvard.edu; acheifet@bidmc.harvard.edu

G.R. Lichtenstein (ed.), *Medical Therapy of Ulcerative Colitis*,
DOI 10.1007/978-1-4939-1677-1_2, © Springer Science+Business Media New York 2014

**Table 2.1** Summary of FDA-approved agents in UC, year of approval, and specific FDA-approved indications

| Drug | FDA approval | FDA-approved indication in ulcerative colitis |
|---|---|---|
| Prednisolone | 1972 | To tide the patient over a critical period of the disease in ulcerative colitis |
| Sulfasalazine | 1977 | Treatment of mild to moderate UC, as adjunctive treatment in severe UC, and for the prolongation of the remission period between acute attacks of UC |
| Mesalamines: | | |
| Asacol | 1992 | Induction and maintenance of clinical and endoscopic remission in mild to moderately active UC |
| Pentasa | 1993 | Induction of clinical and endoscopic remission in mild to moderately active UC |
| Lialda (United States)/ Mezavant (Europe) | 2007 | Induction of clinical and endoscopic remission in mild to moderately active UC |
| Apriso (United States)/ Salofalk (Europe) | 2008 | Maintenance of clinical remission in UC |
| Balsalazide disodium | 2000 | Induction of clinical remission in mild to moderately active UC |
| Infliximab | 2005 | Induction (8 weeks) and maintenance (1 year) of clinical and endoscopic remission in moderate to severely active UC, which is unresponsive to conventional therapy |
| Adalimumab | 2012 | Induction (8 weeks) and maintenance (1 year) of clinical remission in adult patients with moderate to severely active UC which is refractory to steroids, azathioprine, or 6-mercaptopurine |
| Budesonide MMX | 2012 | Treatment of active mild to moderate UC in adults. Licensed for induction of remission (8 weeks) |
| Golimumab | 2013 | Treatment of moderately to severely active UC in adult patients who have demonstrated corticosteroid dependence or who have had an inadequate response to or failed to tolerate oral aminosalicylates, oral corticosteroids, azathioprine, or 6-mercaptopurine. Licensed for induction of clinical remission and maintenance of clinical remission in induction responders |

*UC* ulcerative colitis. *FDA* Food and Drug Administration; data accessed from http://www.accessdata.fda.gov/scripts/cder/drugsatfda/index.cfm

from the market for unsuccessfully demonstrating their efficacy claims [5]. The Kefauver-Harris Amendment also gave the FDA control over advertising for prescription drugs and required that informed consent be obtained from patients participating in clinical trials.

The Food and Drug Administration Modernization Act of 1997 expanded the legislation to include accelerated review of drugs and medical devices, as well as regulation of advertising of unapproved uses (off-label) of approved drugs. Biologic agents, which are medical products derived from living sources, came under the FDA's control in 1972 and later the Center for Biologics Evaluation and Research (CBER). In 2003, the FDA transferred the jurisdiction of many biologics, including monoclonal antibodies, cytokines, novel proteins, immune modulators, and growth factors, to the Center for Drug Evaluation and Research (CDER), which regulates the approval process for most drugs. CBER maintained jurisdiction over other biologics, such as vaccines, blood products, and gene therapy.

## FDA Organization

The FDA is led by the Commissioner of Food and Drugs who is appointed by the President of the United States. The Office of the Commissioner (OC) oversees all the agency's workings and is responsible for implementing the FDA's mission. There are seven centers within the FDA, each with a different product responsibility. The CDER has oversight for all drugs and most biologic therapeutic products. CDER

is responsible for regulating the manufacturing, labeling, and advertising of drug products. Its main objective is to ensure that safe and effective agents are available to improve the health of consumers. The CDER has four functional areas:

- New drug development and review
- Post-market drug surveillance
- Generic drug review
- Over-the-counter drug review

New drug development constitutes a major function of the CDER, as it takes approximately 8 years to study and test a new drug before it is approved for use by the public [6].

## FDA Process of Drug Approval

The Code of Federal Regulations governs the supervision of new drug development by the FDA. The FDA requires three crucial stages for new drug approval: (1) an investigational new drug application (IND), (2) a new drug application (NDA), and (3) post-marketing surveillance (phase IV). Before any trials can take place in humans, an IND is required [7]. The IND is not an application for marketing approval but a request for an exemption from the federal statute that prohibits an unapproved drug from being shipped in interstate commerce. Commercial INDs are applications submitted primarily by companies whose ultimate goal is to obtain marketing approval for a new product. The IND needs to include toxicity data from two animal models and pharmacokinetics and pharmacodynamics. Genotoxicity (DNA mutations) screening is performed, as well as investigations on drug absorption, metabolism, and toxicity of the drug's metabolites [8]. This process can take up to 3 years, but in most cases, it can be completed in 18 months. With some agents, long-term animal studies may continue in parallel with human clinical trials, particularly if the drug is to be used for chronic or recurrent conditions. A sponsor can also demonstrate that a drug is safe by providing data from previous clinical testing or marketing of the drug in the United States or another country. The FDA encourages meetings with the sponsor at this stage to review plans for further testing. Once the IND application has been approved, the drug sponsor can undertake clinical trials in humans. However, the vast majority of INDs are, in fact, filed for noncommercial research. This includes Investigator INDs for research proposals and Emergency Use INDs and Treatment INDs in cases where no other treatments are available for a condition.

The clinical studies process (phase I–III, described below) typically takes up to 10 years to complete and involves hundreds to thousands of patients at a cost of hundreds of millions of dollars. At its completion, the drug sponsor can submit a new drug application (NDA) to the FDA. Once the division director for that therapeutic area signs an approval action letter, the product can be legally marketed in the United States.

## Preclinical Testing

Comprehensive preclinical testing is required but unfortunately does not entirely predict safety of new agents in humans. Systemic allergic reactions can be difficult to predict in preclinical models, as occurred in studies with the anti-CD28 monoclonal antibody TGN1412 [9]. Preclinical studies of immunosuppressive agents are limited to assessing myelosuppression or increased frequency of infections or malignancy in animal models. However, these methods may not detect functional changes in immune function, which needs to be borne in mind when conducting these studies in healthy volunteers and obtaining informed consent at enrollment.

## Investigational New Drug Application

Once the preclinical data collection is completed, the sponsor submits an IND application, as described above. This includes manufacturing information, pharmacological data, and toxicology results. The sponsor nominates principal investigators (PI) who will undertake the clinical trials if the IND is approved. Once the FDA receives the IND, it has 30 days in which to notify the sponsor of concerns that may lead it to place a hold on the process. Otherwise, the IND is effective and clinical studies can begin.

## Clinical Trials

The process of organizing and completing clinical trials is the most time-consuming and expensive element of the FDA approval procedure. Each center that intends to recruit participants is headed by a PI. The PI is responsible for securing and maintaining local institutional review board (IRB) approval and protecting the safety and rights of participants throughout the course of the clinical trial. They must maintain adequate records and submit timely reports relating to study outcomes and adverse events. During the study, the IRB reviews reports of adverse events, as well as reports from the data and safety monitoring committee to decide whether the study may continue based on interim safety reports. In practice, industry-sponsored trials for new agents will often involve contract research organizations (CRO), which assist the investigator in maintaining compliance with the local and federal regulations regarding clinical trials.

## Phase I Studies

The purpose of phase I studies is to establish the safety of a drug and its side effects at various doses in healthy individuals. This process involves obtaining data on the pharmacokinetics, metabolism and excretion, and toxicity by administering the novel agent to healthy human volunteers, starting at subclinical doses. Generally, up to 100 volunteers are recruited over 6–18 months until adequate data are available to design phase II studies. Occasionally phase I studies may involve those with advanced malignancies for whom no other therapies are available. Seventy percent of clinical IND applications advance from phase I to phase II studies [10].

## Phase II Studies

Phase II studies assess the safety and efficacy of a drug in a well-defined group of patients with the relevant disease. The design may comprise phase IIA (open-label trials) followed by phase IIB (randomized controlled trials) or just randomized controlled trials alone.

The primary goal of phase II studies is a proof of concept that the drug is safe and effective in treating a particular disease. Typically, a few hundred patients with strict eligibility criteria are enrolled and followed over a number of years (usually at least 2 years). However, in IBD, most phase II studies occur over 26–52 weeks. Further safety data is also obtained from these studies, as a larger number of participants are involved and adverse events particular to patients with the disease of interest may be highlighted. If the safety and efficacy data are positive, the following step is a phase III study.

An example of a phase II trial in UC is the pediatric UC (T72) trial which was an open-label (phase IIa) study of infliximab use in children, after extrapolation from larger adult studies.

## Phase III Studies

These are the pivotal, large randomized controlled trials whose purpose is to corroborate the findings of phase II studies. Phase III studies further gauge the efficacy, safety, and dosing in diseased patients and controls and typically include hundreds to thousands of patients. These studies often occur over a number of years and are designed to contain sufficient statistical power to detect differences between the agent and placebo or standard of care. Phase III studies are the foundation of the sponsor's new drug application (NDA) to the FDA. Two positive adequately controlled trials (usually phase III or phase IIb) are required to obtain FDA approval for a new drug. These studies form the cornerstone of the prescribing and package insert information. Approximately 30 % of IND applications submitted to the FDA complete phase III studies [10]. Examples of phase III trials in UC include the ULTRA1 and ULTRA2 trials for adalimumab [11, 12] and ACT1 and ACT2 for infliximab [13].

## New Drug Application

The objective of this enormous task is the gathering of sufficient data to submit an NDA to the FDA for approval to market the treatment. The NDA includes a comprehensive evaluation of the characteristics of the drug including physical composition, manufacturing process, pharmacological effects, toxicology, clinical efficacy, and case report data. The NDA is examined by CDER expert panels in each of the areas of interest and with external advisory committees (FDA Advisory Committees) providing further input. The key questions the FDA has to answer are (1) is this drug effective in treating the condition it purports to treat? and (2) do the results support an acceptable benefit-to-risk ratio? Considerations of cost and health economic analyses are not a part of the FDA pre-marketing approval process.

The FDA's evaluation may include inspection of the manufacturing facilities and clinical trial sites to verify the details in the submitted application. The FDA is required to provide an interim evaluation within 6 months; and the average time to a final decision is around 24 months. During this period, the FDA is in regular contact with the drug sponsor to ensure that all additional information or data required by the expert panel is provided. The final decision of the CDER panel is either "approval," "approvable with minor changes," or "not approvable." The majority of NDAs are approved, allowing the sponsor to begin manufacturing and distribution. Those considered not approvable can request an appeal hearing or retract the application and reapply with adjustments.

## Post-marketing Surveillance

Once a drug becomes FDA approved, it is actually the first time it is utilized and studied in patients who were not eligible for the original trials. This may include the elderly, children, women of childbearing age, and patients with significant comorbidities. Ironically, the elderly, who constitute about 70 % of medication recipients, only make up about 30 % of clinical trial participants. In fact, a recent study demonstrated that only 26 % of UC patients seen in everyday clinical practice would have qualified for pivotal clinical trials for infliximab based on the inclusion criteria [14].

Another feature of the post-marketing phase is that the number of people exposed to the drug expands significantly beyond the confines of clinical studies to general practice. As a consequence, rare side effects, adverse events in particular populations, and long-term complications may only become obvious at this juncture. For example, a greater than expected number of cases of tuberculosis (TB) were recognized when infliximab was first used to treat Crohn's disease [15]. Since identifying this increased risk of TB, it is now become standard practice to screen for latent TB prior to initiating an anti-TNF. Other examples are the increased risk of fungal infections with anti-TNF and progressive multifocal leuko-encephalopathy (PML) with natalizumab.

For all of these reasons, the CDER's Office of Drug Safety (ODS) monitors the safety profile of a drug after it has been approved for use. Pharmaceutical companies are required to report all adverse events associated with a new drug. In addition, there is a voluntary system of reporting by health-care workers (MedWatch). The ODS is responsible for updating labeling, notifying the public and physicians of new risks, implementing risk management programs, and rarely withdrawing drugs from the market.

Phase IV studies incorporate such post-marketing surveillance and can be requested by the FDA as part of the approval process, as in the case of infliximab's original license in 2005. The TREAT (Therapy Resource, Evaluation, and Assessment Tool) Registry is an example of an FDA-mandated phase IV trial; and in Europe, the manufacturers of infliximab (Merck) are conducting a post-marketing safety registry for infliximab in collaboration with the European Medicines Agency (EMA). However, once a drug is approved, the FDA cannot enforce this requirement.

The post-marketing surveillance process certainly has its faults, including its dependence on health-care providers and pharmaceutical companies informing the FDA of adverse events. Despite these limitations, 20 % of drugs receive black box warnings after FDA approval, and 4 % of FDA-approved drugs are later withdrawn from the market which demonstrates the positive role of post-marketing surveillance in identifying rare safety signals [16, 17].

The Prescription Drug User Fee Act (PDUFA) was enacted in 1997 and most recently updated and reauthorized in 2012. The Act provides for financial support from pharmaceutical companies to fund the assessment and approval process for new drugs and biologics. The deadlines imposed on the FDA under the Act have led to more expedient approval decisions. However, this process has been criticized by some who feel that the practice may lead to inferior safety monitoring [18], specifically with regard to the discovery of unanticipated post-marketing adverse effects. This area remains of particular relevance to IBD, with case reports of hepatosplenic T-cell lymphoma which appeared after 10 years of antitumor necrosis factor (TNF) use [19]. To offset these concerns, the latest revision of the Act (2012) allowed increased FDA monitoring of adverse events and lengthened the time for FDA review.

## FDA-Approved Medicine in Ulcerative Colitis

Not all therapies utilized for the treatment of UC are FDA approved for this indication, and some (e.g., mercaptopurine, azathioprine) have never been subjected to randomized controlled trials in UC patients. Table 2.1 lists the FDA-approved medications in common use for the treatment of UC along with their dates of approval and details of FDA labels. As the standard of evidence upon which the FDA bases its decision to license a drug for use in the United States has increased in more recent years and the evolution of the randomized controlled trial as the gold standard tool for assessing new medicines, recently licensed treatments for UC have all been approved on this basis. However, some of the older agents such as mercaptopurine and azathioprine were approved before this requirement became standard and, in the case of the former two agents, before the Kefauver-Harris Amendment of 1962, which stated an agent should be proven both effective *and* safe in relation to its directed use [20]. Despite this, there are 50 years of post-marketing surveillance data and multiple meta-analyses supporting the use of these agents for the treatment of UC.

Although all aminosalicylates were FDA approved after the Kefauver-Harris Amendments and on the basis of randomized controlled trials, the actual study endpoints were quite variable. In fact, the various mesalamine formulations have been approved based on either endoscopic endpoints or a combination of clinical and endoscopic variables. No single clinical or endoscopic scoring system has been consistently utilized across trials. This lack of a clear gold-standard scoring system and endpoints limits the physicians' ability to compare the studies and their results. In fact, there are more than ten different scoring systems for UC, most of which have not been appropriately validated [21]. Due to the variability in study design, endpoints, and scoring systems, each drug has a distinctly worded FDA indication (Table 2.1). This has also led to a discrepancy between the FDA-approved indications and/or dose of these medications and what is truly done in clinical practice. For example, the only 5-aminosalicylates FDA approved for maintenance of remission in UC are Asacol (Warner Chilcott), Apriso (Salix), and Lialda (Shire). Additionally, the duration of the maintenance studies is generally no more than 6 months. However, despite FDA labeling, in clinical practice all of the mesalamine products are used to induce and maintain remission in UC [22]. The newer UC medications, such as infliximab and adalimumab, and most recently budesonide MMX and golimumab, have been approved based on more extensive and prolonged phase III trials (Table 2.1) and include both clinical and endoscopic endpoints in their label information.

## Future Treatments for Ulcerative Colitis

The rapid pace of expanding knowledge in the fields of molecular biology and immunology has led to the recognition of many new potential therapeutic targets. Some of the newer drugs at the later stages of development are summarized in Table 2.2. As future pharmacological agents are presented to the FDA for approval in the upcoming years,

**Table 2.2** Therapeutic agents for UC currently at advanced stages of development

| Drug | Mechanism of action | Stage of development |
|---|---|---|
| Vedolizumab [38] | α4β7-integrin cell adhesion molecule (CAM) inhibitor | Phase III |
| Tofacitinib [39] | Oral janus kinase (JAK) inhibitor | Phase III |
| LMW heparin [40] | Orally administered antioxidant | Phase II |
| Etrolizumab [41] | β7-integrin (CAM) inhibitor | Phase II |
| Fecal microbiota transplant[a] | Fecal bacteriotherapy | Phase II |
| Propionyl L-carnitine[a] | Reduces membrane lipid peroxidation in endothelial cells | Phase III |
| DIMS0150[a] | Toll-like receptor 9 activator | Phase III |
| Budesonide rectal foam[a] | Topical steroid | Phase III |
| Tralokinumab[a] | Recombinant human anti-IL-13 antibody | Phase II |
| Bertilimumab[a] | Recombinant human IgG4 antibody | Phase II |

[a]Data from www.clinicaltrials.gov, accessed 7/11/13

increasing use of objective endpoints, such as mucosal healing, CRP and fecal calprotectin, and standardization of clinical endpoints and scoring systems, should be the benchmark upon which approval is based. Existing data suggests UC patients who achieve mucosal healing have better long-term outcomes in terms of future hospitalization, escalation of medical therapy, and colectomy [23, 24]. The data also suggests that mucosal healing can be achieved in similar proportions of patients using mesalamine [25], prednisolone [23], or infliximab [13]. The lack of a single universal and reproducible endoscopic scoring system remains an obstacle to standardization of mucosal healing as a clinical trial endpoint [26]. Surrogate biomarkers for mucosal healing, such as fecal calprotectin, are emerging as a more cost-effective method for assessing outcomes and healing [27]. However, to date, they have yet to be sufficiently validated to allow routine use in clinical trials [28]. Non-pharmacological applications for INDs currently at the clinical trial stage (www.clinicaltrials.gov, accessed 7/11/2013) include fecal transplantation, which has recently shown efficacy in the treatment of *Clostridium difficile* infection [29, 30], and phosphatidylcholine [31].

## Generic Mesalamine and Bioequivalence for Biologic Agents

In 1984, the Congress passed the Hatch-Waxman Act (Drug Price Competition and Patent Term Restoration Act) to improve management options for physicians and patients and avoid replication of previously conducted studies. The act permits sponsors to apply for an abbreviated new drug application (ANDA) for generic drugs. If awarded, the company is required only to prove that the generic medication contains the same active ingredient and is bioequivalent to an FDA-approved therapy. Approval can be granted without having to present independent proof of efficacy and safety of the anticipated generic medication.

However, proving that a generic medication contains the same active ingredient and is bioequivalent has proven to be a controversial area for two groups of common IBD medications: mesalamine and the biologics. Despite these concerns on how to demonstrate bioequivalence, ever increasing pressure to decrease health-care costs has led to legislation for the regulation of generic biologics. The Biologics Price Competition Act forms part of the 2010 Patient Protection and Affordable Care Act and allows for a shortened approval pathway for bio-similars or follow-on biologics. The Act provides for standards for bio-similarity and interchangeability, and there are further provisions for market exclusivity. It is still not clear how the FDA will establish bio-similarity, though it remains of particular interest to the producers of the currently approved biologics [32].

## Further Challenges in Drug Development in IBD

The drug development process is a major undertaking for any drug sponsor. As the regulatory and clinical research environment becomes more complex, challenges persist in providing safe, effective, and affordable therapies to patients with UC in a timely manner [4]. With increasing number of trainees opting for private practice rather than academic medicine, there are limited numbers of gastroenterologists in a position to become involved in clinical trials [6]. Those remaining in academic medicine and wishing to partake in clinical trials are faced with increasing requirements in relation to regulatory compliance, which places a significant time burden on research staff.

Efforts should be made to improve and standardize the design of clinical trials in IBD. Study endpoints should include more objective markers such as mucosal healing and minimally invasive markers of disease activity (such as CRP and fecal calprotectin), together with clinical trial endpoints. Additionally, closer therapeutic monitoring of patients in post-marketing surveillance and in clinical practice is also needed. With this approach one could expect improvement in the approval process, trial data would be easier to interpret, and differences between specific agents could be more easily identified [33]. This would facilitate a more tailored approach to therapy for individual patients. The FDA needs to evolve as clinical trial practice changes and perhaps place an onus on manufacturers to expedite this process of change in clinical trial design.

The many exclusion criteria of sponsored trials have limited the numbers of eligible patients, leading to increased recruitment in South America and Eastern Europe for some recent studies [11]. This raises ethical considerations relating to the practice of conducting clinical trials in settings where other therapeutic options are limited for financial or supply reasons. In addition, very high placebo response rates have been reported in some countries outside of the United States, and this raises questions as to the validity of the results and certainly whether the data from such trials can be generalized to apply in different patient populations [34].

In an effort to confront some of the above issues, the FDA increasingly seeks to engage drug manufacturers at an early stage and has produced multiple guidance documents for industry. Their most recent draft guidelines focus on enrichment strategies for drug and biologic development (http://www.fda.gov/downloads/Drugs/Guidance Compliance Regulatory Information/Guidances/UCM332181.pdf). The FDA encourages increased use of strategies such as prognostic and predictive enrichment of study populations, including the use of genomic and proteomic predictors of response to a treatment. These strategies aim to focus enrollment of patients most likely to respond to a given treatment. It can also decrease the placebo response. One example is the use of HER2/Neu as a biomarker to predict response to Herceptin. Identification of responders in UC has to date focused on patients with higher clinical and endoscopic disease activity (Mayo) scores at enrollment [12, 13]. Use of CRP as an enrichment biomarker has been carried out in a post hoc fashion only [12]. It is expected that using strategies such as these will reduce placebo response rates in UC trials. Given the heterogeneity of the disease, it is likely that discovery of new markers of response likelihood will further streamline the clinical trial process for UC patients. Concerns about the generalizability of results derived from such subgroups can then be allayed by enforcing post-marketing requirements to perform larger studies or very strict labeling identifying the specific groups likely to benefit from the treatment.

As mentioned above, the use of azathioprine in UC has never been subjected to the scrutiny of the FDA approval process. Were it to be the subject of an NDA today, the use of the TPMT assay would be a good example of a means of prognostic enrichment of a UC population, where both response to treatment and risk of adverse effects can be stratified by use of a validated assay [35]. This practice, of course, is common among IBD physicians and is described in clinical guidelines for the management of UC [36].

For the FDA there are strong pressures to approve therapies as rapidly as possible, while comprehensively assessing for potential adverse effects and protecting the public. The more recent renewal and reauthorizations of PDUFA (2007 and 2012) have improved the way FDA regulation responds to the risk and benefits of the drugs [37]. In 2012 the FDA approved 39 new drugs, the largest annual total in 16 years (http://mobile.reuters.com/article/idUSBRE8BU0EK20121231?irpc=932). The FDA Commissioner has previously highlighted the failures of the organization to move and develop with sufficient speed to fully take advantage of advancements in related fields [5], but there is perhaps reason to believe that we may be starting to see improvements in some aspects of the review process. The FDA, the scientific and medical communities, and industry must look increasingly toward collaboration, innovation, and consistency in clinical trial methodology to achieve the goal of timely approval of safe, efficacious, and cost-effective medications.

## Conclusions

The Food and Drug Administration (FDA) has the responsibility to ensure the safety and efficacy of all prescription drugs used in the United States. In IBD, a major role for the FDA is the assessment of new agents as they navigate the drug development pipeline to approval and increasingly in post-marketing surveillance. The role of the FDA continues to expand. Many currently used UC medications have been rigorously studied by the FDA and have proven efficacy and safety profiles in the management of this condition. Certain other medications, while in common use, have no randomized controlled data or FDA license to support their use. For future agents, determining a single validated set of endpoints for clinical trials, and in particular the universal inclusion of objective outcomes, would allow improved studies and direct comparisons of future therapies for IBD. In the coming years, the FDA will need to tackle issues of generic medications and follow-on biologics, in conjunction with the well-recognized and more established issues of timely approval, close safety monitoring, and keeping up with the ever increasingly rapid pace of scientific development.

## References

1. Danese S, Fiocchi C. Ulcerative colitis. N Engl J Med. 2011;365(18):1713–25.
2. Thia KT, Loftus Jr EV, Sandborn WJ, Yang SK. An update on the epidemiology of inflammatory bowel disease in Asia. Am J Gastroenterol. 2008;103(12):3167–82.
3. Longobardi T, Jacobs P, Bernstein CN. Utilization of health care resources by individuals with inflammatory bowel disease in the United States: a profile of time since diagnosis. Am J Gastroenterol. 2004;99(4):650–5.
4. DeMets D, Califf R, Dixon D, Ellenberg S, Fleming T, Held P, et al. Issues in regulatory guidelines for data monitoring committees. Clin Trials. 2004;1(2):162–9.
5. Hamburg MA. Shattuck lecture. Innovation, regulation, and the FDA. N Engl J Med. 2010;363(23):2228–32.
6. Hanauer SB. Another one bites the dust. Nat Clin Pract Gastroenterol Hepatol. 2005;2(10):435.
7. Meadows M. Bringing real life to the table. Patient reps help FDA review products. FDA Consum. 2002;36(1):10–1.
8. Lesko LJ, Salerno RA, Spear BB, Anderson DC, Anderson T, Brazell C, et al. Pharmacogenetics and pharmacogenomics in drug development and regulatory decision making: report of the first FDA-PWG-PhRMA-DruSafe Workshop. J Clin Pharmacol. 2003;43(4):342–58.
9. Suntharalingam G, Perry MR, Ward S, Brett SJ, Castello-Cortes A, Brunner MD, et al. Cytokine storm in a phase 1 trial of the anti-CD28 monoclonal antibody TGN1412. N Engl J Med. 2006;355(10):1018–28.
10. Flieger K. FDA finds new ways to speed treatment to patients. FDA Consum. 1993;27(8):14–8.
11. Reinisch W, Sandborn WJ, Hommes DW, D'Haens G, Hanauer S, Schreiber S, et al. Adalimumab for induction of clinical remission in moderately to severely active ulcerative colitis: results of a randomised controlled trial. Gut. 2011;60(6):780–7.
12. Sandborn WJ, van Assche G, Reinisch W, Colombel JF, D'Haens G, Wolf DC, et al. Adalimumab induces and maintains clinical remission in patients with moderate-to-severe ulcerative colitis. Gastroenterology. 2012;142(2):257–65 e1-3.
13. Rutgeerts P, Sandborn WJ, Feagan BG, Reinisch W, Olson A, Johanns J, et al. Infliximab for induction and maintenance therapy for ulcerative colitis. N Engl J Med. 2005;353(23):2462–76.
14. Ha C, Ullman TA, Siegel CA, Kornbluth A. Patients enrolled in randomized controlled trials do not represent the inflammatory

bowel disease patient population. Clin Gastroenterol Hepatol. 2012;10(9):1002–7. quiz e78.

15. Keane J, Gershon S, Wise RP, Mirabile-Levens E, Kasznica J, Schwieterman WD, et al. Tuberculosis associated with infliximab, a tumor necrosis factor alpha-neutralizing agent. N Engl J Med. 2001;345(15):1098–104.

16. Lasser KE, Allen PD, Woolhandler SJ, Himmelstein DU, Wolfe SM, Bor DH. Timing of new black box warnings and withdrawals for prescription medications. JAMA. 2002;287(17):2215–20.

17. Bakke OM, Manocchia M, de Abajo F, Kaitin KI, Lasagna L. Drug safety discontinuations in the United Kingdom, the United States, and Spain from 1974 through 1993: a regulatory perspective. Clin Pharmacol Ther. 1995;58(1):108–17.

18. Carpenter D, Zucker EJ, Avorn J. Drug-review deadlines and safety problems. N Engl J Med. 2008;358(13):1354–61.

19. Rosh JR, Gross T, Mamula P, Griffiths A, Hyams J. Hepatosplenic T-cell lymphoma in adolescents and young adults with Crohn's disease: a cautionary tale? Inflamm Bowel Dis. 2007;13(8):1024–30.

20. Lahiff C, Kane S, Moss AC. Drug development in inflammatory bowel disease: the role of the FDA. Inflamm Bowel Dis. 2011;17(12):2585–93.

21. Cooney RM, Warren BF, Altman DG, Abreu MT, Travis SP. Outcome measurement in clinical trials for ulcerative colitis: towards standardisation. Trials. 2007;8:17.

22. Fernandez-Becker NQ, Moss AC. Improving delivery of aminosalicylates in ulcerative colitis: effect on patient outcomes. Drugs. 2008;68(8):1089–103.

23. Ardizzone S, Cassinotti A, Duca P, Mazzali C, Penati C, Manes G, et al. Mucosal healing predicts late outcomes after the first course of corticosteroids for newly diagnosed ulcerative colitis. Clin Gastroenterol Hepatol. 2011;9(6):483–9 e3.

24. Colombel JF, Rutgeerts P, Reinisch W, Esser D, Wang Y, Lang Y, et al. Early mucosal healing with infliximab is associated with improved long-term clinical outcomes in ulcerative colitis. Gastroenterology. 2011;141(4):1194–201.

25. Sandborn WJ, Hanauer S, Lichtenstein GR, Safdi M, Edeline M, Scott Harris M. Early symptomatic response and mucosal healing with mesalazine rectal suspension therapy in active distal ulcerative colitis–additional results from two controlled studies. Aliment Pharmacol Ther. 2011;34(7):747–56.

26. Peyrin-Biroulet L, Ferrante M, Magro F, Campbell S, Franchimont D, Fidder H, et al. Results from the 2nd Scientific Workshop of the ECCO. I: impact of mucosal healing on the course of inflammatory bowel disease. J Crohns Colitis. 2011;5(5):477–83.

27. Lahiff C, Safaie P, Awais A, Akbari M, Gashin L, Sheth S, et al. The Crohn's disease activity index (CDAI) is similarly elevated in patients with Crohn's disease and in patients with irritable bowel syndrome. Aliment Pharmacol Ther. 2013;37(8):786–94.

28. Stidham RW, Higgins PD. Value of mucosal assessment and biomarkers in inflammatory bowel disease. Expert Rev Gastroenterol Hepatol. 2010;4(3):285–91.

29. Kelly CP. Fecal microbiota transplantation—an old therapy comes of age. N Engl J Med. 2013;368(5):474–5.

30. Brandt LJ, Aroniadis OC, Mellow M, Kanatzar A, Kelly C, Park T, et al. Long-term follow-up of colonoscopic fecal microbiota transplant for recurrent Clostridium difficile infection. Am J Gastroenterol. 2012;107(7):1079–87.

31. Stremmel W, Hanemann A, Ehehalt R, Karner M, Braun A. Phosphatidylcholine (lecithin) and the mucus layer: evidence of therapeutic efficacy in ulcerative colitis? Dig Dis. 2010;28(3):490–6.

32. Mullard A. Hearing shines spotlight on biosimilar controversies. Nat Rev Drug Discov. 2010;9(12):905–6.

33. Sands BE, Abreu MT, Ferry GD, Griffiths AM, Hanauer SB, Isaacs KL, et al. Design issues and outcomes in IBD clinical trials. Inflamm Bowel Dis. 2005;11 Suppl 1:S22–8.

34. Travis S. Does it all ADA up? Adalimumab for ulcerative colitis. Gut. 2011;60(6):741–2.

35. Gardiner SJ, Gearry RB, Begg EJ, Zhang M, Barclay ML. Thiopurine dose in intermediate and normal metabolizers of thiopurine methyltransferase may differ three-fold. Clin Gastroenterol Hepatol. 2008;6(6):654–60. quiz 04.

36. Kornbluth A, Sachar DB. Ulcerative colitis practice guidelines in adults: American College Of Gastroenterology, Practice Parameters Committee. Am J Gastroenterol. 2010;105(3):501–23. quiz 24.

37. Hennessy S, Strom BL. PDUFA reauthorization - drug safety's golden moment of opportunity? N Engl J Med. 2007;356(17):1703–4.

38. Parikh A, Fox I, Leach T, Xu J, Scholz C, Patella M, et al. Long-term clinical experience with vedolizumab in patients with inflammatory bowel disease. Inflamm Bowel Dis. 2013;19(8):1691–9.

39. Sandborn WJ, Ghosh S, Panes J, Vranic I, Su C, Rousell S, et al. Tofacitinib, an oral Janus kinase inhibitor, in active ulcerative colitis. N Engl J Med. 2012;367(7):616–24.

40. Danese S. New therapies for inflammatory bowel disease: from the bench to the bedside. Gut. 2012;61(6):918–32.

41. Rutgeerts PJ, Fedorak RN, Hommes DW, Sturm A, Baumgart DC, Bressler B, et al. A randomised phase I study of etrolizumab (rhuMAb beta7) in moderate to severe ulcerative colitis. Gut. 2012;62:1122–30.

# The Natural History of Ulcerative Colitis

Sunil Samuel and Edward V. Loftus Jr.

**Keywords**

Natural history • Ulcerative colitis • Phenotype • Location of disease • Clinical activity • Outcome measures • Corticosteroids • Hospitalization • Colorectal cancer risk • Surgery • Mortality • Predictors • Mucosal healing

Studies of the natural history of a disease can shed invaluable information on chronic disabling diseases. Such information can serve as a baseline against which various treatment options need to be developed in order to favorably alter the long-term progress of the debilitating disease. For instance, the data obtained from natural history studies would help to calculate the required number of patients in a clinical trial to demonstrate the presumed efficacy. Similarly, large natural history studies can assist in the management of patients by identifying subsets where disease process may be aggressive or more benign. Such studies can also help to identify predictors of an adverse outcome associated with a chronic disease and thereby help to stratify patients into different groups early during their disease course.

## Phenotype of Ulcerative Colitis

### Location of Disease

The widespread availability of endoscopic modalities to manage IBD has made it possible to accurately chart the extent of ulcerative colitis (UC) and study changes in the extent of

S. Samuel, M.B.B.S., Ph.D.
Department of Gastroenterology, Nottingham University Hospitals NHS Trust, Nottingham City Hospital Campus, Hucknall Road, Nottingham, Nottinghamshire NG5 1PB, UK
e-mail: samuelsunil@hotmail.com

E.V. Loftus Jr., M.D. (✉)
Division of Gastroenterology and Hepatology, Mayo Clinic, 200 First Street SW, Rochester, MN 55905, USA
e-mail: loftus.edward@mayo.edu

disease with time. A commonly employed classification for UC is to stratify patients based on the extent of their colonic disease. The Report of a Working Party of the 2005 World Congress of Gastroenterology in Montreal classified UC into ulcerative proctitis (E1) when the disease was limited to the rectum, left-sided UC (E2) when the disease involved the colorectum distal to the splenic flexure, and extensive UC (E3) when the disease extended proximal to the splenic flexure (also known as pancolitis) [1]. The disease extent in ulcerative colitis is fairly uniformly distributed in population-based studies. In a prospective study of 408 UC patients from Norway, approximately 35 % had extensive disease (disease beyond splenic flexure) at the time of inclusion, and similar numbers had left-sided disease and proctitis (34 % and 32 %, respectively) [2]. UC is characterized by chronic inflammation restricted to the colonic mucosa and traditionally involves contiguous areas of the colon without skip lesions with rectal involvement in most instances [3, 4]. However, rectal sparing and patchy colonic inflammation in patients with established diagnosis of UC are not uncommon during the disease course, especially following therapy [5–7]. In a study of 32 UC patients, Kim et al. found 38 % to have patchiness in their colon inflammation and 44 % to have rectal sparing based on endoscopic and histological evidence during their disease course; these changes were not related to any particular form of UC therapy [5]. A more recent study evaluated the prevalence rates and degree of endoscopic and histological patchiness of inflammation and rectal sparing in a series of 56 UC patients who required colectomy for non-neoplastic reasons [8]. Rectal sparing and disease patchiness were demonstrated endoscopically in 32.1 % and 30.4 % and histologically in 30.4 % and 25 %, respectively; on evaluation

**Fig. 3.1** Graphical representation of the disease activity in 600 UC patients in years 3–7 after diagnosis. 57 % had intermittent activity of which 28 % had a relapse in ≥3 years and 29 % had relapses <3 years. *D* diagnosis. Reprinted with permission from Langholz et al. [17]

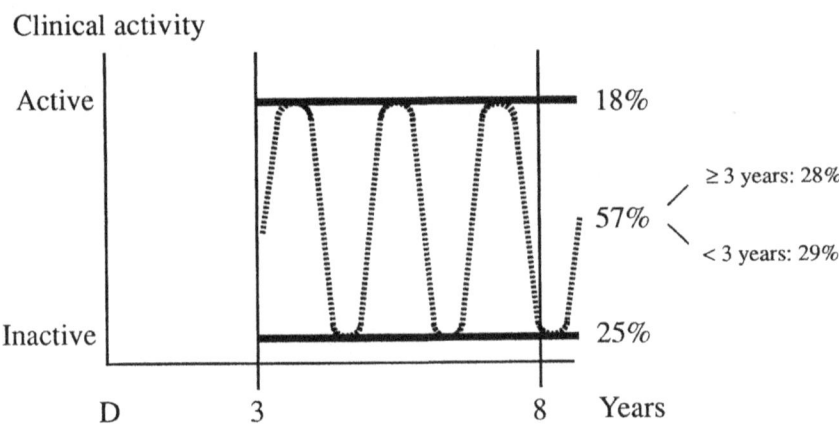

of these patients' colectomy specimens, none had complete absence of rectal involvement, while only 10.7 % had disease patchiness in the colon [8]. It is possible that rectal sparing in adults is probably much more infrequent than previously thought, especially at disease diagnosis. However, in contrast, rectal sparing and disease patchiness may be more common in children; for example, a study by Glickman and colleagues reported a prevalence of 30 % for rectal sparing and 21 % for patchy disease among 73 pediatric patients, compared to 3 % with rectal sparing and none with patchy disease among 38 adults with new-onset UC [9]. Some patients with proven distal UC have simultaneous inflammation in the right colon or the periappendiceal region (cecal patch). These findings, though infrequent, do not appear to have adverse prognostic implications in relation to disease activity or progression [10, 11]. It is generally accepted that UC does not affect the small bowel, but some patients with pancolonic UC can have mucosal inflammation affecting the small bowel proximal to the ileocecal valve termed as "backwash ileitis" [12, 13]. The prevalence of this phenomenon is reported to occur in 10–20 % of patients with pancolitis [14, 15]. The ileal changes of backwash ileitis typically manifest as granularity and erythema [16] and differ from Crohn's disease of the TI by the distinctive lack of deep ulcerations, strictures, or fistula. In those UC patients with associated primary sclerosing cholangitis (PSC), backwash ileitis has been reported to be more common, with a reported prevalence of up to 51 % [16].

## Clinical Activity and Disease Course

The disease course in UC is usually expressed in terms of disease activity, relapses and remissions, and progression and regression of inflammation. A landmark study of 1,161 UC patients from Copenhagen County, Denmark, showed a fairly constant distribution of disease activity during each year of follow-up, with 40–50 % being in remission within a

few years after diagnosis and the proportion of patients with disease activity gradually decreasing with time to 30 % [17]. However, it is important to note that these were not necessarily the same patients remaining in remission or with disease activity from year to year and patients move back and forth between disease states (Fig. 3.1). In the same study, 600 patients had at least 7 full calendar years of follow-up. In years 3–7 after diagnosis, 25 % were in prolonged remission, while 18 % had active disease every year; the remaining 57 % had intermittent disease activity (Fig. 3.1). Thus, for most patients, UC is a condition characterized by relapses interspersed with periods of remission.

The flare-ups of UC are usually unpredictable, but the disease course in the previous year maybe predictive of the disease behavior in subsequent years [17]. In a study of 781 Norwegian patients with UC, an inverse relationship was found between the time to the first relapse and the total number of relapses over a 10-year period [18]. For example, the patients who experienced a relapse in the first year after diagnosis had far greater number of relapses compared to those patients who did not. In the IBD Southeastern Norway (IBSEN) cohort, the 10-year cumulative relapse rate was 83 %, and patients older than 50 years had a significantly reduced risk of relapse compared to those younger than 30 years [19]. The severity of relapses can be variable, with some patients experiencing minimal symptoms while others rapidly progressing to life-threatening fulminant colitis needing emergency colectomy. In a hospital-based study of 115 patients with steroid-refractory acute severe UC (Mayo score [20] ≥10), the colectomy rate approached 60 % by week 54 despite immunosuppressive treatment [21]. This fulminant presentation is particularly seen in young children with UC where there is a lack of response to standard medical treatment [22].

Ulcerative colitis has both the potential to spread to involve previously non-inflamed bowel segments (progression) and also to decrease in the disease extent (regression) with time. Such a change in the disease extent has prognostic implications, since complications such as toxic megacolon and colonic hemorrhage and events such as colectomy are more common in patients with pancolitis at diagnosis when compared to proctitis and left-sided colitis [23, 24]. Langholz et al. reported a cumulative probability of disease progression in 515 patients with proctosigmoiditis (based on rigid sigmoidoscopy and barium enema) of 53 % at 25 years after diagnosis; in the same study, the cumulative probability of disease regression after 25 years in the 207 patients with pancolitis was approximately 76 % [25]. In a prospective study of 399 Norwegian UC patients where colonoscopy was used to evaluate the extent of inflammation, there was progression of inflammation in 14 % of cases, no change in 34 %, and regression in 22 % after 14 months of median follow-up [2]. A similar rate of disease progression was also reported in the IBSEN cohort (17 % had disease progression) [26].

## Outcome Measures in Ulcerative Colitis

### Corticosteroid Usage

Truelove and Witts first described the use of oral corticosteroids in the treatment of ulcerative colitis in 1955 [27] and again demonstrated a similar efficacy with intravenous steroids for the treatment of acute severe colitis [28]. The natural history of patients with UC who require corticosteroids is largely unknown with very few population-based studies. Generally active UC patients requiring steroids show three different patterns of response—one group will have good results achieving steroid-free prolonged remission, a second group will have initial response but lose benefit as treatment is tapered or stopped, and a third group who will have no response to steroids. In Olmsted County, Minnesota, among an inception cohort of 183 UC patients from the prebiologic era, 63 (34 %) received corticosteroid therapy—54 % achieved complete remission, 30 % had partial remission, and 16 % had no response at all after 30 days [29]. Approximately 1 year after corticosteroid initiation, 49 % had noted prolonged response, 22 % were steroid dependent, and 29 % had undergone colectomy [29]. Similar response rates were noted in a hospital-based cohort study of 136 UC patients from Edinburgh, United Kingdom—51, 31, and 18 % had complete, partial, or no response to steroid therapy at 30 days, respectively [30]. A recent Italian study reported early (3 months) and late outcomes (5 years) in 157 patients with UC who required their first systemic steroid therapy within 12 months of diagnosis [31]. Female gender was the only predictor of a better clinical outcome at 3 months, and a complete clinical and endoscopic remission at 3 months after corticosteroid therapy significantly predicted the decreased risk of hospitalizations, immunosuppressive usage, and colectomy at 5 years [31]. It may be relevant therefore to routinely assess the disease response endoscopically after 3 months of corticosteroid therapy in order to risk stratify patients and to plan for early introduction of immunosuppressive treatments in those who fail to achieve endoscopic remission. Antitumor necrosis factor (TNF) agents like infliximab are effective in inducing and maintaining remission in patients with moderately to severely active UC, but the steroid-sparing effects of these biological drugs will need additional prospective studies.

## Hospitalizations

The natural course of ulcerative colitis is that of exacerbation interspersed with periods of remission. Hospitalization therefore accounts for a large part of the costs involved in the care of ulcerative colitis [32, 33]. Recent data from the Nationwide Inpatient Sample suggests that medical hospitalizations for UC in the United States have increased from 56,911 in 1998 to 86,611 in 2007 [34]. In a recent study, patients with UC who required hospitalization for medical reasons were five times more likely to require colectomy, even after adjusting for other factors [35]. Another important factor that may predict hospitalization is the early endoscopic response to corticosteroids. Patients who failed to achieve clinical and endoscopic remission at 3 months after corticosteroid treatment were more likely to undergo hospitalization within 5 years of follow-up (hazard ratio, 3.634; 95 % CI, 2.193–51.039; $P=0.0033$) [31]. Among Olmsted County residents diagnosed with UC between 1970 and 1999, corticosteroids were given during 53 % of UC-related hospitalizations, and 33 % of these patients required more than one hospitalization for inpatient steroids [36]. However, there has been considerable variability in hospitalization rates across North America. In a population-based study from Canada, approximately one-fifth of UC patients had more than one hospital stay every year during the period between 1994 and 2001 [37]. Overall the hospitalization rate for UC was stable at 12.6–13.3 per 100,000 population during the 7-year study period [37]. Approximately 55 % of UC-related hospitalizations involved major surgery, of which the commonest was incision, excision, and anastomosis of the intestine [37]. A multilevel study conducted among 3.2 million members of Kaiser Permanente (Northern California) found that hospitalization rates for UC declined by 29 % between 1998 and 2005 [38]. In the Olmsted County population-based study, 270 UC patients were followed up for 3,458 person-years and 114 (42 %) were hospitalized at least once during the median follow-up of 12.3 years—33 % of all these hospital admissions were surgical [36]. Crude hospitalization rates (per 1,000 patient-years) decreased from 124 for 1970–1980 to 71 for 1990–2001. The 10-year cumulative risk of hospitalization was 49 % in those with

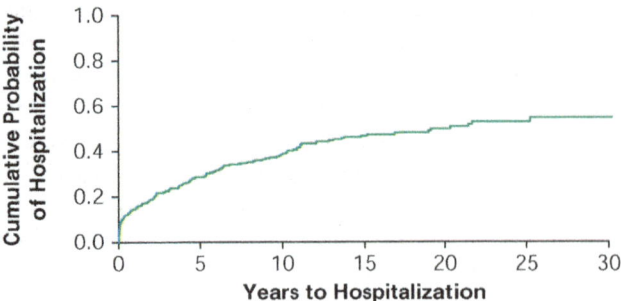

**Fig. 3.2** Overall cumulative incidence of first ulcerative colitis-related hospitalization among an Olmsted County population-based cohort, Minnesota, 1970–2001. Adapted from Ingle et al. [34]

extensive colitis compared to 33 % and 29 % for left-sided disease and proctitis, respectively (Fig. 3.2). Hospitalization data in UC could therefore provide vital information on the cohort of patients that might have an aggressive clinical course and appropriate treatment could be initiated from the outset in these cases.

## Colorectal Cancer (CRC) in Ulcerative Colitis

The cancer risk in UC was recognized as early as the 1920s [39, 40]. Although the true risk of CRC in UC in the modern era remains uncertain, it is probably far lower than previously estimated. The risks reported in studies from tertiary referral centers, which often include patients with disproportionately severe disease, generally overestimate the cancer risk [41–43]. For example, in a 1971 study of 396 children, the risk of colon cancer was 20 % for every decade of life beginning 10 years after the disease diagnosis [43]. A meta-analysis of 116 studies from a wide array centers and geographic sites estimated the cumulative risk of CRC in UC to be 1.6 % at 10 years, 8.3 % at 20 years, and 18.4 % at 30 years [44]. The cumulative increase in CRC risk with time detected in this meta-analysis is probably explained by the inclusion of variety of studies with different designs including referral center studies. Population-based studies from Sweden [45, 46] and Israel [47] have shown increased relative risks of CRC in UC ranging from 1.4 to 6. However, some of these studies have been based on patients diagnosed as far back as the 1920s. Conversely, several recent population-based cohort studies have reported no significant increased risk of CRC when compared to the background population [48–51]. For example, in a population-based study from Copenhagen County, 1,160 UC patients were observed for a total of 22,290 person-years with a median follow-up period of 19 years (range, 1–36 years) and were found to have no increased risk of CRC [48]. A total of 13 patients developed CRC within the study period compared to

the expected number of 12.42 (standardized morbidity ratio, 1.05; 95 % CI, 0.56–1.79) [48]. The cumulative probability of CRC was 0.4 % by 10 years, 1.1 % by 20 years, and 2.1 % by 30 years of disease [48]. Similarly, in Olmsted County, Minnesota, 378 UC patients with 5,567 person-years of follow-up for the study period 1940–2001 had a cumulative incidence of CRC of 0.4 % at 15 years and 2.0 % at 25 years after UC diagnosis [49]. The number of colon cancers was not increased in the study patients when compared to background population [49]. In this same study, none of the patients in Olmsted County who were diagnosed with UC after 1980 had developed CRC [49]. A slightly higher risk of CRC was found in a population study from Hungary—the cumulative risk of CRC was 0.6 % after 10 years, 5.4 % after 20 years, and 7.5 % after 30 years [52]. The presence of dysplasia on any colonic biopsy (before CRC diagnosis), disease duration of over 10 years, extensive colitis, and coexisting PSC all significantly increased the risk of colon cancer [52]. It is obvious that the incidence of CRC in UC is decreasing over time. Whether this is due to the potentially chemoprotective effect of widespread maintenance therapies including aminosalicylates [53], more aggressive endoscopic surveillance regimens, or more aggressive surgical intervention strategies remains unclear.

## Colectomy

Many patients with UC will need surgery during the course of their disease. Early population-based studies from Europe reported 10-year cumulative colectomy rates of over 20 % [23, 24, 50]. In a large inception cohort of 1,586 patients with UC from Stockholm County, the cumulative colectomy rate was 20 % at 5 years, 28 % at 10 years, and 45 % at 25 years [24]. Ten percent of all patients had a colectomy during the first year after diagnosis, while the rates of colectomy decreased in the subsequent years [24]. The extent of disease at diagnosis was the main factor affecting the colectomy rates; the 5-year, 10-year, and 25-year colectomy rates for patients with pancolitis were 32 %, 42 %, and 65 %, respectively [24]. A similar study from Copenhagen County reported a 25-year colectomy rate of 32.4 %, and the disease extent at diagnosis was predictive of subsequent colectomy, with extensive colitis increasing the risk of surgery substantially [50].

In Olmsted County, 316 incident cases of UC were followed up for 3,698 person-years. Overall, 53 patients (17 %) underwent surgery for UC and of these, 70 % underwent more than one surgical procedure [54]. The cumulative risk of colectomy from diagnosis was 16.6 % at 10 years and 19.6 % at 20 years (Fig. 3.3) [54]. Male gender and early need (<90 days) for steroids were significantly associated with time to colectomy. The most common surgeries undertaken

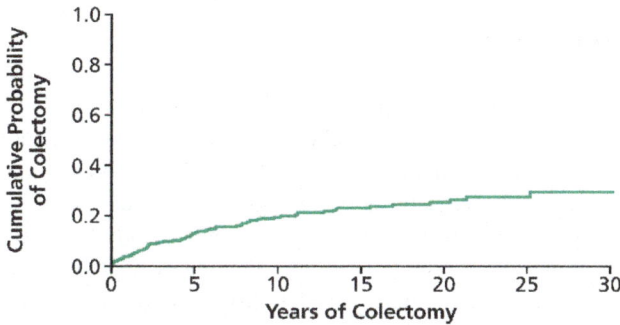

**Fig. 3.3** Overall cumulative incidence of colectomy among a population-based cohort of ulcerative colitis patients from Olmsted County, Minnesota, 1970–2001. Adapted from Ingle et al. [51]

for UC in Olmsted County were total proctocolectomy with ileal pouch-anal anastomosis (TPC-IPAA) (62 %) and TPC with ileostomy (30 %) [54]. The 10-year cumulative risk of subsequent unplanned surgery was 44.1 % overall, but the risk varied depending on the primary surgery undertaken. Patients who underwent TPC-IPAA were almost twice more likely to have unplanned follow-up surgeries when compared to TPC-ileostomy [54]. More recent estimates of 10-year colectomy rates in UC from European population cohorts have been lower than previously reported [19, 55, 56]. Patients in the European Collaborative Study Group of Inflammatory Bowel Disease (EC-IBD) were recruited during a 2-year period between October 1, 1991 and September 30, 1993 from 20 treatment centers and distributed over 12 European countries [55]. The overall cumulative 10-year colectomy rate was 8.7 %; in the northern centers (Denmark, Norway, and Netherlands), the colectomy rates were significantly higher, 10.4 %, compared to 3.9 % in the southern centers of Europe (Greece, Israel, Italy, and Spain) [55]. This geographic difference in colectomy rates could indicate that patients in the northern centers have more severe disease compared to the southern centers (36.3 % of patients in the northern centers had extension of their colitis at follow-up compared to 28.7 % in the southern centers, $P < 0.05$). Among the IBSEN cohort, 423 patients completed 10-year follow-up, and the crude colectomy rate was 3.5 %, 7.6 %, and 9.8 % at 1, 5, and 10 years, respectively [19]. An ESR ≥30 mm and extensive colitis at diagnosis were the only independent risk factors for colectomy [19].

Recent data has suggested that patients who are treated with purine antimetabolites had decreased elective colectomy rates. In contrast, emergent colectomy rates were stable, which was hypothesized to have been due to rapid progression of disease activity [57].

Superimposed infections remain a risk factor for hospitalizations and colectomy in patients with UC. A recent study from the Cleveland Clinic illustrated that patients with *C. difficile* infection had significantly more UC-related emergency room visits in the year following initial infection (37.8 % vs. 4 %) in addition to significantly higher rates of colectomy 1 year following the initial infection associated admission (35.6 % vs. 9.9 %) compared to those patients who did not have infection [58]. Another report from Mount Sinai Hospital in New York highlighted that the rate of UC-related hospitalizations (58 visits vs. 27 visits, $P = 0.001$) and colectomy rates (44.6 % vs. 25 %, $P = 0.04$) 1 year after initial hospitalization were higher in patients who were afflicted with C. difficile [59] infection than those without infection.

## Mortality

Population-based studies on the long-term survival of patients with UC have shown some conflicting data, with older studies reporting a reduced overall survival [60, 61], while newer ones showing either an equivalent or even an improved survival [62–65]. In addition, two large Swedish population-based studies comprised of patients with UC between the 1950s and 1980s reported a slightly increased mortality [66, 67]. In the largest population-based study by Ekbom et al. from Uppsala, Sweden, the standardized mortality ratio (SMR) for UC patients was 1.4 (95 % CI, 1.2–1.5), while the presence of coexisting respiratory diseases like bronchitis, asthma, and emphysema further increased their mortality risk (SMR, 1.5; 95 % CI, 1.1–2.2) [67]. Similar findings were noted by Persson et al. reporting on a cohort of UC patients between 1955 and 1984 from Stockholm, Sweden [66]. However, more recent studies from North America and Europe have shown that the overall mortality from UC is not greater than that of the general population. This may be due to favorable disease pattern or to improvements in the treatment of UC in the recent decades. For example, in Olmsted County, an inception cohort of 378 UC patients had decreased mortality when compared to the general population (SMR, 0.80; 95 % CI, 0.6–1.0) [62]. When stratified by calendar year at diagnosis, survival appeared to improve over time—SMR was 0.80 for patients diagnosed between 1940 and 1959 which improved to 0.50 for the period between 1990 and 2001 [62]. Similarly, an EC-IBD study comprised of UC patients reported an overall mortality risk no higher than the general population (SMR 1.09) [68]. There was, however, a trend toward higher mortality for northern European centers (SMR 1.19) compared to the southern centers (SMR 0.82) [68]. In a meta-analysis of all population-based inception cohort studies in UC, the overall SMR was 1.1 (95 % CI, 0.9–1.2; $P = 0.42$) [69]. Although the overall mortality in UC did not differ from the background population, certain subgroups were at greater risk of dying. Mortality was significantly increased in patients during the first few years after diagnosis, in those with extensive disease and patients from Scandinavian countries [69]. The pooled SMR for the five Scandinavian studies included in the meta-analysis was 1.2, compared to 0.8 for non-Scandinavian studies [69]. The UC-related mortality accounted for 17 % of all deaths, and cause-specific analyses revealed increased mortality from respiratory diseases, colorectal cancer, gastrointestinal, and liver diseases, while mortality from pulmonary cancer was decreased [69]. Similarly, a study on IBD subjects drawn from Kaiser Permanente Medical Care Program, California, found no overall increase in mortality with UC (SMR, 1.0; 95 % CI, 0.9–1.2), but they had a higher risk of dying from digestive diseases other than IBD (SMR, 3.9; 95 % CI, 2.4–6.0) (e.g., liver diseases and colorectal cancer) [70]. Nonetheless those UC patients needing immunosuppressive treatment with azathioprine, 6-mercaptopurine, methotrexate, or infliximab have a higher mortality compared to those who did not, and this probably reflects the increased usage of these treatment regimes in patients with more severe disease [62, 69, 71]. In a study using the General Practice Research Database (GPRD) from the United Kingdom, the mortality in UC patients was increased with current usage (HR, 2.81; 95 % CI, 2.26–3.50) and recent usage (HR, 2.49; 95 % CI, 1.65–3.75) of corticosteroids [71].

## Predictors of Natural History

### Mucosal Healing

Mucosal healing (MH) will likely become an important measure of treatment efficacy for future IBD trials. However, there is considerable disparity in the literature regarding the definition of MH in UC. The International Organization for the Study of Inflammatory Bowel Disease (IOIBD) proposed a definition of MH in UC, which comprised of absence of friability, blood, erosions, and ulcers in all visualized segments of the gastrointestinal mucosa [72]. In a Norwegian population-based cohort of UC patients (IBSEN), education longer than 12 years and extensive disease at diagnosis were significant predictors of MH after 1 year, and the presence of MH decreased the future risks of colectomy [73]. A recent study reported long-term clinical outcomes of patients treated in the Acute Ulcerative Colitis Trials (ACT1 and ACT2) [74]. MH was defined as an absolute Mayo endoscopic subscore of 0 or 1 [20, 74]. The patients who achieved MH at 8 weeks were less likely to progress to colectomy through 54 weeks of follow-up, and the degree of MH correlated with better symptomatic and corticosteroid use at 30 and 54 weeks of follow-up [74]. It is desirable to incorporate MH as a potential goal in clinical practice, but further studies to develop standardized endoscopic scoring indices for MH will need to be performed.

## Conclusion

The majority of UC patients have mild disease, and the prognosis in terms of mortality and CRC occurrence is not significantly different from that of the general population. However, clearly a subset of patients has significant morbidity, and there is a suggestion that in some cohorts there still exists elevated mortality from UC. The treatment goals in UC are rapidly changing from mere control of symptoms to alteration of the natural history of the disease. Further studies are currently necessary to evaluate the long-term outcomes in UC with the changing treatment paradigms.

## References

1. Silverberg MS, et al. Toward an integrated clinical, molecular and serological classification of inflammatory bowel disease: report of a working party of the 2005 Montreal World Congress of gastroenterology. Can J Gastroenterol. 2005;19(Suppl A):5–36.
2. Moum B, et al. Change in the extent of colonoscopic and histological involvement in ulcerative colitis over time. Am J Gastroenterol. 1999;94(6):1564–9.
3. Donnellan WL. Early histological changes in ulcerative colitis. A light and electron microscopic study. Gastroenterology. 1966;50(4):519–40.
4. Waye JD. The role of colonoscopy in the differential diagnosis of inflammatory bowel disease. Gastrointest Endosc. 1977;23(3):150–4.
5. Kim B, et al. Endoscopic and histological patchiness in treated ulcerative colitis. Am J Gastroenterol. 1999;94(11):3258–62.
6. Bernstein CN, et al. Patchiness of mucosal inflammation in treated ulcerative colitis: a prospective study. Gastrointest Endosc. 1995;42(3):232–7.
7. Kleer CG, Appelman HD. Ulcerative colitis: patterns of involvement in colorectal biopsies and changes with time. Am J Surg Pathol. 1998;22(8):983–9.
8. Joo M, Odze RD. Rectal sparing and skip lesions in ulcerative colitis: a comparative study of endoscopic and histologic findings in patients who underwent proctocolectomy. Am J Surg Pathol. 2010;34(5):689–96.
9. Glickman JN, et al. Pediatric patients with untreated ulcerative colitis may present initially with unusual morphologic findings. Am J Surg Pathol. 2004;28(2):190–7.
10. Mutinga ML, et al. The clinical significance of right-sided colonic inflammation in patients with left-sided chronic ulcerative colitis. Inflamm Bowel Dis. 2004;10(3):215–9.
11. Byeon JS, et al. Clinical course of distal ulcerative colitis in relation to appendiceal orifice inflammation status. Inflamm Bowel Dis. 2005;11(4):366–71.
12. McCready FJ, Bargen JA, et al. Involvement of the ileum in chronic ulcerative colitis. N Engl J Med. 1949;240(4):119–27.
13. Saltzstein SL, Rosenberg BF. Ulcerative colitis of the ileum, and regional enteritis of the colon. A comparative histopathologic study. Am J Clin Pathol. 1963;40:610–23.
14. Gustavsson S, Weiland LH, Kelly KA. Relationship of backwash ileitis to ileal pouchitis after ileal pouch-anal anastomosis. Dis Colon Rectum. 1987;30(1):25–8.
15. Schmidt CM, et al. Preoperative terminal ileal and colonic resection histopathology predicts risk of pouchitis in patients after ileoanal pull-through procedure. Ann Surg. 1998;227(5):654–62. discussion 663–5.

16. Loftus Jr EV, et al. PSC-IBD: a unique form of inflammatory bowel disease associated with primary sclerosing cholangitis. Gut. 2005; 54(1):91–6.

17. Langholz E, et al. Course of ulcerative colitis: analysis of changes in disease activity over years. Gastroenterology. 1994;107(1): 3–11.

18. Hoie O, et al. Ulcerative colitis: patient characteristics may predict 10-yr disease recurrence in a European-wide population-based cohort. Am J Gastroenterol. 2007;102(8):1692–701.

19. Solberg IC, et al. Clinical course during the first 10 years of ulcerative colitis: results from a population-based inception cohort (IBSEN Study). Scand J Gastroenterol. 2009;44(4):431–40.

20. Schroeder KW, Tremaine WJ, Ilstrup DM. Coated oral 5-aminosalicylic acid therapy for mildly to moderately active ulcerative colitis. A randomized study. N Engl J Med. 1987; 317(26):1625–9.

21. Seow CH, et al. Trough serum infliximab: a predictive factor of clinical outcome for infliximab treatment in acute ulcerative colitis. Gut. 2010;59(1):49–54.

22. Turner D, et al. Severe paediatric ulcerative colitis: incidence, outcomes and optimal timing for second-line therapy. Gut. 2008; 57(3):331–8.

23. Farmer RG, Easley KA, Rankin GB. Clinical patterns, natural history, and progression of ulcerative colitis. A long-term follow-up of 1116 patients. Dig Dis Sci. 1993;38(6):1137–46.

24. Leijonmarck CE, Persson PG, Hellers G. Factors affecting colectomy rate in ulcerative colitis: an epidemiologic study. Gut. 1990;31(3):329–33.

25. Langholz E, et al. Changes in extent of ulcerative colitis: a study on the course and prognostic factors. Scand J Gastroenterol. 1996;31(3):260–6.

26. Henriksen M, et al. Ulcerative colitis and clinical course: results of a 5-year population-based follow-up study (the IBSEN study). Inflamm Bowel Dis. 2006;12(7):543–50.

27. Truelove SC, Witts LJ. Cortisone in ulcerative colitis; final report on a therapeutic trial. Br Med J. 1955;2(4947):1041–8.

28. Truelove SC, Jewell DP. Intensive intravenous regimen for severe attacks of ulcerative colitis. Lancet. 1974;1(7866):1067–70.

29. Faubion Jr WA, et al. The natural history of corticosteroid therapy for inflammatory bowel disease: a population-based study. Gastroenterology. 2001;121(2):255–60.

30. Ho GT, et al. The efficacy of corticosteroid therapy in inflammatory bowel disease: analysis of a 5-year UK inception cohort. Aliment Pharmacol Ther. 2006;24(2):319–30.

31. Ardizzone S, et al. Mucosal healing predicts late outcomes after the first course of corticosteroids for newly diagnosed ulcerative colitis. Clin Gastroenterol Hepatol. 2011;9(6):483–9 e3.

32. Odes S, et al. Cost analysis and cost determinants in a European inflammatory bowel disease inception cohort with 10 years of follow-up evaluation. Gastroenterology. 2006;131(3):719–28.

33. Kappelman MD, et al. Direct health care costs of Crohn's disease and ulcerative colitis in US children and adults. Gastroenterology. 2008;135(6):1907–13.

34. Ananthakrishnan AN, et al. A nationwide analysis of changes in severity and outcomes of inflammatory bowel disease hospitalizations. J Gastrointest Surg. 2011;15(2):267–76.

35. Ananthakrishnan AN, et al. History of medical hospitalization predicts future need for colectomy in patients with ulcerative colitis. Inflamm Bowel Dis. 2009;15(2):176–81.

36. Ingle SB, et al. Hospitalizations and inpatient corticosteroid usage among ulcerative colitis patients from Olmsted County, Minnesota, 1970–2001. Gastroenterology. 2007;132(Suppl 2, 4): A657–8.

37. Bernstein CN, Nabalamba A. Hospitalization, surgery, and readmission rates of IBD in Canada: a population-based study. Am J Gastroenterol. 2006;101(1):110–8.

38. Herrinton LJ, et al. Time trends in therapies and outcomes for adult inflammatory bowel disease, Northern California, 1998–2005. Gastroenterology. 2009;137(2):502–11.

39. Crohn B, Rosenburg H. The sigmoidoscopic picture of chronic ulcerative colitis. Am J Med Sci. 1925;170:220–8.

40. Bargen JA. Chronic ulcerative colitis associated with malignant disease. Arch Surg. 1928;17:561–76.

41. Greenstein AJ, et al. A comparison of cancer risk in Crohn's disease and ulcerative colitis. Cancer. 1981;48(12):2742–5.

42. Gillen CD, et al. Ulcerative colitis and Crohn's disease: a comparison of the colorectal cancer risk in extensive colitis. Gut. 1994;35(11):1590–2.

43. Devroede GJ, et al. Cancer risk and life expectancy of children with ulcerative colitis. N Engl J Med. 1971;285(1):17–21.

44. Eaden JA, Abrams KR, Mayberry JF. The risk of colorectal cancer in ulcerative colitis: a meta-analysis. Gut. 2001;48(4):526–35.

45. Ekbom A, et al. Ulcerative colitis and colorectal cancer. A population-based study. N Engl J Med. 1990;323(18):1228–33.

46. Karlen P, et al. Increased risk of cancer in ulcerative colitis: a population-based cohort study. Am J Gastroenterol. 1999;94(4): 1047–52.

47. Gilat T, et al. Colorectal cancer in patients with ulcerative colitis. A population study in central Israel. Gastroenterology. 1988; 94(4):870–7.

48. Winther KV, et al. Long-term risk of cancer in ulcerative colitis: a population-based cohort study from Copenhagen County. Clin Gastroenterol Hepatol. 2004;2(12):1088–95.

49. Jess T, et al. Risk of intestinal cancer in inflammatory bowel disease: a population-based study from Olmsted county, Minnesota. Gastroenterology. 2006;130(4):1039–46.

50. Langholz E, et al. Colorectal cancer risk and mortality in patients with ulcerative colitis. Gastroenterology. 1992;103(5):1444–51.

51. Bernstein CN, et al. Cancer risk in patients with inflammatory bowel disease: a population-based study. Cancer. 2001;91(4): 854–62.

52. Lakatos L, et al. Risk factors for ulcerative colitis-associated colorectal cancer in a Hungarian cohort of patients with ulcerative colitis: results of a population-based study. Inflamm Bowel Dis. 2006;12(3):205–11.

53. Eaden J, et al. Colorectal cancer prevention in ulcerative colitis: a case-control study. Aliment Pharmacol Ther. 2000;14(2): 145–53.

54. Ingle SB, et al. Risk factors for ulcerative colitis (UC) surgery in a population-based cohort. Am J Gastroenterol. 2007;102:S480–1.

55. Hoie O, et al. Low colectomy rates in ulcerative colitis in an unselected European cohort followed for 10 years. Gastroenterology. 2007;132(2):507–15.

56. Lakatos L, et al. Incidence, disease phenotype at diagnosis, and early disease course in inflammatory bowel diseases in Western Hungary, 2002–2006. Inflamm Bowel Dis. 2011;17(12):2558–65.

57. Kaplan GG, Seow CH, Ghosh S, et al. Decreasing colectomy rates for ulcerative colitis: a population-based time trend study. Am J Gastroenterol. 2012;107:1879–87.

58. Navaneethan U, Mukewar S, Venkatesh PG, et al. Clostridium difficile infection is associated with worse long term outcome in patients with ulcerative colitis. J Crohns Colitis. 2012;6:330–6.

59. Jodorkovsky D, Young Y, Abreu MT. Clinical outcomes of patients with ulcerative colitis and co-existing Clostridium difficile infection. Dig Dis Sci. 2010;55:415–20.

60. Gyde S, et al. Mortality in ulcerative colitis. Gastroenterology. 1982;83(1 Pt 1):36–43.

61. Edwards FC, Truelove SC. The course and prognosis of ulcerative colitis. Gut. 1963;4:299–315.

62. Jess T, et al. Survival and cause specific mortality in patients with inflammatory bowel disease: a long term outcome study in Olmsted County, Minnesota, 1940–2004. Gut. 2006;55(9):1248–54.

63. Winther KV, et al. Survival and cause-specific mortality in ulcerative colitis: follow-up of a population-based cohort in Copenhagen County. Gastroenterology. 2003;125(6):1576–82.

64. Farrokhyar F, et al. Low mortality in ulcerative colitis and Crohn's disease in three regional centers in England. Am J Gastroenterol. 2001;96(2):501–7.

65. Masala G, et al. Divergent patterns of total and cancer mortality in ulcerative colitis and Crohn's disease patients: the Florence IBD study 1978–2001. Gut. 2004;53(9):1309–13.

66. Persson PG, et al. Survival and cause-specific mortality in inflammatory bowel disease: a population-based cohort study. Gastroenterology. 1996;110(5):1339–45.

67. Ekbom A, et al. Survival and causes of death in patients with inflammatory bowel disease: a population-based study. Gastroenterology. 1992;103(3):954–60.

68. Hoie O, et al. Ulcerative colitis: no rise in mortality in a European-wide population based cohort 10 years after diagnosis. Gut. 2007;56(4):497–503.

69. Jess T, et al. Overall and cause-specific mortality in ulcerative colitis: meta-analysis of population-based inception cohort studies. Am J Gastroenterol. 2007;102(3):609–17.

70. Hutfless SM, et al. Mortality by medication use among patients with inflammatory bowel disease, 1996–2003. Gastroenterology. 2007;133(6):1779–86.

71. Lewis JD, et al. Immunosuppressant medications and mortality in inflammatory bowel disease. Am J Gastroenterol. 2008;103(6):1428–35. quiz 1436.

72. D'Haens G, et al. A review of activity indices and efficacy end points for clinical trials of medical therapy in adults with ulcerative colitis. Gastroenterology. 2007;132(2):763–86.

73. Froslie KF, et al. Mucosal healing in inflammatory bowel disease: results from a Norwegian population-based cohort. Gastroenterology. 2007;133(2):412–22.

74. Colombel JF, et al. Early mucosal healing with infliximab is associated with improved long-term clinical outcomes in ulcerative colitis. Gastroenterology. 2011;141(4):1194–201.

# Principles of Medical Management of Ulcerative Colitis

**4**

Hongha T. Vu and Themistocles Dassopoulos

**Keywords**

Chronic disease management • Ulcerative colitis • Medical therapies • Long-term remission • Inflammatory bowel disease • Disease classification • Activity indices • Corticosteroids • Cyclosporine • Immunomodulators • Monoclonal antibodies against tumor necrosis factor-α • Clinical remission • Quality of life • Prevention of complications • Management of complications • Mucosal healing

## Introduction

Ulcerative colitis (UC) is a chronic inflammatory disease with a relapsing-remitting course. It affects patients in young adulthood, with a mean age of 34.5 years at diagnosis [1], a point in life when the afflicted individuals are completing their higher education, establishing their careers, and starting their families. As patients with UC have a normal lifespan [2], the relapsing course of the disease portends decades of morbidity. The choice of therapy must take into account the long-term issues of compliance and adverse events. In addition, UC is a pervasive disease that can impinge on every aspect of a person's life, from their current functional and mental state to their future reproductive health and risk of malignancy. Optimal management of this chronic condition must therefore be comprehensive in addressing every facet of the disease. This chapter discusses the principles of management of UC patients, with a focus on evidence-based, patient-centered, systematic, and comprehensive therapy.

H.T. Vu, M.D.
Department of Gastroenterology, Barnes Jewish Hospital, Washington University, 918 Woodway Circle, St. Louis, MO 63110, USA

T. Dassopoulos, M.D. (✉)
Department of Medicine, Barnes Jewish Hospital, Washington University, 660 S. Euclid Avenue, Box 8124, St. Louis, MO 63110, USA
e-mail: hvu@dom.wustl.edu; themos@dom.wustl.edu

We provide an overview of the therapeutic options and goals of treatment and provide recommendations for individualizing treatment.

## Ulcerative Colitis as a Model of Chronic Disease Management

The concept of chronic disease management grew out of the realization that the standard, ambulatory care model of acute illness does not meet the needs of patients with chronic illnesses [3, 4]. Models of chronic disease management thus evolved, aiming at improving short- and long-term care, optimizing quality of life, and preventing disease progression and complications. There are several key aspects to the management of UC. These include a coordinated treatment plan for inducing and maintaining remission, a focus on patient function and quality of life, monitoring for and preventing disease and treatment complications, evidence-based care, and behaviorally sophisticated support for the patient in his/her role as self-manager. Coordinating care between multiple providers and/or settings is paramount and is facilitated by regular clinic follow-up and by information systems. Hence, conceptually, patients with UC should benefit from the framework of a structured disease approach.

Central to the chronic disease management model is patient empowerment and involvement. Physicians must establish strong, long-term relationships with their UC patients and provide them with education, support, and open lines of communication. Patients can thus become active

G.R. Lichtenstein (ed.), *Medical Therapy of Ulcerative Colitis*,
DOI 10.1007/978-1-4939-1677-1_4, © Springer Science+Business Media New York 2014

partners in their own health management and achieve better outcomes. In this regard, recent data suggest that patient trust in the physician is associated with improved adherence to IBD therapy [5], which is a surrogate for long-term remission.

Patients with UC need to be well informed regarding their condition and their physician can be instrumental in their education. Education and discussions on the natural course of disease, treatment goals, and patient preferences and expectations allow for individualized management and cultivate effective patient-physician interactions. For example, a patient's wish to avoid surgery may lead them to pursue a more aggressive medical strategy, such as entering a clinical trial. Educational resources and online websites (such as the website of the Crohn's and Colitis Foundation of America; www.ccfa.org) may supplement office discussions and answer questions and concerns not raised in clinic [6]. More knowledgeable patients may take greater personal responsibility for their health and may eventually become comfortable with self-managing certain aspects of their condition. For example, patients may learn to increase doses or start medications when they first develop symptoms of a flare, so that their disease can be controlled at an early stage. Physicians and patients may together devise an action plan to help guide patient self-management. The advantages of this approach were demonstrated in a randomized controlled trial (RCT) that compared guided self-management and patient-directed follow-up to traditional outpatient management [7]. Subjects in the intervention arm had their relapses treated significantly faster and made significantly fewer doctor and hospital visits. Flexible lines of communication may allow patients to update their gastroenterologist on their current clinical status and have simple questions answered. Telecommunication options have expanded so that electronic mail may be used to aid in caring for patients living at a distance or patients more comfortable with this mode of communication. The feasibility and benefits of these approaches were shown in a recent RCT in Danish and Irish patients with mild and moderate ulcerative colitis on 5-aminosalicylate acid treatment [8]. Subjects were randomized to a web group that received disease-specific education and self-treatment or a control group that continued the usual care for 12 months. The web-based group demonstrated significantly better adherence and shorter duration of relapses. The web-based group also had fewer acute and routine visits to the outpatient clinic, leading to cost savings. Among the Danish subjects, general IBD knowledge and disease-specific quality of life was higher in the web-based group, without associated increases in depression and anxiety.

Management of a chronic disease such as UC requires establishment of a high-quality, coordinated health system [9]. Effective care is enhanced through involvement of the primary care physicians who follow patients for health maintenance issues. These include updating vaccinations (influenza annually, pneumococcus, tetanus, meningococcus, hepatitis B, and human papilloma virus in young females), monitoring bone health (including bone densitometry and vitamin D levels), and screening for cancer [10]. Thiopurines increase the risk of nonmelanoma skin cancer, whereas anti-TNF biologics increase the risk of melanoma [11]. Women with IBD receiving corticosteroids and immunosuppressants may have a higher risk of cervical abnormalities [12]. Highlighting the central role of the primary physician, a recent study from Kaiser Permanente, an integrated care organization, showed a significant shift in the outpatient care of UC patients [13]. Between 1998 and 2005, the annual rate of visits to a gastroenterologist for treatment of gastrointestinal disease decreased by 25 % per patient ($P < 0.0001$), whereas the rate of visits to primary care providers increased by 350 % ($P < 0.0001$) (similar significant trends were seen for Crohn's disease).

An emerging trend in the care of UC patients involves the increased use of mid-level providers. Given the rising demands on physicians, as well as the emphasis on health promotion and disease prevention, specialist nurses, nurse practitioners, and physician assistants will inevitably assume greater roles in the management of patients and may even direct care in some domains. The members of these "IBD-dedicated teams" can address straightforward patient concerns without need for an office appointment. They can also answer questions regarding insurance and cost issues and refer patients to social workers or pharmaceutical assistance programs. Studies are beginning to examine the effects of care by IBD-specialist nurses on outcomes. A recent study from Norway found that, in comparison to conventional follow-up, the utilization of a systematic, nurse-led follow-up produced similar outcomes in terms of hospitalizations, surgery, sick leave, performance of endoscopic procedures, and number of additional telephone consultations [14]. Moreover, nurse-led follow-up was associated with a significantly faster treatment upon relapse.

The management of extraintestinal manifestations (EIM) associated with UC frequently requires referral to other specialists, including ophthalmologists, rheumatologists, dermatologists, and hematologists. Concomitant primary sclerosing cholangitis may require management by an advanced endoscopist, general hepatologist, or transplant hepatologist. Stress, depression, and anxiety are also comorbid conditions associated with UC and other chronic diseases. In inflammatory bowel disease, psychiatric comorbidity is associated with poorer clinical outcomes and greater healthcare costs [15–17]. Treatment of these disorders by the primary care physician or the psychiatrist improves disease control and enhances general and emotional well-being [18, 19] and may improve disease outcome [20].

Good communication between the patient and the members of the health care team is critical to the development of an informed, individualized management plan, as well as to the prevention and early detection of complications.

There is surprising variability in the patterns and quality of IBD care, likely reflecting the heterogeneity of the disease but also poor adherence to guidelines [13, 21–23]. This variability mandates efforts to identify specific areas for quality improvement. The American Gastroenterological Association (AGA) has recognized the need to distinguish physicians and practices that deliver high-quality and resource-efficient care for patients with digestive disorders. Using the Physician Consortium for Performance Improvement® (PCPI™) model, the AGA has developed a set of clinical performance measures designed for the purpose of improving IBD quality of care [24]. The performance measures enable the physician to track his/her performance in individual patient care. In the future, reimbursement by insurers may require meeting quality-based targets and outcomes. Ultimately, applying the chronic disease management model in UC should be expected to yield higher-quality health care.

## Classification of Disease

UC is classified by disease extent and severity. This classification is important as disease presentation, outcomes, and therapy depend on these disease characteristics. Disease extent is determined endoscopically. Approximately 40 % of patients have disease limited to the rectum (ulcerative proctitis), and 30–40 % of patients have disease limited to the rectosigmoid (ulcerative proctosigmoiditis) or the left colon (left-sided UC) [25]. 20–30 % of patients have involvement of mucosa proximal to the splenic flexure (extensive colitis) or encompassing the entire colon (pancolitis). Disease extent should be described accurately at the time of the index colonoscopy, as medical therapy (particularly topical therapy) may lead to patchy healing. Topical therapy may explain an atypical finding of rectal sparing in subsequent colonoscopies. A periappendiceal "red patch" and backwash ileitis may also be seen in UC and should not be confused for Crohn's disease.

Patients with distal UC (ulcerative proctitis and proctosigmoiditis) frequently present with the typical symptoms of tenesmus, urgency, and passage of fresh blood. Patients may also complain of constipation, a symptom probably resulting from slower transit in the more proximal colon. More extensive involvement of UC leads to bloody diarrhea, abdominal cramping, and systemic symptoms including, anorexia, weight loss, dehydration, fevers (typically low-grade), and extraintestinal manifestations of UC.

UC is also classified according to disease activity [26]. The American College of Gastroenterology has developed operational definitions. Patients in remission are asymptomatic, with ≤3 stools daily and without rectal bleeding or systemic symptoms. Mild disease is defined as ≤4 stools daily, rare passage of blood or mucus, and no systemic symptoms. Moderate disease is defined as >4 stools daily with daily passage of blood or mucus and minimal systemic symptoms. Severe disease is defined as >6 bloody stools daily with evidence of toxicity including fever, tachycardia, anemia, or elevated erythrocyte sedimentation rate (ESR). Fulminant colitis is characterized by bloody diarrhea with >10 movements daily, continuous bleeding, abdominal pain, and systemic toxicity [27]. Toxic megacolon is defined as systemic toxicity (fever and tachycardia) and colonic dilatation ≥6 cm, which is associated with abdominal distention, hypoactive bowel sounds, and constipation or obstipation [28].

## Activity Indices

Several measures of disease activity have been developed based on clinical symptoms, biochemical data, and endoscopic findings. Most of these indices were developed for the purposes of drug trials and research studies [29]. Nonetheless, the simpler indices may be used in clinical practice. The Truelove and Witts' Severity Index [30] incorporates six variables (number of stools, bleeding, temperature, pulse, hemoglobin, and ESR) to classify patients into three groups (mild, moderate, and severe). Though useful in the general classification of patients, the use of this index has been limited by its qualitative nature. The Powell-Tuck Index [31] uses ten variables (general health, abdominal pain/tenderness, bowel frequency, stool consistency, bleeding, anorexia, nausea/vomiting, temperature, and presence of EIM) to determine a score ranging from 0 to 20. In addition, sigmoidoscopy findings may be added with scores from 0 to 2. The Activity Index (AI) or Seo Index [32] was developed to predict disease severity as classified by the Truelove and Witts' classification. Five quantitative variables (number of stools, number of bloody stools, ESR, hemoglobin, and albumin) were selected after multiple stepwise regressions. The equation (AI = 60 × bloody stools + 13 × number of stools + 0.5 × ESR − 4 × hemoglobin - 15 × albumin + 200) results in a score from 50 to 250. Mild disease is defined as a score <150, moderate as 150–200, and severe as >200. The AI has been shown to predict clinical remission, endoscopic findings, response to infliximab, and need for colectomy [33–36].

Two indices that are frequently used and incorporate endoscopic findings into their determination are the Mayo Clinic Score [37] and the Sutherland Index/UC Disease Activity Index (UC DAI) [38]. The Mayo Score is calculated using four variables (stool frequency, rectal bleeding, flexible sigmoidoscopy findings scored 0–3, and physician global assessment) to determine a score of 0–12. The Mayo Score has been used in multiple studies and has been shown to correlate with quality of life measures. The UC DAI also incorporates four variables (stool frequency, rectal bleeding, endoscopic mucosal appearance, and physician's rating of disease activity) to determine a score ranging from 0 to 12. The UC DAI has been shown to correlate with patient-defined remission [39].

## Medical Therapies

The choice of medical therapy must take into account both disease location and disease activity. Targeted delivery of mesalamine to the inflamed colonic segments leads to optimal effectiveness and minimizes systemic side effects. Systemic therapies are necessary in patients with moderate or severe disease. Therapeutic decisions should also take into consideration the patient's history of response to different therapies, compliance, and comorbidities. Frequent reassessment of the treatment regimen is required given the relapsing-remitting course of the disease and the possibility of worsening activity or proximal progression (Table 4.1).

## Aminosalicylates

The aminosalicylates, sulfasalazine (SASP), and mesalamine (or 5-aminosalicylic acid or 5-ASA) constitute first-line treatment for both the induction of remission and the maintenance of remission in patients with mild to moderate UC. The mechanism of action involves several pathways, including inhibition of activation of transcription factor NF-κB [40], inhibition of prostaglandin synthesis [41], and scavenging of free radicals [42]. SASP (4–6 g/day), the prototype aminosalicylate formulation, contains a sulfapyridine moiety linked by an azo bond to the 5-ASA moiety. Sulfapyridine accounts for most of the adverse effects, whereas 5-ASA accounts for most of the therapeutic benefits. SASP is minimally absorbed by the small intestine and remains intact until reaching the colon, where bacteria cleave the azo bond to release free sulfapyridine and 5-ASA. 5-ASA is poorly absorbed by the colon (and therefore has minimal systemic effects) and has topical (mucosal) anti-inflammatory activity. In effect, sulfapyridine functions as a carrier, delivering the active 5-ASA moiety to the colon. Dose-dependent efficacy and toxicity are observed, mediated by the mesalamine and sulfapyridine moieties, respectively. Up to 40 % of patients may experience dose-related side effects, such as nausea, dyspepsia, headaches, and sperm abnormalities. Idiosyncratic

**Table 4.1** Overview of medical therapies

|         | Induction therapy [1, 2] | Maintenance therapy |
|---------|--------------------------|---------------------|
| Mild    | • Oral 5-ASA<br>• Topical 5-ASA<br>• Topical steroid | • Oral 5-ASA, with or without topical 5-ASA |
| Moderate | • Oral 5-ASA<br>• Topical 5-ASA<br>• Topical steroid<br>• Prednisone in patients with more severe disease or in patients with milder disease who failed oral 5-ASA, topical 5-ASA, and topical steroid<br>• IFX in patients with steroid-refractory disease or intolerance to 5-ASA and thiopurines<br>• ADA in patients with steroid-refractory disease or intolerance to 5-ASA and thiopurines<br>• GOL in patients with steroid-refractory disease or intolerance to 5-ASA and thiopurines | • Oral 5-ASA, with or without topical 5-ASA (in patients who achieved remission on oral 5-ASA, topical 5-ASA or topical steroid<br>• Thiopurines in patients with steroid-dependent disease or patients with frequent flares despite maximal 5-ASA therapy<br>• IFX or IFX-thiopurine combination therapy in patients who achieved remission on IFX and in patients with steroid-dependent disease<br>• ADA or ADA-thiopurine combination therapy in patients who achieved remission on ADA and in patients with steroid-dependent disease<br>• GOL or GOL-thiopurine combination therapy in patients who achieved remission on ADA and in patients with steroid-dependent disease |
| Severe  | • IV corticosteroid (first line)<br>• IV Cyclosporine (first line or after failure of IV steroids)<br>• IFX (first line or after failure of IV steroids) | • Thiopurines in patients who achieved remission on IV corticosteroids or IV cyclosporine<br>• IFX or IFX-thiopurine combination therapy in patients who achieved remission on IFX |

*Notes*: (1) Patients with active distal disease are treated with any combination of topical 5-ASA, oral 5-ASA, and/or topical corticosteroids. (2) Topical therapies are critical in patients with active distal disease. However, they also reduce symptoms of distal disease in patients with extensive UC or pancolitis independent of disease severity side effects are also observed, including bone marrow suppression and hepatotoxicity. SASP inhibits absorption of folate. Advantages of SASP include lower cost than mesalamine and effectiveness against peripheral arthritis. The starting dose is typically 500 mg 2–3 times daily with meals. The dose is gradually increased as tolerated to a maximal dose of 4–6 g/day, taken three times daily with meals. As SASP inhibits folate absorption, folate supplementation is advised.

Oral, sulfa-free aminosalicylates were developed in order to circumvent the side effects of sulfapyridine and now constitute the most commonly prescribed oral therapies. These formulations target 5-ASA release to the site of inflammation along the gastrointestinal tract, differing in the mode of release and site of 5-ASA delivery. Preparations that are available in the USA, the sites of targeted 5-ASA release, and the usual dosages for the treatment of UC are listed below:

- Delzicol® (400 mg) and Asacol HD® (800 mg) (Warner Chilcott, Rockaway, NJ, USA) are mesalamine coated with an acrylic-based resin that dissolves at pH of 7 or greater, releasing the drug in a delayed, pH-dependent manner in the terminal ileum and colon. The usual dose is 2.4–4.8 g/day. In the USA, Delzicol® is approved for the treatment of mildly to moderately active UC and for the maintenance of remission. Asacol HD® is approved for the treatment of moderately active UC.
- Pentasa® (250 and 500 mg; Shire Pharmaceuticals, Wayne, PA, USA) is mesalamine formulated within semipermeable ethyl cellulose microgranules that release the drug in a time-dependent manner throughout the small bowel and colon. The usual dose is 2–4 g/day. In the USA, Pentasa® is approved for the induction of remission and for the treatment of patients with mildly to moderately active UC.
- Lialda® (1,200 mg; Shire Pharmaceuticals, Wayne, PA, USA) is mesalamine coated with a gastro-resistant pH-dependent polymer film, which dissolves at or above pH 7, releasing mesalamine from the tablet core in the terminal ileum and colon. The tablet core contains mesalamine in a multimatrix (MMX) of hydrophilic and lipophilic excipients. The usual dose is 2.4–4.8 g/day. In the USA, Lialda® is approved for the induction of remission in adults with active, mild to moderate UC, and for the maintenance of remission.
- Balsalazide (Colazal® 750 mg; Salix Pharmaceuticals, Raleigh, NC, USA; and generic) consists of 5-ASA in an azo bond with an inert carrier. Colonic bacteria cleave the azo bond to release 5-ASA throughout the colon. The usual dose is 6.75 g/day. Colazal® is approved for the treatment of mildly to moderately active UC.
- Olsalazine (Dipentum®, 250 mg; Pfizer, New York, NY, USA) is a 5-ASA dimer. Colonic bacteria cleave the azo bond to release 5-ASA throughout the colon. The usual dose is 2 g/day. Dipentum® is approved for the maintenance of remission only.
- Apriso® (0.375 g; Salix Pharmaceuticals, Raleigh, NC, USA) is mesalamine with delayed and extended release as granules that dissolve at pH of 6 or greater for delivery throughout the colon. Apriso is approved for the maintenance of remission only. The usual dose is 1.5 g/day.

A recent systematic review included 11 RCTs with 2,086 patients comparing 5-ASA or SASP versus placebo as inductive therapy in active UC [43]. The majority of studies enrolled patients with mild to moderately active UC. There was a strong effect in favor of 5-ASA therapy, with a number needed to treat (NNT) of 6 (95 % confidence interval (CI) 5–8). 40 % of patients achieved remission in the active treatment group, compared with 20 % in the placebo group. The quality of evidence was graded as moderate. There was no difference in efficacy among the different 5-ASA preparations. The systematic review found similar remission rates at low (2.0–2.5 mg/day) versus high doses (>2.5 mg/day). Nonetheless, RCTs and clinical experience are consistent with a dose-response curve with specific oral 5-ASA agents (Asacol®, Pentasa®, Lialda®), with a maximal effect at 4.0–4.8 g/day [44]. In clinical practice, the choice of preparation is usually based on cost and convenience, rather than on claims of superiority of a particular formulation.

The same systematic review also assessed 11 RCTs with 1,502 participants that compared 5-ASA versus placebo in patients with quiescent UC. There was a strong effect in favor of 5-ASA, with a NNT of 4 (95 % CI 3–7). 40 % of patients on 5-ASA relapsed compared with 63 % of patients taking placebo over 6–12 months. The quality of evidence was graded as high. As with active UC, there was no evidence that efficacy varied between different preparations. The optimal maintenance 5-ASA dose appeared to be 2.0–2.4 g/day. Among the seven trials that compared a daily dose of <2 g of 5-ASA with a dose of ≥2 g/day, there was a statistically significant effect in favor of the higher dose (NNT = 10; 95 % CI 5–33). The single trial comparing high versus standard dose (>2.5 g/day vs. 2.0–2.5 g/day; n = 113) found no difference between the two doses. The authors stated that current evidence supports using 2.4 g/day, but conceded that further research is needed to address a possible dose response of 5-ASA in preventing relapse. Again, clinical experience suggests that higher doses (3.6–4.8 g/day) are more effective than lower doses (2.4 g/day) in maintaining remission. In clinical practice, the maintenance dose is frequently the same as the inductive dose.

Only 40 % of patients are compliant with oral 5-ASA therapy [45] and noncompliance is associated with a higher risk of relapse [46]. A study of once daily dosing found lower relapse rates [47]. 5-ASA nephrotoxicity is seen rarely so that renal function should be monitored periodically [48].

Topical forms, either as monotherapy or in conjunction with oral therapies, should be used in patients with distal

UC, as well as patients with more extensive disease but prominent distal symptoms. Topical mesalamine formulations that are available in the USA include:

- Suppositories (Canasa®, Aptalis Pharma, Birmingham, AL, USA), 1,000 mg QD. Suppositories deliver the drug to the distal 10–15 cm of the rectum. Canasa® is approved for the treatment of mild to moderately active ulcerative proctitis.
- Enemas (generic and Rowasa®, Meda Pharmaceuticals, Somerset, NJ, USA) 60 ml daily. Enemas deliver the drug up to the splenic flexure. Rowasa® is approved for the treatment of mild to moderately active distal ulcerative colitis, proctosigmoiditis, or proctitis.

Response is usually seen within 3–4 weeks. Remission rates in distal UC using topical formulations are 50–75 %, superior to those observed with oral 5-ASA monotherapy and with topical steroids [49]. However, the combination of topical and oral 5-ASA is more effective than either agent alone [50, 51]. In addition, the combination of oral 5-ASA and enemas twice a week has been shown to be superior to oral 5-ASA alone in maintaining remission in patients with disease extent greater than proctitis and a history of multiple relapses [52]. Patients on topical therapies may complain of leakage, problems with retention, anal irritation, cramps, and bloating but these symptoms improve over time. Common treatment errors included not maximizing topical therapies in the induction of remission and not utilizing them for maintenance.

## Corticosteroids

Corticosteroids are used for the induction of remission in patients with moderate disease (oral steroids) or severe disease (intravenous steroids). The patient is then transitioned to appropriate maintenance therapy, such 5-ASA (oral and/or topical), thiopurines, or infliximab, depending on the clinical assessment. A subset of patients develops steroid-dependent disease, defined as inability to taper off steroids without experiencing a flare. In these patients, the multitude of steroid toxicities mandates the initiation of steroid-sparing, maintenance therapies. In one population study, approximately one-third of 185 patients with newly diagnosed UC required corticosteroid treatment [53]. Half of these patients went into remission with prolonged response at 1 year. However, 14 (22 %) patients became steroid-dependent and 18 (29 %) required surgery.

Corticosteroids were first shown to be effective in UC in 1955 [54]. Patients with chronic, active UC severe enough to require at least 6 weeks of hospital stay were randomized to cortisone (100 mg orally once daily, $n=109$) versus placebo ($n=101$). In the cortisone group, 58.7 % failed to achieve remission, compared with 84.2 % in the placebo group. The absolute risk reduction was 25.4 % (13.8 % vs. 37.1 %), and the NNT was 4. A recent meta-analysis of RCTs found that 54 % of patients receiving oral steroids failed to achieve remission compared with 79.0 % of patients randomized to placebo. The likelihood of failure to achieve remission was significantly reduced with steroid therapy (relative risk (RR) = 0.65; 95 % CI 0.45–0.93) [55].

Patients with severe UC require hospitalization and intravenous corticosteroids. In a study from Oxford, 49 patients with severe UC were treated with a 5-day course of IV prednisolone (60 mg/day) and rectal hydrocortisone (100 mg twice daily) during the period between 1969 and 1973. Thirty-six patients (74 %) were in complete remission at the end of the 5-day course, 4 (8 %) showed clinical improvement but no remission and required surgery within the next 6 weeks, and 9 (18 %) required emergent surgery after 5 days of treatment [56]. The same group reported their results in an additional 100 courses of the same regimen in 87 patients with severe UC, treated during the period between 1974 and 1978. 60 % of the attacks responded swiftly to the regimen; in 15 %, there was improvement; and in 25 %, failure to respond resulted in emergency colectomy [57]. More recent studies have reported remission rates of 50–61 % [58–60].

A French retrospective study assessed factors predictive of failure of intravenous corticosteroid therapy, defined as colectomy before day 30, intravenous cyclosporine, or death. On multivariate analysis, severe endoscopic lesions (defined as extensive deep ulcerations, mucosal detachment on the edge of these ulcerations, well-like ulcerations, and/or large mucosal abrasions) were associated with an increased risk of failure ($P=0.007$). The presence of Truelove and Witts' criteria for severe disease ($P=0.018$) and an attack that had lasted more than 6 weeks ($P=0.001$) were also independent predictors of failure. Patients with severe endoscopic lesions and Truelove and Witts' criteria for severe disease had a failure rate of 86 %, whereas those with severe endoscopic lesions and moderate disease by the Truelove and Witts' criteria had a failure rate of 50 % [61]. An English prospective study evaluated clinical parameters predictive of surgery in 51 consecutive episodes of severe colitis by the Truelove and Witts' criteria. All patients were treated with intravenous and rectal hydrocortisone. In addition, 14 of 51 patients were treated with intravenous cyclosporine. There was complete response in 21 episodes (<or=3 stools on day 7, without visible blood), incomplete response in 15 (>3 stools or visible blood on day 7, but no colectomy), and colectomy on that admission in 15. Patients with more than eight stools on day 3, or a stool frequency between three and eight together with a CRP >45 mg/l, had an 85 % risk of colectomy during the hospitalization [62].

Corticosteroids are available in oral, intravenous, and topical formulations. Oral corticosteroids are indicated in mild to moderate UC when a patient is flaring despite maximal 5-ASA use [63]. Recommended dosing is prednisone 40–60 mg (or its equivalent) until clinical remission (*not* response) is achieved, usually in 7–14 days [64]. The rapidity of the taper is dictated by how quickly the patient responds. Common errors are starting the prednisone taper as soon as the patient begins to improve, rather than waiting for the patient to achieve clinical remission tapering too quickly in a patient who responded slowly, and tapering too slowly in a patient who promptly entered remission. Generally, prednisone is tapered by 5–10 mg each week until 20 mg, then by 2.5–5 mg each week. However, the importance of individualizing the taper cannot be overemphasized. Patients should not be treated with a "standard" taper and should be instructed to contact their physician periodically regarding the dose changes. On the basis of two RCTs, extended-release budesonide (Uceris® 9 mg; Santarus, San Diego, CA, USA) was recently approved in the USA for the induction of remission in patients with active, mild to moderate UC [65, 66]. The formulation (budesonide in a multimatrix (MMX) of hydrophilic and lipophilic excipients) was designed to deliver the agent to the colon and thus minimize systemic absorption.

Accepted intravenous steroid therapies include methylprednisolone 20 mg every 8 h, hydrocortisone 100 mg every 8 h, or prednisolone 30 mg every 12 h. There is no difference between intravenous bolus delivery and 24-h continuous infusions [67]. Intravenous corticosteroids are administered until clinical remission is achieved—only then should the patient be switched to an oral form. During their hospitalization, patients with severe UC should be monitored for dehydration, electrolyte abnormalities, anemia, and signs of toxicity and megacolon. If no improvement is seen after 5–7 days, then surgical consultation is sought, and the patient is offered the options of cyclosporine, infliximab, or surgery. Common management errors in the hospitalized patient include prematurely switching to oral steroids, not employing topical 5-ASA and steroid therapies, omitting measures to prevent venous thromboembolism, not feeding the patient, underestimating the severity of the disease, and therefore delaying surgical consultation.

Topical corticosteroids are available as foam (hydrocortisone acetate 10 %); each application delivers approximately 900 mg of foam containing 80 mg of hydrocortisone (90 mg of hydrocortisone acetate) and enema (one 60 mL enema delivers 100 mg hydrocortisone) preparations. Topical budesonide formulations are also available in other countries. These options are useful in treating flares in patients with distal or left-sided UC or in those with prominent distal symptoms. The combination of topical 5-ASA and corticosteroids has been shown to be superior to either therapy alone in distal UC [68].

## Cyclosporine

Cyclosporine is a calcineurin inhibitor used as a salvage therapy in patients with severe UC failing intravenous corticosteroids after 5–7 days. In the seminal study by Lichtiger et al. 82 % of patients with severe, steroid-refractory UC treated with intravenous (IV) cyclosporine avoided colectomy in the short term [69]. Based on pooled data from controlled and uncontrolled trials, approximately 80 % of patients respond to IV cyclosporine and avoid colectomy in the short term [70]. However, 88 % of responders will require colectomy at 7 years [71]. Cyclosporine is also effective as first-line therapy in patients with severe UC (in lieu of IV corticosteroids). In a Belgian, double-blind RCT, IV cyclosporine was as effective as IV methylprednisolone in patients with severe UC (response rates of 64 % and 53 %, respectively) [72]. Cyclosporine is administered at a dose of 2 mg/kg/day by continuous IV infusion. The dose is adjusted targeting serum concentrations of 350–500 ng/ml [73]. Dose-dependent toxicities include nephrotoxicity, infection, hypertrichosis, gingival hyperplasia, paresthesias, tremor, and seizures [74]. The risk of seizures is increased in the setting of hypomagnesemia and hypocholesterolemia. Shortly after successful induction with cyclosporine, immunomodulators are started. Steroids are tapered off first, followed by cyclosporine, so that by 4–6 months the patient is in remission on immunomodulators alone. In a study from the University of Chicago, this approach improved long-term success of avoiding colectomy (59 % with vs. 39 % without immunomodulators) [75]. Prophylaxis against *Pneumocystis jiroveci* (*carinii*) with trimethoprim-sulfamethoxazole or dapsone should be administered in cyclosporine-treated patients.

Small, open-label studies of tacrolimus, a calcineurin inhibitor-like cyclosporine, showed effectiveness in preventing colectomy in the short term in two-thirds of patients with refractory UC [76, 77]. In a recent randomized, placebo-controlled trial of oral tacrolimus in hospitalized patients with steroid-refractory UC, tacrolimus therapy improved clinical response at week 2 (50 % vs. 13 %; $P=0.003$) and mucosal healing (44 % vs. 13 %; $P=0.012$) [78].

## Immunomodulators

The thiopurines, 6-mercaptopurine (6-MP) and its pro-drug azathioprine (AZA), modulate immune response through several mechanisms, including inhibition of DNA and RNA synthesis and apoptosis of activated T-cells [79]. 6-MP and AZA are metabolized into the active 6-thioguanine nucleotide (6-TGN) metabolites as well as the inactive metabolites,

6-methylmercaptopurine nucleotides (6-MMPN) and 6-thiouric acid [80]. High 6TGN concentrations lead to leukopenia, where as high 6MMPN concentrations lead to hepatotoxicity. Conversion to the 6-MMPN metabolites is mediated by the enzyme thiopurine methyltransferase (TPMT). The activity of TPMT is largely determined genetically. Alleles conferring high ($TPMT^H$) and low enzyme activity ($TPMT^L$) are inherited in autosomal, codominant fashion. Approximately 89 % of Caucasians carry only $TPMT^H$ alleles ($TPMT^H/TPMT^H$) and have normal TPMT activity, 11 % are heterozygous ($TPMT^H/TPMT^L$) and have intermediate activity, and 0.3 % are homozygous for the same $TPMT^L$ allele ($TPMT^L/TPMT^L$) or are heterozygous with two different low activity alleles ($TPMT^L/TPMT^{L'}$; compound heterozygotes) and have low or undetectable activity. Measurement of TPMT activity is recommended to determine initial optimal dosage and avoid toxicity. Individuals with low or undetectable activity are generally not treated with the thiopurines, as they invariable develop very high 6-TGN concentrations resulting in neutropenia. Individuals with normal activity are treated with standard doses (6-MP 1–1.5 mg/kg/day or AZA 2.0–3.0 mg/kg/day), whereas those with intermediate activity are given half the standard doses (6-MP 0.5 mg/kg/day or AZA 1.0 mg/kg/day) [81].

RCTs [82–84] and observational studies [85–87] have found the thiopurines effective in maintaining steroid-free remission in patients with steroid-dependent UC. The thiopurines are also useful in patients experiencing frequent flares despite maximal 5-ASA therapy. Long-term therapy is required since 87 % of patients with refractory UC relapse once treatment is discontinued [75]. Due to their slow onset of action, the thiopurines are not used as inductive therapies. A recent meta-analysis reported a nonsignificant trend for benefit from thiopurine induction therapy in patients with active UC (RR=0.85; 95 % CI=0.71–1.01) [88].

Leukopenia (frequently, but not always, associated with high 6-TGN concentrations) and transaminitis (frequently, but not always, associated with high 6-MMPN concentrations) are reversible with dose adjustments. Pancreatitis occurs in 1–2 % of patients, usually in the first 6–8 weeks of treatment. Other adverse effects include nausea, emesis, malaise, rash, arthralgias, and myalgias [89]. These may not recur on switching to the alternate thiopurine. Only pancreatitis and fever are absolute contraindications to future use of the alternate thiopurine. Other risks associated with thiopurines include infections (especially in combination with corticosteroids and/or anti-TNF agents) [90] and lymphoma [91].

Oral methotrexate was not effective in a double-blind, randomized, Israeli trial in patients with active, steroid-requiring UC [92]. Mycophenolate mofetil inhibits lymphocyte proliferation by blocking guanine synthesis. Mycophenolate was less effective than AZA in a small, open-label trial in patients with active UC [93].

## Monoclonal Antibodies Against Tumor Necrosis Factor-α

Infliximab (IFX) is a chimeric monoclonal antibody that targets tumor necrosis factor (TNF)-α, an inflammatory cytokine central to IBD pathogenesis. IFX is approved for the induction and maintenance of clinical remission in adults and children with moderately to severely active UC who have had an inadequate response to conventional therapy. IFX is therefore used in patients with (a) steroid-dependent disease failing thiopurines, (b) steroid-refractory disease, (c) intolerance to 5-ASA and thiopurines, and (d) severe UC requiring hospitalization. IFX is administered as an intravenous infusion at a dose of 5 mg/kg at weeks 0, 2, and 6 for induction, and then every 8 weeks for maintenance.

In two large, phase III trials, IFX led to 61–69 % response and 31–47 % remission rates at 8 weeks [94]. This benefit was maintained through 54 weeks with 44–45 % response and 34–35 % remission rates in IFX-treated patients compared to 20 % and 16 % of placebo-treated patients, respectively. Combination IFX and AZA therapy has been shown to result in higher rates of clinical remission in moderate to severe UC compared to monotherapy (40 % vs. 22–24 %) [95]. Similar results were reported with combination therapy in active Crohn's disease [96], likely reflecting the reduced formation of antibodies against IFX in patients also receiving AZA.

IFX has proven effective as salvage therapy in severe, steroid-refractory UC. Treatment with IFX decreased the need for colectomy among hospitalized patients with severe fulminant UC and failing intravenous steroids [97, 98]. Nonetheless half of patients eventually required colectomy at 5 years [99]. In a recent study that compared IFX to cyclosporine in patients with severe, steroid-refractory UC, IFX demonstrated comparable rates of clinical response at 1 week (86 % vs. 84 %) and need for colectomy (23 % vs. 18 %) [100]. IFX may also be used in hospitalized patients as first-line therapy (in lieu of IV corticosteroids) [101].

An important question concerns the possibility of third-line therapy in patients who have failed cyclosporine or IFX. A French retrospective study examined patients treated between 2000 and 2008 with cyclosporine followed by IFX (n=65) and with IFX followed by cyclosporine (n=21) [102]. The median (±standard error) follow-up time was 23 (7) months. During the study period, 49 patients failed to respond to the second-line rescue therapy and underwent a colectomy. The probability of colectomy-free survival (61±5 % at 3 months and 41±6 % at 12 months) was similar in the two groups. Eight serious infections occurred during first-line therapy in seven patients, including two bacterial central-line infections, two cases of *Clostridium difficile* infection, two cases of cytomegalovirus viremia, one viral pericarditis, and one esophageal candidiasis.

All infections had resolved by the time rescue therapy was started. During rescue therapy, nine serious infections occurred in nine patients (cyclosporine → IFX, $n=7$; and IFX → cyclosporine, $n=2$), and there was one fatal pulmonary embolism. In our opinion, the risk-benefit ratio favors colectomy over second-line rescue therapy in patients who have failed cyclosporine or infliximab after also having failed intravenous steroids. Patients who elect second-line therapy should be advised that they have a 60 % chance of colectomy at 1 year and a significant risk of infection.

After successful induction, IFX is continued as scheduled, maintenance therapy. Infusion reactions occur in approximately 10 % of patients and are mitigated by concomitant immunomodulatory therapy or IV hydrocortisone before the infusions [103]. The most important risk concerns infections, particularly opportunistic infections with intracellular pathogens, including *M. tuberculosis*, histoplasmosis, coccidiomycosis, listeriosis, and others. Testing for latent tuberculosis is mandatory before initiation of therapy. Reactivation of the hepatitis B virus may also occur; hence serologies should be evaluated prior to treatment. Other side effects include hepatotoxicity, worsening of heart failure, drug-induced lupus, and demyelinating disorders, such as multiple sclerosis and optic neuritis. The risk of lymphoma does not appear to be increased [104]. Contraindications to treatment include active infection, untreated latent tuberculosis, preexisting demyelinating disorder, moderate to severe heart failure, and current or recent malignancy.

Adalimumab (ADA) is a humanized monoclonal antibody against TNF-α, which was approved after IFX. ADA is administered by subcutaneous injections of 160 mg at week 0 and 80 mg at week 2 for induction, followed by 40 mg every other week for maintenance.

Two small, open-label studies demonstrated that ADA was well tolerated and beneficial for patients with UC including those who had lost response or had developed intolerance to IFX [105, 106]. More recently, two large RCTs evaluated the efficacy of ADA in moderate to severe UC. A multicenter RCT was conducted in North America and Europe in anti-TNF-naïve patients who received ADA 160/80 (160 mg at week 0, 80 mg at week 2, 40 mg at weeks 4 and 6), ADA 80/40 (80 mg at week 0, 40 mg at weeks 2, 4, and 6), or placebo [107]. More patients were in remission at week 8 in the ADA 160/80 group compared to placebo (18.5 % vs. 9.2 %). There was no difference between the ADA 80/40 group compared to placebo (10.0 % vs. 9.2 %). The second RCT evaluated ADA for the induction and maintenance of clinical remission in 494 patients who had moderate to severe UC and an inadequate response to corticosteroids and/or immunosuppressants [108]. Remission rates were higher in the ADA group than in the placebo group at week 8 (16.5 % vs.

9.3 %) and week 52 (17.3 % vs. 8.5 %). Remission rates were lower in patients who had previously received an anti-TNF agent versus those who were anti-TNF naïve. Rates of serious adverse events were similar between ADA and placebo groups in both studies.

ADA is an option in patients who have experienced loss of response to IFX due to the development of antibodies against IFX. ADA may be preferred over IFX by some patients due to its subcutaneous administration. Recent regulatory approval of golimumab offers another treatment option for patients with ulcerative colitis.

Golimumab is a newer, fully human, subcutaneously administered anti-TNF antibody. A randomized placebo-controlled trial evaluated induction therapy with golimumab in anti-TNF-α-naïve patients with moderate to severe ulcerative colitis [144]. Patients had a Mayo Score of 6–12 points (with an endoscopic subscore≥2 points) and had failed conventional medical therapy with oral mesalamine, oral corticosteroids, and AZA/6-mercaptopurine, or had been unable to taper corticosteroids without recurrence of disease activity. Golimumab was more efficacious than placebo in inducing clinical response, clinical remission and mucosal healing at week 6, and in improvising quality of life [144]. Responders from this trial were eligible for the subsequent, 52-week-long maintenance trial [145]. Golimumab was more efficacious than placebo in maintaining clinical response and remission and in achieving mucosal healing and corticosteroid-free clinical remission [145].

## Other Medical Therapies

Controlled trials of antibiotics have demonstrated no therapeutic benefit when added to intravenous steroids [109, 110]. However, protocols outlining treatment regimens for severe colitis generally include broad-spectrum antibiotics for patients with signs of toxicity or with worsening symptoms despite maximal medical therapy [111]. Nicotine transdermal patches are effective in active UC, though less so than 5-ASA [112–114]. There is no evidence for its use as maintenance therapy. Side effects include lightheadedness, dermatitis, and nausea.

Two RCTs found the probiotic preparation VSL#3 (a combination of eight live, freeze-dried bacterial strains, including four strains of *Lactobacilli*, three strains of *Bifidobacterium*, and *Streptococcus thermophilus*) effective in inducing remission in UC patients failing oral 5-ASA [115, 116]. The evidence on other probiotics is more limited. Antidiarrheal agents are useful in decreasing diarrhea but are contraindicated in severe disease given the risk of toxic megacolon. Dietary arachidonic acid may play a role in the development of UC [117]. However, at the present time, there is no recommended diet specific for UC patients. Physicians may suggest that their patients identify foods that aggravate their disease and eliminate them from their diet. Controlled studies of total parenteral nutrition (TPN) for patients with severe colitis have shown no benefit, so that TPN is limited to patients who are unable to eat or have significant malnutrition [118, 119].

## Goals of Therapy

### Clinical Remission

Traditionally, the treatment goal in UC has been the induction and maintenance of steroid-free clinical remission with complete resolution of symptoms. Partial clinical response and reduction in the need for corticosteroids have also been used as endpoints. Symptom-based indices of activity may be used to monitor patients' response to treatment but are influenced by symptoms that are subjective and scoring which may be nonuniform [120].

### Quality of Life

Improved quality of life is an additional goal of UC therapy. In addition to bowel symptoms, UC produces constitutional and extraintestinal symptoms and affects multiple dimensions of patients' lives, including interpersonal relationships, emotional state, work productivity, sexual health, and reproduction decisions. Patient perception of the disease is often incongruent with the physician's perspective, possibly due to variability in symptoms, the waxing and waning nature of UC, and incomplete disclosure of symptoms to the physician. The most common quality of life measure is the McMaster Inflammatory Bowel Disease Questionnaire (IBDQ), which is available in long form and short form [121, 122]. The long form is a 32-item questionnaire used in many study trials. The short form consists of ten questions regarding social, emotional, bowel, and systemic measures of health and is more ideal for clinical use to monitor patients' quality of life.

### Prevention and Management of Complications

An important goal of UC therapy is the prevention and management of disease and drug-related complications. These include anemia, venous thromboembolism, CRC, and the toxicity of steroids and other agents. Anemia is a common but surprisingly undertreated complication [123–125]. Successful treatment of iron-deficiency anemia correlates with improved quality of life [126, 127]. Multiple large studies have demonstrated that IBD patients have a 1.5- to 3.5-fold higher risk of venous thromboembolism when compared with non-IBD patients [128]. The Adult IBD Physician Performance Measures Set developed by the AGA includes a measure on prophylaxis for venous thromboembolism in IBD inpatients [24]. Although the incidence of CRC is increased in the UC population, emerging data suggest that risk may be declining, possibly as a result of surveillance and more effective therapies [129, 130]. Medication toxicity is minimized by patient education and appropriate clinical and laboratory monitoring.

### Mucosal Healing

Demonstration of endoscopic remission was historically not necessary if a patient was asymptomatic. As demonstration of mucosal healing is proof of concept that a drug is effective in UC, assessment of healing has been a secondary endpoint in recent phase II and phase III RCTs. However, there is ongoing debate as to whether mucosal healing should also constitute an endpoint in clinical practice.

Endoscopic healing has been associated with improved long-term outcomes, such as lower rates of relapse and colectomy, decreased steroid use, and improved quality of life [131–136]. Besides endoscopic assessment, mucosal healing can also be assessed histologically. Increased histologic inflammation has been associated with higher rates of relapse, hospitalization, and colectomy [137, 138]. However, at the present time, management driven by endoscopic and/or histologic disease assessment cannot be recommended over management based on simple clinical assessment: There is a good correlation between clinical and endoscopic disease assessment [131, 139]; endoscopy with biopsies is expensive; and there is no evidence that, in patients in clinical remission but with persistent endoscopic or histologic inflammation, escalation of therapy improves outcomes in a cost-effective manner.

Endoscopic and histologic assessment may have a role in stratifying the risk of colorectal (CRC) cancer. The risk of CRC in UC is increased in patients with endoscopic and histologic evidence of active inflammation or evidence of chronic injury (such as colonic strictures, or a foreshortened or tubular colon) [140–142]. Incorporating these findings, the British Society of Gastroenterology has recommended surveillance at 5-year intervals in low-risk patients, including those without endoscopic/histological active inflammation on the previous colonoscopy [143].

## Conclusions

Ulcerative colitis is a life-long disease portending decades of potential morbidity. Effective management requires education and empowerment of patients and a coordinated healthcare system involving primary care physicians, dedicated IBD teams, and other subspecialists. The selection of medical therapy must take into account the severity and extent of the patient's disease but also suit the patient's lifestyle and treatment goals.

5-ASA is first-line therapy in patients with UC and dosing should be maximized with incorporation of topical formulations whenever tolerated. Corticosteroids are only indicated for induction therapy and should be tapered as soon as clinical remission is established. Maintenance therapy with immunomodulators should be considered in steroid-dependent UC as well as in patients with frequent flares, but may require up to 4 months to reach full effectiveness. Tumor necrosis factor antagonists are used (with or without concomitant immunomodulators) in steroid-dependent or refractory UC. These agents, as well as cyclosporine, are options for patients failing intravenous steroids and wishing to avoid colectomy in the short term.

Besides the induction and maintenance of clinical remission, the goals of treatment include improved quality of life and prevention of complications. It is premature to regard mucosal healing as a therapeutic goal in daily clinical practice. The medical therapy of UC patients requires a multifaceted, patient-centered approach that takes into account individual patient preferences.

# References

1. Loftus Jr EV, Silverstein MD, Sandborn WJ, et al. Ulcerative colitis in Olmsted County, Minnesota, 1940–1993: incidence, prevalence, and survival. Gut. 2000;46:336–43.
2. Hoie O, Schouten LJ, Wolters FL, et al. Ulcerative colitis: no rise in mortality in a European-wide population based cohort 10 years after diagnosis. Gut. 2007;56:497–503.
3. Bodenheimer T, Wagner EH, Grumbach IK. Improving primary care for patients with chronic illness. JAMA. 2002;288:1775–9.
4. Bodenheimer T, Wagner EH, Grumbach IK. Improving primary care for patients with chronic illness: the chronic care model, part 2. JAMA. 2002;288:1909–14.
5. Nguyen GC. Patient trust-in-physician and race are predictors of adherence to medical management in inflammatory bowel disease. Inflamm Bowel Dis. 2009;15:1233–9.
6. Bernstein KI, et al. Information needs and preferences of recently diagnosed patients with inflammatory bowel disease. Inflamm Bowel Dis. 2011;17:590–8.
7. Robinson A. Guided self-management and patient-directed follow-up of ulcerative colitis: a randomised trial. Lancet. 2001;358:976–81.
8. Elkjaer M. E-health empowers patients with ulcerative colitis: a randomised controlled trial of the web-guided "Constant-care" approach. Gut. 2010;59(12):1652–61.
9. Wagner EH, Austin BT, Davis C, et al. Improving chronic illness care: translating evidence into action. Health Aff. 2001;20:64–78.
10. Kornbluth A, Sachar DB. Practice Parameters Committee of the American College of Gastroenterology. Ulcerative colitis practice guidelines in adults: American College of Gastroenterology, Practice Parameters Committee. Am J Gastroenterol. 2010;105:501–23.
11. Long MD, Martin CF, Pipkin CA, et al. Risk of melanoma and nonmelanoma skin cancer among patients with inflammatory bowel disease. Gastroenterology. 2012;143:390–9.
12. Singh H. Risk of cervical abnormalities in women with inflammatory bowel disease: a population-based nested case-control study. Gastroenterology. 2009;136(2):451–8.
13. Herrinton LJ, Liu L, Fireman B, et al. Time trends in therapies and outcomes for adult inflammatory bowel disease, Northern California, 1998–2005. Gastroenterology. 2009;137:502–11.
14. Jelsness-Jørgensen LP, Bernklev T, Henriksen M, et al. Is patient reported outcome (PRO) affected by different follow-up regimens in inflammatory bowel disease (IBD)? A one year prospective, longitudinal comparison of nurse-led versus conventional follow-up. J Crohns Colitis. 2012;6(9):887–94.
15. Bitton A, Sewitch MJ, Peppercorn MA, et al. Psychosocial determinants of relapse in ulcerative colitis: a longitudinal study. Am J Gastroenterol. 2003;98:2203–8.
16. Mittermaier C, Dejaco C, Waldhoer T, et al. Impact of depressive mood on relapse in patients with inflammatory bowel disease: a prospective 18-month follow-up study. Psychosom Med. 2004;66:79–84.
17. Persoons P, Vermeire S, Demyttenaere K, et al. The impact of major depressive disorder on the short- and long-term outcome of Crohn's disease treatment with infliximab. Aliment Pharmacol Ther. 2005;22:101–10.
18. Boye B, Lundin KE, Jantschek G, et al. INSPIRE study: does stress management improve the course of inflammatory bowel disease and disease-specific quality of life in distressed patients with ulcerative colitis or Crohn's disease? A randomized controlled trial. Inflamm Bowel Dis. 2011;17:1863–73.
19. Diaz Sibaja MA, Comeche Moreno MI, Mas Hesse B. Protocolized cognitive-behavioural group therapy for inflammatory bowel disease. Rev Esp Enferm Dig. 2007;99:593–8.
20. Goodhand JR, Greig FI, Koodun Y, et al. Do antidepressants influence the disease course in inflammatory bowel disease? A retrospective case-matched observational study. Inflamm Bowel Dis. 2012;18:1232–9.
21. Kappelman MD, Palmer L, Boyle BM, et al. Quality of care in inflammatory bowel disease: a review and discussion. Inflamm Bowel Dis. 2010;16:125–33.
22. Reddy SI, Friedman S, Telford JJ, et al. Are patients with inflammatory bowel disease receiving optimal care? Am J Gastroenterol. 2005;100:1357–61.
23. Mawdsley JE, Irving PM, Makins RJ, et al. Optimizing quality of outpatient care for patients with inflammatory bowel disease: the importance of specialist clinics. Eur J Gastroenterol Hepatol. 2006;18:249–53.
24. American Gastroenterological Association. Adult inflammatory bowel disease physician performance measures set. 2011; http://www.ama-assn.org/resources/doc/pcpi/inflammatory-bowel-disease.pdf.
25. Ekbom A, Helmick C, Zack M, et al. The epidemiology of inflammatory bowel disease: a large, population-based study in Sweden. Gastroenterology. 1991;100:350–8.
26. Kornbluth A, Sachar DB. Practice Parameters Committee of the American College of Gastroenterology. Ulcerative colitis practice guidelines in adults: American College of Gastroenterology, Practice Parameters Committee. Am J Gastroenterol. 2010;105:501–23.
27. Hanauer SB. Inflammatory bowel disease. N Engl J Med. 1996;334:841–8.
28. Gan SI, Beck PL. A new look at toxic megacolon: an update and review of incidence, etiology, pathogenesis, and management. Am J Gastroenterol. 2003;98:2363–71.

29. D'Haens G, Sandborn WJ, Feagan B, et al. A review of activity indices and efficacy end points for clinical trials of medical therapy in adults with ulcerative colitis. Gastroenterology. 2007;132:763–86.

30. Truelove SC, Witts LJ. Cortisone in ulcerative colitis: final report on a therapeutic trial. Br Med J. 1955;2:1041–8.

31. Powell-Tuck J, Bown RL, Lennard-Jones JE. A comparison of oral prednisolone given as single or multiple daily doses for active proctocolitis. Scand J Gastroenterol. 1978;13:833–7.

32. Seo M, Okada M, Yao T, et al. An index of disease activity in patients with ulcerative colitis. Am J Gastroenterol. 1992;87:971–6.

33. Seo M, Okada M, Yao T, et al. Evaluation of disease activity in patients with moderately active ulcerative colitis: comparisons between new activity index and Truelove and Witts classification. Am J Gastroenterol. 1995;90:1759–63.

34. Seo M, Okada M, Yao T, et al. Evaluation of the clinical course of acute attacks in patients with ulcerative colitis through the use of an activity index. J Gastroenterol. 2002;37:29–34.

35. Jarnerot G, Hertervig E, Friis-Liby I, et al. Infliximab as rescue therapy in severe to moderately severe ulcerative colitis: a randomized, placebo-controlled study. Gastroenterology. 2005;128:1805–11.

36. Seo M, Okada M, Maeda K, et al. Correlation between endoscopic severity and clinical activity index in ulcerative colitis. Am J Gastroenterol. 1998;93:2124–9.

37. Schroeder KW, Tremaine WJ, Ilstrup DM. Coated oral 5-aminosalicylic acid therapy for mildly to moderately active ulcerative colitis. N Engl J Med. 1987;317:1625–9.

38. Sutherland LR, Martin F, Greer S, et al. 5-Aminosalicylic acid enema in the treatment of distal ulcerative colitis, proctosigmoiditis, and proctitis. Gastroenterology. 1987;92:1894–8.

39. Higgins PD, Schwartz M, Mapili J, et al. Patient defined dichotomous end points for remission and clinical improvement in ulcerative colitis. Gut. 2005;54:782–8.

40. Rousseaux C, Lefebvre B, Dubuquoy L, et al. Intestinal antiinflammatory effect of 5-aminosalicylic acid is dependent on peroxisome proliferator-activated receptor-gamma. J Exp Med. 2005;201:1205–15.

41. Sharon P, Ligumsky M, Rachmilewitz D, et al. Role of prostaglandins in ulcerative colitis. Enhanced production during active disease and inhibition by sulfasalazine. Gastroenterology. 1978;75:638–40.

42. Ahnfelt-Ronne I, Nielsen OH, Christensen A, et al. Clinical evidence supporting the radical scavenger mechanism of 5-aminosalicylic acid. Gastroenterology. 1990;98:1162–9.

43. Ford AC, Achkar JP, Khan KJ, et al. Efficacy of 5-aminosalicylates in ulcerative colitis: systematic review and meta-analysis. Am J Gastroenterol. 2011;106:601–16.

44. Hanauer SB, Sandborn WJ, Kornbluth A, et al. Delayed-release oral mesalamine at 4.8 g/day (800 mg tablet) for the treatment of moderately active ulcerative colitis: the ASCEND II trial. Am J Gastroenterol. 2005;100:2478–85.

45. Kane S, Cohen RD, Aikens JE, et al. Predictors of non-compliance with mesalamine in quiescent ulcerative colitis. Am J Gastroenterol. 2001;96:2929–32.

46. Kane S, Huo D, Aikens J, et al. Medication nonadherence and the outcomes of patients with quiescent ulcerative colitis. Am J Med. 2003;114:39–43.

47. Kane S, Huo D, Kalyani M. A pilot feasibility study of once daily versus conventional dosing mesalamine for maintenance of ulcerative colitis. Clin Gastroenterol Hepatol. 2003;1:170–3.

48. Gisbert JP, Gonzalez-Lama Y, Mate J. 5-Aminosalicylates and renal function in inflammatory bowel disease: a systematic review. Inflamm Bowel Dis. 2007;13:629–38.

49. Cohen RD, Woseth DM, Thisted RA, et al. A meta-analysis and overview of the literature on treatment options for left-sided ulcerative colitis and ulcerative proctitis. Am J Gastroenterol. 2000;95:1263–76.

50. Safdi M, DeMicco M, Sninsky C, et al. A double-blind comparison of oral versus rectal mesalamine versus combination therapy in the treatment of distal ulcerative colitis. Am J Gastroenterol. 1997;92:1867–71.

51. Marteau P, Probert CS, Lindgren S, et al. Combined oral and enema treatment with Pentasa (mesalamine) is superior to oral therapy alone in patients with extensive mild/moderate active ulcerative colitis: a randomized, double blind, placebo controlled study. Gut. 2005;54:960–5.

52. D'Albasio G, Pacini F, Camarri E, et al. Combination therapy with 5-aminosalicylic acid tablets and enemas for maintaining remission in ulcerative colitis: a randomized double-blind study. Am J Gastroenterol. 1997;92:1143–7.

53. Faubion WA, Loftus EV, Harmsen WS, et al. The natural history of corticosteroid therapy for inflammatory bowel disease: a population-based study. Gastroenterology. 2001;121:255–60.

54. Truelove SC, Witts LJ. Cortisone in ulcerative colitis: final report on a therapeutic trial. Br Med J. 1955;2:1041–8.

55. Ford AC, Bernstein CN, Khan KJ, et al. Glucocorticosteroid therapy in inflammatory bowel disease: a systematic review and meta-analysis. Am J Gastroenterol. 2011;106:590–9.

56. Truelove SC, Jewell DP. Intensive intravenous regimen for severe attacks of ulcerative colitis. Lancet. 1974;1:1067–70.

57. Truelove SC, Willoughby CP, Lee EG, et al. Further experience in the treatment of severe attacks of ulcerative colitis. Lancet. 1978;2:1086–8.

58. Jarnerot G, Rolyn P, Sandberg-Gertzen H. Intensive intravenous treatment of ulcerative colitis. Gastroenterology. 1985;89:1005–13.

59. Abu-Suboh Abadia M, Casellas F, Vilaseca J, et al. Response of first attack of inflammatory bowel disease requiring hospital admission to steroid therapy. Rev Esp Enferm Dig. 2004;96(539–44):544–7.

60. Bossa F, Fiorella S, Caruso N, et al. Continuous versus bolus administration of steroids in severe attacks of ulcerative colitis: a randomized, double-blind trial. Am J Gastroenterol. 2007;102:601–8.

61. Carbonnel F, Gargouri D, Lemann M, et al. Predictive factors of outcome of intensive intravenous treatment for attacks of ulcerative colitis. Aliment Pharmacol Ther. 2000;14:273–9.

62. Travis SP, Farrant JM, Ricketts C, et al. Predicting outcome in severe ulcerative colitis. Gut. 1996;38:905–10.

63. Kornbluth A, Sachar DB. Practice Parameters Committee of the American College of Gastroenterology. Ulcerative colitis practice guidelines in adults: American College of Gastroenterology, Practice Parameters Committee. Am J Gastroenterol. 2010;105:501–23.

64. Baron JH, Connell AM, Kanaglunis TG, et al. Outpatient treatment of ulcerative colitis: comparison between three doses of oral prednisone. Br Med J. 1962;2:441–3.

65. Sandborn WJ, Travis S, Moro L, et al. Once-daily budesonide MMX extended-release tablets induce remission in patients with mild to moderate ulcerative colitis: results from the CORE I study. Gastroenterology. 2012;143:1218–26.

66. Travis SP, Danese S, Kupcinskas L, et al. Once-daily budesonide MMX in active, mild-to-moderate ulcerative colitis: results from the randomised CORE II study. Gut. 2013. [Epub ahead of print].

67. Bossa F, Fiorella S, Caruso N, et al. Continuous versus bolus administration of steroids in severe attacks of ulcerative colitis: a randomized, double-blind trial. Am J Gastroenterol. 2007;102:601–8.

68. Mulder CJ, Fockens P, Meijer DW, et al. Beclomethasone dipropionate (3 mg) versus 5-aminosalicylic acid (2 g) versus the combination of both (3 mg/2 g) as retention enemas in active ulcerative proctitis. Eur J Gastroenterol Hepatol. 1996;8:549–54.

69. Lichtiger S, Present DH, Kornbluth A, et al. Cyclosporine in severe ulcerative colitis refractory to steroid therapy. N Eng J Med. 1994;330:1841–5.

70. Van Assche G, Vermeire S, Rutgeerts P. Management of acute severe ulcerative colitis. Gut. 2011;60:130–3.

71. Moskovitz DN, Van Assche G, Maenhout B, et al. Incidence of colectomy during long-term follow-up after cyclosporine-induced remission of severe ulcerative colitis. Clin Gastroenterol Hepatol. 2006;4:760–5.

72. D'Haens G, Lemmens L, Geboes K, et al. Intravenous cyclosporine versus intravenous corticosteroids as single therapy for severe attacks of ulcerative colitis. Gastroenterology. 2011;120:1323–9.

73. Lichtenstein GR, Abreu MT, Cohen R, et al. American Gastroenterological Association Institute technical review on corticosteroids, immunomodulators, and infliximab in inflammatory bowel disease. Gastroenterology. 2006;130:940–87.

74. Sandborn WJ. A review of immune modifier therapy for inflammatory bowel disease: azathioprine, 6-mercaptopurine, cyclosporine, and methotrexate. Am J Gastroenterol. 1996;91:423–33.

75. Cohen RD, Stein R, Hanauer SB. Intravenous cyclosporine in ulcerative colitis: a five-year experience. Am J Gastroenterol. 1999;94:1587–92.

76. Fellermann K, Tanko Z, Herrlinger KR, et al. Response of refractory colitis to intravenous or oral tacrolimus (FK506). Inflamm Bowel Dis. 2002;8:317–24.

77. Hogenauer C, Wenzl HH, Hinterleitner TA, et al. Effect of oral tacrolimus (FK 506) on steroid-refractory moderate/severe ulcerative colitis. Aliment Pharmacol Ther. 2003;18:415–23.

78. Ogata H, Kato J, Hirai F, et al. Double-blind, placebo-controlled trial of oral tacrolimus (FK506) in the management of hospitalized patients with steroid-refractory ulcerative colitis. Inflamm Bowel Dis. 2012;18:803–8.

79. Atreya I, Neurath MF. Azathioprine in inflammatory bowel disease: improved molecular insights and resulting clinical implications. Expert Rev Gastroenterol Hepatol. 2008;2:23–34.

80. Chouchana L, Narjoz C, Beaune P, et al. Review article: the benefits of pharmacogenetics for improving thiopurine therapy in inflammatory bowel disease. Aliment Pharmacol Ther. 2012;35:15–36.

81. Lennard L. The clinical pharmacology of 6-mercaptopurine. Eur J Clin Pharmacol. 1992;43:329–39.

82. Ardizzone S, Maconi G, Russo A, et al. Randomised controlled trial of azathioprine and 5-aminosalicylic acid for treatment of steroid dependent ulcerative colitis. Gut. 2006;55:47–53.

83. Mantzaris GJ, Sfakianakis M, Archavlis E, et al. A prospective randomized observer-blind 2-year trial of azathioprine monotherapy versus azathioprine and olsalazine for the maintenance of remission of steroid-dependent ulcerative colitis. Am J Gastroenterol. 2004;99:1122–8.

84. Sood A, Midha V, Sood N, et al. Role of azathioprine in severe ulcerative colitis: one-year, placebo-controlled, randomized trial. Indian J Gastroenterol. 2000;19:14–6.

85. George J, Present DH, Pou R, et al. The long-term outcome of ulcerative colitis treated with 5-mercaptopurine. Am J Gastroenterol. 1996;91:1711–4.

86. Ardizzone S, Molteni P, Imbesi V, et al. Azathioprine in steroid-resistant and steroid-dependent ulcerative colitis. J Clin Gastroenterol. 1997;25:330–3.

87. Chebli LA, Chaves LD, Pimentel FF, et al. Azathioprine maintains long-term steroid-free remission through 3 years in patients with steroid-dependent ulcerative colitis. Inflamm Bowel Dis. 2010;16:613–9.

88. Khan KJ, Dubinsky MC, Ford AC, et al. Efficacy of immunosuppressive therapy for inflammatory bowel disease: a systematic review and meta-analysis. Am J Gastroenterol. 2011;106:630–42.

89. Present DH, Meltzer SJ, Krumholz MP, et al. 6-Mercaptopurine in the management of inflammatory bowel disease: short- and long-term toxicity. Ann Intern Med. 1989;111:641–9.

90. Toruner M, Loftus Jr EV, Harmsen WS, et al. Risk factors for opportunistic infections in patients with inflammatory bowel disease. Gastroenterology. 2008;134:929–36.

91. Sokol H, Beaugerie L. Inflammatory bowel disease and lymphoproliferative disorders: the dust is starting to settle. Gut. 2009;58:1427–36.

92. Oren R, Arber N, Odes S, et al. Methotrexate in chronic active ulcerative colitis: a double-blind, randomized, Israeli multicenter trial. Gastroenterology. 1996;110:1416–21.

93. Orth T, Peters M, Schlaak JF, et al. Mycophenolate mofetil versus azathioprine in patients with chronic active ulcerative colitis: a 12-month pilot study. Am J Gastroenterol. 2000;95:1201–7.

94. Rutgeerts P, Sandborn WJ, Feagan BG, et al. Infliximab for induction and maintenance therapy for ulcerative colitis. New Engl J Med. 2005;353:2462–76.

95. Panccione R, Ghosh S, Middleton S, et al. Infliximab, azathioprine, or infliximab + azathioprine for treatment of moderate to severe ulcerative colitis: the UC success trial. Gastroenterology. 2011;140:S-134.

96. Colombel JF, Sandborn WJ, Reinisch W, et al. Infliximab, azathioprine, or combination therapy for Crohn's disease. N Engl J Med. 2010;362:1383–95.

97. Sandborn WJ, Rutgeerts P, Feagan BG, et al. Colectomy rate comparison after treatment of ulcerative colitis with placebo or infliximab. Gastroenterology. 2009;137:1250–60.

98. Jarnerot G, Hertervig E, Friis-Liby I, et al. Infliximab as rescue therapy in severe to moderately severe ulcerative colitis: a randomized, placebo-controlled study. Gastroenterology. 2005;128:1805–11.

99. Gustavsson A, Jarnerot G, Hertervig E, et al. Clinical trial: colectomy after rescue therapy in ulcerative colitis—3-year follow-up of the Swedish-Danish controlled infliximab study. Aliment Pharmacol Ther. 2010;32:984–9.

100. Laharie D, Bourreille A, Branche J, et al. Cyclosporin versus infliximab in severe acute ulcerative colitis refractory to intravenous steroids: a randomized trial. Gastroenterology. 2011;140:S-112.

101. Ochsenkuhn T, Sackmann M, Goke B. Infliximab for acute, not steroid-refractory ulcerative colitis: a randomized pilot study. Eur J Gastroenterol Hepatol. 2004;16:1167–71.

102. Leblanc S, Allez M, Seksik P, et al. Successive treatment with cyclosporine and infliximab in steroid-refractory ulcerative colitis. Am J Gastroenterol. 2011;106:771–7.

103. Farrell RJ, Alsahli M, Jeen YT, et al. Intravenous hydrocortisone premedication reduces antibodies to infliximab in Crohn's disease: a randomized controlled trial. Gastroenterology. 2003;124:917–24.

104. Lichtenstein GR, Feagan BG, Cohen RD, et al. Serious infection and mortality in patients with Crohn's disease: more than 5 years of follow-up in the TREAT registry. Am J Gastroenterol. 2012;107:1409–22.

105. Afif W, Leighton JA, Hanauer SB, et al. Open-label study of adalimumab in patients with ulcerative colitis including those with prior loss of response or intolerance to infliximab. Inflamm Bowel Dis. 2009;15:1302–7.

106. Oussalah A, Laclotte C, Chevaux JB, et al. Long-term outcome of adalimumab therapy for ulcerative colitis with intolerance or lost response to infliximab: a single-centre experience. Aliment Pharmacol Ther. 2008;28:966–72.

107. Reinisch W, Sandborn WJ, Hommes DW, et al. Adalimumab for induction of clinical remission in moderately to severely active ulcerative colitis: results of a randomised controlled trial. Gut. 2011;60:780–7.

108. Sandborn WJ, van Assche G, Reinisch W, et al. Adalimumab induces and maintains clinical remission in patients with moderate-to-severe ulcerative colitis. Gastroenterology. 2012;142: 257–65.

109. Chapman RW, Selby WS, Jewell DP. Controlled trial of intravenous metronidazole as an adjunct to corticosteroids in severe ulcerative colitis. Gut. 1986;27:1210–2.

110. Mantzaris GJ, Hatzis A, Kontogiannis P, et al. Intravenous tobramycin and metronidazole as an adjunct to corticosteroids in acute, severe ulcerative colitis. Am J Gastroenterol. 1994;89:43–6.

111. Kornbluth A, Sachar DB. Practice Parameters Committee of the American College of Gastroenterology. Ulcerative colitis practice guidelines in adults: American College of Gastroenterology, Practice Parameters Committee. Am J Gastroenterol. 2010;105:501–23.

112. Sandborn WJ, Tremaine WJ, Offord KP, et al. Transdermal nicotine for mildly to moderately active ulcerative colitis: a randomized, double-blind, placebo-controlled trial. Ann Intern Med. 1997;126:364–71.

113. Pullan RD, Rhodes J, Ganesh S. Transdermal nicotine for active ulcerative colitis. New Engl J Med. 1994;330:811–5.

114. Thomas GA, Rhodes J, Mani V, et al. Transdermal nicotine as maintenance therapy for ulcerative colitis. N Engl J Med. 1995;332:988–92.

115. Tursi A, Brandimarte G, Papa A, et al. Treatment of relapsing mild-to-moderate ulcerative colitis with the probiotics VSL#3 as adjunctive to a standard pharmaceutical treatment: a double-blind, randomized, placebo-controlled study. Am J Gastroenterol. 2010;105:2218–27.

116. Sood A, Midha V, Makharia GK, et al. The probiotic preparation, VSL#3 induces remission in patients with mild-to-moderately active ulcerative colitis. Clin Gastroenterol Hepatol. 2009;7: 1202–9.

117. de Silva PS, Olsen A, Christensen J, et al. An association between dietary arachidonic acid, measured in adipose tissue, and ulcerative colitis. Gastroenterology. 2010;139:1912–7.

118. Dickinson RJ, Ashton MG, Axon AT, et al. Controlled trial of intravenous hyperalimentation and total bowel rest as an adjunct to the routine therapy of acute colitis. Gastroenterology. 1980;79:1199–204.

119. McIntyre PB, Powell-Tuck J, Wood SR, et al. Controlled trial of bowel rest in the treatment of severe acute colitis. Gut. 1986;27: 481–5.

120. Sands BE, Ooi CJ. A survey of methodological variation in the Crohn's disease activity index. Inflamm Bowel Dis. 2005;11: 133–8.

121. Irvine EJ. Quality of life issues in patients with inflammatory bowel disease. Am J Gastroenterol. 1997;92:18S–24.

122. Jowett SL, Seal CJ, Barton JR, et al. The short inflammatory bowel disease questionnaire is reliable and responsive to clinically important change in ulcerative colitis. Am J Gastroenterol. 2001;96:2921–8.

123. Ott C, Liebold A, Takses A, et al. High prevalence but insufficient treatment of iron-deficiency anemia in patients with inflammatory bowel disease: results of a population-based cohort. Gastroenterol Res Pract. 2012;2012:595970.

124. Goodhand JR, Kamperidis N, Rao A, et al. Prevalence and management of anemia in children, adolescents, and adults with inflammatory bowel disease. Inflamm Bowel Dis. 2012;18: 513–9.

125. Voegtlin M, Vavricka SR, Schoepfer AM, Swiss IBD Cohort Study, et al. Prevalence of anaemia in inflammatory bowel disease in Switzerland: a cross-sectional study in patients from private practices and university hospitals. J Crohns Colitis. 2010;4: 642–8.

126. Gisbert JP, Bermejo F, Pajares R, et al. Oral and intravenous iron treatment in inflammatory bowel disease: hematological response and quality of life improvement. Inflamm Bowel Dis. 2009;15: 1485–91.

127. Wells CW, Lewis S, Barton JR, et al. Effects of changes in hemoglobin level on quality of life and cognitive function in inflammatory bowel disease patients. Inflamm Bowel Dis. 2006;12:123–30.

128. Murthy SK, Nguyen GC. Venous thromboembolism in inflammatory bowel disease: an epidemiological review. Am J Gastroenterol. 2011;106:713–8.

129. Soderlund S, Brandt L, Lapidus A, et al. Decreasing time-trends of colorectal cancer in a large cohort of patients with inflammatory bowel disease. Gastroenterology. 2009;136:1561–7.

130. Jess T, Simonsen J, Jørgensen KT, et al. Decreasing risk of colorectal cancer in patients with inflammatory bowel disease over 30 years. Gastroenterology. 2012;143:375–81.

131. Meucci G, Fasoli R, Saibeni S, et al. Prognostic significance of endoscopic remission in patients with active ulcerative colitis treated with oral and topical mesalazine: a prospective, multicenter study. Inflamm Bowel Dis. 2012;18:1006–10.

132. Froslie KF, Jahnsen J, Moum BA, et al. Mucosal healing in inflammatory bowel disease: results from a Norwegian population-based cohort. Gastroenterology. 2007;133:412–22.

133. Lichtenstein GR, Rutgeerts P. Importance of mucosal healing in ulcerative colitis. Inflamm Bowel Dis. 2010;16:338–46.

134. Rutgeerts P, Vermeire S, van AG. Mucosal healing in inflammatory bowel disease: impossible ideal or therapeutic target? Gut. 2007;56:453–5.

135. Ferrante M, Vermeire S, Fidder H, et al. Long-term outcome after infliximab for refractory ulcerative colitis. J Crohns Colitis. 2008;2:219–25.

136. Colombel JF, Rutgeerts P, Reinisch W, et al. Early mucosal healing with infliximab is associated with improved long-term clinical outcomes in ulcerative colitis. Gastroenterology. 2011;141:1194–201.

137. Riley SA, Mani V, Goodman MJ, et al. Microscopic activity in ulcerative colitis: what does it mean? Gut. 1991;32:174–8.

138. Rubin DT, Huo D, Hetzel JT, et al. Increased degree of histological inflammation predicts colectomy and hospitalization in patients with ulcerative colitis. Gastroenterology. 2007;132:A-19. Abstract 103.

139. Higgins P, Schwartz M, Mapili J, Zimmermann EM. Is endoscopy necessary for the measurement of disease activity in ulcerative colitis. Am J Gastroenterol. 2005;100:355–61.

140. Rutter M, Saunders B, Wilkinson K, et al. Severity of inflammation is a risk factor for colorectal neoplasia in ulcerative colitis. Gastroenterology. 2004;126:451–9.

141. Rutter MD, Saunders BP, Wilkinson KH, et al. Cancer surveillance in longstanding ulcerative colitis: endoscopic appearances help predict cancer risk. Gut. 2004;53:1813–6.

142. Gupta RB, Harpaz N, Itzkowitz S, et al. Histologic inflammation is a risk factor for progression to colorectal neoplasia in ulcerative colitis: a cohort study. Gastroenterology. 2007;133:1099–105. quiz 1340–1.

143. Cairns SR, Scholefield JH, Steele RJ, et al. Guidelines for colorectal cancer screening and surveillance in moderate and high risk groups (update from 2002). Gut. 2010;59:666–89.

144. Sandborn WJ, Feagan BG, Marano C, et al. Subcutaneous golimumab induces clinical response and remission in patients with moderate-to-severe ulcerative colitis. Gastroenterology. 2014;146(1):85–95.

145. Sandborn WJ, Feagan BG, Marano C, et al. Subcutaneous golimumab maintains clinical response in patients with moderate-to-severe ulcerative colitis. Gastroenterology. 2014;146(1):96–109.

# The Importance of Mucosal Healing in Ulcerative Colitis

**5**

Anthony M. Sofia, Sarah R. Goeppinger, and David T. Rubin

**Keywords**

Mucosal healing • Ulcerative colitis • Inflamed rectum • Tenesmus • Incomplete evacuation • Urgency • Bleeding • Hematochezia • Prognostic marker inflammatory damage • Colorectum

## Introduction

Ulcerative colitis (UC) is an idiopathic condition of the colon, in which acute and chronic inflammation results in an injured bowel. Chronic inflammatory damage, confined exclusively to the mucosa of the colorectum, is the hallmark of the disease. The inflammation is characteristically superficial in nature and appears to begin in the rectum with variable extension to more proximal portions of the colon. This inflammation, and subsequent loss of function, is the mechanism underlying the typical symptoms of UC. Although there may be more systemic symptoms, the majority of the symptoms of UC are derived from an inflamed rectum and due to loss of compliance of the rectum, loss of sensation of stool, as well as symptoms of tenesmus incomplete evacuation, urgency, and bleeding with hematochezia. The healed bowel can result in the resolution of symptoms and has been associated with disease control and resolution, but traditional clinical assessment of UC involves symptom management primarily, with the assumption that when bleeding and urgency are improved, adequate disease control has been achieved. However, resolution of bowel inflammation is not always manifest as improved or resolved symptoms, and improved symptoms are not always associated with a healed bowel or durable disease control. This chapter reviews the importance of musical healing as a prognostic marker and therapeutic endpoint in UC.

## Endoscopic Scoring of Mucosal Inflammation in UC

The description of inflammation in UC varies from mild mucosal disruption with loss of vascularity and some edema to more significant diffuse inflammation, with mucopus or even diffuse ulcerations and areas of complete loss of the mucosa. An additional feature of active mucosal inflammation in UC is contact friability or spontaneous bleeding. Although traditionally described as diffuse in its extent and involvement, some patchiness to the endoscopic appearance may be seen during disease onset or with partial treatment by medical therapy (Fig. 5.1).

In an effort to quantify the degree of inflammation, a number of different clinical, endoscopic, and composite scoring systems have been developed over time (Table 5.1). Most frequently embraced is the so-called Mayo endoscopic subscore, which was developed from the previously published "Baron score" and modified in order to be part of a

A.M. Sofia, M.D. (✉)
Department of Internal Medicine, University of Chicago Medicine, 165 N. Canal St. #1030, Chicago, IL 60637, USA
e-mail: masofia@uchicago.edu

S.R. Goeppinger, B.A.
Section of Gastroenterology, Department of Medicine, University of Chicago Medicine, 5841 South Maryland Avenue, MC 4080, Chicago, IL 60637, USA
e-mail: goeppinger@medicine.bsd.uchicago.edu

D.T. Rubin, M.D.
Section of Gastroenterology, Department of Medicine, University of Chicago, 5841 S. Maryland Avenue, MC 4076, Chicago, IL 60637, USA
e-mail: drubin@medicine.bsd.uchicago.edu

G.R. Lichtenstein (ed.), *Medical Therapy of Ulcerative Colitis*,
DOI 10.1007/978-1-4939-1677-1_5, © Springer Science+Business Media New York 2014

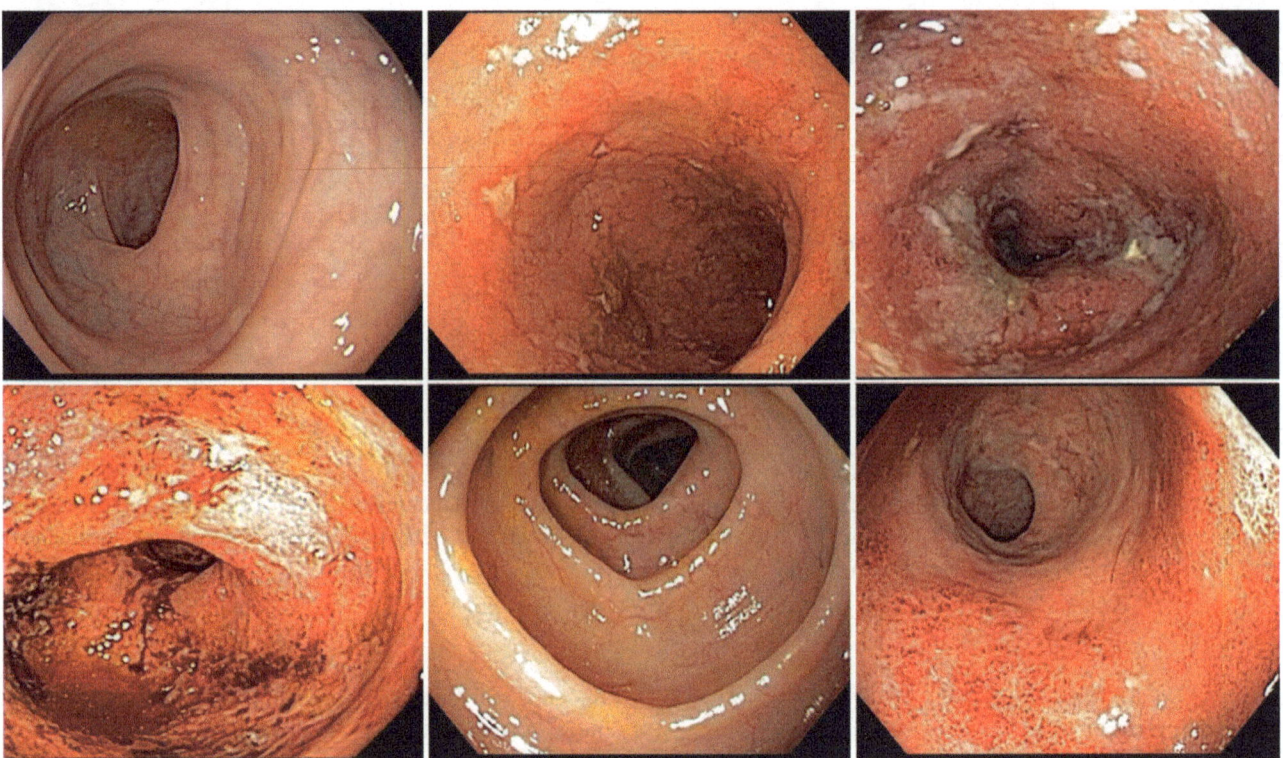

**Fig. 5.1** Variable appearances of mucosa in ulcerative colitis

**Table 5.1** Measuring disease activity in ulcerative colitis

| Based on clinical and biochemical disease activity | Based on endoscopic disease activity | Composite clinical and endoscopic disease activity |
|---|---|---|
| Truelove and Witts severity index (TWSI) | Truelove and Witts sigmoidoscopic assessment | Mayo score (DAI) |
| Powell-Tuck index | Baron score | Sutherland index (DAI, UCDAI) |
| Clinical activity index (CAI) | Powell-Tuck sigmoidoscopic assessment | |
| Activity index (AI or Seo index) | Rachmilewitz endoscopic index | |
| Physician global assessment | Sigmoidoscopic index | |
| Lichtiger index (mTWSI) | Sigmoidoscopic inflammation grade score | |
| Investigators global evaluation | Mayo score flexible proctosigmoidoscopy assessment | |
| Simple clinical colitis activity index (SCCAI) | Sutherland mucosal appearance assessment | |
| Improvement based on individual symptom scores | Modified Baron score | |
| Ulcerative colitis clinical score (UCCS) | UC endoscopic index of severity (UCEIS) | |
| Patient-defined remission | | |

Adapted from D'Haens G, Sandborn WJ, Feagan BG, Geboes K, Hanauer SB, Irvine EJ, Lémann M, Marteau P, Rutgeerts P, Schölmerich J, Sutherland LR. A review of activity indices and efficacy end points for clinical trials of medical therapy in adults with ulcerative colitis. Gastroenterology. 2007 Feb;132(2):763–86 [47]

composite index (the "Mayo score") for the clinical trials of delayed-release mesalamine [1]. In the Mayo endoscopic subscore, the endoscopic appearance is rated from 0 to 3 (Fig. 5.2). A score of 0 is termed "normal," which is defined as an intact mucosa with a preserved vascular pattern and no friability or granularity. A score of 1 represents an abnormal appearance but is not grossly hemorrhagic. The mucosa may appear erythematous and edematous, and the vascular pattern may appear blunted. A score of 2 is moderately hemorrhagic, with bleeding to light touch but without spontaneous bleeding seen ahead of the instrument on initial inspection. In the traditional Mayo scoring, friability is part of a score of 1, but in the modified Mayo scoring (as in the clinical trials with MMX mesalamine), friability is part of a score of 2.

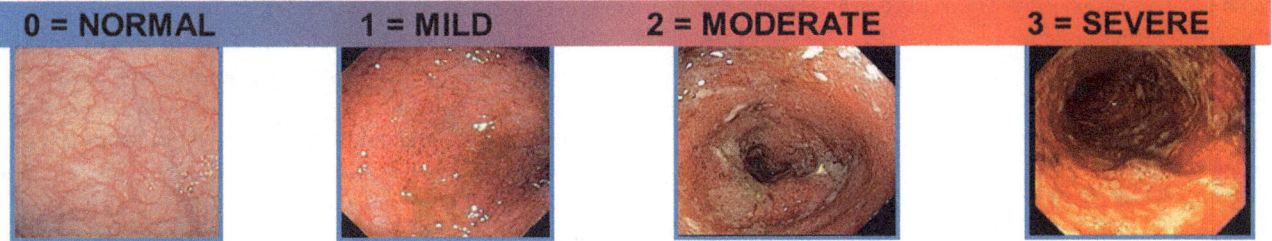

**Fig. 5.2** Representative photos of the Mayo endoscopic subscore. Schroeder KW, Tremaine WJ, Ilstrup DM. Coated oral 5-aminosalicylic acid therapy for mildly to moderately active ulcerative colitis. A randomized study. N Engl J Med. 1987 Dec 24;317(26):1625–9 [46]

A score of 3 is termed "severe," which is defined as having marked erythema, absent vascular markings, granularity, spontaneous bleeding, and ulcerations. In most clinical trials, the term "mucosal healing" has been defined as a Mayo subscore of 0 or 1. The prior definitions of mucosal healing have had limitations, and there has been interest in clarifying endoscopic and histologic definitions for future clinical trials and disease management paradigms. Therefore, in 2007, the International Organization for the Study of Inflammatory Bowel Disease (IOIBD) defined mucosal healing as an absence of friability, blood, erosions, or ulcerations [2, 3].

Most recently, Travis and colleagues have described a novel UC scoring index of severity, the UCEIS (Ulcerative Colitis Endoscopic Index of Severity). In the two-phase development study, a library of 670 video sigmoidoscopies from patients with composite Mayo scores between 0 and 11 were supplemented by 10 videos from 5 people without UC and 5 patients hospitalized with severely active disease. In phase 1, 10 investigators each viewed 16/24 videos to determine agreement on the Baron score with a central reader and agreed definitions of 10 endoscopic descriptors. In phase 2, 30 investigators each rated 25/60 videos for said descriptors and assessed overall severity on an analog scale that ranged from 0 to 100. The study found a 76 % agreement for severe and a 27 % agreement for normal endoscopic appearances. It was concluded that the UCEIS accurately predicted the overall assessment of endoscopic severity in UC; however, additional testing and further validity are needed before use in clinical practice.

For clinical trials, the use of a centralized reader for endoscopic scoring is of interest and has demonstrated significant impact on clinical trial outcomes. Further training of gastroenterologists in particular will be necessary in order to develop reliable approaches to the use of endoscopic mucosal healing as a clinical practice treatment endpoint [4, 5].

Histologic scoring of mucosal healing in UC notably, histologic findings previously have not been part of these definitions of mucosal healing in UC. The IOIBD also defined the two histologic patterns that are consistent with remission. The first is demonstration of chronic inflammation in the lamina propria with regular or irregular glands. The second is a lack of inflammation with an atrophic glandular pattern with short crypts, glands with lateral buddings, dichotomic glands, or an apparently normal glandular pattern [3]. Numerous methods of classifying histologic activity have been proposed, but despite emerging interest by regulatory bodies, these scales have not been validated as clinical trial endpoints or for clinical practice [6]. There remain numerous unanswered questions about whether histologic healing or remission can be a realistic treatment goal for the majority of patients [6, 7].

## Why Mucosal Healing Is Important in UC

Although the obvious connection between the status of the mucosal inflammation and the condition of the patient with UC has long been recognized, it has only been in recent years that a therapeutic goal of mucosal healing could be entertained. This is due to the ability to measure mucosal injury in easier ways, emerging data on clinical outcomes associated with degrees of mucosal inflammation, and the development of many therapies that offer methods of healing the mucosa in patients with UC [2]. It is also due to the appreciation that symptoms similar to active UC can be mimicked by the presence of irritable bowel syndrome or, possibly, injury to the mucosa and submucosa from prior inflammation and chronic changes that occur. In addition, the emerging clinical goal of endoscopic mucosal healing enables further distinction from other conditions such as infections, which also may produce confounding symptoms. Therefore, the adoption of mucosal healing as a therapeutic goal theoretically can reduce the diagnostic reliance on subjective clinical characteristics. Such a therapeutic endpoint also clarifies response to therapy, so that therapeutic adjustments are made with more accurate information. Finally, emerging evidence demonstrates that endoscopic mucosal healing is associated with improved short- and long-term outcomes in UC (Table 5.2).

**Table 5.2** Possible primary and secondary benefits of mucosal healing in ulcerative colitis

| |
|---|
| Reduction of clinical relapse |
| Reduction in surgical rates |
| Reduction in hospitalization |
| Reduction in neoplasia |
| Improvement in quality of life |

Histologic and endoscopic inflammatory activity has been shown to be associated with higher rates of disease relapse in UC. Riley and colleagues evaluated 82 ulcerative colitis patients who were in remission to see if histologic inflammation during remission predicted relapse. Each of the 82 patients were in clinical remission and had rectal biopsies obtained at the beginning of the trial. They were then maintained on sulfasalazine or mesalamine and followed for clinical relapse. The investigators found that a number of histologic findings predicted clinical relapse. The histologic findings predictive of clinical relapse at 12 months were acute inflammatory cell infiltrate, crypt abscesses, mucin depletion, and breached surface epithelium [8]. A more recent study by Meucci and colleagues determined that endoscopic mucosal inflammation during clinical remission predicted disease relapse. The investigators induced clinical remission in ulcerative colitis patients with mesalazine and then performed colonoscopy at 6 weeks of treatment. Patients who had achieved both endoscopic and clinical remission by week 6 had a significantly lower rate of disease relapse in the following 12 months (23 %) than patients who achieved clinical remission alone (80 %, $p < 0.01$) [9].

Active endoscopic inflammation and mucosal healing are also predictive of rates of surgery. Carbonnel and colleagues performed endoscopy on 85 patients with active UC. They found that 93 % of patients with endoscopically severe disease (defined as deep/extensive ulcers, mucosal detachment, large mucosal abrasions, or well-like ulcers) required subsequent colectomy compared to 23 % of the patients with endoscopically moderately active disease (superficial ulcers, deep but not extensive ulcers) [10]. Additional evidence was described by Frøslie and colleagues in the study of a Norwegian observational cohort. Patients were enrolled and had follow-up colonoscopies 1 and 5 years after enrollment. Of the 354 patients who completed the follow-up, those who had achieved mucosal healing after the 1-year colonoscopy were less likely to undergo colectomy by the 5-year follow-up, regardless of treatment exposure (in other words, the healing itself was predictive of the outcome, not how they achieved it). The relative risk of having a colectomy in the patients with mucosal healing was 0.22 (95 % CI: 0.06–0.79) [11].

Increased histologic inflammatory activity is also associated with a higher risk of cancer and dysplasia. Rutter and colleagues first published a case-control study to evaluate the association between severity of inflammation on surveillance colonoscopy and later development of colonic dysplasia. Univariate analysis demonstrated that both endoscopic and histologic inflammation were associated with an increased risk for dysplasia and colorectal cancer. After controlling for other explanatory variables, only histologic inflammation was significantly associated with an increased risk for dysplasia or colorectal cancer. For each one-unit increase in the histologic score, the odds of colorectal neoplasia increased by a factor of 4.69 (95 % CI: 2.10–10.48, $p < 0.001$) [12]. Gupta and colleagues also reviewed a cohort of 418 patients and assessed their histologic activity scores, as reported by their pathologists. Univariate analysis found that mean, maximal, and cumulative severity of histologic inflammation was associated with significant risk for developing advanced neoplasia [13]. Rubin and colleagues performed a case-control study with 59 cases of colorectal neoplasia matched to 141 controls, with prospective regrading of the degrees of histologic inflammation by two expert pathologists. We created a novel expanded histologic grading scale, in order to capture more detail at the lower end of the scale, and included "normalization" of biopsies as well. On multivariate analysis, mean histologic activity index score over the surveillance period was significantly associated with colorectal neoplasia risk (as was male sex). For each one-unit increase in histologic activity index score, there was an adjusted odds ratio of 3.68 (95 % CI, 1.69–7.98; $p = 0.001$) [14]. These studies all demonstrate that increased inflammation over time is a specific and independent risk factor for neoplasia in UC. However, while these studies suggest that altering the course of inflammation may change the likelihood of cancer, there is no direct evidence of this point, and prospective studies to measure such an endpoint will be difficult to perform. Nonetheless, the British Society of Gastroenterology has incorporated a stratification scheme for intervals of surveillance colonoscopy based on the presence of inflammation during the exam [15].

## Achieving Mucosal Healing with Therapy in UC

There are multiple therapeutic avenues by which to achieve mucosal healing in UC. The available therapies for UC include corticosteroids, 5-aminosalicylic acid derivatives, immunomodulators, and biological agents.

Interestingly, corticosteroids have been shown to have some mucosal healing effect for decades. In 1955, Truelove and Witts reported on the use of cortisone in UC. They identified a significant difference between the group treated with oral cortisone and the placebo group, with treated patients having a higher likelihood of achieving a normal or near-normal appearing bowel on sigmoidoscopy [16]. In a later report, they found similar results with intravenous steroids on inducing clinical remission but they did not report on sigmoidoscopic appearance [17]. More recent studies of oral glucocorticoids include a study by Lofberg and colleagues which compared oral budesonide and prednisolone. They used the Mayo endoscopic subscore to determine mucosal response to therapy. They found that 12 % of patients on budesonide and 17 % of patients on prednisolone achieved complete endoscopic remission and there was no significant difference between the two groups [18]. These findings must be interpreted with the additional knowledge that steroids are not effective maintenance therapies in UC and the understanding of the mechanism of steroids on the mucosa of UC, including the inhibition of prostaglandin synthesis, which may in fact impair healing.

Many studies have shown that 5-aminosalicylate therapy can achieve mucosal healing in UC and the majority have used the prior definition of a Mayo endoscopic subscore of 0 or 1. Kamm and colleagues studied mesalazine with Multi Matrix System (MMX) technology (Cosmo, Lainate, Italy) in patients with mild to moderate ulcerative colitis. They determined that 77.6 % of patients on 4.8 g of MMX mesalazine daily, 69.0 % of patients on 2.4 g of MMX mesalazine daily, and 61.6 % of patients on 2.4 g delayed-release mesalamine three times daily were able to achieve mucosal healing at 8 weeks of treatment. This was compared to 46.5 % of patients on placebo, and mucosal healing was defined as a modified Sutherland index less than or equal to 1 [19]. A similar study by Lichtenstein and colleagues studied the percentage of patients who received clinical and endoscopic remission in 8 weeks on MMX mesalamine at a dose of 2.4 g twice per day ($n=93$), 4.8 g once per day ($n=94$), or placebo ($n=93$). This study reported similar results with remission achieved by 34.1 % of patients on a twice-daily dose of MMX mesalamine 2.4 g, 29.2 % on 4.8 g once daily, and 12.9 % on placebo [20]. The combined rate of mucosal healing in both of these studies was 32.0 % of patients on MMX mesalazine 2.4 g daily and 32.2 % of patients on MMX mesalazine 4.8 g daily, compared 15.8 % of patients in the placebo group [21].

In the ASCEND I study, Hanauer and colleagues reported that oral delayed-release mesalamine induced complete remission in 46 % and 36 % of patients with mild to moderate ulcerative colitis for 4.8 g daily and 2.4 g daily, respectively [22]. The ASCEND II study again compared delayed-release mesalamine in 4.8 g daily or 2.4 g daily formulations, limited to patients with moderately active ulcerative colitis. The study found that 20.2 % of the patients on 4.8 g daily and 17.7 % of the patients on 2.4 g daily were able to achieve complete remission [23]. These studies reported patients who achieved complete remission, which required both endoscopic and clinical remission, but did not report on the subset that achieved mucosal healing. A combined analysis of patients with moderate ulcerative colitis from ASCEND I and ASCEND II showed mucosal healing (a score of 0 or 1) at week 3 in 65 % of patients receiving 4.8 g daily of delayed-release mesalazine and 58 % of patients receiving 2.4 g daily. At week 6 they found that mucosal healing rates were significantly higher in patients receiving 4.8 g daily than 2.4 g daily (80 % vs. 68 %, $p=0.012$) [24]. In a subsequent post hoc analysis, Lichtenstein and colleagues reviewed the mucosal healing rates of the ASCEND trials when a Mayo endoscopic subscore of 0 was used and found that the healing rates were substantially lower in those treated with delayed-release mesalamine 2.4 g per day versus 4.8 g/day [24].

In another report, Kruis and colleagues studied once-daily dosing of mesalazine versus three times daily dosing in patients with ulcerative colitis [25]. In this study they measured mucosal healing by a Rachmilewitz endoscopic index of less than 4. Patients achieved mucosal healing in 71 % with once-daily dosing of mesalazine and 70 % of patients with three times daily dosing. These studies show that 5-ASA compounds, despite their different formulations, are capable of inducing mucosal healing (albeit with variable definitions) at significant rates for mild to moderate ulcerative colitis.

There is much less evidence regarding the immunomodulators, azathioprine and 6-mercaptopurine. Ardizzone and colleagues compared the efficacy of azathioprine to oral 5-aminosalicylic acid for inducing remission in steroid-dependent ulcerative colitis. They found that 53 % of patients taking azathioprine achieved both clinical and endoscopic remission compared to 19 % of patients taking oral 5-aminosalicylic acid ($p=0.006$). Additionally, they found that the mean Baron index score for endoscopic activity was significantly lower in the azathioprine group compared to the 5-aminosalicylic acid group at the 3- and 6-month follow-up [26]. Paoluzi and colleagues also performed a trial of azathioprine without a comparison group. They found that 68.7 % of patients achieved endoscopic remission as defined by a Baron index score of 0 [27]. These studies suggest that mucosal healing is achievable with azathioprine, but the results are not directly comparable to other therapies and the exact rate of healing is not known.

The clinical trials of tumor necrosis factor alpha inhibitors have shown that they are capable of inducing mucosal healing (Table 5.3). In contrast to the varied definitions of mucosal healing that studies of the other classes have used, the biologic therapy trials used a Mayo endoscopic subscore of 0 or 1 to define mucosal healing. Infliximab was found in the ACT 1 and ACT 2 trials to achieve mucosal healing at week 8 at rates of 16.5 % on adalimumab versus 9.3 % on placebo. Among those who were anti-TNF-α naïve compared to those who had previously received anti-TNF agents, the rates of remission at week 8 were 21.3 % on adalimumab and 11 % on placebo, and 9.2 % on adalimumab and 6.9 % on placebo, respectively. The significant difference between

**Table 5.3** Mucosal healing rates from trials of biologic therapies for ulcerative colitis

| Drug | Clinical trial | | Reported rates of mucosal healing[a] | | |
| --- | --- | --- | --- | --- | --- |
| Infliximab | ACT1 | | 5 mg | 10 mg | Placebo |
| | | 8 weeks | 62.00 % | 59.00 % | 33.90 % |
| | | p value | <0.001 | <0.001 | |
| | | 30 weeks | 50.40 % | 49.20 % | 24.80 % |
| | | p value | <0.001 | <0.001 | |
| | | 54 weeks | 45.50 % | 46.70 % | 18.20 % |
| | | p value | <0.001 | <0.001 | |
| | ACT2 | | 5 mg | 10 mg | Placebo |
| | | 8 weeks | 60.30 % | 61.70 % | 30.90 % |
| | | p value | <0.001 | <0.001 | |
| | | 30 weeks | 46.30 % | 56.70 % | 30.10 % |
| | | p value | 0.009 | <0.001 | |
| Adalimumab | ULTRA2 | | 160 mg/80 mg/40 mg | | Placebo |
| | | 8 weeks | 41.10 % | | 31.70 % |
| | | p value | 0.032 | | |
| | | 52 weeks | 25.00 % | | 15.40 % |
| | | p value | 0.009 | | |
| Golimumab | PURSUIT-SC | | 400 mg/200 mg | 200 mg/100 mg | Placebo |
| | | 6 weeks | 45.10 % | 42.30 % | 28.70 % |
| | | p value | <0.0001 | 0.0014 | |
| | PURSUIT-M | | 100 mg | 50 mg | Placebo |
| | | 54 weeks | 43.50 % | 41.80 % | 26.90 % |
| | | p value | 0.002 | 0.011 | |
| Vedolizumab | GEMINI-1 | | 300 mg | | Placebo |
| | | 6 weeks | 40.90 % | | 24.80 % |
| | | p value | 0.001 | | |
| | | 52 weeks, dosing every 8 weeks | 41.80 % | | 15.90 % |
| | | p value | <0.001 | | |
| | | 52 weeks, dosing every 4 weeks | 44.80 % | | 15.90 % |
| | | p value | <0.001 | | |

[a]Mucosal healing was defined as a Mayo endoscopic subscore of 0 or 1 for each study included. Dosing schedules are indicated by the first dose, followed by the second and third doses if necessary as reported in the individual studies. Results are reported at various time points after initiating therapy and are accompanied below by their respective p value for comparison with placebo

infliximab dosed at 5 mg/kg, 10 mg/kg, and placebo was also demonstrated at weeks 30 and 54 [28]. In a follow-up post hoc analysis, Colombel and colleagues showed that achieving Mayo endoscopy score of 0 or 1 was associated with a reduction in colectomy [29].

There is also evidence that adalimumab can induce mucosal healing. The ULTRA 1 study was a randomized controlled trial of adalimumab in moderate to severe ulcerative colitis. The results of the induction phase were reported by Reinisch and colleagues. They found that there were no statistically significant differences between the rates of mucosal healing for adalimumab dosed 160 mg followed by 80 mg, adalimumab dosed 80 mg followed by 40 mg, and placebo [30]. This negative result was likely due to an unexpectedly high rate of mucosal healing in the placebo group. In the follow-up study of ULTRA 1, all patients were placed on adalimumab following induction, whether or not they had received adalimumab or placebo. They found that 36.5 % of all patients in the study achieved mucosal healing by week 52 [31]. The ULTRA 2 study was a double-blinded, randomized, placebo-controlled trial of adalimumab. Mucosal healing was achieved in 41.1 % of patients receiving adalimumab at week 8, compared to 31.7 % of patients receiving placebo ($p = 0.032$). At week 52, 25 % of patients receiving adalimumab had achieved mucosal healing, compared to 15.4 % of patients receiving placebo ($p = 0.009$) [32]. In addition to infliximab and adalimumab, a recent phase 2/3 randomized, placebo-controlled trial of golimumab showed that patients were able to achieve mucosal healing using this new TNF-inhibitor therapy. Sandborn and colleagues reported in the PURSUIT-SC study the results of golimumab induction. They found a significant difference in the rate of mucosal healing with 42.3 % of patients receiving the 200 mg/100 mg induction dosing ($p = 0.0014$) and 45.1 % of patients receiving the 400 mg/200 mg induction dosing ($p < 0.0001$) compared to 28.7 % of patients receiving placebo had achieved mucosal healing at week 6 [33]. In the follow-up PURSUIT-M study, Sandborn and colleagues reported significantly higher rates of patients achieving mucosal healing at both 30 and 54 weeks for golimumab than placebo [34]. The patients on golimumab 100 mg achieved mucosal healing at a rate of 42.4 % compared to 26.6 % with placebo ($p = 0.002$). As well, patients on golimumab 50 mg achieved mucosal healing at a rate of 41.7 % ($p = 0.011$).

A new class of biologic medication for ulcerative colitis blocks the leukocyte trafficking from the endothelium to the bowel. Vedolizumab is a humanized monoclonal antibody against the alpha-4-beta-7 integrin. In the GEMINI 1 trial, vedolizumab was found to be capable of inducing mucosal healing in ulcerative colitis [35]. The definition of mucosal healing was the same as in the prior studies of TNF inhibitors, a Mayo endoscopic subscore of 0 or 1. After induction with vedolizumab, 40.9 % of patients achieved mucosal healing, compared to 24.8 % of patients in the placebo arm ($p = 0.001$). Maintenance with vedolizumab was also found to have higher rates of mucosal healing. Vedolizumab dosed every 8 weeks achieved mucosal healing in 51.6 % at 52 weeks of treatment, compared to 56.0 % if it was dosed every 4 weeks, and 19.8 % of the patients in the placebo arm. Both dosing regimens were significantly different from placebo ($p < 0.001$ and $p < 0.001$, respectively), but not statistically significant between each other.

## Challenges to the Adoption of Mucosal Healing into Clinical Practice

The next challenge in mucosal healing is incorporating this new knowledge into clinical practice and addressing barriers to adopting mucosal healing as a goal for therapy. The evidence presented in the previous sections supports the idea that those who achieve mucosal healing would have better outcomes. However, these studies were not performed to compare therapeutic strategies. Currently, there is no prospectively collected evidence that targeting mucosal healing provides a benefit over treating to symptoms and only some emerging information that it can be systematically achieved as a desired clinical endpoint. Additionally, there are important management concerns that have yet to be answered. First, it is unclear if mucosal healing is an achievable endpoint for the majority of patients. Second, there is unclear risk or cost to performing serial endoscopic exams to determine response to therapy. And, importantly, patients' willingness to undergo more frequent invasive testing has not been investigated.

One of the challenges is that the correlation between mucosal healing and clinical remission is not perfect.

Mismatch between symptoms and endoscopic appearance can occur when a patient feels well but has endoscopic inflammation greater than a Mayo endoscopic subscore of 1 or when a patient is still experiencing symptoms despite a Mayo endoscopic subscore of 1 or 0. The choice to adjust therapy based on endoscopic appearance when a patient feels well requires consideration of the risks incurred by the change in therapy and the risk of not achieving mucosal healing despite such therapy adjustments. While there is retrospective evidence to support the long-term benefits of having achieved mucosal healing during the course of treatment, there is not a complete understanding of the near-term risks associated with this pursuit. More frequent invasive testing to assess the status of the mucosa and increased exposure to higher intensity therapies and their side effects are primary concerns that may adversely affect quality of life in the near term, particularly if the patient is symptomatically well. The converse may have implications for management too, although scoping a patient who is still symptomatic but is found to have mucosal healing is the standard of practice in the course of evaluating an actively symptomatic patient.

There is evidence that mismatch between symptoms and mucosal healing is a common clinical problem. The ACT1 trial found a poor correlation between mucosal healing and clinical remission [28]. There are two potential explanations for this observation. First is that the use of a broader definition of mucosal healing (a Mayo endoscopic subscore of 0 or 1) leads to inclusion of patients in the mucosal healing group who actually have clinically active disease. The groups might have appeared more similar if mucosal healing was defined as a Mayo endoscopic subscore of 0 rather than 0 or 1. The second potential explanation is that patients who achieved mucosal healing were experiencing overlap symptoms from irritable bowel syndrome, the side effects from therapy, or another diagnosis, all of which may confound their clinical appearance.

The gold standard for determining the presence or absence of mucosal healing remains endoscopic evaluation. Endoscopy is an invasive test that can provide significant information about the activity of a patient's disease. However, endoscopy requires significant resources, entails risk of patient morbidity, and is limited by interoperator variability [36].

Alternatives to endoscopy for the detection of mucosal healing are being investigated and becoming more widely available to practitioners. The most commonly encountered is a stool test for the quantity of calprotectin. Calprotectin is a prevalent cytosolic protein in granulocytes. The presence of calprotectin in the stool is proportional to neutrophil migration to the gastrointestinal tract and also proportional to the degree of inflammation [37]. Lobaton and colleagues tested a quantitative test for fecal calprotectin and investigated its correlation with endoscopic inflammation. Using a

280 microgram per gram level, they found a sensitivity of 75.4 % and a specificity of 89.1 % for the presence of mucosal healing [37].

Another noninvasive and easily accessible test is the measurement of serum C-reactive protein (CRP) levels. CRP production by hepatocytes increases under conditions of infectious stimuli, inflammatory diseases, neoplasia, and stress among others. While a strong CRP response has been seen in certain inflammatory conditions such as Crohn's disease and rheumatoid arthritis, other conditions like ulcerative colitis produce a much milder effect [38]. The reason for this discrepancy is not yet known. Therefore, the assessment of CRP levels should not be solely used to determine the severity of mucosal inflammation.

Because of its utility as a noninvasive marker of inflammation and the studies showing that mucosal healing can predict clinical course, investigators have been testing the ability of calprotectin levels to make similar predictions. Recently, Lasson and colleagues tested fecal calprotectin levels in the stool of patients at 3 months after being diagnosed with ulcerative colitis and starting treatment. They found that a fecal calprotectin level of 169 micrograms per gram at 3 months after diagnosis predicted those patients who would have more active disease over the following year with a sensitivity of 64.4 % and a specificity of 70.8 %. Similarly, a fecal calprotectin level of 262 micrograms per gram predicted those patients who would have more active disease over the 2- and 3-year follow-up period. The sensitivity and specificity of a cutoff of 262 micrograms per gram were 51 % and 81.8 % at 2 years and 52.2 % and 85.9 % at 3 years [39]. As well, elevated fecal calprotectin levels seem to be able to predict patients at higher risk of disease relapse [40, 41]. De Vos and colleagues studied fecal calprotectin levels in patients receiving treatment with infliximab. Patients with an 80 % decrease in fecal calprotectin level between the baseline measurement and the measurement at 2 weeks or a calprotectin level of less than 50 mg/kg at 2 weeks after initiating therapy were found to have achieved mucosal healing at week 10 of therapy with infliximab with a sensitivity of 54 % and specificity of 67 % [42]. In a separate study of patients receiving infliximab, they found that those patients who achieved deep remission at 52 weeks had consistently very low levels of fecal calprotectin throughout the follow-up period. Additionally, two consecutive fecal calprotectin levels greater than 300 micrograms per gram 1 month apart was predictive of disease relapse while on treatment with a sensitivity of 61.5 % and specificity of 100 % [43].

Fecal calprotectin is an important addition to the management of ulcerative colitis, but it does have limitations. The ability to distinguish active ulcerative colitis from irritable bowel syndrome symptoms is one of the important strengths of using endoscopy to monitor for mucosal healing. Studies have shown that fecal calprotectin is not able to differentiate irritable bowel syndrome symptoms from ulcerative colitis [44, 45]. As well, as demonstrated by the study by Lobaton and colleagues, the test characteristics are good, but the test is not completely able to rule in the presence of mucosal healing or rule out its absence [37]. As a result, if one were to use fecal calprotectin instead of endoscopic evaluation for monitoring disease activity, there would be patients who have achieved mucosal healing that have a negative test and patients who have not achieved mucosal healing who have a positive test. Additionally, the various test characteristics of fecal calprotectin for predicting clinical course are not strong enough to be relied upon with complete certainty [40–43]. They may be able to help guide physician expectations but should be considered within the clinical context.

## Integrating Mucosal Healing into Current UC Management

With the therapeutic goal of mucosal healing, an efficient, practical algorithm for assessing disease response begins with baseline assessment of disease activity. This can be done with the initial endoscopic evaluation. This baseline evaluation can be paired with a surrogate marker, such as CRP if the patient manifests an elevated level, or fecal calprotectin.

After the initial assessment, the first choice of therapy can be based on existing practices and standards for starting medical management of the disease. The therapeutic trial of this initial management is monitored for approximately 3–6 months, with the time to reassessment varying based on the clinical trial data (approximately 3 months for anti-TNF therapies or mesalamine and 6 months for azathioprine/6-mercaptopurine). After this monitoring period, the disease activity is reassessed with either endoscopic evaluation or with surrogate marker testing.

If the endoscopy does not reveal mucosal healing, or the surrogate marker is not consistent with mucosal healing, the next steps are discussed with the patient in a shared decision-making approach. As was previously discussed, the decision to change management based on objective findings can be complicated when the subjective disease activity is discordant. In a subset of patients who do not achieve mucosal healing but who do have symptomatic relief, there may be resistance to escalating beyond therapy that the patient perceives as being effective. For these patients, a comprehensive evaluation of their comorbidities, disease course, and psychosocial factors will help guide discussion. For some patients, the potential reduction in colorectal dysplasia or potential for reduction in hospitalizations may be significant enough to outweigh the risks of increasing medical therapy.

If the endoscopic evaluation reveals mucosal healing, or the surrogate marker is consistent with mucosal healing, then regular clinical follow-up is recommended. During these follow-up visits, disease stability can be measured using standard clinical criteria. After a period of 6–12 months of disease monitoring, the next step is reassessment of disease activity by endoscopy or surrogate marker. Clinical disease monitoring may be complicated by scenarios in which the patient has objectively achieved mucosal healing, but the disease symptoms are still present. Similar to the converse situation, this will require the clinician to pursue alternative diagnoses that can complicate UC. As well, the clinician must have a discussion with the patient about therapeutic options and the reasoning for not escalating therapy in the face of significant symptoms.

## Summary

Objective assessment of mucosal inflammation is clearly associated with improvement in short-term and long-term clinical status of patients with UC and can be obtained with currently available therapies. Emerging indices of inflammatory activity and paradigm shifts in our management strategies are making the adoption of mucosal healing as an endpoint a practical reality. The practicing clinician and clinical scientist need to incorporate this rapidly moving field into their current work.

## References

1. Schroeder KW, Tremaine WJ, Ilstrup DM. Coated oral 5-aminosalicylic acid therapy for mildly to moderately active ulcerative colitis. A randomized study. N Engl J Med. 1987;317:1625–9.
2. Pineton de Chambrun G, Peyrin-Biroulet L, Lemann M, Colombel JF. Clinical implications of mucosal healing for the management of IBD. Nat Rev Gastroenterol Hepatol. 2010;7:15–29.
3. D'Haens G, Sandborn WJ, Feagan BG, et al. A review of activity indices and efficacy end points for clinical trials of medical therapy in adults with ulcerative colitis. Gastroenterology. 2007;132:763–86.
4. Feagan BG, Sandborn WJ, D'Haens G, et al. The role of centralized reading of endoscopy in a randomized controlled trial of mesalamine for ulcerative colitis. Gastroenterology. 2013;145:149–57.e2.
5. Rubin DT. What you see is not always what you get: raising the bar on clinical trial methodology in ulcerative colitis. Gastroenterology. 2013;145:45–7.
6. Peyrin-Biroulet L, Bressenot A, Kampman W. Histologic remission: the ultimate therapeutic goal in ulcerative colitis? Clin Gastroenterol Hepatol. 2013;12:929–34.e2.
7. Cooney RM, Warren BF, Altman DG, Abreu MT, Travis SP. Outcome measurement in clinical trials for Ulcerative Colitis: towards standardisation. Trials. 2007;8:17.
8. Riley SA, Mani V, Goodman MJ, Dutt S, Herd ME. Microscopic activity in ulcerative colitis: what does it mean? Gut. 1991;32:174–8.
9. Meucci G, Fasoli R, Saibeni S, et al. Prognostic significance of endoscopic remission in patients with active ulcerative colitis treated with oral and topical mesalazine: a prospective, multicenter study. Inflamm Bowel Dis. 2012;18:1006–10.
10. Carbonnel F, Lavergne A, Lemann M, et al. Colonoscopy of acute colitis. A safe and reliable tool for assessment of severity. Dig Dis Sci. 1994;39:1550–7.
11. Froslie KF, Jahnsen J, Moum BA, Vatn MH. Mucosal healing in inflammatory bowel disease: results from a Norwegian population-based cohort. Gastroenterology. 2007;133:412–22.
12. Rutter M, Saunders B, Wilkinson K, et al. Severity of inflammation is a risk factor for colorectal neoplasia in ulcerative colitis. Gastroenterology. 2004;126:451–9.
13. Gupta RB, Harpaz N, Itzkowitz S, et al. Histologic inflammation is a risk factor for progression to colorectal neoplasia in ulcerative colitis: a cohort study. Gastroenterology. 2007;133:1099–105. quiz 340–1.
14. Rubin DT, Huo D, Kinnucan JA, et al. Inflammation is an independent risk factor for colonic neoplasia in patients with ulcerative colitis: a case-control study. Clin Gastroenterol Hepatol. 2013;11(12):1601–8.e1–4.
15. Cairns SR, Scholefield JH, Steele RJ, et al. Guidelines for colorectal cancer screening and surveillance in moderate and high risk groups (update from 2002). Gut. 2010;59:666–89.
16. Truelove SC, Witts LJ. Cortisone in ulcerative colitis; final report on a therapeutic trial. Br Med J. 1955;2:1041–8.
17. Truelove SC, Jewell DP. Intensive intravenous regimen for severe attacks of ulcerative colitis. Lancet. 1974;1:1067–70.
18. Lofberg R, Danielsson A, Suhr O, et al. Oral budesonide versus prednisolone in patients with active extensive and left-sided ulcerative colitis. Gastroenterology. 1996;110:1713–8.
19. Kamm MA, Sandborn WJ, Gassull M, et al. Once-daily, high-concentration MMX mesalamine in active ulcerative colitis. Gastroenterology. 2007;132:66–75. quiz 432–3.
20. Lichtenstein GR, Kamm MA, Boddu P, et al. Effect of once- or twice-daily MMX mesalamine (SPD476) for the induction of remission of mild to moderately active ulcerative colitis. Clin Gastroenterol Hepatol. 2007;5:95–102.
21. Sandborn WJ, Kamm MA, Lichtenstein GR, Lyne A, Butler T, Joseph RE. MMX Multi Matrix System mesalazine for the induction of remission in patients with mild-to-moderate ulcerative colitis: a combined analysis of two randomized, double-blind, placebo-controlled trials. Aliment Pharmacol Ther. 2007;26:205–15.
22. Hanauer SB, Sandborn WJ, Dallaire C, et al. Delayed-release oral mesalamine 4.8 g/day (800 mg tablets) compared to 2.4 g/day (400 mg tablets) for the treatment of mildly to moderately active ulcerative colitis: the ASCEND I trial. Can J Gastroenterol. 2007;21:827–34.
23. Hanauer SB, Sandborn WJ, Kornbluth A, et al. Delayed-release oral mesalamine at 4.8 g/day (800 mg tablet) for the treatment of moderately active ulcerative colitis: the ASCEND II trial. Am J Gastroenterol. 2005;100:2478–85.
24. Lichtenstein GR, Ramsey D, Rubin DT. Randomised clinical trial: delayed-release oral mesalazine 4.8 g/day vs. 2.4 g/day in endoscopic mucosal healing—ASCEND I and II combined analysis. Aliment Pharmacol Ther. 2011;33:672–8.
25. Kruis W, Kiudelis G, Racz I, et al. Once daily versus three times daily mesalazine granules in active ulcerative colitis: a double-blind, double-dummy, randomised, non-inferiority trial. Gut. 2009;58:233–40.
26. Ardizzone S, Maconi G, Russo A, Imbesi V, Colombo E, Bianchi PG. Randomised controlled trial of azathioprine and 5-aminosalicylic acid for treatment of steroid dependent ulcerative colitis. Gut. 2006;55:47–53.
27. Paoluzi OA, Pica R, Marcheggiano A, et al. Azathioprine or methotrexate in the treatment of patients with steroid-dependent or steroid-resistant ulcerative colitis: results of an open-label study on

efficacy and tolerability in inducing and maintaining remission. Aliment Pharmacol Ther. 2002;16:1751–9.

28. Rutgeerts P, Sandborn WJ, Feagan BG, et al. Infliximab for induction and maintenance therapy for ulcerative colitis. N Engl J Med. 2005;353:2462–76.

29. Colombel JF, Rutgeerts P, Reinisch W, et al. Early mucosal healing with infliximab is associated with improved long-term clinical outcomes in ulcerative colitis. Gastroenterology. 2011;141:1194–201.

30. Reinisch W, Sandborn WJ, Hommes DW, et al. Adalimumab for induction of clinical remission in moderately to severely active ulcerative colitis: results of a randomised controlled trial. Gut. 2011;60:780–7.

31. Reinisch W, Sandborn WJ, Panaccione R, et al. 52-Week efficacy of adalimumab in patients with moderately to severely active ulcerative colitis who failed corticosteroids and/or immunosuppressants. Inflamm Bowel Dis. 2013;19:1700–9.

32. Sandborn WJ, van Assche G, Reinisch W, et al. Adalimumab induces and maintains clinical remission in patients with moderate-to-severe ulcerative colitis. Gastroenterology. 2012;142:257–65. e1–3.

33. Sandborn WJ, Feagan BG, Marano C, et al. Subcutaneous golimumab induces clinical response and remission in patients with moderate to severe ulcerative colitis. Gastroenterology. 2014;146(1):85–95. quiz e14–5.

34. Sandborn WJ, Feagan BG, Marano C, et al. Subcutaneous golimumab maintains clinical response in patients with moderate-to-severe ulcerative colitis. Gastroenterology. 2014;146:96–109.e1.

35. Feagan BG, Rutgeerts P, Sands BE, et al. Vedolizumab as induction and maintenance therapy for ulcerative colitis. N Engl J Med. 2013;369:699–710.

36. Chen SC, Rex DK. Endoscopist can be more powerful than age and male gender in predicting adenoma detection at colonoscopy. Am J Gastroenterol. 2007;102:856–61.

37. Lobaton T, Rodriguez-Moranta F, Lopez A, Sanchez E, Rodriguez-Alonso L, Guardiola J. A new rapid quantitative test for fecal calprotectin predicts endoscopic activity in ulcerative colitis. Inflamm Bowel Dis. 2013;19:1034–42.

38. Vermeire S, Van Assche G, Rutgeerts P. C-reactive protein as a marker for inflammatory bowel disease. Inflamm Bowel Dis. 2004;10:661–5.

39. Lasson A, Simren M, Stotzer PO, Isaksson S, Ohman L, Strid H. Fecal calprotectin levels predict the clinical course in patients with new onset of ulcerative colitis. Inflamm Bowel Dis. 2013;19:576–81.

40. D'Inca R, Dal Pont E, Di Leo V, et al. Can calprotectin predict relapse risk in inflammatory bowel disease? Am J Gastroenterol. 2008;103:2007–14.

41. Gisbert JP, Bermejo F, Perez-Calle JL, et al. Fecal calprotectin and lactoferrin for the prediction of inflammatory bowel disease relapse. Inflamm Bowel Dis. 2009;15:1190–8.

42. De Vos M, Dewit O, D'Haens G, et al. Fast and sharp decrease in calprotectin predicts remission by infliximab in anti-TNF naive patients with ulcerative colitis. J Crohns Colitis. 2012;6:557–62.

43. De Vos M, Louis EJ, Jahnsen J, et al. Consecutive fecal calprotectin measurements to predict relapse in patients with ulcerative colitis receiving infliximab maintenance therapy. Inflamm Bowel Dis. 2013;19:2111–7.

44. Jonefjall B, Strid H, Ohman L, Svedlund J, Bergstedt A, Simren M. Characterization of IBS-like symptoms in patients with ulcerative colitis in clinical remission. Neurogastroenterol Motil. 2013;25:756–e578.

45. Jelsness-Jorgensen LP, Bernklev T, Moum B. Calprotectin is a useful tool in distinguishing coexisting irritable bowel-like symptoms from that of occult inflammation among inflammatory bowel disease patients in remission. Gastroenterol Res Pract. 2013;2013:620707.

# Oral Mesalamine

**6**

Atsushi Sakuraba

**Keywords**

Mesalamine • Ulcerative colitis • Inflammatory bowel disease

## Introduction

Ulcerative colitis (UC) is a chronic inflammatory bowel disease characterized by a relapsing-remitting course due to recurrent intestinal inflammation [1, 2]. The pathogenesis of UC remains incompletely understood, but the ongoing chronic inflammation has traditionally been the target of treatment. Conventional medications including 5-aminosalicylates (sulfasalazine, olsalazine, balsalazide, and mesalamine formulations), corticosteroids, and immunomodulators such as azathioprine and mercaptopurine have been used for many years in the treatment of UC [3]. More recently, anti-tumor necrosis factor (TNF) agents have brought more options in the medical management of UC [4]. Meanwhile, the goal of treatment remains the same, i.e., successful induction and maintenance of steroid-free remission to improve quality of life and to reduce the risks of future colectomy and/or cancer.

As in any other disorder, successful management of UC begins by accurate diagnosis, evaluation of extent of disease, and assessment of severity of disease. Accurate diagnosis is required to rule out other types of acute or chronic inflammatory bowel diseases, as well as to differentiate infectious causes such as *Clostridium difficile* and cytomegalovirus infections [4]. Evaluation of extent of disease can be accurately and easily measured by endoscopic studies. Based on the most proximal extent of disease, UC can be categorized into proctitis, left-sided colitis, and pancolitis. Microscopic inflammation may occasionally extend beyond the most proximal point of macroscopically visible mucosal inflammation, but the clinical relevance of such microscopic inflammation is unknown. Patients with left-sided colitis or proctitis often have the finding of a patch of cecal inflammation adjacent to the appendiceal orifice called cecal patch. The etiology, as well as the clinical relevance of a cecal patch, is unknown and need not be considered when treating more distal disease. The severity of disease can be assessed by several means. The gross appearance on endoscopy, clinical symptoms, and laboratory data needs to be collected and appropriately assessed. Several indices have been developed to assess disease severity, of which some include all three aforementioned components, whereas some lack the endoscopy parameter [5–9]. Stool frequency, abdominal pain, bleeding, nocturnal stool, and fever are incorporated into most activity indices. Some indices include laboratory parameters like erythrocyte sedimentation rate or hematocrit, but none have incorporated C-reactive protein or stool calprotectin. Extraintestinal manifestations such as arthritis, erythema nodosum, and pyoderma gangrenosum may become present during a flare that may affect the overall health condition of the patient.

After a careful evaluation of the extent of disease and overall disease activity, one must consider the available therapeutic options. Oral mesalamines are the first choice of drug in the management of mild to moderate UC [4]. It can also be given in combination with topical agents for distal colitis, especially in less severe cases. After achieving remission, both oral and topical mesalamine can also be used for maintenance purpose. In outpatients with moderate to severe UC, systemic steroids need to be considered and are usually effective in about two thirds of the patients. In steroid-refractory cases, recent data indicate that infliximab-induced

A. Sakuraba, M.D., Ph.D. (✉)
Department of Medicine, University of Chicago,
5841 S. Maryland Ave. MC4076, Chicago, IL 60637, USA
e-mail: asakurab@medicine.bsd.uchicago.edu

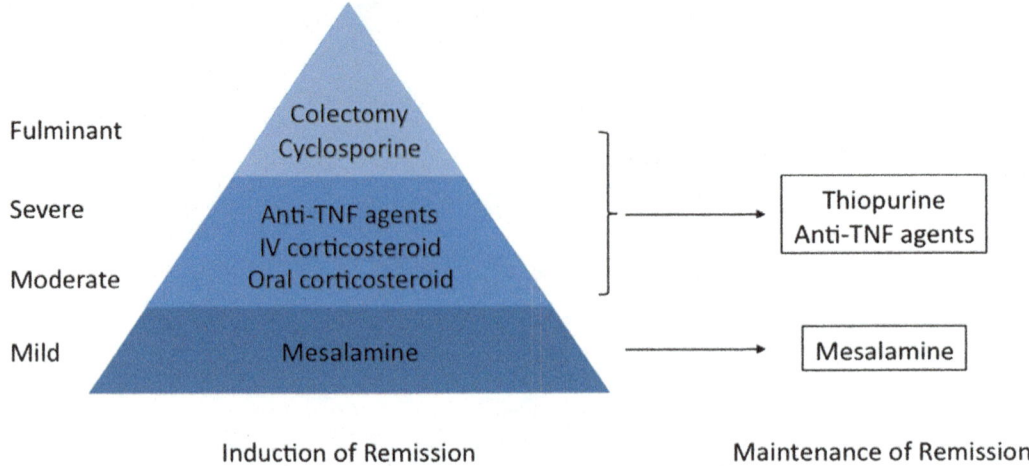

**Fig. 6.1** The potential role of mesalamine in the current treatment algorithm for UC

and maintained remission leads to decreased colectomy rates and fewer hospitalizations [10, 11]. Alternative anti-TNF agents, adalimumab and golimumab, were also recently shown to be effective for induction and maintenance of remission in moderate to severe UC [12–15]. The use of immunosuppressives, such as azathioprine and mercaptopurine, is associated with improved outcome in steroid-dependent UC allowing patients to successfully wean off corticosteroids. In hospitalized patients with steroid-resistant severe UC, infliximab and tacrolimus may be alternatives to cyclosporine in those who are otherwise candidates for colectomy [16–18]. Adequate long-term maintenance therapy with immunosuppressives or anti-TNF therapy is required after rescue therapy for a sustained benefit. The current treatment algorithm for UC, and the position of mesalamines, is summarized in Fig. 6.1.

In the present chapter, we will review the pharmacology, mechanisms of action, and effectiveness of oral mesalamine products in the management of UC.

## 5-Aminosalicylic Acid Formulations

There are currently various 5-aminosalicylic acid (5-ASA [mesalamine]) formulations (sulfasalazine, olsalazine, balsalazide, and mesalamine) available that utilize different methods to increase efficient delivery of the active ingredient to small and/or large intestine [19, 20]. Sulfasalazine was one of the first drugs that were introduced to treat UC. Earlier in the past century, sulfasalazine was started being used to treat rheumatoid arthritis. Swedish investigators initially found that sulfonamides were effective in treating septic arthritis and tried it in rheumatoid arthritis without success. They then coupled sulfonamide with salicylic acid, which was already shown to be effective in treating arthritis, under the assumption that it would actively carry the latter to the inflamed joints. This combination was not shown to be effective for rheumatoid arthritis, but they went on to try a variety of different combinations. One such combination was sulfasalazine, consisting of 5-ASA and sulfapyridine joined together by a diazo-bond. This proved to be effective in treating rheumatoid arthritis, and it then became widely used. Sulfapyridine, which is an antimicrobacterial drug directed against Gram-positive and Gram-negative intestinal bacteria, was already being used to treat UC, but then some physicians used sulfasalazine, and it turned out that it showed a great success in some cases with UC. The use of sulfasalazine gradually increased after the Second World War, and then in 1962, Baron et al. reported the results of a controlled, double-blinded study [21]. They showed that sulfasalazine was effective in the treatment of active UC and later also in maintaining remission of UC [22]. In rheumatoid arthritis, either 5-ASA or sulfapyridine, when given alone, is unlikely to show clinical benefit. 5-ASA is rapidly metabolized and secreted into urine once absorbed from the gastrointestinal tract. Contrary to its effect in inflammatory bowel diseases, studies suggest that the intact sulfasalazine molecule may possess anti-inflammatory properties in rheumatoid arthritis. Furthermore, it is known that about 10–20 % of orally administered sulfasalazine is absorbed systemically and can accumulate in connective tissues of inflamed joints, where it slowly releases 5-ASA, raising the possibility that it also acts as a prodrug in rheumatoid arthritis.

Research into the mechanisms of action of sulfasalazine revealed that it acted as a prodrug, with sulfapyridine working as a carrier and delivering the active component 5-ASA to the colon [23] (Fig. 6.2a). This also led to the discovery that sulfapyridine was responsible for the majority of adverse effects, such as headache, nausea, infertility, hemolytic anemia, and photosensitization. The development of novel drug

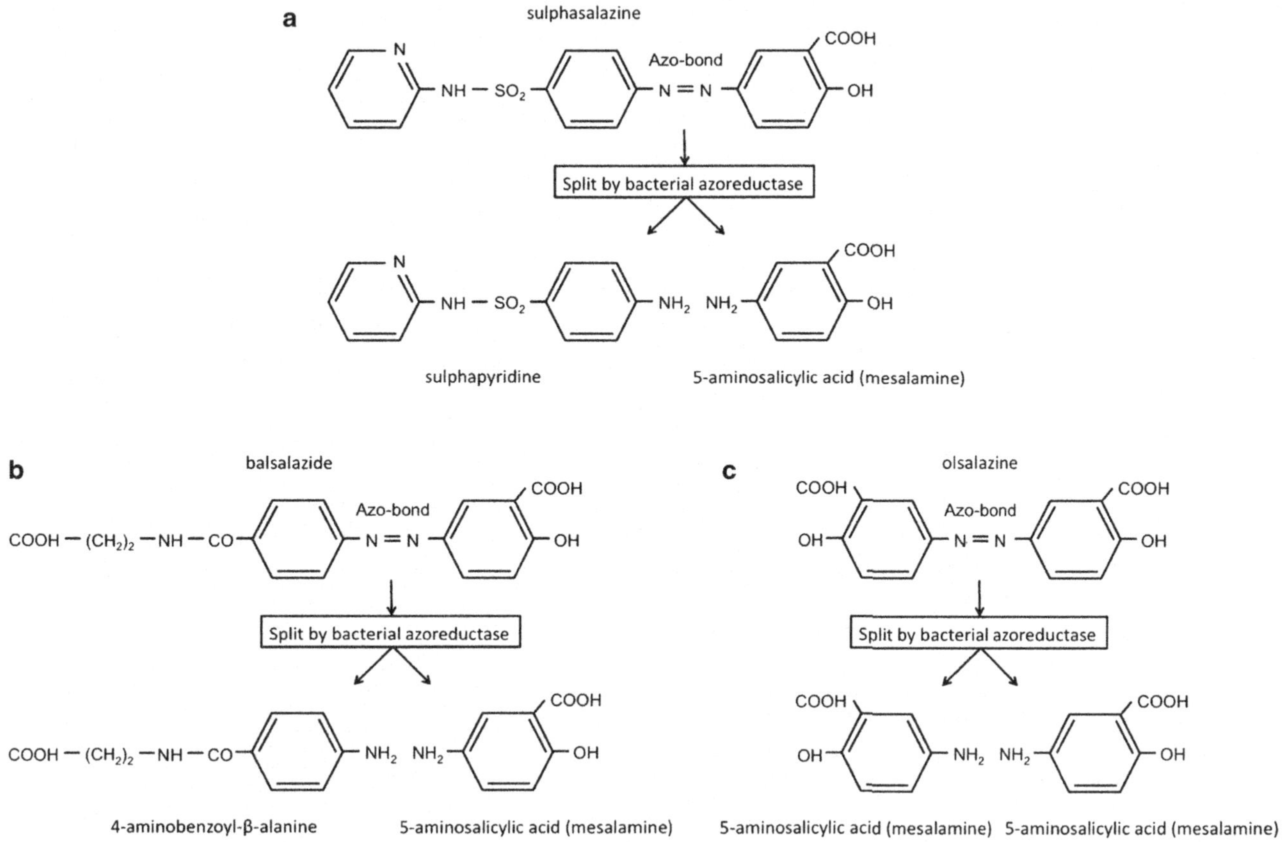

**Fig. 6.2** (**a**) Chemical structure of sulfasalazine and its degradation to sulfapyridine and 5-aminosalicylic acid (mesalamine). (**b**) Chemical structure of balsalazide. (**c**) Chemical structure of olsalazine

delivery systems allowed direct delivery of the active moiety, 5-ASA, to the small bowel and colon. This can be broadly categorized into three groups [24]. The first are those that bind 5-ASA to another carrier, similar to sulfasalazine, which requires splitting of the diazo-bond by the colonic bacterial flora. The other two coat 5-ASA into either a pH-dependent formulation or a microsphere formulation. The oral mesalamine products currently available in the USA are summarized in Table 6.1.

## Prodrugs

Sulfasalazine, balsalazide, and olsalazine work as a prodrug and use a similar mechanism to carry the active moiety, 5-ASA, to the colon. As mentioned above, sulfasalazine consists of 5-ASA and sulfapyridine joined together by a diazo-bond. Sulfasalazine is 40 % 5-ASA, and about 80–90 % reaches the colon, where it is broken down to 5-ASA and sulfapyridine by the azoreductase of the colonic microbiota [23]. The bioavailability of the 5-ASA moiety that is released ranges from 11 to 33 %. Balsalazide instead uses 4-aminobenzoyl-β-alanine as a carrier to

reach the colon [25]; 4-aminobenzoyl-β-alanine and 5-ASA are joined by a diazo-bond (Fig. 6.2b). Balsalazide is 35 % 5-ASA, and nearly the entire dose reaches the colon, where the diazo-bond is uncleaved to release 5-ASA. The bioavailability for balsalazide ranges from 12 to 35 % [26]. Olsalazine is a polymer of two molecules of 5-ASA joined together by a diazo-bond, and it contains about 89 % of 5-ASA [27, 28] (Fig. 6.2c). Approximately 98 % reaches the colon, where it releases two molecules of 5-ASA. The bioavailability of the 5-ASA moiety that is released is about 14–31 %. These three products are all delivered to the colon as an intact form (~about 90–99 %) and are degraded by the bacterial azoreductase to release 5-ASA. Azoreductase is an intracellular enzyme possessed mainly by a wide range of colonic bacteria, which rapidly uncleaves the diazo-bond. Concurrent use of antibiotics that affect the colonic microbiota can decrease the metabolism of these three agents, as can shortened colonic transit time, such as diarrhea, medication, and colectomy. Some studies suggest that during active inflammatory bowel disease, the bioavailability of the bacterial enzymes including azoreductase are compromised, which may interfere with its clinical efficacy [29].

**Table 6.1** Currently available mesalamine formulations in the USA

| Drug name | | Active or prodrug | Characteristics and delivery method | Target site of release | Available tablet | Daily dosage | | Dosing interval | Reference |
| Generic | Trade | | | | | Active UC | Maintenance | | |
|---|---|---|---|---|---|---|---|---|---|
| Sulfasalazine | Azulfidine® Azulfidine EN® | Prodrug | Uses sulfapyridine as a carrier and is degraded by bacterial azoreductase | Colon | 500 mg (200 mg 5-ASA) | 2–6 g | 2–4 g | tid | [19, 73, 74, 96] |
| Balsalazide | Colazal® | Prodrug | Uses 4-aminobenzoyl-β-alanine as a carrier and degraded by bacterial azoreductase | Colon | 750 mg (262 mg 5-ASA) | 2–6.75 g | 2–6.75 g | tid | [71, 75, 76, 97, 98] |
| Olsalazine | Dipentum® | Prodrug | Dimer of 5-ASA and is degraded by bacterial azoreductase | Colon | 250 mg | 2–3 g | 1 g | bid | [25, 77–79, 99–101] |
| Mesalamine (5-ASA) | Pentasa® | Active | Ethyl cellulose coated and controlled release throughout the small bowel and colon | Duodenum-colon | 250, 500, 1000 mg | 2–4 g | 2–4 g | qid | [81, 82, 104, 105] |
| | Delzicol® Asacol HD® | Active | Eudragit-S coated and pH-dependent release at pH≥7 | Terminal ileum-colon | 400, 800 mg | 1.6–4.8 g | 0.8–4.8 g | tid | [5, 70, 80, 85, 102, 103] |
| | Apriso® | Active | Eudragit-L delayed and extended release at pH≥6 | Jejunum-colon | 500 mg | 1.5–4.5 g | 1.5 g | qd | [83, 84, 33] |
| | Lialda® | Active | MMX® delivery and released at pH≥7 | Colon | 1,200 mg | 2.4–4.8 g | 2.4 g | qd | [31, 92, 93] |

## pH-Dependent Formulations

pH-dependent formulations utilize the gradient of pH in the gastrointestinal tract to deliver the active agent into aimed part of the intestine. The pH in the stomach is approximately 2. The pH in the upper small bowel is about 5–6, and in the lower parts of the small bowel including the terminal ileum, it reaches 6–7. Throughout the colon, the pH is maintained close to neutral between 7 and 8 [30]. Asacol® utilizes an acrylic-based resin (Eudragit-S) coating that is soluble at a pH of >7, thus delivering 5-ASA in the terminal ileum and entire colon [31]. Asacol® was recently replaced by Delzicol®, which is a bioequivalent product that does not contain dibutyl phthalate (DBP), a solvent with potential adverse effect on fetal reproductive system [32, 33]. Lialda® is a Multi-Matrix System (MMX®) mesalamine (marketed as Lialda® in the USA and Mezavant® in the European Union) that is designed to deliver 5-ASA throughout the entire colon as a high-strength once-daily dosing tablet [34, 35]. The mechanism of the MMX® delivery system is a double matrix consisting of a lipophilic matrix dispersed within a hydrophilic matrix [36]. 5-ASA is incorporated into microparticles in the lipophilic matrix, contained within the hydrophilic matrix. This double matrices is then covered by a pH-dependent polymer film that delays the release of 5-ASA until the film dissolves when exposed to a pH of >7.0 in the terminal ileum to colon. When the hydrophilic matrix is exposed to the intestinal fluids, it swells and creates a viscous gel mass, theoretically resulting in slow dispersion of 5-ASA. The hydrophilic matrix adheres to the colonic mucosa, which also contributes to targeted drug delivery to the colon. Apriso® utilizes a patented delivery system called Intellicor™ delayed- and extended-release delivery system that provides coverage throughout the colon [37]. It disintegrates at pH 6.0 in the distal jejunum where the 5-ASA begins to be released. This formulation combines delayed and sustained release and allows the 5-ASA to travel through the jejunum to the colon. It provides the convenience of once-daily dosing like the MMX® mesalamines.

## Microsphere Formulation

Pentasa® is currently the only available microsphere formulation of mesalamine [38, 39]. It encapsulates 5-ASA in ethyl cellulose-coated microgranules that gradually starts to release 5-ASA beginning in the duodenum. The release of 5-ASA from the microgranules is not affected by the bowel acidity and occurs in any enteral pH conditions. Thus, the release continues throughout the jejunum, the ileum, and the colon as well as the rectum.

## Mechanisms of Action of Mesalamine

Aspirin and nonsteroidal anti-inflammatory drugs (NSAIDs) have been shown to inhibit prostaglandin synthesis by blocking the effect of cyclooxygenase (COX) enzymes. Similarly to aspirin, its breakdown product salicylate suppresses local prostanoid production at sites of inflammation. 5-ASAs, i.e., mesalamines, are one of the most widely used salicylates, but its pharmacological profile and mechanism of action remains to be fully elucidated. In 1977, Khan et al. demonstrated in a non-placebo-controlled trial that 5-ASA is the active therapeutic moiety of sulfasalazine. Free 5-ASA, if administered orally, is rapidly absorbed from the upper intestine. 5-ASA is poorly absorbed from the colonic mucosa, and about 50 % will be metabolized to acetyl-5-ASA by the intestinal epithelium and luminal bacteria [40]. The absorbed 5-ASA is also metabolized to acetyl-5-ASA in the liver and then excreted into the urine as a mixture of free 5-ASA and acetyl-5ASA. Acetyl 5-ASA is therapeutically inactive, and it is presumed that 5-ASA acts topically on the mucosa of the gastrointestinal tract. This led to the subsequent development of various mesalamine products. After oral or rectal administration into the colon, small amounts of mesalamine is absorbed by the intestinal epithelial cells, but most are passed into the stool in an intact form [40, 41]. The mucosal concentrations of 5-ASA ranged from 3 to 50 ng/mg of wet colonic tissues in patients receiving standard treatment with mesalamine [23]. The therapeutic effect of 5-ASA is dependent on the direct contact of the molecule with the epithelial cells of the intestine than on its tissue concentration, which suggests that a high intraluminal concentration of 5-ASA is required for its action. The proposed mechanisms regarding the effect of mesalamine are summarized in Table 6.2.

Sulfasalazine and mesalamine inhibit the COX and lipoxygenase pathways resulting in reduced production of prostaglandins and leukotrienes, respectively [42, 43]. Prostaglandins and leukotrienes are chemotactic and pro-inflammatory factors that play a major role in the inflammation of inflammatory bowel disease [44, 45], and the anti-inflammatory effect of mesalamine is in part by the

**Table 6.2** Proposed mechanism of action of mesalamine

| Proposed mechanism | Reference |
|---|---|
| Blocking the production of prostaglandin and leukotrienes | [38, 39, 42, 43] |
| Inhibition of pro-inflammatory cytokine production | [44–46] |
| Inhibition of iNO | [50] |
| Free radical scavenger and antioxidant effect | [51–54] |
| Inhibition of the activation of NF-$_\kappa$B | [44, 47, 48] |
| Increasing PPAR-γ expression in epithelial cells | [49] |

effects on their metabolism [46, 47]. Mesalamine also inhibited the transcription of inflammatory mediators in intestinal epithelial cells, which counteracted the antiproliferative effects of TNF-α [48]. Several studies have shown that mesalamine inhibited the production of pro-inflammatory cytokines including interleukin-1 (IL-1) from colonic epithelial cell lines [49, 50]. Egan et al. demonstrated that mesalamine modulated RelA/p65 phosphorylation which ultimately decreased transcriptional activity of NF-κB [51]. Mesalamine also suppressed TNF-α activation of NF-κB by inhibiting the TNF-α-stimulated NF-κB inhibitory protein kinase α (IKKα) activity toward IκBα in intestinal epithelial cells [48, 52]. Peroxisome-proliferator-activated receptor-γ (PPAR-γ) are members of the nuclear receptor superfamily, which are activated by fatty acids. They are involved in the transduction of metabolic and nutritional signals into transcriptional responses. Rousseaux et al. showed that mesalamine increased PPAR-γ expression in epithelial cells. The translocation of PPAR-γ from the cytoplasm to the nucleus was enhanced and resulted in the activation of a peroxisome-proliferator response element-driven gene. These results were likely responsible for the therapeutic effect of mesalamine on colitis induced in wild type, but not PPAR-γ$^{+/-}$ mice [53]. Nitric oxide (NO) is an important final effector of mucosal injury in inflammatory bowel disease. Kennedy et al. showed that mesalamine inhibited inducible NO (iNO) production by human intestinal epithelial cells lines [54]. This was owing to the mesalamine-induced inhibition of the expression of iNO synthetase (iNOS) protein and mRNA and the suppression of cytokine-induced transcriptional upregulation of the iNOS gene. Various studies have also shown that mesalamine prevents tissue damage caused by neutrophil-derived oxidants [55–58]. Greenfield et al. showed that sulfasalazine suppressed the upregulation of HLA molecules on leucocytes, suggesting an immunological effect of mesalamines [59].

## Adverse Effects of Mesalamine

The clinical efficacy of sulfasalazine is dose related; however, not many can tolerate the drug at higher doses due to side effects. The incidence of side effects from sulfasalazine is reported to be about 45 % [40]. The side effect profile of sulfasalazine includes those that are unique to the compound and others, which are common to all mesalamine products. Most of the side effects are intolerance, not allergy, and are related to the sulfapyridine moiety. These include nausea, vomiting, and headache. Symptoms usually occur soon after initiation of sulfasalazine therapy in those patients who are taking higher doses. More severe reactions are uncommon but include allergic responses, various skin eruptions (urticaria, photosensitivity, maculopapular lesions, and epidermal necrolysis), pancreatitis, pulmonary reactions (bronchiolitis obliterans with organizing pneumonia, and eosinophilic pneumonitis, and pleuritis), hepatotoxicity (transaminitis, cholestasis), and arthralgias. Hematologic side effects such as agranulocytosis and immune thrombocytopenia are generally related to the sulfapyridine moiety. Spermatogenic dysfunction such as abnormal sperm counts, motility, and morphology that may contribute to reversible male infertility have also been attributed to sulfapyridine. Sulfasalazine inhibits folate absorption by way of competitive inhibition of folate conjugation. This may cause folate deficiency that hinders DNA synthesis and cell division, affecting most notably the bone marrow. When not many other mesalamine products were available, desensitization was used as a method to overcome allergic reactions to sulfasalazine [60, 61]. This was accomplished by starting at a very low dose of sulfasalazine and gradually increasing its dose after confirming the safeness until the desired dose is reached. This method can also be applied to mesalamine products [62].

Mesalamine is contraindicated in patients who have had hypersensitivity reactions to salicylates in the past. Those who were intolerant or had an allergic reaction with sulfasalazine may be able to take mesalamine without risk of similar reaction. However, of course, introduction of mesalamine should be done with caution in patients with a reported adverse event with sulfasalazine. Renal dysfunctions, including acute and chronic interstitial nephritis and minimal change nephropathy, can occur with sulfasalazine and mesalamine products. We recommend that all patients treated with mesalamine products should have their kidney function evaluated prior to the initiation of therapy and at least annually thereafter. Pulmonary and cardiac hypersensitivity reactions, such as pleuritis, pneumonitis, myocarditis, and pericarditis, have been reported with various mesalamine products. Other minor side effects include alopecia, abdominal distention and flatulence, headache, liver dysfunction, arthritis, skin changes, leucopenia, etc [40, 63, 64].

An acute intolerance syndrome characterized by abdominal pain, diarrhea, and fever may rarely occur with mesalamine therapy [65, 66]. It is difficult to distinguish between a flare of the underlying colitis; however, if intolerance syndrome is suspected, mesalamine should be discontinued immediately. Intolerance syndrome is universal to all mesalamine products, and patients require alternative treatments.

## Drug Interactions

The risk of renal dysfunction may be increased in patients receiving known nephrotoxic agents, such as NSAIDs. Coadministration of azathioprine or mercaptopurine with mesalamine products may result in an increase in blood 6-thioguanine nucleotide concentrations which may lead to leucopenia [67].

## Oral Mesalamine During Pregnancy and Lactation

When sulfasalazine and mesalamine are given orally, the absorbed mesalamine readily crosses the placenta, and mesalamine and its metabolite, acetyl-5ASA, are detected in the cord blood. However, this has not been linked to any fetal abnormalities in several large studies [68, 69]. Female patients taking sulfasalazine who are considering becoming pregnant should take folic acid to decrease the risk of neural tube defects. Animal studies in rodents have not revealed any evidence of impaired fertility or harm to the fetus.

Overall, sulfasalazine and mesalamine products are classified as Food and Drug Administration (FDA) pregnancy Category B, except for Asacol® that is categorized as C. The coating of Asacol® contains dibutyl phthalate (DBP) [70]. In animal studies, DBP was associated with external and skeletal malformations and adverse effects on the male reproductive system at doses >190 times the human dose. Though there are no adequate and well-controlled studies in pregnant women for either sulfasalazine or mesalamine, they can generally be continued safely during any trimester of pregnancy. Low concentrations of mesalamine and higher concentrations of the N-acetyl metabolite have been detected in human breast milk; however, in general, it can be used safely during lactation.

## Therapeutic Efficacy of Mesalamine

### Mesalamine for Active Mild to Moderate UC

The 5-ASA formulations (sulfasalazine, olsalazine, balsalazide, and mesalamine) have long been foundational treatments for mild to moderate UC. Guidelines suggest that combination of oral and topical therapies induces remission in mild to moderately active distal colitis patients and may effectively maintain remission [71–73]. As described above, the therapeutic effect of mesalamine in UC depends on the ability of the active drug to reach the sites of inflammation for topical (not systemic) anti-inflammatory activity. The currently available oral mesalamine preparations each utilize a slightly different method to increase efficient delivery of the active ingredient to small and/or large intestine. These methods include incorporation of mesalamine into a prodrug through covalent azo-bond, incorporation of unmodified mesalamine into a pH-sensitive acrylic coating or moisture-sensitive ethyl cellulose microspheres, and a newer formulation that utilizes both a pH-sensitive acrylic layer and a coating of lipophilic/hydrophilic excipients [19, 39, 74, 75]. All formulations are equally as effective, though the use of sulfasalazine is limited in its use mainly due to patient intolerance [76].

Dating back to the 1950–1960s, several studies demonstrated that sulfasalazine was superior to placebo for the treatment of active UC. In these initial studies, sulfasalazine was used at a dose of 4–6 g daily and was effective in 60–80 % of patients as compared to 30–40 % of the patients treated with placebo [21, 77, 78]. The response was also dose dependent.

Two randomized double-blinded studies demonstrated that balsalazide 6.75 g/day was as effective as sulfasalazine 3 g/day, but with a favorable safety profile [75, 79]. Balsalazide was shown to be superior to mesalamine in a double-blinded randomized trial for active UC. Patients on balsalazide 6.75 g/day showed superior 12-week clinical remission rate as compared to mesalamine 2.4 g/day (62 % vs. 37 %, $p = 0.02$), and it appears that the effect of balsalazide was more rapidly achieved [80]. Several other studies demonstrated similar efficacy between balsalazide and mesalamine [64]. In a double-blinded placebo-controlled trial, olsalazine 2 g/day was superior to placebo in achieving a clinical and endoscopic response [27]. Several studies have shown comparable efficacy between olsalazine 1.5–2 g/day and sulfasalazine 3 g/day for mildly to moderately active UC [81–83].

Asacol® was shown to be superior to placebo at a dose of 1.6 or 2.4 g/day in achieving remission at 6 weeks (43 % and 49 % vs. 23 % of placebo, $p = 0.03$, and 0.003, respectively) [84]. Schroeder et al. showed superior rates of remission with Asacol® 4.8 g/day compared to placebo (24 % vs. 5 %, $p = 0.047$) [5]. The rates of clinical response were more significant in patients with left-sided colitis (75 % vs. 21 %, $p = 0.0001$). Pentasa® was more effective than placebo at 2 or 4 g/day in achieving clinical and endoscopic remission at 8 weeks [85]. A double-blind trial between Pentasa® and sulfasalazine showed that Pentasa® at a dose 2.4 g/day was superior to sulfasalazine 2 g/day in achieving symptomatic and endoscopic improvement at 4 weeks [86].

In a dose-finding study of Apriso®, Kruis et al. demonstrated that doses of 1.5 g, 3 g, or 4.5 g daily were equally as effective for active UC [87]. There were no significant differences in remission rates, time to response, endoscopic improvement, or histological improvement. In another study, 3 g once-daily dosing was as effective as 1 g three times daily, suggesting that once-daily dosing of Apriso® is efficacious [88]. Lialda®, a once-daily mesalamine product, was tested in a randomized clinical trial of 2.4 g, 4.8 g, and placebo for 8 weeks [35]. Remission rates with both doses of Lialda® were significantly superior to placebo, but not different from each other.

More recently, the interest of mesalamine therapy has focused on optimized dosing and once-daily formulations.

## High-Dose Mesalamine

The ASCEND (Assessing the Safety and Clinical Efficacy of a New Dose of 5-ASA) trials aimed to investigate the dose–response effect of mesalamine (Asacol®) in the induction of remission in UC. The ASCEND I trial randomized 301 patients with mildly to moderately active UC to receive either 2.4 g/day or 4.8 g/day of Asacol® [89]. At week 6, similar proportion of patients experienced improvement in each group (51 % vs. 56 %, p=ns). The difference was not significant; however, when results were stratified according to the disease severity, patients with moderate disease had a more substantial response to the 4.8 g/day dose compared to those with mild disease. Based on these results, the ASCEND II trial focused on *moderately* active UC and confirmed that 4.8 g/day of Asacol® led to a greater treatment response than 2.4 g/day (72 % vs. 59 %, p=0.036) [90]. In the ASCEND III trial, 772 patients with moderately active UC were randomized to receive 2.4 g/day or 4.8 g/day doses of Asacol®, and there was no difference between the two groups in terms of overall improvement (complete remission and partial response), but significantly more patients who received 4.8 g/day compared to 2.4 g/day achieved clinical remission at week 3 (p=0.02) and week 6 (p=0.04) [74]. Furthermore, subgroup analysis showed that patients with difficult-to-treat disease, such as those previously treated with steroids, oral mesalamine, rectal therapies, or those taking multiple UC medications, responded better to higher doses than to lower doses.

## Once-Daily Mesalamines

Studies have shown that only about half of the patients are adherent to multidose therapy [91, 92], and in clinical practice, poor adherence often leads to recurrence of disease [93]. Once-daily oral formulations may improve the adherence by decreasing the pill burden and, in fact, are a preferred choice by patients [94, 95]. Lialda® utilizes the MMX® system providing a slow and gradual release of mesalamine throughout the colon that permits once-daily administration [19]. Lichtenstein et al. performed a randomized, double-blind, parallel-group, placebo-controlled multicenter study in patients with mildly to moderately active UC comparing the effect of Lialda® 2.4 g/day given twice daily, 4.8 g/day given once daily, and placebo [96]. Similar proportion of patients achieved clinical remission with 2.4 g/day twice daily or 4.8 g/day once daily (34.1 % and 29.2 % vs. 12.9 % of placebo, p<0.001 and p=0.009, respectively). In another double-blind, placebo-controlled, multicenter trial, the effect of Lialda® 2.4 g once daily and 4.8 g once daily was compared to placebo and a delayed-release mesalamine (Asacol®) 2.4 g daily given three times daily [35]. At week 8, more patients achieved clinical and endoscopic remission in the Lialda® groups compared to placebo (40.5 % and 41.2 % vs. 22.1 %, vs. placebo; p=0.01 and p=0.007, respectively). No significant difference in clinical remission rates between patients receiving Asacol® and placebo was seen (33.7 % vs. 22.1 %, p=0.089); however, it was unclear whether there was a statistical difference between Lialda® and Asacol®. Furthermore, a subsequent study combining the patients that achieved clinical and endoscopic remission in the abovementioned 2 studies evaluated the efficacy of Lialda® 2.4 g daily dosed once or twice daily as maintenance therapy [97]. At 12 months, similar proportion of patients was in clinical and endoscopic remission with once-daily and twice-daily regimen (64.4 % vs. 68.5 %, p=ns). Another once-daily mesalamine preparation (Salofalk®) that is available in Europe was evaluated in a dose-ranging trial and also proved to be efficacious in inducing remission in mildly to moderately active UC [98]. In a randomized, investigator-blinded study, controlled-release mesalamine (Pentasa®) was shown to be more effective when given in once-daily regimen [98]. At 12 months, 73.8 % of patients receiving Pentasa® 2 g once daily maintained remission compared to 63.6 % of patients receiving 1 g twice daily (p=0.024). The study also demonstrated that compliance was better with once-daily regimen.

## Mesalamine for Active Moderate to Severe UC

Corticosteroids have been the primary therapies for the induction of remission in moderate to severe UC [71]. However, patients with left-sided colitis or proctitis may still benefit from topical treatment with mesalamine or glucocorticoid suspensions [3, 99]. Those who fail to respond to treatment with the combination of mesalamine and corticosteroids or who present with severely active UC are candidates for further intensive treatment. Disease activity as well as extent should be reassessed, and prompt decision should be made as to whether the patient needs to be admitted. For patients with moderate to severe UC that can be managed as an outpatient, treatment with biologics (infliximab and adalimumab) has recently emerged. The role of mesalamines in the treatment of severe UC is unclear and likely has no additive effect on corticosteroids and biologics.

## Mesalamine for Maintenance Therapy of UC

The majority of patients with UC have a clinical course that is either relapsing-remitting or chronic continuous. Corticosteroids are effective as a short-term induction agent but lack potential as a maintenance agent and, furthermore, are associated with unfavorable side effects when administered for a long period. Shortly after shown to be effective as an induction agent, several studies aimed to assess the efficacy of sulfasalazine as a maintenance therapy in patients with quiescent UC. Dissanayake et al. showed that 6-month relapse rates were lower with 2 g/day of sulfasalazine compared to placebo (12 % vs. 55 %, $p < 0.001$) [100]. Another study showed that maintenance treatment with sulfasalazine prolonged remission in distal UC [78]. Similar to its effect in active UC, the effect of sulfasalazine in maintaining remission appeared to be dose dependent.

Balsalazide, at a higher dose, was shown to be superior to mesalamine in maintaining remission of UC [101]. Seventy-eight percent of patients on balsalazide 6 g/day were in remission at 26 weeks compared to 44 % on balsalazide 3 g/day and mesalamine 1.5 g/day ($p = 0.006$). Another study demonstrated similar efficacy between high and low dose of balsalazide in maintaining remission of UC [102]. Olsalazine was shown to be superior to placebo in maintaining remission of UC in a randomized controlled trial in patients who were intolerant to sulfasalazine [103]. Olsalazine 1 g/day compared with placebo reduced the relapse rate from 45 to 23 %. Travis et al. showed a dose response of olsalazine in maintaining remission of UC [104]. Olsalazine 2 g/day was more effective than 0.5 or 1 g/day, especially in patients with distal colitis. However, in another study, the rate of maintaining remission was similar between different doses of olsalazine (0.5–2 g/day) and sulfasalazine 2 g/day [105].

Asacol® 0.8 and 1.6 g/day was superior to placebo in maintaining remission of UC for 6 months (63 and 70 % vs. 48 % of placebo, $p = 0.05$ and 0.005, respectively) [106]. Several randomized, double-blind studies have shown that Asacol® was as effective as sulfasalazine in maintaining remission of UC with significantly less drop outs [107]. Miner et al. demonstrated that with Pentasa® 4 g/day significantly more patients were in remission at 12 months compared to placebo (64 % vs. 38 %, $p = 0.0004$) [108]. Pentasa® 1.5 g was equivalent to sulfasalazine 3 g/day in maintaining remission of UC over 12 months period [109]. The effect of Apriso® in maintaining remission of UC has been studied by Lichtenstein et al. who showed that significantly more patients maintained remission over 6 months with Apriso® 1.5 g as compared with placebo (78.9 % vs. 58.3 %, $p < 0.001$) [37]. The once-daily preparation Lialda® has also been evaluated as a maintenance agent. Patients who achieved remission with Lialda® were randomized to either 2.4 g daily dosed once or twice daily as maintenance therapy in an open-label trial [97]. At 12 months, similar proportion of patients were in clinical and endoscopic remission with once-daily and twice-daily regimen (64.4 % vs. 68.5 %, $p = $ ns).

The various mesalamine products appear to be all similarly effective for maintaining remission of UC. Some studies suggest that there is a dose-dependent effect; however, to date, we prefer to continue the dose that was required to induce remission as a maintenance therapy in our clinical practice.

## Therapeutic Equivalence of Various Mesalamine Products

No adequate comparative trials have been conducted with equivalent mesalamine doses to determine if any of the current formulations are superior in the treatment of UC. All of the mesalamine formulations are effective, but they differ in the release and absorption profile, which may influence the outcome in some patients. The prevalence of sulfasalazine intolerance due to sulfapyridine has limited its use in clinical practice, but studies suggest that most mesalamines are equally potent when similar concentrations of mesalamine are provided [76]. The selection of a mesalamine agent should be based on the results of the clinical trials, individual patient characteristics, compliance issues, as well as price, until comparative head-to-head trials are performed.

## Cancer Chemoprevention

Individuals with inflammatory bowel disease, especially those with extensive UC and colonic Crohn's disease, are at increased risk of developing colorectal cancer (CRC) compared with the general population. Previous studies show this risk is strongly associated with dysplasia, extent of disease, duration of disease, and degree of inflammation, while chemoprevention of CRC has less support.

Epidemiologic studies evaluating the effect of mesalamine as a cancer chemopreventive agent have been equivocal [110, 111]. However, Velayos et al. demonstrated, by combining the results of 9 case–control or cohort studies, that the odds ratio for mesalamine's association with CRC was 0.51 (95 % confidence interval 0.29–0.92) [112]. Since adherence to mesalamine medication is an issue for UC patients, both the disease maintenance effect and the cancer chemopreventive effect should be emphasized. The once-daily mesalamine preparations have been shown to be accepted with better compliance with the patients; however, it remains unknown whether they are a preferred agent in this aim.

NSAID groups of compounds, including aspirin, coxibs, and sulindac, have been long studied as possible CRC chemopreventive agents. Pharmacologically, these drugs inhibit COX in various cell types. COX-1 isoform is constitutively expressed, but it is the inducible COX-2 isoform which is thought to play a prominent role in the development of CRC. COX-2 inhibition induces apoptosis and reduced angiogenesis, which leads to inhibition of cell proliferation [113]. Similar to its anti-inflammatory effect, possible mechanisms for mesalamine as a CRC chemopreventive agent include inhibition of COX activity, inactivation of reactive oxygen species (free radicals), increased apoptosis through NF-κB suppression, and activation of PPAR-γ which is an epithelial cell antiproliferative agent.

Balsalazide effectively reduced tumor formation in two rodent models for CRC carcinogenesis [114]. It is suggested that a decrease in proliferation and the induction of apoptosis in colon epithelial cells after the administration of mesalamine may be responsible for the underlying mechanism [115, 116]. Das et al. demonstrated that mesalamine and sulfasalazine, but not sulfapyridine, reduced the cellular expression of TC22, a tropomyosin isoform associated with colonic neoplasia, through modulating PPAR-γ [117]. They also showed that suppression of TC22 by small interfering RNA (siRNA) produced gene level changes on several critical carcinogenic pathways including apoptosis, adhesion, angiogenesis, and tissue remodeling and suggested that these changes may be responsible for the antineoplastic molecular effect of mesalamine. Schoeneck et al. showed that mesalamine inhibited growth of colon cancer cells largely through a mitotic arrest, which has not been reported for NSAIDs so far. Mesalamine also induced apoptosis through partial activation of caspases similar to, although weaker than, established chemopreventive agents [118].

## Conclusion

In summary, mesalamine remains the mainstay in the treatment of mildly to moderately active UC, both as an induction and maintenance of remission agent. Recent studies have shown that moderately active UC and patients with complicated disease may preferentially respond to high-dose mesalamine therapies. Once-daily formulations are as effective as other formulations and, owing to their simplified regimen, may even result in better long-term compliance and outcome. Though the use of more potent biologics and immunomodulators has increased, the value of mesalamine in the management of UC will continue to be recognized.

## References

1. Podolsky DK. Inflammatory bowel disease. N Engl J Med. 2002; 347(6):417–29. PubMed PMID: 12167685, Epub 2002/08/09. eng.
2. Hanauer SB. Update on the etiology, pathogenesis and diagnosis of ulcerative colitis. Nat Clin Pract Gastroenterol Hepatol. 2004;1(1):26–31. PubMed PMID: 16265041, Epub 2005/11/03. eng.
3. Hanauer SB. Medical therapy for ulcerative colitis 2004. Gastroenterology. 2004;126(6):1582–92. PubMed PMID: 15168369, Epub 2004/05/29. eng.
4. Hoentjen F, Sakuraba A, Hanauer S. Update on the management of ulcerative colitis. Curr Gastroenterol Rep. 2011;13(5):475–85. PubMed PMID: 21789495. Epub 2011/07/27. eng.
5. Schroeder KW, Tremaine WJ, Ilstrup DM. Coated oral 5-aminosalicylic acid therapy for mildly to moderately active ulcerative colitis. A randomized study. N Engl J Med. 1987;317(26): 1625–9. PubMed PMID: 3317057, Epub 1987/12/24. eng.
6. D'Haens G, Sandborn WJ, Feagan BG, Geboes K, Hanauer SB, Irvine EJ, et al. A review of activity indices and efficacy end points for clinical trials of medical therapy in adults with ulcerative colitis. Gastroenterology. 2007;132(2):763–86. PubMed PMID: 17258735, Epub 2007/01/30. eng.
7. Truelove SC, Witts LJ. Cortisone in ulcerative colitis; final report on a therapeutic trial. Br Med J. 1955;2(4947):1041–8. PubMed PMID: 13260656, Pubmed Central PMCID: 1981500, Epub 1955/10/29. eng.
8. Baron JH, Connell AM, Lennard-Jones JE. Variation between observers in describing mucosal appearances in proctocolitis. Br Med J. 1964;1(5375):89–92. PubMed PMID: 14075156, Pubmed Central PMCID: 1812908, Epub 1964/01/11. eng.
9. Rachmilewitz D. Coated mesalazine (5-aminosalicylic acid) versus sulphasalazine in the treatment of active ulcerative colitis: a randomised trial. BMJ. 1989;298(6666):82–6. PubMed PMID: 2563951, Pubmed Central PMCID: 1835436, Epub 1989/01/14. eng.
10. Rutgeerts P, Sandborn WJ, Feagan BG, Reinisch W, Olson A, Johanns J, et al. Infliximab for induction and maintenance therapy for ulcerative colitis. N Engl J Med. 2005;353(23):2462–76. PubMed PMID: 16339095, Epub 2005/12/13. eng.
11. Cheifetz AS, Rosenberg L. Infliximab decreases colectomy rates in moderate to severe ulcerative colitis: big news or big deal? Inflamm Bowel Dis. 2011;17(7):1626–8. PubMed PMID: 21053245. Epub 2010/11/06. Eng.
12. Reinisch W, Sandborn WJ, Hommes DW, D'Haens G, Hanauer S, Schreiber S, et al. Adalimumab for induction of clinical remission in moderately to severely active ulcerative colitis: results of a randomised controlled trial. Gut. 2011;60(6):780–7. PubMed PMID: 21209123. Epub 2011/01/07. Eng.
13. Taxonera C, Estelles J, Fernandez-Blanco I, Merino O, Marin-Jimenez I, Barreiro-de Acosta M, et al. Adalimumab induction and maintenance therapy for patients with ulcerative colitis previously treated with infliximab. Aliment Pharmacol Ther. 2011;33(3): 340–8. PubMed PMID: 21133961, Epub 2010/12/08. eng.
14. Sandborn WJ, Feagan BG, Marano C, Zhang H, Strauss R, Johanns J, et al. Subcutaneous golimumab induces clinical response and remission in patients with moderate-to-severe ulcerative colitis. Gastroenterology. 2014;146(1):85–95. quiz e14-5. PubMed PMID: 23735746.
15. Sandborn WJ, Feagan BG, Marano C, Zhang H, Strauss R, Johanns J, et al. Subcutaneous golimumab maintains clinical response in patients with moderate-to-severe ulcerative colitis. Gastroenterology. 2014;146(1):96–109.e1. PubMed PMID: 23770005.
16. Ogata H, Kato J, Hirai F, Hida N, Matsui T, Matsumoto T, et al. Double-blind, placebo-controlled trial of oral tacrolimus (FK506) in the management of hospitalized patients with steroid-refractory ulcerative colitis. Inflamm Bowel Dis. 2012;18(5):803–8. PubMed PMID: 21887732. Epub 2011/09/03. Eng.
17. Ogata H, Matsui T, Nakamura M, Iida M, Takazoe M, Suzuki Y, et al. A randomised dose finding study of oral tacrolimus (FK506) therapy in refractory ulcerative colitis. Gut. 2006;55(9):1255–62. PubMed PMID: 16484504, Pubmed Central PMCID: 1860021, Epub 2006/02/18. eng.
18. Sjoberg M, Walch A, Meshkat M, Gustavsson A, Jarnerot G, Vogelsang H, et al. Infliximab or cyclosporine as rescue therapy in hospitalized patients with steroid-refractory ulcerative colitis: a retrospective observational study. Inflamm Bowel Dis. 2012;18(2):212–8. PubMed PMID: 21438096. Epub 2011/03/26. Eng.
19. Oliveira L, Cohen RD. Maintaining remission in ulcerative colitis—role of once daily extended-release mesalamine. Drug Des Devel Ther. 2011;5:111–6. PubMed PMID: 21448448. Pubmed Central PMCID: 3063115. Epub 2011/03/31. eng.

20. Qureshi AI, Cohen RD. Mesalamine delivery systems: do they really make much difference? Adv Drug Deliv Rev. 2005; 57(2):281–302. PubMed PMID: 15555743, Epub 2004/11/24. eng.

21. Baron JH, Connell AM, Lennard-Jones JE, Jones FA. Sulphasalazine and salicylazosulphadimidine in ulcerative colitis. Lancet. 1962;1(7239):1094–6. PubMed PMID: 13865153, Epub 1962/05/26. eng.

22. Lennard-Jones JE, Misiewicz JJ, Connell AM, Baron JH, Jones FA. Prednisone as maintenance treatment for ulcerative colitis in remission. Lancet. 1965;1(7378):188–9. PubMed PMID: 14238045, Epub 1965/01/23. eng.

23. Azadkhan AK, Truelove SC, Aronson JK. The disposition and metabolism of sulphasalazine (salicylazosulphapyridine) in man. Br J Clin Pharmacol. 1982;13(4):523–8. PubMed PMID: 6121576, Pubmed Central PMCID: 1402052, Epub 1982/04/01. eng.

24. Lichtenstein GR, Kamm MA. Review article: 5-aminosalicylate formulations for the treatment of ulcerative colitis–methods of comparing release rates and delivery of 5-aminosalicylate to the colonic mucosa. Aliment Pharmacol Ther. 2008;28(6):663–73. PubMed PMID: 18532992, Epub 2008/06/06. eng.

25. Chan RP, Pope DJ, Gilbert AP, Sacra PJ, Baron JH, Lennard-Jones JE. Studies of two novel sulfasalazine analogs, ipsalazide and balsalazide. Dig Dis Sci. 1983;28(7):609–15. PubMed PMID: 6345112, Epub 1983/07/01. eng.

26. Wiggins JB, Rajapakse R. Balsalazide: a novel 5-aminosalicylate prodrug for the treatment of active ulcerative colitis. Expert Opin Drug Metab Toxicol. 2009;5(10):1279–84. PubMed PMID: 19743890, Epub 2009/09/12. eng.

27. Selby WS, Barr GD, Ireland A, Mason CH, Jewell DP. Olsalazine in active ulcerative colitis. Br Med J (Clin Res Ed). 1985;291(6506):1373–5. PubMed PMID: 3933675, Pubmed Central PMCID: 1418984, Epub 1985/11/16. eng.

28. Campbell DE, Berglindh T. Pharmacology of olsalazine. Scand J Gastroenterol Suppl. 1988;148:7–12. PubMed PMID: 3067340, Epub 1988/01/01. eng.

29. Carrette O, Favier C, Mizon C, Neut C, Cortot A, Colombel JF, et al. Bacterial enzymes used for colon-specific drug delivery are decreased in active Crohn's disease. Dig Dis Sci. 1995;40(12):2641–6. PubMed PMID: 8536525, Epub 1995/12/01. eng.

30. Fallingborg J, Christensen LA, Ingeman-Nielsen M, Jacobsen BA, Abildgaard K, Rasmussen HH. pH-profile and regional transit times of the normal gut measured by a radiotelemetry device. Aliment Pharmacol Ther. 1989;3(6):605–13. PubMed PMID: 2518873, Epub 1989/12/01. eng.

31. Faber SM, Korelitz BI. Experience with Eudragit-S-coated mesalamine (Asacol) in inflammatory bowel disease. An open study. J Clin Gastroenterol. 1993;17(3):213–8. PubMed PMID: 8228082, Epub 1993/10/01. eng.

32. Shiota K, Mima S. Assessment of the teratogenicity of di(2-ethylhexyl)phthalate and mono(2-ethylhexyl)phthalate in mice. Arch Toxicol. 1985;56(4):263–6. PubMed PMID: 3994510.

33. WarnerChilcott. Delzicol prescribing information. http://www.wcrx.com/pdfs/pi/pi_delzicolpdf

34. Baker DE. MMX mesalamine. Rev Gastroenterol Disord. 2006;6(3):146–52. PubMed PMID: 16957657, Epub 2006/09/08. eng.

35. Kamm MA, Sandborn WJ, Gassull M, Schreiber S, Jackowski L, Butler T, et al. Once-daily, high-concentration MMX mesalamine in active ulcerative colitis. Gastroenterology. 2007;132(1):66–75. PubMed PMID: 17241860, quiz 432–3. Epub 2007/01/24. eng.

36. Tenjarla S, Romasanta V, Zeijdner E, Villa R, Moro L. Release of 5-aminosalicylate from an MMX mesalamine tablet during transit through a simulated gastrointestinal tract system. Adv Ther. 2007;24(4):826–40. PubMed PMID: 17901032. Epub 2007/09/29. eng.

37. Lichtenstein GR, Gordon GL, Zakko S, Murthy U, Sedghi S, Pruitt R, et al. Clinical trial: once-daily mesalamine granules for maintenance of remission of ulcerative colitis—a 6-month placebo-controlled trial. Aliment Pharmacol Ther. 2010;32(8):990–9. PubMed PMID: 20937044, Epub 2010/10/13. eng.

38. Christensen LA, Slot O, Sanchez G, Boserup J, Rasmussen SN, Bondesen S, et al. Release of 5-aminosalicylic acid from Pentasa during normal and accelerated intestinal transit time. Br J Clin Pharmacol. 1987;23(3):365–9. PubMed PMID: 3567055, Pubmed Central PMCID: 1386240, Epub 1987/03/01. eng.

39. Gionchetti P, Campieri M, Belluzzi A, Brignola C, Tampieri M, Iannone P, et al. Pentasa in maintenance treatment of ulcerative colitis. Gastroenterology. 1990;98(1):251. PubMed PMID: 2293593, Epub 1990/01/01. eng.

40. Greenfield SM, Punchard NA, Teare JP, Thompson RP. Review article: the mode of action of the aminosalicylates in inflammatory bowel disease. Aliment Pharmacol Ther. 1993;7(4):369–83. PubMed PMID: 8105984, Epub 1993/08/01. eng.

41. Zhou SY, Fleisher D, Pao LH, Li C, Winward B, Zimmermann EM. Intestinal metabolism and transport of 5-aminosalicylate. Drug Metab Dispos. 1999;27(4):479–85. PubMed PMID: 10101143, Epub 1999/04/02. eng.

42. Rachmilewitz D, Sharon P, Ligumsky M, Zor U. Mechanism of sulphasalazine action in ulcerative colitis. Lancet. 1978;2(8096):946. PubMed PMID: 81963, Epub 1978/10/28. eng.

43. Sharon P, Ligumsky M, Rachmilewitz D, Zor U. Role of prostaglandins in ulcerative colitis. Enhanced production during active disease and inhibition by sulfasalazine. Gastroenterology. 1978;75(4):638–40. PubMed PMID: 30669, Epub 1978/10/01. eng.

44. Gould SR. Letter: prostaglandins, ulcerative colitis, and sulphasalazine. Lancet. 1975;2(7942):988. PubMed PMID: 53480, Epub 1975/11/15. eng.

45. Lauritsen K, Laursen LS, Bukhave K, Rask-Madsen J. Use of colonic eicosanoid concentrations as predictors of relapse in ulcerative colitis: double blind placebo controlled study on sulphasalazine maintenance treatment. Gut. 1988;29(10):1316–21. PubMed PMID: 2904392, Pubmed Central PMCID: 1434004, Epub 1988/10/01. eng.

46. Lauritsen K, Hansen J, Bytzer P, Bukhave K, Rask-Madsen J. Effects of sulphasalazine and disodium azodisalicylate on colonic PGE2 concentrations determined by equilibrium in vivo dialysis of faeces in patients with ulcerative colitis and healthy controls. Gut. 1984;25(11):1271–8. PubMed PMID: 6149981, Pubmed Central PMCID: 1432314, Epub 1984/11/01. eng.

47. Lauritsen K, Staerk Laursen L, Bukhave K, Rask-Madsen J. Longterm olsalazine treatment: pharmacokinetics, tolerance and effects on local eicosanoid formation in ulcerative colitis and Crohn's colitis. Gut. 1988;29(7):974–82. PubMed PMID: 2840367, Pubmed Central PMCID: 1433774, Epub 1988/07/01. eng.

48. Kaiser GC, Yan F, Polk DB. Mesalamine blocks tumor necrosis factor growth inhibition and nuclear factor kappaB activation in mouse colonocytes. Gastroenterology. 1999;116(3):602–9. PubMed PMID: 10029619, Epub 1999/02/25. eng.

49. Rachmilewitz D, Karmeli F, Schwartz LW, Simon PL. Effect of aminophenols (5-ASA and 4-ASA) on colonic interleukin-1 generation. Gut. 1992;33(7):929–32. PubMed PMID: 1353743, Pubmed Central PMCID: 1379406, Epub 1992/07/01. eng.

50. Mahida YR, Lamming CE, Gallagher A, Hawthorne AB, Hawkey CJ. 5-Aminosalicylic acid is a potent inhibitor of interleukin 1 beta production in organ culture of colonic biopsy specimens from patients with inflammatory bowel disease. Gut. 1991;32(1):50–4. PubMed PMID: 1846838, Pubmed Central PMCID: 1379213, Epub 1991/01/01. eng.

51. Egan LJ, Mays DC, Huntoon CJ, Bell MP, Pike MG, Sandborn WJ, et al. Inhibition of interleukin-1-stimulated NF-kappaB RelA/p65 phosphorylation by mesalamine is accompanied by decreased transcriptional activity. J Biol Chem. 1999;274(37):26448–53. PubMed PMID: 10473604, Epub 1999/09/03. eng.

52. Yan F, Polk DB. Aminosalicylic acid inhibits IkappaB kinase alpha phosphorylation of IkappaBalpha in mouse intestinal epithelial cells. J Biol Chem. 1999;274(51):36631–6. PubMed PMID: 10593965, Epub 1999/12/14. eng.

53. Rousseaux C, Lefebvre B, Dubuquoy L, Lefebvre P, Romano O, Auwerx J, et al. Intestinal antiinflammatory effect of 5-aminosalicylic acid is dependent on peroxisome proliferator-activated receptor-gamma. J Exp Med. 2005;201(8):1205–15. PubMed PMID: 15824083, Pubmed Central PMCID: 2213148, Epub 2005/04/13. eng.

54. Kennedy M, Wilson L, Szabo C, Salzman AL. 5-aminosalicylic acid inhibits iNOS transcription in human intestinal epithelial cells. Int J Mol Med. 1999;4(4):437–43. PubMed PMID: 10493988, Epub 1999/09/24. eng.

55. Aruoma OI, Wasil M, Halliwell B, Hoey BM, Butler J. The scavenging of oxidants by sulphasalazine and its metabolites. A possible contribution to their anti-inflammatory effects? Biochem Pharmacol. 1987;36(21):3739–42.

56. Dull BJ, Salata K, Van Langenhove A, Goldman P. 5-Aminosalicylate: oxidation by activated leukocytes and protection of cultured cells from oxidative damage. Biochem Pharmacol. 1987;36(15):2467–72. PubMed PMID: 3038125, Epub 1987/08/01. eng.

57. Ahnfelt-Ronne I, Nielsen OH, Christensen A, Langholz E, Binder V, Riis P. Clinical evidence supporting the radical scavenger mechanism of 5-aminosalicylic acid. Gastroenterology. 1990;98(5 Pt 1):1162–9. PubMed PMID: 1969825, Epub 1990/05/01. eng.

58. Tamai H, Kachur JF, Grisham MB, Gaginella TS. Scavenging effect of 5-aminosalicylic acid on neutrophil-derived oxidants. Possible contribution to the mechanism of action in inflammatory bowel disease. Biochem Pharmacol. 1991;41(6–7):1001–6. PubMed PMID: 1848973. Epub 1991/03/01. eng.

59. Greenfield SM, Hamblin AS, Shakoor ZS, Teare JP, Punchard NA, Thompson RP. Inhibition of leucocyte adhesion molecule upregulation by tumor necrosis factor alpha: a novel mechanism of action of sulphasalazine. Gut. 1993;34(2):252–6. PubMed PMID: 8094364, Pubmed Central PMCID: 1373980, Epub 1993/02/01. eng.

60. Kummerle-Deschner J, Dannecker G. Sulphasalazine desensitization in a paediatric patient with juvenile chronic arthritis. Acta Paediatr. 1995;84(8):952–4. PubMed PMID: 7488828, Epub 1995/08/01. eng.

61. Koski JM. Desensitization to sulphasalazine in patients with arthritis. Clin Exp Rheumatol. 1993;11(2):169–70. PubMed PMID: 8099541. Epub 1993/03/01. eng.

62. Oustamanolakis P, Koutroubakis IE. New desensitization regimen with mesalamine granules in a patient with ulcerative colitis and mesalamine intolerance. Inflamm Bowel Dis. 2010;17(2):E8–9. PubMed PMID: 20848496, Epub 2010/09/18. eng.

63. Fowler BT, Gupta T, Bilal M. Asacol(R)-induced neutropenia resolution without the use of granulocyte colony-stimulating factor. South Med J. 2010;103(11):1167–9. PubMed PMID: 20859250, Epub 2010/09/23. eng.

64. Green JR, Lobo AJ, Holdsworth CD, Leicester RJ, Gibson JA, Kerr GD, et al. Balsalazide is more effective and better tolerated than mesalamine in the treatment of acute ulcerative colitis. The Abacus Investigator Group. Gastroenterology. 1998;114(1):15–22. PubMed PMID: 9428213, Epub 1998/01/15. eng.

65. Sturgeon JB, Bhatia P, Hermens D, Miner Jr PB. Exacerbation of chronic ulcerative colitis with mesalamine. Gastroenterology.

1995;108(6):1889–93. PubMed PMID: 7768395, Epub 1995/06/01. eng.

66. Iofel E, Chawla A, Daum F, Markowitz J. Mesalamine intolerance mimics symptoms of active inflammatory bowel disease. J Pediatr Gastroenterol Nutr. 2002;34(1):73–6. PubMed PMID: 11753169, Epub 2001/12/26. eng.

67. Lowry PW, Franklin CL, Weaver AL, Szumlanski CL, Mays DC, Loftus EV, et al. Leucopenia resulting from a drug interaction between azathioprine or 6-mercaptopurine and mesalamine, sulphasalazine, or balsalazide. Gut. 2001;49(5):656–64. PubMed PMID: 11600468, Pubmed Central PMCID: 1728490, Epub 2001/10/16. eng.

68. Sachar D. Exposure to mesalamine during pregnancy increased preterm deliveries (but not birth defects) and decreased birth weight. Gut. 1998;43(3):316. PubMed PMID: 9863473, Pubmed Central PMCID: 1727248, Epub 1998/12/24. eng.

69. Diav-Citrin O, Park YH, Veerasuntharam G, Polachek H, Bologa M, Pastuszak A, et al. The safety of mesalamine in human pregnancy: a prospective controlled cohort study. Gastroenterology. 1998;114(1):23–8. PubMed PMID: 9428214, Epub 1998/01/15. eng.

70. Asacol HD. Prescribing information. Rockaway, NJ: Warner Chilcott; 2010.

71. Kornbluth A, Sachar DB. Ulcerative colitis practice guidelines in adults: American College Of Gastroenterology Practice Parameters Committee. Am J Gastroenterol. 2010;105(3):501–23. quiz 24. PubMed PMID: 20068560. Epub 2010/01/14. eng.

72. Gionchetti P, Rizzello F, Venturi A, Ferretti M, Brignola C, Miglioli M, et al. Comparison of oral with rectal mesalazine in the treatment of ulcerative proctitis. Dis Colon Rectum. 1998;41(1):93–7. PubMed PMID: 9510317, Epub 1998/03/24. eng.

73. Safdi M, DeMicco M, Sninsky C, Banks P, Wruble L, Deren J, et al. A double-blind comparison of oral versus rectal mesalamine versus combination therapy in the treatment of distal ulcerative colitis. Am J Gastroenterol. 1997;92(10):1867–71. PubMed PMID: 9382054, Epub 1997/10/23. eng.

74. Sandborn WJ, Regula J, Feagan BG, Belousova E, Jojic N, Lukas M, et al. Delayed-release oral mesalamine 4.8 g/day (800-mg tablet) is effective for patients with moderately active ulcerative colitis. Gastroenterology. 2009;137(6):1934–43. e1-3. PubMed PMID: 19766640. Epub 2009/09/22. eng.

75. Green JR, Mansfield JC, Gibson JA, Kerr GD, Thornton PC. A double-blind comparison of balsalazide, 6.75 g daily, and sulfasalazine, 3 g daily, in patients with newly diagnosed or relapsed active ulcerative colitis. Aliment Pharmacol Ther. 2002;16(1):61–8.

76. Sutherland L, Macdonald JK. Oral 5-aminosalicylic acid for induction of remission in ulcerative colitis. Cochrane Database Syst Rev. 2006;2, CD000543. PubMed PMID: 16625536, Epub 2006/04/21. eng.

77. Moertel CG, Bargen JA. A critical analysis of the use of salicylazosulfapyridine in chronic ulcerative colitis. Ann Intern Med. 1959;51:879–89. PubMed PMID: 14423204, Epub 1959/11/01. eng.

78. Dick AP, Grayson MJ, Carpenter RG, Petrie A. Controlled trial of sulphasalazine in the treatment of ulcerative colitis. Gut. 1964;5:437–42. PubMed PMID: 14218553, Pubmed Central PMCID: 1552152, Epub 1964/10/01. eng.

79. Mansfield JC, Giaffer MH, Cann PA, McKenna D, Thornton PC, Holdsworth CD. A double-blind comparison of balsalazide, 6.75 g, and sulfasalazine, 3 g, as sole therapy in the management of ulcerative colitis. Aliment Pharmacol Ther. 2002;16(1):69–77.

80. Levine DS, Riff DS, Pruitt R, Wruble L, Koval G, Sales D, et al. A randomized, double blind, dose–response comparison of balsalazide (6.75 g), balsalazide (2.25 g), and mesalamine (2.4 g) in the

treatment of active, mild-to-moderate ulcerative colitis. Am J Gastroenterol. 2002;97(6):1398–407.

81. Rao SS, Dundas SA, Holdsworth CD, Cann PA, Palmer KR, Corbett CL. Olsalazine or sulphasalazine in first attacks of ulcerative colitis? A double blind study. Gut. 1989;30(5):675–9. PubMed PMID: 2567266, Pubmed Central PMCID: 1434223, Epub 1989/05/01. eng.

82. Ewe K, Eckardt V, Kanzler G. Treatment of ulcerative colitis with olsalazine and sulphasalazine: efficacy and side-effects. Scand J Gastroenterol Suppl. 1988;148:70–5. PubMed PMID: 2906479, Epub 1988/01/01. eng.

83. Kruis W, Brandes JW, Schreiber S, Theuer D, Krakamp B, Schutz E, et al. Olsalazine versus mesalazine in the treatment of mild to moderate ulcerative colitis. Aliment Pharmacol Ther. 1998;12(8):707–15. PubMed PMID: 9726382, Epub 1998/09/03. eng.

84. Sninsky CA, Cort DH, Shanahan F, Powers BJ, Sessions JT, Pruitt RE, et al. Oral mesalamine (Asacol) for mildly to moderately active ulcerative colitis. A multicenter study. Ann Intern Med. 1991; 115(5):350–5. PubMed PMID: 1863024, Epub 1991/09/01. eng.

85. Hanauer S, Schwartz J, Robinson M, Roufail W, Arora S, Cello J, et al. Mesalamine capsules for treatment of active ulcerative colitis: results of a controlled trial. Pentasa Study Group. Am J Gastroenterol. 1993;88(8):1188–97. PubMed PMID: 8338086, Epub 1993/08/01. eng.

86. Riley SA, Mani V, Goodman MJ, Herd ME, Dutt S, Turnberg LA. Comparison of delayed release 5 aminosalicylic acid (mesalazine) and sulphasalazine in the treatment of mild to moderate ulcerative colitis relapse. Gut. 1988;29(5):669–74. PubMed PMID: 2899536, Pubmed Central PMCID: 1433642, Epub 1988/05/01. eng.

87. Kruis W, Bar-Meir S, Feher J, Mickisch O, Mlitz H, Faszczyk M, et al. The optimal dose of 5-aminosalicylic acid in active ulcerative colitis: a dose-finding study with newly developed mesalamine. Clin Gastroenterol Hepatol. 2003;1(1):36–43. PubMed PMID: 15017515, Epub 2004/03/16. eng.

88. Kruis W, Kiudelis G, Racz I, Gorelov IA, Pokrotnieks J, Horynski M, et al. Once daily versus three times daily mesalazine granules in active ulcerative colitis: a double-blind, double-dummy, randomised, non-inferiority trial. Gut. 2009;58(2):233–40. PubMed PMID: 18832520, Epub 2008/10/04. eng.

89. Hanauer SB, Sandborn WJ, Dallaire C, Archambault A, Yacyshyn B, Yeh C, et al. Delayed-release oral mesalamine 4.8 g/day (800 mg tablets) compared to 2.4 g/day (400 mg tablets) for the treatment of mildly to moderately active ulcerative colitis: The ASCEND I trial. Can J Gastroenterol. 2007;21(12):827–34.

90. Hanauer SB, Sandborn WJ, Kornbluth A, Katz S, Safdi M, Woogen S, et al. Delayed-release oral mesalamine at 4.8 g/day (800 mg tablet) for the treatment of moderately active ulcerative colitis: the ASCEND II trial. Am J Gastroenterol. 2005;100(11): 2478–85.

91. Kane SV, Cohen RD, Aikens JE, Hanauer SB. Prevalence of nonadherence with maintenance mesalamine in quiescent ulcerative colitis. Am J Gastroenterol. 2001;96(10):2929–33. PubMed PMID: 11693328, Epub 2001/11/06. eng.

92. Cerveny P, Bortlik M, Kubena A, Vlcek J, Lakatos PL, Lukas M. Nonadherence in inflammatory bowel disease: results of factor analysis. Inflamm Bowel Dis. 2007;13(10):1244–9. PubMed PMID: 17538983, Epub 2007/06/01. eng.

93. Lichtenstein GR, Rubin DT, Sabesin SM, Velayos FS, Vitat P. Maximizing patient adherence and clinical outcomes with mesalamine in mildly-to-moderately active ulcerative colitis. Rev Gastroenterol Disord. 2008;8(1):21–30. PubMed PMID: 18477967, quiz 1–2. Epub 2008/05/15. eng.

94. Hu MY, Peppercorn MA. MMX mesalamine: a novel high-dose, once-daily 5-aminosalicylate formulation for the treatment of ulcerative colitis. Expert Opin Pharmacother. 2008;9(6):1049–58. PubMed PMID: 18377346, Epub 2008/04/02. eng.

95. Kane S, Huo D, Magnanti K. A pilot feasibility study of once daily versus conventional dosing mesalamine for maintenance of ulcerative colitis. Clin Gastroenterol Hepatol. 2003;1(3):170–3. PubMed PMID: 15017487, Epub 2004/03/16. eng.

96. Lichtenstein GR, Kamm MA, Boddu P, Gubergrits N, Lyne A, Butler T, et al. Effect of once- or twice-daily MMX mesalamine (SPD476) for the induction of remission of mild to moderately active ulcerative colitis. Clin Gastroenterol Hepatol. 2007;5(1): 95–102. PubMed PMID: 17234558, Epub 2007/01/20. eng.

97. Kamm MA, Lichtenstein GR, Sandborn WJ, Schreiber S, Lees K, Barrett K, et al. Randomised trial of once- or twice-daily MMX mesalazine for maintenance of remission in ulcerative colitis. Gut. 2008;57(7):893–902. PubMed PMID: 18272546, Pubmed Central PMCID: 2564831, Epub 2008/02/15. eng.

98. Dignass AU, Bokemeyer B, Adamek H, Mross M, Vinter-Jensen L, Borner N, et al. Mesalamine once daily is more effective than twice daily in patients with quiescent ulcerative colitis. Clin Gastroenterol Hepatol. 2009;7(7):762–9. PubMed PMID: 19375519, Epub 2009/04/21. eng.

99. Cobden I, al-Mardini H, Zaitoun A, Record CO. Is topical therapy necessary in acute distal colitis? Double-blind comparison of high-dose oral mesalazine versus steroid enemas in the treatment of active distal ulcerative colitis. Aliment Pharmacol Ther. 1991; 5(5):513–22.

100. Dissanayake AS, Truelove SC. Proceedings: a controlled therapeutic trial of long-term maintenance treatment of ulcerative colitis with sulphasalazine (salazopyrin). Gut. 1973;14(10):818. PubMed PMID: 4148469, Epub 1973/10/01. eng.

101. Kruis W, Schreiber S, Theuer D, Brandes JW, Schutz E, Howaldt S, et al. Low dose balsalazide (1.5 g twice daily) and mesalazine (0.5 g three times daily) maintained remission of ulcerative colitis but high dose balsalazide (3.0 g twice daily) was superior in preventing relapses. Gut. 2001;49(6):783–9. PubMed PMID: 11709512. Pubmed Central PMCID: 1728533. Epub 2001/11/16. eng.

102. Green JR, Gibson JA, Kerr GD, Swarbrick ET, Lobo AJ, Holdsworth CD, et al. Maintenance of remission of ulcerative colitis: a comparison between balsalazide 3 g daily and mesalazine 1.2 g daily over 12 months. ABACUS Investigator group. Aliment Pharmacol Ther. 1998;12(12):1207–16.

103. Sandberg-Gertzen H, Jarnerot G, Kraaz W. Azodisal sodium in the treatment of ulcerative colitis. A study of tolerance and relapse-prevention properties. Gastroenterology. 1986;90(4):1024–30. PubMed PMID: 2868964, Epub 1986/04/01. eng.

104. Travis SP, Tysk C, de Silva HJ, Sandberg-Gertzen H, Jewell DP, Jarnerot G. Optimum dose of olsalazine for maintaining remission in ulcerative colitis. Gut. 1994;35(9):1282–6. PubMed PMID: 7959238, Pubmed Central PMCID: 1375708, Epub 1994/09/01. eng.

105. Kruis W, Judmaier G, Kayasseh L, Stolte M, Theuer D, Scheurlen C, et al. Double-blind dose-finding study of olsalazine versus sulphasalazine as maintenance therapy for ulcerative colitis. Eur J Gastroenterol Hepatol. 1995;7(5):391–6. PubMed PMID: 7614099, Epub 1995/05/01. eng.

106. Hanauer S, Sninsky C, Robinson M, Powers B, McHattie J, Mayle J, et al. An oral preparation of mesalamine as long-term maintenance therapy for ulcerative colitis. A randomized, placebo-controlled trial. The Mesalamine Study Group. Ann Intern Med. 1996;124(2):204–11.

107. Dew MJ, Harries AD, Evans N, Evans BK, Rhodes J. Maintenance of remission in ulcerative colitis with 5-amino salicylic acid in high doses by mouth. Br Med J (Clin Res Ed). 1983;287(6384): 23–4. PubMed PMID: 6134565, Pubmed Central PMCID: 1548114, Epub 1983/07/02. eng.

108. Miner P, Hanauer S, Robinson M, Schwartz J, Arora S. Safety and efficacy of controlled-release mesalamine for maintenance of remission in ulcerative colitis. Pentasa UC Maintenance Study Group. Dig Dis Sci. 1995;40(2):296–304. PubMed PMID: 7851193, Epub 1995/02/01. eng.

109. Mulder CJ, Tytgat GN, Weterman IT, Dekker W, Blok P, Schrijver M, et al. Double-blind comparison of slow-release 5-aminosalicylate and sulfasalazine in remission maintenance in ulcerative colitis. Gastroenterology. 1988;95(6):1449–53. PubMed PMID: 2903110, Epub 1988/12/01. eng.

110. Pinczowski D, Ekbom A, Baron J, Yuen J, Adami HO. Risk factors for colorectal cancer in patients with ulcerative colitis: a case–control study. Gastroenterology. 1994;107(1):117–20. PubMed PMID: 7912678, Epub 1994/07/01. eng.

111. Moody GA, Jayanthi V, Probert CS, Mac Kay H, Mayberry JF. Long-term therapy with sulphasalazine protects against colorectal cancer in ulcerative colitis: a retrospective study of colorectal cancer risk and compliance with treatment in Leicestershire. Eur J Gastroenterol Hepatol. 1996;8(12):1179–83. PubMed PMID: 8980937, Epub 1996/12/01. eng.

112. Velayos FS, Terdiman JP, Walsh JM. Effect of 5-aminosalicylate use on colorectal cancer and dysplasia risk: a systematic review and metaanalysis of observational studies. Am J Gastroenterol. 2005;100(6):1345–53. PubMed PMID: 15929768, Epub 2005/06/03. eng.

113. Moreira L, Castells A. Cyclooxygenase as a target for colorectal cancer chemoprevention. Curr Drug Targets. 2011;12(13):1888–94. PubMed PMID: 21158711. Epub 2010/12/17. Eng.

114. MacGregor DJ, Kim YS, Sleisenger MH, Johnson LK. Chemoprevention of colon cancer carcinogenesis by balsalazide: inhibition of azoxymethane-induced aberrant crypt formation in the rat colon and intestinal tumor formation in the B6-Min/+mouse. Int J Oncol. 2000;17(1):173–9. PubMed PMID: 10853036, Epub 2000/06/15. eng.

115. Ritland SR, Leighton JA, Hirsch RE, Morrow JD, Weaver AL, Gendler SJ. Evaluation of 5-aminosalicylic acid (5-ASA) for cancer chemoprevention: lack of efficacy against nascent adenomatous polyps in the Apc(Min) mouse. Clin Cancer Res. 1999;5(4):855–63. PubMed PMID: 10213222, Epub 1999/04/23. eng.

116. Reinacher-Schick A, Seidensticker F, Petrasch S, Reiser M, Philippou S, Theegarten D, et al. Mesalazine changes apoptosis and proliferation in normal mucosa of patients with sporadic polyps of the large bowel. Endoscopy. 2000;32(3):245–54. PubMed PMID: 10718391, Epub 2000/03/16. eng.

117. Das KK, Bajpai M, Kong Y, Liu J, Geng X, Das KM. Mesalamine suppresses the expression of TC22, a novel tropomyosin isoform associated with colonic neoplasia. Mol Pharmacol. 2009;76(1):183–91. PubMed PMID: 19369484, Pubmed Central PMCID: 2701462, Epub 2009/04/17. eng.

118. Reinacher-Schick A, Schoeneck A, Graeven U, Schwarte-Waldhoff I, Schmiegel W. Mesalazine causes a mitotic arrest and induces caspase-dependent apoptosis in colon carcinoma cells. Carcinogenesis. 2003;24(3):443–51. PubMed PMID: 12663503, Epub 2003/03/29. eng.

# Contrast and Comparison of Mesalamine Derivatives in the Treatment of Ulcerative Colitis

**7**

Prashant R. Mudireddy, Wojciech Blonski, and Gary R. Lichtenstein

**Keywords**

Mesalamine • Ulcerative colitis • 5-Aminosalycylic acid • Remission • Sulfasalazine • Randomized studies

## Introduction

Mesalamine (called mesalazine in Europe) or 5-aminosalicylic acid is the recommended first-line agent for both induction and maintenance of remission in patients with mild to moderately severe ulcerative colitis [1]. Mesalamine is available as both oral and topical formulations. Topical preparations are preferred for distal and left-sided colitis, while oral agents are used for more extensive disease.

Sulfasalazine was the first mesalamine-containing drug used in the treatment of ulcerative colitis. It was developed by Dr. Nana Svartz in the 1940s for the treatment of rheumatoid arthritis, but she noticed that it improved colitis symptoms in patients with ulcerative colitis [2, 3]. Later randomized controlled studies established its efficacy in the treatment of ulcerative colitis [4, 5].

Sulfasalazine contains mesalamine (anti-inflammatory agent) and sulfapyridine (antibiotic) linked by an azo bond.

Peppercorn and his colleagues demonstrated that the azo bond is cleaved by colon bacteria releasing mesalamine and sulfapyridine [6]. In 1977, Azad Khan et al. showed that mesalamine (5-ASA) is the active therapeutic moiety of sulfasalazine, while sulfapyridine acted as the carrier molecule [6]. Despite its efficacy in ulcerative colitis, sulfasalazine is not tolerated in up to 30 % of the patients. The toxicity of sulfasalazine has been attributed to the sulfapyridine, a sulfa compound [7].

In order to decrease the side effects, several oral and topical mesalamine preparations have been developed without the sulfa component. Free mesalamine is rapidly absorbed from the proximal small intestine leaving very little to reach the colon—the site of active inflammation. To prevent this, various mesalamine preparations have been developed to ensure maximal delivery to the colon. Broadly, three different mechanisms have been used to protect mesalamine from metabolism before it reaches the terminal ileum and colon—pH-dependent delayed-release formulations (Asacol, Salofalk, Apriso, Lialda), pH-independent controlled release (Pentasa), and prodrugs which utilize the azo bond (balsalazide, olsalazine) [8].

Topical formulations of mesalamine have the advantage of delivering the drug directly to the site of inflammation [8]. They are available as suppositories, enemas, foams, and gels. Studies have shown that topical mesalamine preparations are very poorly absorbed from the colon [9, 10]. This minimizes their systemic side effects. Also, compared to oral mesalamine, topical mesalamine achieves greater mucosal concentration in the distal colon. In a randomized study, Frieri et al. noted that after 2 weeks of treatment, rectal mucosal concentrations of mesalamine were 20 times greater in those treated with a combination of oral Asacol and mesalamine rectal enema than those treated with oral Asacol alone [11].

P.R. Mudireddy, M.D. (✉)
Department of Gastroenterology, Lennox Hill Hospital, 100 East, 77th St., New York, NY 10075, USA
e-mail: prashantmudireddy@yahoo.com

W. Blonski, M.D., Ph.D.
Department of Internal Medicine, United Health Services, Wilson Memorial Center, 33-57 Harrison St., Picciano Building 4th Floor, Johnson City, NY 13790, USA
e-mail: blonskiw@gmail.com

G.R. Lichtenstein, M.D., F.A.C.P., F.A.C.G., A.G.A.F.
Gastroenterology Division, Hospital of the University of Pennsylvania, University of Pennsylvania School of Medicine, Philadelphia, PA, USA
e-mail: gary.lichtenstein@uphs.upenn.edu

G.R. Lichtenstein (ed.), *Medical Therapy of Ulcerative Colitis*,
DOI 10.1007/978-1-4939-1677-1_7, © Springer Science+Business Media New York 2014

In this chapter, we will discuss various mesalamine preparations currently available and compare and contrast them in their efficacy in the induction of remission, maintenance of remission, and their safety profile. We will also briefly discuss mechanism of action and metabolism of mesalamine.

## Mechanism of Action

The exact mechanism of action of mesalamine is not well understood. Several potential theories have been proposed based on both in vivo and in vitro studies. Mesalamine is thought to exert its effect locally by acting on the inflamed mucosa [8]. Recent studies have shown that mesalamine is peroxisome proliferator-activated receptor-γ agonist (PPAR-γ). The activation of PPAR-γ leads to decreased production of inflammatory cytokines and decreased proliferation of inflammatory cells [12]. Mesalamine inhibits both the cyclooxygenase and 5′-lipooxygenase pathways leading to inhibition of prostaglandin E2 in the inflamed intestine and decreased production of leukotrienes, respectively. Mesalamine is a scavenger of free radicals and thus exhibits antioxidant properties [7]. Mesalamine inhibits antibody production by B cells and interferes with macrophage and neutrophil function [12]. Mesalamine also inhibits the production of several pro-inflammatory cytokines like IL-1, IL-2, TNF-α, and nuclear factor κ-β (NFκ-β) [13].

## Metabolism of Mesalamine and Sulfasalazine

About 30 % of sulfasalazine is absorbed in the proximal intestine, and the rest is cleaved by colon bacteria yielding two byproducts—mesalamine and sulfapyridine. Sulfapyridine is absorbed into the systemic circulation and undergoes acetylation in the *liver* (Fig. 7.1) [12]. Adverse effects of sulfasalazine are due to the sulfa compound and are more pronounced in slow acetylators [7].

The colon epithelial cells absorb mesalamine released in the colon. In the epithelial cells, *N*-acetyl transferase 1 (NAT-1) enzyme metabolizes mesalamine or 5-ASA into *N-Acetyl-5ASA*. This is either secreted back into the lumen and excreted in feces or absorbed into the circulation and excreted in the urine [14]. Some of the 5-ASA is absorbed into the systemic circulation and undergoes acetylation in the liver and is excreted in the urine [14]. A very small portion of 5-ASA undergoes acetylation by colon bacteria and excreted in the feces [14].

Are there any differences in the pharmacokinetic profiles of various oral mesalamine preparations? A recent systematic review by Sandborn and Hanauer showed that the systemic absorption of mesalamine is comparable for all oral preparations. They demonstrated that the urinary and fecal excretion of total 5-ASA was similar among all oral mesalamine preparations [14]. This was also confirmed by a study comparing pharmacokinetic profiles of equimolar doses of Asacol and balsalazide [15].

**Fig. 7.1** Proposed metabolic pathway of 5-ASA after oral administration. The *shaded area* (large intestine) indicates the site of topical action. Unformulated 5-ASA is absorbed rapidly from the small intestine, and many current formulations are designed to delay the release of 5-ASA until the terminal ileum or proximal colon. *5-ASA* 5-aminosalicylic acid, *N-AC-5-ASA* N-acetyl-5-ASA (Reprinted from Lichtenstein GR, Kamm MA. Review article: 5-aminosalicylate formulations for the treatment of ulcerative colitis- methods of comparing release rates and delivery of 5-aminosalicylate to the colonic mucosa. Alimentary Pharmacol Ther 2008; 28 (6): 663-73; Copyright 2008) [73]

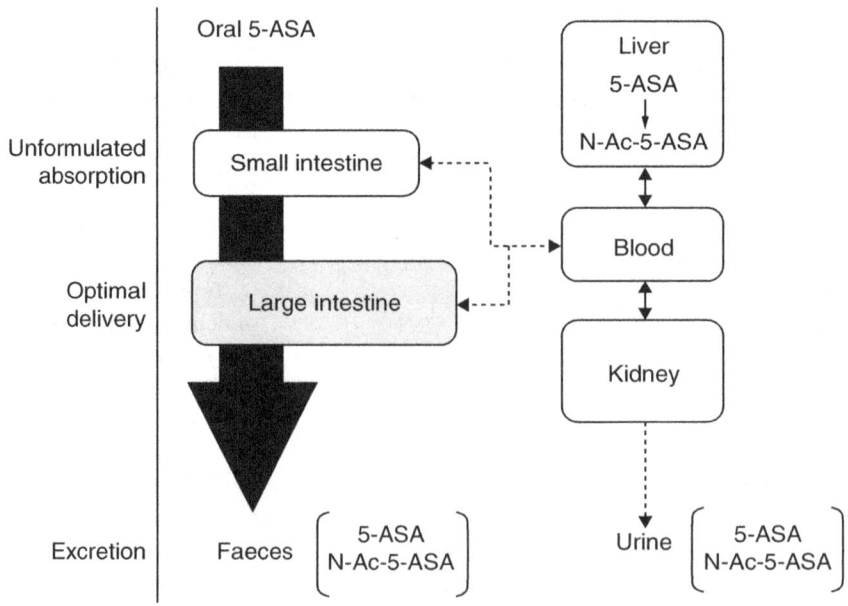

## Mesalamine Formulations and Preparations

A variety of mesalamine formulations have been developed that ensure maximal delivery of active 5-ASA to the terminal ileum and colon. These include both oral and topical mesalamine preparations. While oral preparations ensure maximal 5-ASA concentrations in the proximal colon, topical preparations deliver 5-ASA directly to the left side of the colon. Tables 7.1 and 7.2 summarize various oral and topical 5-ASA preparations currently available, respectively.

## Oral pH-Dependent Formulations

These include Asacol, Ipocol, Claversal, Salofalk, Apriso, and Lialda. In order to prevent proximal absorption, mesalamine is coated with pH-sensitive polymers. The two most common polymers used are Eudragit-S and Eudragit-L [8, 12].

Eudragit-S coating breaks down at pH>7 and releases mesalamine in the terminal ileum and colon [12]. Asacol (Procter and Gamble Pharmaceuticals, Cincinnati, OH, USA) and Ipocol (Sandoz Pharmaceuticals, Bordon, Hampshire, UK) are examples of mesalamine preparations which are enteric coated with Eudragit-S [8, 12, 16]. Asacol is available as 400 and 800 mg tablets and administered 2–3 times per day [17]. Eudragit-L, a derivative of S-polymer, breaks down at a lower pH and releases mesalamine in the jejunum, terminal ileum, and colon [12]. Claversal (Merckle

GMBH, Ulm, Germany) and Salofalk (Axcan Pharma, Mont St. Hilaire, Quebec, Canada, and Falk Pharma, Freiburg, Germany) are examples of mesalamine formulations coated with Eudragit-L [12]. Studies on healthy volunteers and ileostomy patients have demonstrated that Eudragit-L-coated mesalamine preparations are released more proximally than Eudragit-S-coated mesalamine preparations [12].

Apriso (Salix Pharmaceuticals Inc., Morrisville, NC, USA) has been approved by FDA only for the maintenance of remission in ulcerative colitis [8]. It consists of a gelatin capsule containing granules of mesalamine, which are coated with Eudragit-L polymer resin. The capsule dissolves in the stomach and releases the mesalamine granules which in turn break down at pH greater than 6. The granules also contain a polymer matrix, which swells and ensures gradual release of the mesalamine throughout the colon [8]. It is dosed once daily.

MMX mesalamine marketed as Lialda in the USA and Mezavant elsewhere is a novel pH-dependent once-daily mesalamine formulation [8, 12, 16]. FDA has approved it for both induction and maintenance of remission in ulcerative colitis patients. In this formulation, MMX technology is utilized. It contains both hydrophilic and lipophilic matrices, which are in turn coated by pH-sensitive Eudragit-S resin. The Eudragit-S coating delays release of mesalamine until the terminal ileum and colon where pH is greater than 7. The hydrophilic matrix then comes in contact with intestinal fluids and swells forming a viscous gel mass [12, 16]. The viscous gel mass ensures slow release of the mesalamine. The lipophilic core prevents the water from entering the core of

**Table 7.1** 5-ASA formulations and release sites

| Name | Formulation/release site | Dosage |
| --- | --- | --- |
| Sulfasalazine/Azulfidine® | 5-ASA linked to sulfapyridine by an azo bond | 500 mg tablets |
| Asacol®/delayed-release mesalamine | Enclosed in enteric "film" (Eudragit-S) releasing at pH ≥ 7 in the terminal ileum and colon | Asacol, 400 mg<br>Asacol HD, 800 mg |
| Salofalk®, Claversal® | Enclosed Eudragit-L releasing at pH ≥ 6 in the jejunum, ileum, and colon | 250 and 500 mg tablets |
| Pentasa® | Microspheres within a moisture-sensitive, ethyl cellulose, semipermeable membrane releasing mesalamine in the duodenum, jejunum, ileum, and colon | 250 and 500 mg capsules |
| Apriso® | The outer coating (Eudragit-L) dissolves in the jejunum, ileum, and colon (pH ≥ 6), while a polymer matrix core facilitates slow, sustained release throughout the colon | 375 mg |
| Olsalazine/Dipentum® | Two molecules of 5-ASA linked by an azo bond between their amino groups cleaved by azoreductase | 250 mg |
| Balsalazide disodium/Colazal® | 5-ASA linked by an azo bond to 4-amino-benzoyl-β-alanine cleaved by azoreductase | 750 mg |
| Lialda®, Mezavant® | Has lipophilic and hydrophilic matrices to provide delayed release of mesalamine. Has Eudragit-S which enables mesalamine release at pH ≥ 7 in the terminal ileum and continues throughout the colon | 1.2 g |
| Salofalk Granu-Stix® and Pentasa® sachets | Micropellet formulations | 500 mg sachets |

*5-ASA* 5-aminosalicylic acid
With permission from Sonu I, Lin MV, Blonski W, Lichtenstein GR. Clinical pharmacology of 5-ASA compounds in inflammatory bowel disease. Gastroenterol Clin North Am. 2010;39(3):559-99. © Elsevier 2010 [8]

**Table 7.2** Topical 5-ASA preparations

| Formulation | Brand name | Dosages |
| --- | --- | --- |
| Suspension enema | Rowasa, Asacol, Pentasa, Salofalk | 1 g/60 ml, 2 g/60 ml, 4 g/60 ml |
| Suppository | Canasa, Asacol, Claversal, Pentasa | 250, 400, 500, 100 mg |
| Gel | Asacol, Claversal, Salofalk | 1 g/30 ml, 1 g/60 ml, 2 g/60 ml, 2 g/120 ml |
| Foam | Enterasin | 2 g/60 ml |

*5-ASA* 5-aminosalicylic acid

the tablet and dissolving it. This helps to prolong the half-life of the drug [8, 12, 16]. MMX mesalamine is available as 1,200 mg tablets and administered once or twice daily [17].

## Oral pH-Independent Formulations

This includes Pentasa (Shire Pharmaceuticals Inc., Wayne, PA, USA, licensed from Ferring A/S Copenhagen, Denmark), a controlled-release mesalamine formulation. It utilizes a semipermeable, moisture-sensitive ethyl cellulose coating [16]. This allows a slow and sustained release of mesalamine. It also differs from other mesalamine preparations by releasing mesalamine in the duodenum and jejunum, in addition to the terminal ileum. It is estimated that approximately about 20 % of mesalamine is released in the small intestine and the rest in the colon [12]. It is available as 250 and 500 mg tablets and 250 mg capsules. It is administered four times per day.

Both Pentasa and Salofalk are available as sachets (micro-pellet formulations). One of the advantages of micropellet formulations is that it facilitates prolonged release of the mesalamine, thereby allowing less frequent dosing. This has been demonstrated in two studies comparing tablets to micropellets [16].

## Mesalamine Prodrug Formulations

These mesalamine formulations similar to sulfasalazine utilize a diazo bond (Fig. 7.2). The diazo bond is cleaved by colon bacteria's azoreductase enzyme-releasing mesalamine. Balsalazide and olsalazine are examples of prodrugs. Balsalazide/Colazal (Salix Pharmaceutical Inc., Morrisville, NC) utilizes an inert molecule (4-aminobenzoyl-β-alanine) for binding with a single 5-ASA molecule. Balsalazide is available as 750 mg tablets and is administered three times per day [17]. Olsalazine (Alaven Pharmaceuticals, Marietta, GA/Dipentum (UCB Pharma, Brussels, Belgium)) contains two 5-ASA molecules linked by a diazo bond. Olsalazine is available as 250 mg capsules and is administered twice daily [17].

## Topical Mesalamine Formulations

Topical mesalamine preparations deliver 5-ASA directly to the site of inflammation in the distal colon. They are available as suppositories, suspension enemas, gels, and foams. Currently in the USA, only mesalamine suppositories (Canasa) and suspension enemas (Rowasa) are available. Scintigraphy studies have demonstrated that suppositories deliver active drug to the rectum, while suspension enemas can reach as far as the splenic flexure [12].

## Efficacy of Mesalamine in the Induction of Remission in Active UC

The first placebo-controlled study demonstrating sulfasalazine's efficacy in the induction of remission in UC was published by Baron et al. [2]. But due to side effects and intolerance of sulfasalazine, newer mesalamine preparations have been developed in an effort to reduce side effects and improve efficacy. In this section, we will discuss how newer mesalamine preparations compare to placebo and sulfasalazine in the induction of remission and also evaluate if there are any differences among various mesalamine preparations in their ability to induce remission. It is important to recognize that different studies used varied definitions for clinical and endoscopic remissions making comparison between various 5-ASA preparations difficult. Refer to Table 7.3 for randomized double-blind controlled trials comparing therapy with various oral 5-ASA formulations in inducing remission of UC.

## Oral Mesalamine Preparations Versus Placebo

Several randomized controlled studies and meta-analyses have demonstrated superiority of oral mesalamine preparations over placebo in the induction of remission. In one of the recent meta-analyses published by Ford et al. (included 11 RCTs and 2,086 patients), the relative risk of failure to induce remission with mesalamine compared to placebo was 0.79 (95 % CI 0.73–0.85, $p = 0.009$) [18]. This meta-analysis also found that the number needed to treat for mesalamine derivatives was 6 (95 % CI 5–8) [18]. Ford et al. did not find any significant differences between the type of oral mesalamine drug and their efficacy in inducing remission in active UC (Cochrane $Q = 1.11$, $p = 0.77$) [18].

The Cochrane meta-analysis published in 2006 also found that mesalamine preparations were superior to placebo for induction of remission as well as clinical and endoscopic improvement in patients with active UC. In terms of ability to induce clinical or global improvement or remission, the pooled Peto odds ratio between 5-ASA and placebo was 0.40 (95 % CI 0.30–0.53) [19].

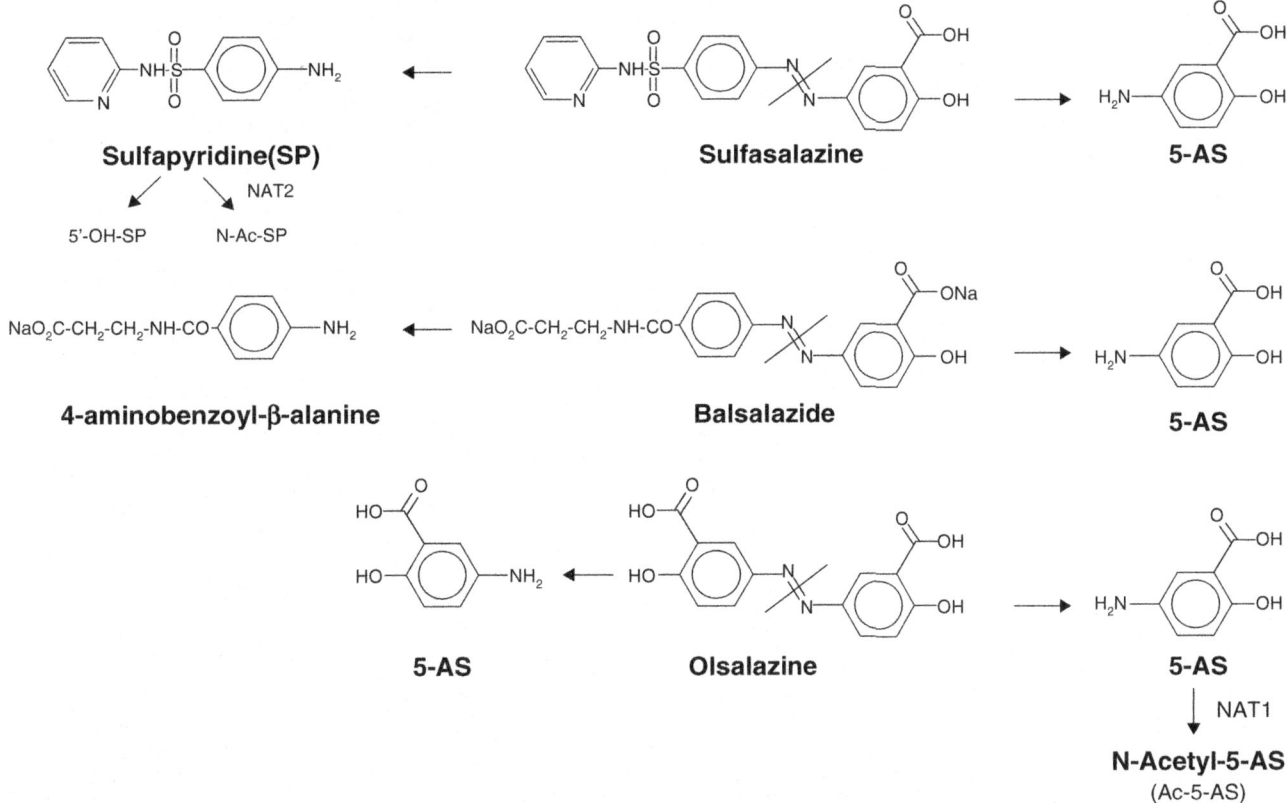

**Fig. 7.2**  Structure of different prodrugs of 5-AS and part of their metabolism. Reprint from Klotz U, Schwab M. Topical delivery of therapeutic agents in the treatment of inflammatory bowel disease. Adv Drug Delivery Rev 2005;57:267–79; © Elsevier 2005) [74]

## Asacol Versus Placebo

Delayed-release mesalamine preparation like Asacol has been shown to be superior to placebo in two RCTs. Schroeder et al. compared 4.8 and 1.6 g/day of Asacol to placebo. Asacol 4.8 g/day produced statistically significant remission compared to placebo ($p < 0.0001$), while 1.6 g/day did not induce significant remission rates compared to placebo ($p = 0.51$) [20]. In another study comparing Asacol to placebo, Snisky found that Asacol 2.4 g/day induced remission in 32 % patients compared to only 9 % by placebo ($p = 0.003$) [21]

## Pentasa Versus Placebo

In a large multicenter double-blind RCT, Pentasa 2 g/day (57 %) and 4 g/day (59 %) produced significantly better clinical improvement compared to placebo, while Pentasa 1 g/day (36 %) could not induce statistically significant remission compared to placebo [22].

## MMX Mesalamine Versus Placebo

Lichtenstein et al. demonstrated that MMX mesalamine is superior to placebo in the induction of both clinical and endoscopic remission. In a large multicenter, double-blind RCT, 280 patients were randomized to either MMX mesalamine 4.8 g/day, MMX mesalamine 2.4 g/day, or placebo. MMX mesalamine 4.8 g/day induced remission in 29.2 % of patients, MMX mesalamine 2.4 g/day in 34.2 % patients, and placebo in 12.4 % patients [23].

## Olsalazine Versus Placebo

In only RCT comparing clinical remission rates between olsalazine and placebo in patients with active UC, olsalazine was not superior to placebo [18, 24]. But if the results of three trials that compared clinical improvement rates (rather than clinical remission) between olsalazine and placebo were to be included in the analysis, then olsalazine would be superior to placebo (RR of no remission or improvement = 0.81, 95 % CI 0.68–0.96) [18, 25–27].

**Table 7.3** Randomized double-blind controlled trials comparing therapy with various oral 5-ASA formulations in inducing remission of ulcerative colitis

| Reference | Treatment arm | Daily dose | # patients | Study duration | Primary end point | Results | AEs | Withdrawals | Comments |
|---|---|---|---|---|---|---|---|---|---|
| Fleig et al. [75] | Sulfasalazine | 3.0 g | 21 | 6 w | Improvement in mean stool frequency (A) and consistency (B) Macroscopic (C) and microscopic (D) appearance of the colonic mucosa measured at w 0 and w 6 | A: 6.9±3.4 vs. 3.0±1.9 ($p<0.05$) B: Significant improvement C: Improvement 8 p No change: 8 p Worsening: 0 p D: improvement: 8 p No change: 7 p Worsening: 2p | Nausea (3 p) Pruritus (1 p) Generalized exanthema (1 p) | Side effects (generalized exanthema) (1 p) | No statistical difference in efficacy between sulfasalazine and benzalazine changes in macroscopic and microscopic appearance of the colonic mucosa |
| | Benzalazine | 2.16 g | 22 | | | A: 6.8±2.1 vs. 4.0±2.7 ($p<0.05$) B: significant improvement C: Improvement 11 p No change: 5 p Worsening: 0 p D: Improvement: 8 p No change: 7 p Worsening: 0 pts | 3 p: nausea and vomiting | Rapid worsening of disease (3 p) Lost to follow-up (2 p) | |
| Riley et al. [76] | Sulfasalazine | 2 g | 19 | 4 w | Improvement in stool frequency, rectal bleeding, and macroscopic and microscopic grade of the colonic mucosa measured at w 0 and w 4 | Significant improvement of macroscopic score above 5 cm at w 4 ($p<0.005$) | Itchy rash (2 p) Headache (6 p) GI symptoms (anorexia, nausea, vomiting, dyspepsia) (4 p) | Itchy rash (2 p) | Improvement in rectal bleeding and macroscopic grade of the colonic mucosa at w 4 was significantly greater in pts treated with high-dose mesalazine than sulfasalazine ($p<0.05$) |
| | Mesalamine | 0.8 g | 20 | | | Significant improvement of rectal bleeding ($p<0.005$), macroscopic ($p<0.01$) and microscopic ($p<0.005$) scores at w 4 | Headache (4 p) GI symptoms (anorexia, nausea, vomiting, dyspepsia) (4 p) | | |
| | Mesalamine | 2.4 g | 21 | | | Significant improvement of stool frequency, ($p<0.01$), rectal bleeding ($p<0.01$), and macroscopic score ($p<0.005$) at w 4 | Headache (5 p) GI symptoms (anorexia, nausea, vomiting, dyspepsia) (7 p) | Up to twofold increase in plasma creatinine (2 p) | |

| Study | Treatment | Dose | N | Duration | Outcome definition | Results | Adverse events | Comments |
|---|---|---|---|---|---|---|---|---|
| Rachmilewitz [77] | Coated mesalamine | 1.5 g | 115 | 8 w | Clinical and endoscopic remission: clinical and endoscopic activity score ≤4 | Clinical remission: w 4: 50/70 pts (71 %) w 8: 37/50 p (74 %) Endoscopic remission: w 8: 20/41 pts (49 %) Clinical remission: w 4: 38/58 p (66 %) ($p=0.338$ vs. coated mesalazine) w 8: 35/43 p (81 %) ($p=0.835$ vs. coated mesalazine) Endoscopic remission: w 8: 18/38 p (47 %) ($p=0.272$ vs. coated mesalazine) | 16/115 p (14 %) Total number of AE: 29 25/105 p (24 %) Total number of adverse events: 47 7/115 p (6 %) 8/105 p (8 %) | 164 patients were included in the efficacy analysis (87 received coated mesalazine and 77 received sulfasalazine) |
| | Sulfasalazine | 3 g | 105 | | | | | |
| Rao et al. [78] | Olsalazine | 2 g | 20 | 4 w | Overall improvement defined as a positive change in at least two of the following criteria: Clinical activity index by Truelove and Witts % of bloody stools Sigmoidoscopic appearance of the colon Histologic appearance of the colonic mucosa | Overall improvement at w 4 vs. w 0 15/18 p (83 %) ($p<0.01$) Proportion of unformed stools (78 % at w 0 vs. 55 % at w 4, $p<0.001$) Bloody stools (61 % at w 0 vs. 22 % at w 4, $p<0.001$) Improvement in sigmoidoscopic score at w 4 vs. w 0: 83 % ($p<0.01$) Improvement in histologic score at w 4 vs. w 0: 44 % ($p<0.01$) Overall improvement at w 4 vs. w 0 9/13 p (69 %) ($p<0.01$) Proportion of unformed stools (72 % at w 0 vs. 28 % at w 4, $p<0.001$) Bloody stools (67 % at w 0 vs. 37 % at w 4, $p<0.001$) Improvement in sigmoidoscopic score at w 4 vs. w 0: 84 % ($p<0.01$) Improvement in histologic score at w 4 vs. w 0: 46 % ($p<0.01$) | Headache and nasal stuffiness (1 p) Diarrhea (1 p) Dyspepsia and nausea (2 p) Exacerbation of bloody diarrhea (1 p) Myalgia, headache, and dizziness (1) 2 4 | No difference in the overall response between treatment arms Significantly greater decrease in proportion of unformed stools at w 4 in patients treated with sulfasalazine vs. olsalazine ($p<0.05$) No difference in tolerance between treatment arms |
| | Sulfasalazine | 3 g | 17 | | | | | |

(continued)

**Table 7.3** (continued)

| Reference | Treatment arm | Daily dose | # patients | Study duration | Primary end point | Results | AEs | Withdrawals | Comments |
|---|---|---|---|---|---|---|---|---|---|
| Munakata et al. [79] | Mesalamine | 1.5 g | 52 | 4 w | Improvement in clinical symptoms and endoscopic findings | Marked and moderate clinical improvement: 30/48 p (63 %) | 6/52 p (11.5 %) | Not reported | No difference in clinical and endoscopic improvement between treatment arms |
| | Sulfasalazine | 3.0 g | 57 | | | Marked and moderate clinical improvement: 32/52 p (62 %) | 16/57 p (28.1 %) | Not reported | General usefulness based on the improvement and safety: mesalazine 65.3 % vs. sulfasalazine 45.6 % ($p = 0.042$) |
| Kruis et al. 1998 [31] | Olsalazine | 3 g | 88 | 12 w | Endoscopic remission: score 0 or 1 on 5-point scale Score 0: normal mucosa with visible vascular pattern, no granularity or friability Score 1: inactive colitis, pink mucosa, no visible blood vessels, faintly granular but no friability | 52.2 % | 41/88 p (46 %) | 11/88 p (13 %) | – |
| | Mesalamine | 3 g | 80 | | | 48.8 % ($p = 0.67$, vs. olsalazine) | 29/80 p (36 %) | 9/80 p (11 %) | |
| Green et al. [80] | Balsalazide | 6.75 g | 50 | 12 w | Complete remission at w 4, 8, and 12: symptomatic remission with no use of relief medication in the previous 4 days and grade 0 or 1 on sigmoidoscopy [Grade 0: normal, vascular pattern clearly visible Grade 1: erythema with loss of vascular pattern] | w 4: 38 % w 8: 54 % w 12: 62 % | 24/50 p (48 %) | 15/50 p (30 %) Treatment failure 6/50 p (12 %) AE: 1/50 p (2 %) | – |
| | Mesalamine | 2.4 g | 49 | | | w 4: 12 % w 8: 22 % w 12: 37 % $p < 0.01$ $p < 0.01$ $p < 0.05$ | 35/49 p (71 %) $p = 0.024$ | 23/49 p (47 %) Treatment failure 16/49 p (33 %) AE: 1/49 p (2 %) $p = 0.068$ $p = 0.015$ | |
| Green et al. [111] | Balsalazide | 6.75 g | 28 | 12 w | Remission rates at the end of study or withdrawal/ remission: return to stool frequency (with or without pain) to that before relapse without the presence of blood and confirmed by biopsy | Completed study in remission: 21/28 p (75 %) | Serious: 2/28 pts (7 %) Minor: 27/28 pts (96 %) | AE: 2/28 pts (7 %) Treatment failure: 1/28 p (4 %) Lost to follow-up: 0/28 (0 %) | |
| | Sulfasalazine | 3 g | 29 | | | Completed study in remission: 17/29 p (69 %) $p = 0.19$ | Serious: 0/29 p (0 %) Minor: 27/29 p (93 %) | AE: 9/29 p (31 %) Treatment failure: 1/29 p (3 %) Lost to follow-up: 1/29 (3 %) $p = 0.041$ $p > 0.2$ $p > 0.2$ | |

| Study | Drug | Dose | N | Duration | Efficacy | Result | AE | Population |
|---|---|---|---|---|---|---|---|---|
| Forbes et al. [82] | Asacol-mesalamine in Eudragit-S coating | 2.4 g | 42 | 8 w | Efficacy based on modified St. Mark's Colitis Score, macroscopic and microscopic appearance of the rectum and (PGA). Clinical remission defined from PGA | Decrease in St. Mark's Colitis Activity Score: −2.3 Clinical remission w 8: 28.6 % Improvement in sigmoidoscopy score: 54.8 % Improvement in histologic score: 31 % | 31/42 p (73.8 %) | 11/42 p (26.1 %) | – |
| | Ipocol-mesalamine in Eudragit-S coating | 2.4 g | 46 | | | Decrease in St. Mark's Colitis Activity Score: −1.5 Clinical remission w 8: 26.1 % Improvement in sigmoidoscopy score: 50.0 % Improvement in histologic score: 30.4 % p=ns p=ns p=ns p=ns | 34/46 p (73.9 %) | 9/46 p (19.6 %) | |
| Pruitt et al. [83] | Balsalazide | 6.75 g | 84 | 8 w | Symptomatic remission: patient functional assessment ratings of normal or mild and absence of rectal bleeding at wk 8 or early completion of treatment | 38/73 p (52 %) 39/84 p (46 %) | 45/84 p (54 %) | AE: 3/84 p (4 %) | 73 p in efficacy-evaluable population 84 p in intention to treat population |
| | Mesalamine | 2.4 g | 89 | | | 38/77 p (49 %) 38/89 p (44 %) | 57/89 p (64 %) | AE: 6/89 p (7 %) | 77 p in efficacy-evaluable population 89 p in intention to treat population |

(continued)

**Table 7.3** (continued)

| Reference | Treatment arm | Daily dose | # patients | Study duration | Primary end point | Results | AEs | Withdrawals | Comments |
|---|---|---|---|---|---|---|---|---|---|
| Levine et al. [84] | Balsalazide | 6.75 g | 53 | 8 w | Improvement in rectal bleeding and in at least one other sign or symptom at w 8 | Improvement in rectal bleeding: 65 %<br><br>Improvement in stool frequency: 59 %<br><br>Improvement in sigmoidoscopic score: 79 %<br><br>Improvement in PGA: 74 %<br>Improvement in overall symptom assessment: 65 %<br>Improvement in patient functional assessment: 71 % | 23/53 p (43 %) | 16/53 p (30 %) | 49 p in efficacy-evaluable population<br><br>53 p in intention to treat population |
| | Balsalazide | 2.25 g | 50 | | | Improvement in rectal bleeding: 32 %<br><br>Improvement in stool frequency: 29 %<br><br>Improvement in sigmoidoscopic score: 53 %<br>Improvement in PGA: 51 %<br><br>$p=0.006$<br>$p=0.006$<br>$p=0.015$<br>$p=0.030$ | 27/50 p (54 %) | 17/50 p (34 %) | 49 p in efficacy-evaluable population<br>50 p in intention to treat population |
| | Mesalamine | 2.4 g | 51 | | | Improvement in rectal bleeding: 53 %<br><br>Improvement in sigmoidoscopic score: 61 %<br>Improvement in PGA: 62 %<br>Improvement in overall symptom assessment: 58 %<br>Improvement in patient functional assessment: 61 %<br><br>$p=$ns<br>$p=$ns<br>$p=$ns<br>$p=$ns<br>$p=$ns | 26/51 p (51 %) | 15/51 p (29 %) | 49 p in efficacy-evaluable population<br>51 p in intention to treat population |

| Study | Treatment | Dose | N | Duration | Remission definition | Remission | | Dropout/AE |
|---|---|---|---|---|---|---|---|---|
| Mansfield et al. [85] | Balsalazide | 6.75 g | 26 | 8 w | Remission defined as stool frequency of ≤2/day without blood and with normal colonic mucosa or minimal erythema on sigmoidoscopy at w 8 | 13/26 p (50 %) | 17/26 p (65 %) | AE: 1/26 p (4 %) Treatment ineffective: 2/26 p (7.5 %) Protocol violation: 2/26 pts (7.5 %) |
| | Sulfasalazine | 3 g | 24 | | | 9/24 p (38 %) | 21/24 p (88 %) | AE: 9/24 p (38 %) Treatment ineffective: 3/24 pt (12 %) Protocol violation: 1/24 p (4 %) |
| | | | | | | $p=0.10$ | | $p=0.004$ |
| Raedler et al. [86] | Mesalamine micropellets | 3 g | 181 | 8 w | Clinical remission: clinical activity index according to Rachmilewitz ≤2 at w 8 | 67 % (intention to treat population) 64.4 % (according to protocol population) | 56/181 p (30.9 %) | Not reported | 179 p in intention to treat population 160 p in according to protocol population 181 p in safety population |
| | Mesalamine tablets | 3 g | 181 | | | 62.9 % (intention to treat population) 64.2 % (according to protocol population) OR=1.199 (95%CI 0.758–1.897) | 43/181 p (23.8 %) | Not reported | 178 p in intention to treat population |
| | | | | | | OR=1.008 (95 % CI 0.623–1.632) | $p=0.43$ | | 162 p in according to protocol population 181 p in safety population |
| Tursi et al. [87] | Balsalazide+VSL #3 | 2.25 g+3 g VSL #3 | 30 | 8 w | Symptomatic remission: patient functional assessment of normal bowel movements and absence of rectal bleeding | 24/30 p (80 %) (95 % CI 59–91) | Not reported | Protocol violation: 1/30 p (3 %) Protocol ineffectiveness: 1/30 p (3 %) |
| | Balsalazide | 4.5 g | 30 | | | 21/30 p (70 %) (95 % CI 43–81) | Not reported | Protocol violation: 1/30 p (3 %) Protocol ineffectiveness: 3/30 p (10 %) |
| | Mesalamine | 2.4 g | 30 | | | 16/30 p (53.3 %) (95%CI 42–62) $p<0.02$ | Not reported | Protocol violation: 2/30 p (6 %) Protocol ineffectiveness: 4/30 p (13 %) AE: 2/30 p (6 %) |

(continued)

**Table 7.3** (continued)

| Reference | Treatment arm | Daily dose | # patients | Study duration | Primary end point | Results | AEs | Withdrawals | Comments |
|---|---|---|---|---|---|---|---|---|---|
| Jiang and Cui [88] | Olsalazine | 1 g | 21 | 8 w | Complete remission: decrease in clinical symptoms with relative normal appearance of the colonic mucosa | Complete remission: 16/21 p (76 %) | Not reported | Not reported | – |
| | Sulfasalazine | 1 g | 21 | | | Complete remission: 10/21 p (48 %) $p<0.05$ | Not reported | Not reported | |
| Marakhouski et al. [89] | Mesalamine pellets | 1.5 g–3.0 g | 115 | 8 w | Clinical remission: clinical activity index ≤4 | At 3 w: 54/114 p (47 %) At 8 w: 76/114 p (67 %) | 36/114 p (32 %) | AE: 1/114 p (0.9 %) | 114 p in intention to treat and safety analysis Daily dose 1.5 g Includes p with dose escalation to 3 g/day in nonresponders to initial dose of 1.5 g/day (n=44) and pts treated with daily dose of 1.5 g (n=70) |
| | Mesalamine tables | 1.5 g–3.0 g | 118 | | | At 3 w: 48/115 p (42 %) At 8 w: 78/115 p (68 %) | 42/118 p (36 %) | 4/118 p (3.4 %) (AE) | 115 p in intention to treat analysis 118 pts in safety analysis Daily dose 1.5 g Includes p with dose escalation to 3 g/day in nonresponders to initial dose of 1.5 g/day (n=52) and p treated with daily dose of 1.5 g (n=63) |
| Gibson et al. [90] | Eudragit-L-coated mesalamine | 3 g | 131 | 8 w | Clinical remission: clinical activity index ≤4 | 69 % | 74/131 p (57 %) | 16/131 p (12 %) | |
| | Ethyl cellulose-coated mesalamine | 3 g | 127 | | | 69 % | 66/127 p (52 %) | 14/127 p (11 %) | |
| Ito et al. [43] | pH-dependent release mesalamine | 2.4 g | 66 | 8 w | Decrease in UC activity index | Mean decrease: 1.5 (95 % CI 0.7, 2.3) | 56/66 p (84.8 %) | Not reported | – |
| | pH-dependent release mesalamine | 3.6 g | 64 | | | Mean decrease: 2.9 (95 % CI 2.3, 3.5) | 53/64 p (82.8 %) | Not reported | |
| | Time-dependent release mesalamine | 2.25 g | 63 | | | 1.3 (95 % CI 0.6, 2.1) $p=0.003$ Difference: 0.2 (95 % CI-0.8, 1.2) | 55/65 p (84.6 %) | Not reported | |

5-ASA 5-aminosalicylic acid, AE adverse events, GI gastrointestinal, PGA physician's global assessment, p patient, w week(s), UC ulcerative colitis

Reprinted from Sonu I, Lin MV, Blonski W, Lichtenstein GR. Clinical pharmacology of 5-ASA compounds in inflammatory bowel disease. Gastroenterol Clin North Am. 2010 Sep: 39(3): 559-99. © Elsevier 2010 [8]

## Balsalazide Versus Placebo

Scherl and colleagues demonstrated that balsalazide (3.3 g twice daily) was better than placebo in achieving remission in patients with mild to moderately active UC. The relative risk of failure to achieve remission between balsalazide and placebo was 0.82 (95 % CI 0.74–0.91) [28].

## Oral Mesalamine Preparations Versus Sulfasalazine

The Cochrane meta-analysis updated in 2006 suggested that the newer mesalamine drugs tended toward therapeutic benefit when compared to sulfasalazine in the induction of remission in patients with active UC [19]. The newer mesalamine preparations in comparison to sulfasalazine had a pooled Peto odds ratio of 0.83 (95 % CI 0.60–1.13) for failure to induce global/clinical improvement or remission and 0.66 (95 % CI 0.42–1.04) for failure to induce endoscopic improvement [19]. Also they noticed that newer mesalamine preparations had fewer side effects compared to sulfasalazine [19].

In another meta-analysis by Nikfar and his colleagues found that none of the new mesalamine formulations were superior to sulfasalazine in inducing overall improvement in patients with active UC (overall improvement defined as a positive change in at least two of the following criteria: sigmoidoscopic appearances, histologic appearances, clinical severity, and percentage of bloody stools) [29]. In four trials (three trials comparing delayed mesalamine and one trial comparing Pentasa to sulfasalazine), the relative risk of overall improvement between sulfasalazine and mesalamine was a nonsignificant value of 1.04 (95 % CI 0.89–1.21). In three trials comparing sulfasalazine and olsalazine, the relative risk for overall improvement was 1.14 (95 % CI 0.91–1.43, $p=0.16$), again a nonsignificant value [29]. In two trials, comparing sulfasalazine and balsalazide, the relative risk of overall improvement was a nonsignificant value of 1.3 (95 % CI 0.93–1.81, $p=0.12$) [29].

## Comparison Between Different Mesalamine Drugs for Induction of Remission

There have been few studies and meta-analyses comparing various oral mesalamine preparations in their ability to induce remission in patients with active UC. A meta-analysis by Rahimi et al. found that balsalazide was superior to mesalamine in the induction of both symptomatic and complete remission [30]. In the pooled analysis of three trials comparing balsalazide to mesalamine in their ability to induce symptomatic remission, the relative risk was 1.23 (95 % CI

1.03–1.47, $p=0.0204$), while the relative risk for ability to induce complete remission was 1.3 (95 % CI 1.002–1.68, $p=0.0481$) [30]. In a meta-analysis by Ford et al., there was no statistically significant difference between the type of mesalamine formulation and their ability to induce remission in patients with active UC (Cochrane $Q=1.11$, $p=0.77$) [18].

In a multicenter, randomized, double-blind trial, olsalazine was similar in efficacy to delayed-release mesalamine in terms of clinical improvement and endoscopic remission in patients with mild to moderately active UC [31]. Kamm et al. compared MMX mesalamine to placebo and delayed-release mesalamine in randomized controlled sphase 3 trial. MMX mesalamine (both 2.4 and 4.8 g/day) was found superior to placebo in the induction of both clinical and endoscopic remission. But delayed-release mesalamine was not superior to both placebo and MMX mesalamine in inducing clinical or endoscopic remission [32].

## Efficacy of Mesalamine in the Maintenance of Remission in UC Patients

Table 7.4 summarizes randomized double-blind controlled trials comparing therapy with various oral 5-ASA formulations in maintaining remission in UC.

## Mesalamine Versus Placebo

The latest Cochrane meta-analysis published in 2006 found that newer mesalamine preparations were superior to placebo in maintaining both clinical and endoscopic remission [33–35]. The Peto odds ratio for failure to maintain clinical or endoscopic remission for mesalamine versus placebo was 0.47 (95 % CI 0.36–0.62) [35]. The number needed to treat to achieve clinical or endoscopic remission was 6 [33].

In the meta-analysis published in 2011 by Ford et al., again mesalamine preparations were shown to be superior to placebo in maintaining remission [18]. A pooled analysis of 11 RCTs and 1,502 patients found that relative risk of relapse for patients on 5-ASAs was 0.65 (95 % CI 0.55–0.76) compared to placebo [18]. The number needed to treat was 4 [18].

## Delayed-Release Mesalamine (Asacol) Versus Placebo

The efficacy of Asacol compared to placebo in maintaining remission in UC patients was studied in two RCTs. Hanauer et al. randomized patients to Asacol 1.6 g/day, Asacol 0.8 g/day, and placebo groups, and they were treated for a period of 6 months. The remission rates in

**Table 7.4** Randomized double-blind controlled trials comparing therapy with various oral 5-ASA formulations in maintaining remission of ulcerative colitis

| Reference | Treatment arms | # pts in each arm | Dosage | Study duration | Primary end point | Results | Efficacy | Adverse events | Withdrawals | Description of S/E |
|---|---|---|---|---|---|---|---|---|---|---|
| McIntyre et al. [91] | Balsalazide Sulfasalazine | 41 38 | 1 g/d 1 g/d | 6 m | To compare balsalazide and sulfasalazine for efficacy and tolerance in the long-term maintenance of remission in patients with UC. A relapse was defined as the recurrence of previous symptoms | 51 % remission 63 % remission | No statistical significance in the maintenance in remissions between the two groups (p=<0.1), thus concluded that coated 5-ASA is a safe, effective therapy for maintaining UC in remission | 2 10 | 0 2 | Rash and abdominal pain |
| Rutgeerts et al. [92] | 5-ASA Sulfasalazine | 131 142 | 0.75 g/d 1.5–2.0 g/d | 12 m | To compare 5-ASA with sulfasalazine in maintaining UC remission. Remission was assessed by symptoms and colonoscopy at investigator's discretion | 28 % relapsed 23 % relapsed | No statistical significance in the cumulative rate of relapse between the two groups. Thus concluded that balsalazide was not significantly different from sulfasalazine in maintaining remission in patients with UC | 24 20 | 9 7 | Diarrhea, nausea, other GI symptoms, skin hypersensitivity, CNS and cardiovascular |
| Mulder et al. [93] | 5-ASA Sulfasalazine | 41 34 | 1,500 mg/d 3 g/d | 12 m | To compare the efficacy and safety of 5-ASA with sulfasalazine for the maintenance of remission in UC. Patients were assessed clinically, endoscopically (recto/sigmoidoscopy), and histologically. Remission was considered when data obtained at each visit were assessed as "normal" or "in remission." Relapse is when patients were prescribed for additional treatment or abnormality in ½ of the assessment groups (clinical, endoscopic a, histology) | 54 % remission 46 % remission | No statistical difference between the remission rates between the two groups (p>0.70), thus concluded that 5-ASA is equally effective as sulfasalazine in the maintenance of remission of UC | 0 4 | 0 4 | Erythroderma, anxiety, backache, laboratory abnormality |

| Study | Drug | N | Dose | Duration | Description | Relapse rate | Conclusion | | | Adverse effects |
|---|---|---|---|---|---|---|---|---|---|---|
| Rijk et al. [94] | Sulfasalazine | 23 | 4 g/d | 48 w | To assess the relapse-preventing properties and the safety of sulfasalazine and olsalazine in patients with UC in remission. A sigmoidoscopy with biopsies was performed to determine whether the colitis was in remission at the inclusion and the 48 w visit | 30.4 % relapse | No statistical significance in the relapse rate between the two groups ($p=0.15$), thus concluded that sulfasalazine and olsalazine are equally effective in maintaining remission of UC with a similar incidence of adverse effects | 7 | 3 | Upper abdominal complaints, rash |
| | Olsalazine | 23 | 2 g/d | | | 26.1 % relapse | | 9 | 3 | Loose stools |
| Küllerich et al. [95] | Olsalazine | 114 | 500 mg b.i.d. | 12 m | The relapse-preventing effect of olsalazine compared with sulfasalazine over 1 year in patients with UC in remission: remission was defined by the following: (1) no visible blood in the stools for more than 3 d within the last week and/or (2) less than 3 stools per day for at least 4 d within the last week and (3) sigmoidoscopy grades 1–2 at admission (no spontaneous bleeding without or with distinct vessels in the mucosa) | 46.9 % relapse rate | The cumulative relapse rate is similar in both groups ($p=0.54$), thus concluded that olsalazine 500 mg b.d. is equally effective and has the same incidence of adverse reactions as sulfasalazine 1 g b.d. in the maintenance therapy of ulcerative colitis | 9 | 9 | Diarrhea, abdominal pain, constipation, urticaria, nausea, dyspepsia |
| | Sulfasalazine | 112 | 1 g b.i.d. | | | 42.4 % relapse rate | | 6 | 6 | Diarrhea, abdominal pain, constipation, urticaria, nausea, dyspepsia |

(continued)

**Table 7.4** (continued)

| Reference | Treatment arms | # pts in each arm | Dosage | Study duration | Primary end point | Results | Efficacy | Adverse events | Withdrawals | Description of S/E |
|---|---|---|---|---|---|---|---|---|---|---|
| Nilsson et al. [96] | Olsalazine | 161 | 1 g/d | 18 m | To compare the relapse-preventing effect of olsalazine and sulfasalazine in patients with UC. Relapse was defined as macroscopic changes in the rectum of grade 3 or 4 | 54.7 % failure rate | No statistical significance in the remission curve ($p=0.19$), thus concluded that the relapse-preventing effect of olsalazine and sulfasalazine did not differ | 39 | 12 | Diarrhea, abdominal pain/cramps, vomiting, eczema, rheumatic symptoms (polyarthritis fever and sacroiliitis), impotence |
| | Sulfasalazine | 161 | 2 g/d | | | 47.2 % failure rate | | 26 | 8 | Diarrhea, eczema, rheumatic symptoms (polyarthritis fever and sacroiliitis), drowsiness, dizziness, vertigo, loss of taste, lack of concentration, psychological discomfort, impotence |
| Ardizzone et al. [97] | 5-ASA | 44 | 0.5 g b.i.d. | 12 m | The prevention of relapse in patients with quiescent UC. Relapse of the disease was defined as appearance of bloody diarrhea with endoscopic signs of inflammation requiring systemic steroids | 20.5 % (6 m) and 38.4 % (12 m) relapse rates | No statistical significant differences in the relapse rate between the two groups after 6 and 12 m ($p=0.32$ and $p=0.18$) thus concluded that 5-ASA is as effective as sulfasalazine in maintaining remission of UC | 5 | 5 | Urticaria and arthralgia |
| | Sulfasalazine | 44 | 1.0 g b.i.d. | | | 27.5 % (6 m) and 51 % (12 m) relapse rates | | 3 | 3 | Severe diarrhea |

| Study | Drug | N | Dose | Duration | Objective | Efficacy | | Outcome | | Side effects |
|---|---|---|---|---|---|---|---|---|---|---|
| Riley et al. [98] | 5-ASA | 48 | 800 mg, 1,200 mg, 1,600 mg/d | 48 w | The long-term efficacy and toxicity of delayed-release mesalamine and enteric-coated sulfasalazine in the maintenance of UC remission. Clinical assessment including sigmoidoscopy and biopsy and symptomatic deterioration (six variables used to assess the severity-stool frequency, rectal bleeding, hemoglobin concentration, ESR, and sigmoidoscopy and histologic grade) | 37.5 % relapse | 20 | No statistical significant differences in the relapse rate or mean time to relapse between the two groups and a better tolerability in the mesalamine group ($p > 0.90$), thus concluded that delayed-release 5-ASA is as effective as sulfasalazine in maintaining remission of UC | 0 | Headache and upper GI upset |
|  | Sulfasalazine | 44 | 2 g, 3 g, 4 g/d |  |  | 38.6 % relapse | 26 |  | 1 | Headache and upper GI upset |
| Green et al. [81] | Balsalazide | 49 | 3 g/d | 12 m | The efficacy and safety of balsalazide (Colazide) compared to mesalazine (Asacol) in maintaining UC remission: symptomatic relapse was defined as the recurrence of moderate or severe symptoms on the patients' overall evaluation | 58 % remission | 30 | Equal proportion of patients in each treatment group remained in remission ($p = 0.4275$) and similar proportion of adverse events ($p = 0.8317$), thus concluded that balsalazide 3 g/d is at least as effective and equally well tolerated and accepted by patients as a long-term maintenance treatment for UC, as delayed-release mesalazine 1.2 g/d | 2 | Headaches, GI symptoms, respiratory infections, abnormal laboratory test, fracture, and hernia |
|  | 5-ASA | 46 | 1.2 g/d |  |  | 58 % remission | 30 |  | 0 | Headaches, GI symptoms, respiratory infections, abnormal laboratory test, suspected UTI, UC complications, cardiac arrest |

(continued)

**Table 7.4** (continued)

| Reference | Treatment arms | # pts in each arm | Dosage | Study duration | Primary end point | Results | Efficacy | Adverse events | Withdrawals | Description of S/E |
|---|---|---|---|---|---|---|---|---|---|---|
| Kruis et al. [99] | Balsalazide (low dose) | 49 | 1.5 g b.i.d. | 26 w | To compare the relapse-preventing effect and safety profile of the two doses of balsalazide and mesalazine. Efficacy assessments were CAI and endoscopic score according to Rachmilewitz and a histologic score | 43.8 % clinical remission | The clinical remission is statistically significant from each other (p=0.006), thus concluded that high-dose balsalazide was superior in maintaining remission in pts with UC. All three treatments were safe and well tolerated | 3 | 3 | Headache, hypertension, malaise, dizziness, abdominal pain, pruritus and skin rashes |
| | Balsalazide (high dose) | 40 | 3.0 g b.i.d. | | | 77.5 % clinical remission | | 2 | 2 | Pancreatitis, gingivitis, alopecia, and nail disorder |
| | 5-ASA | 44 | 0.5 g t.i.d. | | | 56.8 % clinical remission | | 4 | 4 | Palpitation, hypotension, tenesmus, nausea, impotence, diarrhea, and alopecia |
| Mahmud et al. [100] | 5-ASA | 20 | 1.2 g/d | 9 m | To compare/evaluate the renal function (by the measurement of GFR, microalbuminuria and urinary GST activity in patients with UC receiving either mesalazine or olsalazine | GFR, microalbuminuria and urinary GST activity were not statistically different between the two groups | There were no statistical significant differences in GFR and urinary GST activity from the baseline in the two treatment groups (p=ns). The adjusted baseline microalbumin levels were significantly lower in the mesalazine groups (p=0.024), thus concluded that treatment with mesalazine or olsalazine for 9 months had no significant impact on GFR | 2 | 2 | Abdominal pain, abdominal distension, dyspepsia, and nausea |
| | Olsalazine | 20 | 1.0 g/d | | | | | 2 | 2 | Backache, generalized body aches and pains, insomnia, and hypotension |

| Study | Drug | n | Dose | Duration | Objective/definition | Results | Conclusion | | | Adverse events |
|---|---|---|---|---|---|---|---|---|---|---|
| Kohn et al. (abstract) [110] | 5-ASA | 221 | 2.4 g/d | 12 m | To evaluate the efficacy and safety of the two groups: clinical remission was defined as a score of less than or equal to 1 on the UCDAI for at least 1 month, and endoscopic remission was defined as no endoscopic evidence of active disease | 51.4 % clinical remission and 41.9 % clinical and endoscopic remission | There is statistical significant difference between the clinical remission rate ($p=0.026$), but not the clinical and endoscopic remission rate ($p=0.13$), thus concluded that 5-ASA MMX is efficacious as a long-term maintenance therapy in pts with mild to moderate UC (it has a significantly higher number of patients in remission, with a comparable safety profile) | n/a | n/a | |
| | 5-ASA | 221 | 2.4 g/d | | | 36.4 % clinical remission and 31.8 % clinical and endoscopic remission | | n/a | n/a | |
| Prantera et al. [41] | 5-ASA | 162 | 2.4 g/d | 12 m | To assess the proportion of patients in clinical and clinical and endoscopic remission at the end of the study period. Clinical remission was defined as a combined score of less than or equal to 1 on the UCDAI scale, and endoscopic remission was defined as clinical remission, with a normal mucosal appearance upon endoscopic examination | 68 % clinical remission; 60.9 % clinical and endoscopic remission | No statistical significance between both groups in clinical or clinical and endoscopic remission ($p=0.69$), thus concluded that 5-ASA MMX is similarly effective with a comparable safety profile to delayed-release 5-ASA for the maintenance treatment of UC | 92 | 3 | Melena |
| | 5-ASA | 169 | 2.4 g/d | | | 65.9 % clinical remission; 61.7 % clinical and endoscopic remission | | 99 | 3 | Laboratory abnormality and epistaxis |

(continued)

**Table 7.4** (continued)

| Reference | Treatment arms | # pts in each arm | Dosage | Study duration | Primary end point | Results | Efficacy | Adverse events | Withdrawals | Description of S/E |
|---|---|---|---|---|---|---|---|---|---|---|
| Ito et al. [43] | 5-ASA | 65 | 2.4 g/day | 48 w | Percent of patients without bloody stools: each patient would record the condition of their bloody stools, stool frequency, and drug compliance in their diary | 76.9 % without bloody stool | No significant difference in the time to bloody stools ($p=0.27$), thus concluded that the pH- and time-dependent release of mesalamine formulations were similarly safe and effective | 62 | 1 | Nasopharyngitis, diarrhea, abnormal laboratory values |
| | 5-ASA | 66 | 2.25 g/day | | | 69.2 % without bloody stool | | 62 | 3 | Nasopharyngitis, diarrhea, abnormal laboratory values |

5-ASA 5-aminosalicylic acid, GI gastrointestinal, UTI urinary tract infection, GFR glomerular filtration rate, GST glutathione S-transferase, CAI clinical activity index, UC ulcerative colitis, CNS central nervous system, AE adverse events, d day, m months, w week(s), UCDAI ulcerative colitis disease activity index

Reprinted from Sonu I, Lin MV, Blonski W, Lichtenstein GR. Clinical pharmacology of 5-ASA compounds in inflammatory bowel disease. Gastroenterol Clin North Am. 2010 Sep; 39(3): 559-99. © Elsevier 2010 [8]

Asacol 1.6 g/day group, 0.8 g/day group, and placebo were 66 %, 59 %, and 39 %, respectively. Both doses of Asacol maintained significantly better remission rates compared to placebo, but there was no difference in the remission rates of Asacol 1.6 g/day and Asacol 0.8 g/day [34]. In another RCT, Asacol 1.2 g/day for 12 months maintained remission in 77 % of patients compared to 51 % of patients in the placebo group ($p = 0.035$) [35].

## Pentasa Versus Placebo

Miner et al. demonstrated that Pentasa 4 g/day was significantly superior to placebo in maintaining remission at 12 months. Around 36 % of patients receiving Pentasa relapsed compared to 64 % of patients on placebo ($p < 0.05$) [36].

## Apriso Versus Placebo

Lichtenstein and his colleagues demonstrated the superiority of Apriso (mesalamine granules) over placebo in maintaining remission at 6 months. A total of 305 patients were randomized to either Apriso (i = 209) 1.5 g/day or placebo ($n = 96$). The percentage of patients who remained in remission at the end of 6 months was significantly higher in the Apriso group (78.9 %) compared to placebo (58.3 %) ($p < 0.001$) [37].

## Olsalazine Versus Placebo

In two clinical trials comparing olsalazine to placebo, there was no statistically significant difference in their efficacy to maintain remission in patients with inactive UC (RR = 0.72, 95 % CI 0.40–1.30) [38, 39].

## Mesalamine Versus Sulfasalazine

The latest Cochrane meta-analysis demonstrated that sulfasalazine was significant to newer mesalamine preparations in its efficacy to maintain remission [33]. The Peto odds ratio for failure to maintain clinical or endoscopic remission between sulfasalazine and mesalamine formulations was 1.29 (95 % CI 1.05–1.57), with a negative number needed to treat of 19 [35]. Also, the adverse event profile of sulfasalazine and newer 5-ASA drugs was found to be similar (odds ratio 1.16 for sulfasalazine and odds ratio of 1.3 for newer mesalamine preparations). But authors also observed that trials might be biased in favor of sulfasalazine because the patients enrolled in sulfasalazine trials were tolerant to sulfasalazine, and this might have minimized its adverse effects [33].

In meta-analysis by Nikfar et al., there was no statistically significant difference between pH-dependent and pH-independent mesalamine preparations and sulfasalazine relapse rates [29]. The pooled analysis of 6 trials showed nonsignificant relative risk of 0.98 (95 % CI 0.78–1.23, $p = 0.85$) [29]. The pooled analysis of five trials comparing olsalazine and sulfasalazine yielded a nonsignificant relative risk of 0.93 (95 % CI 0.77–1.12, $p = 0.42$), showing no difference in their efficacy to maintain remission. Similarly, pooled analysis of two trials comparing balsalazide to sulfasalazine yielded a nonsignificant relative risk of 1.3 (95 % CI 0.93–1.81, $p = 0.12$) [29].

## Comparison Between Different Mesalamine Drugs for Maintenance of Remission

In a recent meta-analysis, Ford et al. did not find any statistically significant difference between the type of mesalamine preparation and their efficacy in preventing a relapse in patients with inactive UC (Cochrane $Q = 1.23$, $p = 0.54$) [18].

In a meta-analysis by Rahimi et al., balsalazide was superior to mesalamine in maintaining remission in UC patients. A pooled analysis of two trials yielded a nonsignificant relative risk of 0.77 (95 % CI 0.56–1.07, $p = 0.12$) [30]. In an RCT by Courtney et al., olsalazine was found to be superior to mesalamine in maintaining remission. Patients were treated with olsalazine 1 g/day and mesalamine 1.2 g/day for 12 months. The relapse rate was significantly lower in the olsalazine group (12 %) than in the mesalamine group (33 %), with a significant $p$ value of 0.024 [40].

In an RCT, Prantera et al. compared MMX mesalamine and Asacol. A total of 331 patients were randomized to receive either MMX mesalamine ($n = 162$, 2.4 g/day once daily) or Asacol ($n = 169$, 2.4 g/day in two divided doses) for 12 months [41]. Sixty-eight percent (68 %) of patients in the MMX mesalamine group and 66 % of patients in the Asacol group were in clinical remission ($p = 0.69$), while 61 % of patients in the MMX mesalamine group and 62 % of patients in the Asacol group were in clinical and endoscopic remission ($p = 0.89$). This study demonstrated that there was no significant difference in efficacy of MMX mesalamine and Asacol in maintaining remission in UC patients [41]. Similarly, in a recent RCT by D'Haens et al., it was demonstrated that MMX mesalamine and delayed-release mesalamine (Asacol) were similar in their efficacy for the maintenance of endoscopic remission in UC patients. MMX mesalamine (2.4 g/day once daily) maintained endoscopic remission in 83.7 % of per protocol population compared to 81.5 % by delayed-release mesalamine (1.6 g/day twice daily dosage) [42].

In a multicenter randomized, double-blind study, Ito et al. compared efficacy of pH-dependent mesalamine (65 patients) to time-dependent mesalamine (66 patients) preparations in the maintenance of remission. At the end of 48 weeks of treatment, 77 % patients in the pH-dependent 5-ASA group and 69 % of patients in the time-dependent 5-ASA group were in remission. Thus, both preparations were similar in their efficacy of maintaining remission in UC patients [43]. But patients receiving pH-dependent 5-ASA were in remission longer than those receiving time-dependent 5-ASA [43].

## Topical Mesalamine in the Induction of Remission

Several randomized controlled studies and meta-analyses have demonstrated the efficacy of topical mesalamine preparations in the induction of remission in active distal ulcerative colitis (proctitis and left-sided colitis). Current ACG guidelines recommend topical mesalamine as the first-line treatment for patients with mild to moderately active ulcerative proctitis, while combination therapy of oral and topical mesalamine is recommended for active left-sided colitis [1]. But the main disadvantage of rectal therapy seems to be poor patient tolerability. Some of the reasons for this include problems with retention and leakage, difficulty in administration, and patient discomfort.

## Topical Mesalamine Versus Placebo

In several RCTs, mesalamine suppositories and liquid enemas have demonstrated their superiority over placebo in the induction of remission [44–51]. In the most recent meta-analysis by Marshall and his colleagues, rectal 5-ASA was demonstrated to be superior to placebo in all respects, i.e., induction of symptomatic, endoscopic, and histologic improvement and remission [52]. In a pooled analysis of eight trials, the odds ratio in favor of topical mesalamine for symptomatic remission was 8.3 (95 % CI 4.28–16.28, $p < 0.00001$), odds ratio for endoscopic remission was 5.31 (seven trials, 95 % CI 3.15–8.92, $p < 0.00001$), and odds ratio for histologic remission was 6.28 (five trials, 95 % CI 2.74–14.4, $p < 0.0001$) [52].

## Topical Mesalamine Versus Topical Steroids

Meta-analyses and RCTs have shown that rectal mesalamine preparations are superior to rectal steroids in the induction of remission in patients with active UC. In the meta-analysis of seven trials by Marshall et al., the pooled odds ratio in favor of rectal mesalamine for induction of symptomatic improvement was 1.56 (95 % CI 1.15–2.11, $p = 0.004$) and

for induction of symptomatic remission was 1.65 (95 % CI 1.11–2.45, $p = 0.01$) [52].

## Topical Mesalamine Versus Oral Mesalamine or Combination of Oral and Rectal Mesalamine

In the first meta-analysis published by Marshall et al. in 1995, the topical mesalamine was found to be significantly superior to oral mesalamine in the induction of both symptomatic improvement (odds ratio 6.3, 95 % CI 2.7–14.5) and symptomatic remission (odds ratio 4.1, 95 % CI 1.4–10.9) [53]. Several randomized controlled trials have also demonstrated superiority of rectal 5-ASA over oral 5-ASA inactive UC [54–56]. An RCT published by Prantera et al. in 2005 found that MMX mesalamine (1.2 g/day) was superior to mesalamine suspension (4 g/day) after 8 weeks of treatment [57]. But several concerns regarding the design of the trial were raised [58]. The primary end point in this trial was set at 8 weeks in contrast to 3–6 weeks set in other induction of remission studies. The 5-ASA suspension arm was numerically superior to oral 5-ASA groups at 4 weeks (68 % vs. 58 % respectively) [58]. Also results in this study were confounded by high dropout rate of 30 % in the 5-ASA suspension arm. In the latest meta-analysis published by Marshall et al., which included Prantera et al.'s study, the rectal 5-ASA was not found superior to oral 5-ASA. The pooled odds ratio for symptomatic improvement was 2.25 (95 % CI 0.53–19.54, $p = 0.27$) [52].

In another recent meta-analysis published by Ford et al., there was no significant difference between oral and rectal 5-ASA in the induction of remission in patients with mild to moderate UC [59]. In the pooled analysis of four RCTs, the relative risk of failure to achieve remission with topical mesalamine compared to oral mesalamine was 0.82 (95 % CI 0.52–1.28). Ford et al. also demonstrated that combination treatment with rectal and oral mesalamine was significantly superior to oral mesalamine alone in the induction of remission in mild to moderately active UC [59]. The relative risk of failure to achieve remission with combined therapy compared to oral therapy alone was 0.65 (four RCTs, 95 % CI 0.47–0.91). The number needed to treat with combined therapy to achieve remission was 5 [59].

## Comparison Among Various Topical Mesalamine Preparations

In their systematic review, Harris and Lichtenstein concluded that all four rectal mesalamine preparations were equally efficacious in the treatment of proctitis. They also suggested that suspension enemas, gels, and foams were equal in their efficacy for treatment of active distal UC [58].

A study by Campieri et al. demonstrated that mesalamine suspension enema was similar in efficacy to mesalamine suppositories in the treatment of active proctitis [60]. In a single-blind, randomized study, mesalamine foam and gel were equal in efficacy when used in patients with active distal UC. But gel preparation was better tolerated by patients [61]. In another randomized, single-blind study, the response rates were comparable between mesalamine foam arm and mesalamine suspension arm when used in patients with distal UC [62].

## Topical Mesalamine in the Maintenance of Remission

Topical mesalamine has also shown to be effective in the maintenance of remission in distal UC patients up to 1 year [58]. Current American College of Gastroenterology guidelines recommend 5-ASA as the first-line therapy for the maintenance of remission in patients with left-sided inactive UC [1].

## Topical Mesalamine Versus Placebo

In a meta-analysis of seven randomized controlled trials (total 555 patients), topical mesalamine demonstrated its superiority over placebo in the maintenance of remission in quiescent UC. The relative risk of relapse for patients on topical mesalamine compared to those on placebo was 0.60 (95 % CI 0.49–0.73) [63]. The number needed to treat was 3. Since only one trial included patients with extensive colitis, the authors concluded that topical mesalamine was only effective in maintaining remission in patients with inactive distal colitis [63].

## Topical Mesalamine Versus Oral Mesalamine Versus Combination of Oral and Topical Mesalamine

In a meta-analysis of three RCTs (total 129 patients), Ford et al. demonstrated that intermittent therapy with topical mesalamine was superior to oral therapy in the prevention of relapse in those with inactive UC [59]. The relative risk of relapse with topical mesalamine compared to oral mesalamine was 0.64 (95 % CI 0.43–0.95). The number needed to treat with intermittent topical mesalamine therapy was 4 (95 % CI 2–14) [59]. In the same meta-analysis, pooled analysis of two RCTs comparing combined therapy with oral and topical mesalamine to oral mesalamine alone did not show any significant difference in the relapse rates. The relative

risk of relapse with combined therapy compared to oral mesalamine alone was 0.48 (95 % CI 0.17–1.38) [59].

## Adverse Effects/Tolerability of Mesalamine Preparations

Mesalamine preparations are well tolerated compared to sulfasalazine. The most common adverse effects with mesalamine are nausea, vomiting, diarrhea, headache, and rash [14]. These are usually dose related. Less common side effects, which are idiosyncratic, include pancreatitis, hepatitis, pneumonitis, nephrotoxicity, leukopenia, hemolytic anemia, agranulocytosis, and pulmonary fibrosis [7].

Two side effects, which are seen more frequently with mesalamine preparations than sulfasalazine, are worsening of diarrhea and nephrotoxicity [64]. Worsening of diarrhea is particularly more common with olsalazine. In clinical trials of olsalazine approximately 36 % of patients experienced worsening of diarrhea, and about 10–20 % of them had to be withdrawn [64]. Drug-induced diarrhea is characterized by increased diarrhea (usually bloody), urgency, nocturnal diarrhea, fevers, myalgia, and arthralgia. These usually begin within 24–48 h after starting the medication and resolve within 24–48 h after discontinuing the medication [64].

Renal toxicity is a very rare side effect of mesalamine preparations [64]. Though animal studies demonstrated a significant nephrotoxicity with high doses of mesalamine, in clinical practice this is rarely reported [65]. A large British epidemiological study showed that risk of renal toxicity with mesalamine/sulfasalazine is very low, and it can be partly attributed to underlying IBD [66].

## Mesalamine Versus Placebo

In a meta-analysis of ten induction of remission studies, there was no significant difference between mesalamine preparations and placebo in the likelihood of experiencing any adverse event (RR = 1.02, 95 % CI 0.8–1.29) [38]. Also there was no statistically significant difference in the frequency of any individual adverse event except that there was a lower risk of abdominal pain with mesalamine [18].

In a pooled analysis of five maintenance of remission trials, there was no statistically significant difference between mesalamine preparations and placebo in the incidence of total adverse events (RR = 0.98, 95 % CI 0.84–1.15) or individual adverse event like nausea or vomiting or headache [18]. Also there was no significant difference detected in the incidence of adverse events between topical mesalamine and placebo when used to prevent relapse of UC. A pooled analysis of 6 trials yielded an RR of 1.01 (95 % CI 0.59–1.72) [18].

## Mesalamine Versus Sulfasalazine

In Cochrane meta-analysis of the induction of remission trials, sulfasalazine resulted in significantly higher proportion of withdrawals due to adverse events compared to mesalamine preparations [19]. But in the maintenance of remission trials, there was no difference in the number of adverse events between sulfasalazine and mesalamine. Authors noted that there might be a bias in favor of sulfasalazine as most studies included patients who were known to be tolerant to sulfasalazine in the past [33]. In another meta-analysis by Nikfar et al., there was no difference in the incidence of adverse events or withdrawals due to adverse events between sulfasalazine and mesalamine (delayed and controlled release) or sulfasalazine and olsalazine [29]. There were significantly higher withdrawals due to adverse events with sulfasalazine compared to balsalazide [29].

## Comparison Between Mesalamine Preparations

Loftus and his colleagues performed a systematic review of 46 trials to evaluate the difference in the short-term adverse effects of various mesalamine preparations. They concluded that all three mesalamine preparations resulted in similar adverse events in short term [67]. Though olsalazine resulted in higher number of adverse events than placebo, this difference was not statistically significant [67]. Rahimi et al. in their meta-analysis showed that the number of patients with any adverse events and withdrawals due to serious adverse events was similar for balsalazide and mesalamine [30].

## Mesalamine Dosing

The Cochrane meta-analysis demonstrated a trend toward dose-response relationship in the induction of remission trials and no dose-response relationship in the maintenance of remission trials [19, 33].

In ASCEND I (Assessing the Safety and Clinical Efficacy of New Dose of 5-ASA) trial, patients with mild to moderately active UC were randomized to receive either 4.8 or 2.4 g/day of mesalamine. There was significant improvement on the higher-dose mesalamine compared to standard dose in patients with moderately active UC (57 % in 2.4 g/day vs. 72.4 % in 4.8 g/day, $p=0.0384$), but not in those with mild

disease [68]. In ASCEND 2 trial, which only included patients with moderately active UC, patients were randomized to receive 4.8 or 2.4 g/day. There was significant treatment success with 4.8 g/day than 2.4 g/day (72 % vs. 59 %; $p=0.036$) [69]. Thus, results of ASCEND I and ASCEND II trials suggest that dose of 2.4 g/day is sufficient to induce remission in patients with mild disease, while those with moderately active UC benefit from higher dose of 4.8 g/day [69]. The ASCEND III trial, which also compared mesalamine 4.8 g/day to 2.4 g/day in moderately active UC, showed no difference in the efficacy between the two doses. This showed that higher-dose mesalamine (4.8 g/day) is not effective in all patient populations. Indeed, in post hoc analysis, therapeutic benefit of 4.8 g/day over 2.4 g/day dose was seen in patients on multiple UC medications [70].

The meta-analysis by Ford et al. demonstrated that a mesalamine dose of $\geq 2$ g/day was superior to <2 g/day dose both for induction of remission (RR=0.91, 95 % CI 0.85–0.98) and prevention of relapse (RR=0.79, 95 % CI 0.64–0.97) [38]. Also this meta-analysis showed that doses $\geq 2.5$ g/day were not superior to doses between 2 and 2.4 g/day (see Tables 7.5 and 7.6 for details) [18].

Also recent meta-analyses and RCTs have demonstrated that once-daily dosing is at least as effective as conventional dosing [23, 32, 56, 71]. Feagan and Macdonald performed a meta-analysis comparing once-daily dosing of oral mesalamine to conventional dosing. There was no significant difference between once-daily dosing and conventional dosing in terms of clinical remission (RR=0.95, 95 % CI 0.82–1.10), clinical improvement (RR=0.87, 95 % CI 0.68–1.10), or relapse at 6 months (RR=1.10, 95 % CI 0.83–1.46) or 12 months (RR=0.92, 95 % CI 0.83–1.03) [72]. There was no difference in the compliance rates between once-daily dosing and conventional dosing. But authors attributed this to higher compliance observed in clinical trial environment [72]. Similarly, the meta-analysis by Ford et al. showed for the prevention of relapse once daily mesalamine was equally effective as conventional dosing schedules (RR of relapse=0.94; 95 % CI 0.82–1.08) [73]. There was no difference in the frequency of adverse events (RR=1.08, 95%CI 0.97–1.20), but there was no any evidence to suggest that compliance was superior with once-daily dosing (RR=0.87; 95 % CI 0.46–1.66) [73]. See Table 7.7 for details.

## Conclusion

Mesalamine is the first-line agent for both induction of remission and maintenance of remission in patients with mild to moderately severe ulcerative colitis. Topical mesalamine is the preferred treatment for patients with dis-

**Table 7.5** Characteristics of randomized controlled trials of high-dose 5-ASAs vs. standard-dose 5-ASAs in inducing remission in active ulcerative colitis

| Study | Country and number of centers | Disease distribution | Criteria used to define remission | Number of patients | 5-ASA used | Duration of therapy (weeks) | Methodology |
|---|---|---|---|---|---|---|---|
| Miglioli et al. (1990) [101] | Italy, 8 sites | 15 % pancolitis, 42 % left-sided colitis, 43 % proctosigmoiditis | Normal mucosa at colonoscopy | 48 | Mesalamine (Asacol) 800 mg or 1.2 g t.i.d. | 4 | Randomization stated, concealment unclear, double blind |
| Miner et al. (1995) [108] | USA, multiple sites | Not reported | Sigmoidoscopic remission | 168 | Mesalamine (Pentasa) 2 or 4 g daily | 8 | Randomization, concealment, and blinding unclear |
| Hanauer et al. (1996) [22] | USA, 20 sites | 30 % pancolitis, 70 % distal colitis | Sigmoidoscopic score of ≤4 out of 15 | 192 | Mesalamine (Pentasa) 500 mg or 1 g q.i.d. | 8 | Randomization and concealment unclear, double blind |
| Hanauer et al. (1998) [68] | USA and Canada, 55 sites | 20 % pancolitis, 34 % left-sided colitis, 46 % proctosigmoiditis | Clinical and endoscopic remission | 268 | Mesalamine (Asacol) 800 mg t.i.d. or 1.6 g t.i.d. | 6 | Randomization and concealment unclear, double blind |
| D'Haens et al. (2012) [109] | UK, Holland, Belgium, 8 sites | 28 % pancolitis, 72 % left-sided colitis | UCDAI score ≤1 | 25 | Mesalamine (MMX) 2.4 or 4.8 g o.d. | 8 | Randomization and concealment unclear, double blind |
| Hanauer et al. (2007) [68] | USA and Canada, 41 sites | 24 % pancolitis, 30 % left-sided colitis, 46 % proctosigmoiditis | Clinical and endoscopic remission | 301 | Mesalamine (Asacol) 800 mg t.i.d. or 1.6 g t.i.d. | 6 | Randomization and concealment unclear, double blind |
| Kamm et al. (2007) [32] | Multinational, 49 sites | 23 % pancolitis, 77 % distal colitis | Modified sigmoidoscopic score of ≤1 out of 3 with no mucosal friability | 257 | Mesalamine (MMX) 2.4 g or 4.8 g o.d. or mesalamine (Asacol) 800 mg t.i.d. | 8 | Randomization unclear, concealment stated, double blind |
| Lichtenstein et al. (2010) [23] | Multinational, 52 sites | 15 % pancolitis, 85 % distal colitis | Clinical and endoscopic remission | 187 | Mesalamine (MMX) 1.2 g b.i.d. or 4.8 g o.d. | 8 | Randomization unclear, concealment stated, double blind |
| Sandborn et al. 2009 [70] | Multinational, 113 sites | 16 % pancolitis, 35 % left-sided colitis, 48 % proctosigmoiditis | Clinical and endoscopic remission | 772 | Mesalamine (Asacol) 800 mg t.i.d. or 1.6 g t.i.d. | 6 | Randomization unclear, concealment stated, double blind |
| Ito et al. (2010) [43] | Japan, 53 sites | Not reported | UCDAI score ≤2 and a bloody stool score of 0 | 196 | Mesalamine (Asacol) 2.4 or 3.6 g daily, mesalamine (Pentasa) 2.25 g daily | 8 | Randomization unclear, concealment stated, double blind |

5-ASA 5-aminosalicylic acid, b.i.d. twice daily, o.d. once daily, q.i.d. four times daily, RCT randomized controlled trial, t.i.d. three times daily, UC ulcerative colitis, UCDAI ulcerative colitis disease activity index

Reprinted from Ford AC, Achkar JP, Khan KJ, Kane SV, Talley NJ, Marshall JK, Moayyedi P. Efficacy of 5-aminosalicylates in ulcerative colitis: systematic review and meta-analysis. Am J Gastroenterol. 2011 Apr;106(4):601-16. © Nature Publishing Group 2011) [18]

**Table 7.6** Characteristics of randomized controlled trials of high- or standard-dose 5-ASAs vs. low-dose 5-ASAs in preventing relapse in quiescent ulcerative colitis

| Study | Country and number of centers | Disease distribution | Criteria used to define relapse | Number of patients | 5-ASA used | Duration of therapy (months) | Methodology |
|---|---|---|---|---|---|---|---|
| Azad Khan et al. (1977) [7] | UK, 1 site | Not reported | Sigmoidoscopic relapse | 170 | Sulfasalazine 1, 2, or 4 g daily | 6 | Randomization, concealment, and blinding unclear |
| Green et al. (2002) [112] | UK, 4 sites | 33 % pancolitis, 40 % left-sided colitis, 27 % proctosigmoiditis | Increased stool frequency for 1 week and friable mucosa or spontaneous hemorrhage at sigmoidoscopy | 108 | Balsalazide 3 or 6 g daily | 12 | Randomization and concealment unclear, double blind |
| Travis et al. (1994) [102] | UK and Sweden, 2 sites | 35 % pancolitis, 48 % left-sided colitis, 17 % proctosigmoiditis | Increase in bowel frequency with blood or mucus and active disease on sigmoidoscopy | 198 | Olsalazine 500 mg, 1 g, or 2 g daily | 12 | Randomization, concealment, and blinding unclear |
| Fockens et al. (1995) [113] | Holland, 12 sites | 22 % pancolitis, 28 % left-sided colitis, 50 % proctosigmoiditis | Clinical assessment and sigmoidoscopic score of >2 out of 18 | 169 | Mesalamine (Pentasa) 500 mg or 1 g t.i.d. | 12 | Randomization and concealment unclear, double blind |
| Kruis et al. (2001) [99] | Germany, 21 sites | 40 % pancolitis, 34 % left-sided colitis, 24 % proctosigmoiditis | CAI $\geq 6$ and EI >4 | 89 | Balsalazide 1.5 or 3 g b.i.d. | 6 | Randomization and concealment unclear, double blind |
| Paoluzi et al. (2005) [103] | Italy, 1 site | 23 % pancolitis, 77 % left-sided colitis | Clinical or endoscopic relapse | 156 | Mesalamine (Asacol) 400 or 800 mg t.i.d. | 12 | Randomization and concealment unclear, single blind |
| Kruis et al. (2011) [104] | Multinational, 65 sites | Not reported | EI >3 | 648 | Mesalamine (Salofalk) 3 g o.d., 1.5 g o.d., or 500 mg t.i.d. | 12 | Randomization and concealment stated, double blind |

*5-ASA* 5-aminosalicylic acid, *b.i.d.* twice daily, *CAI* clinical activity index, *o.d.* once daily, *EI* endoscopic index, *RCT* randomized controlled trial, *t.i.d.* three times daily, *UC* ulcerative colitis

Reprinted from Ford AC, Achkar JP, Khan KJ, Kane SV, Talley NJ, Marshall JK, Moayyedi P. Efficacy of 5-aminosalicylates in ulcerative colitis: systematic review and meta-analysis. Am J Gastroenterol. 2011 Apr;106(4):601-16. © Nature Publishing Group 2011) [18]

tal disease, and combination of oral and rectal mesalamine is preferred in patients with more extensive disease. Several individual studies and meta-analyses have demonstrated the superiority of mesalamine over placebo. Sulfasalazine was the first mesalamine-containing drug used, but due to its intolerance, several newer mesalamine agents have been developed without the sulfa component. Newer mesalamine preparations have been shown to be equivalent to sulfasalazine in their efficacy to induce remission and maintain remission. Also, various newer mesalamine preparations are similar in their efficacy. Therefore, the choice of initial agent should be based on patient preference, cost-effectiveness, tolerability, and patient's ability to comply with the treatment regimen.

**Table 7.7** Characteristics of randomized controlled trials of once-daily mesalamine dosing vs. a conventional dosing schedule in preventing relapse in quiescent ulcerative colitis

| Study | Country and number of centers | Disease distribution | Criteria used to define relapse | Number of patients | 5-ASA used | Duration of therapy (months) | Methodology |
|---|---|---|---|---|---|---|---|
| | USA, 2 sites | 75 % pancolitis, 20 % left-sided colitis, 5 % proctitis | UCDAI score >3 or an increase >3 | 20 | Mesalamine (Asacol) at a dose between 1.6 and 3.2 g per day once-daily vs. twice-daily dosing | 12 | Randomization and concealment stated, single blind |
| Kamm et al. (2008) [106] | Multinational, 101 sites | Not reported | Clinical or endoscopic relapse | 362 | Mesalamine (MMX) 2.4 g o.d. vs. 1.2 g b.i.d. | 12 | Randomization unclear, concealment stated, unblinded |
| Prantera et al. (2009) [41] | Italy, Poland, and Ukraine, 47 sites | 41.1 % left-sided colitis, 58.9 % proctosigmoiditis | UCDAI score >1 or endoscopic evidence of active disease | 331 | Mesalamine (MMX) 2.4 g o.d. vs. mesalamine (Asacol) 1.6 g in the morning and 800 mg in the evening | 12 | Randomization and concealment stated, double blind |
| Dignass et al. (2009) [107] | Multinational, 68 sites | 28.5 % pancolitis, 71.5 % left-sided colitis | UCDAI score >2 | 362 | Mesalamine (Pentasa) 2 g o.d. vs. 1 g b.i.d. | 12 | Randomization unclear, concealment stated, single blind |
| Sandborn et al. (2010) [114] | USA, Canada, and Puerto Rico, 193 sites | 38.3 % pancolitis, 33.6 % left-sided colitis, 20.1 % proctosigmoiditis | SCCAI >4 | 1,023 | Mesalamine (Asacol) at a dose between 1.6 and 2.4 g per day once-daily vs. twice-daily dosing | 12 | Randomization unclear, concealment stated, single blind |
| Kruis et al. (2011) [104] | Multinational, 65 sites | Not reported | EI >3 | 430 | Mesalamine (Salofalk) 1.5 g o.d. vs. 500 mg t.i.d. | 12 | Randomization and concealment stated, double blind |
| Hawthorne et al. (2011) (CODA) [105] | UK, 32 sites | 30 % pancolitis, 56 % left-sided colitis, 14 % proctitis | Symptoms of relapse with a Baron score of >1 | 213 | Mesalamine (Asacol) 2.4 g o.d. vs. 800 mg t.i.d. | 12 | Randomization and concealment unclear, single blind |

*b.i.d.* twice-daily, *EI* endoscopic index, *o.d.* once daily, *SCCAI* simple clinical colitis activity index, *t.i.d.* three times daily, *UC* ulcerative colitis, *UCDAI* ulcerative colitis disease activity index

With permission from Ford AC, Khan KJ, Sandborn WJ, Kane SV, Moayyedi P. Once-daily dosing vs. conventional dosing schedule of mesalamine and relapse of quiescent ulcerative colitis: systematic review and meta-analysis. Am J Gastroenterol. 2011;106(12):2070-7. © Nature Publishing Group 2011 [18]

# References

1. Kornbluth A, Sachar DB, Practice Parameters Committee of the American College of Gastroenterology. Ulcerative colitis practice guidelines in adults: American College of Gastroenterology, Practice Parameters Committee. Am J Gastroenterol. 2010;105(3): 501–23.
2. Svartz N. Salazopyrin—a new sulfanilamide preparation. A. Therapeutic results in rheumatoid arthritis. B. Therapeutic results in ulcerative colitis. C. Toxic manifestations on treatment with sulfanilamide preparations. Acta Med Scand. 1942;110: 577–90.
3. Svartz N. Sulfasalazine: II. Some notes on the discovery and development of salazopyrin. Am J Gastroenterol. 1988;83: 497–503. 105(3):501–23.
4. Baron JH, Connell AM, Lennard-Jones JE, Jones FA. Sulphasalazine and salicylazosulphadimidine in ulcerative colitis. Lancet. 1962;1(7239):1094–6.
5. Misiewicz J, Lennard-Jones J. Conell et al. Controlled trial of sulphasalazine in maintenance therapy for ulcerative colitis Lancet. 1965;1:185–8.

6. Azad Khan AK, Howes DT, Piris J, et al. Optimum dose of sulphasalazine for maintenance treatment in ulcerative colitis. Gut. 1980;21:232–40.

7. Nielsen OH, Munck LK. Drug insight: aminosalicylates for the treatment of IBD. Nat Clin Pract Gastroenterol Hepatol. 2007;4(3):160–70. Review.

8. Sonu I, Lin MV, Blonski W, Lichtenstein GR. Clinical pharmacology of 5-ASA compounds in inflammatory bowel disease. Gastroenterol Clin North Am. 2010;39(3):559–99. doi:10.1016/j.gtc.2010.08.011.

9. Gionchetti P, Belluzzi A, Campieri M, et al. 5-Aminosalicylic acid in patients with ulcerative colitis in remission: plasma levels after administration of a new rectal enema. Methods Find Exp Clin Pharmacol. 1988;10(10):667–9. PubMed PMID: 3236941. Related citations.

10. Dew MJ, Cardwell M, Kidwai NS, Evans BK, Rhodes J. 5-Aminosalicylic acid in serum and urine after administration by enema to patients with colitis. J Pharm Pharmacol. 1983; 35(5):323–4.

11. Frieri G, Pimpo MT, Palumbo GC, et al. Rectal and colonic mesalazine concentration in ulcerative colitis: oral vs. oral plus topical treatment. Aliment Pharmacol Ther. 1999;13(11):1413–7.

12. Fernandez-Becker NQ, Moss AC. Improving delivery of aminosalicylates in ulcerative colitis: effect on patient outcomes. Drugs. 2008;68(8):1089–103. Review.

13. Prakash A, Markham A. Oral delayed-release mesalazine: a review of its use in ulcerative colitis and Crohn's disease. Drugs. 1999;57(3):383–408. Review.

14. Sandborn WJ, Hanauer SB. Systematic review: the pharmacokinetic profiles of oral mesalazine formulations and mesalazine pro-drugs used in the management of ulcerative colitis. Aliment Pharmacol Ther. 2003;17(1):29–42. Review.

15. Sandborn WJ, Hanauer SB, Buch A. Comparable systemic absorption of 5-ASA and N-AC-5- ASA from U.S. Asacol and Colazal. Am J Gastroenterol. 2002;97:S263.

16. Sandborn WJ. Oral 5-ASA therapy in ulcerative colitis: what are the implications of the new formulations? J Clin Gastroenterol. 2008;42(4):338–44. Review.

17. Sandborn WJ. Treatment of ulcerative colitis with oral mesalamine: advances in drug formulation, efficacy expectations and dose response, compliance, and chemoprevention. Rev Gastroenterol Disord. 2006;6(2):97–105. Spring.

18. Ford AC, Achkar JP, Khan KJ, Kane SV, Talley NJ, Marshall JK, Moayyedi P. Efficacy of 5-aminosalicylates in ulcerative colitis: systematic review and meta-analysis. Am J Gastroenterol. 2011;106(4):601–16. Review.

19. Sutherland L, Macdonald JK. Oral 5-aminosalicylic acid for induction of remission in ulcerative colitis. Cochrane Database Syst Rev. 2006;(2):CD000543. Review.

20. Schroeder KW, Tremaine WJ, Ilstrup DM. Coated oral 5-aminosalicylic acid t therapy for mildly to moderately active ulcerative colitis. A randomized study. N Engl J Med. 1987; 317(26):1625–9.

21. Sninsky CA, Cort DH, Shanahan F, Powers BJ, Sessions JT, Pruitt RE, Jacobs WH, Lo SK, Targan SR, Cerda JJ, et al. Oral mesalamine (Asacol) for mildly to moderately active ulcerative colitis. A multicenter study. Ann Intern Med. 1991;115(5):350–5.

22. Hanauer S, Schwartz J, Robinson M, Roufail W, Arora S, Cello J, Safdi M. Mesalamine capsules for treatment of active ulcerative colitis: results of a controlled trial. Pentasa Study Group. Am J Gastroenterol. 1993;88(8):1188–97.

23. Lichtenstein GR, Kamm MA, Boddu P, Gubergrits N, Lyne A, Butler T, Lees K, Joseph RE, Sandborn WJ. Effect of once- or twice-daily MMX mesalamine (SPD476) for the induction of remission of mild to moderately active ulcerative colitis. Clin Gastroenterol Hepatol. 2007;5(1):95–102.

24. Hetzel DJ, Shearman DJ, Bochner F, et al. Azodisalicylate (olsalazine) in the treatment of active ulcerative colitis. A placebo controlled clinical trial and assessment of drug disposition. J Gastroenterol Hepatol. 1986;1:257–66.

25. Feurle GE, Theuer D, Velasco S, Barry BA, Wördehoff D, Sommer A, Jantschek G, Kruis W. Olsalazine versus placebo in the treatment of mild to moderate ulcerative colitis: a randomised double blind trial. Gut. 1989;30(10):1354–61.

26. Selby WS, Barr GD, Ireland A, Mason CH, Jewell DP. Olsalazine in active ulcerative colitis. Br Med J (Clin Res Ed). 1985; 291(6506):1373–5.

27. Meyers S, Sachar DB, Present DH, Janowitz HD. Olsalazine sodium in the treatment of ulcerative colitis among patients intolerant of sulfasalazine. A prospective, randomized, placebo-controlled, double-blind, dose-ranging clinical trial. Gastroenterology. 1987;93(6):1255–62.

28. Scherl EJ, Pruitt R, Gordon GL, Lamet M, Shaw A, Huang S, Mareya S, Forbes WP. Safety and efficacy of a new 3.3 g b.i.d. tablet formulation in patients with mild-to-moderately-active ulcerative colitis: a multicenter, randomized, double-blind, placebo-controlled study. Am J Gastroenterol. 2009;104(6): 1452–9.

29. Nikfar S, Rahimi R, Rezaie A, Abdollahi M. A meta-analysis of the efficacy of sulfasalazine in comparison with 5-aminosalicylates in the induction of improvement and maintenance of remission in patients with ulcerative colitis. Dig Dis Sci. 2009;54(6):1157–70.

30. Rahimi R, Nikfar S, Rezaie A, Abdollahi M. Comparison of mesalazine and balsalazide in induction and maintenance of remission in patients with ulcerative colitis: a meta-analysis. Dig Dis Sci. 2009;54(4):712–21.

31. Kruis W, Brandes JW, Schreiber S, Theuer D, Krakamp B, Schütz E, Otto P, Lorenz-Mayer H, Ewe K, Judmaier G. Olsalazine versus mesalazine in the treatment of mild to moderate ulcerative colitis. Aliment Pharmacol Ther. 1998;12(8):707–15.

32. Kamm MA, Sandborn WJ, Gassull M, Schreiber S, Jackowski L, Butler T, Lyne A, Stephenson D, Palmen M, Joseph RE. Once-daily, high-concentration MMX mesalamine in active ulcerative colitis. Gastroenterology. 2007;132(1):66–75.

33. Sutherland L, Macdonald JK. Oral 5-aminosalicylic acid for maintenance of remission in ulcerative colitis. Cochrane Database Syst Rev. 2006;(2):CD000544. Review.

34. Hanauer S, Sninsky C, Robinson M, et al. An oral preparation of mesalamine as long-term maintenance therapy for ulcerative colitis. A randomized, placebo-controlled trial. The Mesalamine Study Group. Ann Intern Med. 1996;124(2):204–11.

35. Ardizzone S, Petrillo M, Imbesi V, Cerutti R, Bollani S, Bianchi PG. Is maintenance therapy always necessary for patients with ulcerative colitis in remission? Aliment Pharmacol Ther. 1999;13(3):373–9.

36. Miner P, Hanauer S, Robinson M, Schwartz J, Arora S. Safety and efficacy of controlled-release mesalamine for maintenance of remission in ulcerative colitis. Pentasa UC Maintenance Study Group. Dig Dis Sci. 1995;40(2):296–304.

37. Lichtenstein GR, Gordon GL, Zakko S, Murthy U, Sedghi S, Pruitt R, Merchant K, Shaw A, Bortey E, Forbes WP. Clinical trial: once-daily mesalamine granules for maintenance of remission of ulcerative colitis—a 6-month placebo-controlled trial. Aliment Pharmacol Ther. 2010;32(8):990–9.

38. Sandberg-Gertzén H, Järnerot G, Kraaz W. Azodisal sodium in the treatment of ulcerative colitis. A study of tolerance and relapse-prevention properties. Gastroenterology. 1986;90(4):1024–30.

39. Wright JP, O'Keefe EA, Cuming L, Jaskiewicz K. Olsalazine in maintenance of clinical remission in patients with ulcerative colitis. Dig Dis Sci. 1993;38(10):1837–42.

40. Courtney MG, Nunes DP, Bergin CF, O'Driscoll M, Trimble V, Keeling PW, Weir DG. Randomised comparison of olsalazine and

mesalazine in prevention of relapses in ulcerative colitis. Lancet. 1992;339(8804):1279–81.

41. Prantera C, Kohn A, Campieri M, Caprilli R, Cottone M, Pallone F, Savarino V, Sturniolo GC, Vecchi M, Ardia A, Bellinvia S. Clinical trial: ulcerative colitis maintenance treatment with 5-ASA: a 1-year, randomized multicentre study comparing MMX with Asacol. Aliment Pharmacol Ther. 2009;30(9):908–18.

42. D'Haens G, Sandborn WJ, Barrett K, Hodgson I, Streck P. Once-daily MMX® mesalamine for endoscopic maintenance of remission of ulcerative colitis. Am J Gastroenterol. 2012;107(7):1064–77.

43. Ito H, Iida M, Matsumoto T, Suzuki Y, Sasaki H, Yoshida T, Takano Y, Hibi T. Direct comparison of two different mesalamine formulations for the induction of remission in patients with ulcerative colitis: a double-blind, randomized study. Inflamm Bowel Dis. 2010;16(9):1567–74.

44. Ngô Y, Gélinet JM, Ivanovic A, Kac J, Schénowitz G, Vilotte J, Rambaud JC. Efficacy of a daily application of mesalazine (Pentasa) suppository with progressive release, in the treatment of ulcerative proctitis. A double-blind versus placebo randomized trial. Gastroenterol Clin Biol. 1992;16(10):782–6.

45. Williams CN, Haber G, Aquino JA. Double-blind, placebo-controlled evaluation of 5-ASA suppositories in active distal proctitis and measurement of extent of spread using 99mTc-labeled 5-ASA suppositories. Dig Dis Sci. 1987;32(12 Suppl):71S–5.

46. Campieri M, De Franchis R, Bianchi Porro G, Ranzi T, Brunetti G, Barbara L. Mesalazine (5-aminosalicylic acid) suppositories in the treatment of ulcerative proctitis or distal proctosigmoiditis. A randomized controlled trial. Scand J Gastroenterol. 1990;25(7):663–8.

47. Campieri M, Gionchetti P, Belluzzi A, Brignola C, Tampieri M, Iannone P, Brunetti G, Miglioli M, Barbara L. Topical treatment with 5-aminosalicylic in distal ulcerative colitis by using a new suppository preparation. A double-blind placebo controlled trial. Int J Colorectal Dis. 1990;5(2):79–81.

48. Campieri M, Gionchetti P, Belluzzi A, Brignola C, Tampieri M, Iannone P, Miglioli M, Barbara L. Optimum dosage of 5-aminosalicylic acid as rectal enemas in patients with active ulcerative colitis. Gut. 1991;32(8):929–31.

49. Sutherland LR, Martin F, Greer S, Robinson M, Greenberger N, Saibil F, Martin T, Sparr J, Prokipchuk E, Borgen L. 5-Aminosalicylic acid enema in the treatment of distal ulcerative colitis, proctosigmoiditis, and proctitis. Gastroenterology. 1987;92(6):1894–8.

50. Campieri M, Gionchetti P, Belluzzi A. Sucralfate, 5-aminosalicylic acid, and placebo enemas in the treatment of distal ulcerative colitis. Eur J Gastroenterol Hepatol. 1991;3:41–4.

51. Hanauer SB. Dose-ranging study of mesalamine (PENTASA) enemas in the treatment of acute ulcerative proctosigmoiditis: results of a multicentered placebo-controlled trial. The U.S. PENTASA Enema Study Group. Inflamm Bowel Dis. 1998;4(2):79–83.

52. Marshall JK, Thabane M, Steinhart AH, Newman JR, Anand A, Irvine EJ. Rectal 5-aminosalicylic acid for induction of remission in ulcerative colitis. Cochrane Database Syst Rev. 2010;1, CD004115.

53. Marshall JK, Irvine EJ. Rectal aminosalicylate therapy for distal ulcerative colitis: a meta-analysis. Aliment Pharmacol Ther. 1995;9(3):293–300.

54. Gionchetti P, Rizzello F, Venturi A, et al. Comparison of oral with rectal mesalazine in the treatment of ulcerative proctitis. Dis Colon Rectum. 1998;41(1):93–7.

55. Safdi M, DeMicco M, Sninsky C, et al. A double-blind comparison of oral versus rectal mesalamine versus combination therapy in the treatment of distal ulcerative colitis. Am J Gastroenterol. 1997;92(10):1867–71.

56. Kam L, Cohen H, Dooley C, et al. A comparison of mesalamine suspension enema and oral sulfasalazine for treatment of active distal ulcerative colitis in adults. Am J Gastroenterol. 1996;91(7):1338–42.

57. Prantera C, Viscido A, Biancone L, Francavilla A, Giglio L, Campieri M. A new oral delivery system for 5-ASA: preliminary clinical findings for MMx. Inflamm Bowel Dis. 2005;11(5):421–7.

58. Harris MS, Lichtenstein GR. Review article: delivery and efficacy of topical 5-aminosalicylic acid (mesalazine) therapy in the treatment of ulcerative colitis. Aliment Pharmacol Ther. 2011;33(9):996–1009.

59. Ford AC, Khan KJ, Achkar JP, Moayyedi P. Efficacy of oral vs. topical, or combined oral and topical 5-aminosalicylates, in Ulcerative Colitis: systematic review and meta-analysis. Am J Gastroenterol. 2012;107(2):167–76.

60. Campieri M, Gionchetti P, Belluzzi A, et al. 5-Aminosalicylic acid as enemas or suppositories in distal ulcerative colitis? J Clin Gastroenterol. 1988;10(4):406–9.

61. Gionchetti P, Ardizzone S, Benvenuti ME, et al. A new mesalazine gel enema in the treatment of left-sided ulcerative colitis: a randomized controlled multicentre trial. Aliment Pharmacol Ther. 1999;13(3):381–8.

62. Campieri M, Paoluzi P, D'Albasio G, et al. Better quality of therapy with 5-ASA colonic foam in active ulcerative colitis. A multicenter comparative trial with 5-ASA enema. Dig Dis Sci. 1993;38(10):1843–50.

63. Ford AC, Khan KJ, Sandborn WJ, Hanauer SB, Moayyedi P. Efficacy of topical 5-aminosalicylates in preventing relapse of quiescent ulcerative colitis: a meta-analysis. Clin Gastroenterol Hepatol. 2012;10(5):513–9.

64. Nathanson JW, Cohen RD. Current and future topical mesalamine derivatives in ulcerative colitis. In: Lichtenstein GR, editor. Ulcerative colitis: the complete guide to medical management. Thorofare, NJ: Slack Inc.; 2011. p. 157–72.

65. Schroeder KW. Role of mesalazine in acute and long-term treatment of ulcerative colitis and its complications. Scand J Gastroenterol Suppl. 2002;(236):42–7. Review.

66. Van Staa TP, Travis S, Leufkens HG, Logan RF. 5-Aminosalicylic acids and the risk of renal disease: a large British epidemiologic study. Gastroenterology. 2004;126(7):1733–9.

67. Loftus Jr EV, Kane SV, Bjorkman D. Systematic review: short-term adverse effects of 5-aminosalicylic acid agents in the treatment of ulcerative colitis. Aliment Pharmacol Ther. 2004;19(2):179–89. Review.

68. Hanauer SB, Sandborn WJ, Dallaire C, et al. Delayed-release oral mesalamine 4.8 g/day (800 mg tablets) compared to 2.4 g/day (400 mg tablets) for the treatment of mildly to moderately active ulcerative colitis: the ASCEND I trial. Can J Gastroenterol. 2007;21(12):827–34.

69. Hanauer SB, Sandborn WJ, Kornbluth A, et al. Delayed-release oral mesalamine at 4.8 g/day (800 mg tablet) for the treatment of moderately active ulcerative colitis: the ASCEND II trial. Am J Gastroenterol. 2005;100(11):2478–85.

70. Sandborn WJ, Regula J, Feagan BG, Belousova E, Jojic N, Lukas M, Yacyshyn B, Krzeski P, Yeh CH, Messer CA, Hanauer SB. Delayed-release oral mesalamine 4.8 g/day (800-mg tablet) is effective for patients with moderately active ulcerative colitis. Gastroenterology. 2009;137(6):1934–43.e1-3.

71. Brunner M, Greinwald R, Kletter K, Kvaternik H, Corrado ME, Eichler HG, Müller M. Gastrointestinal transit and release of 5-aminosalicylic acid from 153Sm-labelled mesalazine pellets vs. tablets in male healthy volunteers. Aliment Pharmacol Ther. 2003;17(9):1163–9.

72. Feagan BG, MacDonald JK. Once daily oral mesalamine compared to conventional dosing for induction and maintenance of

remission in ulcerative colitis: a systematic review and meta-analysis. Inflamm Bowel Dis. 2012;18(9):1785–94.

73. Lichtenstein GR, Kamm MA. Review article: 5-aminosalicylate formulations for the treatment of ulcerative colitis- methods of comparing release rates and delivery of 5-aminosalicylate to the colonic mucosa. Aliment Pharmacol Ther. 2008;28(6):663–73.

74. Klotz U, Schwab M. Topical delivery of therapeutic agents in the treatment of inflammatory bowel disease. Adv Drug Del Rev. 2005;57:267–79.

75. Fleig WE, Laudage G, Sommer H, Wellmann W, Stange EF, Riemann J. Prospective, randomized, double-blind comparison of benzalazine and sulfasalazine in the treatment of active ulcerative colitis. Digestion. 1988;40(3):173–80.

76. Riley SA, Mani V, Goodman MJ, Herd ME, Dutt S, Turnberg LA. Comparison of delayed release 5 aminosalicylic acid (mesalazine) and sulphasalazine in the treatment of mild to moderate ulcerative colitis relapse. Gut. 1988;29(5):669–74.

77. Rachmilewitz D. Coated mesalazine (5-aminosalicylic acid) versus sulphasalazine in the treatment of active ulcerative colitis: a randomised trial. BMJ. 1989;298(6666):82–6.

78. Rao SS, Dundas SA, Holdsworth CD, Cann PA, Palmer KR, Corbett CL. Olsalazine or sulphasalazine in first attacks of ulcerative colitis? A double blind study. Gut. 1989;30(5):675–9.

79. Munakata A, Yoshida Y, Muto T, Tsuchiya S, Fukushima T, Hiwatashi N, Kobayashi K, Kitano A, Shimoyama T, Inoue M, et al. Double-blind comparative study of sulfasalazine and controlled-release mesalazine tablets in the treatment of active ulcerative colitis. J Gastroenterol. 1995;30 Suppl 8:108–11.

80. Green JR, Lobo AJ, Holdsworth CD, Leicester RJ, Gibson JA, Kerr GD, Hodgson HJ, Parkins KJ, Taylor MD. Balsalazide is more effective and better tolerated than mesalamine in the treatment of acute ulcerative colitis. The Abacus Investigator Group. Gastroenterology. 1998;114(1):15–22.

81. Green JR, Gibson JA, Kerr GD, et al. Maintenance of remission of ulcerative colitis: a comparison between balsalazide 3 g daily and mesalazine 1.2 g daily over 12 months. ABACUS Investigator group. Aliment Pharmacol Ther. 1998;12:1207–16.

82. Forbes A, Al-Damluji A, Ashworth S, Bramble M, Herbert K, Ho J, Kang JY, Przemioslo R, Shetty A. Multicentre randomized-controlled clinical trial of Ipocol, a new enteric-coated form of mesalazine, in comparison with Asacol in the treatment of ulcerative colitis. Aliment Pharmacol Ther. 2005;21(9):1099–104.

83. Pruitt R, Hanson J, Safdi M, Wruble L, Hardi R, Johanson J, Koval G, Riff D, Winston B, Cross A, Doty P, Johnson LK. Balsalazide is superior to mesalamine in the time to improvement of signs and symptoms of acute mild-to-moderate ulcerative colitis. Am J Gastroenterol. 2002;97(12):3078–86.

84. Levine DS, Riff DS, Pruitt R, Wruble L, Koval G, Sales D, Bell JK, Johnson LK. A randomized, double blind, dose-response comparison of balsalazide (6.75 g), balsalazide (2.25 g), and mesalamine (2.4 g) in the treatment of active, mild-to-moderate ulcerative colitis. Am J Gastroenterol. 2002;97(6):1398–407.

85. Mansfield JC, Giaffer MH, Cann PA, McKenna D, Thornton PC, Holdsworth CD. A double-blind comparison of balsalazide, 6.75 g, and sulfasalazine, 3 g, as sole therapy in the management of ulcerative colitis. Aliment Pharmacol Ther. 2002;16(1):69–77.

86. Raedler A, Behrens C, Bias P. Mesalazine (5-aminosalicylic acid) micropellets show similar efficacy and tolerability to mesalazine tablets in patients with ulcerative colitis–results from a randomized-controlled trial. Aliment Pharmacol Ther. 2004;20(11–12):1353–63.

87. Tursi A, Brandimarte G, Giorgetti GM, Forti G, Modeo ME, Gigliobianco A. Low-dose balsalazide plus a high-potency probiotic preparation is more effective than balsalazide alone or mesalazine in the treatment of acute mild-to-moderate ulcerative colitis. Med Sci Monit. 2004;10(11):PI126–31. Epub 2004 Oct 26.

88. Jiang XL, Cui HF. Different therapy for different types of ulcerative colitis in China. World J Gastroenterol. 2004;10(10):1513–20.

89. Marakhouski Y, Fixa B, Holomán J, Hulek P, Lukas M, Bátovský M, Rumyantsev VG, Grigoryeva G, Stolte M, Vieth M. Greinwald R; International Salofalk Study GroupA double-blind dose-escalating trial comparing novel mesalazine pellets with mesalazine tablets in active ulcerative colitis. Aliment Pharmacol Ther. 2005;21(2):133–40.

90. Gibson PR, Fixa B, Pekárková B, Bátovský M, Radford-Smith G, Tibitanzl J, Gabalec L, Florin TH, Greinwald R. Comparison of the efficacy and safety of Eudragit-L-coated mesalazine tablets with ethylcellulose-coated mesalazine tablets in patients with mild to moderately active ulcerative colitis. Aliment Pharmacol Ther. 2006;23(7):1017–26.

91. McIntyre PB, Rodrigues CA, Lennard-Jones JE, Barrison IG, Walker JG, Baron JH, Thornton PC. Balsalazide in the maintenance treatment of patients with ulcerative colitis, a double-blind comparison with sulphasalazine. Aliment Pharmacol Ther. 1988;2(3):237–43.

92. Rutgeerts P. Comparative efficacy of coated, oral 5-aminosalicylic acid (Claversal) and sulphasalazine for maintaining remission of ulcerative colitis. International Study Group. Aliment Pharmacol Ther. 1989;3(2):183–91.

93. Mulder CJ, Tytgat GN, Dekker W, Blok P, Schrijver M, van der Heide H. Double-blind comparison of slow-release 5-aminosalicylate and sulfasalazine in remission maintenance in ulcerative colitis. Gastroenterology. 1988;95(6):1449–53.

94. Rijk MC, van Lier HJ, van Tongeren JH. Relapse-preventing effect and safety of sulfasalazine and olsalazine in patients with ulcerative colitis in remission: a prospective, double-blind, randomized multicenter study. The Ulcerative Colitis Multicenter Study Group. Am J Gastroenterol. 1992;87(4):438–42.

95. Kiilerich S, Ladefoged K, Rannem T, Ranløv PJ. Prophylactic effects of olsalazine v sulphasalazine during 12 months maintenance treatment of ulcerative colitis. The Danish Olsalazine Study Group. Gut. 1992;33(2):252–5.

96. Nilsson A, Danielsson A, Löfberg R, Benno P, Bergman L, Fausa O, Florholmen J, Karvonen AL, Kildebo S, Kollberg B, et al. Olsalazine versus sulphasalazine for relapse prevention in ulcerative colitis: a multicenter study. Am J Gastroenterol. 1995;90(3):381–7.

97. Ardizzone S, Petrillo M, Molteni P, Desideri S, Bianchi PG. Coated oral 5-aminosalicylic acid (Claversal) is equivalent to sulfasalazine for remission maintenance in ulcerative colitis. A double-blind study. J Clin Gastroenterol. 1995;21(4):287–9.

98. Riley SA, Mani V, Goodman MJ, et al. Comparison of delayed-release 5-aminosalicylic acid (mesalazine) and sulfasalazine as maintenance treatment for patients with ulcerative colitis. Gastroenterology. 1988;94:1383–9.

99. Kruis W, Schreiber S, Theuer D, Brandes JW, Schütz E, Howaldt S, Krakamp B, Hämling J, Mönnikes H, Koop I, Stolte M, Pallant D, Ewald U. Low dose balsalazide (1.5 g twice daily) and mesalazine (0.5 g three times daily) maintained remission of ulcerative colitis but high dose balsalazide (3.0 g twice daily) was superior in preventing relapses. Gut. 2001;49(6):783–9.

100. Mahmud N, O'Toole D, O'Hare N, Freyne PJ, Weir DG, Kelleher D. Evaluation of renal function following treatment with 5-aminosalicylic acid derivatives in patients with ulcerative colitis. Aliment Pharmacol Ther. 2002;16(2):207–15.

101. Miglioli M, Bianchi Porro G, Brunetti G, et al. Delayed release mesalazine in the treatment of mild ulcerative colitis: a dose ranging study. Eur J Gastroenterol Hepatol. 1990;2:229–34.

102. Travis SP, Tysk C, de Silva HJ, Sandberg-Gertzén H, Jewell DP, Järnerot G. Optimum dose of olsalazine for maintaining remission in ulcerative colitis. Gut. 1994;35(9):1282–6.

103. Paoluzi OA, Iacopini F, Pica R, Crispino P, Marcheggiano A, Consolazio A, Rivera M, Paoluzi P. Comparison of two different daily dosages (2.4 vs. 1.2 g) of oral mesalazine in maintenance of remission in ulcerative colitis patients: 1-year follow-up study. Aliment Pharmacol Ther. 2005;21(9):1111–9.

104. Kruis W, Jonaitis L, Pokrotnieks J, Mikhailova TL, Horynski M, Bátovský M, Lozynsky YS, Zakharash Y, Rácz I, Kull K, Vcev A, Faszczyk M, Dilger K, Greinwald R, Mueller R, International Salofalk OD Study Group. Randomised clinical trial: a comparative dose-finding study of three arms of dual release mesalazine for maintaining remission in ulcerative colitis. Aliment Pharmacol Ther. 2011;33(3):313–22.

105. Hawthorne AB, Stenson R, Gillespie D, Swarbrick ET, Dhar A, Kapur KC, Hood K, Probert CS. One-year investigator-blind randomized multicenter trial comparing Asacol 2.4 g once daily with 800 mg three times daily for maintenance of remission in ulcerative colitis. Inflamm Bowel Dis. 2012;18(10):1885–93.

106. Kamm MA, Lichtenstein GR, Sandborn WJ, Schreiber S, Lees K, Barrett K, Joseph R. Randomised trial of once- or twice-daily MMX mesalazine for maintenance of remission in ulcerative colitis. Gut. 2008;57(7):893–902.

107. Dignass AU, Bokemeyer B, Adamek H, Mross M, Vinter-Jensen L, Börner N, Silvennoinen J, Tan G, Pool MO, Stijnen T, Dietel P, Klugmann T, Vermeire S, Bhatt A, Veerman H. Mesalamine once daily is more effective than twice daily in patients with quiescent ulcerative colitis. Clin Gastroenterol Hepatol. 2009;7(7):762–9.

108. Miner P, Nostrant T, Wruble L, et al. Multicenter trial of Pentasa for active ulcerative colitis. Gastroenterology. 1991;100(Suppl):A231.

109. D'Haens G, Hommes D, Engels L, et al. Once daily MMX mesalazine for the treatment of mild-to-moderate ulcerative colitis: a phase II, dose-ranging study. Aliment Pharmacol Ther. 2006; 24:1087–97.

110. Kohn A, Prantera C, Caprilli R, et al. Maintenance treatment of ulcerative colitis with 5-aminosalicylic acid (5-ASA): Results from the Italian population of a one year, randomized, multinational study comparing MMx_ with Asacol_. Gastroenterology. 2009;136 Suppl 1:A65.

111. Green JR, Mansfield JC, Gibson JA, et al. A double-blind comparison of balsalazide, 6.75 g daily, and sulfasalazine, 3 g daily, in patients with newly diagnosed or relapsed active ulcerative colitis. Aliment Pharmacol Ther. 2002;16:61–8.

112. Green JRB, Swan CHJ, Rowlinson A, et al. Short report: comparison of two doses of balsalazide in maintaining ulcerative colitis in remission over 12 months. Aliment Pharmacol Ther. 1992;6:647–52.

113. Fockens P, Mulder CJJ, Tytgat GNJ, et al. Comparison of the efficacy and safety of 1.5 compared with 3.0 g oral slow-release mesalazine (Pentasa) in the maintenance treatment of ulcerative colitis. Eur J Gastroenterol Hepatol. 1995;7:1025–30.

114. Sandborn WJ, Korzenik J, Lashner B, et al. Once-daily dosing of delayed-release oral mesalamine (400-mg tablet) is as effective as twice-daily dosing for maintenance of remission of ulcerative colitis. Gastroenterology. 2010;138:1286–96.

# Topical Mesalamine

## Sushila Dalal and Russell D. Cohen

**Keywords**

Topical mesalamine • Ulcerative colitis • Treatment • Proctitis • Colon • Oral mesalamine

## Introduction

Proctitis and left-sided colitis represent the majority of newly diagnosed ulcerative colitis (UC) cases [1–3]. Affected patients, with inflammation limited to the distal 60 cm of the colon, can be effectively treated with both oral and topical mesalamine formulations. The current 2010 American College of Gastroenterology guidelines state that for mild to moderate distal ulcerative colitis, topical mesalamine is superior to oral mesalamine or topical steroids [4]. Furthermore, the combination of oral and topical mesalamine is more effective than either agent alone.

## Rationale for Topical Mesalamine Use in Ulcerative Colitis

Professor Nanna Svartz first described the use of sulfasalazine in the treatment of ulcerative colitis in 1941, though the first report of a placebo-controlled trial of the medication for ulcerative colitis did not occur until 1962 [5–7]. Still, the mechanism of the medication's efficacy remained uninvestigated until the 1977 study by Azad Khan, Piris,

S. Dalal, M.D. (✉)
Department of Medicine, Section of Gastroenterology,
The University of Chicago Medical Center, Chicago, IL, USA
e-mail: sushila.dalal@uchospitals.edu

R.D. Cohen, M.D.
Gastroenterology Division, Section of Gastroenterology,
Department of Medicine, Inflammatory Bowel Disease Center,
The University of Chicago Medical Center,
5841 S. Maryland Ave., MC4076, Chicago 60637-1463, IL, USA
e-mail: rcohen@medicine.bsd.uchicago.edu

and Truelove [8]. Sulfasalazine is a conjugate of 5-aminosalicylic acid (5-ASA) and sulfapyridine, linked by an azo bond. About 1/3 of the drug is absorbed in the upper GI tract [9]. Upon delivery of the drug to the colon, colonic bacteria cleave the azo bond, releasing 5-ASA and sulfapyridine [10]. While most of the sulfapyridine is absorbed, very little of the 5-ASA is absorbed [11].

Azad Khan, Piris, and Truelove investigated whether sulfasalazine's therapeutic efficacy was provided by the parent compound itself or one of the two products found in the colon: 5-ASA or sulfapyridine [8]. The authors noted that when given as individual oral medications, 5-ASA and sulfapyridine were almost completely absorbed in the small intestine. Thus, their study could not compare the effects of oral sulfasalazine to oral 5-ASA and sulfapyridine. Instead, the authors formulated retention enemas containing sulfasalazine, 5-ASA, and sulfapyridine to determine the direct effects of these compounds on the colonic mucosa.

In patients receiving enema formulations of these compounds for 2 weeks, 30 % of the patients receiving topical sulfasalazine or 5-ASA had histologic improvement of colonic inflammation on flexible sigmoidoscopy biopsies, while only 5 % of those receiving sulfapyridine improved [8]. Thus, this study demonstrated that 5-ASA was the active component of sulfasalazine. Furthermore, this study demonstrated the efficacy of topical treatment with 5-ASA and sulfasalazine in ulcerative colitis.

This study was soon followed by several other studies of sulfasalazine enemas. Palmer, Goepel, and Holdsworth found improvement in 70 % of patients taking a 3 g sulfasalazine enema for 2 weeks versus improvement in 11 % of those taking placebo in a double-blind study [12]. Frimberger et al. found a 73.6 % response rate in a double-blind study of 33 patients with left-sided ulcerative colitis on 3 % sulfasalazine enemas [13].

Early studies, such as the one by Palmer et al., describe the need to evaluate topical sulfasalazine therapy because of many patients' inability to tolerate oral sulfasalazine due to nausea and vomiting [12]. A further rationale for the use of topical mesalamine to target this medication to the distal colon has been the variability of 5-ASA concentrations in this area after ingestion of oral 5-ASA. The achieved mucosal concentration of 5-ASA in the distal colon when delivered orally is dependent on several variables such as pH and colonic transit, with evidence that the highest 5-ASA concentrations are found in the proximal colon [14–16].

Topical therapy increases mucosal mesalamine concentration up to the splenic flexure. In a study of 22 patients with mild to moderate ulcerative colitis that were randomized to receive 2.4 g of oral mesalamine plus 4 g/day of topical mesalamine or 2.4 g of oral mesalamine alone, biopsies were taken from the rectum and from the descending colon, just distal to the splenic flexure, after 2 weeks of therapy [17]. High performance liquid chromatography analysis of these biopsies showed that mucosal levels of mesalamine in the rectum were significantly higher in the group that received oral plus topical therapy than in the group that received oral therapy alone (52.1 ng/mg, range 13.6–122.1 ng/mg, vs. 0.2 ng/mg, range 0.2–9.7 ng/mg; $p < 0.0001$). Mucosal mesalamine levels in the descending colon were also significantly higher in patients who received oral plus topical therapy as compared to those who received oral therapy alone (46.6 ng/mg, range 6–112.6 ng/mg, vs. 15.9 ng/mg, range 2.3–42.4 ng/mg; $p = 0.01$) [17].

Furthermore, higher mucosal levels of 5-ASA do appear to correlate with improvements in colonic inflammation. A group of 24 ulcerative colitis patients receiving 2.4–3.2 g of oral mesalamine per day, of which 4 patients were also receiving topical 5-ASA treatment at 2 g/day, underwent endoscopic biopsies of the rectum [18]. 5-ASA concentrations in the biopsies were measured by high performance liquid chromatography. Higher mucosal concentrations of 5-ASA were associated with significantly lower endoscopic scores of inflammation severity as well as with lower scores of histologic inflammation [18].

## Topical Mesalamine Formulations

Suppositories, enemas (liquid suspensions), gels, and foam formulations of topical mesalamine have been developed, though only suppositories and enemas are currently commercially available in the United States.

5-ASA suppositories are efficacious in treating rectal and sigmoid colon inflammation. In a study of six patients with inflammatory bowel disease (IBD) compared with six healthy controls, $^{99m}$Tc 5-ASA suppositories localized to the sigmoid colon and rectum over a 3-h study period (Fig. 8.1) [19]. A double-blind, placebo-controlled trial of patients with 9–10 cm of proctitis using 500 mg 5-ASA or placebo suppositories three times daily resulted in remission in 78.6 % (11/14) of the treatment group after 6 weeks [19]. None of the 11 patients remaining in the placebo group at the end of 6 weeks achieved remission. More recently, a single-center, single-blind trial of 403 patients with mild to moder-

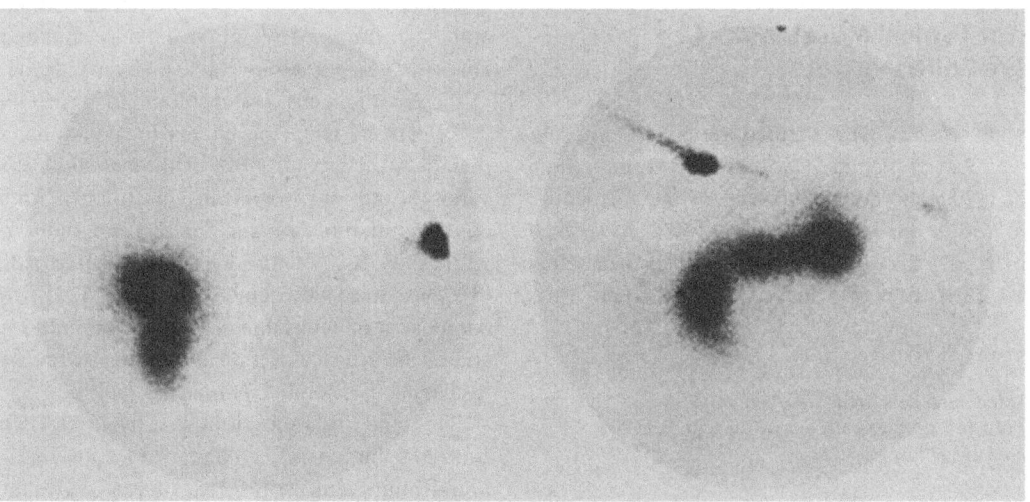

**Fig. 8.1** Distribution of 5-ASA suppository in a patient with ulcerative proctitis. $^{99m}$Tc-labeled 5-ASA suppository was given to a patient with refractory ulcerative proctitis. The medication spread to the sigmoid colon after 3.5 h in (**a**) *anterior view* and (**b**) *right lateral view. From Williams CN, Haber G, Aquino JA. Double-blind, placebo-controlled evaluation of 5-ASA suppositories in active distal proctitis and measurement of extent of spread using $^{99m}$Tc-labeled 5-ASA suppositories. Dig Dis Sci. 1987;32(12 Suppl):71S–75S. With permission from Springer © 1987* [19]

ately active proctitis taking 1 g 5-ASA suppositories administered nightly as compared to 500 mg suppositories given three times daily showed non-inferiority for the once-daily dosing, with clinical remission rates of 87.9 % and 90.7 %, respectively, in a per protocol analysis [20].

Mesalamine foam is also useful in the treatment of left-sided ulcerative colitis. In a randomized, double-blind, placebo-controlled study of 2 g of mesalamine foam vs. placebo in 111 patients with mild to moderately active proctitis, proctosigmoiditis, or left-sided ulcerative colitis over a 6-week period, 65 % in the treatment group versus 40 % in the placebo group achieved clinical remission, 57 % vs. 37 % achieved endoscopic remission, and 59 % vs. 41 % had improved histologic indices [21]. The treatment group utilized two 1 g 5-ASA foam enemas. In a subgroup analysis, the clinical benefit of treatment was seen in the group with mild disease (with a clinical disease activity index of eight or less), but was not seen in the smaller group of 16 patients with moderate disease activity. In terms of disease location, patients with proctosigmoiditis had the highest response rate to treatment (61 %), as compared to those with proctitis (54 %) or left-sided colitis (40 %).

A crossover study of 10 patients compared a $^{99m}$Tc-labeled preparation of 4 g 5-ASA in 20 mL foam vs. 4 g 5-ASA in 100 mL suspension enemas [22]. In vitro studies of the foam suggested that the 4 g foam expanded to 180–200 mL after being expelled with a propellant gas. Study subjects were asked to lie supine for 4 h after administration. After 120 min, 6/10 patients receiving the 5-ASA foam had homogenous coverage of the medication in the descending colon, 3/10 had nonhomogenous spread in the descending colon, and 1/10 had no drug coverage in the descending colon. In the 5-ASA enema group, 7/10 had nonhomogenous coverage in the descending colon, while 3/10 had no coverage.

The total foam volume does not appear to determine efficacy. A 2007 study by Eliakim et al. reported remission rates of 77 % after 6 weeks of twice-daily treatment with either a 30 mL or a 60 mL 1 g mesalamine foam [23].

A gel formulation of mesalamine has also been designed with the hope for efficacy with easier tolerability and less "messy" application. Unlike the mesalamine foam, a propellant gas is not instilled into the colon with the gel formulation. A 4 g/60 mL 5-ASA gel was tested in a study of 12 patients with mild to moderately active ulcerative colitis [24]. In this open-label study, patients were asked to lie on their left side for 4 h after administration of a $^{99m}$Tc-labeled gel. 11/12 (92 %) of patients had spread of the gel beyond the sigmoid colon, while 6/12 (50 %) had coverage past the splenic flexure [24]. In a randomized, multicenter, investigator-blind trial of 103 patients with mild to moderate left-sided ulcerative colitis or proctosigmoiditis, the efficacy of a 2 g/60 mL 5-ASA gel enema was compared to a 2 g/120 mL 5-ASA foam enema over a 4-week treatment

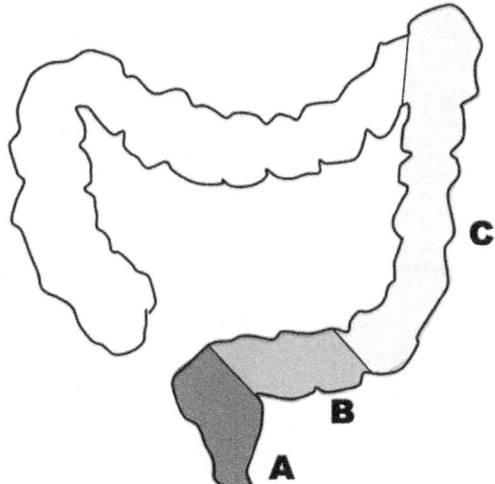

**Fig. 8.2** Expected distribution of topical mesalamine formulations. (**a**) Suppositories reach the rectum. (**b**) Foam reaches the rectum and sigmoid colon. (**c**) Liquid and gel enemas can reach the splenic flexure. *From Marshall JK, Irvine EJ. Putting rectal 5-aminosalicylic acid in its place: The role in distal ulcerative colitis. Am J Gastroenterol. 2000;95(7):1628–1636* [57]

period [25]. After 4 weeks of therapy, clinical remission was observed in 76 % of patients using the gel and 69 % using the foam. Endoscopic remission was achieved in 51 % using the gel and 52 % using the foam. Patients using the foam reported more difficulty in retention (25 % vs. 6 %), more bloating (50 % vs. 26 %), and more discomfort (48 % vs. 26 %) [25].

The distribution of all of the topical mesalamine formulations is variable and is partially dependent on patient factors, such as severity of inflammation and ability to lie on their left side for an extended time after administration. In general, suppositories are expected to reach the rectum, foams are expected to reach the rectum and sigmoid, and gel and liquid enemas can reach the splenic flexure (Fig. 8.2).

## Topical 5-ASA for Induction of Left-Sided Ulcerative Colitis Remission

Marshall et al. published a Cochrane Database systematic review of rectal 5-aminosalicylic acid for induction of remission in ulcerative colitis, evaluating randomized trials comparing rectal 5-ASA to placebo or another active therapy in patients with ulcerative colitis with a distal disease margin 60 cm from the anal verge or distal to the splenic flexure [26]. The authors conducted a search of the MEDLINE database (1966–2008), the Cochrane Central Register of Controlled Trials and the Cochrane IBD/FBD Group Specialized Trials Register, as well as manual reviews of reference listings and conference proceedings. Thirty-eight trials fulfilled the inclusion criteria. This group found that

**Table 8.1** Summary of results from trials included in the Marshall et al. meta-analyses of studies comparing rectal 5-ASA to placebo for clinical remission, endoscopic remission, and histologic remission [26]

| Study | Medication | Disease location | Duration | Remission or response and data |
|---|---|---|---|---|
| Campieri et al. [28] | 1 and 1.5 g 5-ASA suppositories vs. placebo | Less than 20 cm from the anal verge | 4 Weeks | *Clinical remission*: 69 % 5-ASA 1 g/day vs. 74 % 5-ASA 1.5 g/day vs. 39 % placebo |
| | | | | *Endoscopic remission*: 55 % 5-ASA 1 g/day vs. 59 % 5-ASA 1.5 g/day vs. 23 % placebo |
| | | | | *Histologic remission*: 10 % 5-ASA 1 g/day vs. 16 % 5-ASA 1.5 g/day vs. 6 % placebo |
| Campieri et al. [30] | 1.5 g 5-ASA suppositories vs. placebo | Less than 20 cm from the anal verge | 30 Days | *Clinical remission*: 56 % 5-ASA vs. 7 % placebo |
| | | | | *Endoscopic remission*: 41 % 5-ASA vs. 7 % placebo |
| | | | | *Histologic remission*: 28 % 5-ASA vs. 3 % placebo |
| Campieri et al. [59] | Sucralfate 10 g vs. 5-ASA 2 g vs. placebo in 100 mL enemas | Mild to moderate activity no further than splenic flexure | 30 Days | *Clinical improvement*: 22 % sucralfate vs. 94 % 5-ASA vs. 14 % placebo |
| | | | | *Endoscopic improvement*: 22 % sucralfate vs. 88 % 5-ASA vs. 14 % placebo |
| | | | | *Histologic improvement*: 17 % sucralfate vs. 83 % 5-ASA vs. 7 % placebo |
| Campieri et al. [60] | 1, 2, and 4 g 5-ASA enemas vs. placebo | Mild to moderate UC distal to the splenic flexure | 4 Weeks | *Clinical remission*: 85 % 5-ASA 1 g vs. 83 % 5-ASA 2 g vs. 86 % 5-ASA 4 g vs. 41 % placebo |
| | | | | *Endoscopic remission*: 74 % 5-ASA 1 g vs. 73 % 5-ASA 2 g vs. 79 % 5-ASA 4 g vs. 30 % placebo |
| | | | | *Histologic remission*: 63 % 5-ASA 1 g vs. 70 % 5-ASA 2 g vs. 76 % 5-ASA 4 g vs. 15 % placebo |
| Hanauer et al. [58] | 1, 2, or 4 g 5-ASA enema vs. placebo | Mild to moderate UC extending less than 30 cm from the anal verge | 8 Weeks | *Clinical remission*: vs. 47 % 5-ASA 1 g vs. 49 % 5-ASA 2 g vs. 44 % 5-ASA 4 g vs. 14 % placebo |
| | | | | *Endoscopic remission*: 59 % 5-ASA 1 g vs. 65 % 5-ASA 2 g vs. 66 % 5-ASA 4 g vs. 24 % placebo |
| | | | | *Histologic remission*: 42 % 5-ASA 1 g vs. 49 % 5-ASA 2 g vs. 55 % 5-ASA 4 g vs. 16 % placebo |
| Moller et al. [61] | 3 g sulfasalazine enema vs. placebo | Extending less than 15 cm from the anal verge | 2 Weeks | *Symptomatic response*: 81 % excellent response (no symptoms) with sulfasalazine vs. 14 % excellent response with placebo |
| | | | | *Endoscopic response*: 75 % excellent response (full endoscopic remission) with sulfasalazine vs. 21 % excellent response with placebo |
| Pokrotneiks et al. [21] | 2 g 5-ASA foam enema vs. placebo | Mild to moderate UC distal to the splenic flexure | 6 Weeks | *Clinical remission*: 65 % 5-ASA vs. 40 % placebo |
| | | | | *Endoscopic remission*: 57 % 5-ASA vs. 37 % placebo |
| | | | | *Histologic improvement*: 59 % 5-ASA vs. 41 % placebo |
| Williams et al. [19] | 5-ASA suppositories 500 mg TID vs. placebo | Extending less than 15 cm from the anal verge | 6 Weeks | Mean DAI treatment group was 0.4 ± 0.9 compared to 5.4 ± 3.4 in the placebo |
| | | | | Remission achieved by 79 % on 5-ASA compared to 8 % placebo |

topical 5-ASA was superior to placebo for inducing remission, with a pooled odds ratio for eight trials of 8.30 for symptomatic remission (95 % CI 4.28–16.12, $p < 0.00001$). The pooled odds ratio for seven of the same eight trials for endoscopic remission was 5.31 (95 % CI 3.15–8.92, $p < 0.00001$). Furthermore, the pooled odds ratio for histologic remission was 6.28 (5 trials, 95 % CI 2.74–14.40; $p < 0.0001$) (Table 8.1).

Our group at the University of Chicago conducted a meta-analysis and overview of the mesalamine literature

from 1958 to 1997 on treatment options for left-sided ulcerative colitis and ulcerative proctitis [27]. This overview reported that in placebo-controlled trials studying mesalamine enemas in active left-sided ulcerative colitis, mesalamine enemas showed a duration, but not dose response, in achieving remission.

In the University of Chicago study, meta-analyses were conducted for studies examining mesalamine suppository treatment for ulcerative proctitis. One of these meta-analyses included two studies of 1 g mesalamine suppositories

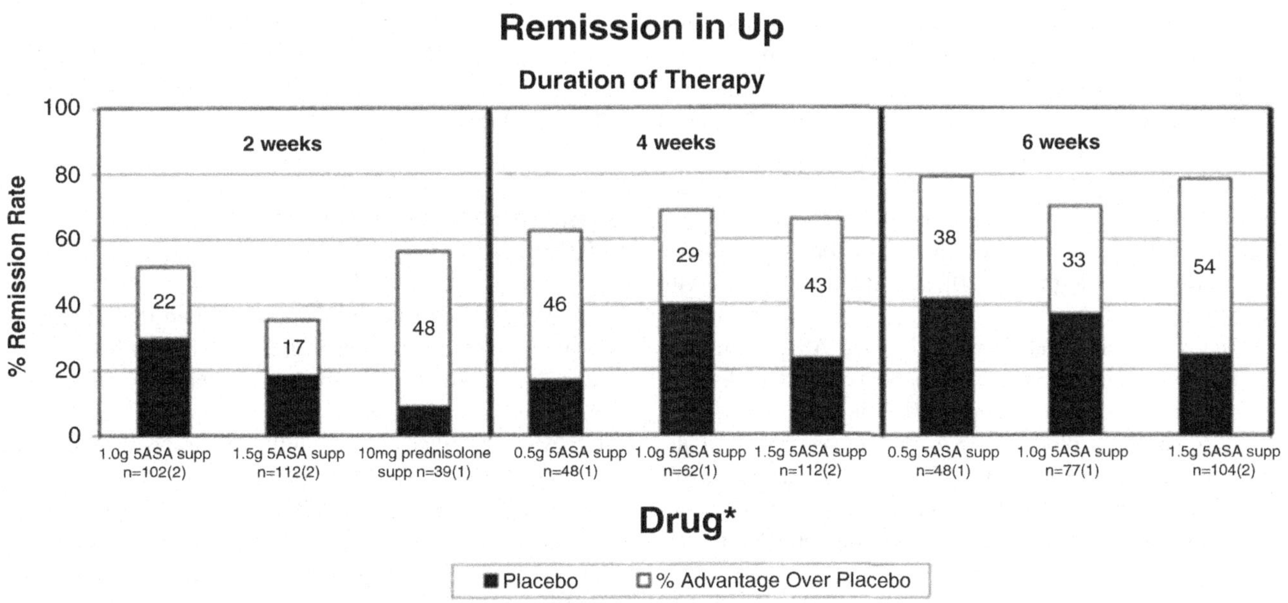

## Remission in Up

### Duration of Therapy

**Fig. 8.3** Comparison of mesalamine suppositories for treatment of ulcerative proctitis. Numbers within bar graphs are percent advantage over placebo. *N* is the number of patients; the number of studies is in parentheses. *From Cohen RD, Woseth DM, Thisted RA, Hanauer SB. A* *Meta-analysis and Overview of the Literature on Treatment Options for Left-Sided Ulcerative Colitis and Ulcerative Proctitis. Am J Gastroenterol. 2000;95(5):1263–1276* [27]

examining clinical and endoscopic remission at 2 weeks [28, 29]. Meta-analysis of these two studies showed a pooled advantage of mesalamine suppositories over placebo of 23.6 % for clinical remission with the 95 % confidence interval crossing zero (−8.8. to 56.0). The pooled advantage for endoscopic remission was 32.7 % with a CI of 15.3–50.1. The University of Chicago group performed a separate meta-analysis of two studies of 1.5 g mesalamine suppositories for 4 weeks and two studies of 1.5 g mesalamine suppositories for 6 weeks, which showed a pooled advantage over placebo in inducing clinical remission of 44.3 % (CI 29.4–59.1) at 4 weeks and 57.9 % (CI 36.1–79.7) at 6 weeks [19, 28, 30, 31]. The pooled advantage in achieving endoscopic remission at 4 weeks was 33.3 % higher in the treatment group (CI 18.5–48) and the pooled advantage over placebo in achieving clinical remission at 4 weeks was 52 % (CI 37.8–66.3). Overall review of mesalamine suppository studies for ulcerative proctitis revealed a duration, but not dose response (Fig. 8.3).

## Comparison of Topical Mesalamine to Topical Corticosteroids

The Marshall et al. 2010 meta-analysis included a study of rectal 5-ASA as compared to rectal corticosteroids [26]. This analysis showed that rectal 5-ASA was superior to rectal corticosteroids for inducing symptomatic remission. A comparison of six trials showed a pooled odds ratio of 1.65 (95 % CI 1.11–2.45, *p*=0.01) for symptomatic remission.

Lee et al. compared 2 g 5-ASA foam to 20 mg prednisolone foam in a 4-week trial of 295 patients in 36 centers in the United Kingdom with mild to moderately active UC [32]. The 5-ASA group achieved a significantly higher rate of clinical remission than the prednisolone group (52 % vs. 31 %, *p*<0.001). The rates of endoscopic and histologic remission did not differ between groups. In a separate study, the Danish 5-ASA group reported a double-blind, multi-center trial of 1 g/day 5-ASA enemas compared to 25 mg/day prednisolone enemas for 4 weeks in 123 patients [33]. The overall response to therapy was defined as the sum of the clinical and endoscopic effects. Though no significant difference in clinical and endoscopic improvement occurred in the groups after 2 weeks, rates of remission did significantly differ, with 51 % in the 5-ASA group and 31 % in the prednisolone group achieving remission (*p*<0.05).

Two studies compared 5-ASA foam or enema to beclomethasone foam or enema [34, 35]. Biancone et al. found, in a randomized, multicenter, double-blind trial, that 3 mg beclomethasone dipropionate foam or enema vs. 2 g 5-ASA foam or enema did not have significantly different rates of remission (24 % vs. 28 % at 4 weeks and 36 % vs. 52 % at 8 weeks) [34]. Gionchetti et al. also reported on a single-center, randomized, investigator-blind trial which demonstrated that patients with active distal UC receiving 1 g 5-ASA enemas or 3 mg beclomethasone propionate enemas for 6 weeks both had significantly improved disease activity indices but no statistically significant difference in the rates of clinical remission [35].

Farup et al. compared 5-ASA suppositories 500 mg twice daily to hydrocortisone foam 178 mg twice daily for 4 weeks [36]. Remission rates at 2 and 4 weeks did not significantly differ between treatments. A nonsignificant trend towards more histologic improvement with 5-ASA suppositories at 2 and 4 weeks (70 and 78 % vs. 50 and 61 %, respectively) was noted. Patients on 5-ASA suppositories had a greater mean increase in DAI than those on hydrocortisone foam, which was attributed to improved efficacy in the subgroup with proctitis.

Finally, Leman et al. compared 1 g 5-ASA enemas to 2.3 mg budesonide enemas in 97 patients with UC distal to the splenic flexure at endoscopy [37]. Clinical remission was achieved in 60 % of the 5-ASA patients vs. 38 % of the budesonide patients ($p = 0.03$), although there was no statistical difference in the rates of endoscopic improvement, histologic improvement, or histologic remission between the two groups.

## Efficacy of Topical vs. Oral Mesalamine in Achieving Remission

Ford et al. have recently performed a systematic review and meta-analysis examining the efficacy of oral vs. topical, or combined oral and topical 5-ASA in ulcerative colitis [38]. Four randomized, controlled trials with endpoints between 4 and 8 weeks compared topical 5-ASA to oral 5-ASA for induction of remission in mild to moderate UC [39–42]. One trial, by Gionchetti et al., studied only patients with proctitis on 400 mg 5-ASA suppositories three times daily, while the other three studies examined the use of 4 g 5-ASA enemas. Overall, 49.5 % of patients taking topical 5-ASA alone failed to achieve remission compared to 58.7 % of patients on oral 5-ASA alone. The relative risk of failure to achieve remission with topical 5-ASA was 0.82 (95 % CI = 0.52–1.28). Statistically significant heterogeneity between studies was noted. When the Gionchetti study of patients with proctitis was removed from the analysis, the relative risk of remission with topical vs. oral 5-ASA was 1.04 (95 % CI 0.79–1.37).

Ford et al. also identified four randomized, controlled trials studying oral and topical mesalamine vs. oral mesalamine alone [42–45]. In a meta-analysis, 37.3 % of patients on combined therapy and 55.1 % of patients on oral therapy alone failed to achieve remission. The relative risk of failure to achieve remission with combination therapy as compared to oral therapy alone was 0.65 (95 % CI = 0.47–0.91) with no significant heterogeneity between studies. The number needed to treat with combined therapy to prevent one failure of remission was five (95 % CI 3–13). The Vecchi et al. study did include equivalent doses of 5-ASA in the combined therapy and oral therapy alone groups, while the other trials had a higher total 5-ASA dose in the combination therapy group [45]. When only the three trials with higher total 5-ASA dose

in the combination therapy group were analyzed, combination therapy was no longer superior to oral 5-ASA, with a relative risk of failure to achieve remission of 0.51 (CI = 0.26–1.00).

## Topical Mesalamine for Maintenance of Remission

Placebo-controlled trials have demonstrated the efficacy of topical mesalamine in maintaining remission for distal ulcerative colitis. Ford et al. performed a meta-analysis of seven randomized, controlled trials that examined the use of topical 5-ASA or placebo in adult patients with quiescent ulcerative colitis [38]. Three of these trials included only patients with ulcerative proctitis using mesalamine suppositories or placebo [29, 46, 47]. One study included patients with proctitis or proctosigmoiditis using mesalamine suppositories or placebo [48]. Two studies included only patients with left-sided colitis using mesalamine enemas or placebo [49, 50]. The seventh trial studied a mixture of patients with pancolitis, left-sided colitis, and proctosigmoiditis who were on mesalamine enemas and placebo [51]. This 1997 d'Albasio trial also compared combined oral and topical 5-ASA therapy to oral therapy with placebo as a topical therapy. One of the three trials including only patients with proctitis, by Marteau et al., allowed the continued use of stable-dose, previously prescribed oral 5-ASA medications. The other five trials in the meta-analysis compared patients on topical 5-ASA alone to patients on placebo. The duration of therapy ranged from 6 to 24 months.

The Ford meta-analysis found that 36.9 % of patients on topical mesalamine and 68.3 % of those on placebo experienced a relapse of disease. The relative risk of relapse with topical mesalamine compared to placebo was 0.60 (95 % CI 0.49–0.73). The number needed to treat with topical mesalamine to prevent one relapse was 3 (95 % CI 2–5). No significant heterogeneity was detected between the trials.

Ford et al. have reported a separate meta-analysis of two studies examining the efficacy of combined oral and topical 5-ASA vs. oral 5-ASA in preventing relapse in quiescent ulcerative colitis [38]. One of the two trials included was also the 1997 d'Albasio study, which included a mixture of patients with pancolitis, left-sided colitis, and proctosigmoiditis on mesalamine enemas 4 g twice weekly and oral mesalamine 1.6 g a day vs. oral mesalamine alone 1.6 g a day [51]. The 2007 study by Yokoyama et al. also evaluated a mixture of patients with pancolitis, left-sided colitis, and proctitis. The two study groups took oral mesalamine 3 g a day with or without mesalamine enema 1 g twice weekly [52]. In total, 42.6 % of patients on combination therapy and 73.5 % of patients on oral 5-ASA relapsed. The relative risk of relapse with combination therapy as compared with oral 5-ASA therapy alone was 0.48 (95 % CI = 0.17–1.38).

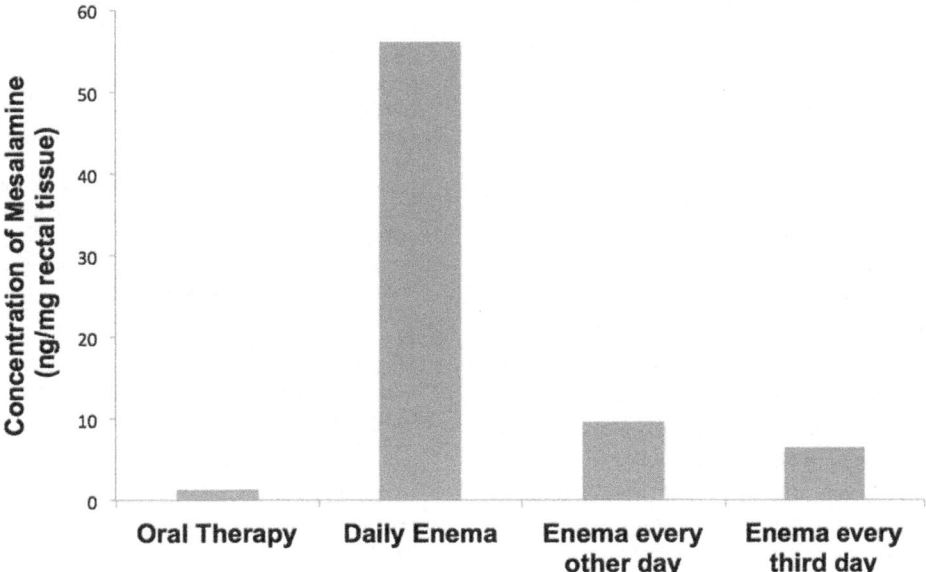

**Fig. 8.4** Comparison of rectal mucosal mesalamine concentrations after oral mesalamine therapy and 1, 2, and 3 days after a 4 g mesalamine enema administration. Statistical significance reached for 1 day vs. 2 days after enema, 2 and 3 days after enema vs. oral therapy, and 3 days after enema vs. oral therapy. *From Pimpo MT, Galletti B, Palumbo G, et al. Mesalazine vanishing time from rectal mucosa following its topical administration. J Crohns Colitis. 2010;4(1):102–105* [53]

Notably, several of these trials examining the use of topical mesalamine in the maintenance of remission utilized an intermittent dosing frequency, with use of 5-ASA enemas several times per week. Continuous versus intermittent dosing of topical mesalamine has not been compared in the literature. However, Pimpo et al. reported that mesalamine does remain in the rectal mucosa for several days beyond the day of dosing [53]. This study investigated 45 patients with ulcerative colitis in remission (16 with pancolitis and 29 with distal colitis) on oral 5-ASA therapy alone who were placed on 4 g mesalamine enemas every day, every other day, or every three days. Two rectal biopsies were taken for high performance liquid chromatography to measure mesalamine concentrations. The concentration of mesalamine in nanograms per milligram of rectal tissue was $1.32 \pm 1.41$ for oral therapy alone, $56.1 \pm 39.2$ for daily enema therapy, $9.65 \pm 6.60$ for enema therapy every other day, and $6.39 \pm 5.03$ for enema therapy every third day. Thus, while mucosal concentrations of mesalamine in the rectum rapidly decreased 2 days after topical therapy dosing, levels were still higher than with oral therapy alone (Fig. 8.4).

## Role of Mesalamine in Extensive Ulcerative Colitis

While topical mesalamine therapy does not reliably extend beyond the splenic flexure, many symptoms, even in patients with pancolitis, may come from the disease activity in the distal colon. Frequency, bleeding, and urgency are often due to inflammation in the distal colon. Marteau et al. found significantly higher rates of remission in patients with mild to moderate ulcerative colitis extending proximal to the splenic flexure who were on combination therapy with topical and oral mesalamine as compared to those on oral mesalamine alone after 8 weeks [43]. Each patient in this study received 4 g per day of oral mesalamine. For the first 4 weeks of the study, the patients received a 1 g mesalamine enema or a placebo enema. After 4 weeks, remission rates were 44 % for the combined therapy group (95 % CI 31–58 %) and 34 % (95 % CI 21–49 %) for the oral monotherapy group ($p = 0.31$). Clinical improvement was achieved in 89 % of the combined therapy group (95 % CI 78–96) and 62 % of the oral monotherapy group (95 % CI 46–75), with $p = 0.0008$.

At 8 weeks, 64 % of the combined therapy group (95 % CI 50–76 %) and 43 % (95 % CI 53–81) of the oral monotherapy group had achieved remission ($p = 0.03$). Clinical improvement was achieved in 86 % of the combined therapy group (95 % CI 75–94) and 68 % of the patients on oral monotherapy alone (95 % CI 53–81), with $p = 0.026$. Thus, the addition of topical therapy to oral therapy in patients with extensive disease did improve remission outcomes at 8 weeks and also improved clinical improvement after 4 and 8 weeks.

## Acceptability of Topical Therapy to Patients

Although topical mesalamine therapy is effective, the market share has fallen in the past two decades [54]. From 1992 to 2009, total 5-ASA prescriptions increased by 72 %, while relative to the total 5-ASA use, the market share of topical mesalamine fell from 11 to 9 % during this time period. The choice to use topical therapy is based not only on the physician's knowledge of its usefulness but also on the physician's perceptions of patient preferences and actual patient preferences.

Data on patient compliance with topical therapy is mixed. Kane et al. performed a retrospective cohort study of 3,574 patients with ulcerative colitis who were followed up to assess their medication adherence over 12 months [55]. Rectal 5-ASA use was associated with improved medication persistence at 12 months. The authors speculated that rectal 5-ASA use may correlate with disease severity and that patients with more severe disease were more likely to take their prescribed medical therapy. A study of 485 inflammatory bowel disease patients in Padua, Italy, who were given a questionnaire to determine treatment adherence, reported that the patients were more adherent with oral therapies than rectal therapy (60 % vs. 32 %, $p = 0.001$) [56]. While assumptions regarding the patient's willingness to accept topical therapy may affect prescription, a formal study of informed patients' thoughts and opinions on this matter has not been extensively addressed.

## Conclusions

Topical mesalamine therapy is an effective means of delivering 5-ASA to the distal colon. However, several different formulations and modes of delivery designed to target different extents of the distal colon are available. These medications are effective in achieving endoscopic, clinical, and histologic remission in patients with left-sided ulcerative colitis. Topical mesalamine is superior to topical steroids in several studies, and the combination of topical and oral mesalamine is more effective than oral therapy alone in inducing remission.

Topical therapy is also effective in preventing relapse. Though these medications do only reliably reach the left colon, they can be helpful in the management of symptoms in patients with extensive disease as well. While the effectiveness of topical mesalamine has been established, ultimately their use is dictated by the physicians' offering of these therapies to patients and by the patients' willingness to accept them.

## References

1. Ekbom A, Helmick C, Zack M, Adami HO. Ulcerative proctitis in central Sweden 1965-1983. A population-based epidemiological study. Dig Dis Sci. 1991;36(1):97–102.
2. Jess T, Riis L, Vind I, et al. Changes in clinical characteristics, course, and prognosis of inflammatory bowel disease during the last 5 decades: a population-based study from Copenhagen, Denmark. Inflamm Bowel Dis. 2007;13(4):481–9.
3. Langholz E. Ulcerative colitis. An epidemiological study based on a regional inception cohort, with special reference to disease course and prognosis. Dan Med Bull. 1999;46(5):400–15.
4. Kornbluth A, Sachar DB, Practice Parameters Committee of the American College of Gastroenterology. Ulcerative colitis practice guidelines in adults: American College of Gastroenterology, Practice Parameters Committee. Am J Gastroenterol. 2010;105(3): 501–23.
5. Baron JH, Connell AM, Lennard-Jones JE, Jones FA. Sulphasalazine and salicylazosulphadimidine in ulcerative colitis. Lancet. 1962; 1(7239):1094–6.
6. Svartz N. Salazopyrin, a new sulfanilamide preparation. Acta Medica Scand. 1942;110:577.
7. Svartz N. Behandlund der ulzerosen kolitis mit salazopyrin. Gastroenterologia. 1941/1942;66:312.
8. Azad Khan AK, Piris J, Truelove SC. An experiment to determine the active therapeutic moiety of sulphasalazine. Lancet. 1977;2(8044):892–5.
9. Peppercorn MA. Sulfasalazine. Pharmacology, clinical use, toxicity, and related new drug development. Ann Intern Med. 1984; 101(3):377–86.
10. Peppercorn MA, Goldman P. The role of intestinal bacteria in the metabolism of salicylazosulfapyridine. J Pharmacol Exp Ther. 1972;181(3):555–62.
11. Campieri M, Lanfranchi GA, Bazzocchi G, et al. Treatment of ulcerative colitis with high-dose 5-aminosalicylic acid enemas. Lancet. 1981;2(8241):270–1.
12. Palmer KR, Goepel JR, Holdsworth CD. Sulphasalazine retention enemas in ulcerative colitis: a double-blind trial. Br Med J (Clin Res Ed). 1981;282(6276):1571–3.
13. Frimberger E, Fruhmorgen P, Kuhner W, Ottenjann R. Sulfasalazine enema in acute left-sided ulcerative colitis (author's transl). MMW Munch Med Wochenschr. 1980;122(36):1233–5.
14. De Vos M, Verdievel H, Schoonjans R, Praet M, Bogaert M, Barbier F. Concentrations of 5-ASA and ac-5-ASA in human ileocolonic biopsy homogenates after oral 5-ASA preparations. Gut. 1992;33(10):1338–42.
15. Nugent SG, Kumar D, Rampton DS, Evans DF. Intestinal luminal pH in inflammatory bowel disease: possible determinants and implications for therapy with aminosalicylates and other drugs. Gut. 2001;48(4):571–7.
16. Haddish-Berhane N, Farhadi A, Nyquist C, Haghighi K, Keshavarzian A. Biological variability and targeted delivery of therapeutics for inflammatory bowel diseases: an in silico approach. Inflamm Allergy Drug Targets. 2007;6(1):47–55.
17. Frieri G, Pimpo MT, Palumbo GC, et al. Rectal and colonic mesalazine concentration in ulcerative colitis: oral vs. oral plus topical treatment. Aliment Pharmacol Ther. 1999;13(11):1413–7.
18. Frieri G, Giacomelli R, Pimpo M, et al. Mucosal 5-aminosalicylic acid concentration inversely correlates with severity of colonic inflammation in patients with ulcerative colitis. Gut. 2000; 47(3):410–4.
19. Williams CN, Haber G, Aquino JA. Double-blind, placebo-controlled evaluation of 5-ASA suppositories in active distal proctitis and measurement of extent of spread using $^{99m}$Tc-labeled 5-ASA suppositories. Dig Dis Sci. 1987;32(12 Suppl):71S–5.
20. Andus T, Kocjan A, Muser M, et al. Clinical trial: A novel high-dose 1 g mesalamine suppository (Salofalk) once daily is as efficacious as a 500-mg suppository thrice daily in active ulcerative proctitis. Inflamm Bowel Dis. 2010;16(11):1947–56.
21. Pokrotnieks J, Marlicz K, Paradowski L, Margus B, Zaborowski P, Greinwald R. Efficacy and tolerability of mesalazine foam enema (Salofalk foam) for distal ulcerative colitis: a double-blind,

randomized, placebo-controlled study. Aliment Pharmacol Ther. 2000;14(9):1191–8.

22. Campieri M, Corbelli C, Gionchetti P, et al. Spread and distribution of 5-ASA colonic foam and 5-ASA enema in patients with ulcerative colitis. Dig Dis Sci. 1992;37(12):1890–7.

23. Eliakim R, Tulassay Z, Kupcinskas L. Clinical trial: randomized-controlled clinical study comparing the efficacy and safety of a low-volume vs. a high-volume mesalazine foam in active distal ulcerative colitis. Aliment Pharmacol Ther. 2007;26(9):1237–49.

24. Gionchetti P, Venturi A, Rizzello F, et al. Retrograde colonic spread of a new mesalazine rectal enema in patients with distal ulcerative colitis. Aliment Pharmacol Ther. 1997;11(4):679–84.

25. Gionchetti P, Ardizzone S, Benvenuti ME, et al. A new mesalazine gel enema in the treatment of left-sided ulcerative colitis: a randomized controlled multicentre trial. Aliment Pharmacol Ther. 1999;13(3):381–8.

26. Marshall JK, Thabane M, Steinhart AH, Newman JR, Anand A, Irvine EJ. Rectal 5-aminosalicylic acid for induction of remission in ulcerative colitis. Cochrane Database Syst Rev. 2010;1, CD004115.

27. Cohen RD, Woseth DM, Thisted RA, Hanauer SB. A meta-analysis and overview of the literature on treatment options for left-sided ulcerative colitis and ulcerative proctitis. Am J Gastroenterol. 2000;95(5):1263–76.

28. Campieri M, De Franchis R, Bianchi Porro G, Ranzi T, Brunetti G, Barbara L. Mesalazine (5-aminosalicylic acid) suppositories in the treatment of ulcerative proctitis or distal proctosigmoiditis. A randomized controlled trial. Scand J Gastroenterol. 1990;25(7):663–8.

29. d'Albasio G, Paoluzi P, Campieri M, et al. Maintenance treatment of ulcerative proctitis with mesalazine suppositories: a double-blind placebo-controlled trial. The Italian IBD study group. Am J Gastroenterol. 1998;93(5):799–803.

30. Campieri M, Gionchetti P, Belluzzi A, et al. Topical treatment with 5-aminosalicylic in distal ulcerative colitis by using a new suppository preparation. A double-blind placebo controlled trial. Int J Colorectal Dis. 1990;5(2):79–81.

31. Williams CN. Efficacy and tolerance of 5-aminosalicylic acid suppositories in the treatment of ulcerative proctitis: a review of two double-blind placebo controlled trials. Can J Gastroenterol. 1990;4:472.

32. Lee FI, Jewell DP, Mani V, et al. A randomised trial comparing mesalazine and prednisolone foam enemas in patients with acute distal ulcerative colitis. Gut. 1996;38(2):229–33.

33. Danish 5-ASA Group. Topical 5-aminosalicylic acid versus prednisolone in ulcerative proctosigmoiditis. A randomized, double-blind multicenter trial. Dig Dis Sci. 1987;32(6):598–602.

34. Biancone L, Gionchetti P, Blanco Gdel V, et al. Beclomethasone dipropionate versus mesalazine in distal ulcerative colitis: a multicenter, randomized, double-blind study. Dig Liver Dis. 2007;39(4):329–37.

35. Gionchetti P, D'Arienzo A, Rizzello F, et al. Topical treatment of distal active ulcerative colitis with beclomethasone dipropionate or mesalamine: a single-blind randomized controlled trial. J Clin Gastroenterol. 2005;39(4):291–7.

36. Farup PG, Hovde O, Halvorsen FA, Raknerud N, Brodin U. Mesalazine suppositories versus hydrocortisone foam in patients with distal ulcerative colitis. A comparison of the efficacy and practicality of two topical treatment regimens. Scand J Gastroenterol. 1995;30(2):164–70.

37. Lemann M, Galian A, Rutgeerts P, et al. Comparison of budesonide and 5-aminosalicylic acid enemas in active distal ulcerative colitis. Aliment Pharmacol Ther. 1995;9(5):557–62.

38. Ford AC, Khan KJ, Achkar JP, Moayyedi P. Efficacy of oral vs. topical, or combined oral and topical 5-aminosalicylates, in ulcerative colitis: systematic review and meta-analysis. Am J Gastroenterol. 2012;107(2):167–76.

39. Gionchetti P, Rizzello F, Venturi A, et al. Comparison of oral with rectal mesalazine in the treatment of ulcerative proctitis. Dis Colon Rectum. 1998;41(1):93–7.

40. Kam L, Cohen H, Dooley C, Rubin P, Orchard J. A comparison of mesalamine suspension enema and oral sulfasalazine for treatment of active distal ulcerative colitis in adults. Am J Gastroenterol. 1996;91(7):1338–42.

41. Prantera C, Viscido A, Biancone L, Francavilla A, Giglio L, Campieri M. A new oral delivery system for 5-ASA: preliminary clinical findings for MMx. Inflamm Bowel Dis. 2005;11(5):421–7.

42. Safdi M, DeMicco M, Sninsky C, et al. A double-blind comparison of oral versus rectal mesalamine versus combination therapy in the treatment of distal ulcerative colitis. Am J Gastroenterol. 1997;92(10):1867–71.

43. Marteau P, Probert CS, Lindgren S, et al. Combined oral and enema treatment with Pentasa (mesalazine) is superior to oral therapy alone in patients with extensive mild/moderate active ulcerative colitis: a randomised, double blind, placebo controlled study. Gut. 2005;54(7):960–5.

44. Fruhmorgen P, Demling L. On the efficacy of ready-made-up commercially available salicylazosulphapyridine enemas in the treatment of proctitis, proctosigmoiditis and ulcerative colitis involving rectum, sigmoid and descending colon. Hepatogastroenterology. 1980;27(6):473–6.

45. Vecchi M, Meucci G, Gionchetti P, et al. Oral versus combination mesalazine therapy in active ulcerative colitis: a double-blind, double-dummy, randomized multicentre study. Aliment Pharmacol Ther. 2001;15(2):251–6.

46. Marteau P, Crand J, Foucault M, Rambaud JC. Use of mesalazine slow release suppositories 1 g three times per week to maintain remission of ulcerative proctitis: a randomised double blind placebo controlled multicentre study. Gut. 1998;42(2):195–9.

47. Hanauer S, Good LI, Goodman MW, et al. Long-term use of mesalamine (Rowasa) suppositories in remission maintenance of ulcerative proctitis. Am J Gastroenterol. 2000;95(7):1749–54.

48. D'Arienzo A, Panarese A, D'Armiento FP, et al. 5-aminosalicylic acid suppositories in the maintenance of remission in idiopathic proctitis or proctosigmoiditis: a double-blind placebo-controlled clinical trial. Am J Gastroenterol. 1990;85(9):1079–82.

49. Biddle WL, Greenberger NJ, Swan JT, McPhee MS, Miner Jr PB. 5-aminosalicylic acid enemas: effective agent in maintaining remission in left-sided ulcerative colitis. Gastroenterology. 1988;94(4):1075–9.

50. Miner P, Daly R, Nester T. The effect of varying dose intervals of mesalamine enemas for the prevention of relapse in distal ulcerative colitis. Gastroenterology. 1994;106 Suppl 2:A736.

51. d'Albasio G, Pacini F, Camarri E, et al. Combined therapy with 5-aminosalicylic acid tablets and enemas for maintaining remission in ulcerative colitis: a randomized double-blind study. Am J Gastroenterol. 1997;92(7):1143–7.

52. Yokoyama H, Takagi S, Kuriyama S, et al. Effect of weekend 5-aminosalicylic acid (mesalazine) enema as maintenance therapy for ulcerative colitis: results from a randomized controlled study. Inflamm Bowel Dis. 2007;13(9):1115–20.

53. Pimpo MT, Galletti B, Palumbo G, et al. Mesalazine vanishing time from rectal mucosa following its topical administration. J Crohns Colitis. 2010;4(1):102–5.

54. Harris MS, Lichtenstein GR. Review article: delivery and efficacy of topical 5-aminosalicylic acid (mesalazine) therapy in the treatment of ulcerative colitis. Aliment Pharmacol Ther. 2011;33(9):996–1009.

55. Kane SV, Accortt NA, Magowan S, Brixner D. Predictors of persistence with 5-aminosalicylic acid therapy for ulcerative colitis. Aliment Pharmacol Ther. 2009;29(8):855–62.

56. D'Inca R, Bertomoro P, Mazzocco K, Vettorato MG, Rumiati R, Sturniolo GC. Risk factors for non-adherence to medication in

inflammatory bowel disease patients. Aliment Pharmacol Ther. 2008;27(2):166–72.

57. Marshall JK, Irvine EJ. Putting rectal 5-aminosalicylic acid in its place: the role in distal ulcerative colitis. Am J Gastroenterol. 2000;95(7):1628–36.

58. Hanauer SB, Robinson M, Pruitt R, et al. Budesonide enema for the treatment of active, distal ulcerative colitis and proctitis: a dose-ranging study. U.S. Budesonide Enema Study Group. Gastroenterology. 1998;115(3):525–32.

59. Campieri M, Gionchetti P, Beluzzi A, et al. Sucralfate 5-aminosalicylic acid and placebo enemas in the treatment of ulcerative colitis. Eur J Gastroenterol Hepatol. 1991;3:41–4.

60. Campieri M, Gionchetti P, Belluzi A, et al. Optimum dosage of 5-aminosalicylic acid as rectal enemas in patients with active ulcerative colitis. Gut. 1991;32(8):929–31.

61. Moller C, Kiviluoto O, Santavirta S. Local treatment of ulcerative proctitis with Salicylazosulphapyridine (Salazopyrin) enema. Clin Trials J. 1978;15(6):199–203.

# Oral and Parenteral Corticosteroid Therapy in Ulcerative Colitis

Anita Afzali, Chelle L. Wheat, and Scott D. Lee

**Keywords**

Corticosteroids • Ulcerative colitis • Oral • Parenteral • Glucocorticosteroids • Corticosteroid mechanism of action • Efficacy • Remission • Patient selection • Disease severity • Extent of disease • Mild-to-moderate ulcerative colitis • Severe-to-fulminant ulcerative colitis • Maintenance therapy • Corticosteroid dose • Route adjustment • Predictors of nonresponders • Colectomy • Adverse effects

## Introduction

Over the past 50 years, the widespread use of corticosteroids in the management of active ulcerative colitis (UC) has resulted in a dramatic mortality reduction. In the 1930s, mortality from UC was estimated to be up to 75 % [1], and this has decreased to less than 1 % in the twenty-first century [2]. Similarly to other drugs used to treat autoimmune inflammatory disorders, corticosteroids were first used in the treatment of rheumatoid arthritis and then applied to inflammatory bowel disease.

In 1949, Edward C. Kendall and Philip S. Hench, two American chemists, identified "Compound E" which would later become known as cortisone [3]. They introduced "Compound E" to the rheumatology community and found

that the wonder drug, when injected into rheumatoid arthritic joints, allowed for marked pain relief, as well as decreased inflammation and recovery. Their contribution was recognized in 1950, when they, along with Tadeus Reichstein, were awarded a Nobel Prize for Physiology and Medicine for their introduction and discovery of adrenal cortex hormones [4].

Glucocorticosteroids are a class of steroid hormones synthesized in the adrenal cortex, and cortisol (or hydrocortisone) is the most important human glucocorticosteroid. There are a variety of synthetic glucocorticosteroids, and they are grouped into classes based on chemical structure, route of administration, and pharmacokinetics. Corticosteroids can be administered orally (e.g., prednisone, prednisolone, and budesonide), parenterally (e.g., intravenous methylprednisolone and hydrocortisone), and topically or rectally (e.g., hydrocortisone suppositories or foam). This chapter will focus on the oral and parenteral use of conventional corticosteroids in ulcerative colitis.

The initial controlled trials demonstrating efficacy of oral corticosteroids in patients with ulcerative colitis was published in 1955 by Truelove and Witts [5], and the mainstay of intravenous corticosteroid use was established in 1974 [6] for the treatment of severe disease exacerbations. Acute severe ulcerative colitis is potentially a life-threatening condition, and systemic corticosteroids remain the gold standard for the treatment of acute moderate and severe colitis. While there have been significant advances in the number of therapies proven to be effective for both induction and maintenance of remission of UC, corticosteroids

A. Afzali, M.D., M.P.H. (✉)
Division of Gastroenterology, Department of Internal Medicine, University of Washington, 1959 NE Pacific Street, Suite AA-103, P.O. Box 356424, Seattle, WA 98195, USA
e-mail: anitaa@medicine.washington.edu

C.L. Wheat, M.P.H.
Department of Inflammatory Bowel Disease, University of Washington, 1959 NE Pacific Street, Ste AA-103, UW Box 356424, Seattle, WA 98195, USA

S.D. Lee, M.D.
Division of Gastroenterology, Department of Inflammatory Bowel Disease Program, University of Washington, 1959 NE Pacific Street, Suite AA103, UW Box 356424, Seattle, WA 98195, USA

remain a critical line of therapy that many if not most UC patients will be exposed to at some point during their disease course. It is important for physicians to clearly understand how best to employ corticosteroids and the risks associated with their use.

## Corticosteroid Mechanism of Action

The use of corticosteroids in inflammatory bowel disease is based on its ability to modulate the immune response and suppress inflammation. It is known that corticosteroids function partly by the induction of anti-inflammatory genes such as secretory leukocyte proteinase inhibitor and lipocortin-1 and interleukin-1 receptor antagonists [7]. However, the primary function of corticosteroids is repression of inflammatory genes by binding to cytosolic glucocorticoid receptor (GR) that on activation translocates to the cell nucleus. GR activation then either induces or represses the expression of

responsive genes [8]. By switching off the inflammatory genes that are activated by pro-inflammatory transcription factors and encoding anti-inflammatory proteins, corticosteroids inhibit the expression of adhesion molecules and minimize the trafficking of inflammatory cells to tissue, including the intestines [9]. They also induce apoptosis of activated lymphocytes and decrease inflammatory cytokine release [10–12]. A schematic representation of the mechanism of action of corticosteroids on the immune system is described in Fig. 9.1.

Although corticosteroids can suppress inflammatory genes, they also inhibit the transcription of other genes, including osteocalcin, keratin, proopiomelanocortin (POMC), and corticotropin-releasing factor (CRF-1) [8]. These genes are associated with some of the known side effects of long-term corticosteroid use and include osteoporosis, poor wound healing, adrenal insufficiency, and diabetes.

Corticosteroid binding protein (Bs) transports corticosteroid molecules (Ss) into the cell cytoplasm, while dissociated

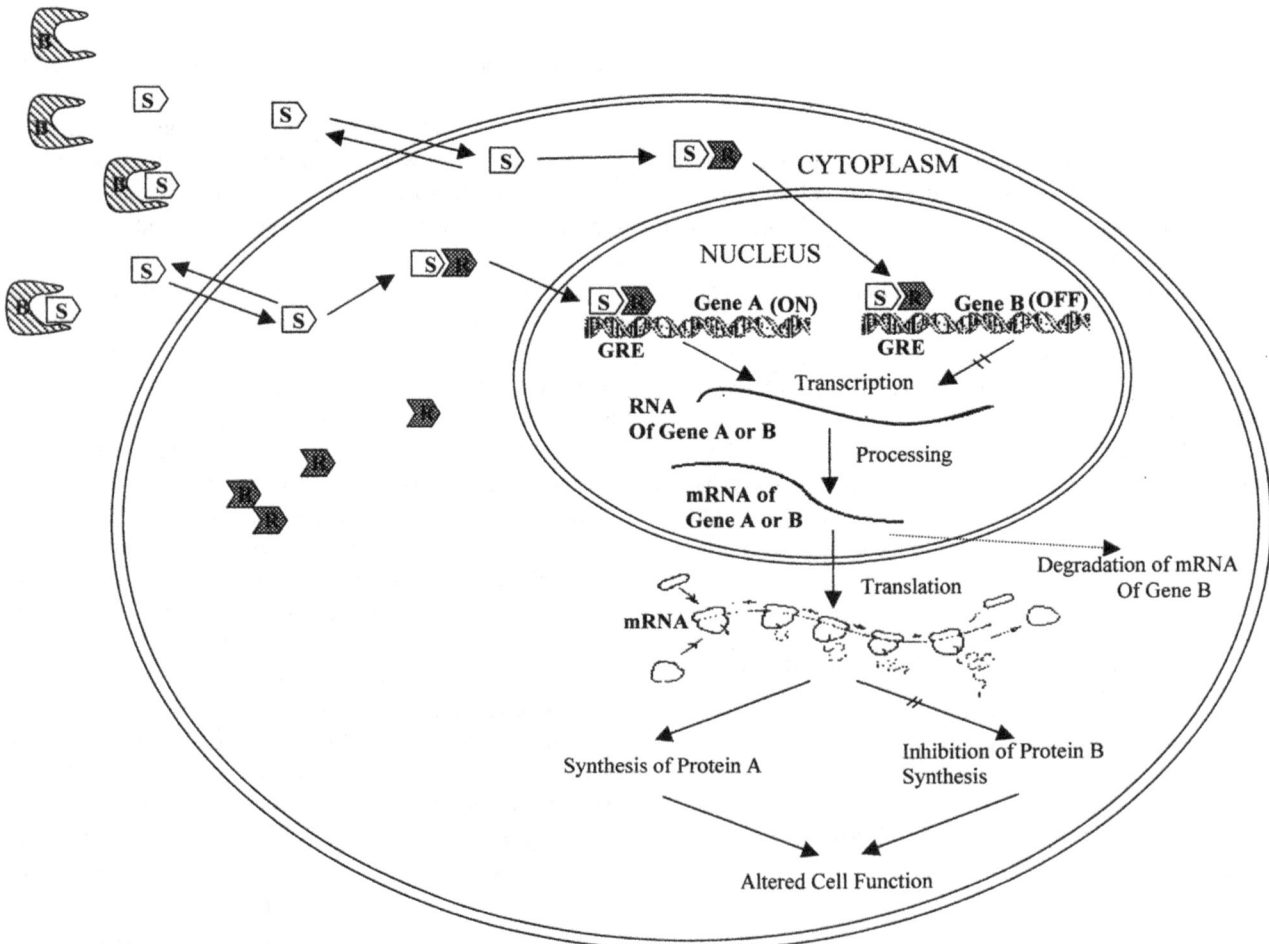

**Fig. 9.1** The mechanism of action of corticosteroids on the immune system

corticosteroid molecules can also cross the cell membrane freely. Once inside the cytoplasm, they bind to their receptors (Rs), and the corticosteroid/receptor complex then translocates into the nucleus and bind to the glucocorticoid response elements (GREs). GREs are located in the promoter region of steroid-responsive target genes and can either promote (ON) or suppress (OFF) the transcription of a gene. This in turn may also decrease the synthesis of proteins (protein A or B) and posttranscription of the gene (gene A or B). Adapted from Yang and Lichtenstein [13].

## Efficacy of Corticosteroids in Induction of Remission

Truelove and Witts [5] were the first investigators to suggest the addition of corticosteroid use in the medical treatment of ulcerative colitis in 1955. Their preliminary findings in 1954 [14] included 210 patients from five different hospitals with chronic ulcerative colitis that would normally have received 6 weeks of treatment in the hospital. Of those patients, 109 were treated with oral cortisone (up to 100 mg per day) compared to placebo ($n = 101$) for 6 weeks. At the end of the study period, patients were classified into three categories: clinical remission, improved, and no change or worse. Clinical remission was defined as one or two nonbloody stools daily, weight gain, and without fever or tachycardia. Hemoglobin and ESR values were also either normal or returning to normal. The improved group included all intermediate cases, and the no change or worse group is self-explanatory. Cortisone-treated patients appeared to do better than placebo-treated patients and were more likely to be in clinical remission (41.3 % vs. 15.8 %) at the end of the 6-week study ($p$-value <0.001). These findings held particularly true in patients treated with cortisone on their first attack of disease but also true of disease relapse as well as all grades of disease severity. In a subset of patients, sigmoidoscopic or barium enema examinations were also assessed at the end of treatment and seemed to suggest that the cortisone-treated group did better than the control group; however, the numbers of patients in these groups were a small sample of the total patients and therefore only a preliminary conclusion [5].

In 1974, it was discovered that a 5-day intensive intravenous cortisone regimen for treatment of severe attacks similarly resulted in higher remission rates [6]. A total of 49 patients over a 5-year period received intravenous prednisolone 60 mg in divided doses for 5 days. Nearly 75 % ($n = 36$) of the patients experienced rapid improvement and were symptom-free after 5 days, and 92 % ($n = 33$) of these patients remained without symptoms during the next 6 weeks. The patients were followed on an average of 3 years, and approximately 50 % remained in remission ($p$-value <0.02). Factors that influenced the success of the intravenous regimen included patients who were treated during their first attack and those with radiological evidence of extensive or distal disease. The authors also concluded that complete failure to respond to intravenous therapy or deterioration during the 5-day course of treatment was an absolute indication for emergency surgery in patients with severe disease.

A number of subsequent studies have also demonstrated similar remission rates in patients treated with corticosteroid therapy. Furthermore, a recent systematic review [9] identified five randomized controlled trials (RCTs) [5, 15–18], which involved 445 patients and determined the efficacy and safety of corticosteroid therapy in ulcerative colitis. Of the 226 patients that received corticosteroids, 46 % achieved remission compared to 21 % of the 219 patients that were treated with placebo after 2–8 weeks. Corticosteroids induced remission in active UC with a number needed to treat (NNT) of 3 (95 % CI 2–9). When oral corticosteroids that were thought to act mainly topically and therefore poorly absorbed, such as oral fluticasone or beclomethasone, were excluded, there were three remaining trials [5, 16, 17] with a NNT of 2 (95 % CI 1.4–6) [19]. Similarly, intravenous corticosteroids were also successful at inducing remission [20], but given the route of administration and short duration therapy, it was not included in the meta-analysis.

## Who Should Receive Corticosteroid Therapy?

Severity and extent of disease is based on both clinical and endoscopic findings and is characterized as mild, moderate, severe, as well as fulminant colitis [21]. Although the natural history of ulcerative colitis is variable, it is estimated that approximately 15 % of UC patients will develop severe symptoms that require hospitalization and intensive medical therapy [22]. Acute severe colitis is potentially a life-threatening condition that requires early appropriate medical therapy with a primary goal to induce remission and decrease the risk for colectomy. Indeed, corticosteroids have helped decrease the mortality risk associated with severe or fulminant colitis from 75 % in the 1930s [1] to less than 1 % in the twenty-first century [2]; however, since the introduction and widespread use of corticosteroids, there has been no significant change in colectomy rates over the last 30 years [2].

### Mild-to-Moderate Ulcerative Colitis

Based on the recent American College of Gastroenterology (ACG) practice guidelines for the management of ulcerative colitis in adult patients, oral or parenteral corticosteroid therapy should be reserved for patients with moderate or severe disease activity [23]. The exception would include patients who have failed first-line therapy for their colitis. For example, patients with mild-to-moderate distal colitis who have failed oral aminosalicylates, topical mesalamine, and topical steroids or who are refractory to these therapies and have also failed mesalamine enemas or suppositories should receive a course of oral corticosteroid therapy. Similarly, patients with mild-to-moderate extensive colitis that have failed oral sulfasalazine or aminosalicylates, have a course of corticosteroids if refractory to other therapy, or have systemic symptoms that require rapid improvement should be considered [23]. Corticosteroid therapy in these circumstances, and in fact in almost all cases, should be indicated primarily for short-term induction of remission and not as maintenance therapy [24].

## Severe-to-Fulminant Ulcerative Colitis

Severe colitis has been previously defined by the Truelove and Witts criteria [5] and includes bloody stool frequency of six or more per day with evidence of toxicity as shown by tachycardia (>90 bpm), temperature >37.8 °C, anemia (hemoglobin <10.5 g/dL), or an elevated erythrocyte sedimentation rate (ESR) of >30 mm/h.

Patients with severe colitis should receive oral corticosteroids (the equivalent of 40–60 mg of prednisone) daily with a goal to induce remission [23]. Those that are refractory to maximum oral prednisone, oral aminosalicylates, and topical medications or that have systemic signs of toxicity should be hospitalized for intravenous corticosteroid therapy. Although there have been no comparative head-to-head studies that have determined any differences in the efficacy of different parenteral corticosteroids, the most commonly prescribed parenteral corticosteroid is in the form of methylprednisolone (40–60 mg), since it has decreased mineralocorticoid properties as compared to hydrocortisone (300–400 mg daily) [24].

## Maintenance Therapy in Ulcerative Colitis

Corticosteroids have not been shown to be beneficial in the maintenance of remission in ulcerative colitis and therefore should not be used for this indication [25].

Following the original large-scale therapeutic trials of oral cortisone [5] that demonstrated its effectiveness in the induction of disease remission, a follow-up trial assessed if small cortisone maintenance doses would sustain a patient in clinical remission [26]. A total of 68 patients were randomized to receive oral cortisone, 25 mg orally twice per day ($n = 37$) compared to placebo ($n = 31$). Patients were observed for 1 year, and the study determined that maintenance treatment with cortisone had no beneficial effect on the course of

disease. In fact, cortisone-treated patients suffered a higher rate of relapse (48.6 %) compared to the placebo arm (41.9 %), although this difference was not statistically significant ($p$-value >0.05).

Similarly, in another randomized trial, oral prednisone (5 mg orally three times per day) was given for 6 months in patients with ulcerative colitis in remission and compared to placebo [27]. The study determined no difference in the number of patients that remained in remission (12/32 in the treatment arm compared to 12/30 in the placebo arm) or had disease relapse (18/32 in the treatment arm compared to 17/30 in the placebo arm) at the end of the study period. Furthermore, prednisone-treated patients experienced more side effects.

In a double-blind crossover trial ($n = 24$) that compared prednisone (40 mg orally given on alternate days) to placebo for maintenance treatment in ulcerative colitis, there was a reduced number of patients that experienced disease relapse when treated with corticosteroids over a period of 3 months ($p$-value <0.01) [28]. However, this was again at the expense of a larger number of corticosteroid-related side effects. While this trial did show benefit of using corticosteroids over a 3-month period, given that UC is a lifelong disease with no known medical cure and the fact that by modern standards the length of this trial would not be an adequate period of time to be considered a maintenance trial, it must be emphasized that corticosteroids should not be used as a maintenance treatment [24].

## Corticosteroid Dose and Route Adjustment

Once the decision to use corticosteroids has been made, there is unfortunately little evidence-based data available to indicate the optimal dose and route for corticosteroid administration in management of active colitis.

In one study of outpatients with moderate ulcerative colitis treated with corticosteroids (oral prednisone 20, 40, and 60 mg), remission was achieved in two-thirds of the patients who received 40 or 60 mg but only in one-third of those given 20 mg daily. In addition, the side effects were more frequent in patients that received 60 mg daily than 40 mg and with no significantly greater efficacy [29].

Another randomized trial performed on patients with active proctocolitis found no difference in response rate or side effects produced in those that received oral prednisolone at 10 mg four times a day or 40 mg as once per day dosing [30].

With the lack of evidence that doses higher than 60 mg per day result in significantly higher efficacy, we recommend that patients with moderate-to-severe active colitis that require corticosteroid use for active disease be treated with a course of prednisone 40–60 mg orally once per day. In addition to lack of evidence that higher doses result in higher efficacy, higher doses of corticosteroids result in significantly more frequent and severe adverse effects. Finally, another reason to use a single daily dosing regimen is that studies have shown that lowering the daily frequency of any given medication increases compliance rates. Thus, given the lack of evidence regarding improved efficacy over single daily dosing regimen, in all likelihood this dose regimen will increase compliance and hence increase the likelihood of efficacy.

As noted above, there are a significant percentage of UC patients whose disease is nonresponsive to corticosteroid therapy. Prior to diagnosing a UC patient as steroid-resistant or nonresponsive, a trial of corticosteroids is administered in intravenous form when there is a lack of response to oral treatment at 40–60 mg daily [31] or when there are systemic signs of toxicity, and the patient requires hospitalized care. This is based on the pharmacokinetics of oral versus parenteral corticosteroids. It has been demonstrated that peak plasma levels of oral corticosteroid absorption is delayed in patients with active colitis [32], and parenteral corticosteroid administration as a continuous infusion is associated with a higher plasma concentrations and less variability in plasma levels [33]. Hence, changing patients from oral to intravenous steroids will insure that the lack of response is not due to any issues with absorption of oral corticosteroids.

If there is no clinical improvement with the initial oral corticosteroid regimen after 5–7 days, or if there are systemic signs of toxicity or evidence of fulminant colitis, then the patient requires hospitalization for parenteral corticosteroid treatment, commonly methylprednisolone at a dose equivalent to 1 mg/kg per body weight. If significant clinical improvement is achieved following administration of parenteral treatment, then the intravenous corticosteroid therapy can be transitioned to oral form, and a similar taper schedule as outlined above can be followed [24].

While a continuous infusion results in less variability in plasma concentrations, there is no improved efficacy of continuous corticosteroid infusion compared to a single intravenous daily bolus. In a double-blind randomized trial of patients with severe ulcerative colitis that either received 1 mg/kg/day of methylprednisolone administered as continuous infusion or given as a bolus dose, no significant difference in the efficacy or safety profile is found [20].

In a systematic review [2] of 32 cohort and controlled clinical trials assessing the efficacy of corticosteroids in severe ulcerative colitis, 24 studies reported the dose administered of intravenous corticosteroids, standardized as methylprednisolone equivalent (using mean adult weight 70 kg). In this meta-regression analysis that controlled for disease severity, there was no correlation found between corticosteroid dose used and colectomy rate ($R^2 < 0.01$, $p$-value 0.98). Further, the risk for colectomy did not decrease any further when corticosteroid doses beyond 60 mg daily were used.

In patients that have received systemic steroid therapy for active colitis and achieved clinical improvement, physicians should at this point implement a plan to discontinue corticosteroids since there is no benefit for its use in maintenance therapy and long-term use results in a higher risk of adverse effects [24]. As there is a very high rate of disease relapse after corticosteroids are stopped, discontinuation of corticosteroids should be done with a plan to implement a steroid-sparing maintenance medication.

There are no randomized trials that have studied an optimal corticosteroid taper schedule after clinical symptoms improve in a patient with active disease. We recommend that if oral prednisone 40–60 mg daily for moderate-to-severe active colitis is given and if there is significant clinical improvement, a taper dose schedule can then be initiated with 5–10 mg taper weekly until 20 mg daily dose is reached [24]. Then, tapering should proceed by 2.5–5.0 mg per week. In addition to concerns regarding relapse of disease, clinicians should be cautious of the development of symptoms secondary to adrenal insufficiency, especially in those patients that have been on corticosteroids for a prolonged time. Adrenal insufficiency may manifest up to 9 months after steroid cessation, particularly in times of stress [34].

## Predictors of Corticosteroid Nonresponders

It is estimated that one-third of patients hospitalized with severe ulcerative colitis will fail to respond to corticosteroid therapy and may require urgent colectomy [2]. The development of predictive measures for identifying patients that are nonrespondent to corticosteroid treatment has helped determine who may be suitable for second-line medical therapy (calcineurin inhibitors such as cyclosporine or antitumor necrosis factor antibodies such as infliximab) or colectomy. Since much of the morbidity and mortality associated with severe UC is related to delayed surgery, it is prudent to identify early which patients are likely to fail corticosteroid treatment and determine when to initiate other rescue medical therapy, so that if surgery is necessary, it is not inappropriately delayed [35, 36].

There are two predictive models that have helped determine which patients may need early colectomy. In one prospective study by Travis et al. [37], patients with severe colitis defined as 8 stools per day or 3–8 stools per day and an elevated C-reactive protein (CRP) of >45 mg/L on the third day of intravenous therapy had a positive predictive value (PPV) of 85 % for colectomy. Similarly, Lindgren et al. [36] developed a regression formula to predict the likelihood of medical failure (fulminant colitis index = number stool frequency/day + 0.14 × CRP mg/L) and found that a cutoff score greater than 8 at day 3 had a PPV of 72 % for colectomy.

More recently, Ho et al. [38] developed predictive factors of nonresponse to corticosteroid therapy and a risk score to help identify patients within the first 3 days of medical therapy for either early second-line medical therapy or early surgery. This was developed from a retrospective chart review of 167 patients with severe ulcerative colitis. The scoring system was based on a 0–9 point scale and included an assessment of mean stool frequency (<4, 4–6, 7–9, >9), presence of colonic dilation (>4 cm), and hypoalbuminemia (<30 g/L). Patients with a score of 0–1 had a low likelihood of medical therapy failure (11 % risk), and those with a score of 2–3 had an intermediate likelihood of failure to medical therapy (43 % risk). A score of ≥4 predicted a high likelihood of nonresponse to medical therapy failure with a sensitivity of 85 % and specificity of 75 % (AUC, area under the curve 0.88).

Clinical evaluation after 3 days of systemic corticosteroid therapy appears to be the best tool in assessing the short-term prognosis of active colitis in a patient [39]. These are some clinical parameters described that may be used when assessing for treatment response and consideration for second-line medical therapy or surgery. We recommend that if the patient has not responded after 3–5 days of intravenous corticosteroids, considerations be given toward the aforementioned options and importantly steroids be tapered as rapidly as feasible, as the patient will still develop the inherent side effects from the ongoing corticosteroid use without benefit.

## Corticosteroid Use and Rate of Colectomy

The lifetime colectomy risk in severe colitis is estimated to be 30–35 % [2, 31]. Based on well-established clinical parameters, the general response to parenteral corticosteroid treatment in short-term studies (5–14 days) is reported between 45 and 80 % [24]. Patients are typically deemed steroid refractory if there is a lack of response to intensive intravenous corticosteroid treatment at adequate doses (1 mg/kg/day) for 7–10 days [40]. The prolongation of corticosteroid therapy beyond 10 days did not improve remission rates. In fact, longer corticosteroid treatment may result in more deleterious outcomes as surgery is delayed in the patient with severe colitis. Unfortunately and despite our current medical therapy, the short-term colectomy rate in severe colitis has not changed over the past three decades in a systematic review from 1974 to 2006 [2].

In a large population-based Olmsted County cohort [41], patients with ulcerative colitis that did not respond to corticosteroids in the short term (less than 30 days) had a 90 % colectomy rate. However, even among the patients that initially responded to corticosteroid treatment in the short term, only 49 % of the patients maintained remission without surgery or prolonged corticosteroid use over the following 1-year study period. The data also approximated that a quarter of patients with UC are steroid dependent at the end of 1 year.

These findings raise concern for the less than optimal long-term outcomes in some patients with active colitis that require a course of systemic corticosteroids and also highlight the high risk for colectomy in patients nonresponsive to corticosteroids. Other medical treatment modalities and surgery should be considered once it is determined that a patient is steroid refractory. These data also emphasize that even those patients that respond to corticosteroids are still at significant risk for colectomy. Thus, once a patient has had improvement in symptoms, while the patient is beginning to taper corticosteroids, he or she should also be placed on a long-term maintenance non-corticosteroid therapy.

## Adverse Effects Related to Corticosteroid Therapy

The potential for adverse effects related to corticosteroids is both dose and duration of therapy dependent. Corticosteroids resulted in side effects in over 50 % of patients that were receiving high-dose steroid treatment and in 30 % of patients on prophylactic doses [42].

Early side effects related to supraphysiologic corticosteroid doses include moon facies, acne, edema, glucose intolerance, sleep and mood disturbances, and dyspepsia [24]. The effects from prolonged use (usually >12 weeks) are believed to be due to the corticosteroid effects of gene induction [8]. As a result, adverse events such as posterior sublenticular cataracts, osteoporosis, osteonecrosis, myopathy, hypertension, and hyperlipidemia may occur [8, 24, 43]. In a review paper [44] on communicating risks associated with IBD therapy to patients, an estimated frequency for a number of adverse events associated with corticosteroid therapy was determined and described in Table 9.1.

Most of the side effects related to corticosteroid use are best treated with withdrawing the steroid and substituting with other therapy. The risk for osteopenia and osteoporosis in patients with UC can be reduced by keeping the dose of corticosteroids minimal. Further, factors that contribute to osteoporosis in the non-IBD population may also play a role in patients with IBD and include sedentary lifestyles, low body weight, hypogonadism, poor dietary intake of vitamin D and calcium, smoking, and corticosteroid use [45].

Bone mineral density (BMD) testing has been recommended for patients on corticosteroids for greater than 3 months in a year. If osteoporosis, defined by a $T$-score ≤2.5 SDs below normal is present, then bisphosphonate therapy should be initiated [46, 47]. Patients that are postmenopausal or with a history of a previous fracture in which corticosteroid therapy will be initiated or have remained on therapy

**Table 9.1** Estimated frequency of adverse events related to corticosteroid therapy

| Adverse event | Estimated frequency (%) |
| --- | --- |
| Any side effect leading to discontinuation of corticosteroid | 55 |
| Acne | 50 |
| Facial swelling | 35 |
| Osteoporosis | 33 |
| Increased eye pressure | 22 |
| Infections | 13 |
| Hypertension | 13 |
| Ankle edema | 11 |
| Cataracts | 9 |
| Memory problems | 7 |
| Easy bruising | 7 |
| Psychosis, confusion or agitation | 1 |
| Other including diabetes, severe hip/bone damage, and adrenal insufficiency | Uncertain frequency |

Modified from Siegel CA. Review article: Explaining the risks of inflammatory bowel disease therapy to patients. Alimentary Pharmacology and Therapeutics 2011; 33: 23–32 [44]

for >3 months should also be on prophylactic bisphosphonate therapy [24]. Daily vitamin D (400–800 IU/day) and calcium (1,200–1,500 mg/day) are also advised for patients on chronic steroid therapy [24].

Given the associated risk for the development of cataracts and glaucoma with corticosteroid exposure, annual ophthalmologic examinations are recommended for patients with long-term corticosteroid use [24].

Corticosteroid-induced metabolic disturbances such as hyperglycemia, sodium and fluid retention, metabolic alkalosis, and hyperlipidemia may also occur [23]. Patients should be monitored for these metabolic abnormalities. There is an increased risk for adrenal insufficiency, particularly in patients on chronic corticosteroids when the steroids are discontinued or tapered too rapidly, especially following surgery. In addition, stress-dose corticosteroids may be needed perioperatively [48].

Patients with IBD and corticosteroid exposure are at significant increased risk for the development of opportunistic infections (OR 3.4; 95 % CI 1.8–6.2) [49]. Most commonly, corticosteroid use is associated with increased infections in the mouth, pharynx, or esophagus with candidiasis. Furthermore, this risk is synergistically increased when corticosteroids are used concomitantly with thiopurines or infliximab [49]. A similarly increased risk for infectious complications was found in a retrospective cohort study of IBD patients ($n = 159$) that underwent elective bowel surgery and received corticosteroid treatment (OR 3.69, 95 % CI 1.24–10.97) [50].

Despite the fact that previous literature of patients with solid organ transplants or human immunodeficiency syndrome (HIV) has demonstrated utility in prophylaxis against potential opportunistic infections, there are no current well-defined guidelines for infection prophylaxis in patients with inflammatory bowel disease on immunomodulators or immunosuppressants [51–53].

Studies have found that a lymphocyte count <600/mm$^3$ and a CD4 count <300/mm$^3$ are predictive for particular opportunistic infections (OIs), such as *Pneumocystis jiroveci* (formerly *Pneumocystis carinii*, PCP) [54, 55]. This is of particular concern for long-term corticosteroid exposure (>1 month) as it is associated with dose-dependent lymphocyte depletion and when used concomitantly with other immunosuppressive agents has additional risk for lymphocytopenia [52].

One of the first case reports of patients with underlying inflammatory bowel disease that developed PCP was described in two patients with ulcerative colitis while on high-dose corticosteroids [56]. Since then, although data on PCP prophylaxis in patients with IBD is limited, it is suggested that prophylaxis should be provided to patients on chronic treatment with at least two immunosuppressant agents, including corticosteroids and to patients with a lymphocyte count <600/mm$^3$ and a CD4 count <300/mm$^3$ [52]. Prophylaxis treatment options include trimethoprim-sulfamethoxazole (TMP-SMZ) or if not tolerated, then alternatives include dapsone, aerosolized pentamidine, and atovaquone.

Given the increased susceptibility for infections, patients that display systemic symptoms of infection, such as fever, must always be evaluated. More importantly, all patients with IBD should have a thorough review of their vaccination history and risk assessment at the time of their initial IBD consultation and before any immunosuppressive therapy is initiated. A rigorous and standardized vaccination program may help decrease some of the infectious complications associated with IBD therapy, including corticosteroids (Table 9.2) [57].

## Conclusion

Although corticosteroids contribute morbidity, especially in regard to infectious complications, and potential mortality to the ulcerative colitis patient, they continue to have a place for the treatment of severe and fulminant disease in the short term. In those patients that respond, the effect is rapid and corticosteroids are widely available and very inexpensive. Evidence from multiple investigational studies supports their efficacy for the management of acute severe disease exacerbation; however, among this patient population, it is estimated that up to one-third of patients will fail therapy and still require colectomy. In addition, while there are no definitive studies that provide evidence to the optimal dosage,

**Table 9.2** Management recommendations for patients receiving long-term corticosteroid therapy

- DEXA scan
- Daily vitamin D and calcium supplementation
- Annual ophthalmologic examinations
- Routine laboratory studies to include comprehensive metabolic panel and complete blood count every 3–6 months
- General vaccination considerations

  *If vaccination history unknown, check the following titers at first clinic visit:*
  - MMR
  - Varicella
  - Hepatitis A
  - Hepatitis B

  *Vaccinations to consider administrating:*
  - Tdap
  - HPV
  - Influenza
  - Pneumococcal
  - Hepatitis A
  - Hepatitis B
  - Meningococcal

*MMR* measles, mumps, rubella. *Tdap* tetanus, diphtheria, pertussis. *HPV* human papilloma virus
Modified from Wasan SK, Baker SE, Skolnik PR et al. A practical guide to vaccinating the inflammatory bowel disease patient. American Journal of Gastroenterology 2010; 105: 1231–1238 [57]

currently available evidence suggests that 40–60 mg once daily (prednisone equivalent) is likely the most effective dose, and higher doses do not result in improved response but do result in more side effects.

Given the side effects associated with corticosteroid use, they should be used with caution along with careful monitoring and only in this narrowly defined patient subpopulation. Once the decision has been made to use corticosteroids, if there is not a prompt improvement in symptoms with oral corticosteroids, the patient should be given a trial of parenteral forms to eliminate any issues of absorption and provide stable plasma levels. Failing this, they should be tapered rapidly and discontinued with consideration given to rescue medical therapies or surgical discussion. If patients do respond, definitive long-term steroid-sparing maintenance medical therapy should be considered while the steroids are being tapered because most patients will flare once steroids are discontinued and are still at very high risk for colectomy.

It is worthwhile stressing that corticosteroids have no long-term role in the maintenance of UC, as its prolonged use does not result in maintenance of remission. In addition, the longer the duration that the patient remains on corticosteroids, the higher the likelihood that the patient will develop a significant and even life-threatening complication. Finally, it is critical that all patients on any dose or route of corticosteroids receive all appropriate immunizations and be evaluated for the need for BMD prophylaxis and possible chemoprophylaxis against opportunistic infections.

# References

1. Hardy TL, Bulmer E. Ulcerative colitis: a survey of ninety-five cases. Br Med J. 1933;2:812–5.
2. Turner D, Walsh CM, Steinhart AH, Griffiths AM. Response to corticosteroids in severe ulcerative colitis: a systematic review of the literature and meta-regression. Clin Gastroenterol Hepatol. 2007;5:103–10.
3. Hench PS, Kendall ED, Slocumb CH, et al. The effects of the adrenal cortical hormone 17-hydroxy-11-dehydrocorticosterone (compound E) on the acute phase of rheumatic fever; preliminary report. Mayo Clin Proc. 1949;24:277–97.
4. Raju TN. The nobel chronicles. 1950: Edward Calving Kendall (1886–1972); Philip Showalter Hench (1896–1965); and Tadeus Reichstein (1897–1996). Lancet. 1999;353:1370.
5. Truelove SC, Witts LJ. Cortisone in ulcerative colitis: final report on a therapeutic trial. Br Med J. 1955;4947:1041–8.
6. Truelove SC, Jewell DP. Intensive intravenous regimen for severe attacks of ulcerative colitis. Lancet. 1974;1:1067–70.
7. Hayashi R, Wada H, Ito K, et al. Effects of glucocorticoids on gene transcription. Eur J Pharmacol. 2004;500:51–62.
8. Barnes PJ. How corticosteroids control inflammation: quintiles prize lecture 2005. Br J Pharmacol. 2006;148:245–54.
9. Ford AC, Bernstein CN, Khan KJ, et al. Glucocorticosteroid therapy in inflammatory bowel disease: systematic review and meta-analysis. Am J Gastroenterol. 2011;106:590–9.
10. De Bosscher K, Vanden Berghe W, Haegeman G. The interplay between the glucocorticoid receptor and nuclear factor-kappaB or activator protein-1: molecular mechanisms for gene repression. Endocr Rev. 2003;24:488–522.
11. Kagoshima M, Ito K, Cosio B, et al. Glucocorticoid suppression of nuclear factor-kappa B: a role for histone modifications. Biochem Soc Trans. 2003;31:60–5.
12. Buttgereit F, Saag KG, Cutolo M, et al. The molecular basis for the effectiveness, toxicity, and resistance to glucocorticoids: focus on the treatment of rheumatoid arthritis. Scand J Rheumatol. 2005;34:14–21.
13. Yang YX, Lichtenstein GR. Corticosteroids in Crohn's disease. Am J Gastroenterol. 2002;97:803–23.
14. Truelove SC, Witts LJ. Cortisone in ulcerative colitis: preliminary report on a therapeutic trial. Br Med J. 1954;2:375–8.
15. Angus P, Snook JA, Reid M, et al. Oral fluticasone propionate in active distal ulcerative colitis. Gut. 1992;33:711–4.
16. Bossa F, Latiano A, Rossi L, et al. Erythrocyte-mediated delivery of dexamethasone in patients with mild-to-moderate ulcerative colitis, refractory to mesalamine: a randomized, controlled study. Am J Gastroenterol. 2008;103:2509–16.
17. Lennard-Jones JE, Longmore AJ, Newell AC, et al. An assessment of prednisone, salazopyrin, and topical hydrocortisone hemisuccinate used as out-patient treatment for ulcerative colitis. Gut. 1960;1:217–22.
18. Rizzello F, Gionchetti P, Galeazzi R, et al. Oral beclomethasone dipropionate in patients with mild to moderate ulcerative colitis: a dose-finding study. Adv Ther. 2001;18:261–71.
19. Talley NJ, Abreu MT, Achkar JP, et al. An evidence-based systematic review on medical therapies for inflammatory bowel disease. Am J Gastroenterol. 2011;106:S2–5.
20. Bossa F, Fiorella S, Caruso N, et al. Continuous infusion versus bolus administration of steroids in severe attacks of ulcerative colitis: A randomized, double-blind trial. Am J Gastroenterol. 2007;102:601–8.
21. Hanauer SB. Inflammatory bowel disease. N Engl J Med. 1996;334:841–8.
22. Edwards FC, Truelove SC. The course and prognosis of ulcerative colitis. Part I: short-term prognosis. Gut. 1963;4:300–8.
23. Kornbluth A, Sachar DB. Ulcerative colitis practice guidelines in adults: American College of Gastroenterology, Practice Parameters Committee. Am J Gastroenterol. 2010;105:501–23.

24. Lichtenstein GR, Abreu MT, Cohen R, et al. American Gastroenterological Association Institute technical review on corticosteroids, immunomodulators, and infliximab in inflammatory bowel disease. Gastroenterology. 2006;130:940–87.
25. Sachar DB. Maintenance therapy in ulcerative colitis and Crohn's disease. J Clin Gastroenterol. 1995;20:117–22.
26. Truelove SC. Cortisone and corticotrophin in ulcerative colitis. Br Med J. 1959;34:387–94.
27. Lennard-Jones JE, Mickiewicz JJ, Connell AM, et al. Prednisone as maintenance treatment for ulcerative colitis in remission. Lancet. 1965;1:188–90.
28. Powell-Tuck J, Bown RL, Chambers TJ, et al. A controlled trial of alternate day prednisolone as a maintenance treatment for ulcerative colitis in remission. Digestion. 1981;22:263–70.
29. Baron JH, Connell AM, Kanaghinis TG, et al. Out-patient treatment of ulcerative colitis: comparison between three doses of oral prednisone. Br Med J. 1962;2:441–3.
30. Powell-Tuck J, Bown RL, Lennard-Jones JE. A comparison of oral prednisolone given as single or multiple daily doses for active proctocolitis. Scand J Gastroenterol. 1978;13:833–7.
31. Esteve M, Gisbert JP. Severe ulcerative colitis: at what point should we define resistance to steroids? World J Gastroenterol. 2008; 14:5504–7.
32. Elliott PR, Powell-Tuck J, Gillespie PE, et al. Prednisone absorption in acute colitis. Gut. 1980;21:49–51.
33. Berghouse LM, Elliot PR, Lennard-Jones JE. Plasma prednisolone levels during intravenous therapy in acute colitis. Gut. 1982;23: 980–3.
34. Buchman AL. Side effects of corticosteroid therapy. J Clin Gastroenterol. 2001;33:289–94.
35. Hyde GM, Jewell DP. Review article: the management of severe ulcerative colitis. Aliment Pharmacol Ther. 1997;11:419–24.
36. Lindgren SC, Flood LM, Kilander AF, et al. Early predictors of glucocorticosteroid treatment failure in severe and moderately severe attacks of ulcerative colitis. Eur J Gastroenterol Hepatol. 1998;10:831–5.
37. Travis SP, Farrant JM, Ricketts C, et al. Predicting outcome in severe ulcerative colitis. Gut. 1996;38:905–10.
38. Ho GT, Mowat C, Goddard CJ, et al. Predicting the outcome of severe ulcerative colitis: development of a novel risk score to aid early selection of patients for second-line medical therapy or surgery. Aliment Pharmacol Ther. 2004;19:1079–87.
39. Bernal I, Manosa M, Domenech E, et al. Predictors of clinical response to systemic steroids in active ulcerative colitis. Dig Dis Sci. 2006;51:1434–8.
40. Meyers S, Level PK, Feuer EJ, et al. Predicting the outcome of corticoid therapy for acute ulcerative colitis. Results of a prospective randomized, double-blind trial. J Clin Gastroenterol. 1987;9: 50–4.
41. Faubion Jr WA, Loftus Jr EV, Harmsen WS, et al. The natural history of corticosteroid therapy for inflammatory bowel disease: a population-based study. Gastroenterology. 2001;121:255–60.
42. Singleton JW, Law DH, Kelley Jr ML, et al. National cooperative Crohn's disease study: adverse reactions to study drugs. Gastroenterology. 1979;77:870–82.
43. Simon TD. How do you avoid and treat steroid side effects? Inflamm Bowel Dis. 2008;14:S214–5.
44. Siegel CA. Review article: explaining the risks of inflammatory bowel disease therapy to patients. Aliment Pharmacol Ther. 2011; 33:23–32.
45. Bernstein CN, Leslie WD, Leboff MS. AGA technical review on osteoporosis in gastrointestinal diseases. Gastroenterology. 2003; 124:795–841.
46. Lichtenstein GR, Sands BE, Pazianas M. Prevention and treatment of osteoporosis in inflammatory bowel disease. Inflamm Bowel Dis. 2006;12:797–813.
47. Compston J. Osteoporosis in inflammatory bowel disease. Gut. 2003;52:63–4.
48. Cooper MS, Stewart PM. Corticosteroid insufficiency in acutely ill patients. N Engl J Med. 2003;348:727–34.
49. Toruner M, Loftus Jr EV, Harmsen WS, et al. Risk factors for opportunistic infections in patients with inflammatory bowel disease. Gastroenterology. 2008;134:929–36.
50. Aberra FN, Lewis HD, Hass D, et al. Corticosteroids and immunomodulators: postoperative infectious complication risk in inflammatory bowel disease patients. Gastroenterology. 2003;125:320–7.
51. Poppers DM, Scherl EJ. Prophylaxis against pneumocystis pneumonia in patients with inflammatory bowel disease: toward a standard of care. Inflamm Bowel Dis. 2008;14:106–13.
52. Viget N, Vernier-Massouille G, Salmon-Ceron D, et al. Opportunistic infections in patients with inflammatory bowel disease: prevention and diagnosis. Gut. 2008;57:549–58.
53. Rahier JF, Yazdanpanah Y, Colombel JF, et al. The European (ECCO) Consensus on infection in IBD: What does it change for the clinician? Gut. 2009;58:1313–5.
54. Gluck T, Kiefmann B, Grohmann M, et al. Immune status and risk for infection in patients receiving chronic immunosuppressive therapy. J Rheumatol. 2005;32:1473–80.
55. Mansharamani NG, Balachandran D, Vernovsky I, et al. Peripheral blood CD4+ T-Lymphocyte counts during Pneumocystis carinii pneumonia in immunocompromised patients without HIV infection. Chest. 2000;118:712–20.
56. Bernstein CN, Kolodny M, Block E, et al. Pneumocystis carinii pneumonia in patients with ulcerative colitis treated with corticosteroids. Am J Gastroenterol. 1993;88:574–7.
57. Wasan SK, Baker SE, Skolnik PR, et al. A practical guide to vaccinating the inflammatory bowel disease patient. Am J Gastroenterol. 2010;105:1231–8.

# Rectal Glucocorticoid Use in Ulcerative Colitis

Seymour Katz

**Keywords**

Rectal glucocorticoids • Ulcerative colitis • Rectal therapy • 5-ASA • First-pass metabolism feature • Pouchitis • Topical budesonide • Mechanism of action • Glucocorticoid resistance

## Introduction

Topical therapy in ulcerative colitis (UC) has had an unappreciated if not neglected role in UC management. Often relegated to the proctitis and proctosigmoiditis patient, little attention has been paid to a topical therapy in more extensive disease or pancolitis in which urgency and tenesmus are prime problems amenable to topical corticosteroid foams or suppository therapy. Topical glucocorticosteroids (GCS) have a long track record of efficacy, but rectal 5-ASA has had a comparably better experience with less damaging adverse events. Nevertheless clinicians often utilize an alternating regimen of GCS every other day with 5-ASA to induce remission and then limit further use of GCS.

Glucocorticoid enemas were first shown to be effective 51 years ago in the United Kingdom by Truelove [1] and by Bargen [2] at the Mayo Clinic and have become a standard component of UC therapy [3].

Rectal delivery of glucocorticoids by liquid enemas can extend to the splenic flexure [4] and occasionally more proximally [5]. Rectal foam dispenses medication to the rectum and distal descending colon [6], whereas suppositories release their drug only locally in the rectum [7].

This chapter will detail the experience with such agents, including the pharmacology of glucocorticoids given rectally as well as the topically active first-pass metabolism corticosteroids budesonide and beclomethasone dipropionate (BDP).

The efficacy of topical delivery of therapeutic agents (5-ASA, glucocorticoids) is influenced by multiple factors including colonic motility, intraluminal pH, extent and characteristics of IBD, and the vagaries of drug dispersion. Clinical response rates can vary from 35 to 75 %. Ideally, first-pass metabolism corticosteroids would seem the best option to avoid extensive bioavailability with fewer resultant systemic side effects [3, 8]. Budesonide is the most extensively studied in enema, foam, and suppository of the topical nonsystemic glucocorticoid therapy (Table 10.1).

## Glucocorticoids

### Mechanisms of Action

Glucocorticoid activity is dependent on specific glucocorticoid receptors (GR) found on chromosome 5. The GR-α isoform is a physiologically important form. GR-β does not bind glucocorticoids [9, 10], and GR-γ is a variant that may alter GR-α activity. Glucocorticoids bind to GR-α as a homodimer to specific glucocorticoid response elements (GREs) which activate gene expression. DNA binding of the GR, which activates gene expression, may be repressed by monomer protein-protein interactions that are also capable of DNA binding. This GRE pathway is crucial to survival [11]. Many glucocorticoid effects (e.g., anti-inflammatory and immunosuppressive) require the interaction of the GR with activating protein 1 (AP-1) and NF-κB transcription

S. Katz, M.D. (✉)
New York University of Medicine, Great Neck, NY 11021, USA
e-mail: seymourkatz.md@gmail.com

**Table 10.1** Topical corticosteroids

| Systemic |
| --- |
| Hydrocortisone (in alcohol or as a hemisuccinate sodium) |
| Prednisolone-21 phosphate |
| Betamethasone |
| Nonsystemic steroids |
| Prednisolone metasulfobenzoate |
| Beclomethasone dipropionate |
| Budesonide |

factors. These transcription factors are also capable of regressing GR-dependent transcription. The overall expected effect is GR-dependent transcription and activation of lymphocytes to result in apoptosis and anti-inflammatory effects [12].

High levels of the CXC-chemokines, growth-related oncogene (GRO)-$\alpha$/CXCL1, IL-8, and gamma-interferon (MIG)/CXCL9 were detected in active ulcerative colitis when compared with controls ($p=0.02$, 0.005, and 0.03, respectively). During treatment with corticosteroids, both GRO-$\alpha$ and MIG decreased [13]. HLA class II allele DRB1*0103 may be a "surrogate" marker for steroid resistance since it is associated with severe disease and high risk for colectomy.

## Glucocorticoid Resistance

Thirty percent of patients given glucocorticoids will not enter remission and are considered steroid resistant. Lymphocyte steroid resistance may be the key for glucocorticoid failure in UC [14], but this conclusion is hampered by varied lymphocyte sensitivity in normal subjects as well [15].

The impact of steroid resistance has been detailed in studies from the Mayo Clinic and Scandinavia. Faubion et al. [16] recorded a complete 30-day steroid-induced remission in 58 %, partial in 26 % (84 % total), and a failure in 16 %. One-year follow-up revealed 38 % of CD patients so treated required surgery as did 24 % of UC patients. Munkholm et al. [17] had reported a similar steroid-induced remission at 30 days (48 % complete, 38 % partial, total 80 %) and no response in 20 %. Interestingly, the failure of steroid responsiveness was not related to the severity of disease (i.e., remission rates of 48 % in severe versus 35 % in moderate disease) in the initial oral cortisone study [18].

There may be a rare familial disorder of altered glucocorticoid receptors resulting in mutations that encode GR [19–21]. These patients lack functional glucocorticoid receptors in target organs, yet counterintuitively these patients with poor glucocorticoid responses still suffer the ravages of glucocorticoid adverse events. Such glucocorticoid resistance appears unrelated to abnormalities in steroid absorption, metabolism, or number of glucocorticoid receptors. GR isoform variations may play a role, i.e., a greater preponderance of GR-$\beta$ isoforms that do not bind glucocorticoids have been found in steroid-resistant UC patients [22]. The actual concentration of GR-$\beta$ is small compared to GR-$\alpha$ [23]. GR-$\gamma$ may affect glucocorticoid binding as an alternative theory of glucocorticoid resistance [24, 25]. Other thoughts on glucocorticoid resistance include impaired binding or a reduced number of receptors available for binding of DNA resulting in a GR-ligand complex failure to activate the appropriate genes [26].

Glucocorticoids modulate transcription factors and cytokines. IL-4/IL-2 promotes steroid resistance in vitro [27] and in murine cell lines [28]. IL-2 reduces nuclear translocation of GR by adding a Janus kinase (JAK) inhibitor. JAK inhibitors block IL-2 receptor signaling and restore responsiveness to glucocorticoids. STAT5 is associated with nuclear GR and when phosphorylated by IL-2 binding will inhibit nuclear translocations of GR. In a STAT5 knockout mouse model, IL-2 fails to induce steroid resistance [27]. IL-2 and IL-4 cytokines increase p38 mitogen-activated protein (MAP) kinase which phosphorylates GRs associated with steroid resistance [29] and reduces antiproliferative glucocorticoid activity [27]. Steroid-resistant patients usually produce more IL-2 than steroid-sensitive patients.

NF-$\kappa$B regulates cytokine synthesis with a peculiar epithelial cell distribution in steroid-resistant patients, yet this is also found in lamina propria macrophages in steroid-sensitive patients [30]. The conclusion seems inescapable that lymphocyte resistance to glucocorticoids results from signaling pathways activated by IL-2. Conceivably inhibiting IL-2 overcomes this resistance. Unfortunately, in vitro-activated lymphocyte studies show a surprisingly low IL-2 production which was not correlated with steroid sensitivity.

Membrane cytokine binding activates transcription factor in the receptor complex and produces inflammation. Glucocorticoids oppose this process by promoting apoptosis to lessen inflammation [31].

Genetic factors add to the glucocorticoid receptor disorders with steroid resistance. These include the multidrug resistance 1(MDR1) gene. The MDR1 gene product, a P-glycoprotein 170 found in colonic and jejunal tissue [32], transports glucocorticoids and reduces intracellular fluid drug and glucocorticoid concentrations. High levels of P-glycoprotein 170 are protective in UC but may be downregulated by inflammation [33]. It is uncertain if MDR1 polymorphisms are related to steroid resistance (Table 10.2).

**Table 10.2** Mechanism of steroid resistance

Genetic

- GR mutations
- MDR1 gene
- HLA class II DRB1*0103

Acquired

- Abnormal steroid absorption or metabolism—not proven
- Altered glucocorticoid receptor concentrations—not proven
- Greater presence of GR-β and GR-γ isoforms—possible
- Lessened affinity of ligand for glucocorticoid receptors—not proven
- Reduced glucocorticoid receptor affinity to bind DNA—possible
- Altered expressions of transcription factors/cytokines

Adapted from Creed TJ, Probert CS. Steroid resistance in inflammatory bowel disease—mechanisms and therapeutic strategies. *Aliment Pharmacol Ther.* 2007;25:111–122 [31]

## Other Mechanisms of Action

The actual benefit of glucocorticoids in controlling diarrhea in IBD may also include the significant stimulation of ATPase activity and the number of ATPase molecules and apical $5'$-nucleotidase, all of which precede the observable morphologic effect on inflammation as detected by endoscopy or histology [34, 35].

Rectal potential differences (PDs) as a measure of ion transport across the rectal mucosa improved after glucocorticoids (both topical and systemic therapy) as well as with 5-ASA enemas. The clinical utility and significance of this observation remains unexplored [36].

## Glucocorticoid Absorption from the Rectocolon

Glucocorticoid receptors are present in most human cells. This widespread receptor presence may well explain the systemic glucocorticoids adverse event history [37]. Rectal glucocorticoids are presumed to provide lesser systemic bioavailability and plasma concentration than oral glucocorticoids. Nevertheless plasma concentrations of prednisolone given rectally have been reported as equivalent to orally administered glucocorticoids [37, 38].

The bioavailability is further reduced with foam preparations (2 %) with even lower plasma peak levels (Table 10.3) [39].

Although decreased glucocorticoid receptor sites are reported in PMN leukocytes of prior steroid-treated patients, similar reduced receptor sites have been reported in glucocorticoid-naïve and normal control patients [40]. Topical glucocorticoids are effective, but systemic absorption does occur [41] but may be lessened with rapidly metabolized budesonide. These were effective with maintenance of normal ACTH levels in 90 % of patients at 6 weeks [42].

**Table 10.3** Rectal hydrocortisone pharmacology

|  | Ulcerative colitis | Controls |
|---|---|---|
| Bioavailability (%) | $16.4 \pm 14.8$ | $30.0 \pm 15.1$ |
| $C_{max}$ (nM) | $277 \pm 215$ | $610 \pm 334$ |

With food bioavailability, 2 %; $C_{max}$, 35 ng/ml
Adapted from Petitjean O, Wendling JL, Tod M, et al. Pharmacokinetics and absolute rectal bioavailability of hydrocortisone acetate in distal colitis. *Aliment Pharmacol Ther.* 1992;6:351–357 [131]

## Clinical Experience with Topical Glucocorticoids

In 1997, Marshall and Irvine reported a meta-analysis of 33 reviewed rectal corticosteroids studies that met their "strict" inclusion criteria of 83 published reports [43]. Inclusion criteria required randomization, disease distal to splenic flexure, a predefined symptom score, and no inclusion of Crohn's patients or duplicate reporting of trial data. The response rates based on symptomatic, endoscopic, and histological criteria for conventional oral glucocorticoids (hydrocortisone, prednisolone, or betamethasone) were 77, 66, and 58 % with remission rates of 45, 34, and 29 %. The response to topical corticosteroids (budesonide, BDP, or prednisolone) was 73, 69, and 55 % with remission rates of 46, 31, and 23 %.

In this analysis, 5-ASA preparations resulted in improvement in 81, 75, and 65 % with remission recorded as 58, 41, and 38 %. Placebo response rates were 34 % symptom and 38 % endoscopic improvement, and remission rates of symptomatic and endoscopic criteria of 9 and 17 %.

Although topical corticosteroids were 32 % superior to placebo, seven trials proved 5-ASA to be superior to corticosteroids when considering clinical, endoscopic, and histological standard of remission. The result of pooled odds ratio (2.42 95 % CI 1.7–3.41) favored 5-ASA for symptomatic remission, as well as endoscopic (1.89 95 % CI 1.26–2.96) and histological (2.03 95 % CI 1.28–3.2) remission. This occurred even with discrepant volumes of instilled medication (e.g., 30 cc prednisolone foam versus 120 cc 5-ASA foam) [44]. Furthermore a Cochrane analysis of 38 studies reaffirmed rectal 5-ASA superiority over rectal corticosteroids for inducing symptomatic improvement and remission [45].

Throughout all these analyses, a placebo benefit of 30 % and a remission placebo rate of 10 % must be kept in mind when evaluating efficacy [46]. Foam and suppositories will provide a higher response rate in distal UC [42] and better patient compliance [47]. As anticipated, higher endoscopic and histological remission rates accrued with longer treatment duration [44, 48–61] and with lower relapse rates [62, 63].

The Marshall and Irvine meta-analysis concluded that rectal 5-ASA is comparable to rectal glucocorticoids for improvement, but better for inducing remission. This was

**Table 10.4** Randomized controlled trials of treatment for active L-UC: topically active corticosteroids

| Author year | Study design | Treatment 1 compared to | Treatment 2 | Results |
|---|---|---|---|---|
| Lofberg et al. 1996 [129] | RCT, double blind ($n=72$) | Oral budesonide 10 mg | Prednisolone 40 mg | Endoscopic scores: budesonide comparable efficacy to prednisolone after 9 weeks |
| Campieri et al. 1998 [116] | RCT, double blind ($n=157$) | BDP enema (3 mg/60 ml) | PSP enema (30 mg/60 ml) | Clinical and endoscopic remission with BDP 29 % and PSP 25 % at 4 weeks ($p=$NS) |
| Hanauer et al. 1998 [42] | RCT, double blind ($n=233$) | Budesonide enema, varying strengths: 0.5, 2.0, 8.0 mg/100 ml | Placebo | Remission at 6 weeks: Budesonide 0.5 mg/ 100 ml, 7 % ($p=$NS) Budesonide 2.0 mg/100 ml, 19 % ($p \leq 0.05$) Budesonide 8.0 mg/100 ml, 27 % ($p<0.001$) |
| Lindgren et al. 2002 [99] | RCT, double blind ($n=149$) | Budesonide enema, varying strengths: induction, 2.0, 4.0 mg/100 ml; remission, 2.0 mg/100 ml | Placebo | 2 mg dose induces remission; no effect on maintenance of remission |
| Bar-Meir et al. 2003 [125] | RCT, open label ($n=251$) | Budesonide foam 2 mg (Budenofalk) | Hydrocortisone acetate foam 100 mg (Colifoam) | Remission rates: BDP 55 % and hydrocortisone acetate 51 % at 8 weeks |
| Hammond et al. 2004 [126] | RCT, open label ($n=38$) | Budesonide 2 mg/50 ml foam | Betamethasone 5 mg/100 ml | Mean life quality index score at 4 weeks: budesonide foam 2.9 and betamethasone enema 2.1 ($p<0.09$) |

Adapted from Regueiro M, Loftus Jr EV, Steinhart AH, et al. Medical management of left-sided ulcerative colitis and ulcerative proctitis; critical evaluation of therapeutic trials. *Inflamm Bowel Dis.* 2006;12:979–994 [67]
*BDP* beclomethasone dipropionate, *PSP* prednisolone sodium phosphate, *RCT* randomized controlled trial

consistent across symptomatic, endoscopic, and histological outcomes. However, 5-ASA was as effective as budesonide in two trials regarding improvement and remission but failed to meet all end points. Adverse events were comparable for all rectal preparations of budesonide albeit with less endogenous cortisol suppression than conventional glucocorticoids based on serum cortisol determinations.

The role of rectal corticosteroids is an alternative distal colitis treatment in patients failing or intolerant to 5-ASA preparations. 5-ASA preparations were superior to glucocorticoids in active disease as well as maintenance of remission (Table 10.4).

In 2000, Cohen et al. [64] visited therapy for left-sided UC and proctitis via a meta-analysis of the accumulated literature through 1997 and concluded that topical 5-ASA again was superior to oral therapies or topical glucocorticoids. In left-sided disease, 5-ASA's higher remission rate over glucocorticoid enemas was not dose dependent. Similarly 5-ASA suppositories were superior to glucocorticoid topical therapy in ulcerative proctitis, but no dose response could be established. Overall, the authors concluded remission and improvement rates of 10–80 % with 5-ASA enemas over oral 5-ASA and glucocorticoid enemas.

Confounding features of meta-analyses open to criticism include different study populations, methodologies, and variation in study design. Odds ratios can be exaggerated by

17 % if studies are not double blinded [65], 30 % if lacking randomization [66], 41 % if inadequate concealment of treatment allocation, or 30 % if unclear concealment [65].

In a detailed analytic review of therapeutic trials for left-sided ulcerative proctitis, Regueiro et al. in 2006 evaluated the literature from 1995 through September 2005 [67]. Their assessment required multiple high-quality, randomized, controlled trials with consistent results to merit "A+" grade down to "D" for expert opinion only. Trials were excellent only if specifically designed for left-sided disease, with positive results compared to placebo or a comparative drug.

Rectally administered corticosteroids rated A+ on evidence and excellent efficacy with a clear advantage of 4–5 times more likely to have symptomatic and endoscopic improvement than placebo. Pooled OR was 0.21 (95 % CI 0.07–0.71) for symptom and 0.27 (95 % CI 0.10–0.77) for endoscopic improvement [68].

Rectal glucocorticoids for maintenance of remission fare poorly and should be considered ineffective for this indication; in addition, there are the added adverse effects that it carries (osteoporosis, cataracts, avascular necrosis, etc.). Indeed there was no value or gain of oral glucocorticoids over placebo after 6 months (as noted in the earliest study in 1965) [69]. The oral steroid therapy data from the Mayo Clinic are clearly unfavorable for any sustained benefit, i.e., the 1-month combined partial and complete remission note of 84 % diminished to 49 % without glucocorticoids at 1 year, 22 % of patients became dependent on glucocorticoids, and 29 % required colectomy [16].

No benefit was noted with a maintenance dose of rectal hydrocortisone 100 mg biweekly for 6 months [70]. No rectal budesonide (2 mg biweekly) maintenance benefit versus placebo could be established [71].

Proctitis may become a vexing problem when active. 5-ASA or glucocorticoid suppositories given 2–3 times daily may be helpful even with the expected difficulty of retaining them with refractory disease [67].

5-ASA or glucocorticoid enemas and glucocorticoid foam have been the mainstays of topical therapy for rectosigmoid UC. Occasionally enema preparations may skip (or bypass) the inflamed irritable rectal sigmoid due to instillation with the patient on his or her left side. Suppositories are recommended 2–3 times daily as supplemental rectal medication until relief is achieved [71].

## Nonsystemic First-Pass Metabolism Glucocorticoids

### Budesonide

#### Pharmacokinetics

Budesonide is a nonhalogenated corticosteroid that has the highest known affinity for the glucocorticoid receptor, yet with a remarkably low rate of corticosteroid systemic side effects. It is a 1:1 mixture of epimers (22R)- and (22S)- which are quickly metabolized with a half-life of $2.7 \pm 0.6$ h. Budesonide's metabolism requires hydroxylation mainly by cytochrome P450 isoenzyme CYP3A4 found in highest concentration in the hepatocytes and intestinal epithelium [72] and is 88 % protein bound. Since oral budesonide is cleared significantly in the intestinal mucosa and as a first pass through the liver (at a rate approaching hepatic blood flow), the resultant bioavailability borders on 10 % [73, 74]. When given rectally, budesonide may reach the splenic flexure [75] with a reported bioavailability up to 15 % in proctitis or left-sided UC patients [76]. Elimination is correlated with drug exposure concentration and duration of surface contact which will vary with inducers of CYP3A4 (e.g., rifampicin, Dilantin) and inhibitors (grapefruit juice, ketoconazole, etc.) [77]. Hepatic disease (e.g., cirrhosis) reduces budesonide metabolism and raises its plasma level up to $2.5\times$ normal [78]. Its use in the elderly has not been studied.

In one study, no ill effects were recorded when taken during pregnancy [79]. Budesonide is a category "C" drug, i.e., category with A/E in animals versus no controlled studies in pregnant women. No data is available of budesonide levels in breast milk nor evidence of fetal adrenal insufficiency, but safety issues with inhaled budesonide in lactating patients caution against its use when breastfeeding.

Topical budesonide enemas can reach the splenic flexure within 15 min of administration. Maximal plasma levels from absorption of this route occurred within 1–3 h ($1.5 \pm 0.9$ h) [80]. An 8-week use of European pH-released budesonide formulation (Budenofalk) resulted in identifiable drug levels in the descending colon, sigmoid, and rectal mucosa (15–60 ng/g) in biopsies from UC patients [81].

Budesonide has demonstrated efficacy both orally and rectally with the advantage of fewer corticosteroid side effects due to its low (systemic) bioavailability. Budesonide enema therapy at 6 weeks was significantly more effective in one study than placebo with maintenance of normal ACTH levels [42].

There is a predominant impression that rectal steroid use is diminishing based on reports of successful 5-ASA therapy in 80 % of UC patients [82]. The Mayo Clinic's analysis recorded only 34 % of UC patients requiring steroids [16]. Rectal therapy fares better than oral therapy in most cases of distal colitis [83], particularly so when combined with oral therapy than either given as sole therapy [84–86]. Revisiting two prior rectal and oral 5-ASA studies noted time to resolution of rectal bleeding to be as early as 2 days with a median time of 8 days. Time for mucosal healing and clinical remission were higher as well with combined therapy by week 3, all making the case for the value of combined therapy. However considerable improvement in bleeding, bowel motion frequency, and mucosal healing in left-sided disease and proctitis has been noted with high-dose oral 5-ASA alone (ASCEND data). 5-ASA preparations are more effective than topical corticosteroids [87].

Once-daily 3 g mesalazine administered as granules is superior to 9 mg [88] budesonide once daily administered as capsules for achieving remission in mild-to-moderately active UC, i.e., fewer patients achieved clinical remission at week 8 with budesonide 9 mg (39.5 %) versus with 5-ASA granules (54.5 %). However it is noteworthy that remission of UC was attained in about 40 % of budesonide-treated patients with a rapid onset of resolution [88].

Budesonide enemas are as effective as prednisone enemas and significantly better than placebo (Table 10.5) [42, 48–50, 89–91].

5-ASA remains the "workhorse," i.e., the mainstay of therapy in mild to moderate UC. Rectal formulations given alone or with oral preparations are most effective in proctitis or left side UC. Rectal corticosteroids (hydrocortisone, budesonide, beclomethasone) have a benefit albeit less than 5-ASA [92]. When given as a foam or enema, it is anticipated that 60–66 % remission can be achieved after 4 weeks [93]. Yet rectal 5-ASA was superior to rectal budesonide with greater remission rate, quality of life parameters, and endoscopic and histological improvement [93, 94]. A Cochrane review of oral budesonide's role in UC revealed it to be no better than placebo and definitely less effective than 5-ASA [95–97]. Further concerns with budesonide

**Table 10.5** Budesonide enemas for active distal ulcerative colitis [48, 49, 92]

| | Budesonide, 2 mg (N=20) | Placebo (N=20) | Budesonide, 2 mg (N=28) | Prednisolone, 31 mg (N=28) |
|---|---|---|---|---|
| Failure (%) | 35 | 80* | | |
| Plasma cortisol | | | | |
| After 4 weeks (mmol/L) | 446±91 | 447±89 | | |
| Complete remission (%) | | | 52 | 24* |
| Objective improvement (%) | | | 93 | 75* |
| Δ Plasma cortisol (mmol/L) | | | +11 | −127 |

Adapted from Schölmerich J. Review article: systemic and topical steroids in inflammatory bowel disease. *Aliment Pharmacol Ther*. 2004;20(suppl 4):66–74 [92]

*$p < 0.05$ versus budesonide

**Table 10.6** Results of budesonide versus placebo [110, 111]

| Modified ITT (N=410) | Bud-MMX 9 mg | Bud-MMX 6 mg | Entocort 9 mg | Placebo |
|---|---|---|---|---|
| Study population | 109 | 109 | 103 | 89 |
| UCDAI remission, n(%) | 19(17.4) | 9(8.3) | 13(12.6) | 4(4.5) |
| Δ vs. placebo | 12.9 | 3.8 | 8.1 | – |
| 95 % CI | 4.6, 21.3 | −3.0, 10.5 | 0.4, 15.9 | – |
| p-Value[a] | 0.0047 | 0.2876 | 0.0481 | – |

[a]Chi-square test for remission versus placebo

involved a 50 % reduction in morning cortisol level versus placebo budesonide formulation [98]. *Comment*: Budesonide in oral controlled ileal release pH-dependent or rectal formulations is less effective than 5-ASA for induction of remission in UC. The added burden of adverse adrenal events lessens the value of budesonide.

The budesonide enema experience is equally discouraging in the maintenance of remission of UC with no difference in relapse rates compared to PBO, and an additional concern of budesonide is induced higher rate of adrenal symptoms [98]. Nevertheless budesonides' fewer corticosteroid adverse events compared to prednisolone are of value with lesser budesonide-related adrenal insufficiency compared to conventional GCS [98–104]. There is a concern of budesonides' impact on growth in pediatric patients, i.e., adolescents with adrenal suppression [105] if used for prolonged periods [106, 107]. Overall GCS clinical side effects were not statistically different than PBO (Table 10.5) [108, 109].

Further study of Budesonide MMX® 9 mg in UC patients presumed to deliver active drug throughout the colon resulted in 17.4 % of patients entering remission over 8 weeks versus 7.4 % in placebo ($p = 0.0143$); no statistical significance occurred for the 6 mg group but no adverse event differences between drug and placebo [110]. Budesonide MMX® 9 mg administered once daily was found to be safe and effective at inducing a "modest" remission in patients with mild to moderate UC (Table 10.6) [111].

Prior experience with budesonide enemas showed efficacy comparable to metronidazole in a double-blind randomized controlled trial (RCT). Whether this response is sustained with maintenance therapy in the 10–15 % of patients developing chronic pouchitis will await further long-term trials.

## Beclomethasone Dipropionate

Using this first-pass metabolized steroid, *beclomethasone dipropionate* (BDP), in 177 UC patients, the clinical remission rate was virtually identical (63 %) to that achieved by 5-ASA (62.5 %). Although a more favorable improvement in disease activity indices occurred in patients with more extensive disease with BDP, the plasma cortisol levels were significantly reduced in the BDP group. This was not a placebo-controlled trial [112]. BDP was found to be as effective as 5-ASA by inducing improvement on remission in 70 % (148 patients) of patients versus 65.3 % (143 patients) given 5-ASA, when given topically (foam/enema) in 488 patients culled from four clinical trials. BDP's high first-pass hepatic elimination provides significantly less systemic bioavailability with reduced GCS side effects while maintaining efficacy [113]. Mild-to-moderately active UC patients did best with oral beclomethasone dipropionate but less so was achieved in proctitis patients. Of the 394 UC patients not in remission, when given oral 5-ASA, rectal 5-ASA, or rectal steroids, 81.7, 39.8, or 9.4 %, respectively, occurred with remission; BDP at 5 or 10 mg/day resulted in remission in 44.4 %, response in 22.3 %, and failure in 33.7 %. Adverse events included headache and nausea in 7.6 %. 6.6 % required hospitalization and 1 % went to colectomy [114].

BDP's safety was evaluated in 8 UC patients using the 1 mg ACTH test of the pituitary-adrenal axis reserve. Fasting and peak cortisol responses to ACTH were suppressed in 6/8 patients. One patient with suppressed fasting cortisol and another with a "blunted" ACTH response were noted as well 2 weeks after initiation of BDP therapy. One month after cessation of BDP, 7/8 patients' ACTH tests were normal. *Comment*: BDP in an enema formulation is capable of significant suppression of the pituitary-adrenal axis [115].

Two hundred and seventeen UC patients entered a single-blind, randomized, controlled trial of either BDP 3 mg enema o.d. or 5-ASA 1 g enema daily for 6 weeks. A significant Disease Activity Index (DAI) decrease ($p < 0.05$) occurred in 36.7 % BDP- versus 29.2 % 5-ASA-treated patients. An initial problem in interpretation (other than lacking a placebo arm) was a 15.7 % (34 patients) dropout rate: 18 in the BDP group (16.2 %) and 16 (15.1 %) in the 5-ASA

**Table 10.7** BDP versus 5-ASA enema versus combination in distal ulcerative colitis

| 4 Weeks | BDP, 3 mg (N=20) | 5-ASA, 1 g (N=21) | Combination (N=20) |
|---|---|---|---|
| Endoscopic remission (%) | 30 | 10 | 37 |
| Clinical improvement (%) | 70 | 76 | 100 |
| Endoscopic improvement (%) | 75 | 71 | 100 |

Adapted from Ulder CJ, Fockens P, Meijer JW, et al. Beclomethasone dipropionate (3 mg) versus 5-aminosalicylic acid (2 g) versus the combination of both (3 mg/2 g) as retention enemas in active ulcerative proctitis. *Eur J Gastreonterol Hepatol.* 1996;8:549–553 [132]

group. A total of 203 patients were eventually included in the ITT analysis. Both agents were equivalent in efficacy (i.e., DAI score), and sigmoidoscopic appearance with BDP was better for the moderate UC patients (DAI 7–10; i.e., 28.8 % remission versus 5.9 % 5-ASA), especially in left-sided disease. There was no adrenal suppression, and morning plasma cortisol levels were unchanged. Both budesonide and BDP appear effective and safe with their first-pass metabolism feature [116]. BDP enemas were as effective as conventional glucocorticoids both with a diminished effect on plasma cortisol [117]. BDP enema in combination with oral 5-ASA was better than either drug alone (Table 10.7) [117].

Another study of beclomethasone liquid enema or foam versus 2 g 5-ASA liquid enema or foam which was given once daily for 8 weeks had comparable remission rates for all four formulations. Any adverse events were related to disease exacerbations. Serum cortisol levels were stable in 86 % of patients before and after study completion [118]. A four random controlled trial meta-analysis comparing rectal BDP to rectal 5-ASA (1 foam, 3 enemas) again confirmed similar efficacy (69.9 % 5-ASA versus 65.3 % BDP OR 1.23, CI 0.82–1.85) [113].

In general, distal versus left-sided UC when refractory to 5-ASA can be treated with glucocorticoid enemas, but for a limited period of time. Topical budesonide (enemas or foam) is a reasonable alternative to standard steroid enema therapy.

The risk of corticosteroid systemic effects is considerably reduced when using first-pass metabolism agents such as budesonide or beclomethasone dipropionate (BDP). Yet the anti-inflammatory activity is retained [119–122]. BDP has been useful when combined with oral 5-ASA as well [123].

*Prednisolone metasulfobenzoate* (PMB), a poorly absorbed GCS, was studied at 40 mg/day dosage of 60 mg/day for 6 months versus prednisolone 40 mg/day for 2 weeks and then tapered over 8 weeks. Fewer A/E occurred with PMB group (8 % mood changes versus 46 % with prednisolone). Remission rates at 6 months were 51 % and 35 % for the 40 mg and 60 mg PMB group and 32 % in prednisolone group. There was no dose response [124]. This benefit was not sustained in a random controlled study, which was discontinued due to lack of efficacy.

## Foam Preparations

Further experience with a steroid foam (Cortifoam® 100 mg/5 ml) appeared comparable to hydrocortisone enemas (Cortenemas® 100 mg/60 ml) in 30 patients yet 53 % (8/15) of the enema group reported difficulties with enema retention versus 0 % (0/15) in the foam group [47]. A budesonide foam (Budenofalk® 2 mg/ml) was compared to a PBO liquid enema and budesonide liquid enema (Entocort® 2 mg/100 cc) in 541 patients over 4 weeks with proctitis or proctosigmoiditis with remission rates of 60 % in budesonide foam versus 66 % in liquid enema group yet 84 % of patients preferred foam [93]. In a trial of 251 ulcerative proctosigmoiditis patients given hydrocortisone foam (Colifoam® 100 mg/15 cc) versus budesonide foam (Budenofalk® 2 mg/20 cc), both groups achieved comparable remission rates (53 % budesonide and 52 % hydrocortisone group) with similar endoscopic and histological improvements. Strangely 3 % of the budesonide group had a degree of adrenal suppression with cortisol levels <5 μg/ml, yet none of the hydrocortisone patients experienced adrenal suppression. Again, patients preferred foam over enema therapy [125]. A significantly greater degree of adrenal suppression (87 %) occurred with betamethasone liquid enema (5 mg/100 cc) versus a budesonide foam (2 mg/50 ml) of 22 % [126].

5-ASA again asserted its superiority over steroid topical therapy in a 245-patient 4-week study comparing prednisolone foam (Predfoam® 20 mg/30 cc) achieving remission of 31 % and 5-ASA foam (Asacol® 2gm/120 cc) remission of 52 %. 5-ASA foam achieved a greater endoscopic remission as well (5-ASA 40 % versus 31 %) [44].

Budesonide foam is equivalent in efficacy to hydrocortisone foam [125], but 5-ASA enemas may have better efficacy than budesonide or standard glucocorticoid enemas [51, 52]. Budesonide foam is comparable in efficacy to 5-ASA enemas [127] and not different than betamethasone enema therapy [126].

In one study, 23/44 (52 %) budesonide foam (2 mg) patients entered remission versus 14/38 (37 %) receiving hydrocortisone foam (hydrocortisone acetate 100 mg). Although numerically greater, the budesonide foam group's results did not achieve statistical significance. Three percent of the budesonide foam group had low plasma cortisol levels. There were no significant adverse events. Remission criteria were strict, corresponding to a DAI of 0 in this 8-week study [125].

## Budesonide Foam Versus Enema in Active Ulcerative Colitis and Proctosigmoiditis

A large 449-patient randomized, controlled trial revealed a 60 % remission rate with budesonide foam versus 66 % rate with budesonide enema on a per protocol basis ($p = 0.02$) for non-inferiority foam. Eighty-four percent of patients preferred the easier application and tolerability of foam. Given a 15 % non-inferiority margin, 541 patients had to be enrolled, making this the largest rectal therapy trial for distal UC. Interestingly, the patients with a Rachmilewitz clinical DAI >8 score had a significantly lesser remission rate as did patients with a prior failure with oral or rectal 5-ASA. Still 49 % and 41 % budesonide foam and 50 and 68 % budesonide enema treated, patients previously given oral and rectal 5-ASA non-responders achieved remission. There were high rates of endoscopic (50 % foam, 54 % budesonide) and histological (51 % foam, 57 % enema) remission [68].

A rectal budesonide foam remission rate of 60 % is comparable to rectal 5-ASA remission (53 %) and considerably higher than placebo in published studies. Greater acceptance of the foam (84 %) over enema (6 %) was impressive but predictable. Although increased flatulence with foam preparations has been reported [128], this may be related to incorrect usage of product variation regarding volume and pressure effects.

The role of oral budesonide in the therapy of pouchitis was revisited in an Italian study of 20 patients given budesonide CIR 9 mg daily for 8 weeks [128]. Fifteen of 20 patients entered remission with a median drop in their Pouchitis Disease Activity Index (PDAI) from 14 to 3 (remission defined as ≤4 PDAI and improved IBDQ score (102 rising to 182)). These patients were unresponsive to a prior 4-week course of antibiotics.

## Conclusion

Rectal therapy with glucocorticoids and 5-ASA is effective in inducing remission in ulcerative proctitis and left-sided ulcerative colitis (Table 10.8). 5-ASAs orally and rectally are preferred. Glucocorticoid enemas are effective, but there are concerns regarding systemic absorption albeit less so with first-pass metabolism corticosteroids (budesonide or BDP). There is little to no support for rectal glucocorticoids for maintenance of remission as exists for rectal 5-ASA. Rectal glucocorticoids or rectal 5-ASA in combination with oral 5-ASA is more effective than monotherapy [129, 130]. Figure 10.1 shows a management algorithm for treatment of ulcerative proctitis.

**Table 10.8** Corticosteroids foam preparations for ulcerative colitis

| Rectal steroid foams vs. liquid enemas | Ruddell et al. 1980 [47] | Hydrocortisone foam 100 mg/5 ml vs. hydrocortisone liquid enema 100 mg/60 ml administered twice daily | Randomized investigator-blinded single center | 30 | Proctosigmoiditis | 2 weeks | Clinical improvements equivalent Difficulty with enema retention lower in the foam group |
|---|---|---|---|---|---|---|---|
| | Gross et al. 2006 [93] | Budesonide foam 2 mg/25 ml + placebo enema vs. budesonide enema 2 mg/100 ml + placebo administered once daily | Randomized double-blind multicenter | 541 | Proctitis or proctosigmoiditis | 4 weeks | Clinical remission equivalent Majority preferred foam |
| Newer generation rectal corticosteroids compared to standard steroid formulation | Hammond et al. 2004 [126] | Budesonide foam 2 mg/20 ml vs. hydrocortisone foam 100 mg/15 ml administered once daily | Randomized open-label multicenter | 251 | Proctitis or proctosigmoiditis | 4 weeks | Clinical remission equivalent Adrenal suppression rates similar |
| Steroid foam vs. 5-ASA | Lee et al. 1996 [44] | 5-ASA foam 2 g/120 ml vs. prednisolone 20 mg/30 ml administered once daily | Randomized investigator-blinded multicenter | 295 | Left-sided UC | 4 weeks | Clinical remission favors 5-ASA |
| | Biancone et al. 2007 [118] | 4 arms: BDP liquid enema 3 mg vs. BDP foam 3 mg vs. 5-ASA foam 2 g vs. 5-ASA liquid enema 2 g | Randomized double-blind multicenter | 99 | Mild-moderate proctitis or proctosigmoiditis | 8 weeks | Remission rates equivalent in all 4 arms including combined BDP vs. combined 5-ASA groups Serum cortisol similar |

Adapted from Loen BL, Siegel C. Foam Preparations For Treatment of Ulcerative Colitis, Current Drug Deliver 2011;8(No. 5)1–7 [133]

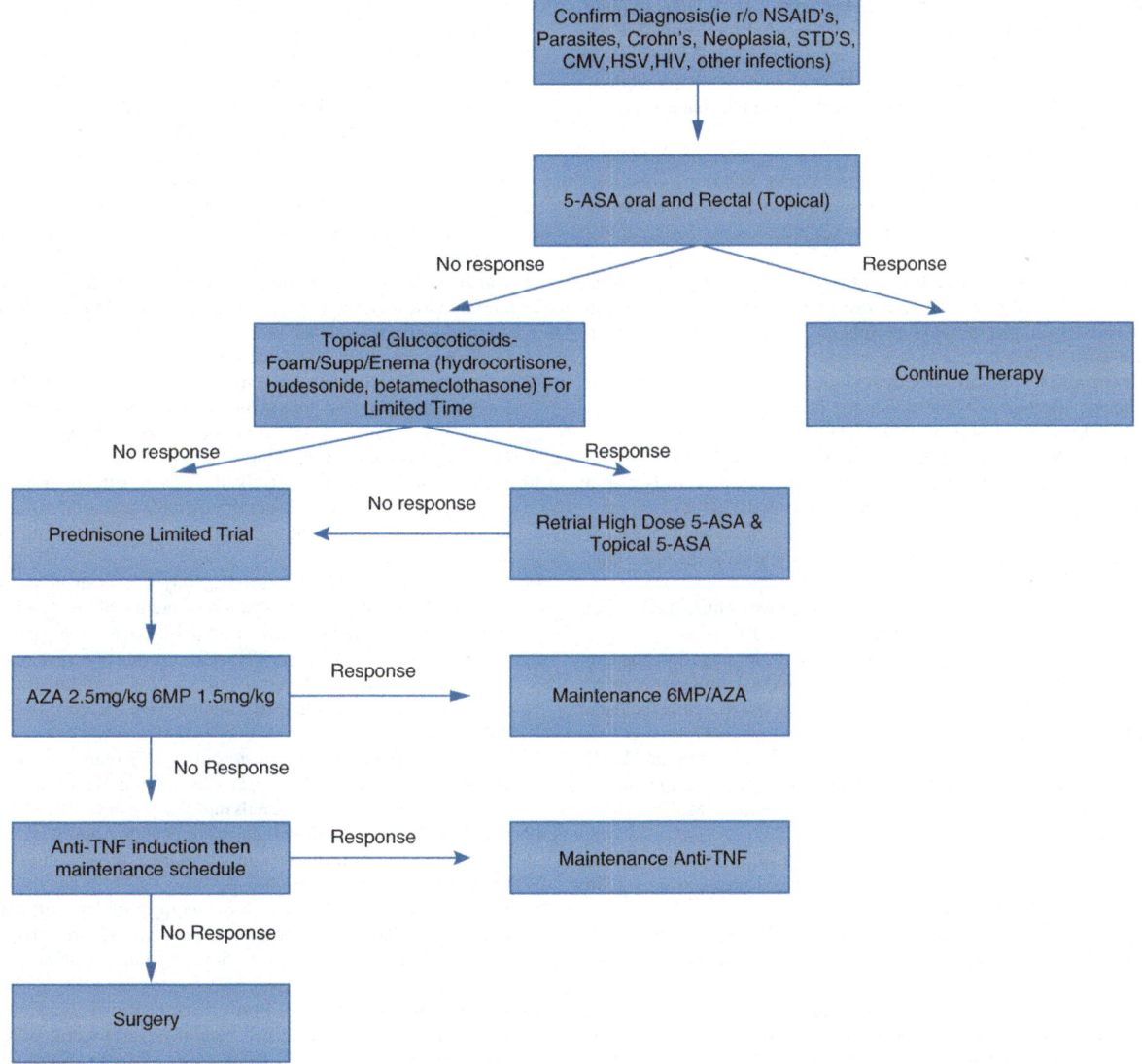

**Fig. 10.1** Management algorithm for ulcerative proctitis/proctosigmoiditis. *NSAIDS* nonsteroidal anti-inflammatory drugs, *STDs* sexually transmitted diseases, *CMV* cytomegalovirus, *HSV* herpes simplex virus, *HIV* human immunodeficiency virus

**Acknowledgment** The author is grateful to Seth Lipka, M.D., for the technical assistance.

## References

1. Truelove SC. Treatment of ulcerative colitis with local hydrocortisone. BMJ. 1956;2:1267–72.
2. Bargen JA. Chronic Ulcerative Colitis: A Lifelong Study. Charles C. Thomas: Springfield, IL; 1969.
3. Mulder CJ, Tygat GN. Review article: topical corticosteroids in inflammatory bowel disease. Aliment Pharmacol Ther. 1993;7: 125–30.
4. Jay M, Digenis GA, Foster TS, et al. Retrograde spreading of hydrocortisone enema in inflammatory bowel disease. Dig Dis Sci. 1986;31:139–44.
5. Swarbrick ET, Loose H, Lennard-Jones JE. Enema volume as an important factor in successful topical corticosteroid treatment of colitis. Proc R Soc Med. 1974;67(8):753–4.
6. Farthering MJ, Rutland MD, Clark ML. Retrograde spread of hydrocortisone containing foam given intrarectally in ulcerative colitis. Br Med J. 1979;2:822–4.
7. Jay M, Beihn RM, Digenis GA, et al. Disposition of radiolabelled suppositories in humans. J Pharm Pharmacol. 1985;37:266–8.
8. Friend DR. Review article: issues in oral administration of locally acting glucocorticosteroids for treatment of inflammatory bowel disease. Aliment Pharmacol Ther. 1998;12(7):591–603.
9. Hollenberg SM, Weinberger C, Ong ES, et al. Primary structure and expression of a functional human glucocorticoid receptor cDNA. Nature. 1985;318:635–41.
10. Encío IJ, Detera-Wadleigh SD. The genomic structure of the human glucocorticoid receptor. J Biol Chem. 1991;266(11): 7182–8.

11. Reichardt HM, Kaestner KH, Tuckermann J, et al. DNA binding of the glucocorticoid receptor is not essential for survival. Cell. 1998;93(4):531–41.

12. Stöcklin E, Wissler M, Goiulleux M, et al. Functional interactions between Stat5 and the glucocorticoid receptor. Nature. 1996; 383:726–8.

13. Egesten A, Eliasson M, Olin AI, et al. The proinflammatory CXC-chemokines GRO-alpha/CXCL1 and MIG/CXCL9 are concomitantly expressed in ulcerative colitis and decrease during treatment with topical corticosteroids. Int J Colorectal Dis. 2007;22(12): 1421–7.

14. Hearing SD, Norman M, Probert CS, et al. Predicting therapeutic outcome in severe ulcerative colitis by measuring in vitro steroid sensitivity of proliferating peripheral blood lymphocytes. Gut. 1999;45(3):382–8.

15. Hearing SD, Norman M, Smyth C, et al. Wide variation in lymphocyte steroid sensitivity among healthy human volunteers. J Clin Endocrinol Metab. 1999;84:4149–54.

16. Faubion WAJ, Loftus Jr EV, Harmsen WS, et al. The natural history of corticosteroid therapy for inflammatory bowel disease: a population-based study. Gastroenterology. 2001;121(2):255–60.

17. Munkholm P, Langholz E, Davidsen M, et al. Frequency of glucocorticoid resistance and dependency in Crohn's disease. Gut. 1994;35(3):360–2.

18. Truelove SC, Witts LJ. Cortisone in ulcerative colitis; final report on a therapeutic trial. Br Med J. 1955;2(4947):1041–8.

19. Hurley DM, Accili D, Stratakis CA, et al. Point mutation causing a single amino acid substitution in the hormone binding domain of the glucocorticoid receptor in familial glucocorticoid resistance. J Clin Invest. 1991;87(2):680–6.

20. Karl M, Lamberts SW, Detera-Wadleigh SD, et al. Familial glucocorticoid resistance caused by a splice site deletion in the human glucocorticoid receptor gene. J Clin Enocrinol Metab. 1993; 76(3):683–9.

21. Malchoff DM, Brufsky A, Reardon G, et al. A mutation of the glucocorticoid receptor in primary cortisol resistance. J Clin Invest. 1993;91(5):1918–25.

22. Bantel H, Domschke W, Schulze-Osthoff K. Molecular mechanisms of glucocorticoid resistance. Gastroenterology. 2000; 119(4):1178–9.

23. Matthews JG, Ito K, Barnes PJ, et al. Defective glucocorticoid receptor nuclear translocation and altered histone acetylation patterns in glucocorticoid-resistant patients. J Allergy Clin Immunol. 2004;113(6):1100–8.

24. Ray DW, Davis JR, White A, et al. Glucocorticoid receptor structure and function in glucocorticoid-resistant small cell lung carcinoma cells. Cancer Res. 1996;56(14):3276–80.

25. Rivers C, Levy A, Hancock J, et al. Insertion of an amino acid in the DNA-binding domain of the glucocorticoid receptor as a result of alternative splicing. J Clin Endocrinol Metab. 1999;84(11): 4283–6.

26. Kam JC, Szefler SJ, Surs W, et al. Combination IL-2 and IL-4 reduces glucocorticoid receptor-binding affinity and T cell response to glucocorticoids. J Immunol. 1993;151(7):3460–6.

27. Goleva E, Kisich KO, Leung DY. A role for STAT5 in the pathogenesis of IL-2 induced glucocorticoid resistance. J Immunol. 2002;169(10):5934–40.

28. Bantel H, Domschke W, Shulze-Osthoff K, et al. Abnormal activation of transcription factor NF-kappaB involved in steroid resistance in chronic inflammatory bowel disease. Am J Gastroenterol. 2000;95(7):1845–6.

29. Walker KB, Potter JM, House AK. Variable inhibition of mitogen-induced blastogenesis in human lymphocytes by prednisolone in vitro. Transplant Proc. 1985;17(2):1675–8.

30. Irusen E, Matthews JG, Takahashi A, et al. p38 Mitogen-activated protein kinase-induced glucocorticoid receptor phosphorylation reduces its activity: role in steroid-insensitive asthma. J Allergy Clin Immunol. 2002;109(4):649–57.

31. Creed TJ, Probert CS. Review article: steroid resistance in inflammatory bowel disease-mechanisms and therapeutic strategies. Aliment Pharmacol Ther. 2007;25(2):111–22.

32. Ho GT, Nimmo ER, Tenesa A, et al. Allelic variations of the multidrug resistance gene determine susceptibility and disease behavior in ulcerative colitis. Gastroenterology. 2005;128(2):288–96.

33. Bouma G, Crusius JB, García-González M. Genetic markers in clinically well defined patients with ulcerative colitis. Clin Exp Immunol. 1999;115(2):294–300.

34. Hanauer SB, Sandor WJ, Kornbluth A, et al. Delayed-release oral mesalamine at 4.8 g/day(800 mg tablet) for the treatment of moderately active ulcerative colitis: the ASCEND II Trial. Am J Gastroenterol. 2005;100(11):2478–85.

35. Schuerlen C, Allgayer H, Hardt M, et al. Effect of short-term topical corticosteroid treatment on mucosal enzyme systems in patients with distal inflammatory bowel disease. Hepatogastroenterology. 1998;45(23):1539–45.

36. Pienkowski P, Fioramonti J, Skalli F, et al. Effects of corticoids, 5-aminosalycilic acid and sucralfate on the potential difference of the rectum in inflammatory colitis in man. Gastroenterol Clin Biol. 1989;13(2):202–7.

37. Powell-Tuck J, Lennard-Jones JE, May CS, et al. Plasma prednisolone levels after administration of prednisolone-21 phosphate as a retention enema in colitis. Br Med J. 1976;1(6003):193–5.

38. Lee DA, Taylor GM, James VH, et al. Plasma prednisolone levels and adrenocortical responsiveness after administration of prednisolone-21-phosphate as a retention enema. Gut. 1979;20(5): 349–55.

39. Andus T, Targan SR. Corticosteroids. In: Targan S, Shanahan F, editors. Inflammatory Bowel Disease: From Bench to Bedside. Baltimore, MD: Williams&Wilkins; 1993. p. 487–502.

40. Campieri M, Gionchetti P, Belluzzi A, et al. 5-Aminosalicylic acid as enemas or suppositories in distal ulcerative colitis? J Clin Gastroenterol. 1988;10(4):406–9.

41. Hanauer SB, Kane S. The pharmacology of anti-inflammatory drugs in inflammatory bowel disease. In: Kirsner JB, editor. Inflammatory bowel disease. 5th ed. Philadelphia, PA: WB Saunders Co; 2000.

42. Hanauer SB, Robinson M, Pruitt R, et al. Budesonide enema for the treatment of active, distal ulcerative colitis and proctitis: a dose-ranging study. US Budesonide Enema Study Group. Gastroenterology. 1998;115(3):525–32.

43. Marshall JK, Irvine EJ. Rectal corticosteroids versus alternative treatments in ulcerative colitis: a meta-analysis. Gut. 1997;40(6): 775–81.

44. Lee FI, Jewell DP, Mani V, et al. A randomised trial comparing mesalazine and prednisolone foam enemas in patients with acute distal ulcerative colitis. Gut. 1996;38(2):229–33.

45. Marshall JK, Thabane M, Steinhart AH, et al. Rectal 5-Aminosalicylic acid for induction of remission in ulcerative colitis. Cochrane Database Syst Rev. 2010;1:CD004115.

46. Ilnycki A, Shanahan F, Anton PA, et al. The placebo response in ulcerative colitis [abstract]. Gastroenterology. 1996;110:929.

47. Ruddell WS, Dickinson RJ, Dixon MF, et al. Treatment of distal ulcerative colitis (proctosigmoiditis) in relapse: comparison of hydrocortisone enemas and rectal hydrocortisone foam. Gut. 1980;21(10):885–9.

48. Danielsson A, Hellers G, Lyrenäs E, et al. A controlled randomized trial of budesonide versus prednisolone retention enemas in active distal ulcerative colitis. Scand J Gastroenterol. 1987;22(8):987–92.

49. Danielsson A, Löfberg R, Persson T, et al. A steroid enema, budesonide, lacking systemic effects for the treatment of distal ulcerative colitis or proctitis. Scand J Gastroenterol. 1992;27(1): 9–12.

50. Löfberg R, Ostergaard-Thomsen O, Langholz E, et al. Budesonide versus prednisolone retention enemas in active distal ulcerative colitis. Aliment Pharmacol Ther. 1994;8(6):623–9.

51. Lémann M, Galian A, Rutgeerts P, et al. Comparison of budesonide and 5-aminosalicylic acid enemas in active distal ulcerative colitis. Aliment Pharmacol Ther. 1995;9(5):557–62.

52. Lamers C, Meijer J, Engels L, et al. Comparative study of the topically acting glucocorticosteroid budesonide and 5-aminosalicylic acid enema therapy of proctitis and proctosigmoiditis [abstract]. Gastroenterology. 1991;100:A223.

53. Farup PG, Hovde O, Halvorsen FA, et al. Mesalazine suppositories versus hydrocortisone foam in patients with distal ulcerative colitis. A comparison of the efficacy and practicality of two topical treatment regimens. Scand J Gastroenterol. 1995;30(2):164–70.

54. Sharma MP, Duphare HV, Dasarathy S. A prospective randomized double blind trial comparing prednisolone and 4-aminosalicylic acid enemas in acute distal ulcerative colitis. J Gastroenterol Hepatol. 1992;7(2):173–7.

55. Friedman LS, Richter JM, Kirkham SE, et al. 5-Aminosalicylic acid enemas in refractory distal ulcerative colitis; a randomized controlled trial. Am J Gastroenterol. 1986;81(6):412–8.

56. Mulder CJ, Tytgat GN, Wiltink EH, et al. Comparison of 5-aminosalicylic acid(3 g) and prednisolone phosphate sodium enemas (30 mg) in the treatment of distal ulcerative colitis: a prospective, randomized, double-blind trial. Scand J Gastroenterol. 1988;23(8):1005–8.

57. O'Donnell LJ, Arvind AS, Cameron D, et al. Double blind, controlled trial of 4-aminosalicylic acid and prednisolone enemas in distal ulcerative colitis. Gut. 1992;33(7):947–9.

58. Tarpila S, Turunen U, Seppälä K, et al. Budesonide enema in active haemorrhagic proctitis – a controlled trial against hydrocortisone foam enema. Aliment Pharmacol Ther. 1994;8(6):591–5.

59. Cobden I, al-Mardini H, Zaitoun A, et al. Is topical therapy necessary in acute distal ulcerative colitis? Double-blind comparison of high-dose oral mesalazine versus steroid enemas in the treatment of active distal ulcerative colitis. Aliment Pharmacol Ther. 1991;5(5):513–22.

60. Grace RH, Gent AE, Hellier MD. Comparative trial of sodium cromoglycate enemas with prednisolone enemas in the treatment of ulcerative colitis. Gut. 1987;28(1):88–92.

61. Halpern Z, Sold O, Baratz M, et al. A controlled trial of beclomethasone versus betamethasone enemas in distal ulcerative colitis. J Clin Gastroenterol. 1991;13(1):38–41.

62. Meyers S, Janowitz HD. The "natural history" of ulcerative colitis: an analysis of the placebo response. J Clin Gastroenterol. 1989;11(1):33–7.

63. Riley SA, Mani V, Goodman MJ, et al. Microscopic activity in ulcerative colitis: what does it mean? Gut. 1991;32(2):174–8.

64. Cohen RD, Woseth DM, Thisted RA, et al. A meta-analysis and overview of the literature on treatment options for left-sided ulcerative colitis and ulcerative proctitis. Am J Gastroenterol. 2000;95(5):1263–76.

65. Schulz KF, Chalmers I, Hayes RJ, et al. Empirical evidence of bias. Dimensions of methodological quality associated with estimates of treatment effects in controlled trials. JAMA. 1995;273(5):408–12.

66. Peto R. Why do we need systematic overviews of randomized trials? Stat Med. 1987;6(3):233–44.

67. Regueiro M, Loftus Jr EV, Steinhart AH, et al. Medical management of left-sided ulcerative colitis and ulcerative proctitis: critical evaluation of therapeutic trials. Inflamm Bowel Dis. 2006;12(10):979–94.

68. Malchow H, Gertz B, The CLAFOAM Study Group. A new mesalazine foam enema (claversal foam) compared with a standard liquid enema in patients with active distal ulcerative colitis. Aliment Pharmacol Ther. 2002;16(3):415–23.

69. Rizzello F, Gionchetti P, D'Arienzo A, et al. Oral beclometasone dipropionate in the treatment of active ulcerative colitis: a double-blind placebo-controlled study. Aliment Pharmacol Ther. 2002;16(6):1109–16.

70. Truelove SC, Hambling MH. Treatment of ulcerative colitis with local hydrocortisone hemisuccinate sodium; a report on a controlled therapeutic trial. Br Med J. 1958;2(5104):1072–7.

71. Lindgren S, Suhr O, Persson T, et al. Treatment of active distal ulcerative colitis (UC) and maintenance of remission with Entocort enema: a randomized controlled dosage study. Gut. 1997;41:223.

72. Jönsson G, Aström A, Andersson P. Budesonide is metabolized by cytochrome P450 3A (CYP3A) enzymes in human liver. Drug Metab Dispos. 1995;23(1):137–42.

73. Spencer CM, McTavish D. Budesonide: a review of its pharmacological properties and therapeutic efficacy in inflammatory bowel disease. Drugs. 1995;50(5):854–72.

74. McKeage K, Goa KL. Budesonide (Entocort ® EC Capsules): a review of its therapeutic use in the management of active Crohn's disease in adults. Drugs. 2002;62(15):2263–82.

75. Nilsson M, Edsbäcker S, Larsson P, et al. Dose-proportional kinetics of budesonide controlled ileal release (CIR) capsules. Gastroenterology 1994;1783P(abstract).

76. Danielsson A, Edsbäcker S, Löfberg R, et al. Pharmacokinetics of budesonide enema in patients with distal ulcerative colitis or proctitis. Aliment Pharmacol Ther. 1993;7(4):401–7.

77. Seidegåd J. Reduction of the inhibitory effect on ketoconazole on budesonide pharmacokinetics by separation of their time of administration. Clin Pharmacol Ther. 2000;68(1):13–7.

78. Edsbacker S, Anderson T. Pharmacokinetics of budesonide (Entocort EC) capsules for Crohn's disease. Clin Pharmacokinet. 2004;43(12):803–21.

79. Beaulieu DB, Ananthakrishna AN, Issa M, et al. Budesonide induction and maintenance therapy for Crohn's disease during pregnancy. Inflamm Bowel Dis. 2009;15(1):25–8.

80. Nyman-Pantelidis M, Nilsson A, Wagner ZG, et al. Pharmacokinetics and retrograde colonic spread of budesonide enemas in patients with distal ulcerative colitis. Aliment Pharmacol Ther. 1994;8(6):617–22.

81. Peña AS, Kolkman JJ, Greinwald R, et al. Pharmacokinetics after single and multiple oral dosing of budesonide pH-modified-release capsules in patients with distal ulcerative colitis. In: Buhr HJ, Dignass A, Gross V, et al., editors. Topical steroids in gastroenterology and hepatology. Dordrecht: Kluwer; 2004. p. 30–5.

82. Sutherland LR, May GR, Shaffer EA. Sulfasalazine revisited: a meta-analysis of 5-aminosalicylic acid in the treatment of ulcerative colitis. Ann Intern Med. 1993;118(7):540–59.

83. Hamilton I, Pinder IF, Dickinson RJ, et al. A comparison of prednisolone enemas with low-dose oral prednisolone in the treatment of acute distal ulcerative colitis. Dis Colon Rectum. 1984;27(11):701–2.

84. Marteau P, Probert CS, Lingren S, et al. Combined oral and enema treatment with Pentasa (mesalazine) is superior to oral therapy alone in patients with extensive mild/moderate active ulcerative colitis: a randomised, double blind, placebo controlled study. Gut. 2005;54(7):960–5.

85. Sandborn WJ, Hanauer S, Lichtenstein GR, et al. Early symptomatic response and mucosal healing with mesalamine rectal suspension therapy in the treatment of active distal ulcerative colitis (UC): additional results from two controlled, randomized trials. Aliment Pharmacol Ther. 2011;34(7):747–56.

86. Safdi M, DeMicco M, Sninsky C, et al. A double-blind comparison of oral versus rectal mesalamine versus combination therapy

in the treatment of distal ulcerative colitis. Am J Gastroenterol. 1997;92(10):8167–71.

87. Kornbluth AA, Salomon P, Sacks HS, et al. Meta-analysis o the effectiveness of current drug therapy of Ulcerative colitis. J Clin Gastroenterol. 1993;16(3):215–8.

88. Gross V, Bunganic I, Belousova EA, et al. 3 g mesalazine granules are superior to 9 mg budesonide for achieving remission in active ulcerative colitis: a double-blind, double-dummy, randomised trial. J Crohns Colitis. 2011;5(2):129–38.

89. The Danish Budesonide Study Group. Budesonide enema in distal ulcerative colitis. A randomized dose-response trial with prednisolone enema as positive control. Scand J Gastroenterol. 1991; 26(112):1225–30.

90. Bianchi Porro G, Prantera C, Campieri M, et al. Comparative trial of methylprednisolone and budesonide enemas in active distal ulcerative colitis. Eur J Gastroenterol Hepatol. 1994;6:125–30.

91. Bayless T, Sninsky C, for the U.S. Budesonide Enema Study Group. Budesonide enema is effective alternative to hydrocortisone enema in active distal ulcerative colitis [abstract]. Gastroenterology. 1995;108:A778.

92. Schölmerich J. Review article: systematic and topical steroids in inflammatory bowel disease. Aliment Pharmacol Ther. 2004;20 Suppl 4:66–74.

93. Gross V, Bar-Meir S, Lavy A, et al. Budesonide foam versus budesonide enema in active ulcerative proctitis and proctosigmoiditis. Aliment Pharmacol Ther. 2006;23(2):303–12.

94. Hartmann F, Stein J, BudMesa-Study Group. Clinical trial: controlled, open, randomized multicentre study comparing the effects of treatment on quality of life, safety, and efficacy of budesonide or mesalazine enemas in active let-sided ulcerative colitis. Aliment Pharmacol Ther. 2010;32(3):368–76.

95. Sherlock ME, Seow CH, Steinhart AH, et al. Oral budesonide for induction of remission in ulcerative colitis. Cochrane Database Syst Rev. 2010;10:CD007698.

96. D'Haens GR, Kovács A, Vergauwe P, et al. Clinical trial: preliminary efficacy and safety study of a new Budesonide-MMX® 9 mg extended-release tablets in patients with active left sided ulcerative colitis. J Crohn Colitis. 2010;4(2):153–60.

97. Gross V, Bunganic I, Mikhailova TL, et al. Efficacy and tolerability of a once daily treatment with budesonide capsules versus mesalamine granules for the treatment of active ulcerative colitis: a randomized, double-blind, double-dummy, multicenter study. Gastroenterology. 2009;136(5):A-15.

98. Seow CH, Benchimol EL, Griffiths AM, et al. Budesonide for Induction of remission in Crohn's disease. Cochrane Database Syst Rev. 2008;3, CD000296.

99. Lindgren S, Löfberg R, Bergholm L, et al. Effect of budesonide enema on remission and relapse rate in distal ulcerative colitis and proctitis. Scand J Gastroenterol. 2002;37(6):705–10.

100. Rutgeerts P, Löfberg R, Malchow H, et al. A comparison of budesonide with prednisolone for active Crohn's disease. N Eng J Med. 1994;331(13):842–5.

101. Bar Meir S, Chowers Y, Lavy A, et al. Budesonide versus prednisone in the treatment of active Crohn's disease. The Israeli Budesonide study group. Gastroenterology. 1998;115(4):835–40.

102. Levine A, Weizman Z, Broid E, et al. A comparison of budesonide and prednisone for the treatment of active pediatric Crohn's disease. J Pediatr Gastroenterol Nutr. 2003;36(2):248–52.

103. Escher JC, European Collaborative Research Group on Budesonide in Paediatric IBD. Budesonide versus prednisolone for the treatment of active Crohn's disease in children: a randomized, double blind, controlled, multicentre trial. Eur J Gastroenterol Hepatol. 2004;16(1):47–54.

104. Tursi A, Giorgetti GM, Brandmarte G, et al. Beclomethasone dipropionate for the treatment of mild-to-moderate Crohn's disease: an open-label, budesonide-controlled, randomized study. Med Sci Monit. 2006;12(6):129–32.

105. Levine A, Kori M, Dinari G, et al. Comparison of two dosing methods for induction of response and remission with oral budesonide in active pediatric Crohn's disease: a randomized placebo-controlled trial. Inflamm Bowel Dis. 2009;15(7): 1055–61.

106. Heuschkel R, Salvestrini C, Beattie RM, et al. Guidelines for the management of growth failure in childhood. Inflamm Bowl Dis. 2008;14(6):839–49.

107. Kundhal O, Zachos M, Holmes JL, Griffiths AM. Controlled ileal release budesonide in pediatric Crohn disease: efficacy and effect on growth. J Pediatr Gastroenterol Nutr. 2001;33(1):75–80.

108. Greenberg GR, Feagan BG, Martin F, et al. Oral budesonide for the active Crohn's disease. Canadian Inflammatory Bowel Disease Study Group. N Engl J Med. 1994;331(13):836–41.

109. Tremaine WJ, Hanauer SB, Katz S, et al. Budesonide CIR capsules(once or twice daily divided dose) in active Crohn's disease: a randomized placebo-controlled study in the United States. Am J Gastroenterol. 2002;97(7):1748–54.

110. Sandborn WJ, Travis S, Moro L, et al. Budesonide MMX ® 9 mg for the induction of remission of mild-to-moderate ulcerative colitis (UC): data from a multicenter, randomized, double-blind placebo-controlled study in North America and India. DDW. 2011;Abstract 746.

111. Sandborn WJ, Travis S, Danese S, et al. Budesonide MMX ® 9 mg for induction of remission of placebo-controlled study in the Europe, Russia, Israel, and Australia. DDW. 2011;Abstract 292.

112. Campieri M, Adamo S, Valpiani D, et al. Oral beclometasone dipropionate in the treatment of extensive and left-sided active ulcerative colitis: a multicenter randomized study. Aliment Pharmacol Ther. 2003;17(12):1471–80.

113. Manguso F, Balzano A. Meta-analysis: the efficacy of rectal beclomethasone dipropionate vs. 5-aminosalicylic acid in mild to moderate distal ulcerative colitis. Aliment Pharmacol Ther. 2007;26(1):21–9.

114. Nunes T, Barreiro-de Acosta M, Nos P, et al. Usefulness of oral beclometasone dipropionate to induce remission in active ulcerative colitis patients: results from the RECLICU study. DDW. 2010;New Orleans Abstracts W1301.

115. Luboshitzky R, Rachelis Z, Nussensone E, et al. Beclomethasone dipropionate enema in ulcerative colitis: is it safe? Endocr Pract. 2009;2:1–18.

116. Campieri M, Cottone M, Miglio F, et al. Beclomethasone dipropionate enemas versus prednisolone sodium phosphate enemas in the treatment of distal ulcerative colitis. Aliment Pharmacol Ther. 1998;12(4):361–6.

117. Mulder CJ, Fockens P, Meijer JW, et al. Beclomethasone dipropionate (3 mg) versus 5-aminosalicylic acid (2 g) versus the combination of both (3 mg/2 g) as retention enemas in active ulcerative proctitis. Eur J Gastroenterol Hepatol. 1996;8(6):549–53.

118. Biancone L, Gionchetti P, Blanco Gdel V, et al. Beclomethasone dipropionate versus mesalazine in distal ulcerative colitis: a multicenter, randomized, double-blind study. Dig Liver Dis. 2007; 39(4):329–37.

119. Kumana CR, Seaton T, Meghji M, et al. Beclomethasone dipropionate enemas for treating inflammatory bowel disease without producing Cushing's syndrome or hypothalamic pituitary adrenal suppression. Lancet. 1982;1(8272):579–83.

120. Bansky G, Bühler H, Stamm B, et al. Treatment of distal ulcerative colitis with beclomethasone enemas: high therapeutic efficacy without endocrine side effects: a prospective, randomized, double blind trial. Dis Colon Rectum. 1987;30(4):288–92.

121. Harris DM. Some properties of beclomethasone dipropionate and related steroids in man. Postrad Med J. 1975;51 Suppl 4:20–5.

122. D'Azrienzo A, Manguso F, Castiglione GN, et al. Beclomethasone dipropionate (3 mg) enemas combined with oral 5-ASA (2.4 g) in the treatment of ulcerative colitis not responsive to oral 5-ASA alone. Ital J Gastroenterol Hepatol. 1998;30(3):254–7.

123. Gionchetti P, D'Arienzo A, Rizzello F, et al. Topical treatment of distal active ulcerative colitis with beclomethasone dipropionate or mesalamine: a single-blind randomized controlled trial. J Clin Gastroenterol. 2005;39(4):291–7.

124. Rhodes JM, Robinson R, Beales I, et al. Clinical trial: oral prednisolone metasulfobenzoate (Predocol) vs. oral prednisolone for active ulcerative colitis. Aliment Pharmacol Ther. 2008;27(3):228–40.

125. Bar-Meir S, Fidder HH, Faszczyk M, et al. Budesonide foam vs hydrocortisone acetate foam in the treatment of active ulcerative proctosigmoiditis. Dis Colon Rectum. 2003;46(7):929–36.

126. Hammond A, Anrus T, Gierand M, et al. Controlled, open, randomized multicenter trial comparing the effects of treatment on quality of life, safety and efficacy of budesonide foam and betamethasone enemas in patients with active distal ulcerative colitis. Hepatogastroenterology. 2004;51(59):1345–9.

127. Rufle W, Frühmorgen P, Huber W, et al. Budesonide foam as a new therapeutic principle in distal ulcerative colitis in comparison with mesalazine enema: an open, controlled, randomized and prospective multicenter pilot study. Z Gastroenterol. 2000;38(4): 287–93.

128. Gionchetti P, Rizzello F, Poggioli G, et al. Oral budesonide in the treatment of chronic refractory pouchitis. Aliment Pharmacol Ther. 2007;25(10):1231–6.

129. MacDermott RP, Green JA. Refractory ulcerative colitis treatment. Gastroenterol Hepatol (NY). 2007;3(1):64–9.

130. Löfberg R, Danielsson A, Suhr O, et al. Oral budesonide versus prednisolone in patients with active extensive and left-sided ulcerative colitis. Gastroenterology. 1996;10(6):1713–8.

131. Petitjean O, Wendling JL, Tod M, et al. Pharmacokinetics and absolute rectal bioavailability of hydrocortisone acetate in distal colitis. Aliment Pharmacol Ther. 1992;6:351–7.

132. Ulder CJ, Fockens P, Meijer JW, et al. Beclomethasone dipropionate (3 mg) versus 5-aminosalicylic acid (2 g) versus the combination of both (3 mg/2 g) as retention enemas in active ulcerative proctitis. Eur J Gastroenterol Hepatol. 1996;8: 549–53.

133. Loen BL, Siegel C. Foam preparations for treatment of ulcerative colitis. Curr Drug Deliv. 2011;8(5):1–7.

# Antimetabolite Therapy in Ulcerative Colitis: Azathioprine, 6-Mercaptopurine, and Methotrexate

## 11

María Chaparro and Javier P. Gisbert

**Keywords**

Thiopurines • Azathioprine • Mercaptopurine • Methotrexate • Ulcerative colitis

## Introduction

Ulcerative colitis (UC) is a lifelong, immune-mediated inflammatory condition of the colonic mucosa, which is characterized by a relapsing and remitting course [1]. The primary goals of therapy in the treatment of UC are to induce remission of patient's symptoms as rapidly as possible and maintain remission on a long-term basis. By reducing the episodes of relapse, it is possible to reduce the risk of long-term complications and improve patient quality of life.

Corticosteroids remain one of the most effective therapies for inducing remission in patients with moderate to severe UC. However, approximately 50–80 % of patients in whom corticosteroids are prescribed will experience a rapid relapse of symptoms. Antimetabolite therapy has found widespread use for corticosteroid-dependent patients in clinical practice, although the data supporting the use of thiopurines—azathioprine and mercaptopurine—and methotrexate are more robust in the steroid-dependent Crohn's disease than in UC. This chapter will review the current state of the art regarding the thiopurine drugs and methotrexate for the treatment of UC.

## Thiopurines for the Treatment of Ulcerative Colitis Patients

### What Is the Mechanism of Action of the Thiopurine Drugs?

The metabolism of azathioprine and mercaptopurine is complex [2]. Azathioprine is nonenzymatically converted to mercaptopurine after oral administration and absorption. Both azathioprine and mercaptopurine are prodrugs. Mercaptopurine can then be metabolized to an active metabolite, thioguanine. Thioguanine is incorporated into ribonucleotides, thereby exerting an antiproliferative effect on mitotically active lymphocyte populations [3]. Thiopurine methyltransferase (TPMT) metabolizes mercaptopurine into an inactive 6-methylmercaptopurine. Therefore, reduction in TPMT activity predisposes to the development of adverse effects such as bone marrow suppression due to preferential metabolism of mercaptopurine to thioguanine nucleotides. Azathioprine and mercaptopurine also may possess direct anti-inflammatory properties by inhibiting a cytotoxic T cell and natural killer cell function and inducing apoptosis of T cells. Although it has been speculated that azathioprine may possess immunosuppressive and metabolic benefits beyond that of mercaptopurine, these drugs are used interchangeably in clinical practice [4].

### What are the Indications for the Treatment with Thiopurines in UC Patients?

At present, thiopurine treatment is recommended in steroid-dependent and steroid-refractory UC patients [5]. For an arbitrary but practical reason, the "European Crohn's and

M. Chaparro, M.D., Ph.D. (✉) • J.P. Gisbert, M.D., Ph.D.
Department of Gastroenterology, La Princesa University Hospital,
Diego de Leon 62, Madrid 28006, Spain
e-mail: javier.p.gisbert@gmail.com

G.R. Lichtenstein (ed.), *Medical Therapy of Ulcerative Colitis*,
DOI 10.1007/978-1-4939-1677-1_11, © Springer Science+Business Media New York 2014

Colitis Organization" proposes several scenarios where thiopurine treatment in UC should be recommended [5]: (a) patients who have a severe relapse, (b) those who require two or more corticosteroid courses within a 12-month period, (c) those whose disease relapses as the steroid dose is reduced below an arbitrary 15 mg, and (d) those whose disease relapses within 3 months of stopping steroids.

## What Is the Recommended Dosage of Thiopurines for the Treatment of UC Patients?

The choice of azathioprine and mercaptopurine dosage is generally based on the weight of the patient, with the intention of achieving the highest therapeutic efficacy and, at the same time, reducing the incidence of adverse effects. Several clinical trials have shown that the adequate azathioprine dosage in Crohn's disease patients is 2–3 mg/kg/day. Azathioprine is 55 % mercaptopurine by molecular weight, and 88 % of azathioprine is converted to mercaptopurine. When changing from mercaptopurine to azathioprine, a conversion factor of 2.07 can be used [6]; thus, the equivalent dosage of mercaptopurine is approximately 1.5 mg/kg/day [7].

Strategies for initiating treatment with thiopurines vary and range from slow titration to immediately starting at the full weight-based dose [7]. A theoretical rationale behind slow titration is to carefully monitor for clinical signs of toxicity. However, dose-dependent toxicities (such as hepatitis and delayed myelotoxicity) are unlikely until a significant cumulative dose has been given. On the other hand, idiosyncratic reactions such as pancreatitis, fever, rash, nausea/vomiting, diarrhea, and arthralgias, which are dose independent, would not be avoided by giving lower doses of the drug. Therefore, slow titration may further delay an already lengthy period before therapeutic effects are seen [7].

In conclusion, as long as TPMT activity is normal, treatment can be started at an adequate dosage (i.e., 2–3 mg/kg/day for azathioprine and 1.5 mg/kg/day for mercaptopurine) with monitoring of clinical side effects, biweekly blood count, and liver function tests for 2 months and then every 3–6 months for the entire duration of the treatment [7].

## Are Thiopurines Effective in the Treatment of UC Patients?

### Are They Effective in Inducing Remission in UC?

There are two randomized and controlled trials that evaluated the efficacy of azathioprine in inducing remission in UC. The first one included 80 patients with active UC that were randomized to receive azathioprine (2.5 mg/kg) or placebo [8]. Both groups were similar considering the primary end point, which was the remission rate after 1 month of treatment. The second trial comprised 50 UC patients who were treated with sulfasalazine, steroids, and azathioprine (2 mg/kg) or sulfasalazine, steroids, and placebo [9]. The remission rates were similar in both groups after 4 months of treatment [9].

Data from the studies assessing the efficacy of thiopurines in inducing and maintaining remission in UC have been pooled in two meta-analyses. The first one by Gisbert et al. included studies comparing thiopurines with placebo or 5-aminosalicylates [10]. The second meta-analysis, recently published by Kahn et al., only included clinical trials comparing azathioprine or mercaptopurine with placebo [11]. Both meta-analyses provide relevant information regarding the efficacy of thiopurines in UC. Although there seems to be a trend towards the benefit of azathioprine when compared with placebo in inducing remission, it did not achieve statistical significance.

Nevertheless, it has been suggested that, in all studies that assess the effectiveness of thiopurines in inducing remission in UC patients, the evaluation of response to the treatment is too early considering the delayed (approximately 4 weeks) onset of action of these drugs.

In summary, thiopurines do not seem to be effective in inducing remission in UC patients.

### Are Thiopurines Effective in Maintaining Remission in UC?

Three clinical trials assessing the efficacy of azathioprine in the maintenance of remission in UC have been published [8, 12, 13]. In these studies, patients with quiescent UC under thiopurine treatment were included, and they were followed up during within 9–12 months to estimate the risk of relapsing. All of them showed that azathioprine is effective in maintaining remission in UC.

In the abovementioned meta-analysis by Gisbert et al., the mean efficacy with thiopurines was 60 and 37 % in the control group (including both 5-aminosalicylates and placebo groups) [10]. The *odds ratio* (OR) for this comparison was 2.56. When only the three studies comparing azathioprine/mercaptopurine with placebo were considered, the OR was 2.59 [10]. Another meta-analysis by Timmer et al. demonstrated that azathioprine therapy appears to be more effective than placebo for the maintenance of remission in ulcerative colitis [14].

In conclusion, thiopurines are effective in maintaining remission in UC patients.

### Are Thiopurines as Effective in UC as They Are in Crohn's Disease?

Few studies have directly compared the efficacy of thiopurines in UC and Crohn's disease. Kull et al. compared the

6-month efficacy of azathioprine in both diseases [15]. The authors found that clinical remission rates were slightly higher for UC than for Crohn's disease patients (77 % vs. 70 %); furthermore, complete corticosteroid weaning was obtained significantly more often in UC than in Crohn's disease patients (59 % vs. 30 %). Verhave et al. concluded that patients with UC treated with thiopurines responded similarly to their Crohn's disease counterparts; moreover, they determined that the beneficial effect occurred 1 month sooner in UC than in Crohn's disease patients [16]. Finally, Fraser et al. demonstrated that azathioprine was more likely to achieve remission in patients with UC than with Crohn's disease (58 % vs. 45 %) but was equally effective for maintenance of remission [17].

In the study by Bastida et al., the beneficial effect of azathioprine was independent of the type of inflammatory bowel disease (IBD), Crohn's disease, or UC [18]. Finally, Gisbert et al. found in a recent prospective study that azathioprine was similarly effective for both IBD types, as remission was achieved in 49 % of Crohn's disease patients and in 42 % of UC patients; furthermore, azathioprine treatment resulted in a similar reduction in the number of surgical procedures and hospitalizations in both diseases [19].

The number needed to treat (NNT) to prevent one relapse with azathioprine, when compared with placebo, has been calculated to be 5, which compares favorably with the NNT of 7 reported with azathioprine in Crohn's disease [10]. Furthermore, some authors have suggested that this effect of thiopurines might occur sooner in UC than in Crohn's disease [16].

In summary, it could be concluded that thiopurines are at least as effective in UC as in Crohn's disease patients.

## Is Treatment with Thiopurines Safe, Specifically in UC Patients?

Unfortunately, more than one-third of IBD patients have to discontinue thiopurine therapy during the course of the disease, the main reason being the occurrence of intolerable adverse events, which are reported in 10–30 % of the IBD patients using thiopurines. The side effects of thiopurines can be divided into dose-independent and pharmacologically explainable dose-dependent events. Among the dose-independent events, idiosyncratic or allergic reactions are rash, fever, arthralgias, pancreatitis, and hepatitis. The dose-dependent toxicity of thiopurines may largely be explained by the complex metabolism of thiopurines, which results in a number of potentially effective or toxic metabolites. Hepatotoxicity and myelotoxicity are usually considered dose-dependent reactions [20, 21].

Nausea is usually the most frequent thiopurine-related adverse event. Although it is not a life-threatening adverse effect, it severely limits treatment with thiopurines, as more than 80 % of patients with nausea have to discontinue the treatment with these drugs. Infection is a relatively common indirect toxicity, being observed in approximately 7 % of patients [4]. In addition to bacterial infections, viral infections are associated with use of azathioprine and mercaptopurine. The herpesviruses, specifically Epstein-Barr virus, cytomegalovirus, varicella-zoster virus, and herpes simplex virus, have all been reported to cause some rare but serious complications in IBD patients receiving azathioprine/mercaptopurine. Most herpesvirus infections are probably unrecognized and manifest as self-limited viral syndromes, but life-threatening complications such as disseminated varicella-zoster, pneumonitis, and viral-mediated hemophagocytic syndrome have been reported [4].

In the same way, it has been suggested that there is an increased risk for the development of some malignancies in IBD patients under thiopurine therapy. The relationship between thiopurines and development of cancer, especially hematological malignancies such as lymphomas, remains a controversial topic. A meta-analysis of the risk of malignancy associated with the use of immunosuppressive drugs suggested that the administration of immunosuppressive drugs in IBD patients probably does not confer a significantly increased risk of malignancy compared with patients with IBD who are not receiving these agents [22]. There was not a significant difference when the authors analyzed the length of exposure to immunosuppressants or whether the patients had Crohn's disease or UC.

The issue of the relationship between lymphoma and IBD is complex due to the effects caused by the disease per se and by the disease activity and because different IBD therapies clearly overlap. A meta-analysis of Kandiel et al. identified six cohort studies with azathioprine or mercaptopurine exposure that have been specifically designed to evaluate cancer as adverse outcome [23]. The total number of observed cases was 11, with a pooled relative risk of 4.18. Recently, results from the very large French population-based CESAME study suggest a doubling of the risk of lymphoma in patients with IBD, with the majority of cases occurring in association with immunosuppressive therapy [24]. However, because these data were obtained from observational studies, it is not possible to exclude the possibility that disease severity is a confounding factor. Another recent meta-analysis by Kotlyar et al. found that there is a higher risk for lymphoma in patients using azathioprine or 6-MP [25]. The overall Standard Incidence Ratio (SIR) for lymphoma was 4.49 (95 % CI, 2.81–7.17), ranging from 2.43 (95 % CI, 1.50–3.92) in eight population studies to 9.16 (95 % CI, 5.03–16.7) in ten referral studies. Population studies demonstrated an increased risk among current users (SIR = 5.71; 95 % CI, 3.72–10.1), but not in former users of azathioprine or 6-mercaptopurine (SIR = 1.42; 95 % CI, 0.86–2.34).

The level of risk became significant after 1 year of exposure to azathioprine or 6-mercaptopurine. Also, men have greater risk than women (RR=2.05; P<.05); both sexes were at increased risk for lymphoma (SIR for men=3.60; 95 % CI, 2.68–4.83; SIR for women=1.76, 95 % CI, 1.08–2.87). Also, there was found to be an age-dependent risk for lymphoma with patients younger than 30 years having the highest RR (SIR=6.99; CI, 2.99–16.4); younger men had the highest risk. The absolute risk was highest in patients older than 50 years (1:377 cases per patient-year).

As an overall conclusion, the consensus about the relationship between immunosuppressants and lymphoma is that the risk is of small magnitude and, in any case, the beneficial effects exerted by these drugs on IBD patient outcomes would clearly outweigh the risk caused by the drug itself.

In addition to lymphoma, there has been a concern that azathioprine may be related to other malignancies. However, this association remains controversial. Azathioprine and mercaptopurine do not increase the risk of colorectal cancer; moreover, it seems to have a protector effect by controlling mucosal inflammation [26]. On the other hand, an increased risk of nonmelanoma skin cancer is well recognized in the immunosuppressed transplant population as well, and it has also been reported in IBD [27, 28]. A recent meta-analysis has reinforced this association. However, this finding has not been confirmed by all authors [29].

## How Can Thiopurine Therapy Be Optimized in UC Patients?

Determining TPMT genotype or enzyme activity phenotype prior to initiating azathioprine therapy has the potential to reduce myelosuppression by 25–50 %. Approximately, 90 % of the population has a wild-type genotype with a normal activity of the enzyme; about 11 % of the population has intermediate activity and 0.3 % of the population has low activity [30, 31]. However, some patients will still experience myelosuppression despite a normal TPMT activity, and thus, all patients undergoing thiopurine treatment will need regular complete blood count monitoring during follow-up [32]. Nevertheless, determination of TPMT activity prior to the administration of these drugs would allow for identification of those patients who should avoid thiopurine treatment due to a very high risk of severe myelotoxicity. This has been proven to be a cost-benefit strategy [33, 34].

Inosine triphosphate pyrophosphatase (ITPA) is another enzyme involved in the metabolism of thiopurines. The deficient function of this enzyme leads to an abnormal accumulation of potential toxic metabolites. Indeed, some authors have reported that ITPA polymorphisms are associated with allergic reactions to thiopurines. However, this association has not been confirmed by all authors. Until further studies confirm the utility of ITPA testing, its use cannot be recommended in clinical practice [4].

The measurement of serum thiopurine metabolite levels has been proposed by some authors as a useful tool to optimize treatment with azathioprine and mercaptopurine [35, 36]. However, the utility of this strategy has been debated in the literature and even referred to as the "metabolite controversy." In 2000, Dubinsky et al. showed that, in children, higher thioguanine levels corresponded to a higher frequency of response [37]. In fact, 65 % of patients with thioguanine levels in the therapeutic range had a beneficial response as opposed to the 27 % with suboptimal levels [37]. Similar results have been reported by others, but this has not been consistent among all groups [38–40]. As an example, a recent large multicenter trial did not support the determination of thioguanine levels to predict treatment outcomes, and no useful serum metabolites threshold value to adjust the drug's dose was identified [40].

In summary, although thioguanine is an important metabolite associated with both the efficacy and toxicity of azathioprine/mercaptopurine, other metabolites are likely to also play an essential role. At the current time, we believe that the data are insufficient to support routine monitoring of mercaptopurine and thiopurine metabolites.

## How Long Should Thiopurine Therapy be Maintained in UC Patients?

As thiopurine therapy is associated with a wide range of adverse events, more data are required to determine the optimal duration of therapy, particularly for patients in remission. Data regarding the long-term efficacy of thiopurines and about IBD patient outcomes after the cessation of these drugs are scarce. Several trials have shown that, irrespective of the duration of remission, withdrawing thiopurine therapy increases the risk of relapse in Crohn's disease patients [41].

In the case of UC, Holtman et al. performed a multicenter retrospective study aiming to evaluate the long-term efficacy of thiopurine therapy [42]. Data from 358 UC patients were analyzed according to the duration of the treatment (less than 3 years, 3–4 years, and longer than 4 years). In this study, the risk of relapse and the need for steroid treatment were significantly lower after initiating thiopurine treatment. The authors found that discontinuation of the thiopurines after 3 years of treatment was associated with a high risk of relapse. Therefore, authors concluded that treatment with these drugs should be maintained for at least 4 years [42].

These benefits of the long-term treatment with thiopurines have been confirmed by other authors. In this respect, in a study performed on 622 IBD patients (346 UC), it was found that the beneficial effect of azathioprine remains at least after 5 years of treatment [43]. In the same way, Chebli et al. evaluated the efficacy of azathioprine on a cohort of 42 UC patients who had been on this drug for at least 3 years. They found that the remission rate and the steroid-sparing effect were maintained at the end of follow-up [43].

The consequences of the discontinuation of thiopurine treatment in UC patients were evaluated by Hawthorne et al. [44]. Seventy-nine UC patients who had been taking azathioprine for at least 6 months were included. Patients were randomized to receive azathioprine or placebo for 12 months. This study showed that the protective effect of azathioprine in the maintenance of remission in UC lasts for at least 2 years in patients who have achieved remission while taking the drug. Moreover, discontinuation of the treatment led to a double-risk of relapse, when compared with patients who maintained treatment (36 % in the azathioprine group vs. 56 % in the placebo group).

Similar results were reported by Cassinotti et al. [45]. These authors included 127 patients who were in steroid-free remission at the time of azathioprine withdrawal, and they were followed-up for a median of 55 months or until relapse. Sixty-seven percent of patients relapsed at a median of 12 months after withdrawal of the drug. Several predictive factors for relapse were identified in this study: lack of sustained remission during azathioprine maintenance, extensive colitis, and treatment duration, with a higher risk of relapse among those patients who had received short treatments (3–6 months) compared with those who had been under thiopurines for longer than 48 months.

All these data suggest that the efficacy of azathioprine in UC patients remains in long-term treatment and that withdrawal of the drug in patients who were in remission is associated with a high risk of relapse. Therefore, in the same sense as in transplant patients, thiopurine therapy should probably be indefinitely maintained once the remission is reached in UC patients.

In conclusion, thiopurine withdrawal trials have shown that, irrespective of the duration of remission, withdrawing thiopurine therapy increases the risk of relapse both in CD and UC. Given these results, continuation may be favorable in the majority of patients. Nevertheless, there remain a minority who needlessly continue thiopurine therapy and are exposed to the associated risks. Accordingly, the identification of patients who, despite cessation of thiopurine therapy, will be at a low risk of relapse is of particular interest.

## Methotrexate in the Treatment of Ulcerative Colitis

### What Is the Clinical Pharmacology of Methotrexate?

Methotrexate was initially used for the treatment of leukemia in children, at which time it was noticed that those with concomitant psoriasis or rheumatoid arthritis showed improvement in these conditions [46]. Subsequent studies confirmed efficacy in these two diseases, which led to trials in IBD. Methotrexate is an analog of folic acid and of aminopterin, which is also a folic acid antagonist. One of the main mechanisms of its action is the inhibition of dihydrofolate reductase, the enzyme involved in de novo synthetic pathway for purines and pyrimidines. The rationale for the use of high-dose methotrexate in the treatment of cancer is that rapidly proliferating malignant cells become starved of purine and pyrimidine precursors and therefore are unable to sufficiently maintain DNA and RNA synthesis, leading to decreased proliferation. The underlying anti-inflammatory effect of low-dose methotrexate in inflammatory diseases such as IBD is less clear, as the antiproliferative activity of low-dose methotrexate is minimal [47].

### What Is the Preferred Route of Administration of Methotrexate?

Methotrexate can be administered orally, intramuscularly, or subcutaneously. The parenteral route is preferred as the threshold absorption rate, when it is administered orally, can be decreased by 30–70 %. Intramuscular and subcutaneous administration result in similar bioavailability of the drug, but subcutaneous administration is normally better tolerated [48]. The majority of the drug, between 65 and 80 %, is excreted by the kidneys and the rest is secreted in the bile [49]. A correlation has not been found between metabolites in serum and clinical efficacy, suggesting that there is no clinical value in monitoring these levels.

The optimal dose of methotrexate in UC has not been established. However, based on the recommendations for Crohn's disease, the majority of authors suggest administering 25 mg subcutaneously weekly for the treatment of active disease with, perhaps, a dose reduction to 15 mg subcutaneously weekly for the maintenance of remission [50].

Time to onset of action is probably earlier than thiopurines. The only head-to-head study comparing methotrexate with azathioprine was not sufficiently powered to address the question of rapidity of onset of action, but there was a suggestion that methotrexate may provide clinical benefit earlier than thiopurines [46].

### What Is the Effectiveness of Methotrexate in UC?

A relevant proportion of UC will require the use of immunosuppressants during the course of the disease. Unfortunately, up to one-third of patients do not respond to thiopurines and a further 15 % are unable to tolerate these agents. Methotrexate is an established alternative to thiopurines in the management of Crohn's disease. However, prospective studies evaluating the effectiveness of methotrexate in UC patients are scarce, especially in a dose range demonstrated to be effective in the treatment of Crohn's disease. The first retrospective case series assessing the effectiveness of methotrexate in UC was published by Kozakek et al. [51]. The authors observed that five of seven patients treated with methotrexate, 25 mg intramuscularly on a weekly basis, achieved remission. The same group later described a cohort that comprised 30 patients with steroid-refractory UC and 70 % response rate after 12 weeks of 25 mg intramuscularly/ week and a long-term response of 40 % on oral methotrexate at a dose 7.5–15 mg/week.

The initial clinical observations, along with the significant therapeutic effectiveness of methotrexate in patients with Crohn's disease, led to the first and only prospective, placebo-controlled trial investigating the efficacy of oral methotrexate therapy for the induction and maintenance of remission in patients with UC [52]. This trial was performed by Oren et al. and included patients with at least moderately active UC who were randomized to receive either methotrexate at a dose of 12.5 mg per week orally (i.e., probably subtherapeutic) or placebo for 9 months. Thirty-seven patients received placebo and 30 received methotrexate. There were no significant differences among the groups with regard to the primary outcomes, monthly steroid use or clinical Mayo score, or the sigmoidoscopy scores for inflammation. Interestingly, dropout rates were four times higher among placebo-treated patients than in the methotrexate-treated patients. This could reflect partial improvement benefit with methotrexate [52]. In conclusion, methotrexate administered orally did not prove to be more effective in inducing and maintaining remission than placebo.

Three prospective open-label studies have investigated the effectiveness of methotrexate compared to mercaptopurine or 5-aminosalicylates. The one performed by Mate et al. included UC patients with at least moderately active UC who were randomized to either one of the following therapeutic regimens: mercaptopurine 1.5 mg/kg/day, oral methotrexate 15 mg/week, or 5-ASA 3 g/day [53]. The remission rates after 30 weeks of therapy were 78.6 %, 58 %, and 25 %, respectively. Patients who had achieved remission on their respective drug regimen were continued on them in a 106-week follow-up study. At this time point, only one of seven patients on methotrexate maintained remission compared to 7 of 11 in the mercaptopurine group. Although this study failed to show the benefit of methotrexate in UC, it has been criticized for its poor methodological quality.

Egan et al. compared the effectiveness of two different doses of parenteral methotrexate [54]. Sixteen Crohn's disease and 14 UC patients were included, and the authors did not provide a breakdown of results by diagnosis. After 16 weeks, a total of 17 % (3/18 in the 15-mg group and 2/12 in the 25-mg group) achieved remission. Paoluzi et al.

report the results of short- and long-term methotrexate therapy (12.5 mg/week intramuscularly) in ten steroid-dependent UC patients who were intolerant or resistant to thiopurines. After 6 months, all ten patients were in clinical remission [55].

Several retrospective series have also been published [51, 56–59], comprising a limited number of patients. Most had failed or been intolerant to AZA and were treated with methotrexate at various dosages and routes of administration. The response or remission rates ranged from 40 to 75 %, suggesting that some patients with UC may respond well to methotrexate. One study distinguished between patients given methotrexate for azathioprine intolerance and azathioprine failure [59]. Methotrexate (median oral dose 20 mg/week) was tolerated by 27 of 31 (87 %) patients who had been unable to tolerate azathioprine. Of those treated with methotrexate after failure with azathioprine, 5 of 11 patients had a colectomy vs. 5 of 31 patients who were intolerant of azathioprine ($p < 0.05$) [59]. The results are heterogeneous and it is possible that the dose and the route of administration of methotrexate are important determinants of efficacy.

Currently, there are no published prospective, placebo-controlled data regarding the clinical value of parenteral methotrexate in patients with UC in a dose range demonstrated to be effective in the treatment of Crohn's disease. In this respect, two clinical trials to assess the efficacy of methotrexate in UC are under way. An investigator-initiated trial in France, "Comparison of methotrexate vs. placebo in steroid-refractory ulcerative colitis (METEOR)," is currently assessing the efficacy of 25 mg methotrexate/week administered subcutaneously compared to placebo in inducing clinical remission (ClinicalTrials.gov Identifier: NCT00498589). The "Randomized, double-blind, prospective trial investigating the efficacy of methotrexate in induction and maintenance of steroid-free remission in ulcerative colitis (MERIT-UC)" is the second study which is also hopefully going to answer the question of the usefulness of methotrexate in UC (ClinicalTrials.gov Identifier: NCT01393405).

In summary, when viewed in its totality, data from uncontrolled studies regarding the effectiveness of methotrexate in UC suggest that, if it is given at a similar dosage (25 mg/ week) and in a similar manner (intramuscular or subcutaneous) as in CD, it may be a clinically useful therapy for steroid-dependant UC patients, including patients who did not tolerate or did not respond to thiopurines. However, there is currently insufficient evidence to recommend methotrexate for UC.

## How Is the Safety Profile of Methotrexate?

The most commonly observed adverse events related to methotrexate therapy are associated with the gastrointestinal tract, including nausea, anorexia, and less often stomatitis or diarrhea [47]. Nausea can usually be minimized by changing the time of dosing (before bedtime), ensuring adequate intake of folic acid and, if needed, adding antiemetic around the time of the weekly dose [47].

More serious adverse events include hepatotoxicity, bone marrow suppression, and, rarely, hypersensitivity pneumonitis and opportunistic infections. Elevation of liver functions tests is relatively frequent in patients on methotrexate therapy. However, the development of hepatic fibrosis, which is believed to be related to intrahepatic accumulation of methotrexate metabolites, is a rare event [47, 60, 61]. Alcohol consumption, diabetes mellitus, obesity, and viral hepatitis can increase the risk of developing hepatotoxicity [4]. In patients with psoriasis, liver toxicity related to methotrexate is frequently seen: nearly a quarter of patients had either active hepatitis or cirrhosis on follow-up liver biopsy after more than 3.4 years of treatment [62]. However, the incidence of hepatotoxicity from methotrexate in patients with IBD is thought to be significantly lower than in psoriasis [63].

Hypersensitivity pneumonitis has been reported in about 1 % of patients, and risk factors include advanced age, diabetes, and rheumatoid lung disease [62, 64]. Rare cases have been reported in patients with IBD [51, 65]. Pretreatment chest X-ray or pulmonary function tests are not routinely ordered, but a high clinical suspicion is essential if pulmonary symptoms begin during treatment.

Methotrexate is a known teratogen and a known abortifacient and thus is contraindicated during pregnancy. In addition, methotrexate may be toxic to sperm [66, 67]. For these reasons, it has been recommended to stop methotrexate at least 3 months before planned pregnancy in both men and women and not to use methotrexate during pregnancy or breast-feeding.

Once treatment with methotrexate has started, laboratory controls should be performed to evaluate for pancytopenia and hepatotoxicity. Pancytopenia is uncommon and there have not been severe episodes in studies with methotrexate [50, 68]. Nevertheless, this complication has been reported and can be life threatening [69]. A full blood count and a liver test should be obtained monthly for the first 2 months and every 2–3 months for the duration of the therapy.

## Conclusions

Azathioprine and mercaptopurine are effective in maintaining remission in UC, at least as effective as for Crohn's disease. The efficacy of thiopurines in UC patients remains in long-term treatment, and withdrawal of the drug in patients who were in remission is associated with a high risk of relapse. Therefore, in the same sense as in transplanted patients, thiopurine therapy should probably be indefinitely maintained once remission is reached in IBD patients. With respect to methotrexate, there is currently insufficient evidence to recommend its use for UC.

**Acknowledgment** CIBERehd is funded by the Instituto de Salud Carlos III.

## References

1. Sandborn WJ. Current directions in IBD therapy: what goals are feasible with biological modifiers? Gastroenterology. 2008;135(5): 1442–7.
2. Nielsen OH, Vainer B, Rask-Madsen J. Review article: the treatment of inflammatory bowel disease with 6-mercaptopurine or azathioprine. Aliment Pharmacol Ther. 2001;15(11):1699–708.
3. Gisbert JP, Gomollon F, Mate J, Pajares JM. [Individualized therapy with azathioprine or 6-mercaptopurine by monitoring thiopurine methyl-transferase (TPMT) activity]. Rev Clin Esp. 2002;202(10):555–62.
4. Siegel CA, Sands BE. Review article: practical management of inflammatory bowel disease patients taking immunomodulators. Aliment Pharmacol Ther. 2005;22(1):1–16.
5. Travis SP, Stange EF, Lemann M, Oresland T, Bemelman WA, Chowers Y, et al. European evidence-based Consensus on the management of ulcerative colitis: Current management. J Crohns Colitis. 2008;2(1):24–62.
6. Gisbert JP, Gomollon F, Mate J, Pajares JM. [Questions and answers on the role of azathioprine and 6-mercaptopurine in the treatment of inflammatory bowel disease]. Gastroenterol Hepatol. 2002;25(6): 401–15.
7. Prefontaine E, Sutherland LR, Macdonald JK, Cepoiu M. Azathioprine or 6-mercaptopurine for maintenance of remission in Crohn's disease. Cochrane Database Syst Rev. 2009;1, CD000067.
8. Jewell DP, Truelove SC. Azathioprine in ulcerative colitis: final report on controlled therapeutic trial. Br Med J. 1974;4(5945):627–30.
9. Caprilli R, Carratu R, Babbini M. Double-blind comparison of the effectiveness of azathioprine and sulfasalazine in idiopathic proctocolitis. Preliminary report. Am J Dig Dis. 1975;20(2):115–20.
10. Gisbert JP, Linares PM, McNicholl AG, Mate J, Gomollon F. Meta-analysis: the efficacy of azathioprine and mercaptopurine in ulcerative colitis. Aliment Pharmacol Ther. 2009;30(2):126–37.
11. Khan KJ, Dubinsky MC, Ford AC, Ullman TA, Talley NJ, Moayyedi P. Efficacy of immunosuppressive therapy for inflammatory bowel disease: a systematic review and meta-analysis. Am J Gastroenterol. 2012;106(4):630–42.
12. Sood A, Midha V, Sood N, Kaushal V. Role of azathioprine in severe ulcerative colitis: one-year, placebo-controlled, randomized trial. Indian J Gastroenterol. 2000;19(1):14–6.
13. Sood A, Kaushal V, Midha V, Bhatia KL, Sood N, Malhotra V. The beneficial effect of azathioprine on maintenance of remission in severe ulcerative colitis. J Gastroenterol. 2002;37(4):270–4.
14. Timer AL, Mcdonald JW, Tsoulis DJ, Macdonald JK. Azathioprine and 6-mercaptopurine for maintenance of remission in ulcerative colitis. Cochrane Database Syst Rev. 2012;9:CD000478. doi:10.1002/14651858.CD000478.pub3.
15. Kull E, Beau P. [Compared azathioprine efficacy in ulcerative colitis and in Crohn's disease]. Gastroenterol Clin Biol. 2002;26(4):367–71.
16. Verhave M, Winter HS, Grand RJ. Azathioprine in the treatment of children with inflammatory bowel disease. J Pediatr. 1990;117(5): 809–14.
17. Fraser AG, Orchard TR, Jewell DP. The efficacy of azathioprine for the treatment of inflammatory bowel disease: a 30 year review. Gut. 2002;50(4):485–9.

18. Bastida G, Nos Mateu P, Aguas Peris M, Beltrán Niclós B, Rodríguez Soler M, Ponce GJ. Optimization of immunomodulatory treatment with azathioprine or 6-mercaptopurine in inflammatory bowel disease. Gastroenterol Hepatol. 2007;30:511–6.

19. Gisbert JP, Nino P, Cara C, Rodrigo L. Comparative effectiveness of azathioprine in Crohn's disease and ulcerative colitis: prospective, long-term, follow-up study of 394 patients. Aliment Pharmacol Ther. 2008;28(2):228–38.

20. Gisbert JP, Gomollon F. Thiopurine-induced myelotoxicity in patients with inflammatory bowel disease: a review. Am J Gastroenterol. 2008;103(7):1783–800.

21. Gisbert JP, Gonzalez-Lama Y, Mate J. Thiopurine-induced liver injury in patients with inflammatory bowel disease: a systematic review. Am J Gastroenterol. 2007;102(7):1518–27.

22. Masunaga Y, Ohno K, Ogawa R, Hashiguchi M, Echizen H, Ogata H. Meta-analysis of risk of malignancy with immunosuppressive drugs in inflammatory bowel disease. Ann Pharmacother. 2007; 41(1):21–8.

23. Kandiel A, Fraser AG, Korelitz BI, Brensinger C, Lewis JD. Increased risk of lymphoma among inflammatory bowel disease patients treated with azathioprine and 6-mercaptopurine. Gut. 2005;54(8):1121–5.

24. Beaugerie L, Brousse N, Bouvier AM, Colombel JF, Lemann M, Cosnes J, et al. Lymphoproliferative disorders in patients receiving thiopurines for inflammatory bowel disease: a prospective observational cohort study. Lancet. 2009;374(9701):1617–25.

25. Kotlyar DS, Lewis JD, Beaugerie L, Tierney A, Brensinger CM, Gisbert JP, Loftus EV Jr, Peyrin-Biroulet L, Blonski WC, Van Domselaar M, Chaparro M, Sandilya S, Bewtra M, Beigel F, Biancone L, Lichtenstein GR. Risk of lymphoma in patients with inflammatory bowel disease treated with azathioprine and 6-mercaptopurine: a meta-analysis. Clin Gastroenterol Hepatol. 2014. pii: S1542-3565(14)00767-8. doi: 10.1016/j.cgh.2014.05.015. (Epub ahead of print).

26. van Schaik FD, van Oijen MG, Smeets HM, van der Heijden GJ, Siersema PD, Oldenburg B. Thiopurines prevent advanced colorectal neoplasia in patients with inflammatory bowel disease. Gut. 2012;61(2):235–40.

27. Peyrin-Biroulet L, Khosrotehrani K, Carrat F, Bouvier AM, Chevaux JB, Simon T, et al. Increased risk for nonmelanoma skin cancers in patients who receive thiopurines for inflammatory bowel disease. Gastroenterology. 2011;141(5):1621–28 e1-5.

28. Singh H, Nugent Z, Demers AA, Bernstein CN. Increased risk of nonmelanoma skin cancers among individuals with inflammatory bowel disease. Gastroenterology. 2011;141(5):1612–20.

29. Ariyaratnam J, Subramanian V. Association between thiopurine use and nonmelanoma skin cancers in patients with inflammatory bowel disease: a meta-analysis. Am J Gastroenterol. 2014;109(2):163–9. doi:10.1038/ajg.2013.451.. Epub 2014 Jan 14. Review.

30. Vuchetich JP, Weinshilboum RM, Price RA. Segregation analysis of human red blood cell thiopurine methyltransferase activity. Genet Epidemiol. 1995;12(1):1–11.

31. Gisbert JP, Gomollon F, Cara C, Luna M, Gonzalez-Lama Y, Pajares JM, et al. Thiopurine methyltransferase activity in Spain: a study of 14,545 patients. Dig Dis Sci. 2007;52(5):1262–9.

32. Sandborn WJ. State-of-the-art: immunosuppression and biologic therapy. Dig Dis. 2010;28(3):536–42.

33. Winter J, Walker A, Shapiro D, Gaffney D, Spooner RJ, Mills PR. Cost-effectiveness of thiopurine methyltransferase genotype screening in patients about to commence azathioprine therapy for treatment of inflammatory bowel disease. Aliment Pharmacol Ther. 2004;20(6):593–9.

34. Dubinsky MC, Lamothe S, Yang HY, Targan SR, Sinnett D, Theoret Y, et al. Pharmacogenomics and metabolite measurement for 6-mercaptopurine therapy in inflammatory bowel disease. Gastroenterology. 2000;118(4):705–13.

35. Osterman MT, Kundu R, Lichtenstein GR, Lewis JD. Association of 6-thioguanine nucleotide levels and inflammatory bowel disease activity: a meta-analysis. Gastroenterology. 2006;130(4):1047–53.

36. Gisbert JP, Gonzalez-Lama Y, Mate J. [Monitoring of thiopurine methyltransferase and thiopurine metabolites to optimize azathioprine therapy in inflammatory bowel disease]. Gastroenterol Hepatol. 2006;29(9):568–83.

37. Dubinsky MC, Reyes E, Ofman J, Chiou CF, Wade S, Sandborn WJ. A cost-effectiveness analysis of alternative disease management strategies in patients with Crohn's disease treated with azathioprine or 6-mercaptopurine. Am J Gastroenterol. 2005;100(10): 2239–47.

38. Lowry PW, Franklin CL, Weaver AL, Pike MG, Mays DC, Tremaine WJ, et al. Measurement of thiopurine methyltransferase activity and azathioprine metabolites in patients with inflammatory bowel disease. Gut. 2001;49(5):665–70.

39. Reuther LO, Sonne J, Larsen NE, Larsen B, Christensen S, Rasmussen SN, et al. Pharmacological monitoring of azathioprine therapy. Scand J Gastroenterol. 2003;38(9):972–7.

40. Gonzalez-Lama Y, Bermejo F, Lopez-Sanroman A, Garcia-Sanchez V, Esteve M, Cabriada JL, et al. Thiopurine methyl-transferase activity and azathioprine metabolite concentrations do not predict clinical outcome in thiopurine-treated inflammatory bowel disease patients. Aliment Pharmacol Ther. 2011;34(5):544–54.

41. Gisbert J, Chaparro M, Gomollón F. Common misconceptions about 5-aminosalicylates and thiopurines in inflammatory bowel disease. World J Gastroenterol. 2011;17:3467–78.

42. Holtmann MH, Krummenauer F, Claas C, Kremeyer K, Lorenz D, Rainer O, et al. Long-term effectiveness of azathioprine in IBD beyond 4 years: a European multicenter study in 1176 patients. Dig Dis Sci. 2006;51(9):1516–24.

43. Chebli LA, Chaves LD, Pimentel FF, Guerra DM, Barros RM, Gaburri PD, et al. Azathioprine maintains long-term steroid-free remission through 3 years in patients with steroid-dependent ulcerative colitis. Inflamm Bowel Dis. 2010;16(4):613–9.

44. Hawthorne AB, Logan RF, Hawkey CJ, Foster PN, Axon AT, Swarbrick ET, et al. Randomised controlled trial of azathioprine withdrawal in ulcerative colitis. BMJ. 1992;305(6844):20–2.

45. Cassinotti A, Actis GC, Duca P, Massari A, Colombo E, Gai E, et al. Maintenance treatment with azathioprine in ulcerative colitis: outcome and predictive factors after drug withdrawal. Am J Gastroenterol. 2009;104(11):2760–7.

46. Feagan BG, Alfadhli A. Methotrexate in inflammatory bowel disease. Gastroenterol Clin North Am. 2004;33(2):407–20 xi.

47. Herfarth HH, Osterman MT, Isaacs KL, Lewis JD, Sands BE. Efficacy of methotrexate in ulcerative colitis: failure or promise. Inflamm Bowel Dis. 2010;16(8):1421–30.

48. Kurnik D, Loebstein R, Fishbein E, Almog S, Halkin H, Bar-Meir S, et al. Bioavailability of oral vs subcutaneous low-dose methotrexate in patients with Crohn's disease. Aliment Pharmacol Ther. 2003;18(1):57–63.

49. Aberra FN, Lichtenstein GR. Review article: monitoring of immunomodulators in inflammatory bowel disease. Aliment Pharmacol Ther. 2005;21(4):307–19.

50. Feagan BG, Fedorak RN, Irvine EJ, Wild G, Sutherland L, Steinhart AH, et al. A comparison of methotrexate with placebo for the maintenance of remission in Crohn's disease. North American Crohn's Study Group Investigators. N Engl J Med. 2000;342(22):1627–32.

51. Kozarek RA, Patterson DJ, Gelfand MD, Botoman VA, Ball TJ, Wilske KR. Methotrexate induces clinical and histologic remission in patients with refractory inflammatory bowel disease. Ann Intern Med. 1989;110(5):353–6.

52. Oren R, Arber N, Odes S, Moshkowitz M, Keter D, Pomeranz I, et al. Methotrexate in chronic active ulcerative colitis: a double-blind, randomized, Israeli multicenter trial. Gastroenterology. 1996;110(5):1416–21.

53. Mate-Jimenez J, Hermida C, Cantero-Perona J, Moreno-Otero R. 6-mercaptopurine or methotrexate added to prednisone induces and maintains remission in steroid-dependent inflammatory bowel disease. Eur J Gastroenterol Hepatol. 2000;12(11):1227–33.

54. Egan LJ, Sandborn WJ, Tremaine WJ, Leighton JA, Mays DC, Pike MG, et al. A randomized dose-response and pharmacokinetic study of methotrexate for refractory inflammatory Crohn's disease and ulcerative colitis. Aliment Pharmacol Ther. 1999;13(12):1597–604.

55. Paoluzi OA, Pica R, Marcheggiano A, Crispino P, Iacopini F, Iannoni C, et al. Azathioprine or methotrexate in the treatment of patients with steroid-dependent or steroid-resistant ulcerative colitis: results of an open-label study on efficacy and tolerability in inducing and maintaining remission. Aliment Pharmacol Ther. 2002;16(10):1751–9.

56. Fraser AG, Morton D, McGovern D, Travis S, Jewell DP. The efficacy of methotrexate for maintaining remission in inflammatory bowel disease. Aliment Pharmacol Ther. 2002;16(4):693–7.

57. Siveke JT, Folwaczny C. Methotrexate in ulcerative colitis. Aliment Pharmacol Ther. 2003;17(3):479–80.

58. Manosa M, Garcia V, Castro L, Garcia-Bosch O, Chaparro M, Barreiro-de Acosta M, et al. Methotrexate in ulcerative colitis: a Spanish multicentric study on clinical use and efficacy. J Crohns Colitis. 2011;5(5):397–401.

59. Cummings JR, Herrlinger KR, Travis SP, Gorard DA, McIntyre AS, Jewell DP. Oral methotrexate in ulcerative colitis. Aliment Pharmacol Ther. 2005;21(4):385–9.

60. Barbero-Villares A, Mendoza J, Trapero-Marugan M, Gonzalez-Alvaro I, Dauden E, Gisbert JP, et al. Evaluation of liver fibrosis by transient elastography in methotrexate treated patients. Med Clin (Barc). 2011;137(14):637–9.

61. Barbero-Villares A, Mendoza J, Taxonera C, López-Sanromán A, Pajares R, Bermejo F, et al. Evaluation of liver fibrosis by transient elastography (Fibroscan) in patients with inflammatory bowel disease treated with methotrexate: a multicentric trial. Scand J Gastroenterol. 2012;47(5):575–9.

62. Malatjalian DA, Ross JB, Williams CN, Colwell SJ, Eastwood BJ. Methotrexate hepatotoxicity in psoriatics: report of 104 patients from Nova Scotia, with analysis of risks from obesity, diabetes and alcohol consumption during long term follow-up. Can J Gastroenterol. 1996;10(6):369–75.

63. Te HS, Schiano TD, Kuan SF, Hanauer SB, Conjeevaram HS, Baker AL. Hepatic effects of long-term methotrexate use in the treatment of inflammatory bowel disease. Am J Gastroenterol. 2000;95(11):3150–6.

64. Alarcon GS, Kremer JM, Macaluso M, Weinblatt ME, Cannon GW, Palmer WR, et al. Risk factors for methotrexate-induced lung injury in patients with rheumatoid arthritis. A multicenter, case-control study. Methotrexate-Lung Study Group. Ann Intern Med. 1997;127(5):356–64.

65. Bohon P, Dugernier T, Debongnie JC, Pirenne B. [Hypersensitivity interstitial pneumopathy and ulcero-hemorrhagic rectocolitis: role of methotrexate]. Acta Gastroenterol Belg. 1993;56(5–6):352–7.

66. Sussman A, Leonard JM. Psoriasis, methotrexate, and oligospermia. Arch Dermatol. 1980;116(2):215–7.

67. Morris LF, Harrod MJ, Menter MA, Silverman AK. Methotrexate and reproduction in men: case report and recommendations. J Am Acad Dermatol. 1993;29(5 Pt 2):913–6.

68. Feagan BG, Rochon J, Fedorak RN, Irvine EJ, Wild G, Sutherland L, et al. Methotrexate for the treatment of Crohn's disease. The North American Crohn's Study Group Investigators. N Engl J Med. 1995;332(5):292–7.

69. al-Awadhi A, Dale P, McKendry RJ. Pancytopenia associated with low dose methotrexate therapy. A regional survey. J Rheumatol. 1993;20(7):1121–5.

# Azathioprine/6-Mercaptopurine Metabolism in Ulcerative Colitis: A Guide to Metabolite Assessment—An Evidence-Based Approach

Carmen Cuffari

**Keywords**

Azathioprine • 6-Mercaptopurine metabolism • Ulcerative colitis • Metabolite assessment • Evidence-based

## Introduction (Box 12.1)

Ulcerative colitis (UC) and Crohn's disease are chronic relapsing idiopathic inflammatory bowel disorders affecting over 1.7 million individuals in North America; about half have unremitting disease with symptoms of abdominal pain and diarrhea that impact patient's quality of life and work-related productivity [1, 2]. It stands to reason that the major goal of therapy for physicians caring for patients with inflammatory bowel disease (IBD) is to achieve and sustain a long-term disease remission with effective evidence-based corticosteroid-sparing therapeutic approaches that minimize the risk of drug-related toxicity.

Although 6-mercaptopurine (6-MP) and its prodrug azathioprine (AZA) have proven efficacy in the treatment of UC, the interpretation of clinical studies is often complicated by the heterogeneous nature of this bowel disorder [3] and the inter-investigator variability in the therapeutic end points used in monitoring clinical responsiveness to treatment. Over the last half century, a number of scoring systems have been developed to measure disease activity in patients with UC [4]. Most of these systems are based on a combination of clinical symptoms and endoscopic findings that are difficult to validate because of the myriad of symptoms overlapping with disease behavior [5]. Furthermore, the importance of tissue healing has become clinically relevant in light of recent reports correlating disease activity with a patient's

overall risk of disease relapse and colorectal cancer [6]. Indeed, mucosal healing has now become an important predictor of clinical outcome, to the extent that all future-controlled clinical trials must now establish stringent primary end points of disease remission to include tissue healing in assessing treatment efficacy [4].

With the advent of pharmacogenomics and 6-MP metabolite monitoring in clinical practice, gastroenterologists have also found discordance between antimetabolite levels and their own assessment of disease activity [7–9]. The recent purported mucosal healing effect on AZA therapy in patients with UC [10] may require that clinicians redefine the therapeutic window of treatment efficacy based on the measurement of these antimetabolite levels. This review focuses on the role of antimetabolite therapy in sustaining long-term remission in patients with UC, as well as providing a guide on how to apply pharmacogenomics and metabolite monitoring in clinical practice based on a review of the literature.

## Pharmacogenetics of 6-Mercaptopurine

Pharmacogenomics deals with the influence of genetic variation on drug response by correlating gene expression with a drug's efficacy or toxicity. Although the terms pharmacogenomics and pharmacogenetics tend to be used interchangeably, pharmacogenetics is generally regarded as the study or clinical testing of genetic variation that gives rise to differing responses to drugs, as it applies to either a single or at most a few gene polymorphisms.

Over the last 20 years, much has been learned about the pharmacogenetics of AZA and 6-MP metabolism in the clinical management of patients with leukemia and in

C. Cuffari, M.D. (✉)
Department of Pediatrics, Division of Pediatric Gastroenterology and Nutrition, The Johns Hopkins University School of Medicine, 600N. Wolfe St. CMSC 2-123, Baltimore 21287, MD, USA
e-mail: ccuffari@jhmi.edu

G.R. Lichtenstein (ed.), *Medical Therapy of Ulcerative Colitis*, DOI 10.1007/978-1-4939-1677-1_12, © Springer Science+Business Media New York 2014

**Fig. 12.1** Azathioprine (AZA) metabolism. *XO* xanthine oxidase, *6-TU* 6-thiouric acid, and *6-TIMP* 6-thioinosine monophosphate

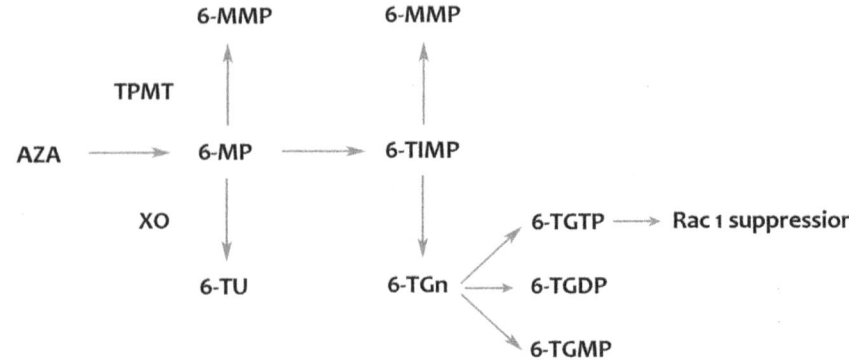

IBD. Although most of our understanding has focused on the polymorphisms of thiopurine methyltransferase (TPMT) enzyme activity, recent studies have now also introduced potential polymorphisms in intracellular antimetabolite transport that influences clinical response despite presumed therapeutic drug dosing and metabolite levels [11].

Once absorbed into the plasma, AZA is rapidly converted to 6-MP by a nonenzymatic reaction. 6-MP is then taken up by a variety of actively replicating cells and tissues, including erythrocytes, T- and B-cell lymphocytes, as well as the bone marrow. The uptake of 6-MP is believed to be a rapid process. Once inside the cell, the metabolism of 6-MP occurs intracellularly along the competing routes catalyzed by hypoxanthine phosphoribosyltransferase and thiopurine S-methyltransferase (TPMT), giving rise to 6-thioguanine nucleotides (6-TGn) and 6-methyl-mercaptopurine (6-MMP), respectively (Fig. 12.1) [12]. 6-TGN is the active ribonucleotide of 6-MP that functions as a purine antagonist inducing lymphocytotoxicity and immunosuppression [13–15].

An apparent genetic polymorphism has been observed in TPMT activity in both the Caucasian and African-American population. Negligible activity is noted in 0.3 % of individuals and low levels (<5 U/mL of blood) in 11 % of individuals. TPMT enzyme deficiency is inherited as an autosomal recessive trait, and to date, 10 mutant alleles and several silent and intronic mutations have been described. In patients with the heterozygous TPMT genotype, 6-MP metabolism is shunted preferentially into the production of 6-TG nucleotides. Although 6-TG nucleotides are thought to be lymphocytotoxic and beneficial in the treatment of patients with leukemia and lymphoma, patients with low (<5) TPMT activity are at risk for bone marrow suppression by achieving potentially toxic erythrocyte 6-TGN levels on standard doses of 6-MP [16]. Despite low TPMT enzyme activity levels, presumed therapeutic erythrocyte 6-TGN metabolite levels can still be achieved without untoward cytotoxicity by lowering the dose of 6-MP 10- to 15-fold [17].

6-TGNs are active ribonucleotides that collectively function as purine antagonists, incorporating into DNA, thereby interfering with the ribonucleotide replication. Recent studies have also shown that one of these 6-TGN ribonucleotides, 6-TGTP, induces the apoptosis of both peripheral blood and intestinal lamina propria T-cell lymphocytes through the inhibition of Rac1, a GTPase that inhibits apoptosis. The specific blockade of CD28-dependent Rac1 activation by 6-TGTP is the proposed molecular target of 6-MP and its prodrug AZA (Fig. 12.1) [18].

The intracellular buildup of this specific 6-TGN metabolite may also be dependent on others, as yet undefined inherent genetic polymorphisms. Our recent studies have also proposed that there may also exist pharmacogenetic differences in the intracellular transport of 6-MP in peripheral blood lymphocytes that could potentially affect responsiveness to antimetabolite therapy. Our studies have shown an inherent variability in the transport of 6-MP in immortalized lymphocytes derived from patients with IBD. In these studies, seven inward and eight outward transporters were tested. One patient demonstrated the least amount of intracellular transport of 6-MP that correlated with the lowest susceptibility to 6-MP cytotoxicity. In this particular patient, multiple inward transporters, including the concentrative nucleoside transporters CNT-1, CNT-3, and the equilibrative nucleoside transporters ENT-3 and ENT-4 were notably low in expression. In comparison, a second patient exhibited robust 6-MP transport, an increased susceptibility to 6-MP cytotoxicity, and an increased expression of all influx transporters (except CNT-1), and equilibrative transporter ENT-4. Although no single transporter was either under- or overexpressed to explain these patterns of 6-MP transport, a correlation was shown between intracellular drug levels and the in vitro susceptibility to 6-MP-induced cytotoxicity. Interestingly, these differences were independent of 6-MP dose or erythrocyte 6-MP metabolite levels that were monitored clinically. Ongoing studies will also attempt to correlate these differences in drug transport with clinical responsiveness to antimetabolite therapy and drug metabolite levels. Identification of such transporters prior to initiating therapy may allow physicians to tailor therapy more effectively in patients with steroid-dependent IBD [11].

## Clinical Application of Metabolite Testing

In patients with UC, the aim is to optimize antimetabolite therapy early in the course of the disease in order to minimize the overall risk for disease progression. The factor with the most significant direct correlation with disease progression is severity of colitis early in the course of the illness [5]. In a large population-based cohort study, patients with severe active UC were 14.8 times more likely to have disease progression compared to patients without severe colitis. Patients with left-sided colitis at diagnosis are 2.5 times more likely to progress to extensive colitis than patients with isolated proctitis progressing to either extensive colitis or left-sided disease [19]. Although disease progression can occur in patients of all age groups, most children will present clinically with extensive colitis at diagnosis, while those children presenting with either proctosigmoiditis or left-sided disease will rapidly progress to pancolitis within 6 years of the diagnosis [20]. In general, pediatricians regard ulcerative colitis as a rapidly progressive disease in children, with an associated increased likelihood of requiring proctocolectomy. The rapid induction and maintenance of disease remission remain the primary goal therapy in patients with UC. Using a Markov model, there is an 80–90 % probability that a patient with clinically inactive disease would remain in remission for a year, with a 20 % chance of relapse in the following year. By contrast, data from patients with clinically active disease demonstrate a 70 % probability of having a relapse during the year following diagnosis [21]. The same results were shown within the post hoc analysis of the combined ACT I and ACT II data among the infliximab-treated patients. Interestingly, mucosal healing was the primary end point of long-term remission in those studies [22]. The importance of tissue healing was also underscored by Froslie and coworkers. In that study, patients with UC that achieved tissue healing at 1 year were less likely to require colectomy in the subsequent 5-year follow-up period [23].

Although 6-MP and AZA have clinical efficacy in maintaining disease remission in patients with UC, the wide therapeutic dosing range used in clinical practice today would suggest that pharmacokinetic differences in drug metabolism may also influence responsiveness to therapy. Moreover, a true separation between immunosuppression and cytotoxicity has yet to be defined since the dosing of 6-MP and azathioprine has been based largely on clinical outcome. Indeed, the wide range in azathioprine dose used in clinical practice would suggest that a safe and established therapeutic dose has yet to be determined. The situation is further complicated with recent evidence that would suggest that mucosal healing of the affected bowel decreases the risk of disease relapse and progression.

**Table 12.1** Clinical responsiveness to 6-MP and AZA therapy based on threshold (235–250[a]) erythrocyte 6-TGN metabolite levels

| Study | Patients (response) | 6-TGN response threshold | | Odds ratio |
| --- | --- | --- | --- | --- |
| | | Above | Below | |
| Dubinsky [26] | 92 (30) | 0.78 | 0.40 | 5.0 |
| Gupta [27] | 101 (47) | 0.56 | 0.43 | 1.7 |
| Belaiche [28] | 28 (19) | 0.75 | 0.65 | 1.6 |
| Cuffari [7] | 82 (47) | 0.86 | 0.35 | 11.6 |
| Achkar [8] | 60 (24) | 0.51 | 0.22 | 3.8 |
| Lowry [9] | 170 (114) | 0.64 | 0.68 | 0.9 |
| Goldenberg [29] | 74 (14) | 0.24 | 0.18 | 1.5 |

[a]pmoles/8 $\times$ 10$^8$ RBCs

Conventional dosing strategies must now be redefined based on these new end points of clinical remission that includes mucosal healing. Nevertheless, immunosuppression is not without its risk. The clinician must always remain aware of potential adverse effects, including allergic reactions, hepatitis, pancreatitis, bone marrow suppression, and lymphoma while attempting to achieve an optimal therapeutic response irrespective on how the physician chooses to define it clinically [24, 25].

The measurement of erythrocyte 6-TG and 6-MMP metabolite levels by means of high-pressure liquid chromatography (HPLC) has now become a useful clinical tool for documenting patients' compliance to therapy. In our preliminary study, erythrocyte 6-TG metabolite levels showed a strong inverse correlation with disease activity, where the lack of clinical response was clearly associated with low (<50) erythrocyte 6-TGN metabolite levels. To date, a number of studies in both the pediatric and adult literature have supported the notion of therapeutic drug monitoring in patients with IBD. However, a uniform consensus has not yet been reached on account of the absence of well-controlled clinical trials (Table 12.1) [7–9, 26–29]. Although a meta-analysis by Osterman and colleagues has shown that higher metabolite levels correlated with a more favorable clinical response, no clearly defined therapeutic window of efficacy and toxicity has been established based on 6-MP metabolite levels [30]. Since mucosal healing has now become the salient end point for clinical remission, metabolite testing should now be considered just as a guide to therapy. The notion of using the existing threshold 6-TGN metabolite levels would seem antiquated. At present, the existing technology should only be used in identifying pharmacogenomic differences in drug metabolism, monitoring patient compliance with antimetabolite therapy, and avoiding excessive immunosuppression in patient with recalcitrant disease, high (>400) 6-TGN levels, and normal white blood cell counts.

## TPMT Testing

### Low and Intermediate (<5 U/mL Blood) TPMT

Eleven percent of the population is considered heterozygous carriers of the TPMT-deficient allele and potentially at risk for drug-induced leukopenia. In the patient who is homozygous recessive with absent TPMT enzyme activity, there is the added risk of severe, irreversible bone marrow suppression. Since then, there have been a number of similar cases of irreversible bone marrow suppression both in patients with IBD on maintenance azathioprine therapy and in patients with leukemia on standard doses of 6-MP. It remains the author's opinion that these patients should not be considered candidates for antimetabolite therapy.

A number of secondary malignancies, including acute myelogenous leukemia and brain tumors, have been insinuated to be related to the use of maintenance 6-MP therapy in patients with leukemia and the heterozygous TPMT genotype. Although 6-TG and 6-MMP metabolites were not measured in these patients, it may be assumed that these patients were potentially exposed to high-maintenance 6-TG metabolite levels despite presumed therapeutic 6-MP dosing and were thus overly immunosuppressed.

In IBD, Black and coworkers showed that patients with Crohn's disease and a "mutant" TPMT allele also incurred significant drug-induced leukopenia on standard doses of azathioprine therapy and were compelled to discontinue treatment. In contrast, patients with the wild-type allele achieved a good clinical response while on azathioprine therapy without untoward cytotoxicity [31]. This study and others would suggest that all patients with the heterozygous allele are at an increased risk for drug toxicity and should not be prescribed azathioprine or 6-MP therapy. However, this would exclude 11 % of the population who could potentially benefit from 6-MP therapy. It has been shown in prospective open-label clinical trials that by identifying these patients prior to initiating AZA therapy and adopting a moderate dosing strategy (6-MP, 0.5–1 mg/kg/day; AZA, 1–1.5 mg/kg/day), most patients may achieve a favorable clinical response while avoiding potential bone marrow suppression. It remains the author's opinion that these patients be monitored carefully with serial CBCs.

### High (>16 U/mL Blood) TPMT

The genetic polymorphism in TPMT activity observed in the general population may also have far-reaching implications regarding patient responsiveness to therapy and clinical response time. Twenty percent of the population is considered to be rapid (>16) metabolizers of 6-MP and AZA and in

theory would require larger than the standard doses of drug in order to achieve any therapeutic drug benefit [21]. In these patients, 6-MP metabolism is shunted away from 6-TGN production and into the formation of 6-MMP (Fig. 12.1). In patients with leukemia, high TPMT activity is associated with an increased risk for disease recurrence [17].

In a prospective open-label study in adults, just 20 % of patients with either UC or Crohn's disease and erythrocyte TPMT levels >16 U/mL of blood responded to AZA therapy despite therapeutic drug dosing (2 mg/kg/day). In comparison, 30 % of patients with TPMT levels between 12 and 16 U/mL blood responded to therapy. These were also more likely to require higher dosages (2 mg/kg/day) of AZA from the outset in order to optimize their erythrocyte 6-TGN metabolite levels [21].

In comparison, patients with TPMT activity levels ≤12 U/mL blood achieved high (>250) mean erythrocyte 6-TG levels after 16 weeks of induction AZA. This occurred even though both groups received a similar dosage of AZA. In this patient population, 69 % of patients achieved a favorable clinical response with presumed therapeutic erythrocyte 6-TGN metabolite levels after 4 months of continuous AZA therapy [21].

High hepatic TPMT activity may draw most of the 6-MP from the plasma, thereby limiting the amount of substrate available for the bone marrow and peripheral leukocytes. This concept of rapid AZA metabolism interfering with therapeutic response could explain the low response rate in a controlled clinical trial in Crohn's disease that compared high-dose oral (2 mg/kg/day) azathioprine therapy with and without initiating a short course of high-dose intravenous (1.6 g/36 h infusion) AZA therapy. That study was confined to individuals with upper normal or high levels of TPMT enzyme activity so that the intravenous azathioprine treatment group could be studied safely. Even at 2 mg/kg/day of oral azathioprine therapy, only 20 % of these rapid metabolizers in both groups achieved clinical remission, a clinical response that is lower than that reported in most consecutive patient publications [32].

Furthermore, high (>15) erythrocyte TPMT levels may also explain the rather low clinical response noted in the AZA treatment arm of the SONIC trials. In that study, despite optimized induction dosages (2.5 mg/kg/day) of AZA, just 30 % of patients responded to therapy [33], a clinical response that is lower than what has been generally concluded from the Cochrane meta-analyses of AZA therapy in treating patients with IBD [34].

## Clinical Application of TPMT Testing

Most physicians will monitor CBC and serum aminotransferases monthly during the first 3 months of initiating therapy. Although TPMT measurement has been shown to predict leukopenia in up to 20 % of patients, TPMT monitoring may be used clinically to increase the level of physician comfort in prescribing antimetabolite therapy, in general, and in minimizing the perceived need for monitoring CBC, and for dose titration, all of which may increase clinical response time.

For example, knowing the TPMT status in a patient may aid the physician in utilizing a variable AZA dosing strategy in patients with IBD. Patients with absent TPMT should not receive AZA therapy. Those with very low (<5) TPMT activity can be effectively treated with 1.0–1.5 mg/kg/day of AZA while monitoring CBC and erythrocyte 6-TG levels. Patients with TPMT activity between 5 and 12 U/mL blood have an increased likelihood of responding to a more moderate dosing strategy, such as 1.5–2.0 mg/kg/day. In patients with above average (>12) TPMT activity, AZA therapy may have to be started at 2.0 mg/kg/day in order to achieve a favorable clinical response. However, higher dosages, such as 2.5 mg/kg/day, may be needed for those with very high (>16) TPMT enzyme activity. Physicians must be cognizant of the potential refractoriness to antimetabolite therapy among those patients with high TPMT enzyme activity despite presumed therapeutic drug dosing. It remains the author's opinion that although empiric drug dosing remains an acceptable standard of care based on TPMT genetic polymorphisms, the clinician must be sensitive to potential phenotypic differences in TPMT activity that may influence responsiveness and or toxicity to antimetabolite therapy. Among those patients with either recalcitrant disease or drug-induced toxicity, the measurement of erythrocyte 6-MP metabolites may facilitate a more cogent clinician response to therapy (Textbox).

---

**Box 12.1: Key Summary**
1. Measure TPMT genotype/phenotype prior to initiating anti-metabolite therapy;
2. TPMT:
   (a) homozygous recessive—consider an alternate therapy;
   (b) heterozygous—consider 1.0–1.5 mg/kg/day of AZA;
   (c) homozygous dominant—consider 2.0–2.5 mg/kg/day of AZA;
3. Follow CBC q2weeks ×2, then q4weeks ×2, then with each follow-up;
4. If after 2 months patient remains either steroid dependent or has a disease exacerbation, check 6-TGn/6MMP metabolites (please see Table 12.2);

(continued)

---

5. Toxicity:
   (a) Pancreatitis—discontinue anti-metabolite therapy (idiosyncratic reaction to anti-metabolites);
   (b) Hepatitis (ALT>3×N)—if 6-MMP/6-TGn ratio > 1/50 lower dose of AZA by 25 mg/day and repeat ALT in 2 weeks;
   (c) Leukopenia: high 6-TGn (>250)—consider lowering dose of AZA by 25 mg/day and repeat WBC in 2 weeks.

*Disclaimer: This is a suggestion by the author and has not been assessed in prospective randomized placebo-controlled trials.*

---

**Table 12.2** Metabolite profiles, clinical impression, and therapeutic decision

| Group A | Absent/very low (<50) 6-TGN absent 6-MMP | Nonadherence | Patient education |
|---|---|---|---|
| Group B | Low (<250) 6-TGN Low (<2,500) 6-MMP | Sub-therapeutic dose | Dose titration |
| Group C | Low (<250) 6-TGN High (>5,700) 6-MMP | Rapid metabolizer | Switch therapy vs allopurinol |
| Group D | High (>400) 6-TGN High (>5,700) 6-MMP | Thiopurine resistant | Switch therapy |

While TPMT testing may guide the physician's initial dosing practices, metabolite testing will allow them to clinically respond to patient's refractoriness to therapy despite presumed therapeutic dosing (Table 12.2). Patients that are clearly noncompliant (Group A) with low metabolite (6TGN, 6-MMP) levels should be educated and have the need for improved adherence to the therapy reinforced. Patients that are nonresponding and clearly sub-therapeutic (Group B) should have their dose of AZA titrated to improve overall clinical response. Previous studies have shown this approach to be highly effective in improving overall clinical response while avoiding unnecessary toxicity. In a study of 25 adult patients refractory to AZA and low (<250) erythrocyte 6-TGN metabolite levels, 18 were pushed into clinical remission by having their dose of AZA increased by 25 mg/day [21]. Among patients that are deemed rapid metabolizer (Group C), the possibility of changing the pharmacokinetics through the addition of allopurinol may be considered. However, the physician will need to be aware of the potential risk of toxicity [35]. It remains the author's opinion that this therapeutic approach be restricted to tertiary care centers experienced with this approach and accessible to metabolite monitoring. Lastly, those patients clearly refractory to AZA despite therapeutic drug dosing should be considered for alternative therapies (Group D).

## Combination Therapy

It has been the practice in many institutions, including our own, to initiate maintenance anti-TNF-α therapy in patients that have shown clear refractoriness to either long-term 6-MP or AZA therapy. All of the studies, including ACCENT, CHARM, and PRECISE, did not show a therapeutic benefit with combination therapy (anti-TNF-α with antimetabolite) to just anti-TNF-α therapy alone in maintaining disease remission in patients with moderate to severe Crohn's disease. In comparison, the SONIC study focused its attention on patients who were naïve to anti-TNF-α therapies and either naïve or had stopped (>3 months) AZA therapy prior to recruitment. In that study, combination therapy was shown to be superior to either infliximab or AZA monotherapy [33].

A similarly designed study was recently presented in abstract form in patients with moderate to severe UC. In that 16-week study, 40 % of patients on combination therapy achieved a steroid-free remission, significantly higher than those patients on monotherapy alone (22 % infliximab; 24 % AZA). Both the combination and the infliximab-only treatment arms were superior to AZA monotherapy in overall clinical response and mucosal healing [36].

The purported benefit of combination therapy in SONIC and the above-referenced study in patients with moderate to severe UC is balanced with the increasing concern of hepatic T-cell lymphoma among young (<18 years) patients on combination therapy. This concern has led many physicians to consider discontinuing either 6-MP or AZA with the introduction of biological therapy despite the potential for reducing antibody to infliximab formation. Although all anti-TNF-α have antigenic properties, thereby rendering patients susceptible to antibody formation, those patients on infliximab are most vulnerable. The concurrent use of immunosuppressive therapy has in the past been shown by Rutgeerts and coworkers to maintain a favorable clinical response to maintenance infliximab therapy, presumably due to the prevention of antibody formation. In that study, 75 % (12/16) of patients on concurrent 6-mercaptopurine maintained a favorable clinical response compared to 50 % (9/18) on no concurrent immunosuppressive therapy [37]. In the ACCENT 1 study, only 18 % of the patients on neither concurrent prednisone nor immunosuppressive drug therapy developed antibody to infliximab compared to just 10 % of patients on concurrent azathioprine or methotrexate therapy [38].

In a previously presented study of adult patients with IBD on combination therapy, high 6-TGN levels associated with an improved clinical responsiveness to maintenance anti-TNF therapy. In that study, patients in remission had higher (>300) median erythrocyte 6-TGN metabolite levels compared to patients (<100) with either a partial clinical response or ongoing corticosteroid dependency. Interestingly, patients with anti-TNF-associated side effects (SE) also had low (<100) median 6-TGN levels [39]. Although the concurrent use of either AZA or 6-MP may allow for a more protracted clinical response, the precise mechanism of action is unclear. Whether this purported benefit would justify the increased risk of hepatic T-cell lymphoma is debatable, especially since adalimumab and certolizumab pegol have proven efficacy of salvaging patients refractory to infliximab. Unfortunately, TPMT and 6-MP metabolite levels have shown no correlation with the 36 reported cases to date of hepatic T-cell lymphoma [40].

## Conclusions

6-MP and AZA have proven efficacy in the maintenance of disease remission in patients with IBD. The application of pharmacogenetics and metabolite testing in clinical practice may improve the overall clinical response to antimetabolite therapy and reduce the risk of antimetabolite-induced side effects. The careful monitoring of complete blood counts and erythrocyte 6-TG metabolite levels is indicated in patients with either low (<5) or above average (>16) TPMT levels, and it remains the authors' opinion that relying on either total leukocyte counts or mean corpuscular volume as the sole measure of dosing adequacy should be used with caution.

## References

1. Sandler RS, Everhart JE, Donowitz M, et al. The burden of selected digestive diseases in the United States. Gastroenterology. 2002; 122:1500–11.
2. Lichtenstein G, Yan S, Bala M, Hanauer S. Remission in patients with Crohn's disease associated with improvement in employment and quality of life and decrease in hospitalization and surgeries. Am J Gastroenterol. 2004;99:91–6.
3. Farmer R, Easley K, Rankin G. Clinical patterns, natural history, and progression of ulcerative colitis. A long-term follow-up of 1116 patients. Dig Dis Sci. 1993;38:1137–46.
4. Sands BE, Abreu MT, Ferry GD, et al. Design issues and outcomes in IBD clinical trials. Inflamm Bowel Dis. 2005;11:S22–8.
5. Farrell R, Peppercorn M. Endoscopy in inflammatory bowel disease. In: Sartor R, Sandborn W, editors. Kirsner's Inflammatory Bowel Diseases. 6th ed. Philadelphia, Pa: WB Saunders; 2004. p. 380–98.
6. Eaden J, Abrams K, Mayberry J. The risk of colorectal cancer in ulcerative colitis: a meta-analysis. Gut. 2001;48:526–35.

7. Cuffari C, Hunt S, Bayless TM. Utilization of erythrocyte 6-thioguanine metabolite levels to optimize therapy in IBD. Gut. 2001;48:642–6.

8. Achar JP, Stevens T, Brzezinski A, Seidner D, Lashner B. 6-Thioguanine levels versus white blood cell counts in guiding 6-mercaptopruine and azathioprine therapy. Am J Gastroenterol. 2000;95:A272.

9. Lowry PW, Franklin CL, Weaver AL, Szumlanski C, Mays DC, Loftus EV, Tremaine WJ, Lipsky JJ, Weinshilboum RM, Sandborn WJ. Leukopenia resulting from a drug interaction between azathioprine or 6-mercaptopurine and mesalamine, sulphasalazine or balsalazide. Gut. 2001;49:656–64.

10. Actis GC, Pellicano R, Ezio D, Sapino A. Azathioprine, mucosal healing in ulcerative colitis, and the chemoprevention of colitic cancer: a clinical-practice-based forecast. Inflamm Allergy Drug Targets. 2010;9:6–9.

11. Conklin L, Cuffari C, Li X. 6-MP transport in lymphocyte: correlation with toxicity. J Dig Dis. 2012;13(2):82–93.

12. Weinshilboum RN, Sladek SL. Mercaptopurine pharmacogenetics: monogenic inheritance of erythrocyte thiopurine methyl transferase activity. Am J Hum Genet. 1980;32:651–62.

13. Christie NT, Drake S, Meyn RE. 6-thioguanine induced DNA damage as a determinant of cytotoxicity in cultured hamster ovary cells. Cancer Res. 1986;44:3665–71.

14. Fairchild CR, Maybaum J, Kennedy KA. Concurrent unilateral chromatid damage and DNA strand breaks in response to 6-thioguanine treatment. Biochem Pharmacol. 1986;35:3533–41.

15. Brogan M, Hiserot J, Olicer M. The effects of 6-mercaptopurine on natural killer cell activities in Crohn's disease. J Clin Immunol. 1985;5:204–11.

16. Evans WE, Horner M, Chu YQ, et al. Altered mercaptopurine metabolism, toxic effects, and dosage requirements in a thiopurine methyltransferase deficient child with acute lymphoblastic leukemia. J Pediatr. 1991;119:985–9.

17. Lennard L. The clinical pharmacology of 6-mercaptopurine in acute lymphoblastic leukemia. Eur J Clin Pharmacol. 1992;43:329–39.

18. Tiede I, Fritz G, Strand S, Poppe D, Dvorsky R, Strand D, Lehr HA, Wirtz S, Becker C, Atreya R, Mudter J, Hildner K, Bartsch B, Holtmann M, Blumberg R, Walczak H, Iven H, Galle PR, Ahmadian MR, Neurath MF. CD28-dependent Rac1 activation is the molecular target of azathioprine in primary human CD4+ T lymphocytes. J Clin Invest. 2003;111(8):1133–45.

19. Langholz E, Munkholm P, Davidsen M, et al. Changes in extent of ulcerative colitis—a study on the course and prognostic factors. Scand J Gastroenterol. 1996;31:260–6.

20. Seidman EG. Inflammatory bowel disease. In: Roy CC, Silverman A, Alagille A, editors. Clinical Pediatric Gastroenterology, edition 4. Philadelphia, Pa: Mosby; 1993.

21. Cuffari C, Bayless TM, Hanauer SB, Lichtenstein G, Present DH. Optimizing therapy in patients with pancolitis. Inflamm Bowel Dis. 2005;11:937–46.

22. Reinisch W, Sandborn WJ, Rutgeerts P, Feagan BG, Rachmilewitz D, Hanauer SB, Lichtenstein GR, de Villiers WJ, Blank M, Lang Y, Johanns J, Colombel JF, Present D, Sands BE. Long-term infliximab maintenance therapy for ulcerative colitis: the ACT-1 and -2 extension studies. Inflamm Bowel Dis. 2012;18:201–11.

23. Frøslie KF, Jahnsen J, Moum BA, Vatn MH, IBSEN Group. Mucosal healing in inflammatory bowel disease: results from a Norwegian population-based cohort. Gastroenterology. 2007;133(2):412–22.

24. Present DH, Meltzer SJ, Krumholz MP, et al. 6-mercaptopurine in the management of inflammatory bowel disease: short and long-term toxicity. Ann Intern Med. 1995;111:641–9.

25. Present DH, Korelitz BI, Wisch N, et al. Treatment of Crohn's disease with 6-mercaptopurine. A long-term, randomized, double-blind study. N Engl J Med. 1980;302:981–7.

26. Dubinsky MC, Lamothe S, Yang HY, Targan SR, Sinnett D, Theoret Y, Seidman EG. Pharmacogenomics and metabolite measurement for 6-mercaptopurine therapy in inflammatory bowel disease. Gastroenterology. 2000;118:705–13.

27. Gupta P, Gokhlae R, Kirschner BS. 6-mercaptopurine metabolite levels in children with inflammatory bowel disease. J Pediatr Gastroenterol Nutr. 2001;33:450–4.

28. Belaiche J, Desager JP, Horsman Y, Louis E. Therapeutic drug monitoring of azathioprine and 6-mercaptopurine metabolites in Crohn's disease. Scand J Gastroenterol. 2001;36:71–6.

29. Goldenberg BA, Rawsthorne P, Bernstein CN. The utility of 6-thioguanine metabolite levels in managing patients with inflammatory bowel disease. Am J Gastroenterol. 2004;99(9):1744–8.

30. Osterman MT, Kundu R, Lichtenstein GR, Lewis JD. Association of 6-thioguanine nucleotide levels and inflammatory bowel disease activity: a meta-analysis. Gastroenterology. 2006;130(4):1047–53.

31. Black AJ, McLeod HL, Capell HA, Powrie RH, Matowe LK, Pritchard SC, Collie-Duguid ES, Reid DM. Thiopurine methyltransferase genotype predicts therapy-limiting severe toxicity from azathioprine. Ann Intern Med. 1998;129:716–8.

32. Sandborn WJ, Tremaine WJ, Wolf DC, Targan SR, Sninsky CA, Sutherland LR, Hanauer SB, McDonald JW, Feagan BG, Fedorak RN, Isaacs KL, Pike MG, Mays DC, Lipsky JJ, Gordon S, Kleoudis CS, Murdock Jr RH. Lack of effect of intravenous administration on time to respond to azathioprine for steroid-treated Crohn's disease. North American Azathioprine Study Group. Gastroenterology. 1999;117(3):527–35.

33. Colombel JF, Sandborn WJ, Reinisch W, Mantzaris GJ, Kornbluth A, Rachmilewitz D, Lichtiger S, D'Haens G, Diamond RH, Broussard DL, Tang KL, van der Woude CJ, Rutgeerts P, SONIC Study Group. Sonic Infliximab, azathioprine, or combination therapy for Crohn's disease. N Engl J Med. 2010;362(15):1383–95.

34. Prefontaine E, Macdonald JK, Sutherland LR. Azathioprine or 6-mercaptopurine for induction of remission in Crohn's disease. Cochrane Database Syst Rev. 2010;6, CD000545. Review.

35. Sparrow MP, Hande SA, Friedman S, Lim WC, Reddy SI, Cao D, Hanauer SB. Allopurinol safely and effectively optimizes thioguanine metabolites in inflammatory bowel disease patients not responding to azathioprine and mercaptopurine. Aliment Pharmacol Ther. 2005;22(5):441–6.

36. Panccione R, Ghosh S, Middleton S, et al. Infliximab, azathioprine or infliximab plus azathioprine for treatment of moderate to severe ulcerative colitis: the UC success trial. Gastroenterology. 2011;A385.

37. Vermeire S, Noman M, Van Assche G, Baert F, D'Haens G, Rutgeerts P. Effectiveness of concomitant immunosuppressive therapy in suppressing the formation of antibodies to infliximab in Crohn's disease. Gut. 2007;56(9):1226–31.

38. Hanauer SB, Feagan BG, Lichtenstein GR, Mayer LF, Schreiber S, Colombel JF, Rachmilewitz D, Wolf DC, Olson A, Bao W, Rutgeerts P, ACCENT I Study Group. Maintenance infliximab for Crohn's disease: the ACCENT I randomised trial. Lancet. 2002; 359(9317):1541–9.

39. Cuffari C, Harris M, Bayless TM. 6-mercaptopurine metabolites levels correlate with a favorable clinical response to long-term infliximab therapy. Gastroenterology. 2007;A234.

40. Jones JL, Loftus Jr EV. Lymphoma risk in inflammatory bowel disease: is it the disease or its treatment? Inflamm Bowel Dis. 2007;13(10):1299–307. Review.

# Cyclosporine for Ulcerative Colitis

13

Gregory P. Botta, Wojciech Blonski,
and Gary R. Lichtenstein

**Keywords**

Ulcerative colitis • Inflammatory disorder • Cyclosporine • Immune response • Pharmacology • Rescue therapy • Clinical trials • Adverse events • Cyclosporine-refractory ulcerative colitis

## Introduction

Ulcerative colitis (UC) is an idiopathic inflammatory disorder of unknown etiology that affects the mucosa and the submucosa of the colon. The inflamed epithelium extends continuously from the rectum and involves part or all (pancolitis) of the colon. Symptomatically, patients exhibit increased, bloody, bowel movements with fecal urgency, diarrhea, abdominal cramping, abdominal pain, hematochezia, and fever. These characteristics can have a gradual or an acute onset with variable durations of flare and remission. Population cohort studies have shown that during the lifetime of their disease, 10–40 % of patients with ulcerative colitis will ultimately require a colectomy [1–3].

## Epidemiology

Increasing in incidence and prevalence across the globe, UC is stratified based on geographic location. Incidence averages are now 6.3 (Asia and the Middle East), 19.2 (North America), and 24.3 (Europe) cases per 100,000. Further, UC incidence is higher in men, peaks between the ages of 30 and 40 years, and, although data is scarce, appears to be rising within developing nations signifying its emergence as a truly global disease [4]. UC's prevalence averages between 249 and 505 cases per 100,000 with a large majority occurring in industrialized, northern latitudes of North America and Europe [4, 5]. A genetic component exists in UC where first-degree relatives of UC patients increase their risk of harboring the same disease process by 10- to 15-fold [6]. Genome-wide association and candidate gene studies have identified over 163 inflammatory bowel disease (IBD)-related loci with 23 genes specific for UC and 30 specific for Crohn's disease (CD) using meta-analysis. As expected, candidate genes synchronize with interleukin expression as well as the JAK-STAT inflammatory pathway and the interferon regulatory family. Further, considerable overlap exists with other immune-related disease states including psoriasis, ankylosing spondylitis, and mycobacterial infection [7, 8].

## Immune Response

Ulcerative colitis is a result of innate and acquired autoimmunologic responses and a possible loss of tolerance to the bacteria of the gut. Innate responses by resident macrophages and neutrophils are increased and activated within the lining

G.P. Botta, M.D., Ph.D. (✉)
Division of Gastroenterology, University of Pennsylvania
Perelman School of Medicine, 415 Curie Boulevard, 950
Biomedical Research Building II/III Philadelphia, PA 19104, USA
e-mail: gregory.botta@gmail.com

W. Blonski, M.D., Ph.D.
Internal Medicine, United Health Services, Wilson Memorial
Center, 33-57 Harrison St., Picciano Building 4th Floor,
Johnson City, NY 13790, USA
e-mail: blonskiw@gmail.com

G.R. Lichtenstein, M.D., F.A.C.P., F.A.C.G., A.G.A.F.
Division of Gastroenterology, Hospital of the University of
Pennsylvania, University of Pennsylvania School of Medicine,
3400 Spruce Street 3rd Floor, Philadelphia, PA 19104, USA
e-mail: grl@uphs.upenn.edu

G.R. Lichtenstein (ed.), *Medical Therapy of Ulcerative Colitis*,
DOI 10.1007/978-1-4939-1677-1_13, © Springer Science+Business Media New York 2014

153

of the gut of UC patients. This activation releases cytokines such as IL-1 and IL-2 resulting in an inflammatory microenvironment. Secondary to the cytokine response, monocytes and more granulocytes extravasate into the gut lining adding to the proinflammatory niche of UC [9]. In addition to the local macrophages within the lamina propria of the gut, resident dendritic cells are present within immunologic Peyer's patches. After inflammatory signals from an autoimmune reaction to local antigen or normal enteric bacteria, the dendritic cells activate and stimulate T cells. The stimulation of T cells occurs by direct co-stimulatory binding of CD40, CD80, or CTLA4 (among others) and by release of IL-5 and IL-13 (among others) [10]. Upon activation, effector and regulatory T cells migrate to the gut and produce more of an atypical TH2 response but with the addition of some TH1 cytotoxicity. Successively, populations of B cells increase in this TH2 response, and plasma cells begin to release IgG1, IgG4, and IgE antibodies directed against normal tissue as well as autoantibodies against p-ANCA and tropomyosin [11, 12].

## Pharmacologic Options

### Acute Disease

Current medical therapy aims to palliate the inflammatory process by inducing and maintaining remission. While doing so, it is expected that there will be mucosal healing with concurrent abatement of the intestinal symptoms and improvement in the quality of life of our patients. Patients initially presenting with mild-to-moderate colitis and without prior pharmacologic intervention are generally started on a regimen of aminosalicylates such as mesalamine [13]. When patients reach the stage of severe colitis, current treatments now include steroids, anti-TNF therapies, and calcineurin inhibitors such as infliximab and cyclosporine.

One of the main predisposing factors to UC is an overactive immune-mediated inflammatory response. Aminosalicylates represent the first-line treatment in mild-to-moderate disease [13, 14]. When patients present with severe ulcerative colitis, an attempt to avoid the use of antidiarrheal medication, analgesics containing opioids, and anticholinergic should be made. Each of these interventions inhibits gastrointestinal motility and increases the potential risk of toxic, dilated bowels and subsequent perforation [15, 16].

Many different measures have been used to define an acute, severe UC flare, each a variation of the Truelove and Witts criteria (greater than 6 stools per day with either large amounts of blood in each stool, a hemoglobin less than 10.5 g/dL, a body temperature over 37.8 °C, a pulse rate over 90 beats per minute, or an ESR of more than 30 mm/h) [17, 18]. The current definition of UC as outlined in the American College of Gastroenterology 2010 guidelines note that "any patient presenting with persistent bloody diarrhea, rectal urgency, or tenesmus, [we recommend that] stool examinations and sigmoidoscopy or colonoscopy and biopsy should be performed to confirm the presence of colitis and to exclude the presence of infectious and noninfectious etiologies" [19]. Any patient meeting the clinical criteria of severe ulcerative colitis should be immediately hospitalized and considered a medical emergency. Initially, patients should be evaluated for enteric pathogens, cytomegalovirus, and *Clostridium difficile* within the stool and have these pathogens excluded on a mucosal biopsy after a flexible sigmoidoscopy. Visualization of the colon will show the hallmark characteristics of an acute, severe UC flare: granularity, ulceration, friability, and the attenuation of vascularity [19]. These pathologic findings, combined with clinical presentation and the exclusion of pathogens, underscore a diagnosis of ulcerative colitis. At the onset, patients should receive daily IV corticosteroids such as hydrocortisone (300 mg) or methylprednisolone (60 mg) to induce remission. Glucocorticoids have a rapid onset of action (within 48 h) and effectively reduce the inflammatory response in 80 % of patients. Furthermore, patients who receive steroids for treatment of UC may experience side effects ranging from psychosis to hypertension and diabetes as well as osteoporosis and avascular necrosis. Long-term use of corticosteroids is not advocated given the significant adverse event profile that can occur. The use of rescue immunosuppressive medications such as calcineurin inhibitors (cyclosporine, tacrolimus) or anti-TNF medications (infliximab, adalimumab, golimumab) has been advocated in this scenario. In addition the use of calcineurin inhibitors (cyclosporine, tacrolimus) and infliximab has been clinically evaluated in patients with even, severe steroid-refractory disease (Fig. 13.1).

### Rescue Therapy

Immunomodulation of the inflammatory microenvironment with calcineurin inhibitors has been used as salvage therapy for steroid-refractory UC patients. It is thought that "refractoriness" derives from an overwhelming proinflammatory milieu that reduces the anti-inflammatory affinity of steroids to its receptor and attenuates its effects. A patient is defined as refractory to steroids when their use has not decreased UC symptoms (increased stool urgency, frequency, hematochezia, colonic dilation, tenesmus, fever) within 3–5 days. It is important for the clinician to exclude the presence of pseudo-refractory states that are not appropriately managed with the use of corticosteroids prior to initiating rescue therapies. These would include symptoms related to the presence of adhesions, fibrotic intestinal strictures, abscesses, small intestinal bacterial overgrowth, *Clostridium difficile*-related colitis, opportunistic viral infections (cytomegalovirus), or lactose intolerance. These are clinical scenarios that simulate the presence of UC-like

**Fig. 13.1** Pharmacologic mechanism of calcineurin and mTOR inhibitors. Similar mechanisms of action group cyclosporine, tacrolimus, and sirolimus into dependent inhibitors (see Chap. 14 for further information). Each is capable of negating the action of a transcription factor/activator by cooperative binding with either cyclophilin or FK506. Importantly, these attenuating mechanisms reside within the immunologic regulation of T cells

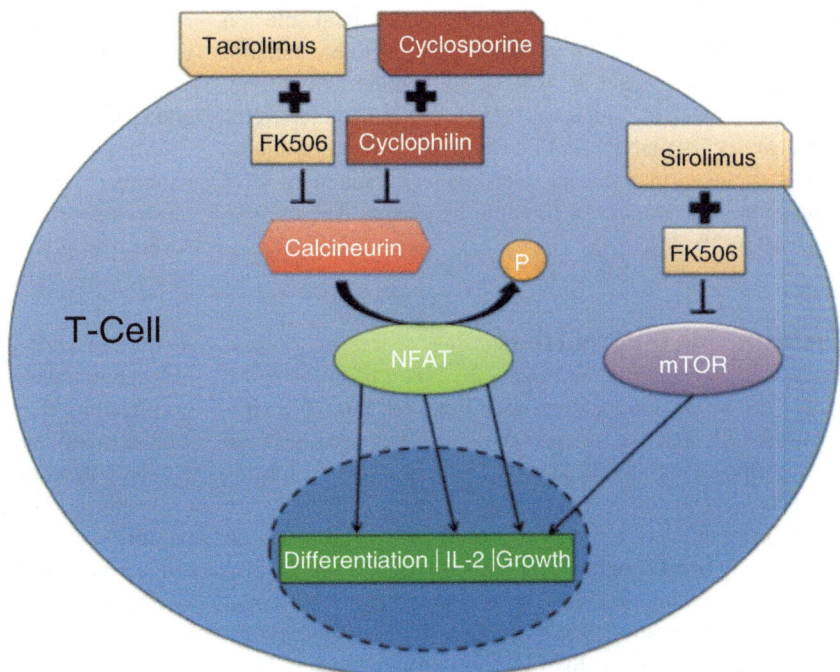

symptoms often indistinguishable from those in patients with actual, active ulcerative colitis.

After a patient is deemed truly refractory and documented to have active UC, options to further treatment include immunomodulators such as azathioprine (AZA), 6-mercaptopurine (6-MP), and mycophenolate; the calcineurin/mTOR inhibitors tacrolimus and cyclosporine (CSA); and biologic agents like infliximab, adalimumab, and, more recently, golimumab [20].

The use of azathioprine (AZA) or 6-mercaptopurine (6-MP) is not typically used acutely and is not particularly helpful for patients with active, refractory UC given the long duration of time that is required for the onset of action. Two commonly prescribed calcineurin inhibitors include tacrolimus and cyclosporine, both of which downregulate T cell activation and chemokine production without significant myelosuppression (Fig. 13.1). Specifically, the calcineurin inhibitors bind to immunophilins and inhibit the calcineurin-dependent dephosphorylation and activation of nuclear factor of activated T cells (NFAT) [21]. Whereas tacrolimus attaches to the FK506 binding protein, cyclosporine binds to cyclophilin, and both ultimately inhibit NFAT transcription of differentiation, growth, and chemokine genes. Cyclosporine harbors a long history of clinical use as an antirejection drug in solid-organ transplantation as well as in rheumatoid arthritis [22]. It has a quick onset of action that results in severe UC improvement within 1–2 weeks at a dose between 2 and 4 mg/kg/day via continuous intravenous (IV) infusion [23]. Recent evidence suggests oral formulations may be as effective as IV administration and is described below.

Two other medications, sirolimus and mycophenolate mofetil, target immune cell proliferation but are not currently recommended as a standard of therapy for patients with UC pending clinical trials. Sirolimus also binds to the immunophilin FK506 binding protein but instead downregulates mammalian target of rapamycin (mTOR) attenuating T cell proliferation [21]. Mycophenolate mofetil acts as a prodrug that is hydrolyzed to mycophenolic acid, inhibiting the inosine monophosphate dehydrogenase enzyme. As such, guanine nucleotide synthesis and proliferation are downregulated specifically in B and T cells as they are incapable of rescue purine synthesis. Of note, only tacrolimus and cyclosporine harbor enough clinical data to warrant their recommended use in severe, steroid-refractory UC.

## Cyclosporine Pharmacology

A fungal metabolite, cyclosporine is a lipophilic, cyclic peptide that is poorly soluble in water and must be either in an emulsion or a suspension prior to oral or IV use [24]. As such, there is a very narrow therapeutic window where levels below specific blood concentrations do not assist in attenuating the immunologic response, while levels above advance adverse effects. Additionally, the IV pharmacokinetic profile is variable and highly dependent on the patient's cytochrome P450 profile within the liver, gut, and kidney as well as bile excretion dynamics. Importantly, high bile excretion (after a high-fat meal) will aid in the bioavailable absorption of cyclosporine but also in its excretion [25, 26].

As the cyclosporine microemulsion increases contact with the plasma, its pharmacokinetic profile is less variable and more regulated. This variation reaches peak plasma levels in approximately 2 h but has a highly variable half-life ranging between 9 and 27 h [27]. Its hepatic cytochrome P450 metabolism is similar to IV cyclosporine and its excretion also occurs mainly via bile excretion. After oral ingestion of cyclosporine, plasma levels achieve a maximal level (Cmax) in an average of 4 h, while its plasma half-life can reach 19 h [25, 28].

## Cyclosporine Clinical Trials

The first landmark randomized, double-blind, placebo-controlled prospective trial assigned 20 patients with severe UC not improving after at least 7 days of IV corticosteroids (equivalent to 300 of IV hydrocortisone or equivalent dose in other formulations) to receive either IV cyclosporine at 4 mg/kg/day ($n=11$) or placebo ($n=9$) for up to 14 days [29]. Response was defined as improvement on a numerical Lichtiger scale from 0 (no symptoms) to 21 (severe symptoms) with a score of less than 10 on 2 consecutive days [29]. The active treatment arm had 9/11 (82 %) of patients with a validated response within a mean of 7 days when compared to 0/9 (0 %) of patients in the placebo arm ($p<0.001$) [29]. Nonresponders, two patients in cyclosporine arm and four patients in placebo arm, underwent colectomy, while five remaining nonresponders in the placebo arm crossed over to open-label treatment with IV cyclosporine [29]. In all five placebo patients that crossed over to IV cyclosporine, a clinical response was observed within a mean of 7 days with a decrease in their mean Lichtiger score from 11 to 7 [29]. Importantly, the mean disease activity index within the treatment group was decreased by more than 50 %, permitting all cyclosporine-treated patients to have successful hospital discharges [29]. The small number of enrolled patients in this study was in part due to the hospital's safety committee stopping the trial early due to the observation of statistically significant responses in the active treatment group [29]. The initial trial was planned with the intent to enroll 42 total patients.

A subsequent randomized, double-blind controlled trial published in 2001 observed that IV cyclosporine had comparable efficacy to IV methylprednisolone alone in severe UC flares [20]. There were 29 patients who were randomly assigned to an 8-day course of either IV cyclosporine (4 mg/kg/day) or IV methylprednisolone (40 mg/day) [20]. Patients who demonstrated responses at day 8 (defined as a Lichtiger score of less than 10 on days 7 and 8 with a decrease in the Lichtiger score from day 1 to day 8 of at least three points and the possibility to discharge the patient) received the same medication orally in an open-label fashion (cyclosporine 8 mg/kg or methylprednisolone 32 mg/day) combined with oral azathioprine 2–2.5 mg/kg/day [20, 29]. Oral methylprednisolone was given at a dose of 32 mg/day for the first

3 weeks with a subsequent taper by 4 mg/week until discontinuation, whereas oral cyclosporine was continued for 3 months and then discontinued [20]. Oral azathioprine was continued for up to 12 months [20].

After the initial 8 days of IV therapy, 8/15 (53 %) of patients on methylprednisolone and 9/14 (64 %) of patients on cyclosporine had a response ($p=0.4$) to therapy without severe, drug-related toxicity observed, suggesting similar efficacy of cyclosporine and glucocorticosteroids in severe attacks of UC [20].

Further, 7/9 (78 %) of patients with a cyclosporine-induced response maintained UC remission at 12 months on oral azathioprine when compared to 3/8 (37 %) of patients with a methylprednisolone-induced response [20]. Overall, 1-year colectomy rates were 36 % (5/14 patients) in the cyclosporine group and 40 % (6/15 patients) in the methylprednisolone group [20]. Cyclosporine was shown to be an efficacious alternative to glucocorticosteroids in inducing a response in patients with severe UC and also as a bridging agent to oral azathioprine after achievement of a clinical response [20].

Of further clinical importance, applying cyclosporine to UC patients while attenuating steroid exposure can benefit patients who are sensitive to avascular necrosis, osteoporosis, or immune deficiency.

A single-center, randomized double-blind controlled trial compared the efficacy and safety of an 8-day treatment with IV cyclosporine 4 mg/kg versus IV cyclosporine 2 mg/kg in patients with an acute, severe UC flare [30]. Following the Lichtiger clinical activity index as described above [29], 73 patients with a severe UC flare were enrolled and followed for 8 days on either the 4 mg/kg or 2 mg/kg IV cyclosporine dosage [30]. The following concomitant medications were allowed: (1) IV corticosteroids (stable dose for at least 5 days without clinical response prior to enrollment and during the 8 days of the trial), (2) oral corticosteroids (initiated at least 14 days from inclusion without clinical benefit) which were switched to IV corticosteroids on day 1 of the trial with subsequent transition to oral corticosteroids on day 8 with a taper by 5 mg of prednisone per week, (3) AZA/6-MP (started at least 3 months prior to inclusion with a stable dose 4 weeks prior to admission), (4) both oral and rectal aminosalicylates (continued at stable doses for the first 8 days), and (5) antibiotics (continued at inclusion if clinically necessary and during the trial for infections) [30]. Of note, patients who were not on azathioprine at the time of trial onset started receiving azathioprine 2–2.5 mg/kg orally on day 8 [30].

Clinical response rates (defined as a Lichtiger clinical activity index (CAI) score less than 10 at day 8 with a drop of at least three from baseline) were 84.2 % for the 4 mg/kg arm and 85.7 % for the 2 mg/kg arm ($p>0.05$) with a median time to clinical response of 4 days in both arms, signifying that the lower dose was as efficacious as the higher [30].

Coordinately, the blood levels of cyclosporine correlated with their dosing amounts such that 2 mg/kg had a blood level of $237 \pm 33$, while $332 \pm 43$ ng/mL was observed in the 4 mg/kg group ($p < 0.0001$) [30]. Short-term colectomy rates were not statistically significantly different between the 4 mg/kg group and the 2 mg/kg group (13.1 % vs. 8.6 %, $p > 0.05$) [30]. The multivariate logistic regression analysis determined that, from several variables such as active smoking, mean cyclosporine dose, patient's age, location of UC (left-sided vs. pancolitis), and concomitant corticosteroids and azathioprine use, only active smoking was inversely associated with clinical response (OR 0.06, 95 % CI 0.008–0.407) [30].

There were no statistically significant differences between the treatment arms (4 mg/kg vs. 2 mg/kg) in the proportion of patients experiencing adverse events such as tremor or paresthesia (7.9 % vs. 5.7 %, $p$-value not reported), increase of serum creatinine by at least 10 % (18.4 % vs. 17.1 %, $p$-value not reported), fever (7.9 % vs. 2.9 %, $p$-value not reported), or diabetes mellitus (2.6 % vs. 0 %, $p$-value not reported) [30]. However, a trend toward a greater proportion of novel hypertension in the higher cyclosporine arm was observed (23.7 % vs. 8.6 %, $p < 0.08$) [30]. It was suggested that lower doses of cyclosporine should be used in patients with acute, severe UC given the comparable efficacy to higher doses and better safety profile [30]. There was a suggestion that active smokers with severe UC may become refractory to all medical treatment, but the small number of smokers in this study precludes the definitive interpretation of this finding [30].

A retrospective cohort analysis examined 142 patients admitted to a tertiary medical center with an acute, severe UC flare. These patients were stratified to either treated with IV cyclosporine (2–4 mg/kg/day) in conjunction with IV glucocorticosteroids for 7 days after they deteriorated or not responding to 5–7 days of prior treatment with IV glucocorticosteroids (methylprednisolone 40 mg/day) [31]. Patients whose condition worsened or did not improve while on IV

cyclosporine for 7–10 days underwent immediate colectomy [31]. Those patients who responded to IV cyclosporine (83 %, 118/142 patients) were then switched to a tapering dose of oral glucocorticosteroids and 3 months of oral cyclosporine emulsions (Neoral, Novartis) at an initial dose of 8 mg/kg/day that was adjusted to blood cyclosporine levels ranging between 150 and 250 ng/mL, with addition of azathioprine (2.5 mg/kg/day) or 6-mercaptopurine (1.5 mg/kg/day) [31]. Of the 142 patients, 44 were already on azathioprine at the time of their severe flare, 74 were started on azathioprine de novo, and 24 patients did not receive azathioprine/6-mercaptopurine [31]. However, it is unclear when azathioprine de novo was initiated as the authors initially stated it occurred after achieving responses to IV cyclosporine with subsequent statements noting that azathioprine was initiated at the time of onset of IV cyclosporine therapy [31].

Among 118 patients who avoided initial colectomy, 41 (35 %) underwent a future colectomy within a mean of 542 days [31]. According to the life table analysis, overall 1-year and 7-year colectomy rates were 33 % and 88 %, respectively [31]. Subgroup analysis showed that the proportion of patients who underwent colectomy was statistically and significantly ($p < 0.05$) greater among those patients who were already on azathioprine (59 %, 26/44 patients) at the time of the severe flare when compared to those who were started de novo on azathioprine at the time of treatment with IV cyclosporine (32 %, 24/74 patients). This observation suggests that prior failure of azathioprine to maintain a state of remission predicted poor treatment success with cyclosporine for severe UC flares [31]. In other words, patients who failed prior therapy with azathioprine and who presented with severe activity mandating the use of cyclosporine had poorer outcomes than those individuals who were azathioprine naïve at the time they received the cyclosporine for refractory disease (Fig. 13.2). Furthermore, of the 26 patients who were already on azathioprine and required colectomy, 23 (88 %) underwent colectomy within 1 year after an initially

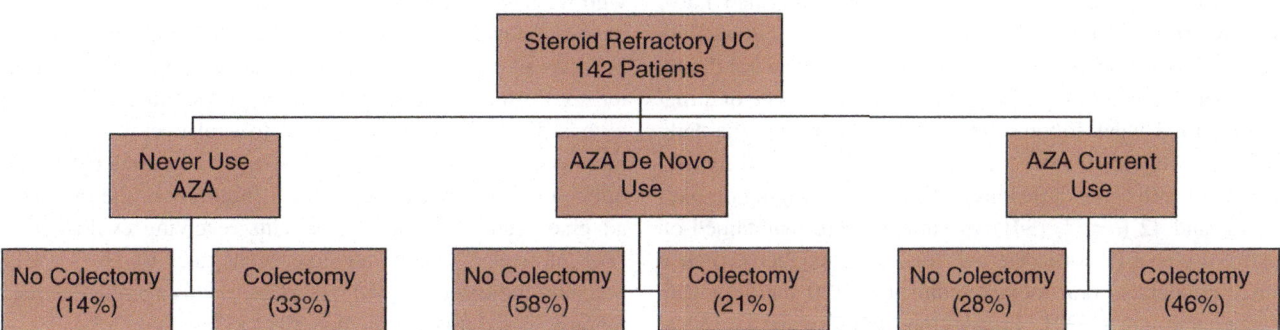

**Fig. 13.2** Cyclosporine-responsive patients without prior thiopurine usage have the highest success of avoiding colectomy. Stratifying by chronology of azathioprine dosing (never with cyclosporine (de novo) or before cyclosporine (current)). Patients naïve to AZA and co-dosed with cyclosporine at the same time avoid colectomy at the highest rate (58 %) compared to those on cyclosporine who do not receive AZA (14 %) or those who had prior AZA therapy prior to cyclosporine treatment (28 %) [31]

successful treatment with cyclosporine. This can be compared to a 50 % 1-year colectomy rate (12/24 patients) in the subgroup of patients who were started on azathioprine de novo and required colectomy [31].

The authors concluded that cyclosporine is indeed effective in the short term and that AZA-naïve patients show better outcome prior to beginning cyclosporine therapy [31]. It was suggested that IV cyclosporine should be used as a bridge to long-term treatment with immune modulators or colectomy.

Further, a prior retrospective study including 42 patients with severe UC treated with IV cyclosporine 4 mg/kg/day for a mean of 10 days and 31 patients continuing oral cyclosporine at 8 mg/kg/day for a mean of 20 weeks showed that the combination of cyclosporine and azathioprine/6-mercaptopurine was associated with a significantly higher probability of avoiding colectomy at 5.5 years than cyclosporine monotherapy (66 % vs. 40 %, $p=0.04$) [32]. Colectomy-free rates were 62 % for all patients, 72 % for responders to cyclosporine, and 80 % for responders to cyclosporine on concomitant azathioprine/6-mercaptopurine. Further, life table analysis demonstrated colectomy-free rates at 5.5 years of 58 %, 70 %, and 71 %, respectively [32]. The results of both studies should be interpreted with caution due to their retrospective design and low number of patients enrolled [31, 32].

Recent meta-analysis of six retrospective cohort studies comparing treatment with infliximab versus cyclosporine in 321 patients with acute, severe corticosteroid-refractory UC demonstrated comparable therapeutic profiles of both agents in terms of rescue therapy [33]. No statistically significant difference was observed in the 3-month (OR=0.86, 95 % CI 0.31–2.41, $p=0.775$) and 12-month colectomy rates (OR=0.60, 95 % CI=0.19–1.89, $p=0.381$), in adverse drug reactions (OR=0.76, 95 % CI=0.34–1.70, $p=0.508$), or in postoperative complications (OR=1.66, 95 % CI=0.26–10.50, $p=0.591$) between infliximab and cyclosporine [33]. These data were further supported by a recent multicenter, parallel, open-label randomized controlled trial designed by GETAID in which 115 cyclosporine and infliximab naïve patients from 27 medical centers in Europe presenting with severe UC refractory to IV corticosteroids were randomly assigned to receive either IV cyclosporine at the dose of 2 mg/kg/day for 1 week followed by oral cyclosporine at the daily dose of 4 mg/kg for 91 days (goal trough 150–250 ng/mL, $n=58$) or infliximab infusions at the dose of 5 mg/kg on days 0, 14, and 42 ($n=57$) [34]. All patients were maintained on stable doses of IV corticosteroids for 7 days and then switched in responders to oral methylprednisolone (30 mg/day) with subsequent taper [34]. In addition, those with a clinical response at day 7 were started on azathioprine 2–2.5 mg/kg/day or were continued on azathioprine if it was initiated within 4 weeks before trial onset [34]. Primary efficacy end points included treatment failure defined as presence of any of six

predefined criteria: (1) no clinical response within the first 7 days, (2) clinical relapse (increase in Lichtiger score by at least three points sustained for 3 consecutive days) between days 7 and 98, (3) absence of corticosteroid-free remission on day 98 (Mayo disease activity index of less than 2 and an endoscopically defined subscore of less than 1), (4) interruption of treatment secondary to severe adverse events, (5) need for colectomy, or (6) patient's death [34]. The proportion of patients who experienced treatment failure was similar between the two treatment arms (60 % in cyclosporine arm vs. 54 % in infliximab arm, $p=0.52$) [34]. Multivariate analysis adjusted for independent predictors of treatment failure (age greater than 40 years and hemoglobin concentration 95–125 g/L) showed a nonsignificant increased odds ratio for treatment failure with cyclosporine versus infliximab at 1.4 (95 % CI 0.6–3.2, $p=0.36$) [34]. The authors suggested that given comparable efficacy, treatment choice with either cyclosporine or infliximab should be based on the physician's or medical center's experience [34]. Furthermore, data from a small retrospective study of 19 patients with severe corticosteroid-refractory UC who were treated with IV cyclosporine after failing to respond clinically to infliximab or with infliximab after failing to respond clinically to IV cyclosporine suggested that cyclosporine and infliximab might be efficacious salvage agents for each other in this patient population [35]. In that study, remission was achieved by 40 % of patients receiving infliximab salvage therapy with mean duration of 10.4 months and 33 % of patients receiving cyclosporine salvage therapy with mean duration of 28.5 months [35]. Caution should be exercised when implementing this strategy immediately after failure of one agent and reserved after a "resting period" to avoid infectious complications resulting from massive immunosuppression [19].

A prospective study of 83 consecutive patients presenting with corticosteroid-refractory severe UC who received salvage therapy with either IV cyclosporine ($n=45$) or infliximab ($n=38$) showed that 84 % of patients who received a single dose of infliximab (5 mg/kg) versus 56 % of patients who received at least 72 h of IV cyclosporine (2–4 mg/kg/day) avoided colectomy ($p=0.006$) [36]. Similarly, the proportions of patients who avoided short-term and medium-term colectomy were significantly greater in those treated with infliximab when compared to oral cyclosporine at 3 months (76 % vs. 53 %, $p=0.04$) and 12 months (65 % vs. 42 %, $p=0.04$), respectively [36]. In addition, the only two adverse events occurred in patients receiving cyclosporine [36]. However, serious adverse event rates of 16 % (3/19 patients) indicated that the risk of using this agent as salvage therapy may outweigh the benefits [35].

The most recently published retrospective cohort study of 78 patients with severe corticosteroid-refractory UC who underwent colectomy following treatment with IV corticosteroids alone or combined with either IV cyclosporine or infliximab at a tertiary university center suggested that neither cyclosporine nor infliximab was associated with an increased risk of postoperative complications [37]. No difference in total postoperative complications was observed between patients who received cyclosporine (RR = 0.63, 95 % CI 0.33–1.23) or infliximab (RR = 0.65, 95 % CI, 0.36–1.17) in conjunction with IV corticosteroids and those receiving IV corticosteroid monotherapy [37]. Furthermore, no significantly increased risk of infectious (cyclosporine with IV corticosteroids, RR = 0.54, 95 % CI, 0.17–1.76; infliximab with IV corticosteroids, RR = 0.86, 95 % CI, 0.36–2.09) or noninfectious (cyclosporine with IV corticosteroids, RR = 0.88, 95 % CI, 0.43–1.80; infliximab with IV corticosteroids, RR = 0.40, 95 % CI, 0.15–1.07) postoperative complications was observed in patients treated with cyclosporine or infliximab combined with IV corticosteroids when compared with IV corticosteroids alone [37].

According to a recent systematic review of the literature, remission rates achieved with IV cyclosporine were 91.4 % in four controlled trials and 71.4 % in 18 uncontrolled trials with the lower 2 mg/kg/day dose being safer and as efficacious as the higher, standard 4 mg/kg/day dose [38]. The Cochrane meta-analysis on the efficacy of cyclosporine in severe UC published in 2005 [23] was not able to provide pooled data due to significant differences in design and patient populations in the two randomized controlled trials [20, 29] that were included in the final analysis. Further, they suggested that there is limited evidence supporting superiority of efficacy with short-term treatment with cyclosporine than standard treatment alone for severe UC [23]. It was also suggested that long-term treatment with cyclosporine has unclear benefits due to the risk of adverse events, in particular nephrotoxicity [23]. Recent data from studies comparing cyclosporine and infliximab in severe UC suggest that there is not enough strong evidence to prefer one agent over the other and that results from ongoing randomized controlled trials will likely help to determine the best agent for medical salvage therapy [39]. In the end, early discussions of benefits of surgery with your patient are recommended due to the fact that a delay in offering surgery to a patient may increase the risk of complications, and this population is recognized to carry a 2.8 % mortality given the fact that they have already failed first-line treatment options [39].

There is consensus that cyclosporine therapy should be initiated by experienced physicians who are faced with patients unresponsive to corticosteroids, within the initial week of the flare, and tailored to symptomatology and blood tests.

## Analysis of Long-Term Cyclosporine Therapy

Small prospective and larger retrospective analyses have analyzed the long-term side effects of cyclosporine therapy

prior to subsequent relapse or colectomy [40, 41]. Campbell et al. constructed the largest retrospective database of 76 patients with acute corticosteroid-refractory UC who required treatment with either IV (4 mg/kg/day) or oral (5 mg/kg/day) cyclosporine for a median of 4 days or 4 weeks [40]. Patients who responded (<3 bowel movements/day and C-reactive protein <45 mg/L) to IV or oral cyclosporine rescue therapy underwent long-term treatment with oral cyclosporine for a median of 6 weeks with an initial daily dose of 5 mg/kg that was later titrated to a trough blood level of 150–300 ng/L and were followed for a median of 2.9 years [40]. As soon as patients' corticosteroids were discontinued, treatment with oral azathioprine was initiated concomitantly with oral cyclosporine [40]. Although, overall, an initial remission was achieved by 74 % (56/76) of patients, only 35 % of initial responders maintained their remission by 12 months and 10 % by 36 months, and only 42 % of initial responders were colectomy-free after 84 months of follow-up [40]. Neither duration of treatment with IV hydrocortisone prior to treatment with cyclosporine nor addition of azathioprine to cyclosporine improved time to first relapse or time to surgery [40]. On the other hand, time to the first relapse ($p < 0.01$) and time to the colectomy ($p < 0.05$) were significantly greater in patients treated with oral cyclosporine when compared to IV [40].

These data were further supported by a recent retrospective analysis of the records of 36 patients (38 episodes of cyclosporine use) presenting with acute corticosteroid-refractory UC who, within a median of 8 days after hospitalization, were primarily started on oral cyclosporine (32/38 episodes) at the initial dose of 4.5–8.3 mg/kg/day (six patients were started on IV cyclosporine 2–5 mg/kg/day and switched to oral formulation after 2–8 days). These data showed that 30.5 % (11/36) of the patients immediately failed to respond to cyclosporine within a mean of 6.1 days and underwent colectomy [41]. Among 25 patients who initially responded to cyclosporine and were subsequently discharged on oral cyclosporine (85 % were started on azathioprine within a median of 5 weeks after discharge), 84 % were colectomy-free after a median follow-up of 3.8 years [41].

Another small cohort study evaluated 23 patients treated with oral microemulsion cyclosporine (5 mg/kg/day titrated to blood trough concentration 200 ng/mL) for 3 months due to corticosteroid-refractory or corticosteroid-dependent UC and demonstrated a 70 % clinical response (at least 50 % reduction in clinical activity) rate (16/23 patients) at 3 months [42]. Those who responded to oral cyclosporine were switched to oral azathioprine at the daily dose of 2 mg/kg for a median of 24 months, while nonresponders underwent colectomy [42]. After a median follow-up of 12 months among initial responders, 11 patients were colectomy-free, while 5 underwent colectomy with a chronic response rate of 47 % (11/23 patients) [42]. The study also compared their results with data from the five largest published studies. Their series evaluated 210 patients with ulcerative colitis treated with IV cyclosporine followed by oral formulation with an acute response of 68 % and a chronic response of 42 % [32, 42–46]. It was therefore proposed that the oral microemulsion formulation of cyclosporine may replace IV cyclosporine in treating patients with acute, severe corticosteroid-refractory or corticosteroid-dependent UC [42]. These observations suggest that cyclosporine therapy may have long-term successful outcomes in avoiding colectomy when doses and blood levels are monitored and adverse effects are dealt with on a patient-by-patient basis.

## Alternative Routes of Administration

### Microemulsions

Neoral (Novartis) is an oral microemulsion variant of cyclosporine that has a history of being used in solid-organ transplant immunosuppression in combination with azathioprine and corticosteroids. Similar to IV cyclosporine, this agent has an ability to achieve therapeutic blood concentrations between 150 and 250 ng/dL. When studies have compared these agents, it has been demonstrated that Neoral has similar efficacy with a lower toxicity profile. A short-term open-label retrospective trial was carried out on 40 patients with severe UC. Initial patient dosages followed a 2 mg/kg/day of continuous IV cyclosporine until response was achieved or for a maximum of 14 days with responders being switched to 6–8 mg/kg of oral cyclosporine (Neoral) for 6 months of maintenance treatment [47]. All of the patient's fasting blood levels of cyclosporine were sustained at between 150 and 300 ng/mL for 3–6 months on the oral formula which correlated with their previous IV administration of cyclosporine blood levels [47]. The authors also retrospectively analyzed the cohort of 15 patients with severe, acute corticosteroid-resistant UC who were treated with oral microemulsion cyclosporine at a dose of 5 mg/kg/day for 3 months [47]. In both cohorts, IV cyclosporine followed by oral cyclosporine or oral cyclosporine alone had similar disease severity with equal distribution of left-sided UC and borderline statistically significant differences in frequency of blood transfusions and total parenteral nutrition [47]. On the other hand, all patients treated with IV cyclosporine did not respond to the prior high dose of IV corticosteroids, whereas 43 % of those who were treated only with oral cyclosporine chronically relapsed on a high dose of oral corticosteroids [47]. When comparing oral versus IV cyclosporine only, the patients treated with oral cyclosporine achieved a significantly higher UC remission rate in the short-term (100 % vs 65 %, $p=0.011$), a similar rate of treatment failure (42 % vs 42 %), and a lower, albeit non-significant, decrease in adverse events (0 % vs 17 %, $p=0.171$).

## Enemas

The pharmacokinetics of cyclosporine-retention enemas was assessed in a prospective crossover study that determined that cyclosporine enemas achieve high concentrations within distal colonic tissue with negligible systemic absorption after a single dose in healthy subjects [48]. Initially two small, uncontrolled trials regarding the administration of cyclosporine via enemas were performed in an effort to minimize its systemic toxicity [49, 50]. Data from an open-label study on ten patients presenting with treatment-resistant, left-sided UC showed significant improvement in 50 % of the patients during a 4-week treatment with nightly retention enemas of cyclosporine (350 mg) [49]. Similarly, a small study on 12 patients with distal, refractory UC showed strong correlation between clinical and histologic improvement ($p<0.005$) and a 58 % rate of clinical improvement [50]. However, limited efficacy was observed due to the fact that the continuous UC of many patients from rectum to right-sided colon outpaced the volumetric expansion of the enema.

To deduce if localized UC could benefit from enemas, one controlled trial of 40 patients with mild-to-moderate left-sided colitis was undertaken [51]. This trial observed no clinical benefit from cyclosporine enemas (8 of 20 patients, 40 %) over placebo (9 of 20 patients, 45 %) when dosed at 350 mg/day for 4 weeks [51]. Based on available data, cyclosporine enemas for mild, moderate, or severe UC are not recommended at this time.

## Adverse Events

Many adverse effects seen with cyclosporine are dose dependent and can be reduced or avoided with dosage adjustment. Physicians should remain mindful of these potential complications and have pharmacologic and/or surgical options readily available should the patient's condition necessitate these interventions.

## Infection

Opportunistic infections secondary to immune suppression are a common concern with calcineurin inhibitors such as cyclosporine and regimens that often include steroids as well as azathioprine. Suppressed T cell regulation coupled with a reduction in the inflammatory cytokine response permits *Pneumocystis jiroveci* (*carnii*) (PCP) and community acquired pneumonia (CAP) as well as reactivated cytomegalovirus (CMV) and *Clostridium difficile* (*C. difficile*) infections within patients [52–55]. Considering many severe UC patients will have repetitive hospital admissions, steroid dosing, and concurrent antibiotic therapy in addition to extended immuno-suppression, their risk of infection is increased substantially [56]. CMV reactivation in patients with UC results in a more rapid clinical degradation and higher rates of colectomy [57]. As a result, all patients should have a thorough review of their vaccination history, including Hepatitis B, and risk analysis of possible chronic infections [58]. All live vaccines or prophy-lactic antibiotic dosing should occur prior to immunosuppres-sion with all patients receiving both influenza and pneumococcal vaccines [59–61]. General recommendations include a trimethoprim-sulfamethoxazole dosing schedule (160–800 mg, three times a week) or dapsone, if sulfa allergic, in an effort to ward off infection during treatment, similar to other CD4+-depleted patients [62].

## Diabetes Mellitus

For decades, calcineurin inhibitors have been recognized for their potential to incite new onset diabetes mellitus in trans-plant patients [63]. Although this diabetogenic effect is far less than immunosuppression with steroids, it is still higher than with azathioprine alone [64, 65]. Cyclosporine and other calcineurin inhibitors target intercellular NFAT, the cAMP response element binding (CREB) protein, and the PI3K/Akt (among other) pathways within the beta cells of the pancreas [66]. Inhibition of NFAT has been associated with distur-bances in the gene transcription necessary for insulin release, insulin resistance, and metabolism [64, 67]. Beta-cell toxicity and CREB-activated glucagon-like peptide (GLP-1) have also been implicated in cyclosporine-related diabetes forma-tion [68, 69]. In addition, cyclosporine has been shown to affect both glucose signaling and insulin secretion within beta cells [70]. Despite these disturbances in endocrine pancreas function, the increased induction of diabetes is favorably lowered with a linear decrease in cyclosporine concentration [68].

## Seizures

Seizures should be monitored with high IV drug levels of cyclosporine as they have been appreciated in clinical studies [71]. Seizure onset was witnessed with lower patient choles-terol levels (corresponding with decreased solubility and higher free drug concentration) or seizure threshold-lowering hypomagnesemia [72]. It is necessary to decrease cyclospo-rine dosage to 2 mg/kg in these situations [73]. Additionally, the use of total parenteral nutrition (TPN) with intralipids has been used with the intention of elevating serum lipids. Control of hypertension, correction of hypomagnesemia, and following blood concentration levels of those with hypocho-lesterolemia can greatly reduce seizure risk.

## Nephrotoxicity

Structural and functional nephrotoxicity is a major concern of patients taking cyclosporine [63]. Watchful surveillance of age-related nephrotoxicity is necessary when doses approach 5 mg/kg/day of oral cyclosporine [74]. These increased doses correlate with higher blood concentrations, and studies have found that an increase of more than 30 % in serum creatinine can be used as a predictor of cyclosporine-induced nephropa-thy [73]. Serum creatinine levels can be reduced immediately with a reduction in cyclosporine dosages and blood concen-tration to minimum efficacy levels that induce clinical response (150 ng/dL) [73]. In addition, secondary to the genetic uniqueness of patients, histologic nephrotoxicity can occur even at low, chronic doses [73]. One can consider avoidance of cyclosporine altogether in those patients with preexisting renal disease as reduced doses preclude cyclospo-rine efficacy.

## Miscellaneous

Various studies evaluating adverse reactions to patients treated with cyclosporine noted dose-dependent side effects that included: paresthesias, hyper- and hypotrichosis, increased liver enzymes, hypertension, tremor, headache, nausea and vomiting, hypomagnesemia, hypokalemia, and myalgias [9, 20, 23, 29, 62]. Each of these adverse reactions can be monitored and cyclosporine dosages can be adjusted to minimum trough blood levels of 150 ng/dL. It is important to recognize that different studies report cyclosporine con-centration results by different assays: (1) a monoclonal assay, (2) a polyclonal assay, and (3) an HPLC assay. Secondary therapies can be initiated to reduce these side effects while still harboring the benefits of cyclosporine. Hypertension is generally treated with calcium channel blockers, specifically diltiazem, due to its renal perfusion characteristics. Importantly, diltiazem inhibits cyclosporine liver metabolism so blood cyclosporine concentrations should be monitored and dosage reduced if necessary [73, 75]. Hair loss/gain is reversible with cessation as are headache, nausea, and vomit-ing. If a patient is found to have gingival hyperplasia, an experienced dentist can be consulted to examine its extent and determine the necessity of cyclosporine cessation.

## Outcomes and Long-Term Prognosis

### Maintenance Therapy

To date, most studies of cyclosporine center on the premise of acute symptomatic alleviation. There is limited evidence for maintenance of remission with long-term use of cyclosporine in any patient population. Further, prolonged cyclosporine use in solid-organ transplant antirejection literature mimics the adverse effects seen in UC clinical trials: serious infection risks, nephrotoxicity, hypertension, metabolic effects, and neuropathy [25, 26, 65, 71, 75, 76]. Should remission of a flare occur after the acute use of cyclosporine, maintenance therapy is recommended to prevent further inflammation and relapse of UC. Maintenance therapy is generally a gradual attenuation of steroids to less than 20 mg/day combined with cyclosporine and the addition of azathioprine. Importantly, between 40 and 50 % of patients will avoid colectomy within 2 years when cyclosporine is used prior to maintenance with azathioprine [77]. However, once cyclosporine therapy has been initiated in thiopurine-naïve UC patients, the addition of azathioprine may be necessary to maintain their remission for a minimum of 6 months. Indeed, 2 mg/kg/day of AZA added (if TPMT [thiopurine methyltransferase] enzyme activity is not low) after IV-induced cyclosporine remission of severe, steroid-refractory UC has shown to reduce patient colectomy rates from 60 to 26 % [78, 79]. Should a patient have maximized thiopurine therapy prior to treatment with cyclosporine, a consensus recommends that anti-TNF inhibitors should instead be implemented and the use of cyclosporine should not be considered [31].

## Cyclosporine Refractory Ulcerative Colitis

### Pharmacologic

Up to 48 % of patients initially responding to cyclosporine for acute colitis may become refractory to its immunosuppressive benefits over the long term and proceed to colectomy [41]. Retrospective studies suggest that these patients may benefit from antitumor necrosis factor (TNF) agents as is the case in Crohn's disease (given the lack of demonstrated benefit for cyclosporine in patients with Crohn's disease) [34]. Individuals who attempt the use of cyclosporine initially are not immediate candidates for anti-TNF therapy if they fail given that there has been a high rate of infectious complications observed when implementing this strategy. Similarly, if failure of anti-TNF therapy occurs, cyclosporine use should not be contemplated immediately afterward as similar complications may ensue [19].

### Colectomy

It is important to make an early decision regarding curative surgery or beginning rescue therapy as detailed above. Foremost, experienced physicians can determine if the risk of rescue therapy failure is high enough to proceed with an immediate colectomy with the assistance of a skilled gastrointestinal or colorectal surgeon. While old data prior to the introduction of anti-TNF therapy demonstrated that the evidence is strong that more than eight stools per day stratifies 85 % of patients into an immediate colectomy, this is no longer the case given the advent of cyclosporine and subsequent anti-TNF therapy in our patient population [40].

Up to 80 % of acute steroid-refractory UC flares can be controlled with cyclosporine alone and, if naïve to azathioprine, can avoid colectomy up to 58 % of the time (Fig. 13.2) [31, 34]. A variety of studies have shown that a majority of patients will choose cyclosporine therapy initially to avoid colectomy and that these patients have a better quality of life compared to surgery [80, 81]. Those who fail to suppress severe UC flares and who have maximized thiopurine usage therapy already have the highest risk for colectomy (Fig. 13.2) [31]. The prior use of thiopurines may expose patients to inherent infectious risks and toxicities leading to cyclosporine failure and ultimately colectomy as well [31]. Thus it is recommended that in severe steroid-refractory UC, cyclosporine initiation should be considered a bridge to thiopurine modulation de novo in naïve patients in an effort to decrease colectomy rates in this population (Fig. 13.3) [31].

## Conclusions

Intravenous and oral cyclosporines are each established therapeutic options in corticosteroid-refractory ulcerative colitis and are not inferior to therapy with corticosteroids or infliximab. Both formulations can more successfully delay colectomy in patients with severely active UC, who are also azathioprine naïve and respond to therapy.

It is important for physicians to first recognize if their patient is in an acute, severe UC flare and initially treat the patients with corticosteroids (Fig. 13.4). If the patient has many comorbid conditions (see algorithm) or poor performance status due to age, a colectomy should be considered immediately [77]. If the patient does not respond to steroids within 3–5 days or their UC becomes fulminant based upon any clinical assessment (any variation of Truelove and Witts or Lichtiger scoring) and is fit for potential immunosuppressive therapy, the physician should consider oral or IV cyclosporine, especially in AZA-naïve individuals (AZA-exposed patients can be considered for infliximab therapy). Blood trough levels should be monitored for concentrations ideally between 150 and 250 ng/dL by any of the three measurement assays. In addition, the physician should remain cognizant of symptoms and blood tests that may point toward adverse effects and attenuate cyclosporine dosages accordingly. Should the patient not respond after 5 days, a colectomy should be discussed with the patient and the surgical team. If remission should occur within the first week of cyclosporine therapy, steroids should be tapered, and the patient can be

**Fig. 13.3** Cyclosporine responders avoid colectomy when naïve to thiopurine at higher rates. Stratifying azathioprine (AZA) use by cyclosporine (CSA) response and colectomy. Compared to patients never started on AZA or those who have already been on AZA, patients with steroid-refractory UC and begun on cyclosporine have the highest rates of colectomy avoidance when AZA is started de novo [31]

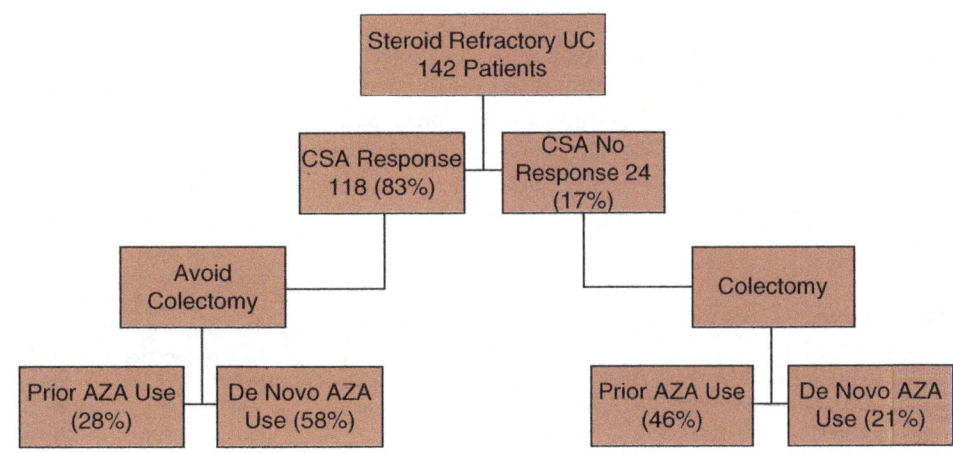

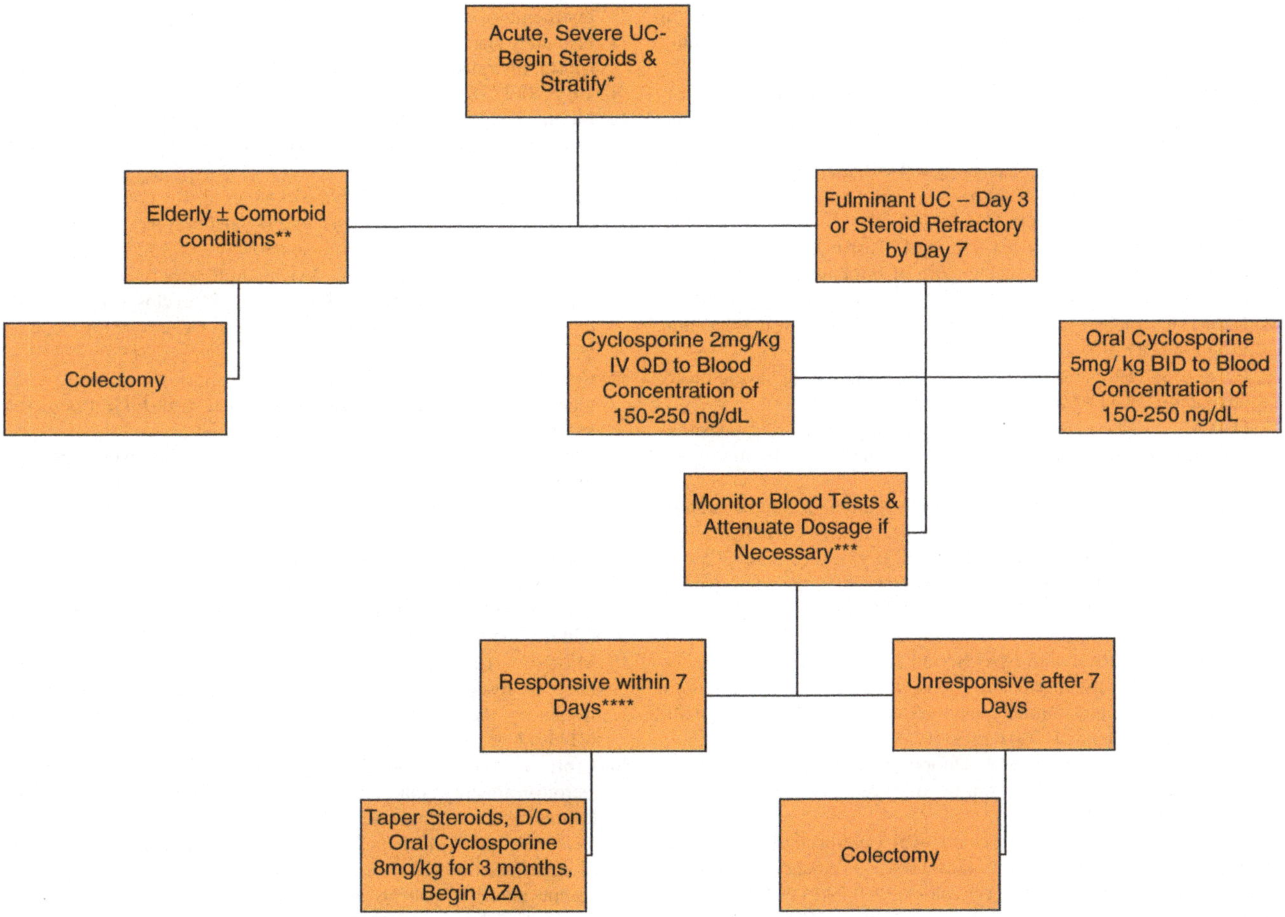

**Fig. 13.4** Recommendation for cyclosporine therapy. Collective recommendation derived from multiple clinical studies. *Stratification of patients based upon acuity, performance status, blood tests, and symptoms. **Comorbid conditions to consider include: renal impairment, active infection, frailty, poor nutrition, and malignancy [77]. ***Blood tests to consider include: cyclosporine trough levels, creatinine, magnesium, cholesterol, and electrolytes. Urine should be tested if necessary in nephrotoxicity cases. ****Responsive is defined as a decrease in frequency of stool, change in consistency of stool, cessation of blood in stool, and decrease in pain associated with bowel movements (Adapted from overall summation of studies included within this chapter)

discharged on oral cyclosporine, 6–8 mg/kg/daily for 3 months, with concomitant AZA, 2 mg/kg/day for up to 6 months.

In summary, bridging corticosteroids to cyclosporine or infliximab plus azathioprine appears to be a potent anti-inflammatory combination in our UC patient population that decreases their symptoms, time in the hospital, and colectomy rates while improving their quality of life.

## References

1. Farmer RG, Easley KA, Rankin GB. Clinical patterns, natural history, and progression of ulcerative colitis. A long-term follow-up of 1116 patients. Dig Dis Sci. 1993;38:1137–46.
2. Doherty GA, Cheifetz AS. Management of acute severe ulcerative colitis. Expert Rev Gastroenterol Hepatol. 2009;3:395–405.
3. Solberg IC, Lygren I, Jahnsen J, et al. Clinical course during the first 10 years of ulcerative colitis: results from a population-based inception cohort (IBSEN Study). Scand J Gastroenterol. 2009;44:431–40.
4. Molodecky NA, Soon IS, Rabi DM, et al. Increasing incidence and prevalence of the inflammatory bowel diseases with time, based on systematic review. Gastroenterology. 2012;142(1):46–54.e42. quiz e30. doi:10.1053/j.gastro.2011.10.001. Epub 2011 Oct 14.
5. Hanauer SB. Inflammatory bowel disease: epidemiology, pathogenesis, and therapeutic opportunities. Inflamm Bowel Dis. 2006;12 Suppl 1:3–9.
6. Lichtenstein GR. Inflammatory bowel disease. In: Goldman L, Schafer AI, editors. Goldman's Cecil medicine. 24th ed. Philadelphia, PA: Elsevier; 2012. p. 913–21.
7. Jostins L, Ripke S, Weersma RK, et al. Host-microbe interactions have shaped the genetic architecture of inflammatory bowel disease. Nature. 2012;491(7422):119–24. doi:10.1038/nature11582.
8. Kerner C, Lichtenstein GR. Digestive Diseases Self-Education Program (DDSEP). 2014. 7.
9. Pham CQD, Efros CB, Berardi RR. Cyclosporine for severe ulcerative colitis. Ann Pharmacother. 2006;41(1):96–101.
10. Hart AL, Al-Hassi HO, Rigby RJ, et al. Characteristics of intestinal dendritic cells in inflammatory bowel diseases. Gastroenterology. 2005;129(1):50–65.
11. Biancone L, Monteleone G, Marasco R, Pallone F. Autoimmunity to tropomyosin isoforms in ulcerative colitis (UC) patients and unaffected relatives. Clin Exp Immunol. 1998;113(2):198–205.
12. Strober W, Fuss IJ. Proinflammatory cytokines in the pathogenesis of inflammatory bowel diseases. Gastroenterology. 2011;140(6):1756–67.
13. Lichtenstein GR, Kamm MA, Boddu P, et al. Effect of once- or twice-daily MMX mesalamine (SPD476) for the induction of remission of mild-to-moderately active ulcerative colitis. Clin Gastroenterol Hepatol. 2007;5:95–102.
14. La Nauze RJ, Sparrow MP. Thiopurine immunomodulators in ulcerative colitis: moving forward with current evidence. Curr Drug Targets. 2011;12(10):1406–12.
15. Dickinson RJ, Ashton MG, Axon AT, et al. Controlled trial of intravenous hyperalimentation and total bowel rest as an adjunct to the routine therapy of acute colitis. Gastroenterology. 1980;79:1199–204.
16. McIntyre PB, Powell-Tuck J, Wood SR, et al. Controlled trial of bowel rest in the treatment of severe acute colitis. Gut. 1986;27:481–5.
17. Truelove SC, Witts LJ. Cortisone in ulcerative colitis; preliminary report on a therapeutic trial. Br Med J. 1954;2:375–8.
18. Truelove SC, Witts LJ. Cortisone in ulcerative colitis; final report on a therapeutic trial. Br Med J. 1955;2:1041–8.
19. Kornbluth A, Sachar DB. Ulcerative colitis practice guidelines in adults: American College Of Gastroenterology, Practice Parameters Committee. Am J Gastroenterol. 2010;105(3):501–23. doi:10.1038/ajg.2009.727. quiz 524.
20. D'Haens G, Lemmens L, Geboes K, et al. Intravenous cyclosporine versus intravenous corticosteroids as single therapy for severe attacks of ulcerative colitis. Gastroenterology. 2001;120(6):1323–9.
21. Martínez-Martínez S, Redondo JM. Inhibitors of the calcineurin/NFAT pathway. Curr Med Chem. 2004;11(8):997–1007.
22. Borel JF, Kis ZL. The discovery and development of cyclosporine (Sandimmune). Transplant Proc. 1991;23(2):1867–74.
23. Shibolet O, Regushevskaya E, Brezis M, Soares-Weiser K. Cyclosporine A for induction of remission in severe ulcerative colitis. Cochrane Database Syst Rev. 2005;1, CD004277.
24. Von Wartburg A, Traber R. Cyclosporins, fungal metabolites with immunosuppressive activities. Prog Med Chem. 1988;25:1–33.
25. Kapturczak MH, Meier-Kriesche HU, Kaplan B. Pharmacology of calcineurin antagonists. Transplant Proc. 2004;36(2 Suppl):25S–32.
26. Venkataramanan R, Starzl TE, Yang S, et al. Biliary excretion of cyclosporine in liver transplant patients. Transplant Proc. 1985;17(1):286–9.
27. Kovarik JM, Mueller EA, van Bree JB, et al. Reduced inter- and intraindividual variability in cyclosporine pharmacokinetics from a microemulsion formulation. J Pharm Sci. 1994;83(3):444–6.
28. Friman S, Bäckman L. A new microemulsion formulation of cyclosporin: pharmacokinetic and clinical features. Clin Pharmacokinet. 1996;30(3):181–93.
29. Lichtiger S, Present DH, Kornbluth A, et al. Cyclosporine in severe ulcerative colitis refractory to steroid therapy. N Engl J Med. 1994;330:1841–5.
30. Van Assche G, D'Haens G, Noman M, et al. Randomized, double-blind comparison of 4 mg/kg versus 2 mg/kg intravenous cyclosporine in severe ulcerative colitis. Gastroenterology. 2003;125:1025–31.
31. Moskovitz DN, Van Assche G, Maenhout B, et al. Incidence of colectomy during long-term follow-up after cyclosporine-induced remission of severe ulcerative colitis. Clin Gastroenterol Hepatol. 2006;4:760–5.
32. Cohen RD, Stein R, Hanauer SB. Intravenous cyclosporin in ulcerative colitis: a five-year experience. Am J Gastroenterol. 1999;94:1587–92.
33. Chang KH, Burke JP, Coffey JC. Infliximab versus cyclosporine as rescue therapy in acute severe steroid-refractory ulcerative colitis: a systematic review and meta-analysis. Int J Colorectal Dis. 2013;28:287–93.
34. Laharie D, Bourreille A, Branche J, et al. Ciclosporin versus infliximab in patients with severe ulcerative colitis refractory to intravenous steroids: a parallel, open-label randomised controlled trial. Lancet. 2012;380:1909–15.
35. Maser EA, Deconda D, Lichtiger S, et al. Cyclosporine and infliximab as rescue therapy for each other in patients with steroid-refractory ulcerative colitis. Clin Gastroenterol Hepatol. 2008;6:1112–6.
36. Croft A, Walsh A, Doecke J. Outcomes of salvage therapy for steroid-refractory acute severe ulcerative colitis: ciclosporin vs infliximab. Aliment Pharmacol Ther. 2013;38:294–302.
37. Nelson R, Liao C, Fichera A, et al. Rescue therapy with cyclosporine or infliximab is not associated with an increased risk for postoperative complications in patients hospitalized for severe steroid-refractory ulcerative colitis. Inflamm Bowel Dis. 2014;20:14–20.
38. Garcia-Lopez S, Gomollon-Garcia F, Perez-Gisbert J. Cyclosporine in the treatment of severe attack of ulcerative colitis: a systematic review. Gastroenterol Hepatol. 2005;28:607–14.
39. Rolny P, Vatn M. Cyclosporine in patients with severe steroid refractory ulcerative colitis in the era of infliximab. Scand J Gastroenterol. 2013;48:131–5.

40. Campbell S, Travis S, Jewell D. Ciclosporin use in acute ulcerative colitis: a long-term experience. Eur J Gastroenterol Hepatol. 2005;17:79–84.

41. Sharkey L, Bredin F, Nightingale A, et al. The use of Cyclosporin A in acute steroid-refractory ulcerative colitis: long term outcomes. J Crohns Colitis. 2011;5:91–4.

42. Actis GC, Lagget M, Rizzetto M, et al. Long-term efficacy of oral microemulsion cyclosporin for refractory ulcerative colitis. Minerva Med. 2004;95:65–70.

43. Actis GC, Pinna-Pintor M. An audit of the immunosuppressive management of ulcerative colitis. A retrospective chart review from a referral Day-Hospital of Gastroenterology. Minerva Gastroenterol Dietol. 2002;48:115–20.

44. Carbonnel F, Boruchowicz A, Duclos B, et al. Intravenous cyclosporine in attacks of ulcerative colitis: short-term and long-term responses. Dig Dis Sci. 1996;41:2471–6.

45. Hyde GM, Thillainayagam AV, Jewell DP. Intravenous cyclosporin as rescue therapy in severe ulcerative colitis: time for a reappraisal? Eur J Gastroenterol Hepatol. 1998;10:411–3.

46. McCormack G, McCormick PA, Hyland JM, et al. Cyclosporin therapy in severe ulcerative colitis: is it worth the effort? Dis Colon Rectum. 2002;45:1200–5.

47. Actis GC, Aimo G, Priolo G, et al. Efficacy and efficiency of oral microemulsion cyclosporin versus intravenous and soft gelatin capsule cyclosporin in the treatment of severe steroid-refractory ulcerative colitis: an open-label retrospective trial. Inflamm Bowel Dis. 1998;4:276–9.

48. Sandborn WJ, Strong RM, Forland SC, et al. The pharmacokinetics and colonic tissue concentrations of cyclosporine after i.v., oral, and enema administration. J Clin Pharmacol. 1991;31:76–80.

49. Sandborn WJ, Tremaine WJ, Schroeder KW, et al. Cyclosporine enemas for treatment-resistant, mildly to moderately active, left-sided ulcerative colitis. Am J Gastroenterol. 1993;88:640–5.

50. Winter TA, Dalton HR, Merrett MN, et al. Cyclosporin A retention enemas in refractory distal ulcerative colitis and 'pouchitis'. Scand J Gastroenterol. 1993;28:701–4.

51. Sandborn WJ, Tremaine WJ, Schroeder KW, et al. A placebo-controlled trial of cyclosporine enemas for mildly to moderately active left-sided ulcerative colitis. Gastroenterology. 1994;106:1429–35.

52. de Saussure P, Lavergne-Slove A, Mazeron MC, et al. A prospective assessment of cytomegalovirus infection in active inflammatory bowel disease. Aliment Pharmacol Ther. 2004;20:1323–7.

53. Takahashi Y, Tange T. Prevalence of cytomegalovirus infection in inflammatory bowel disease patients. Dis Colon Rectum. 2004;47:722–6.

54. Issa M, Vijayapal A, Graham MB, et al. Impact of Clostridium difficile on inflammatory bowel disease. Clin Gastroenterol Hepatol. 2007;5:345–51.

55. Schneeweiss S, Korzenik J, Solomon DH, et al. Infliximab and other immunomodulating drugs in patients with inflammatory bowel disease and the risk of serious bacterial infections. Aliment Pharmacol Ther. 2009;30:253–64.

56. Nguyen GC, Kaplan GG, Harris ML, Brant SR. A national survey of the prevalence and impact of Clostridium difficile infection among hospitalized inflammatory bowel disease patients. Am J Gastroenterol. 2008;103:1443–50.

57. Minami M, Ohta M, Ohkura T, et al. Cytomegalovirus infection in severe ulcerative colitis patients undergoing continuous intravenous cyclosporine treatment in Japan. World J Gastroenterol. 2007;13(5):754–60.

58. Melmed GY. Vaccination strategies for patients with inflammatory bowel disease on immunomodulators and biologics. Inflamm Bowel Dis. 2009;15:1410–6.

59. Melmed GY, Agarwal N, Frenck RW, et al. Immunosuppression impairs response to pneumococcal polysaccharide vaccination in patients with inflammatory bowel disease. Am J Gastroenterol. 2010;105:148–54.

60. Sands BE, Cuffari C, Katz J, et al. Guidelines for immunizations in patients with inflammatory bowel disease. Inflamm Bowel Dis. 2004;10:677–92. 485.

61. Esteve M, Saro C, Gonzalez-Huix F, et al. Chronic hepatitis B reactivation following infliximab therapy in Crohn's disease patients: need for primary prophylaxis. Gut. 2004;53:1363–5.

62. Cheifetz AS, Stern J, Garud S, et al. Cyclosporine is safe and effective in patients with severe ulcerative colitis. J Clin Gastroenterol. 2011;45:107–12.

63. Azzi JR, Sayegh MH, Mallat SG. Calcineurin inhibitors: 40 years later, can't live without. J Immunol. 2013;191(12):5785–91. doi:10.4049/jimmunol.1390055.

64. Heisel O, Heisel R, Balshaw R, Keown P. New onset diabetes mellitus in patients receiving calcineurin inhibitors: a systematic review and meta-analysis. Am J Transplant. 2004;4(4):583–95. doi:10.1046/j.1600-6143.2003.00372.x.

65. Yoshimura N, Nakai I, Ohmori Y, et al. Effect of cyclosporine on the endocrine and exocrine pancreas in kidney transplant recipients. Am J Kidney Dis. 1998;12(1):11–7.

66. Demozay D, Tsunekawa S, Briaud I, et al. Specific glucose-induced control of insulin receptor substrate-2 expression is mediated via Ca2+-dependent calcineurin/NFAT signaling in primary pancreatic islet β-cells. Diabetes. 2011;60(11):2892–902. doi:10.2337/db11-034.

67. Weir MR, Fink JC. Risk for posttransplant diabetes mellitus with current immunosuppressive medications. Am J Kidney Dis. 1999;34(1):1–13. doi:10.1053/AJKD03400001.

68. Hahn HJ, Dunger A, Laube F, et al. Reversibility of the acute toxic effect of cyclosporin A on pancreatic B cells of Wistar rats. Diabetologia. 1986;29(8):489–94.

69. Arnette D, Gibson TB, Lawrence MC, et al. Regulation of ERK1 and ERK2 by glucose and peptide hormones in pancreatic beta cells. J Biol Chem. 2003;278(35):32517–25. doi:10.1074/jbc.M301174200.

70. Nielsen JH, Mandrup-Poulsen T, Nerup J. Direct effects of cyclosporin A on human pancreatic beta-cells. Diabetes. 1986;35(9):1049–52.

71. Wijdicks EF, Wiesner RH, Krom RA. Neurotoxicity in liver transplant recipients with cyclosporine immunosuppression. Neurology. 1995;45(11):1962–4.

72. Miller LW. Cyclosporine-associated neurotoxicity: the need for a better guide for immunosuppressive therapy. Circulation. 1996;94(6):1209–11. doi:10.1161/01.CIR.94.6.1209.

73. Sternthal MB, Murphy SJ, George J, et al. Adverse events associated with the use of cyclosporine in patients with inflammatory bowel disease. Am J Gastroenterol. 2008;103:937–43.

74. Kubo M, Kiyohara Y, Kato I, et al. Risk factors for renal glomerular and vascular changes in an autopsy-based population survey: the Hisayama study. Kidney Int. 2003;63:1508–15.

75. Bleck JS, Thiesemann C, Kliem V, et al. Diltiazem increases blood concentrations of cyclized cyclosporine metabolites resulting in different cyclosporine metabolite patterns in stable male and female renal allograft recipients. Br J Clin Pharmacol. 1996;41(6):551–6.

76. Krentz AJ, Dousset B, Mayer D, et al. Metabolic effects of cyclosporin A and FK 506 in liver transplant recipients. Diabetes. 1993;42(12):1753–9.

77. Durai D, Hawthorne AB. Review article: how and when to use ciclosporin in ulcerative colitis. Aliment Pharmacol Ther. 2005;22:907–16.

78. Fernandez-Banares F, Bertran X, Esteve-Comas M, et al. Azathioprine is useful in maintaining long-term remission induced by intravenous cyclosporine in steroid-refractory severe ulcerative colitis. Am J Gastroenterol. 1996;91:2498–9.

79. Maser EA, Deconda D, Lichtiger S, et al. Cyclosporine and infliximab as rescue therapy for each other in patients with steroid-refractory ulcerative colitis. Clin Gastroenterol Hepatol. 2008;6(10):1112–6.

80. Siegel CA, Schwartz LM, Woloshin S, et al. When should ulcerative colitis patients undergo colectomy for dysplasia? Mismatch between patient preferences and physician recommendations. Inflamm Bowel Dis. 2010;16(10):1658–62. doi:10.1002/ibd.21233.

81. Kaplan GG, Seow CH, Ghosh S, et al. Decreasing colectomy rates for ulcerative colitis: a population-based time trend study. Am J Gastroenterol. 2012;107(12):1879–87. doi:10.1038/ajg.2012.333.

# Tacrolimus, Sirolimus, and Mycophenolate Mofetil

Andreas Fischer and Daniel C. Baumgart

**Keywords**

Tacrolimus • Sirolimus • Mycophenolate mofetil • Ulcerative colitis • Corticosteroid-refractory ulcerative colitis • Medical therapy • Calcineurin inhibitors

## Tacrolimus

When cyclosporine was introduced as rescue therapy for corticosteroid-refractory ulcerative colitis in the early 1990s, this marked a turning point in the management of these patients, for many of which colectomy had been the only remaining therapeutic option [1, 2]. Since then, the value of cyclosporine has been confirmed in numerous studies [3], and a recent randomized controlled trial carried out at 27 European inflammatory bowel disease centers found that its efficacy for inducing remission in severe ulcerative colitis refractory to intravenous steroids equaled that of infliximab [4]. However, the safety profile of cyclosporine, especially in the long run, appears rather unfavorable. Neurological side effects such as paresthesias, nephrotoxicity, hypertension, headache, and gingival hyperplasia have been reported in up to one third of patients [2, 3]. In addition, intravenous administration with therapeutic drug monitoring is generally required, although an oral formulation of cyclosporine exists.

As a consequence, an intense search for novel calcineurin inhibitors commenced which led to the isolation of a macro-

lide produced by *Streptomyces tsukubaensis* initially termed FK-506 in 1987 that was later renamed into tacrolimus (for Tsukuba macrolide immunosuppressant) [5]. Similar to cyclosporine, tacrolimus acts by inhibiting calcineurin, a phosphatase required for the translocation of the transcription factor NFAT (nuclear factor of activated T cells) into the nucleus, where it controls production of interleukin-2 in T lymphocytes. In addition, inhibition of other transcription factors such as NF-κB or Oct-1 has been demonstrated for these compounds, and consequently, both cyclosporine and tacrolimus act primarily by inhibiting T cell activation, although direct effects on B cell activation have been reported as well [6, 7].

While cyclosporine and tacrolimus exert similar effects, their mechanism of action differs with cyclosporine binding to cyclophilin and tacrolimus to a protein termed FKBP (for FK binding protein) that belongs to a group of cytosolic peptidylprolyl isomerases called immunophilins [7]. Due to this differential mode of action, the immunosuppressive potency of tacrolimus vastly exceeds that of cyclosporine [5, 6]. Moreover, both compounds exhibit important differences in terms of pharmacokinetics, and oral absorption of tacrolimus is more reliable compared to cyclosporine as it does not depend on bile flow or integrity of the intestinal mucosa. As a consequence, tacrolimus gradually replaced cyclosporine in many indications within transplantation medicine, which consequently piqued an interest in its potential usability in ulcerative colitis.

This development was paralleled by encouraging data obtained in animal models of IBD [8–11] and an anecdotal series with tacrolimus treatment of Crohn's disease and ulcerative colitis as early as 1993 [6]. However, it was not

A. Fischer, M.D. • D.C. Baumgart, M.D., Ph.D. (✉)
Department of Medicine, Division of Gastroenterology and
Hepatology Charité Medical Center - Virchow Hospital
Medical School of the Humboldt- University of Berlin,
Augustenburger Platz 1, 13353 Berlin, Germany
e-mail: andi.fischer@charite.de; daniel.baumgart@charite.de

G.R. Lichtenstein (ed.), *Medical Therapy of Ulcerative Colitis*,
DOI 10.1007/978-1-4939-1677-1_14, © Springer Science+Business Media New York 2014

until 1998 that a first detailed description of its use in adults was published in a form of a small open-label, uncontrolled pilot study. In this trial, 11 patients suffering from acute flares of ulcerative colitis or Crohn's disease refractory to a standard therapy consisting of corticosteroids, azathioprine, and mesalamine received intravenous tacrolimus after about a week of unsuccessful intravenous steroid treatment [12]. Within 10 days, 9 out of the 11 patients displayed a favorable response, whereas the remaining 2 patients underwent colectomy. Subsequent case series involving 9–40 ulcerative colitis patients confirmed these data [13–15], and as a consequence, a first randomized multicenter trial on the use of tacrolimus in ulcerative colitis was published in 2006 [16]. This study compared two arms with low (5–10 ng/ml) and high (10–15 ng/ml) trough levels to a placebo group in a total of 60 hospitalized patients with moderately or severely active left-sided colitis or pancolitis and was carried out in 17 centers in Japan. Response as indicated by a drop in the disease activity score of more than 4 was observed in 68 % of patients in the high-dose group as compared to 10 % in the placebo group ($p<0.001$) within 2 weeks of therapy. Similarly, more patients receiving the low dose displayed a clinical response (38 %), although statistical significance was not met in this group, most likely due to the small number of patients analyzed. Although this study has been criticized for its low number of patients and the potential inclusion of patients with less severe disease [17], it provided the first data on the short-term efficacy of tacrolimus in a randomized design.

Later on, the same group published results from a second double-blind placebo-controlled trial that involved 62 hospitalized patients with steroid-dependent or steroid-refractory disease and employed target tacrolimus trough levels of 10–15 ng/ml. Again, the primary endpoint was clinical response after 2 weeks of therapy as indicated by a drop in the disease activity index of at least 4 points which was met by 50 % in the tacrolimus group as opposed to 13.3 % in the placebo group ($p=0.003$). Rates for mucosal healing (44 % vs. 13 %) and clinical remission (9 % vs. 0 %) were also higher in the tacrolimus group, although the latter difference was not statistically significant. None of the patients required colectomy during a 12-week open-label extension, which again raised objections on whether disease severity might have been lower than in other case series that reported colectomy rates between 10 and 50 % [18]. Although the incidence of adverse events in both prospective trials was reported to be not significantly different between the tacrolimus and placebo groups, experiences coming from the use of tacrolimus in other indications demonstrated that it is associated with infections, nephrotoxicity, changes in glucose metabolism, and neurological adverse events such as tremor or paresthesias [19, 20], suggesting that the apparent lack of relevant side effects in these trials might have been due to the short time of treatment and/or follow-up. Data from uncontrolled observational studies furthermore suggest that even when used for short times, tacrolimus therapy might be associated with side effects in up to 50 % of patients, although, in these series, the majority of adverse reactions were mild and very rarely required discontinuation of therapy [13–21].

In summary, the available evidence provides support for tacrolimus in the induction of remission when treatment with corticosteroids has failed. However, head-to-head comparison studies with infliximab and/or cyclosporine have not been conducted to date. Nonetheless, national and international professional societies have adopted tacrolimus into their current treatment guidelines for refractory ulcerative colitis [22, 23]. A target serum trough concentration of 10–15 ng/ml is supported by both Ogata trials, although several case series including more than 100 patients have demonstrated efficacy for trough levels below 10 ng/ml as well [13, 21, 24]. Thus, further appropriately designed trials will be required to determine the optimal dose of tacrolimus.

When administering the drug orally, target levels will be reached faster when therapy is started with higher doses (0.1–0.2 mg/kg daily divided into two doses), especially when patients are allowed to eat [3]. However, special caution has to be exercised in this scenario, and monitoring of drug serum levels is advised daily for the first days of therapy in order to avoid adverse effects due to overdosage. Alternatively, tacrolimus therapy can be initiated by continuous intravenous infusion in hospitalized patients in order to reach target levels faster. As a result of its narrow therapeutic window and its metabolization via the cytochrome C system (in particular CYP3A4), special caution is advised with respect to potential drug interactions, e.g., with macrolide antibiotics, certain antiepileptic and antifungal drugs, and antiretroviral medications [25].

Given the substantial risk of adverse reactions associated with systemic immunosuppression, strategies aimed at delivering pharmaceutical compounds selectively to sites of inflammation could pose an important improvement to the therapeutic options in ulcerative colitis. So far, both direct rectal application and use of carriers that facilitate drug release specifically to areas of inflamed mucosa have been tested. With respect to the first strategy, a report published in 2008 presented data from a total of eight patients suffering from either ulcerative proctitis, left-sided colitis, or extensive ulcerative colitis that had failed previous treatment with oral and rectal mesalamine, immunomodulators, and steroids [26]. After 8 weeks of rectal tacrolimus, remission was achieved in six out of these eight patients, and steroids could be reduced or discontinued in seven patients. Trough serum levels varied between undetectable and concentrations as high as 7 ng/ml, and no systemic adverse effects were reported. A second case series described a total of 17 patients treated with suppositories or enemas prepared from tacrolimus capsules. After 4 weeks of therapy, a clinical response was observed in 10 out of 12 (83 %) patients suffering from proctitis refractory to conventional therapy and 3 out of 5 (60 %)

patients with left-sided colitis with a total of 5 patients showing mucosal healing by the end of therapy [27]. Again, no systemic side effects were observed with average whole blood trough levels of 2.5 and 0.7 ng/ml in patients receiving enemas or suppositories containing 2 mg tacrolimus, respectively, whereas peak tacrolimus concentrations measured in mucosal biopsies exceeded 100 ng/ml on an average. Taken together, these data suggest that topical application of tacrolimus might constitute a promising approach in particular for ulcerative proctitis refractory to standard therapy and further prospective, randomized studies in this challenging group of patients would be highly desirable.

It is conceivable, however, that the value of rectally administered tacrolimus will be limited when disease extends beyond the left flexure and strategies to modify pharmacokinetics in a way that allows selective release of the drug in areas of inflamed mucosa might represent an approach better suited for these cases. In this respect, it has been noted that mucus production is increased in inflamed mucosa, and evidence has been provided that this results in increased adhesion and selective accumulation of nanoparticle carriers in these areas [28]. As in addition, both paracellular permeability and local density of lymphocytes increase with active inflammation; these changes might provide a basis for the development of carriers able to selectively release immunomodulators to inflamed mucosa. Pilot studies with tacrolimus entrapped into nanoparticles yielded promising results in two animal models of colitis and demonstrated significantly increased concentrations of the drug in inflamed tissue as compared to healthy mucosa [29]. Modifications of this approach include coupling of nanoparticles with pH-sensitive microspheres to further increase specificity of drug delivery to areas of actively inflamed mucosa, and although up to now no clinical data are available for this approach, animal models provided first encouraging results supporting this concept [30, 31].

A key drawback of most studies on the use of tacrolimus in ulcerative colitis is the lack of data concerning its long-term safety and efficacy, and neither of the prospective randomized trials described above reported follow-up data beyond 12 weeks. Several case series tried to address this issue by investigating the long-term outcomes of patients in which remission was induced by tacrolimus and reported colectomy-free rates between 66 and 77.5 % within up to 39 months [13, 32, 33]. While these data indicate that colectomy can be avoided or at least delayed in a substantial percentage of patients who achieve remission upon treatment with tacrolimus, they do not allow for an assessment of its impact on maintaining remission as the majority of patients in these studies received maintenance therapy with thiopurines or biologics. To date, the only study investigating a potential role for tacrolimus in the maintenance of remission is a case series with 24 patients who were either thiopurine naive or intolerant (15 patients) or had previously failed

maintenance therapy with thiopurines (9 patients). Treatment with tacrolimus for up to 3 years was compared to a retrospective control group of 34 patients receiving thiopurines as the standard therapy [34]. Among the subgroup naive or intolerant to thiopurines, remission (as defined by a Truelove-Witts severity index of 4 or less) was maintained after 1 and 3 years in 51 % and 19 %, respectively, as compared to 59 % and 36 % in patients receiving maintenance therapy with azathioprine or 6-MP. Although this difference did not reach statistical significance, again presumably due to the insufficient number of patients included, these observations seem to favor the use of thiopurines for maintenance of remission over tacrolimus in patients tolerating these compounds. Remission rates were even lower for patients who previously failed azathioprine therapy (25 % and 0 % after 1 and 3 years, respectively) with a significantly lower relapse-free survival compared to the control group receiving thiopurines for maintenance of remission. Adverse events requiring drug withdrawal occurred in 16.7 % of patients receiving tacrolimus compared to 14.7 % patients in the thiopurine group for infections (one patient receiving a combination of tacrolimus and azathioprine), rise in serum creatinine levels (tacrolimus), or leukopenia, pancreatitis, or nausea (thiopurine group). Other side effects observed with long-term tacrolimus therapy included tremor and impaired renal function (21 % and 17 %, respectively). Another small series demonstrated that tacrolimus therapy was effective for inducing clinical and endoscopic remission of steroid-refractory/steroid-dependent UC [35]. Endoscopic improvement was associated with favorable medium- and long-term prognosis. This study was retrospective and evaluated the medical records of 51 patients treated with tacrolimus for ulcerative colitis. Clinical remission and improvement were defined as a Lichtiger score of 4 or less and as a Lichtiger score of ≤10 and a reduction in the score of ≥3 compared with the baseline score, respectively. Endoscopic findings were evaluated based on the endoscopic activity index and Mayo endoscopic score. The endpoint, termed "clinical effectiveness" (as measured by a combination of clinical remission and improvement), was seen in 62.7 % of the patients at 3 months. Thirty-six patients underwent colonoscopy at 3 months, with 33.3 % (12 patients) and 27.8 % (10 patients) showing Mayo endoscopic scores of 0 and 1, respectively. On Kaplan-Meier analysis, the overall percentage of event-free survivors, who did not require colectomy nor switching to other induction therapy such as infliximab, was 73.0 % at 6 months, 49.9 % at 1 year, and 37.8 % at 2 years. Patients with a Mayo endoscopic score of 0–1 at 3 months showed significantly better medium- and long-term prognosis than those with a score of 2–3 (p<0.01). Thus the finding of early mucosal healing was associated with a better long-term prognosis.

Therefore, although data are sparse, it appears that tacrolimus, while showing short-term efficacy, has only limited value for maintaining remission. Based on the current evidence, its place within the therapeutic armamentarium therefore resembles that of cyclosporine. It can be used to quickly induce remission in severe steroid-refractory ulcerative colitis and serve as a bridging agent until thiopurines started in parallel become effective. Caution and tight monitoring are needed with this strategy as patients receiving combined immunosuppression are particularly prone to infection [36, 37].

## Sirolimus

Sirolimus, another macrolide, was originally named rapamycin after its isolation from a soil sample derived from Easter Island (or Rapa Nui in the native language). It is produced by *Streptomyces hygroscopicus* and was initially characterized as a powerful antifungal compound [38, 39]. Further analyses, however, revealed its potent cytostatic and immunosuppressive activities, and as a result, sirolimus and its derivative everolimus are currently being used or evaluated for the treatment of a variety of pathological conditions including certain cancers [40], graft-versus-host disease [41], and polycystic kidney disease [42]. Although sirolimus resembles tacrolimus structurally and binds to the same intracellular target FKBP12, its mode of action does not involve inhibition of calcineurin signaling. Instead, the sirolimus-FKBP12 complex inhibits a serine/threonine kinase termed mTOR (for mammalian target of rapamycin) that is of pivotal importance for a variety of key developmental and cell biological functions [7, 43]. A fast growing body of evidence has revealed that this inhibition results in impaired function of dendritic cells and reduced T cell proliferation and associated mTOR signaling with the control of T cell antigen responsiveness [44]. In addition, mTOR has been demonstrated to have a key role in the regulation of autophagy [45] which in turn emerged as a pivotal component in the pathogenesis of inflammatory bowel diseases [46]. Thus, from a pathophysiological point of view, mTOR inhibition might hold some potential in the treatment of inflammatory bowel diseases. This is furthermore supported by results from animal studies in which sirolimus and P2281, a novel mTOR inhibitor, effectively improved histologic inflammation in the DSS model of colitis [47, 48]. Moreover, the rapamycin derivative everolimus significantly ameliorated colitis in the IL10$^{-/-}$ model [49]. However, while case reports published in 2008 described significant improvement of two Crohn's disease patients who previously failed established therapies upon treatment with sirolimus [50] and everolimus [51], a prospective randomized double-blind trial comparing everolimus to placebo and azathioprine for the treatment of moderately to severely active Crohn's disease was prematurely terminated for lack of efficacy [52]. In this study, a total of 144 patients were enrolled when an interim analysis after 7 months suggested that everolimus was not superior to placebo for inducing a steroid-free remission. In addition, everolimus did not exert a positive effect on disease activity markers or quality of life, and 66 % of patients receiving the drug discontinued therapy, mostly for lack of efficacy. Given these results, it appears rather unlikely that future studies will further investigate mTOR inhibitors in the therapy of ulcerative colitis or Crohn's disease.

## Mycophenolate Mofetil

Mycophenolate mofetil (MMF) is the oral ester prodrug of mycophenolic acid (MPA), a compound synthesized by *Penicillium brevicompactum* and related species [53]. MPA acts by reversibly inhibiting inosine-5′-monophosphate dehydrogenase (IMPDH), thereby preventing de novo guanosine synthesis. The resulting deprivation of deoxyguanosine triphosphate ultimately leads to reduced DNA synthesis [54]. Importantly, MPA preferentially inhibits the type II isoform of IMPDH that is almost exclusively expressed in activated T and B lymphocytes. As, in addition, lymphocytes critically depend on the de novo synthesis of guanosine triphosphate whereas salvage pathways exist in most other cells, MPA is relatively specific in its immunosuppressive mode of action and has been widely employed for the prevention of allograft rejection following solid organ transplantation [55].

A potential role for MMF in the treatment of inflammatory bowel diseases was first studied in Crohn's disease. A small open-label single-center randomized trial published in 1999 found that treatment of patients suffering from moderately active Crohn's disease with a combination of corticosteroids and MMF induced a Crohn's disease activity index (CDAI) drop comparable to that observed with a combination of corticosteroids and azathioprine [56]. In contrast, patients with an initial CDAI > 300 displayed a significantly greater decrease in CDAI during the first month of treatment with MMF and prednisolone compared with the azathioprine/prednisolone group. This advantage, however, was lost as treatment continued, probably reflecting the delayed onset of action of azathioprine. Subsequent studies failed to demonstrate a significant benefit in the treatment of Crohn's disease [57–59], and a multicenter, international, randomized, double-blind, controlled trial to evaluate the efficacy of MMF in refractory Crohn's disease was prematurely terminated by the sponsor (officially citing slow recruitment) [59].

In ulcerative colitis, only a single prospective trial investigating the impact of MMF was published. In this open-label study, 24 patients with active ulcerative colitis were randomly assigned to receive a combination of prednisolone with either MMF or azathioprine for up to 1 year. Remission rates were found to be higher in the azathioprine group throughout the study, and fewer patients receiving MMF were able to discontinue steroid treatment. In addition, while no severe adverse events were recorded in patients receiving azathioprine, 2 out of 12 patients had to be withdrawn from the trial in the MMF group for recurrent upper airway infections and a case of bacterial meningitis [60].

Experiences with MMF in patients refractory or intolerant to azathioprine were described in a retrospective series coming from a single center in the UK. In this study, 6 out of 19 patients (31 %) treated with MMF achieved steroid-free remission, whereas 11 (58 %) failed therapy and 2 (11 %) had to discontinue treatment because of side effects. No details on the duration of therapy or the frequency of relapses among ulcerative colitis patients were given in this report [61].

While these data, although sparse, might suggest that MMF is inferior to azathioprine in the treatment of ulcerative colitis but could represent an alternative option for patients intolerant or refractory to thiopurines, long-standing experiences with MMF in transplantation medicine revealed several key issues excluding its use in inflammatory bowel diseases. Most importantly, MMF has long been known to harbor the risk of intestinal mucosal damage itself, which includes the induction of colonic ulcerations [62]. Among kidney transplant patients receiving MMF as part of their immunosuppressive regime, afebrile, chronic diarrhea occurs as one of the most frequent adverse and difficult to manage events, many times resulting in discontinuation of the drug [63]. Prospective trials investigating this phenomenon found that while opportunistic infections were responsible in about 60 % of cases, the rest of the patients exhibited an erosive enterocolitis with a Crohn's disease-like pattern that correlated with MPA trough levels and resolved upon cessation of MMF (which, however, led to allograft rejection in a considerable percentage of these patients) [64]. Endoscopic and histologic evaluation of colonic biopsies from such patients frequently revealed signs of mucosal damage with focal crypt distortion, cryptitis, and increased apoptosis being the predominant pattern of injury [64–66]. These findings might not be confined to patients having received a transplant as illustrated by a case series describing the appearance of an atypical colitis in two out of five ulcerative colitis patients treated with MMF. Histologic evaluation of biopsies from these patients that received MMF doses much lower than that employed in transplant medicine revealed features not typical for inflammatory bowel disease but suggestive of a drug-induced colitis similar to that described in transplant patients [67]. Furthermore, MMF treatment has been associated with a higher incidence of lymphoproliferative disorders compared to azathioprine [68], and substantial evidence points to a teratogenic potential of this compound [69]. Taken together, MMF should not be used in inflammatory bowel disease.

# References

1. Lichtiger S, Present DH, Kornbluth A, et al. Cyclosporine in severe ulcerative colitis refractory to steroid therapy. N Engl J Med. 1994;330:1841–5.
2. Lichtiger S, Present DH. Preliminary report: cyclosporin in treatment of severe active ulcerative colitis. Lancet. 1990;336:16–9.
3. Naganuma M, Fujii T, Watanabe M. The use of traditional and newer calcineurin inhibitors in inflammatory bowel disease. J Gastroenterol. 2011;46:129–37.
4. Laharie D, Bourreille A, Branchè J, et al. Ciclosporin versus infliximab in patients with severe ulcerative colitis refractory to intravenous steroids: a parallel, open-label randomised controlled trial. Lancet. 2012;380:1909–15.
5. Kino T, Hatanaka H, Hashimoto M, et al. FK-506, a novel immunosuppressant isolated from a Streptomyces. I. Fermentation, isolation, and physico-chemical and biological characteristics. J Antibiot (Tokyo). 1987;40:1249–55.
6. Thomson AW, Carroll PB, McCauley J, et al. FK 506: a novel immunosuppressant for treatment of autoimmune disease. Rationale and preliminary clinical experience at the University of Pittsburgh. Springer Semin Immunopathol. 1993;14:323–44.
7. Sigal NH, Dumont FJ. Cyclosporin A, FK-506, and rapamycin: pharmacologic probes of lymphocyte signal transduction. Annu Rev Immunol. 1992;10:519–60.
8. Aiko S, Conner EM, Fuseler JA, Grisham MB. Effects of cyclosporine or FK506 in chronic colitis. J Pharmacol Exp Ther. 1997;280:1075–84.
9. Hoshino H, Goto H, Sugiyama S, Hayakawa T, Ozawa T. Effects of FK506 on an experimental model of colitis in rats. Aliment Pharmacol Ther. 1995;9:301–7.
10. Higa A, McKnight GW, Wallace JL. Attenuation of epithelial injury in acute experimental colitis by immunomodulators. Eur J Pharmacol. 1993;239:171–6.
11. Takizawa H, Shintani N, Natsui M, et al. Activated immunocompetent cells in rat colitis mucosa induced by dextran sulfate sodium and not complete but partial suppression of colitis by FK506. Digestion. 1995;56:259–64.
12. Fellermann K, Ludwig D, Stahl M, David-Walek T, Stange EF. Steroid-unresponsive acute attacks of inflammatory bowel disease: immunomodulation by tacrolimus (FK506). Am J Gastroenterol. 1998;93:1860–6.
13. Baumgart DC, Pintoffl JP, Sturm A, Wiedenmann B, Dignass AU. Tacrolimus is safe and effective in patients with severe steroid-refractory or steroid-dependent inflammatory bowel disease—a long-term follow-up. Am J Gastroenterol. 2006;101:1048–56.
14. Baumgart DC, Wiedenmann B, Dignass AU. Rescue therapy with tacrolimus is effective in patients with severe and refractory inflammatory bowel disease. Aliment Pharmacol Ther. 2003;17:1273–81.
15. Högenauer C, Wenzl HH, Hinterleitner TA, Petritsch W. Effect of oral tacrolimus (FK 506) on steroid-refractory moderate/severe ulcerative colitis. Aliment Pharmacol Ther. 2003;18:415–23.
16. Ogata H, Matsui T, Nakamura M, et al. A randomised dose finding study of oral tacrolimus (FK506) therapy in refractory ulcerative colitis. Gut. 2006;55:1255–62.
17. Baumgart DC, Macdonald JK, Feagan B. Tacrolimus (FK506) for induction of remission in refractory ulcerative colitis. Cochrane Database Syst Rev. 2008;CD007216.
18. Annunziata ML, Hanauer SB. Calcineurin inhibition in severe ulcerative colitis: lost in translation? Inflamm Bowel Dis. 2012;18:809–11.
19. Mayer AD, Dmitrewski J, Squifflet JP, et al. Multicenter randomized trial comparing tacrolimus (FK506) and cyclosporine in the

prevention of renal allograft rejection: a report of the European Tacrolimus Multicenter Renal Study Group. Transplantation. 1997;64:436–43.

20. McSharry K, Dalzell AM, Leiper K, El-Matary W. Systematic review: the role of tacrolimus in the management of Crohn's disease. Aliment Pharmacol Ther. 2011;34:1282–94.

21. Schmidt KJ, Herrlinger KR, Emmrich J, et al. Short-term efficacy of tacrolimus in steroid-refractory ulcerative colitis—experience in 130 patients. Aliment Pharmacol Ther. 2013;37:129–36.

22. Dignass A, Preiss JC, Aust DE, et al. Updated German guideline on diagnosis and treatment of ulcerative colitis, 2011. Z Gastroenterol. 2011;49:1276–341.

23. Dignass A, Lindsay JO, Sturm A, et al. Second European evidence-based consensus on the diagnosis and management of ulcerative colitis part 2: current management. J Crohns Colitis. 2012;6: 991–1030.

24. Romano C, Comito D, Famiani A, Fries W. Oral tacrolimus (FK 506) in refractory paediatric ulcerative colitis. Aliment Pharmacol Ther. 2010;31:676–7.

25. Chow DK, Leong RW. The use of tacrolimus in the treatment of inflammatory bowel disease. Expert Opin Drug Saf. 2007;6:479–85.

26. Lawrance IC, Copeland TS. Rectal tacrolimus in the treatment of resistant ulcerative proctitis. Aliment Pharmacol Ther. 2008; 28:1214–20.

27. van Dieren JM, van Bodegraven AA, Kuipers EJ, et al. Local application of tacrolimus in distal colitis: feasible and safe. Inflamm Bowel Dis. 2009;15:193–8.

28. Lamprecht A, Schafer U, Lehr CM. Size-dependent bioadhesion of micro- and nanoparticulate carriers to the inflamed colonic mucosa. Pharm Res. 2001;18:788–93.

29. Lamprecht A, Yamamoto H, Takeuchi H, Kawashima Y. Nanoparticles enhance therapeutic efficiency by selectively increased local drug dose in experimental colitis in rats. J Pharmacol Exp Ther. 2005;315:196–202.

30. Lamprecht A, Yamamoto H, Takeuchi H, Kawashima Y. A pH-sensitive microsphere system for the colon delivery of tacrolimus containing nanoparticles. J Control Release. 2005;104:337–46.

31. Lamprecht A, Yamamoto H, Ubrich N, Takeuchi H, Maincent P, Kawashima Y. FK506 microparticles mitigate experimental colitis with minor renal calcineurin suppression. Pharm Res. 2005;22: 193–9.

32. Fellermann K, Tanko Z, Herrlinger KR, et al. Response of refractory colitis to intravenous or oral tacrolimus (FK506). Inflamm Bowel Dis. 2002;8:317–24.

33. Yamamoto S, Nakase H, Mikami S, et al. Long-term effect of tacrolimus therapy in patients with refractory ulcerative colitis. Aliment Pharmacol Ther. 2008;28:589–97.

34. Yamamoto S, Nakase H, Matsuura M, Masuda S, Inui K, Chiba T. Tacrolimus therapy as an alternative to thiopurines for maintaining remission in patients with refractory ulcerative colitis. J Clin Gastroenterol. 2011;45:526–30.

35. Miyoshi J, Matsuoka K, Inoue N, Hisamatsu T, Ichikawa R, Yajima T, Okamoto S, Naganuma M, Sato T, Kanai T, Ogata H, Iwao Y, Hibi T. Mucosal healing with oral tacrolimus is associated with favorable medium- and long-term prognosis in steroid-refractory/dependent ulcerative colitis patients. J Crohns Colitis. 2013;7(12):e609–14. doi:10.1016/j.crohns.2013.04.018. Epub 2013 May 14.

36. Bhorade S, Ahya VN, Baz MA, et al. Comparison of sirolimus with azathioprine in a tacrolimus-based immunosuppressive regimen in lung transplantation. Am J Respir Crit Care Med. 2011;183:379–87.

37. Escher M, Stange EF, Herrlinger KR. Two cases of fatal Pneumocystis jirovecii pneumonia as a complication of tacrolimus therapy in ulcerative colitis—a need for prophylaxis. J Crohns Colitis. 2010;4:606–9.

38. Sehgal SN, Baker H, Vezina C. Rapamycin (AY-22,989), a new antifungal antibiotic. II. Fermentation, isolation and characterization. J Antibiot (Tokyo). 1975;28:727–32.

39. Vezina C, Kudelski A, Sehgal SN. Rapamycin (AY-22,989), a new antifungal antibiotic. I. Taxonomy of the producing streptomycete and isolation of the active principle. J Antibiot (Tokyo). 1975;28:721–6.

40. Sabatini DM. mTOR and cancer: insights into a complex relationship. Nat Rev Cancer. 2006;6:729–34.

41. Armand P, Gannamaneni S, Kim HT, et al. Improved survival in lymphoma patients receiving sirolimus for graft-versus-host disease prophylaxis after allogeneic hematopoietic stem-cell transplantation with reduced-intensity conditioning. J Clin Oncol. 2008;26:5767–74.

42. Walz G, Budde K, Mannaa M, et al. Everolimus in patients with autosomal dominant polycystic kidney disease. N Engl J Med. 2010;363:830–40.

43. Wullschleger S, Loewith R, Hall MN. TOR signaling in growth and metabolism. Cell. 2006;124:471–84.

44. Thomson AW, Turnquist HR, Raimondi G. Immunoregulatory functions of mTOR inhibition. Nat Rev Immunol. 2009;9:324–37.

45. Janku F, McConkey DJ, Hong DS, Kurzrock R. Autophagy as a target for anticancer therapy. Nat Rev Clin Oncol. 2011;8:528–39.

46. Khor B, Gardet A, Xavier RJ. Genetics and pathogenesis of inflammatory bowel disease. Nature. 2011;474:307–17.

47. Farkas S, Hornung M, Sattler C, et al. Rapamycin decreases leukocyte migration in vivo and effectively reduces experimentally induced chronic colitis. Int J Colorectal Dis. 2006;21:747–53.

48. Bhonde MR, Gupte RD, Dadarkar SD, et al. A novel mTOR inhibitor is efficacious in a murine model of colitis. Am J Physiol Gastrointest Liver Physiol. 2008;295:G1237–45.

49. Matsuda C, Ito T, Song J, et al. Therapeutic effect of a new immunosuppressive agent, everolimus, on interleukin-10 gene-deficient mice with colitis. Clin Exp Immunol. 2007;148:348–59.

50. Massey DC, Bredin F, Parkes M. Use of sirolimus (rapamycin) to treat refractory Crohn's disease. Gut. 2008;57:1294–6.

51. Dumortier J, Lapalus MG, Guillaud O, et al. Everolimus for refractory Crohn's disease: a case report. Inflamm Bowel Dis. 2008; 14:874–7.

52. Reinisch W, Panes J, Lemann M, et al. A multicenter, randomized, double-blind trial of everolimus versus azathioprine and placebo to maintain steroid-induced remission in patients with moderate-to-severe active Crohn's disease. Am J Gastroenterol. 2008;103: 2284–92.

53. Florey H, Jennings M. Mycophenolic acid; an antibiotic from Penicillium brevicompactum Dlerckx. Lancet. 1946;1:46–9.

54. Allison AC, Eugui EM. Mycophenolate mofetil and its mechanisms of action. Immunopharmacology. 2000;47:85–118.

55. Lipsky JJ. Mycophenolate mofetil. Lancet. 1996;348:1357–9.

56. Neurath MF, Wanitschke R, Peters M, Krummenauer F, Meyer zum Buschenfelde KH, Schlaak JF. Randomised trial of mycophenolate mofetil versus azathioprine for treatment of chronic active Crohn's disease. Gut. 1999;44:625–8.

57. Fellermann K, Steffen M, Stein J, et al. Mycophenolate mofetil: lack of efficacy in chronic active inflammatory bowel disease. Aliment Pharmacol Ther. 2000;14:171–6.

58. Hassard PV, Vasiliauskas EA, Kam LY, Targan SR, Abreu MT. Efficacy of mycophenolate mofetil in patients failing 6-mercaptopurine or azathioprine therapy for Crohn's disease. Inflamm Bowel Dis. 2000;6:16–20.

59. Rampton DS, Neurath MF, Almer S, D'Haens G, Petritsch W, Stange EF. Mycophenolate mofetil in Crohn's disease. Lancet. 2000;356:163–4.

60. Orth T, Peters M, Schlaak JF, et al. Mycophenolate mofetil versus azathioprine in patients with chronic active ulcerative colitis: a 12-month pilot study. Am J Gastroenterol. 2000;95:1201–7.

61. Palaniappan S, Ford AC, Greer D, et al. Mycophenolate mofetil therapy for refractory inflammatory bowel disease. Inflamm Bowel Dis. 2007;13:1488–92.

62. Golconda MS, Valente JF, Bejarano P, Gilinsky N, First MR. Mycophenolate mofetil-induced colonic ulceration in renal transplant recipients. Transplant Proc. 1999;31:272–3.

63. Dalle IJ, Maes BD, Geboes KP, Lemahieu W, Geboes K. Crohn's-like changes in the colon due to mycophenolate? Colorectal Dis. 2005;7:27–34.

64. Maes BD, Dalle I, Geboes K, et al. Erosive enterocolitis in mycophenolate mofetil-treated renal-transplant recipients with persistent afebrile diarrhea. Transplantation. 2003;75:665–72.

65. Papadimitriou JC, Cangro CB, Lustberg A, et al. Histologic features of mycophenolate mofetil-related colitis: a graft-versus-host disease-like pattern. Int J Surg Pathol. 2003;11:295–302.

66. Lee S, de Boer WB, Subramaniam K, Kumarasinghe MP. Pointers and pitfalls of mycophenolate-associated colitis. J Clin Pathol. 2012;66(1):8–11.

67. Skelly MM, Logan RF, Jenkins D, Mahida YR, Hawkey CJ. Toxicity of mycophenolate mofetil in patients with inflammatory bowel disease. Inflamm Bowel Dis. 2002;8:93–7.

68. Mathew TH. A blinded, long-term, randomized multicenter study of mycophenolate mofetil in cadaveric renal transplantation: results at three years. Tricontinental Mycophenolate Mofetil Renal Transplantation Study Group. Transplantation. 1998;65:1450–4.

69. Hoeltzenbein M, Elefant E, Vial T, et al. Teratogenicity of mycophenolate confirmed in a prospective study of the European Network of Teratology Information Services. Am J Med Genet A. 2012;158A:588–96.

# Infliximab for Ulcerative Colitis

Marc Ferrante, Séverine Vermeire, Gert Van Assche, and Paul Rutgeerts

**Keywords**

Ulcerative colitis • Infliximab • 5-ASA • Corticosteroids • Immunodilators • 6-MP • Colectomy • Cyclosporine

## Introduction

Ulcerative colitis (UC) is characterized by recurring episodes of inflammation limited to the mucosal layer of the colon. Inflammatory episodes give rise to rectal bleeding, diarrhea, and abdominal pain. Most patients with UC can be treated successfully with a symptom-focused step-up approach comprising 5-aminosalicylates, corticosteroids (CS), and immunomodulators, such as azathioprine (AZA) and 6-mercaptopurine (6-MP) [1]. However, a population-based cohort study in 1994 showed that with these treatment modalities, UC remained active in up to 50 % of patients throughout follow-up and approximately 20 % required colectomy [2]. Furthermore, approximately 15 % of UC patients will have a severe UC attack requiring hospitalization during their illness and are treated primarily with high doses of intravenous (IV) CS [3, 4]. Despite IV CS, patients with severe attacks have a high colectomy rate varying from 38 to 47 % [5, 6]. In addition, cyclosporine A (CsA) has been validated as an efficacious treatment in acute severe IV steroid-refractory UC, but its use is frequently associated with toxicity and only seems to postpone an inevitable colectomy [7–9]. In the past decade, agents directed against tumor necrosis factor (TNF) have been introduced successfully in the treatment of patients with moderate-to-severe and acute severe IV steroid-refractory UC.

Most studies with infliximab (IFX) have focused on Crohn's disease (CD), which is believed to be a typical T-helper 1-type disease driven by proinflammatory cytokines such as IL12, IFN-γ (gamma), and TNF. In contrast to CD, UC has historically been considered a T-helper 2-driven disease, with a less prominent role for TNF. However, two lines of evidence suggest an important role of TNF in UC pathogenesis. First, increased levels of TNF and/or TNF receptors were found in colonic mucosa, colon perfusates, rectal dialysate, stools, serum, and urine of patients with active UC [10–18]. Second, CDP571, a monoclonal antibody directed against human TNF-α (alpha), significantly improved UC-like colitis in the cotton-top tamarin [19]. Therefore, several investigators started clinical trials to evaluate the efficacy of IFX in patients with UC.

This chapter will focus on the experience with IFX in the management of UC. Data on the use of IFX during pregnancy (Chap. 24), the use of IFX in a pediatric setting (Chap. 26), the use of IFX for CD-related complications of the pouch (Chap. 31), the perioperative use of IFX (Chap. 34), and other safety issues (Chap. 27) are reported elsewhere in this handbook.

## Open-Label Randomized Corticosteroids-Controlled Trials of Infliximab in UC

Several open-label clinical trials evaluated the efficacy of IFX in UC, providing a rational for subsequent randomized controlled trials (Fig. 15.1) [20–24]. Two small randomized

M. Ferrante, M.D., Ph.D. (✉) • S. Vermeire, M.D., Ph.D.
• G. Van Assche, M.D., Ph.D. • P. Rutgeerts, M.D., Ph.D., F.R.C.P.
Department of Gastroenterology, University Hospitals Leuven, Herestraat 49, Leuven B3000, Belgium
e-mail: marc.ferrante@uzleuven.be; severine.vermeire@uzleuven.be; gert.vanassche@uzleuven.be; paul.rutgeerts@uzleuven.be

G.R. Lichtenstein (ed.), *Medical Therapy of Ulcerative Colitis*,
DOI 10.1007/978-1-4939-1677-1_15, © Springer Science+Business Media New York 2014

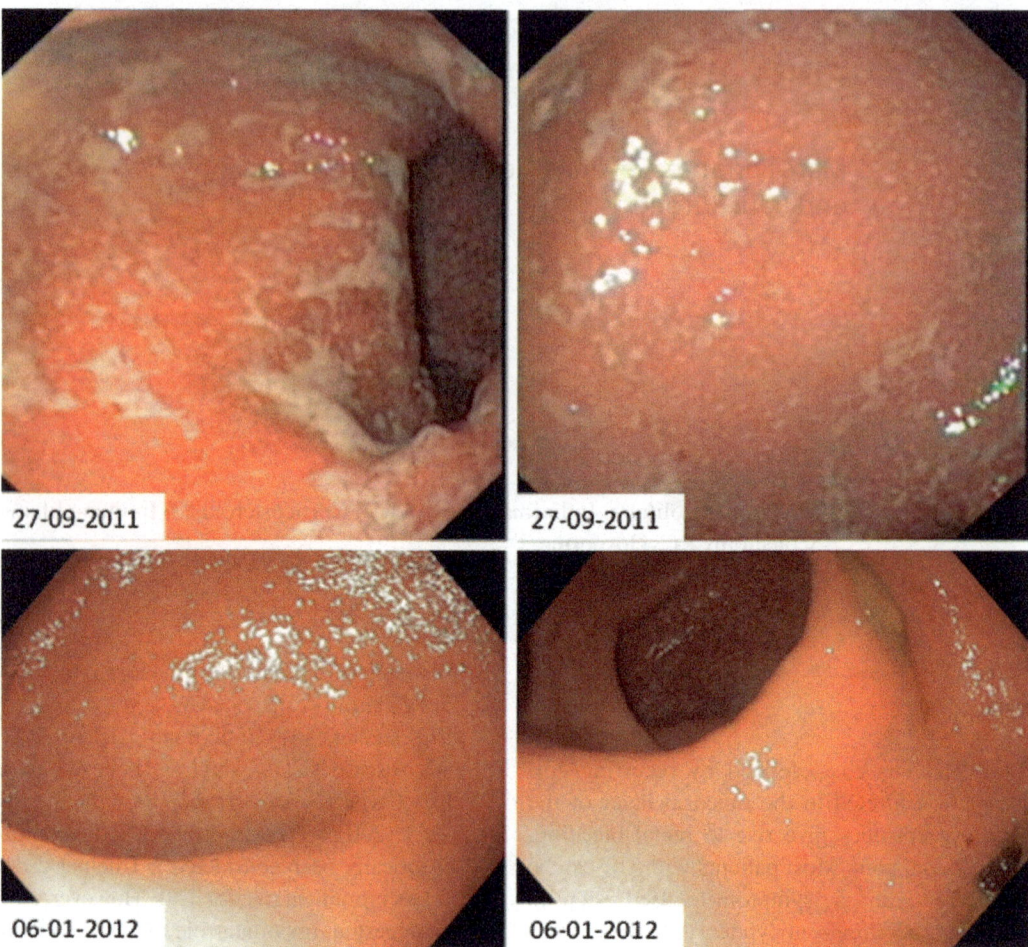

**Fig. 15.1** Mucosal healing 14 weeks after introduction of infliximab. Endoscopic images of the sigmoid at baseline (*upper panel*) and at week 14 (*lower panel*) in a patient receiving infliximab 5 mg/kg body weight at baseline, week 2 and week 6

open-label trials compared IFX with CS for the treatment of UC. In an Italian paper by Armuzzi et al. IFX was as effective as CS for the management of 20 patients with steroid-dependent moderate-to-severe UC [25]. In a German paper by Ochsenkuhn et al. 13 patients with acute severe UC were able to achieve remission if started on IFX [26]. Drawing conclusions from these two studies is difficult, since they both were clearly underpowered.

## Initial Randomized Placebo-Controlled Trials with Infliximab in UC

Between 2000 and 2005, five randomized double-blind placebo-controlled trials with IFX in patients with moderate-to-severe UC were published [27–30]. The initial three trials provided conflicting results, but were underpowered mainly due to slow patient enrollment [31]. Furthermore, comparison between the different trials is difficult due to the heterogeneous patient populations and the different endpoints used.

In a pilot study by Sands et al. 11 (of 60 planned) patients with severe, active IV steroid-refractory UC were randomized to receive a single intravenous infusion of placebo or IFX at a dose of 5, 10, or 20 mg/kg body weight [27]. Patients had to have active disease for at least 2 weeks (modified Truelove and Witts >10) and have received at least 5 days of IV CS prior to randomization. The primary endpoint used in this trial was treatment failure at week 2, defined as absence of clinical response (modified Truelove and Witts <5 and 5 point reduction compared to baseline), increase in CS dosage, addition of immunosuppressive agents, colectomy, or death. Treatment failure occurred in all three patients randomized to placebo, compared to four out of eight patients randomized to IFX. No significant adverse events were observed.

A second randomized placebo-controlled trial by Probert et al. was conducted in 43 patients with active UC (ulcerative colitis symptom score or UCSS ≥6 and Baron endoscopy score ≥2) who failed treatment with CS (≥30 mg prednisolone or equivalent) for at least 1 week [28]. Patients were randomized to receive an infusion with IFX 5 mg/kg body weight or placebo at week 0 and 2. Clinical remission was defined as a UCSS ≤2, while sigmoidoscopic remission was defined as a Baron score of 0. At week 6, no significant difference was observed in clinical (39 % vs. 30 %, p = 0.76) or sigmoidoscopic remission rates (26 % vs. 30 %, p = 0.96) between the IFX and placebo groups. Furthermore, no significant difference was observed in sigmoidoscopic remission. The two reported serious adverse events (sepsis and colectomy) occurred in the placebo group.

A third trial by Jarnerot et al. included 45 (of the 70 planned) patients with severe to moderately severe UC [29]. Patients were randomized to one single infusion of IFX at a dose of 4–5 mg/kg body weight or placebo either at day 4 after initiation of CS treatment if they fulfilled the index criteria for fulminant UC on day 3 (fulminant colitis index ≥8, n = 28) or on days 6–8 if they fulfilled index criteria for a severe or moderately severe acute attack of UC on days 5–7 (Seo index >150, n = 17). Within 90 days after randomization, colectomy occurred less frequently in patients randomized to IFX compared to placebo (29 % vs. 67 %, p = 0.017). After 3 years of follow-up, colectomy was observed in 50 % of patients randomized to IFX compared to 76 % randomized to placebo (p = 0.012) [32]. Of note, sub-analysis of the initial data showed that the difference was only significant in the patients with a severe or moderately severe attack of UC randomized on days 6–8 [29]. Interestingly, none of the eight patients achieving endoscopic remission at 3 months underwent colectomy within the 2-year follow-up period compared to 50 % of patients who did not achieve endoscopic remission (p = 0.02) [32].

## The ACT1 and ACT2 Trials

The two largest studies in patients with moderate-to-severe UC, the active ulcerative colitis trials 1 and 2 (ACT1 and ACT2), were conducted in parallel and published in 2005 by Rutgeerts et al. [30]. In each study, 364 outpatients with moderate-to-severe colitis (total Mayo score ≥6 points with an endoscopic sub-score of ≥2) were included. Patients were refractory to CS and/or thiopurines (ACT1) or refractory to at least one standard therapy including 5-aminosalicylates, CS, and/or thiopurines (ACT2).

Patients were randomized to receive IV placebo or IFX 5 or 10 mg/kg body weight for 22 weeks in ACT2 or 46 weeks in ACT1. Clinical response was defined as a decrease from baseline in total Mayo score of ≥3 points and ≥30 % with an accompanying decrease in the sub-score for rectal bleeding of ≥1 point or absolute rectal bleeding sub-score ≤1 point. Clinical remission was defined as a total Mayo score of ≤2 points, with no individual sub-score exceeding 1 point. Mucosal healing was defined as an absolute endoscopic sub-score of 0 or 1 point.

As depicted in Table 15.1, both in ACT1 and ACT2, clinical response, clinical remission, and mucosal healing were significantly more frequently observed at week 8 in patients randomized to IFX (both 5 and 10 mg/kg body weight) compared to placebo. Furthermore, differences remained significant at week 30 (ACT1 and ACT2) and week 54 (ACT1). Of note, the proportion of serious adverse events was similar in all groups (Table 15.2).

Further studies using the ACT1 and ACT2 study population clearly showed that IFX is able to alter the course of UC with an improvement in hospitalization rates, colectomy rates, and quality of life. Sandborn et al. reported on the

**Table 15.1** Clinical response rates and mucosal healing rates in the ACT (active ulcerative colitis) trials

| | ACT1 | | | ACT2 | | |
|---|---|---|---|---|---|---|
| | Placebo (n = 121) | IFX 5 mg/kg (n = 121) | IFX 10 mg/kg (n = 122) | Placebo (n = 123) | IFX 5 mg/kg (n = 121) | IFX 10 mg/kg (n = 120) |
| *Clinical response* | | | | | | |
| Week 8 | 37.2 % | 69.4 % | 61.5 % | 29.3 % | 64.5 % | 69.2 % |
| Week 30 | 29.8 % | 52.1 % | 50.8 % | 26.0 % | 47.1 % | 60.0 % |
| Week 54 | 19.8 % | 45.5 % | 44.3 % | – | – | – |
| *Clinical remission* | | | | | | |
| Week 8 | 14.9 % | 38.8 % | 32.0 % | 5.7 % | 33.9 % | 27.5 % |
| Week 30 | 15.7 % | 33.9 % | 36.9 % | 10.6 % | 25.6 % | 35.8 % |
| Week 54 | 16.5 % | 34.7 % | 34.4 % | – | – | – |
| *Mucosal healing* | | | | | | |
| Week 8 | 33.9 % | 62.0 % | 59.0 % | 30.9 % | 60.3 % | 61.7 % |
| Week 30 | 24.8 % | 50.4 % | 49.2 % | 30.1 % | 46.3 % | 56.7 % |
| Week 54 | 18.2 % | 45.5 % | 46.7 % | – | – | – |

*IFX* infliximab

Adapted from: Rutgeerts P, Sandborn WJ, Feagan BG et al. Infliximab for induction and maintenance therapy for ulcerative colitis. N Engl J Med 2005;353:2462–76 [30]

**Table 15.2** UC-related hospitalization, colectomy, quality of life, and adverse events in the ACT (active ulcerative colitis) trials

| | Pooled ACT1 and ACT2 | | | |
| --- | --- | --- | --- | --- |
| | Placebo ($n=244$) | IFX 5 mg/kg ($n=242$) | IFX 10 mg/kg ($n=242$) | Combined IFX ($n=484$) |
| *UC-related hospitalization* | | | | |
| Within 54 weeks (%) | 25 % | 16 % | 15 % | 16 % |
| Events per 100 patient-years (n) | 40 | 21 | 19 | 20 |
| *Colectomy* | | | | |
| Within 54 weeks (%) | 17 % | 12 % | 8 % | 10 % |
| *Mean ± SD change in IBDQ week 8* | | | | |
| Bowel | 7.9±9.7 | 14.5±11.7 | 13.0±11.8 | 13.7±11.8 |
| Emotional | 6.2±10.6 | 12.7±12.6 | 11.3±12.6 | 12.0±12.6 |
| Systemic | 3.0±4.8 | 5.7±5.9 | 5.2±5.8 | 5.4±5.9 |
| Social | 3.8±6.0 | 7.4±8.0 | 6.2±7.1 | 6.8±7.5 |
| *Mean ± SD change in SF-36 week 8* | | | | |
| Physical functioning | 6.0±17.3 | 12.8±19.3 | 9.1±18.3 | 11.0±18.9 |
| Role-physical | 22.4±39.7 | 29.6±41.0 | 32.6±44.1 | 31.1±42.5 |
| Bodily pain | 13.1±24.7 | 20.2±22.5 | 19.8±24.3 | 20.0±23.4 |
| General health | 5.6±15.8 | 10.0±16.9 | 10.8±19.4 | 10.4±18.1 |
| Vitality | 11.5±20.7 | 16.6±22.0 | 20.0±22.7 | 18.3±22.3 |
| Social functioning | 15.8±24.8 | 21.2±24.8 | 20.9±27.1 | 21.0±25.9 |
| Role-emotional | 12.4±47.6 | 15.5±46.1 | 21.1±44.7 | 18.2±45.4 |
| Mental health | 5.0±18.4 | 10.6±17.5 | 10.4±18.8 | 10.5±18.2 |
| *Adverse events within 54 weeks* | | | | |
| Any adverse event (%) | 196 (80) | 208 (86) | 209 (86) | 417 (86) |
| Any serious adverse event (%) | 57 (23) | 43 (18) | 46 (19) | 89 (18) |
| Any infection (%) | 80 (33) | 94 (39) | 100 (41) | 194 (40) |
| Any serious infection (%) | 6 (2) | 7 (3) | 12 (5) | 19 (4) |

Adapted from Colombel JF, Rutgeerts P, Reinisch W et al. Early mucosal healing with infliximab is associated with improved long-term clinical outcomes in ulcerative colitis. Gastroenterology 2011;141:1194–201 [35]

1-year colectomy and hospitalization rates (Table 15.2) [33]. Complete follow-up was available in 87 % of the patients. The cumulative incidence of colectomy through week 54 was 10 % for the combined IFX group and 17 % for the placebo group ($p=0.02$). Looking at the subgroups, the difference was only significant between IFX 10 mg/kg body weight and placebo ($p=0.007$). However, one should take into account that patients were allowed to receive rescue commercial IFX. Commercial IFX was used by 11 % of patients in the placebo group compared with 6 % in the combined IFX group. Therefore, rescue therapy with commercial IFX was evaluated as a potential confounder to the colectomy analysis. Post hoc analysis of the time to colectomy or use of commercial IFX demonstrated that both IFX 5 mg/kg and 10 mg/kg body weight significantly reduced the incidence rates of colectomy or the use of commercial IFX compared with placebo ($p=0.001$ and $p<0.001$, respectively). Furthermore, a significantly reduced number of UC-related hospitalizations per 100 patient-years was observed for both IFX groups compared with placebo (21 for IFX 5 mg/kg, 19 for IFX 10 mg/kg body weight, and 40 for placebo, $p=0.02$ and $p=0.007$).

Further analysis of the ACT1 and ACT2 data showed a significant and rapid improvement in health-related quality of life evaluated by both the Inflammatory Bowel Disease Questionnaire (IBDQ) and the 36-item short form health survey (SF-36) [34]. Improvement in all components of the IBDQ and SF-36 were significantly greater in both IFX groups compared to the placebo group (Table 15.2). Furthermore, continued improvement in health-related quality of life was maintained throughout the study period (54 weeks in ACT1 and 30 weeks in ACT2).

A recently published sub-analysis by Colombel et al. highlighted the benefit of achieving early mucosal healing [35]. Lower endoscopy sub-scores at week 8 were associated with increased rates of symptomatic remission, steroid-free symptomatic remission, mucosal healing, and colectomy-free survival at weeks 30 and 54 (Table 15.3). The Kaplan–Meier curves for colectomy survival separated as early as 8 weeks for IFX-treated patients who achieved mucosal healing at week 8 (Mayo endoscopic sub-score 0 or 1) when compared with those who did not ($p<0.001$). No significant separation was observed between patients with a sub-score of 0 and those with a sub-score of 1 ($p=0.87$), suggesting

**Table 15.3** Short-term endoscopic response as predictor of long-term outcome in the ACT (active ulcerative colitis) trials

| | Mayo endoscopic sub-score at week 8 | | | | |
|---|---|---|---|---|---|
| | Score 0 (n = 120) | Score 1 (n = 175) | Score 2 (n = 127) | Score 3 (n = 62) | p-value |
| *Outcome week 30 IFX-treated patients* | | | | | |
| Clinical remission | 71 % | 51 % | 23 % | 10 % | <0.0001 |
| Steroid-free clinical remission | 46 % | 34 % | 11 % | 7 % | <0.0001 |
| Mucosal healing | 83 % | 67 % | 26 % | 10 % | <0.0001 |
| *Outcome week 54 IFX-treated patients* | | | | | |
| Clinical remission | 73 % | 47 % | 24 % | 10 % | <0.0001 |
| Steroid-free clinical remission | 47 % | 35 % | 5 % | 5 % | <0.0001 |
| Sustained mucosal healing (week 30 and 54) | 77 % | 54 % | 21 % | 7 % | <0.0001 |
| Colectomy-free survival | 95 % | 95 % | 87 % | 80 % | =0.0004 |
| Colectomy-and commercial IFX-free survival | 92 % | 92 % | 84 % | 69 % | <0.0001 |

$p < 0.005$ compared with the placebo group; *IFX* infliximab
Adapted from Rutgeerts P, Sandborn WJ, Feagan BG et al. Infliximab for induction and maintenance therapy for ulcerative colitis. N Engl J Med 2005;353:2462–76 [30], Sandborn WJ, Rutgeerts P, Feagan BG et al. Colectomy rate comparison after treatment of ulcerative colitis with placebo or infliximab. Gastroenterology 2009;137:1250–60 [33], Feagan BG, Reinisch W, Rutgeerts P et al. The effects of infliximab therapy on health-related quality of life in ulcerative colitis patients. Am J Gastroenterol 2007;102:794–802 [34]

that achieving complete mucosal healing (absence of all endoscopic abnormalities) may not be mandatory to alter the course of the disease.

A total of 229 of 484 IFX-treated patients from the ACT1 and ACT2 trials entered a long-term extension cohort study published by Reinisch et al. [36]. During a median follow-up of 128 weeks, 70 patients who entered the extension phase (31 %) discontinued IFX administration. In 12 patients, this was due to a lack of efficacy (5 %), while 24 patients discontinued IFX due to adverse events (10 %). During this extension phase, no new or unexpected safety signals were observed.

## The Benefit of Combination Therapy in UC

In patients with CD naïve to immunomodulatory and biological therapy, the SONIC trial has clearly shown a benefit of using combination therapy with both IFX and AZA in inducing CS-free clinical remission and mucosal healing [37]. In UC such a benefit is less clear. The unpublished double-blind randomized controlled UC success trial included 231 patients with moderate-to-severe UC (Mayo score ≥6) who had failed CS and were either naïve to AZA

or had stopped AZA ≥3 months prior to inclusion [38]. Patients were randomized to receive AZA monotherapy, IFX monotherapy, or a combination therapy with both AZA and IFX. At week 8, nonresponders (Mayo score reduction <1 point) in the AZA arm were eligible for rescue therapy with IFX. At week 16, a significantly greater proportion of patients in the combination group achieved steroid-free remission (total Mayo score ≤2), clinical response (decrease in total Mayo score of ≥3 points and ≥30 %), and mucosal healing (Mayo endoscopic sub-score 0 or 1) compared to the AZA group. A difference between combination therapy with IFX and AZA and monotherapy with IFX was only seen for steroid-free clinical remission (40 % vs. 22 %, $p = 0.017$), but not for clinical response (77 % vs. 69 %, $p = 0.514$) or mucosal healing (63 % vs. 55 %, $p = 0.295$). Based on these data, an early introduction of IFX in combination with a thiopurine could be advocated in UC. However, overtreatment with possible severe adverse events warrants further characterization of a population at risk for a more complicated disease behavior. In contrast to CD, risk factors for a more complicated disease behavior are poorly defined in UC.

## Long-Term Outcome in Open-Label Cohort Studies

Several investigators evaluated the long-term outcome including colectomy-free survival in UC patients treated with IFX (Table 15.4). In the first long-term outcome study from Oxford, 30 patients receiving IFX for UC were followed for a median of 13 months [39]. During follow-up, 16 patients (53 %) needed colectomy, while only five achieved steroid-free clinical remission. However, no fixed maintenance IFX treatment was provided in these patients.

A large cohort from Leuven included 217 consecutive patients who received IFX for moderate-to-severe UC or acute IV steroid-refractory UC [40]. Initial response to IFX was observed in 73 % of patients. After a median follow-up of 43 months, 50 % of patients showed sustained clinical response, while 18 % needed colectomy. Furthermore, 70 % of patients under CS therapy at baseline were able to stop this therapy by the end of follow-up.

In a French retrospective multicentric study, 191 UC patients receiving IFX therapy were followed for a median of 18 months [41]. Primary nonresponse was observed in 22 % of patients. IFX optimization was required in 45 % of patients on maintenance therapy with IFX. In the end, 36 patients (19 %) underwent colectomy.

In a retrospective Danish study including UC patients from three different hospitals, 39 % of 56 patients treated with IFX for steroid-refractory UC needed colectomy during a median follow-up of 538 days [42]. Most patients, however, did not receive complete induction (IFX weeks 0, 2,

**Table 15.4** Long-term outcome and predictors of colectomy

| Center | Number of patients | Indication | Median follow-up | Colectomy | Predictors of colectomy |
|---|---|---|---|---|---|
| Oxford, UK [39] | 30 | All UC | 13 months | 53.3 % | 1. Younger age at diagnosis |
| Leuven, Belgium [40] | 217 | All UC | 43 months | 18.4 % | 1. Baseline CRP ≥5 mg/L<br>2. Absence of short-term clinical response<br>3. Absence of short-term mucosal healing<br>4. Absence of short-term CRP normalization L<br>5. Previous IV treatment with CS or CsA<br>6. A MDR1 3435TT genotype |
| Multicentric, France [41] | 191 | All UC | 18 months | 18.8 % | 1. Absence of short-term clinical response<br>2. Baseline CRP ≥10 mg/L<br>3. Previous treatment with CsA<br>4. IFX for acute severe UC |
| Multicentric, Spain [45] | 47 | All UC | 5 months | 10.6 % | 1. More extensive disease |
| Herlev, Denmark [43] | 52 | All UC | 22 months | 26.9 % | None identified |
| Multicentric, Denmark [42] | 56 | Acute severe UC | 18 months | 39.3 % | None identified |
| Multicentric, Italy [44] | 83 | Acute severe UC | 23 months | 30.1 % | None identified |
| Multicentric, Scotland [49] | 39 | Acute severe UC | 7 months | 38.4 % | None identified |

*UC* ulcerative colitis

and 6) or maintenance therapy with IFX every 8 weeks. In a similar study from the Herlev Hospital in Denmark, colectomy was observed in 27 % of 52 patients after a median follow-up of 22 months [43].

In a retrospective multicentric Italian study including 83 patients with acute severe IV steroid-refractory colitis, 25 patients (30 %) needed colectomy during a median follow-up of 23 months [44]. Finally, in a rather short-term retrospective multicentric Spanish study, 10.6 % of 47 patients treated with IFX for UC needed colectomy during a median follow-up of 5 months [45].

## Predictors of Short-Term Outcome

In a monocentric retrospective study including the first 100 UC patients treated with IFX in Leuven, independent predictors of absence of short-term response were a pANCA+/ASCA- status and an older age at first IFX infusion [46]. However, these predictors could not be confirmed in an update of this cohort [40, 47]. In a French retrospective multicentric study, a baseline hemoglobin level ≤9.4 g/dL was an independent predictor of primary nonresponse to IFX [41]. In a German study including 90 patients with UC treated with IFX, a low clinical activity index at baseline, presence of ANCA antibodies, and presence of IL23R variants were independent predictors of absence of short-term response to IFX [48].

In a Scottish trial evaluating the efficacy of IFX in patients with acute severe IV steroid-refractory UC, higher colectomy rates at day of discharge were observed in patients with a serum albumin level <34 g/L at day 3 of IV CS [49].

The predictive value of fecal calprotectin (FC) levels was evaluated in a prospective multicentric Belgian study including 53 patients with active UC treated with IFX 5 mg/kg body weight at weeks 0, 2, and 6 [50]. A significant decrease of FC levels between baseline and week 2 was predictive of endoscopic remission at week 10 (Mayo endoscopic sub-score 0 or 1).

Finally, by using Affymetrix Human Genome microarrays, Arijs et al. compared the colonic mucosal gene expression from patients with UC responding and not responding to an induction therapy with IFX [51]. Among the top five differentially expressed genes were IL13Rα2 (alpha2) and IL11 which were both significantly higher expressed at baseline in UC short-term nonresponders compared to responders (Mayo endoscopic sub-score 0 or 1 and histological activity score 0 or 1). The authors could not confirm the previously reported higher mean baseline colorectal TNF-α (alpha) expression in patients not achieving clinical remission [52]. Recently, Rismo et al. observed higher gene expression levels of IL17A and IFN-γ (gamma) in the colonic mucosa of UC patients who achieved remission (UC-DAI <3 with endoscopic sub-score 0 or 1) after three IFX infusions [53].

Importantly, none of the proposed predictors of short-term outcome have been confirmed in other trials.

## Predictors of Long-Term Outcome

Proposed predictors of long-term colectomy risk are depicted in Table 15.4. Several investigators showed that in outpatients with moderate-to-severe colitis as well as in hospitalized patients treated with IFX for acute severe IV steroid-refractory colitis, both clinical response and mucosal healing on the short-term were predictive of colectomy-free survival on the long term [32, 35, 40, 41].

Furthermore, there is direct and indirect evidence that patients with more severe UC have a worse outcome. In a French retrospective multicentric study, IFX administered for acute severe IV steroid-refractory colitis was a predictor for both UC-related hospitalization and colectomy [41]. An elevated baseline CRP and the absence of a normalization of CRP levels on the short-term have been associated with the need for colectomy on the long term [40, 41, 47]. Furthermore, the previous need of IV CS and/or CsA has also been associated with a higher colectomy risk [40, 41, 47].

In the French retrospective multicentric study, a shorter disease duration prior to start of IFX was associated with a worse outcome as suggested by a higher hospitalization but not colectomy rate [41]. Finally, in a Spanish retrospective study, extent of disease was predictive of colectomy [45]. However, in the larger Belgian and French long-term cohort studies, extent of disease was not a risk factor.

As in CD, higher IFX serum levels have been reported to be associated with a better long-term outcome of IFX-treated patients. In a Canadian trial by Seow et al. 115 patients with UC were followed for a median of 5 months. Detectable serum IFX levels were associated with higher clinical remission rates (69 % vs. 15 %, $p < 0.001$), higher endoscopic improvement rates (76 % vs. 28 %, $p < 0.001$), and lower colectomy rates (7 % vs. 55 %, $p < 0.001$) [54]. Further studies are ongoing to conclude on the predictive role of measuring serum IFX levels.

In addition, a Finnish study showed that a normalization of FC levels ($\leq 100$ µg/g) after induction therapy with anti-TNF agents was predictive of sustained clinical remission after 1 year [55].

## Cyclosporine Versus Infliximab for Acute Severe IV Steroid-Refractory Colitis

The landmark Scandinavian data by Jarnerot et al. suggested a benefit of IFX in patients with acute severe IV steroid-refractory colitis [29]. However, sub-analysis of the provided data showed that the difference was only significant in patients with a severe or moderately severe attack of UC randomized on days 6–8 but not in those with fulminant colitis. Furthermore, a multicentric retrospective observational study suggested a better short-term colectomy-free survival in patients treated with CsA compared to those treated with a single infusion of IFX [56]. Based on these data, some investigators advocate the use of CsA over IFX in patients with acute severe IV steroid-refractory colitis. However, other investigators prefer to use IFX due to the high long-term col-

ectomy rates and the risk of severe adverse events in patients treated with CsA [7–9].

The first head-to-head comparison of IV CsA and maintenance IFX was recently reported by Laharie et al. [57]. In this open-label CYS-IFX trial, 111 patients were randomized to (1) receive IV CsA at an initial dose of 2 mg per kg body weight, adapted to serum levels between 150 and 250 ng/mL which was switched to oral treatment in patients with clinical response at day 7, or (2) infuse with IFX 5 mg per kg body weight, followed by sequent infusions at weeks 2 and 6 in patients with clinical response at day 7. In both arms, CS were switched to oral therapy and progressively tapered once the patient achieved clinical response, while AZA was added at day 8 in those not yet on thiopurines. The composite primary endpoint was treatment failure defined by (1) absence of clinical response at day 7; (2) relapse between days 7 and 98; (3) mortality, colectomy, or any other severe adverse event leading to treatment interruption between days 0 and day 98; and (4) absence of steroid-free remission at day 98. The primary endpoint was achieved in 60 % of the patients randomized to CsA and 54 % of patient randomized to IFX, a difference which was not significantly different ($p = 0.49$). Furthermore, response rate at day 7 was similar (85 % CsA vs. 86 % IFX, $p = 0.97$) as well as the colectomy-free survival during the first 98 days ($p = 0.66$) and the occurrence of severe adverse events.

In our center, the use of IFX is preferred over CsA based on the available long-term efficacy and safety data and the better outcome in patients previously having failed AZA [58].

Finally, sequential use of both CsA and IFX should not be recommended because of the significant potential toxicity [59, 60]. Concomitant therapy with both these drugs is contraindicated for the same reason.

## Managing Loss of Response to Infliximab

In randomized controlled trials, primary nonresponse to IFX was present in 10–30 % of patients. A key question is the time point and the method for defining nonresponse. We advocate to perform a sigmoidoscopy no later than at week 14 prior to the fourth infusion of IFX and this regardless of the presence of clinical symptoms. Although there is clear evidence that mucosal healing on the short-term has a significant influence on the long-term outcome [35, 40], it needs to be explored if IFX therapy should be intensified in asymptomatic patients who did not achieve mucosal healing on the short term. As mentioned below, we advocate the use of serum IFX levels to guide treatment intensification in such a scenario.

Secondary nonresponse affects approximately 30 % of patients during the first year of therapy and may be due to altered clearance of drug, neutralizing antibodies or biological escape mechanisms. In our center, the optimal strategy in patients with loss of response to IFX depends on the results of serial measurements of IFX serum levels and antibodies to IFX (ATI) [61]. In patients with low IFX serum levels (<3 µg/mL) and absent or low ATI antibodies (<8 µg/mL), IFX therapy can be optimized by increasing the dose (up to 10 mg/kg body weight in adults) or shortening the interval between IFX infusion (up to every 4 weeks). In symptomatic patients with normal or high IFX serum levels, disease activity should be confirmed by sigmoidoscopy and if present, a switch to a non-anti-TNF agent is warranted. Finally, in patients with high ATI antibodies, switch to another anti-TNF agent or a non-anti-TNF agent is necessary.

Patients with UC who had to switch from IFX to adalimumab (ADA) due to loss of response or intolerance seem to have somewhat lower clinical remission rates after initiation of ADA therapy than patients who were anti-TNF naïve. In ULTRA 2, patients with moderate-to-severe UC (total Mayo score ≥6 points with an endoscopic sub-score of ≥2) were randomized to receive either ADA 160 mg at week 0, 80 mg at week 2, and then 40 mg every other week or placebo [62]. In 295 anti-TNF patients, clinical remission (Mayo score ≤2 with no individual sub-score >1) at week 8 and week 52 was observed in 21.3 % and 22.0 % of ADA-treated patients, while in 199 patients previously exposed to anti-TNF, clinical remission at week 8 and week 52 was observed in 9.2 % and 10.2 % of ADA-treated patients. In a cohort study from Leuven including 50 UC patients who had to switch from IFX to ADA for loss of response or intolerance, 52 % patients achieved a durable response, while 20 % needed colectomy during a median follow-up of 23 months [63].

## When to Stop Infliximab?

Once started with maintenance anti-TNF therapy, it is not clear when this therapy can be stopped. In CD, the STORI trial showed a relapse rate of 50 % in patients who had been treated with IFX for at least 1 year and continued their immunomodulatory agent [64]. However, a group of CD patients with a low risk of relapse could be identified (absence of surgical resections, low leukocyte count, low CRP, low FC, mucosal healing). A similar stratification still needs to be explored for patients with UC.

## Conclusion

The results from the ACT trials were a major breakthrough for the treatment of patients with moderate-to-severe UC. It was shown that patients under IFX were not only able to achieve and maintain clinical remission; IFX use was also associated with higher mucosal healing rates leading to lower hospitalization and lower surgery rates.

In parallel, there is increasing evidence for the use of IFX in patients with acute severe IV steroid-refractory colitis. However, more controlled data with a longer follow-up are awaited to conclude superiority over CsA in this setting.

Finally, in independent long-term cohort studies, it was shown that patients with a higher disease activity (suggested by CRP at baseline and previous treatment with IV CS and/or CsA) and patients with absence of short-term clinical, biological, or endoscopic response were more at risk for colectomy. Therefore, in patients with UC treated with IFX, we suggest to perform a sigmoidoscopy early. In patients who do not achieve mucosal healing by week 14 and display good serum IFX levels, the drug should be discontinued.

## References

1. Hanauer SB. Medical therapy for ulcerative colitis 2004. Gastroenterology. 2004;126:1582–92.
2. Langholz E, Munkholm P, Davidsen M, Binder V. Course of ulcerative colitis: analysis of changes in disease activity over years. Gastroenterology. 1994;107:3–11.
3. Edwards FC, Truelove SC. The course and prognosis of ulcerative colitis. Gut. 1963;41:299–315.
4. Truelove SC, Witts LJ. Cortisone in ulcerative colitis; final report on a therapeutic trial. Br Med J. 1955;1(4947):1041–8.
5. Jarnerot G, Rolny P, Sandberg-Gertzen H. Intensive intravenous treatment of ulcerative colitis. Gastroenterology. 1985;89:1005–13.
6. Truelove SC, Jewell DP. Intensive intravenous regimen for severe attacks of ulcerative colitis. Lancet. 1974;1:1067–70.
7. Campbell S, Travis S, Jewell D. Ciclosporin use in acute ulcerative colitis: a long-term experience. Eur J Gastroenterol Hepatol. 2005;17:79–84.
8. Lichtiger S, Present DH, Kornbluth A, et al. Cyclosporine in severe ulcerative colitis refractory to steroid therapy. N Engl J Med. 1994;330:1841–5.
9. Moskovitz DN, Van Assche G, Maenhout B, et al. Incidence of colectomy during long-term follow-up after cyclosporine-induced remission of severe ulcerative colitis. Clin Gastroenterol Hepatol. 2006;4:760–5.
10. Hadziselimovic F, Emmons LR, Gallati H. Soluble tumour necrosis factor receptors p55 and p75 in the urine monitor disease activity and the efficacy of treatment of inflammatory bowel disease. Gut. 1995;37:260–3.
11. Guimbaud R, Bertrand V, Chauvelot-Moachon L, et al. Network of inflammatory cytokines and correlation with disease activity in ulcerative colitis. Am J Gastroenterol. 1998;93:2397–404.
12. Nielsen OH, Gionchetti P, Ainsworth M, et al. Rectal dialysate and fecal concentrations of neutrophil gelatinase-associated lipocalin, interleukin-8, and tumor necrosis factor-alpha in ulcerative colitis. Am J Gastroenterol. 1999;94:2923–8.
13. Tsukada Y, Nakamura T, Iimura M, Iizuka BE, Hayashi N. Cytokine profile in colonic mucosa of ulcerative colitis correlates with disease activity and response to granulocytapheresis. Am J Gastroenterol. 2002;97:2820–8.
14. MacDonald TT, Hutchings P, Choy MY, Murch S, Cooke A. Tumour necrosis factor-alpha and interferon-gamma production measured at the single cell level in normal and inflamed human intestine. Clin Exp Immunol. 1990;81:301–5.
15. Murch SH, Braegger CP, Walker-Smith JA, MacDonald TT. Location of tumour necrosis factor alpha by immunohistochemistry in chronic inflammatory bowel disease. Gut. 1993;34:1705–9.

16. Braegger CP, Nicholls S, Murch SH, Stephens S, MacDonald TT. Tumour necrosis factor alpha in stool as a marker of intestinal inflammation. Lancet. 1992;339:89–91.

17. Spoettl T, Hausmann M, Klebl F, et al. Serum soluble TNF receptor I and II levels correlate with disease activity in IBD patients. Inflamm Bowel Dis. 2007;13:727–32.

18. Hanai H, Watanabe F, Yamada M, et al. Correlation of serum soluble TNF-alpha receptors I and II levels with disease activity in patients with ulcerative colitis. Am J Gastroenterol. 2004;99: 1532–8.

19. Watkins PE, Warren BF, Stephens S, Ward P, Foulkes R. Treatment of ulcerative colitis in the cottontop tamarin using antibody to tumour necrosis factor alpha. Gut. 1997;40:628–33.

20. Actis GC, Bruno M, Pinna-Pintor M, Rossini FP, Rizzetto M. Infliximab for treatment of steroid-refractory ulcerative colitis. Dig Liver Dis. 2002;34:631–4.

21. Chey WY, Hussain A, Ryan C, Potter GD, Shah A. Infliximab for refractory ulcerative colitis. Am J Gastroenterol. 2001;96: 2373–81.

22. Gornet JM, Couve S, Hassani Z, et al. Infliximab for refractory ulcerative colitis or indeterminate colitis: an open-label multicentre study. Aliment Pharmacol Ther. 2003;18:175–81.

23. Kaser A, Mairinger T, Vogel W, Tilg H. Infliximab in severe steroid-refractory ulcerative colitis: a pilot study. Wien Klin Wochenschr. 2001;113:930–3.

24. Su C, Salzberg BA, Lewis JD, et al. Efficacy of anti-tumor necrosis factor therapy in patients with ulcerative colitis. Am J Gastroenterol. 2002;97:2577–84.

25. Armuzzi A, De PB, Lupascu A, et al. Infliximab in the treatment of steroid-dependent ulcerative colitis. Eur Rev Med Pharmacol Sci. 2004;8:231–3.

26. Ochsenkuhn T, Sackmann M, Goke B. Infliximab for acute, not steroid-refractory ulcerative colitis: a randomized pilot study. Eur J Gastroenterol Hepatol. 2004;16:1167–71.

27. Sands BE, Tremaine WJ, Sandborn WJ, et al. Infliximab in the treatment of severe, steroid-refractory ulcerative colitis: a pilot study. Inflamm Bowel Dis. 2001;7:83–8.

28. Probert CS, Hearing SD, Schreiber S, et al. Infliximab in moderately severe glucocorticoid resistant ulcerative colitis: a randomised controlled trial. Gut. 2003;52:998–1002.

29. Jarnerot G, Hertervig E, Friis-Liby I, et al. Infliximab as rescue therapy in severe to moderately severe ulcerative colitis: a randomized, placebo-controlled study. Gastroenterology. 2005;128: 1805–11.

30. Rutgeerts P, Sandborn WJ, Feagan BG, et al. Infliximab for induction and maintenance therapy for ulcerative colitis. N Engl J Med. 2005;353:2462–76.

31. Rutgeerts P. Infliximab for ulcerative colitis: the need for adequately powered placebo-controlled trials. Am J Gastroenterol. 2002;97:2488–9.

32. Gustavsson A, Jarnerot G, Hertervig E, et al. Clinical trial: colectomy after rescue therapy in ulcerative colitis – 3-year follow-up of the Swedish-Danish controlled infliximab study. Aliment Pharmacol Ther. 2010;32:984–9.

33. Sandborn WJ, Rutgeerts P, Feagan BG, et al. Colectomy rate comparison after treatment of ulcerative colitis with placebo or infliximab. Gastroenterology. 2009;137:1250–60.

34. Feagan BG, Reinisch W, Rutgeerts P, et al. The effects of infliximab therapy on health-related quality of life in ulcerative colitis patients. Am J Gastroenterol. 2007;102:794–802.

35. Colombel JF, Rutgeerts P, Reinisch W, et al. Early mucosal healing with infliximab is associated with improved long-term clinical outcomes in ulcerative colitis. Gastroenterology. 2011;141:1194–201.

36. Reinisch W, Sandborn WJ, Rutgeerts P, et al. Long-term infliximab maintenance therapy for ulcerative colitis: the ACT-1 and -2 extension studies. Inflamm Bowel Dis. 2012;18:201–11.

37. Colombel JF, Rutgeerts P, Reinisch W, et al. SONIC: a randomized, double-blind, controlled trial comparing infliximab and infliximab plus azathioprine to azathioprine in patients with Crohn's disease naive to immunomodulators and biological therapy. Gut. 2009; 57:A1.

38. Panaccione R, Ghosh S, Middleton S, Márquez JR, Scott BB, Flint L, van Hoogstraten HJ, Chen AC, Zheng H, Danese S, Rutgeerts P. Combination therapy with infliximab and azathioprine is superior to monotherapy with either agent in ulcerative colitis. Gastroenterology. 2014;146(2):392–400.e3.

39. Jakobovits SL, Jewell DP, Travis SPL. Infliximab for the treatment of ulcerative colitis: outcomes in Oxford from 2000 to 2006. Aliment Pharmacol Ther. 2007;25:1055–60.

40. Ferrante M, Drobne D, Vermeire S, et al. Long-term outcome of infliximab in patients with ulcerative colitis. Gut. 2010;2010:A193.

41. Oussalah A, Evesque L, Laharie D, et al. A multicenter experience with infliximab for ulcerative colitis: outcomes and predictors of response, optimization, colectomy, and hospitalization. Am J Gastroenterol. 2010;105:2617–25.

42. Mortensen C, Caspersen S, Christensen NL, et al. Treatment of acute ulcerative colitis with infliximab, a retrospective study from three Danish hospitals. J Crohns Colitis. 2011;5:28–33.

43. Teisner AS, Ainsworth MA, Brynskov J. Long-term effects and colectomy rates in ulcerative colitis patients treated with infliximab: a Danish single center experience. Scand J Gastroenterol. 2010;45:1457–63.

44. Kohn A, Daperno M, Armuzzi A, et al. Infliximab in severe ulcerative colitis: short-term results of different infusion regimens and long-term follow-up. Aliment Pharmacol Ther. 2007;26:747–56.

45. Gonzalez-Lama Y, Fernandez-Blanco I, Lopez-Sanroman A, et al. Open-label infliximab therapy in ulcerative colitis: a multicenter survey of results and predictors of response. Hepatogastroenterology. 2008;55:1609–14.

46. Ferrante M, Vermeire S, Katsanos KH, et al. Predictors of early response to infliximab in patients with ulcerative colitis. Inflamm Bowel Dis. 2007;13:123–8.

47. Ferrante M, Vermeire S, Fidder H, et al. Long-term outcome after infliximab for refractory ulcerative colitis. J Crohn's Colitis. 2008;2:219–25.

48. Jurgens M, Laubender RP, Hartl F, et al. Disease activity, ANCA, and IL23R genotype status determine early response to infliximab in patients with ulcerative colitis. Am J Gastroenterol. 2010;105: 1811–9.

49. Lees CW, Heys D, Ho GT, et al. A retrospective analysis of the efficacy and safety of infliximab as rescue therapy in acute severe ulcerative colitis. Aliment Pharmacol Ther. 2007;26:411–9.

50. De Vos M, Dewit O, D'Haens G, et al. Fast and sharp decrease in calprotectin predicts remission by infliximab in anti-TNF naive patients with ulcerative colitis. J Crohns Colitis. 2012;6:557–62.

51. Arijs I, Li K, Toedter G, et al. Mucosal gene signatures to predict response to infliximab in patients with ulcerative colitis. Gut. 2009;58:1612–9.

52. Olsen T, Goll R, Cui G, Christiansen I, Florholmen J. TNF-alpha gene expression in colorectal mucosa as a predictor of remission after induction therapy with infliximab in ulcerative colitis. Cytokine. 2009;46:222–7.

53. Rismo R, Olsen T, Cui GL, Christiansen I, Florholmen J, Goll R. Mucosal cytokine gene expression profiles as biomarkers of response to infliximab in ulcerative colitis. Scand J Gastroenterol. 2012;47:538–47.

54. Seow CH, Newman A, Irwin SP, Steinhart AH, Silverberg MS, Greenberg GR. Trough serum infliximab: a predictive factor of clinical outcome for infliximab treatment in acute ulcerative colitis. Gut. 2010;59:49–54.

55. Molander P, Af Bjorkesten CG, Mustonen H, et al. Fecal calprotectin concentration predicts outcome in inflammatory bowel disease

after induction therapy with TNFalpha blocking agents. Inflamm Bowel Dis. 2012;18(11):2011–7.

56. Sjoberg M, Walch A, Meshkat M, et al. Infliximab or cyclosporine as rescue therapy in hospitalized patients with steroid-refractory ulcerative colitis: a retrospective observational study. Inflamm Bowel Dis. 2012;18:212–8.

57. Laharie D, Bourreille A, Branche J, et al. Ciclosporin versus infliximab in acute severe ulcerative colitis refractory to intravenous steroids: a randomized study. J Crohn's Colitis. 2011; 5:S8.

58. Van Assche G, Vermeire S, Rutgeerts P. Management of acute severe ulcerative colitis. Gut. 2011;60:130–3.

59. Chaparro M, Burgueno P, Iglesias E, et al. Infliximab salvage therapy after failure of ciclosporin in corticosteroid-refractory ulcerative colitis: a multicentre study. Aliment Pharmacol Ther. 2012;35:275–83.

60. Leblanc S, Allez M, Seksik P, et al. Successive treatment with cyclosporine and infliximab in steroid-refractory ulcerative colitis. Am J Gastroenterol. 2011;106:771–7.

61. Rutgeerts P, Vermeire S, Van Assche G. Predicting the response to infliximab from trough serum levels. Gut. 2010;59:7–8.

62. Sandborn WJ, Van Assche G, Reinisch W, et al. Adalimumab induces and maintains clinical remission in patients with moderate-to-severe ulcerative colitis. Gastroenterology. 2012;142:257–65.

63. Ferrante M, Karmiris K, Compernolle G, et al. Efficacy of adalimumab in patients with ulcerative colitis: restoration of serum levels after dose escalation results in a better long-term outcome. Gut. 2011;60:A72.

64. Louis E, Mary JY, Vernier-Massouille G, et al. Maintenance of remission among patients with Crohn's disease on antimetabolite therapy after infliximab therapy is stopped. Gastroenterology. 2012;142:63–70.

# Beyond Infliximab: Other Anti-TNF Therapies for Ulcerative Colitis

Ming-Hsi Wang and Jean-Paul Achkar

**Keywords**

Infliximab • Anti-TNF therapies • Ulcerative colitis • Chimeric monoclonal antibody • Tumor necrosis factor-alpha (TNF-α) • Remission • Adalimumab • Golimumab

The era of biologic therapy for inflammatory bowel disease (IBD) was launched in 1998 with the Food and Drug Administration's (FDA) approval of infliximab (IFX), a chimeric monoclonal antibody to tumor necrosis factor-alpha (TNF-α), for Crohn's disease (CD) [1]. However, it was not until 2005, after the results of several open-label clinical studies [2–5] and of the ACT1 and ACT2 trials [6] of IFX for treatment of moderate to severe ulcerative colitis (UC), that this agent was approved for therapy of UC. In a recent meta-analysis, it was estimated that the number of patients with UC needed to treat with IFX to achieve one remission was only four [7]. However, as experience with using anti-TNF-α agents in CD has shown, the development of loss of response or intolerance to an initial anti-TNF-α agent, partly due to immunogenic effects, is a real problem and having other choices for blocking TNF-α is advantageous [8–10]. Since 2012, the FDA has approved two other anti-TNF-α antibodies, adalimumab and golimumab, for the treatment of UC. In this chapter, we will review the evidence supporting the use of these agents for UC therapy.

## Adalimumab for Ulcerative Colitis

Adalimumab (Humira, Abbott Laboratories, Abbott Park, IL) (ADA) is a fully humanized recombinant monoclonal antibody (human IgG1 heavy chain and kappa light chain variable regions) with specific and high-affinity binding to soluble and transmembrane forms of TNF-α. Clinical trials demonstrated that ADA was effective in inducing and maintaining remission in CD including in patients who were naïve to IFX or had previously responded to IFX and then lost response or became intolerant [11–18]. The FDA had previously approved ADA to treat rheumatoid arthritis (2002), psoriatic arthritis (2005), ankylosing spondylitis (2006), CD (2007), plaque psoriasis (2008), and juvenile idiopathic arthritis (2008) and then approved it for the treatment of UC in September 2012.

Initial descriptions of efficacy of ADA for UC came from case reports and small open-label trials in UC patients who had previously been exposed to IFX [19–21]. In an open-label 4-week clinical trial of ten patients with mild to moderate UC who had lost response to or become intolerant of IFX [19], four patients (40 %) benefited from subsequent ADA therapy (a loading dose of 160 mg ADA subcutaneously at week 0 followed by 80 mg at week 2) with one achieving clinical remission and three having clinical improvement at week 4. Among the six patients who did not respond, two underwent colectomy. In another small, single center, open-label trial of 13 patients with mild to moderate UC who had lost response to or become intolerant of IFX [22], long-term treatment with ADA (median 42 weeks; starting with ADA 160 mg subcutaneously at week 0, 80 mg at week 2, and then 40 mg every other week) was well tolerated with no serious toxicities and was effective in maintaining clinical remission in a subgroup of UC patients,

M.-H. Wang, M.D., Ph.D. (✉)
Department of Gastroenterology and Hepatology, Cleveland Clinic, 9500 Euclid Avenue, Cleveland, OH 44195, USA
e-mail: wangm3@ccf.org

J.-P. Achkar, M.D., F.A.C.G.
Department of Gastroenterology and Hepatology,
Cleveland Clinic, 9500 Euclid Avenue, Desk A31,
Cleveland, OH 44195, USA
e-mail: achkarj@ccf.org

G.R. Lichtenstein (ed.), *Medical Therapy of Ulcerative Colitis*,
DOI 10.1007/978-1-4939-1677-1_16, © Springer Science+Business Media New York 2014

potentially avoiding colectomy in about half of the patients. Finally, Afif et al. [20] conducted a 24-week open-label clinical trial of ADA 160 mg on week 0, 80 mg on week 2, then 40 mg every other week starting week 4 in 20 patients with moderate to severe UC including 13 patients who had lost response or developed intolerance to IFX. Disease activity was assessed using the Mayo score. At week 8, clinical response (defined as decrease in Mayo score of >30 % from baseline and a decrease of ≥3 points plus a decrease in the rectal bleeding subscore of ≥1 or a rectal bleeding subscore of 0 or 1) was 25 %, clinical remission (defined as Mayo score ≤2 with no individual score >1) was 5 %, and mucosal healing (defined as decrease of the Mayo endoscopy subscore from 2 or 3 to 0 or 1) was 30 %. At week 24, based on a partial Mayo score, 50 % had clinical response and 25 % were in clinical remission. The authors concluded that ADA was well tolerated and provided a clinically beneficial option for UC patients who had lost response to or could not tolerate IFX [20]. However, although these early studies suggested efficacy of ADA in patients with mild to moderate UC who had lost response or become intolerant to IFX, results needed to be interpreted with caution due to factors such as non-blinding/open-label dosing, no comparison groups, and small sample sizes.

The first randomized, placebo-controlled trial of ADA in UC was named ULTRA1 [23] and aimed to assess the efficacy and safety of ADA in anti-TNF naïve patients with moderately to severely active UC. In this 8-week trial, 390 adult patients with moderate to severe UC as defined by a Mayo score of ≥6 points and an endoscopic subscore of 2–3 points despite treatment with corticosteroids and/or immunomodulators were randomized to one of three arms: (1) ADA 160/80 (160 mg at week 0, 80 mg at week 2, 40 mg at weeks 4 and 6), (2) ADA 80/40 (80 mg at week 0, 40 mg at weeks 2, 4, and 6), or (3) placebo. It is important to note that the study was originally designed to compare only the ADA 160/80 and placebo groups, but after initiation of the study and recruitment of the first 186 subjects, the study design was amended to include the ADA 80/40 group as required by European regulatory agencies. The primary endpoint of clinical remission at week 8 as defined by a Mayo score ≤2 with no individual subscore >1, ranked secondary endpoints, and safety of treatment were assessed. At week 8, 9.2 % of those in the placebo group had achieved clinical remission as compared to 18.5 % of patients in the ADA 160/80 group ($p = 0.03$) and 10.0 % in the ADA 80/40 group ($p = 0.83$). Serious adverse effects occurred in 7.6, 3.8, and 4.0 % of patients in the placebo, ADA 80/40, and ADA 160/80 groups respectively, but these differences were not statistically significant. A total of two malignancies occurred, both in placebo-treated patients (one basal cell carcinoma and one breast cancer). One opportunistic infection (esophageal candidiasis) occurred in the ADA 160/80 group. There were no cases of tuberculosis or death. For the secondary endpoints including clinical response, mucosal healing, rectal bleeding, physician global assessment, and stool frequency, there were

minimal statistically significant differences due to unusually high response rates in the placebo group. Interestingly, however, there were marked regional differences in these placebo response rates at week 8, reaching 54 % in Canada and 57 % in Eastern Europe compared to 31 % in the United States/ Puerto Rico and 31 % in Western Europe.

The dosing of ADA used in the ULTRA1 trial was based on the ADA doses known to be safe and effective in CD [14, 15, 18]. Based on subgroup analyses of body weight (<82 kg vs. ≥82 kg) and CRP, the authors suggested that UC patients may require a higher dose of ADA to induce remission compared to CD patients [23]. In addition, on analysis of sequential partial Mayo score data, the authors made an observation that plateau efficacy may not have been reached at week 8, indicating that a longer exposure of ADA may be required to induce remission in UC patients.

Subsequently, a long-term 52-week randomized placebo-controlled trial named ULTRA2 [24] was conducted to assess if ADA 160/80 (160 mg at week 0, 80 mg at week 2, and then 40 mg every other week) could induce and maintain clinical remission in 494 adults with moderate to severe UC. Patients in this trial had active disease despite treatment with corticosteroids and/or 6-mercaptopurine or azathioprine. Of note 40 % of subjects had previously received anti-TNF treatment. The two co-primary endpoints were clinical remission at week 8 and clinical remission at week 52 defined as a Mayo score of 2 or less with no subscore greater than 1. At week 8, 16.5 % in the ADA group versus 9.3 % in the placebo group had achieved clinical remission ($p = 0.02$), and at week 52, the corresponding numbers were 17.3 % for ADA versus 8.5 % for placebo ($p = 0.004$). In terms of secondary endpoints, clinical response rates at week 52 were 30.2 % in the ADA group compared to 18.3 % in the placebo group ($p = 0.002$) while mucosal healing rates at week 52 were 25.0 % in the ADA group and 15.4 % in the placebo group ($p = 0.009$). In a subgroup analysis, patients with prior anti-TNF exposure had twofold lower remission rates compared to the anti-TNF naïve group: 9.2 % at week 8 and 10.2 % at week 52 for prior anti-TNF exposure compared to 21.3 % at week 8 and 22 % at week 52. The remission rates in the anti-TNF naïve group are comparable to the effects reported with IFX in patients with UC who were naïve to anti-TNF therapy (Table 16.1).

ADA treatment was generally well tolerated and the overall safety profile was comparable with placebo. Malignancies occurred in two ADA-treated patients (one skin squamous cell carcinoma and one gastric cancer) compared to none in the placebo group. There was no significant difference in serious adverse events between the ADA- (12.3 %) and placebo-treated (12.1 %) groups. Greater proportions of reported injection site reactions (12.1 % in ADA group vs. 3.8 % in placebo group, $p < 0.001$) and hematological-related adverse events (1.9 % in ADA group vs. 0 % in placebo group, $p = 0.03$) were observed in ADA-treated patients. The development of antibodies to ADA was detected in 2.9 % (7 of 245) of patients in the ADA 160/80 treatment

**Table 16.1** Comparisons of efficacy of IFX (infliximab), ADA (adalimumab), and GLM (golimumab) treatments in moderate-to-severe UC

| Clinical trials | ACT1/ACT2 | | | ULTRA1/ULTRA2 | | | PURSUIT-SC | | | |
|---|---|---|---|---|---|---|---|---|---|---|
| | Placebo (n=121/123) | IFX 5 mg/kg (n=121/121) | IFX 10 mg/kg (n=122/120) | Placebo (n=130/246) | ADA 80/40 (n=130/-) | ADA 160/80 (n=130/248) | Placebo (n=331) | GLM 100/50 (n=72) | GLM 200/100 (n=331) | GLM 400/200 (n=331) |
| Study design | ACT1: moderate-to-severe active UC despite concurrent CS alone or CS+AZA/6-MP: randomized to placebo or IFX (5 or 10 mg/kg) at week 0, 2, and 6 then every 8 week through week 46. ACT2: moderate-to-severe active UC despite concurrent CS alone or CS+AZA/6-MP and 5-ASA; randomized to placebo or IFX (5 or 10 mg/kg) at week 0, 2, and 6 then every 8 week through week 22 | | | ULTRA1: moderate-to-severe active UC despite CS and/or AZA/6-MP; anti-TNF naïve; randomized to placebo or ADA (80/40: 80 mg at week 0, 40 mg at week 2, 4 and 6; 160/80: 160 mg at week 0, 80 mg at week 2, 40 mg at week 4 and 6) through week 8. ULTRA2: moderate-to-severe active UC with concurrent CS and/or AZA/MP; 40 % had previous treatment of anti-TNF; randomized to placebo or ADA (160 mg at week 0, 80 mg at week 2, 40 mg every other week) through week 52 | | | Pursuit-SC induction: moderate-to-severe active UC despite CS and/or AZA/6-MP, or CS dependent; anti-TNF naïve; randomized to placebo or GLM (100/50: 100 mg at week 0, 50 mg at week 2; 200/100: 200 mg at week 0, 100 mg at week 2; 400/200: 400 mg at week 0, 200 mg at week2) through week 6. Pursuit-SC maintenance: patients who responded to induction therapy with GLM were randomized to placebo, GLM 50 mg, GLM 100 mg every 4 weeks through week 52 | | | |
| **Clinical response** | | | | | | | | | | |
| Week 8[a] | 37.2 %/29.3 % | 69.4 %/64.5 % | 61.5 %/69.2 % | 44.6 %/34.6 % | 52.5 %/- | 54.6 %/50.4 % | 29.7 % | - | 51.8 % | 55.0 % |
| Week 54[b] | 19.8 %/- | 45.5 %/- | 44.3 %/- | -/18.3 % | -/- | -/30.2 % | 31 % | 47 % | 51 % | - |
| **Clinical remission** | | | | | | | | | | |
| Week 8[a] | 14.9 %/5.7 % | 38.8 %/33.9 % | 32.0 %/27.5 % | 9.2 %/9.3 % | 10.0 %/- | 18.5 %/16.5 % | 6.3 % | - | 18.7 % | 17.8 % |
| Week 54[b] | 16.5 %/- | 34.7 %/- | 34.4 %/- | -/8.5 % | -/- | -/17.3 % | 15 % | 24 % | 29 % | - |
| **Mucosal healing** | | | | | | | | | | |
| Week 8[a] | 33.9 %/30.9 % | 62.0 %/60.3 % | 59.0 %/61.7 % | 41.5 %/31.7 % | 37.7 %/- | 46.9 %/41.1 % | 28.5 % | - | 43.2 % | 45.3 % |
| Week 54[b] | 18.2 %/- | 45.5 %/- | 46.7 %/- | -/15.4 % | -/- | -/25 % | 27 % | 42 % | 44 % | - |
| **Adverse event** | | | | | | | | | | |
| Any AE (%) | 103 (85.1)/90 (73.2) | 106 (87.6)/99 (81.8) | 111 (91.0)/96 (80.0) | 108 (48.4)/218 (83.8) | 70 (53.8)/- | 112 (50.2)/213 (82.9) | 126 (38.3 %)/103 (66.0 %) | 34 (47.9 %)/112 (72.7 %) | 124 (37.5 %)/113 (73.4) | 129 (38.9 %)/- |
| Any serious AE (%) | 31 (25.6)/24 (19.5) | 26 (21.5)/13 (10.7) | 29 (23.8)/11 (9.2) | 17 (7.6)/32 (12.3) | 5 (3.8 %)/- | 9 (4.0 %)/31 (12.1) | 20 (6.1 %)/12 (7.7 %) | 2 (2.8 %)/13 (8.4 %) | 9 (2.7 %)/22 (14.3 %) | 5 (1.5 %)/- |
| Serious infection (%) | 5 (4.1)/1 (0.8) | 3 (2.5)/2 (1.7) | 8 (6.6)/3 (2.5) | 3 (1.3)/5 (1.9) | 2 (1.5)/- | 0 (0)/4 (1.6) | 6 (1.8 %)/3 (1.9 %) | 0 (0.0 %)/5 (3.2 %) | 1 (0.3 %)/5 (3.2 %) | 3 (0.9 %)/- |
| Malignancies (%) | 0 (0)/1 (0.3) | 2 (0.6)/1 (0.3) | 1 (0.3)/0 (0) | 2 (0.9)/0 (0) | 0 (0)/- | 0 (0)/2 (0.8) | -/1 (0.4 %) | -/0 (0 %) | -/1 (0.3 %) | -/- |

[a]Week 6 for PURSUIT-SC induction trial

[b]Week 52 for ULTRA1/2 trials; CS corticosteroids, AZA azathioprine, 6-MP 6-mercaptopurine

group; all seven patients had received ADA monotherapy. Similar to reports with other anti-TNF antibodies, the development of anti-ADA antibodies was lower in patients receiving combination therapy with ADA and an immunosuppressive agent [25]. Serum trough ADA concentrations for remitters were numerically higher than those for non-remitters throughout the duration of the study. This correlation is consistent with observations in other studies [26].

Of note, in the ULTRA2 trial, greater proportions of ADA-treated patients achieved almost all secondary endpoints at week 8 (clinical response, mucosal healing, physician global assessment, rectal bleeding subscore, corticosteroid-free remission, IBDQ score). This is in contrast to the ULTRA1 trial in which only rectal bleeding and physician global assessment subscores were significantly better in ADA-treated patients. This discrepancy might be due to the relatively high placebo response rates observed in ULTRA1 as noted above. In summary, evidence from these trials demonstrates that ADA is effective in inducing and maintaining clinical remission and clinical response in patients with moderate to severe UC failing conventional treatment with corticosteroids and/or immunomodulators.

## Golimumab (SIMPONI) for UC

Golimumab (GLM) is a human IgG1κ monoclonal antibody specific for human TNF-α which was genetically engineered using mice immunized with human TNF. It was approved by the FDA in May 2013 for the induction and maintenance of clinical response and remission in UC as well as for improving endoscopic mucosal appearance during induction therapy. The approved dosing is induction with a 200 mg subcutaneous injection at week 0 followed by a 100 mg injection at week 2 and then maintenance therapy dosed at 100 mg every 4 weeks.

A combined phase 2 and phase 3 placebo-controlled randomized trial [27] called the "PURSUIT-SC" trial was conducted to assess the dosing and dose-response relationship of GLM and to evaluate the safety and efficacy of GLM induction therapy in patients with moderate to severe UC. Patients included in this study had active UC with failure to respond to or inability to tolerate treatment with oral mesalamine, oral corticosteroids, 6-mercaptopurine, and/or azathioprine, or were corticosteroid dependent; all patients were naïve to anti-TNF therapy. In the phase 2 portion of the study, 169 patients were randomized and an additional 122 patients were enrolled while the phase 2 data were analyzed. Based on findings of a trend to a dose-response relationship and a correlation between higher GLM serum concentrations and clinical response parameters, the phase 3 portion of this study randomized 774 patients to treatment at weeks 0 and 2 with placebo ($n=258$), GLM 200/100 ($n=258$, 200 mg at week 0 and 100 mg at week 2), or GLM 400/200 ($n=258$, 400 mg at week 0 and 200 mg at week 2). The primary end-

point was clinical response at week 6, defined as a decrease in Mayo score of both $\geq 30\%$ and $\geq 3$ points along with an improvement in the rectal bleeding subscore. Secondary endpoints included clinical remission, mucosal healing, and change from baseline IBDQ. At week 6, patients who received GLM did significantly better than placebo-treated patients in terms of clinical response rates (51.8 % in GLM 200/100 and 55.0 % in GLM 400/200 vs. 29.7 % in placebo; $p < 0.0001$ for both GLM group comparisons to placebo), clinical remission rates (18.7 % in GLM 200/100 and 17.8 % in GLM 400/200 vs. 6.3 % in placebo, $p < 0.0001$ for both GLM group comparisons to placebo), mucosal healing rates (43.2 % in GLM 200/100 vs. 28.5 % in placebo, $p = 0.0005$; 45.3 % in GLM 400/200 vs. 28.5 % in placebo, $p < 0.0001$), and improvement in IBDQ scores from baseline (27.4 points in GLM 200/100 and 27.0 points in GLM 400/200 vs. 14.6 points in placebo; $p < 0.0001$ for both GLM group comparisons to placebo). Similar to the phase 2 findings, there was a correlation between higher serum GLM concentrations and clinical response parameters.

Among all treated patients in the phase 2 and 3 studies, adverse events occurred in 39.1 % of the GLM groups compared to 38.2 % in the placebo group; serious adverse events occurred in 3.0 % of the GLM groups and 6.1 % of the placebo group. One death and one case of demyelination occurred, both in patients from the GLM 400/200 group.

A follow-up phase 3 placebo-controlled, randomized, double blind, withdrawal study called "PURSUIT-M" [28] was conducted to evaluate the safety and efficacy of subcutaneous (SC) GLM maintenance therapy among moderate to severe active UC patients who had responded to GLM induction therapy. Four hundred and sixty-four patients who had responded to induction therapy with either intravenous or subcutaneous GLM were randomized to receive placebo, GLM 50 mg, or GLM 100 mg at week 0 and then every 4 weeks through week 52. The primary endpoint was clinical response maintained through week 54 as assessed by partial Mayo scores every 4 weeks and full Mayo scores at weeks 30 and 54. Secondary endpoints included clinical remission at both weeks 30 and 54, mucosal healing at both weeks 30 and 54, maintenance of clinical remission among those who entered the study in remission, and corticosteroid-free clinical remission among those who were on steroids at baseline. The primary endpoint was achieved in 31.4 % of placebo-treated patients, 47.1 % of GLM 50 mg treated patients ($p = 0.01$ vs. placebo), and 50.6 % of GLM 100 mg treated patients ($p < 0.001$ vs. placebo). Clinical remission at both week 30 and week 54 was 15.4 % for placebo, 23.5 % for GLM 50 mg ($p = 0.09$ vs. placebo), and 28.6 % for GLM 100 mg ($p = 0.003$ vs. placebo), while mucosal healing at both week 30 and week 54 was 26.9 % for placebo, 43.5 % for 41.8 % for GLM 50 mg ($p = 0.01$ vs. placebo), and GLM 100 mg ($p = 0.001$ vs. placebo). Among patients who were in clinical remission at baseline of the PURSUIT-M study, greater proportions of those treated with GLM maintained clinical remission (40.4 % of GLM 100 mg and 36.5 % of GLM 50 mg) compared to those treated with placebo (24.1 %), but these differences did not reach statistical significance. Among patients who were on corticosteroids at baseline of the PURSUIT-M study, there were no significant differences between groups in achieving corticosteroid-free clinical remission at week 54.

Through week 54, the proportions of any adverse event were 66.0, 72.7, and 73.4 % and of serious adverse events 7.7, 8.4, and 14.3 % in the placebo, GLM 50 mg, and GLM 100 mg groups respectively. There were four cases of active TB among patients from India, Poland, and South Africa, all of whom were on GLM. Three deaths occurred through week 54, all in the GLM 100 mg group, and another 6 deaths were reported after week 54, 1 from the placebo group and 5 from the GLM groups. Malignancy rates were 0.4, 0.0, and 0.3 % in placebo, GLM 50 mg, and GLM 100 mg, respectively. The authors concluded that the safety of GLM in UC was similar to GLM experience in other labeled rheumatological indications and with other anti-TNFs.

## Certolizumab (Cimzia) for UC

Certolizumab pegol is a humanized monoclonal antibody Fab fragment linked to polyethylene glycol, which increases its plasma half-life and reduces the requirement for frequent dosing. Based on in vitro studies [29], certolizumab pegol has higher binding affinity for TNF than ADA or IFX and does not activate complement pathway, cell- or antibody-mediated cytotoxicity, or apoptosis due to lack of the Fc portion of the immunoglobulin molecule. Certolizumab pegol was approved by the FDA in 2008 for the treatment and maintenance of response in adults with moderate to severe CD. The use of certolizumab pegol for moderate to severe UC is currently under study in a phase 2 clinical trial [30].

## Positioning Adalimumab, Golimumab, and Infliximab Use in Ulcerative Colitis

Table 16.1 shows side-by-side comparisons of study design and results for the IFX (ACT1/2), ADA (ULTRA1/2), and GLM (PURSUIT-SC/PURSUIT-M) in UC trials. On initial review, IFX appears to have higher rates of clinical response, clinical remission, and mucosal healing compared to the other two agents. Although these agents have the same mechanism of action, one can theorize whether factors such as intravenous versus subcutaneous administration or higher dose requirements play more of a role in UC as compared to CD. However, because there are no head-to-head trials, one cannot directly compare these response rates between IFX, ADA, and GLM. In addition, although the study designs are similar for the three agents, there are some differences that may partially explain different results between trials. For example, the ULTRA2 trial included subjects who had received prior anti-TNF therapy whereas this was an exclusion factor for all the other studies. In that trial, patients with prior anti-TNF exposure had much lower response, remission, and mucosal healing rates compared to the anti-TNF naïve group so this had an effect on overall response/remission rates. Also, in the ULTRA1 and ULTRA2 trials, there was a suggestion that higher doses of ADA may be needed in UC compared to CD. In the PURSUIT-M study, there was a more stringent definition for the primary endpoint of clinical response through week 54, with a requirement that patients needed to be in continuous clinical response through week 54 with assessments every 4 weeks. Finally, when reviewing Table 16.1, one of the most notable differences between study agents is in clinical remission rates. At week 6/8, remission rates for IFX 5 mg/kg were 39 % as compared to 17–19 % for ADA 160/80 and 19 % for GLM 200/100. Interestingly, however, the numbers for the placebo groups were also very different with placebo remission rates of 15 % in the IFX study as compared to 9 % for the ADA study and 6 % for the GLM study. Such variability could be due to factors such as differences in patient characteristics across studies or to systematic differences in assessment and scoring of the measures used to assess remission. This latter point is highlighted by the findings from a mesalamine study that interobserver differences in endoscopic assessment in UC trials can affect study results [31]. For future studies, centralized review of endoscopic images in UC trials will likely play an important role.

## Conclusion

After the FDA approval of IFX for the treatment of UC in 2005, there was a 7-year time interval during which it was the only anti-TNF agent approved for UC therapy. However, between September 2012 and May 2013, both ADA and GLM were approved for UC therapy, thus currently providing clinicians with 3 options for anti-TNF therapy in UC. At this point, choosing between these agents should depend on factors such as patient preference for intravenous versus subcutaneous administration, physician experience in prescribing each of the agents, and medical insurance coverage for formulary drugs.

However, similar to the experience and the learning curve with anti-TNF agents in CD, many questions remain. Chief among these are the role of top-down therapy in UC, whether concomitant immune modulators should be added when starting anti-TNF therapy, and determining the effectiveness of a second or third anti-TNF agent after loss of response or intolerance of a first or second course of anti-TNF therapy. In addition, although there is some information for IFX, assessment of outcomes such as rates of hospitalization and colectomy and long-term sustainability of response and remission for IFX, ADA, and GLM are needed.

## References

1. Kornbluth A. Infliximab approved for use in Crohn's disease: a report on the FDA GI Advisory Committee conference. Inflamm Bowel Dis. 1998;4:328–9.

2. Chey WY, Hussain A, Ryan C, Potter GD, Shah A. Infliximab for refractory ulcerative colitis. Am J Gastroenterol. 2001;96:2373–81.

3. Kaser A, Mairinger T, Vogel W, Tilg H. Infliximab in severe steroid-refractory ulcerative colitis: a pilot study. Wien Klin Wochenschr. 2001;113:930–3.

4. Su C, Salzberg BA, Lewis JD, Deren JJ, Kornbluth A, Katzka DA, Stein RB, Adler DR, Lichtenstein GR. Efficacy of anti-tumor necrosis factor therapy in patients with ulcerative colitis. Am J Gastroenterol. 2002;97:2577–84.

5. Gornet JM, Couve S, Hassani Z, Delchier JC, Marteau P, Cosnes J, Bouhnik Y, Dupas JL, Modigliani R, Taillard F, Lemann M. Infliximab for refractory ulcerative colitis or indeterminate colitis: an open-label multicentre study. Aliment Pharmacol Ther. 2003;18:175–81.

6. Rutgeerts P, Sandborn WJ, Feagan BG, Reinisch W, Olson A, Johanns J, Travers S, Rachmilewitz D, Hanauer SB, Lichtenstein GR, de Villiers WJ, Present D, Sands BE, Colombel JF. Infliximab for induction and maintenance therapy for ulcerative colitis. N Engl J Med. 2005;353:2462–76.

7. Ford AC, Sandborn WJ, Khan KJ, Hanauer SB, Talley NJ, Moayyedi P. Efficacy of biological therapies in inflammatory bowel disease: systematic review and meta-analysis. Am J Gastroenterol. 2011;106:644–59. quiz.

8. Baert F, Noman M, Vermeire S, Van AG, D'Haens G, Carbonez A, Rutgeerts P. Influence of immunogenicity on the long-term efficacy of infliximab in Crohn's disease. N Engl J Med. 2003;348:601–8.

9. Farrell RJ, Alsahli M, Jeen YT, Falchuk KR, Peppercorn MA, Michetti P. Intravenous hydrocortisone premedication reduces antibodies to infliximab in Crohn's disease: a randomized controlled trial. Gastroenterology. 2003;124:917–24.

10. Hanauer SB, Wagner CL, Bala M, Mayer L, Travers S, Diamond RH, Olson A, Bao W, Rutgeerts P. Incidence and importance of antibody responses to infliximab after maintenance or episodic treatment in Crohn's disease. Clin Gastroenterol Hepatol. 2004;2:542–53.

11. Papadakis KA, Shaye OA, Vasiliauskas EA, Ippoliti A, Dubinsky MC, Birt J, Paavola J, Lee SK, Price J, Targan SR, Abreu MT. Safety and efficacy of adalimumab (D2E7) in Crohn's disease patients with an attenuated response to infliximab. Am J Gastroenterol. 2005;100:75–9.

12. Sandborn WJ, Hanauer S, Loftus Jr EV, Tremaine WJ, Kane S, Cohen R, Hanson K, Johnson T, Schmitt D, Jeche R. An open-label study of the human anti-TNF monoclonal antibody adalimumab in subjects with prior loss of response or intolerance to infliximab for Crohn's disease. Am J Gastroenterol. 2004;99:1984–9.

13. Peyrin-Biroulet L, Laclotte C, Bigard MA. Adalimumab maintenance therapy for Crohn's disease with intolerance or lost response to infliximab: an open-label study. Aliment Pharmacol Ther. 2007;25:675–80.

14. Sandborn WJ, Rutgeerts P, Enns R, Hanauer SB, Colombel JF, Panaccione R, D'Haens G, Li J, Rosenfeld MR, Kent JD, Pollack PF. Adalimumab induction therapy for Crohn disease previously treated with infliximab: a randomized trial. Ann Intern Med. 2007;146:829–38.

15. Colombel JF, Sandborn WJ, Rutgeerts P, Enns R, Hanauer SB, Panaccione R, Schreiber S, Byczkowski D, Li J, Kent JD, Pollack PF. Adalimumab for maintenance of clinical response and remission in patients with Crohn's disease: the CHARM trial. Gastroenterology. 2007;132:52–65.

16. Sandborn WJ, Hanauer SB, Rutgeerts P, Fedorak RN, Lukas M, MacIntosh DG, Panaccione R, Wolf D, Kent JD, Bittle B, Li J, Pollack PF. Adalimumab for maintenance treatment of Crohn's disease: results of the CLASSIC II trial. Gut. 2007;56:1232–9.

17. Youdim A, Vasiliauskas EA, Targan SR, Papadakis KA, Ippoliti A, Dubinsky MC, Lechago J, Paavola J, Loane J, Lee SK, Gaiennie J, Smith K, Do J, Abreu MT. A pilot study of adalimumab in infliximab-allergic patients. Inflamm Bowel Dis. 2004;10:333–8.

18. Hanauer SB, Sandborn WJ, Rutgeerts P, Fedorak RN, Lukas M, MacIntosh D, Panaccione R, Wolf D, Pollack P. Human anti-tumor necrosis factor monoclonal antibody (adalimumab) in Crohn's disease: the CLASSIC-I trial. Gastroenterology. 2006;130:323–33.

19. Peyrin-Biroulet L, Laclotte C, Roblin X, Bigard MA. Adalimumab induction therapy for ulcerative colitis with intolerance or lost response to infliximab: an open-label study. World J Gastroenterol. 2007;13:2328–32.

20. Afif W, Leighton JA, Hanauer SB, Loftus Jr EV, Faubion WA, Pardi DS, Tremaine WJ, Kane SV, Bruining DH, Cohen RD, Rubin DT, Hanson KA, Sandborn WJ. Open-label study of adalimumab in patients with ulcerative colitis including those with prior loss of response or intolerance to infliximab. Inflamm Bowel Dis. 2009;15:1302–7.

21. Barreiro-de AM, Lorenzo A, Dominguez-Munoz JE. Adalimumab in ulcerative colitis: two cases of mucosal healing and clinical response at two years. World J Gastroenterol. 2009;15:3814–6.

22. Oussalah A, Laclotte C, Chevaux JB, Bensenane M, Babouri A, Serre AA, Boucekkine T, Roblin X, Bigard MA, Peyrin-Biroulet L. Long-term outcome of adalimumab therapy for ulcerative colitis with intolerance or lost response to infliximab: a single-centre experience. Aliment Pharmacol Ther. 2008;28:966–72.

23. Reinisch W, Sandborn WJ, Hommes DW, D'Haens G, Hanauer S, Schreiber S, Panaccione R, Fedorak RN, Tighe MB, Huang B, Kampman W, Lazar A, Thakkar R. Adalimumab for induction of clinical remission in moderately to severely active ulcerative colitis: results of a randomised controlled trial. Gut. 2011;60:780–7.

24. Sandborn WJ, van AG, Reinisch W, Colombel JF, D'Haens G, Wolf DC, Kron M, Tighe MB, Lazar A, Thakkar RB. Adalimumab induces and maintains clinical remission in patients with moderate-to-severe ulcerative colitis. Gastroenterology. 2012;142:257–65.

25. Colombel JF, Sandborn WJ, Reinisch W, Mantzaris GJ, Kornbluth A, Rachmilewitz D, Lichtiger S, D'Haens G, Diamond RH, Broussard DL, Tang KL, van der Woude CJ, Rutgeerts P. Infliximab, azathioprine, or combination therapy for Crohn's disease. N Engl J Med. 2010;362:1383–95.

26. Chaparro M, Guerra I, Munoz-Linares P, Gisbert JP. Systematic review: antibodies and anti-TNF-alpha levels in inflammatory bowel disease. Aliment Pharmacol Ther. 2012;35:971–86.

27. Sandborn WJ, Feagan BG, Marano C, Zhang H, Strauss R, Johanns J, Adedokun OJ, Guzzo C, Colombel JF, Reinisch W, Gibson PR, Collins J, Jarnerot G, Hibi T, Rutgeerts P. Subcutaneous golimumab induces clinical response and remission in patients with moderate to severe ulcerative colitis. Gastroenterology 2013; doi:pii: S0016-5085(13)00846-9. 10.1053/j.gastro.2013.05.048. [Epub ahead of print].

28. Sandborn WJ, Feagan BG, Marano C, Zhang H, Strauss R, Johanns J, Adedokun OJ, Guzzo C, Colombel JF, Reinisch W, Gibson PR, Collins J, Jarnerot G, Rutgeerts P. Subcutaneous golimumab maintains clinical response in patients with moderate-to-severe ulcerative colitis. Gastroenterology 2013; doi:pii: S0016-5085(13)00886-X. 10.1053/j.gastro.2013.06.010. [Epub ahead of print].

29. Nesbitt A, Fossati G, Bergin M, Stephens P, Stephens S, Foulkes R, Brown D, Robinson M, Bourne T. Mechanism of action of certolizumab pegol (CDP870): in vitro comparison with other anti-tumor necrosis factor alpha agents. Inflamm Bowel Dis. 2007;13: 1323–32.

30. Clinical Trials.gov. Study of Cimzia for the treatment of ulcerative colitis (UC CIMZIA) (http://clinicaltrials.gov/ct2/show/NCT01090154). 2012.

31. Feagan BG, Sandborn WJ, D'Haens G, Pola S, McDonald JW, Rutgeerts P, Munkholm P, Mittmann U, King D, Wong CJ, Zou G, Donner A, Shackelton LM, Gilgen D, Nelson S, Vandervoort MK, Fahmy M, Loftus Jr EV, Panaccione R, Travis SP, Van Assche GA, Vermeire S, Levesque BG. The role of centralized reading of endoscopy in a randomized controlled trial of mesalamine for ulcerative colitis. Gastroenterology. 2013;145:149–57.

# Novel Biologics for the Treatment of Ulcerative Colitis

Farzana Rashid and Gary R. Lichtenstein

**Keywords**

Mucosal ulcerative colitis • Biological agents • Anti-TNF • Janus kinase inhibitors • Corticosteroids

## Introduction

At present we have agents effective for the treatment of patients with ulcerative colitis; however, no treatment available is considered to be ideal. The characteristics of an ideal treatment for ulcerative colitis (UC) would include an ability for patients treated to achieve normal bowel function and normal quality of life, and this medication should have an ability to induce clinical remission rapidly and maintain remission over an extended period of time while achieving mucosal healing with minimal side effects. The ideal agent should be cheap and easy to administer and eliminate the need for steroids, hospitalizations, and surgeries while preventing the long-term complication of colon cancer development.

Several therapies are currently available for the treatment of UC, and they have been shown to be effective for the induction, maintenance of remission, and/or mucosal healing. These medications include aminosalicylates, corticosteroids, antimetabolites (azathioprine, mercaptopurine), cyclosporine, and biologic agents (infliximab, adalimumab, and golimumab). However, the rate of primary nonresponders and secondary loss of response to the currently available therapy is still relatively high. The side effects of some of these agents (cyclosporine, mercaptopurine/azathioprine) can also be very significant.

Biologic agents include naturally occurring or modified biologic compounds, recombinant proteins or peptides, monoclonal antibodies and fusion proteins, and antisense oligonucleotides to nucleic acids. As they are more "natural" or similar to the human body's own products, they have the potential to provide more effective and safe treatments for human diseases like UC.

There has been significant progress in understanding the pathophysiology of UC, and this has led to the development of new therapies that target key molecules and immunological mechanisms. This chapter will discuss several new treatments being evaluated for the treatment of UC. Table 17.1 outlines the general characteristics of phase I, II, and III trials in drug development. Table 17.2 outlines the therapies in the pipeline for the treatment of UC.

## Treatments Aimed at Blocking Proinflammatory Cytokines

### Anti-tumor Necrosis Factor (Anti-TNF) Agents

#### Golimumab (Formerly Known as CNTO 148)

There are currently several therapies on the market for UC targeting TNF-α including infliximab, adalimumab, and golimumab. Golimumab is a fully humanized monoclonal immunoglobulin also directed against TNF-α. Genetically engineered mice were immunized with human anti-TNFα resulting in an antibody with a human-derived variable and

F. Rashid, M.D. (✉)
Department of Gastroenterology, The University of Pennsylvania School of Medicine, 218 Wright Saunders Building, 51 North 39th Street, Philadelphia 19104, PA, USA
e-mail: farzana.rashid@uphs.upenn.edu

G.R. Lichtenstein, M.D., F.A.C.P., F.A.C.G., A.G.A.F.
Gastroenterology Division, Hospital of the University of Pennsylvania, University of Pennsylvania School of Medicine, Philadelphia, PA, USA
e-mail: gary.lichtenstein@uphs.upenn.edu

regions that are constant. The variable region of golimumab binds to both the soluble and transmembrane bioactive forms of TNF-α and as a result inhibits the biological activity of TNF-α. Golimumab has been shown in vitro to modulate the biological effects mediated by TNF including the expression of adhesion proteins responsible for leukocyte infiltration (E-selectin, ICAM-1, and VCAM-1) and the secretion of pro-inflammatory cytokines (IL-6, IL-8, G-CSF, and GM-CSF).

**Table 17.1** FDA (Food and Drug Administration) categories for describing the clinical trial of a drug, based on the study's characteristics (www.clinicaltrials.gov) (http://www.fda.gov/drugs/resourcesforyou/consumers/ucm143534.htm)

| Phase | Definition |
|---|---|
| 0 | Exploratory study involving very limited human exposure to the drug, with no therapeutic or diagnostic goals (e.g., screening studies, microdose studies) |
| 1 | Studies that are usually conducted with healthy volunteers and that emphasize safety. The goal is to find out what the drug's most frequent and serious adverse events are and, often, how the drug is metabolized and excreted |
| 2 | Studies that gather preliminary data on effectiveness (whether the drug works in people who have a certain disease or condition). For example, participants receiving the drug may be compared with similar participants receiving a different treatment, usually an inactive substance (called a placebo) or a different drug. Safety continues to be evaluated, and short-term adverse events are studied |
| 3 | Studies that gather more information about safety and effectiveness by studying different populations and different dosages and by using the drug in combination with other drugs |
| 4 | Studies occurring after FDA has approved a drug for marketing. These including postmarket requirement and commitment studies that are required of or agreed to by the sponsor. These studies gather additional information about a drug's safety, efficacy, or optimal use |

Golimumab has been approved by the Food and Drug Administration in the United States to treat moderately to severely active rheumatoid arthritis (RA), active psoriatic arthritis, and active ankylosing spondylitis (AS) and recently gained regulatory approval in 2013 for the treatment of moderate to severe UC patients who have had an inadequate response or intolerance to prior conventional treatments or who require continuous steroid therapy. Golimumab is given subcutaneously, and for UC the dosage recommended is 200 mg initially at week 0 and then 100 mg at week 2 and then 100 mg every 4 weeks. Serum golimumab concentrations reach steady-state pharmacokinetics by week 8 after the first maintenance dose. Treatment with 100 mg golimumab subcutaneously every 4 weeks during maintenance resulted in a mean steady-state trough serum concentration of $1.8 \pm 1.1$ μg/ml [1].

A combined double-blind, placebo-controlled, phase II dose-finding and phase III dose-confirmation trials demonstrated golimumab's efficacy for induction of a clinical response and remission in patients with moderate to severe ulcerative colitis (PURSUIT). There were 1,064 adults with UC (Mayo score, 6–12, endoscopy subscore ≥2). Patients were randomly assigned to groups given golimumab doses of 100 mg and then 50 mg (phase II only), 200 mg and then 100 mg, and 400 mg and then 200 mg, 2 weeks apart. The phase III primary endpoint was a clinical response at week 6. The secondary endpoints included clinical remission, mucosal healing, and IBDQ score change at week 6. In phase II, median changes from baseline in the Mayo score were −1.0, −3.0, −2.0, and −3.0 in placebo and 100 mg/50 mg, 200 mg/100 mg, 400 mg/200 mg golimumab, respectively. In phase III, rates of clinical response at week 6 were 51.8 %

**Table 17.2** Novel therapies for the treatment of ulcerative colitis

| Drug | Mechanism of action | Route | Status |
|---|---|---|---|
| Golimumab (Simponi) | TNFα antagonist | SC | Approved for UC |
| Biosimilar | TNFα antagonist | | |
| Tofacitinib (Xeljanz) | Janus kinase inhibitor | Oral | Phase II completed |
| Basiliximab (Simulect) | IL-2 antagonist suppressing lymphocyte activity and reducing corticosteroid resistance | IV | |
| Vedolizumab | Specifically targets the α4β7 integrin (inhibits leukocyte adhesion) | IV | Phase III |
| PF-547659 | Monoclonal antibody to MAdCAM-1 (inhibits leukocyte adhesion) | IV/SC | Phase I and II ongoing |
| AJM300 | α4-integrin inhibitor (inhibits leukocyte adhesion) | Oral | Phase I |
| Etrolizumab | β7-integrin inhibitor (inhibits leukocyte adhesion) | IV/SC | Phase II |
| Alicaforsen | Decrease in the production of ICAM-1 (inhibits leukocyte adhesion) | Enema | |
| BMS-936557 | Antibody to CXCL 10 (chemokine antagonist) | IV | Phase III |
| SB-656933 | CXCR2 antagonist (chemokine antagonist) | | Phase II terminated; no further drug development |
| Abatacept | Competes with CD28 for CD80 and CD86 binding | IV | |
| FMT | Alteration of microbiome | NG, NJ, PR | Clinical trials ongoing |
| HMPL-004 | Inhibitory activity against TNF-α, IL-1β, and NF-κB | Oral | Phase II completed |

*SC* subcutaneous, *IV* intravenous, *NG* nasogastric, *NJ* nasojejunal, *PR* per rectum, *FMT* fecal microbiota transplantation, *TNFα* tumor necrosis factor α, *MAdCAM-1* mucosal addressin cell adhesion molecule, *ICAM-1* intercellular adhesion molecule 1, *CXCL 10* CXC-motif chemokine 10, *CXCR2* CXC chemokine receptor type 2, *NF-κB* nuclear factor kappa beta and 55 % among patients given 200 mg/100 mg and 400 mg/200 mg golimumab respectively vs. 29.7 % in the placebo group ($P<0.0001$). Rates of clinical remission and mucosal healing and mean changes in the IBDQ scores were significantly greater in both the golimumab groups compared to placebo group ($P \leq 0.0005$). Rates of serious adverse events were 6.1 % and 3.0 %, and rates of serious infection were 1.8 % and 0.5 % in the placebo and golimumab groups, respectively. One patient in the 400/200 mg group died from surgical complications of an ischiorectal abscess.

In the phase III, double-blind trial evaluating golimumab in the maintenance of a clinical response in patients with moderate to severe UC, patients who responded to the initial golimumab induction therapy were randomly assigned to groups given placebo or injections of 50 or 100 mg of golimumab every 4 weeks through week 52 [2]. Four hundred sixty-four patients were included in this study. Patients who responded to placebo in the induction study continued to receive placebo. Nonresponders in the induction study received 100 mg golimumab. The primary outcome was clinical response maintained through week 54, and secondary outcomes included clinical remission and mucosal healing at week 30 and week 54. Clinical response was found to be maintained in 47.0 % receiving 50 mg golimumab, 49.7%receiving 100 mg golimumab, and 31.2 % receiving placebo ($P=0.010$ and $P<0.001$, respectively). At weeks 30 and 54, 27.8 % patients who received 100 mg golimumab were in clinical remission, and 42.4 % had mucosal healing compared to placebo (15.6 % and 26.6 %, $P=0.004$ and $P=0.002$, respectively) or 50 mg golimumab (23.2 and 41.7 %). Serious adverse events occurred in 7.7 %, 8.4 %, and 14.3 % of patients given placebo, 50 mg or 100 mg golimumab, respectively. Serious infections occurred in 1.9 %, 3.2 %, and 3.2 % in placebo, 50 mg or 100 mg golimumab, respectively. Among all patients who received golimumab, three died and four developed active tuberculosis. Of those that died, they all received 100 mg golimumab and died from sepsis, tuberculosis, and cardiac failure.

In controlled phase III trials through week 16 in patients with rheumatoid arthritis, psoriasis, and ankylosing spondylitis, serious infections were observed in 1.4 % of golimumab-treated patients and 1.3 % of control patients. In these trials, the incidence of serious infections per 100 patient years of follow-up was 5.7 (95 % CI: 3.8, 8.2) for the golimumab group and 4.2 (95 % CI 1.8, 8.2) for the placebo group. In the controlled phase II/III trial through week 6 of golimumab induction in UC, the incidence of serious infections in the golimumab 200/100 mg-treated patients was similar to the incidence of serious infections in placebo-treated patients. Through week 60, the incidence of serious infections was similar between patients who received golimumab induction and 100 mg maintenance compared to those who received golimumab induction and placebo for maintenance.

Serious infections in golimumab patients included sepsis, pneumonia, cellulitis, abscess, tuberculosis, invasive fungal infections, and hepatitis B infection [1].

During controlled portions of the phase II trial in RA and the phase III trials in rheumatoid arthritis, psoriasis, and ankylosing spondylitis, the incidence of malignancies other than lymphoma per 1,000 patient years of follow-up was not higher in the combined golimumab group compared to placebo group and was similar to that expected in the general US population according to the SEER database. In the phase II/III trials in UC, the incidence of non-lymphoma malignancies was also similar between the drug and placebo groups [1].

In UC trials, 3 % [34], 28 % (341), and 69 % (823) of golimumab-treated patients were positive, negative, and inconclusive for antibody development. No definitive conclusions regarding the relationship between antibodies to golimumab and clinical efficacy or safety measures could be drawn due to small sample size [1].

Golimumab has just been approved in 2013 in the United States and is available for the treatment of UC [3–7].

## Anti-TNF Biosimilars

The Biologics Price Competition and Innovation Act (BPCI Act) was signed into law by President Obama as part of healthcare reform (Affordable Care Act) to encourage the development of biosimilars and interchangeable biological products which ultimately may lead to better patient access and a lower cost to consumers [8].

A biosimilar is a biotherapeutic product which is similar in terms of quality, safety, and efficacy to an already licensed reference biotherapeutic product [9]. To establish the biosimilarity, the US FDA requires that clinical studies must show that there are no clinically meaningful differences between the biosimilar and the reference product in terms of safety, purity, and potency. The drugs must be shown to have the same pharmacokinetics and pharmacodynamics and for the most part equivalent efficacy and safety to the reference product.

The BPCI Act provides an abbreviated licensure pathway for biosimilar and interchangeable biological products under section 351(k) of the Public Health Service Act (PHS Act). As a result, a biosimilar that is demonstrated to be highly similar to the reference product may rely on existing scientific knowledge about the safety, purity, and potency of the reference product and as a result may not be required to provide full product-specific nonclinical and clinical data in order to be licensed [8].

The patent of infliximab (the first anti-TNF-α used in UC) expires between 2013 and 2015 which has opened up the market for the development of biosimilar drugs. Thus far, no single biosimilar has been reported to be tested for UC.

## Janus Kinase Inhibitors

### Tofacitinib (CP 690550)

Janus kinases (JAK) 1, 2, and 3 are extremely important in cytokine signaling that is involved in lymphocyte survival, proliferation, differentiation, and apoptosis [10]. JAK3 is found only in hematopoietic cells and is part of the signaling pathway activated by IL-2, IL-4, IL-7, IL-9, IL-15, and IL-21 which is crucial in the activation, function, and proliferation of lymphocytes (Fig. 17.1) [11].

Tofacitinib is an oral small molecule inhibitor of JAK1 and 3. In vitro studies have shown that it interferes with Th2 and Th17 cell differentiation and blocks the production of IL-17 and IL-22 [12].

In a phase II double-blind, placebo-controlled trial, the efficacy of tofacitinib in 194 adults with moderately to severely active ulcerative colitis was evaluated [13]. Patients were randomly assigned to receive tofacitinib at a dose of 0.5, 3, 10, or 15 mg or placebo twice daily for 8 weeks. The primary outcome was a clinical response at 8 weeks and occurred in 32 %, 48 %, 61 %, and 78 % of patients receiving tofacitinib at a dose of 0.5 mg ($P=0.39$), 3 mg ($P=0.55$), 10 mg ($P=0.10$), and 15 mg ($P<0.001$), respectively—compared with 42 % of patients receiving placebo. Clinical

remission (Mayo score $\leq 2$ with no subscore >1) at 8 weeks occurred in 13 %, 33 %, 48 %, and 41 % of patients receiving tofacitinib at a dose of 0.5 mg ($P=0.76$), 3 mg ($P=0.01$), 10 mg ($P<0.001$), and 15 mg ($P<0.001$), respectively, as compared with 10 % of patients receiving placebo. Treatment with the drug resulted in reduced C-reactive protein and fecal calprotectin levels.

Tofacitinib has generally been well tolerated in clinical trials. The most commonly reported adverse events related to infection reported by Sandborn and colleagues were influenza and nasopharyngitis [13]. Two patients receiving the 10 mg dose twice daily had serious adverse events from infection (postoperative abscess, anal abscess). Of significance but uncertain long-term consequence, a dose-dependent increase in low-density and high-density lipoprotein cholesterol was seen after 8 weeks of treatment which were reversible after discontinuing the studied drugs [13]. Three patients treated with tofacitinib (one at dose of 10 mg twice daily and two at dose of 15 mg twice daily) had an absolute neutrophil count of less than 1,500 (with none being <1,000) [13]. Tofacitinib is a true immunosuppressant and will most likely be used as monotherapy, and there is a concern for increased risk of infections and lymphoma with using this drug compared to other biologics.

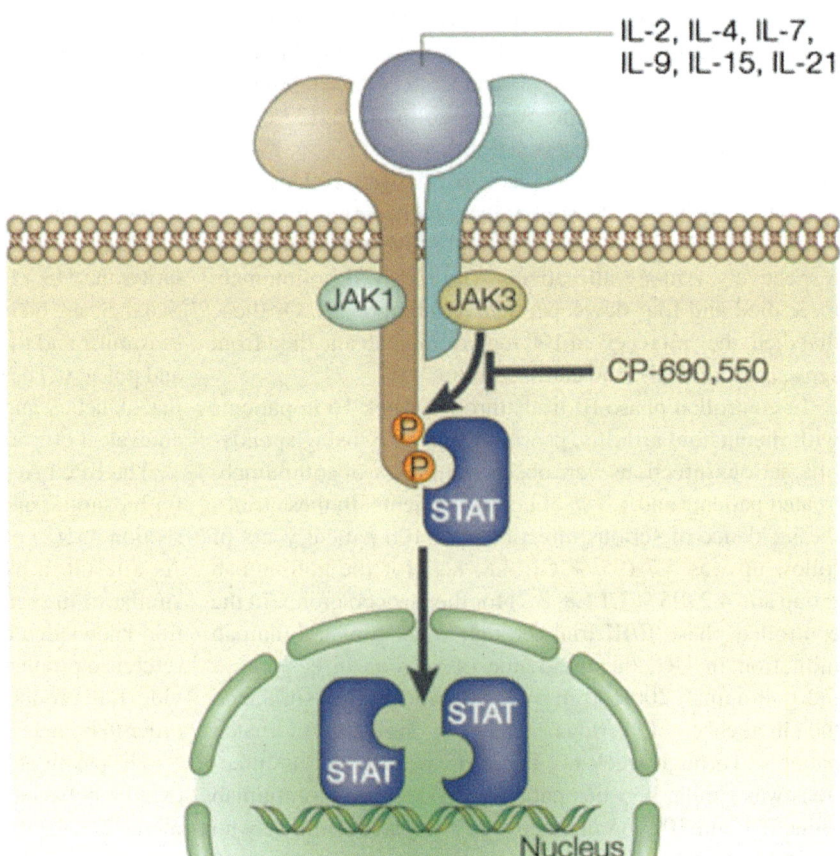

**Fig. 17.1** Tofacitinib. With permission from O'Shea, J, Pesu M, Borie DC, Changelian PS. A new modality for immunosuppression: targeting the JAK/STAT pathway. Nature Reviews 2004;4:555–564. © Nature Publishing Group 2004

There is currently an ongoing multicenter, randomized, double-blind placebo-controlled parallel group study evaluating tofacitinib as a maintenance therapy in patients with ulcerative colitis [14]. Patients will either be given placebo orally twice daily, tofacitinib 5 mg orally twice daily, or tofacitinib 10 mg orally twice daily. The primary endpoint is the proportion of subjects in remission at week 52. Secondary outcomes that will be measured are the proportion of patients with mucosal healing at week 52 and number of patients in sustained steroid free remission [14].

## Adjunct Therapy in Corticosteroid Resistance

### Basiliximab

Interleukin (IL)-2 is a T-cell autocrine growth factor that has been demonstrated to antagonize the action of steroids, thus contributing to the resistance of lymphocytes to corticosteroids. The high-affinity receptor for IL-2 is CD25 [15–18].

Basiliximab is a chimeric IgG1 monoclonal antibody that binds to the IL-2 receptor (CD25) and has been studied as an agent for the treatment of steroid-resistant ulcerative colitis.

An initial open-label, uncontrolled, 24-week trial was performed with basiliximab in ten patients with steroid-resistant UC. Patients were given a single bolus of 40 mg of intravenous basiliximab plus steroid treatment. The outcomes were assessed using the UC Symptom Score (UCSS), rectal biopsy, and IBDQ. Lymphocyte steroid sensitivity was measured in vitro in 39 subjects in the presence or absence of basiliximab. Nine achieved clinical remission within 8 weeks. Eight of the nine initial responders relapsed (median, 9 weeks), but remission was re-achieved with corticosteroids and azathioprine. Seven patients were in clinical remission at 24 weeks, and five were off of all steroid therapy. In vitro measurement of lymphocyte steroid sensitivity showed steroid resistance in 22 %. All however were rendered steroid sensitive with basiliximab [19].

A further open-label uncontrolled clinical trial was performed in 20 patients with moderate ($n = 13$) to severe ($n = 7$) steroid-resistant UC. Patients were given a single dose of 40 mg basiliximab with standard steroid therapy. The primary endpoint was clinical remission within 8 weeks (UCSS). Fifty percent achieved clinical remission within 8 weeks (seven of the moderate, three of the severe) and 65 % at 24 weeks. Five patients required colectomy (four severe and one moderate UC), and one required rescue cyclosporine (moderate UC). Two patients developed herpes zoster. Otherwise, the treatment was well tolerated [20].

However, in contrast, in a study by Sands et al., 149 patients with moderate to severe UC despite treatment with oral prednisone for 14 days were randomly assigned to groups that were given 20 mg ($n = 46$) or 40 mg ($n = 52$) basiliximab or placebo ($n = 51$) at weeks 0, 2, and 4 [21].

All subjects received 30 mg/day prednisone through week 2; the dose was reduced by 5 mg each week to 20 mg/day, which was maintained until week 8. At week 8, rates of clinical remission were compared for patients given basiliximab and placebo. Twenty-eight percent of patients given placebo, 29 % of those given the 40 mg dose of basiliximab, and 26 % of those given the 20 mg dose of basiliximab achieved clinical remission ($P = 1.00$ vs. placebo for each dose). Six subjects who received basiliximab had serious adverse events (6.1 %) compared with two who received placebo (3.9 %; $P = 0.72$). Therefore, contrary to the prior open-label trials, this study did not demonstrate the efficacy of basiliximab in increasing the effect of corticosteroids to help induce remission in outpatients with corticosteroid-resistant moderate to severe UC.

## Treatments That Target Leukocyte Migration and Adhesion

### Adhesion Molecule Blockers

Intercellular adhesion molecules play a role in leukocyte adhesion and migration, local lymphocyte stimulation, and T lymphocyte trafficking in the intestine. These molecules are upregulated in the presence of inflammation.

### Vedolizumab (Previously Known as LDP02, MLN02, and MLN0002)

In UC, there is an ongoing inflammatory response with activation of T cells, cytokine production, upregulation of the normal lymphocyte homing response, and recruitment of high numbers of T cells to the intestinal mucosa. The $\alpha_4\beta_7$ integrin molecule is found on circulating T lymphocytes and is involved in the recruitment of leukocytes to the gastrointestinal tract. The $\alpha_4\beta_7$ integrin is activated on the lymphocyte surface membrane and binds with its ligand (mucosal addressin cell adhesion molecule-1—MAdCAM-1) on the endothelial cell surface membranes. This ligand binds lymphocytes from the endothelial lumen as they pass, and once bound, the lymphocytes migrate into the lamina propria and tissue. Studies have shown significantly higher levels of $\alpha_4\beta_7$ integrin and MAdCAM-1 in colons of IBD patients. The binding of these molecules results in the homing of gut-associated lymphocytes to areas of inflamed and normal colonic mucosa (Figs. 17.2 and 17.3).

Natalizumab is a humanized monoclonal antibody directed against the $\alpha_4$ integrin on leukocytes (specifically lymphocytes). Because it is a nonselective inhibitor of the alpha 4 integrin which directs leukocytes not only to the intestinal mucosa but also to the central nervous system, there has been a fatal rarely occurring side effect of the drug—the risk of progressive multifocal leukoencephalopathy.

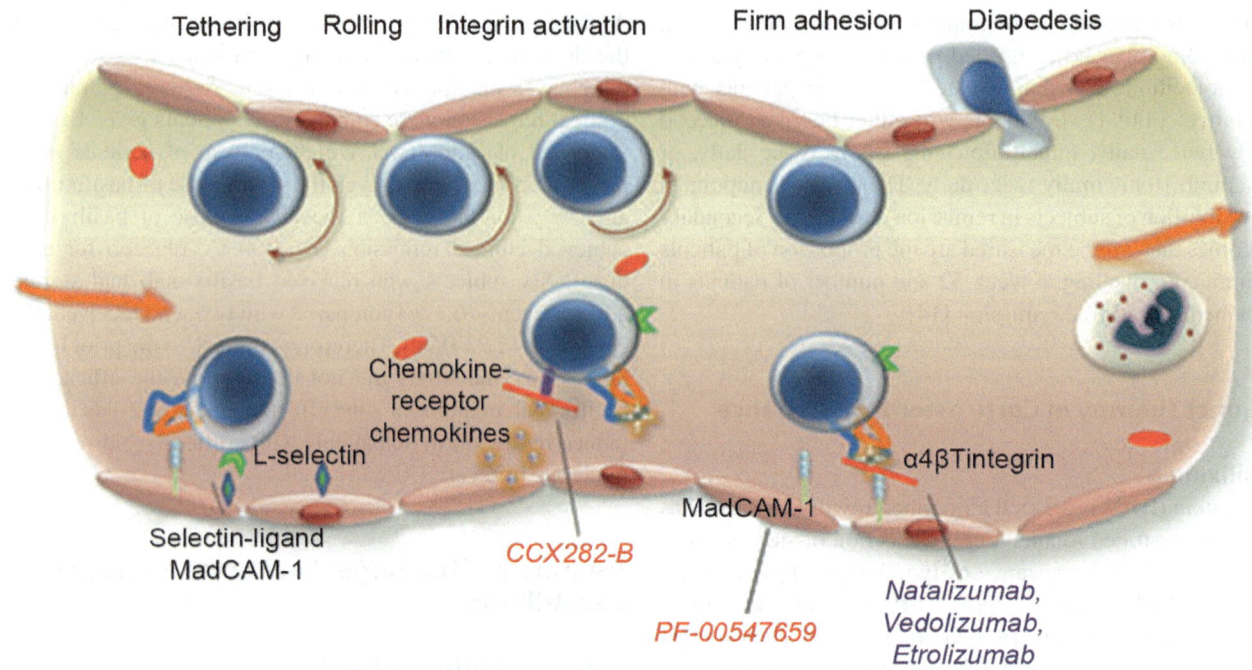

**Fig. 17.2** Mechanism of action of adhesion molecules in the intestinal endothelium and their blockage by anti-adhesion drugs. With permission from Lobatón T1, Ve`rmeire S, Van Assche G, Rutgeerts P. Review article: anti-adhesion therapies for inflammatory bowel disease. Aliment Pharmacol Ther. 2014 Mar;39(6):579–94. © 2014 John Wiley & Sons Ltd. [35]

By contrast, vedolizumab is a recombinant IgG1-humanized monoclonal antibody that specifically targets the $\alpha_4\beta_7$ integrin heterodimer which is expressed in essence exclusively in the gut. This selectively blocks the interaction between $\alpha_4\beta_7$ and MAdCAM-1 in the gut, thereby inhibiting leukocyte migration to the intestinal mucosa. Vedolizumab is administered intravenously every 4 weeks.

In 1996, a monoclonal antibody against $\alpha_4\beta_7$ integrin was used to demonstrate resolution of colitis in cotton-top tamarin monkeys. A monoclonal antibody to the $\alpha_4\beta_7$ integrin or a nontherapeutic monoclonal antibody via intramuscular injection was given to eight monkeys with chronic colitis. The control animals showed no improvement, but those receiving the antibody demonstrated clinical and histological response. Animal studies have also shown that inhibition of MAdCAM-1 prevents the development of ileitis in mice by preventing T-cell adhesion to ileal endothelium [22].

In 2000, a phase I double-blind, placebo-controlled trial using humanized $\alpha_4\beta_7$ antibody was reported in abstract form [23]. There were 29 patients with moderately severe UC. A single dose of the humanized antibody was given to participants consisting of 0.15 mg/kg subcutaneously (SC), 0.15 mg/kg intravenously (IV), 0.5 mg/kg IV, and 3 mg/kg IV or placebo. A dose of 0.5 mg/kg was found sufficient to completely saturate the antibody receptors. Complete endoscopic and clinical remission were seen 40 % (two patients) receiving 0.5 mg/kg.

A phase II randomized, double-blind, placebo-controlled trial using the $\alpha_4\beta_7$ antibody (MLN02) was performed over 6 weeks evaluating the drug's efficacy [24]. One hundred eighty-one adults with moderately or severely active UC (disease extent >25 cm from anal verge, UC clinical score (UCCS) 5–9 points with a score of at least 1 for stool frequency or rectal bleeding, and a modified Baron score of at least grade 2 on sigmoidoscopy) were randomly assigned to receive either placebo, MLN02 0.5 mg/kg IV, or MLN02 2 mg/kg IV. Each patient received two infusions (day 1 and day 29). At week 6, the primary outcome of clinical remission (UCCS of 0–1 and a modified Baron grade of 0–1 with no evidence of rectal bleeding) was seen in 14 %, 33 %, and 32 % in the placebo, 0.5 mg/kg ($P=0.02$), and 2 mg/kg ($P=0.02$) groups, respectively. Secondary outcomes of clinical response were also higher in the MLN02 0.5 mg/kg and 2 mg/kg groups compared to the placebo groups with 66 %, 53 %, and 33 %, $P=0.002$, respectively. Endoscopic remission was seen in 28 %, 12 %, and 8 % of those receiving 0.5 mg/kg, 2 mg/kg, and placebo, respectively.

Later, a phase II randomized controlled trial evaluating increasing doses of vedolizumab was performed using a new formulation developed from using the Chinese hamster ovary cell-based system [25]. Patients were randomized to receive 2, 6, or 10 mg/kg of the new drug or placebo. Patients received four infusions—one on days 1, 15, 29, and 85. Safety, pharmacokinetics, pharmacodynamics, and immunogenicity

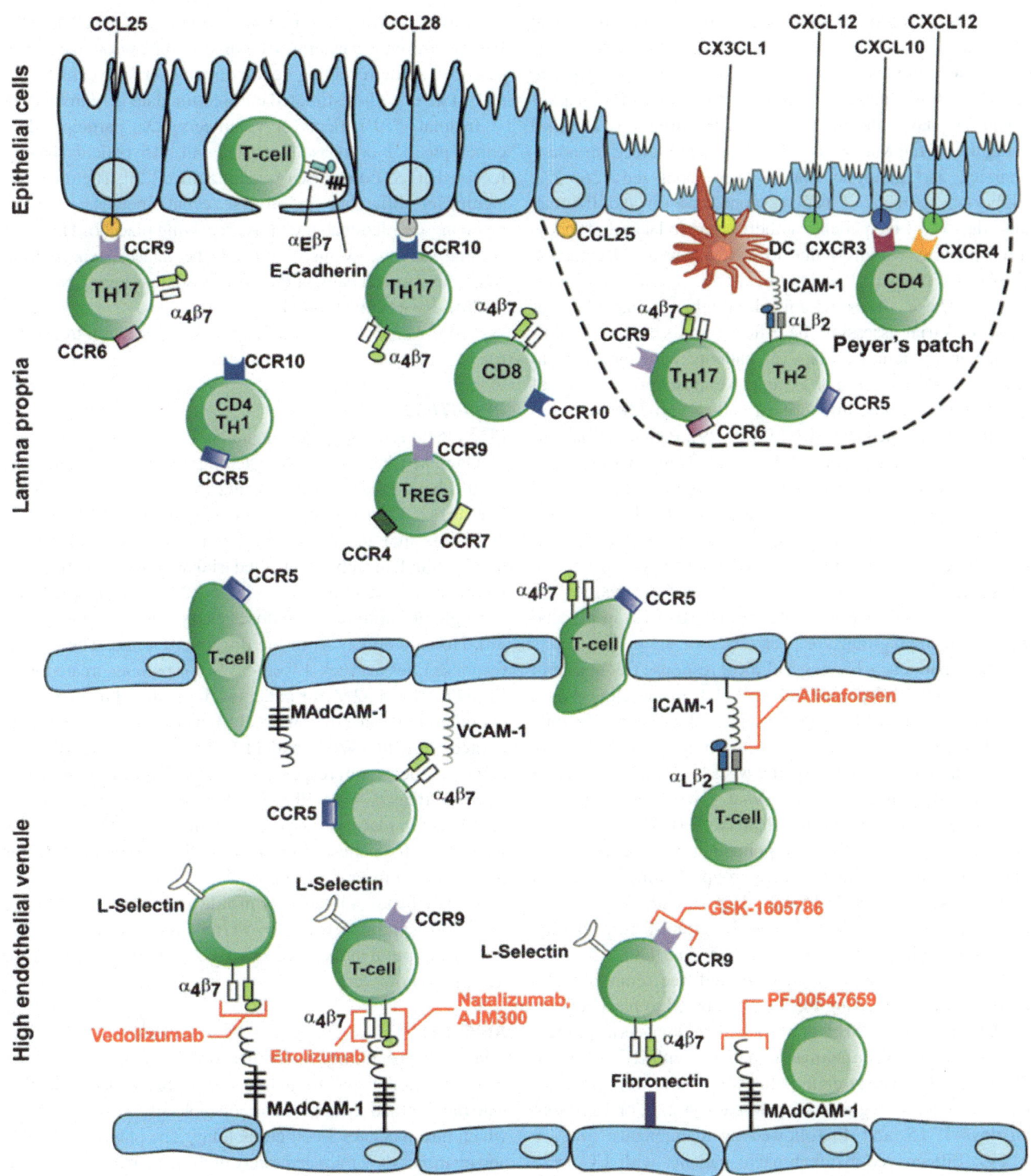

**Fig. 17.3** Mechanism of action of adhesion molecules in the intestinal endothelium and their blockage by anti-adhesion drugs. With permission from Thomas S, Baumgart DC. Targeting leukocyte migration and adhesion in Crohn's disease and ulcerative colitis. Inflammopharmacol 2012;20:1–18. © Springer 2012 [33]

evaluations were performed at multiple time points to day 253. Forty-six patients (9 placebo and 37 vedolizumab) received at least one dose of study medication. Vedolizumab maximally saturated the a4b7 receptors on peripheral serum lymphocytes at all measurable serum concentrations. Vedolizumab was well tolerated. At every assessment from day 29 to 253,

>50 % of the vedolizumab-treated patients were in clinical response; placebo response rates were 22–33 %. After this study was completed, some patients were then assigned to receive vedolizumab 2 or 6 mg/kg every 8 weeks for an additional 547 days, and the efficacy of the drug was assessed using the partial Mayo score (PMS), and the safety, immunogenicity, and pharmacokinetics were analyzed [26, 27]. Eighty-one percent of patients continued on vedolizumab until day 547. Five patients withdrew due to lack of efficacy; three patients withdrew due to adverse events. Remission rates were between 70 and 80 %.

The phase III randomized, double-blind, placebo-controlled trial assessing the efficacy and safety of vedolizumab in induction therapy in patients with moderate to severe UC (Mayo score of $\geq 6$ and an endoscopic subscore of $\geq 2$ despite steroids, thiopurines, and/or anti-TNF therapy) was then performed (GEMINI I) [28, 29]. Patients were randomized to receive either vedolizumab 300 mg IV or placebo on days 1 and 15. Two hundred twenty-four patients received vedolizumab and 149 patients received placebo. Of note, 39 % in the vedolizumab group had previous anti-TNF failure. The clinical response, remission, and mucosal healing rates were 25.5 % vs. 47.1 % ($P<0.0001$), 5.4 % vs. 16.9 % ($P=0.0009$), and 24.8 % vs. 40.9 % ($P=0.0012$) in placebo vs. vedolizumab groups, respectively.

Those patients achieving a clinical response (reduction in Mayo score of $\geq 3$ points and $\geq 30$ % from baseline plus a decrease in rectal bleeding subscore $\geq 1$ point or absolute rectal bleeding subscore of $\leq 1$ point) in the GEMINI I study after induction therapy at 0 and 2 weeks were randomized to receive vedolizumab 300 mg IV at 4 week intervals or 8 week intervals or placebo for 46 weeks [30, 31]. Three hundred seventy-three patients responded at 6 weeks and were randomized into the maintenance groups. Clinical remission at 52 weeks was seen in 15.9 %, 41.8 %, and 44.8 % in the placebo, 8 weekly, and 4 weekly groups, respectively. Mucosal healing at 52 weeks was seen in 19.8 %, 51.6 %, and 56 %, respectively. Glucocorticoid-free remission was higher in those receiving the drug compared to placebo.

Parikh et al. in 2013 published their long-term clinical experience with vedolizumab in patients with IBD for up to 78 weeks [32]. Thirty-eight patients with UC were randomized to a loading regimen of vedolizumab 2, 6, or 10 mg/kg on days 1, 15, and 43 followed by maintenance every 8 weeks. Fifteen vedolizumab-naïve patients with UC were randomized to vedolizumab in the same dosing/schedule. Seventy-two patients were dosed (53 UC and 19 CD) and 52 (72 %) completed the study. Twenty-one of 53 UC patients achieved clinical response, and 38 of 53 UC patients achieved clinical remission. Mean partial Mayo scores declined from baseline through day 155 both in treatment-naïve patients with UC and rollover patients with UC. No deaths or systemic opportunistic infections were reported, and the adverse event profile was similar to previously observed.

A longer-term phase III trial is ongoing (GEMINI LTS). Patients from the earlier trials will have the option to enter an extended study receiving vedolizumab every 4 weeks for up to 100 weeks. The estimated completion date is March 2016.

In total, 579 patients or volunteers have participated in either phase I or phase II trials with 415 patients having received at least one dose of vedolizumab [22]. There was no significant difference in adverse events between patients receiving vedolizumab and those receiving placebo. The most common adverse events were headache, nausea, exacerbation of UC, abdominal pain, fatigue, and nasopharyngitis. No cases of PML have been reported.

Vedolizumab is a promising new upcoming treatment for UC.

### PF-547659

PF-547659 is a monoclonal antibody to MAdCAM-1. By blocking MAdCAM-1, leukocyte migration to the gut mucosa should be altered, thus decreasing the inflammation in UC. See section discussing vedolizumab (Figs. 17.2 and 17.3).

In this first in-human study which was a randomized, double-blind, placebo-controlled trial, 80 patients with active UC received placebo or PF-547659 (0.03–10 mg/kg IV/sc) in single or multiple (three doses every 4 weeks) doses [33–36]. No side effects from the drug were noted. The overall response rates at week 4 were 52 % for patients treated with PF-547659 and 32 % for patients administered placebo. The overall remission rates at week 4 were 13 % for patients treated with PF-547659 and 11 % for patients administered placebo. The overall response rates at week 12 were 42 % for patients treated with PF-547659 and 21 % for patients administered placebo. The overall remission rates at week 12 were 22 % for patients treated with PF-547659 and 0 % for patients administered placebo.

Due to the favorable safety profile and efficacy findings in the aforementioned trial, PF-547659 may be a promising treatment option in the future for UC. Further larger trials are necessary, however.

### AMG 181

AMG 181 specifically targets the $\alpha4\beta7$ integrin heterodimer (similar to vedolizumab) and as a result blocks its interaction with mucosal addressin cell adhesion molecule-1 (MAdCAM-1) which thus mediates T-cell gut homing. The pharmacokinetics and pharmacodynamics and safety of the drug were first studied in cynomolgus monkeys [37]. Pan and colleagues also evaluated the same in health volunteers and patients with both Crohn's disease and UC in a randomized, double-blinded, placebo-controlled ascending multiple-dose study [38, 39].

Phase II studies (a 360-patient trial) had to be suspended for "inaccuracy in study documents required correction for future enrollees." This was also the reason given for the suspension of another placebo-controlled trial that aimed at recruiting 252 patients [40–43].

## AJM300 ($\alpha_4$-Integrin Inhibitor)

AJM300 is a small molecule administered orally and targeting the $\alpha_4$-integrin subunit and as a result prevents mainly adhesion and infiltration of lymphocytes into an area of gastrointestinal inflammation (Figs. 17.2 and 17.3).

On November 6, 2013, the company that is developing AJM300, Ajinomoto Pharmaceuticals Co., Ltd., has released data showing efficacy of AJM300 in the treatment of UC [44]. This phase II, randomized, double-blind comparative study was performed for patients with moderately active ulcerative colitis and included 102 patients in 42 Japanese sites. The primary endpoint was clinical response rate at 8 week post-administration for the aim to induce remission and which was significantly higher in the AJM300 treatment group compared to patients receiving placebo. These preliminary studies suggest that AJM300 could provide an oral option for UC, but further investigative studies are needed.

## Etrolizumab (rhuMAb-Beta7 or $\beta_7$-Integrin Inhibitor)

Etrolizumab is a humanized monoclonal antibody targeting the integrin subunit $\beta_7$ and as such blocks both $\alpha_4\beta_7$ and $\alpha_E\beta_7$ integrins thus targeting the gastrointestinal system and avoiding effects on the central nervous system (Figs. 17.2 and 17.3).

Stefanich et al. in 2011 evaluated anti-$\beta_7$ in cynomolgus monkeys and demonstrated inhibition of lymphocyte homing to the inflamed colons in severe combined immunodeficient and CD45RB$^{high}$ CD4$^+$ T-cell transfer models of inflammatory bowel disease. The results also suggested that etrolizumab selectively blocked lymphocyte homing to the gastrointestinal tract without affecting lymphocyte trafficking to non-mucosal tissues [33].

In a phase I double-blind randomized within cohort, placebo-controlled study by Rutgeerts and colleagues published in *Gut* (2013) involving 48 outpatients with moderate to severe UC, the safety and pharmacology of etrolizumab were evaluated [45, 46]. A single-ascending dose (SAD) stage followed by a multidose (MD) stage was involved. A single dose of etrolizumab (0.3, 1.0, 3.0, 10 mg/kg IV, 3.0 mg/kg SC) or placebo was given in a 4:1 ratio to each group. This was followed by a MD stage in a different group of patients in which three doses of etrolizumab (0.5, 1.5, 3.0 mg/kg SC, 4 mg/kg IV) or placebo were given monthly in a 4:1 ratio to each group. The Mayo score was evaluated on day 29 after the study drug administration in the SAD and after days 43 and 71 in the MD stage. The drug was well tolerated. Headache was the most common adverse event occurring more often in actively treated patients. Eight patients had serious adverse events—seven were in the SAD stage (six treated with etrolizumab and one in the placebo group) and one was in the MD stage (etrolizumab treated). The most common serious adverse event was exacerbation of UC. In the SAD stage, two patients had impaired wound healing after an urgent colectomy for exacerbation of UC. A clinical response was observed in 12/18 patients and clinical remission was seen in 3/18 patients treated with etrolizumab in the MD stage compared to 4/5 and 1/5 patients treated with placebo. Two patients (one SAD stage, one MD stage) developed transient low level of JCV shedding but neither developed any symptoms or signs of progressive multifocal leukoencephalopathy.

A phase II randomized, double-blind, placebo-controlled induction study (EUCALYPTUS trial) by Vermeire and colleagues was published as an abstract [47]. This study's aim was to evaluate the efficacy and safety of etrolizumab in outpatients with refractory moderately to severely active UC. The primary efficacy endpoint was the proportion of patients in clinical remission at week 10, and the secondary endpoint was endoscopic remission. Patients were randomized to receive either two dose levels of etrolizumab (100 mg monthly SC or 300 mg monthly SC+loading dose (LD) of 420 mg SC between weeks 0 and 2) or placebo for three doses. The Mayo score was evaluated at weeks 0, 6, and 10. Etrolizumab showed significantly higher rates of clinical remission compared to placebo (100 mg dose 20.5 % and 300 mg+LD dose 10.3 % vs. 0 % ($P=0.004$ and 0.049, respectively). In the anti-TNF naive subgroup, the rates of clinical remission at week 10 were significantly higher in the 100 mg dose group compared with placebo (43.8 % vs. 0 %, $P=0.007$). Endoscopic remission of 10.3 % (100 mg dose) and 7.7 % (300 mg+LD) was seen compared to 0 % in the placebo group. In the anti-TNF naive subgroup, endoscopic remission was 25 % (100 mg) and 16.7 % (300 mg+LD) vs. 0 %, respectively ($P=0.058$ vs. placebo for the 100 mg dose group). Rates of adverse events were comparable. One etrolizumab-treated patient developed a rash and headache after the first dose and was admitted to the hospital for observation. Four actively treated patients (all in the 300 mg+LD dose group) developed with mild injection site reactions.

In summary, etrolizumab is a promising treatment for moderately to severely active UC, and further phase III studies are needed.

## Alicaforsen (ISIS 2302)

Alicaforsen is a 20 base phosphorothioate oligodeoxynucleotide that hybridizes to a sequence in the 3′ untranslated region of intercellular adhesion molecule 1 (ICAM-1) mRNA. The translated oligonucleotide RNA serves as a substrate for the nuclease RNase-H. This results in a decrease in the production of ICAM-1 altering the intestinal inflammation found in UC.

Initially, alicaforsen was tried intravenously and subcutaneously in Crohn's disease and was found to produce a rapid and persistent clinical response in a pilot trial of 15 patients. However, two larger trials in steroid-dependent moderate CD did not show any greater effect than placebo. A thought was this because the drug could not reach the intestinal tissue from the bloodstream. Therefore, an enema formulation was developed.

In an open-label uncontrolled study, 12 patients with chronic, unremitting pouchitis were treated with 240 mg alicaforsen enemas nightly for 6 weeks [48, 49]. Clinical evaluation and pouchoscopy with biopsy were performed at baseline and at weeks 3, 6, and 10. The primary endpoint was reduction from the baseline of the pouchitis disease activity index (PDAI) at week 6. Secondary endpoints included the PDAI at week 10. A statistically significant reduction in the PDAI from baseline to week 6 was observed (11.42–6.83, $P=0.001$). Mean reductions in the endoscopy and clinical symptom subscore from baseline to week 3 and week 6 were seen and were statistically significant. Ten of 12 patients achieved a mucosal appearance score of 0 or 1 on endoscopy. By week 6, 58 % were in remission as defined by PDAI <7. The enemas were well tolerated.

In 2004, van Deventer et al. evaluated the safety and efficacy of alicaforsen enemas in a randomized, placebo-controlled, double-blind escalating dose multicenter study after 1, 3, and 6 months [50]. There were 40 patients with mild to moderately active distal UC. Patients received 60 ml enema once daily for 28 consecutive days of different doses—0.1, 0.5, 2, or 4 mg/ml. At day 29, the alicaforsen enema resulted in dose-dependent improvement in disease activity index (DAI) ($P=0.003$). The 4 mg/ml enema improved disease activity index by 70 % compared with the placebo response of 28 % ($P=0.004$). At month 3, the groups using the 2 and 4 mg/ml drug enemas improved DAI by 72 % and 68 % compared with a placebo (11.5 %) ($P=0.016$ and 0.021, respectively). None of the patients in the 4 mg/ml group compared with 50 % of the placebo group required additional medical or surgical intervention over baseline during the 6-month period. The drug appeared safe.

In an open-label study in patients with UC published by Miner and colleagues in 2006, 15 patients with active UC received nightly enemas of ISIS 230 (240 mg) for 6 weeks [51]. There was a 46 % reduction in the mean DAI at the end of the 6-week treatment period; 5/15 (33 %) demonstrated complete mucosal healing. No serious adverse events occurred in the study.

Miner and colleagues in 2006 evaluated the effects of the alicaforsen enema to standard mesalamine enemas in patients with mild to moderately active left-sided UC in a randomized, double-blind, active-controlled, multicenter clinical trial [52]. Patients received 120 mg alicaforsen, 240 mg alicaforsen, or 4 g mesalamine enema every night for 6 weeks followed by a monitoring period of 24 weeks. The primary endpoint was the DAI at week 6 with clinical improvement, remission, and relapse as secondary endpoints. No significant differences were seen in the DAI at week 6 between the groups. However, the median duration of response with the alicaforsen enema was two- to threefold longer (128 and 146 days)

compared to mesalamine (54 days). Complete mucosal healing occurred in 24 % of the 240 mg alicaforsen group compared to 17 % in the mesalamine group. The authors concluded that the alicaforsen enema had a more durable response compared to mesalamine enemas but otherwise had a profile similar to mesalamine enemas.

A randomized, placebo-controlled, double-blind, two-dose multicenter study involving 112 subjects was performed in 2006 [53]. Patients were randomized to receive one of four alicaforsen enemas or placebo daily for 6 weeks. The primary endpoint was DAI at week 6. Secondary endpoints were clinical improvement, relapse rates, and durability of response. In this study, no difference was observed between the treatment arms and placebo in terms of DAI at week 6. However, there was a reduction in the mean DAI compared to baseline in the 240 mg alicaforsen enema group compared to placebo from week 18 to week 30 (51 % vs. 18 % $P=0.04$, 50 % vs. 11 % $P=0.03$).

Finally, Vegter and colleagues performed a meta-analysis using individual patient data to evaluate the efficacy and durability of alicaforsen enemas compared to placebo or high-dose mesalamine in patients with moderate or severe UC or disease up to 40 cm from the anal verge [54]. Efficacy was analyzed for short-term (week 6–10) and long-term (week 30) outcomes. Alicaforsen showed superior efficacy compared to placebo in patients with disease extent up to 40 cm, patients with moderate and severe diseases, and especially when patients had either moderate or severe disease that extended up to 40 cm from the anal verge. Mesalamine showed short-term efficacy, but at week 30, the efficacy of mesalamine decreased and alicaforsen became significantly more efficacious.

## Therapies That Target Chemokines and Chemokine Receptors

Chemokines promote the directed chemotaxis of leukocytes. Specifically, CXC chemokines are notable for their role in the initiation and amplification of inflammatory diseases such as inflammatory bowel disease, and targeting chemokines and chemokine receptors are a novel mechanism in which to treat inflammatory bowel disease [55, 56].

### BMS-936557 (Previously Termed MDX-1100)

Interferon-$\gamma$-inducible protein-10 (IP-10 or CXCL10) is a chemokine that plays an important role in the migration of cells into sites of inflammation by influencing activation and migration of activated T cells, monocytes, eosinophils, natural killers, and epithelial and endothelial cells [57, 58]. The receptor for CXCL10 is CXCR3 but IL-10 also seems to modulate cellular function independently of CXCR3 [57]. CXCL10 has been found to be expressed in higher levels in the colonic tissue and plasma of patients with UC [59, 60]. In animal models of UC, blocking CXCL10 has been shown to modify disease progression [58, 61–64]. BMS-936557 is a fully human, monoclonal antibody to CXCL10.

A phase I open-label, dose-escalation study of MDX-1100 has been performed in patients with UC using MDX-1100 [65]. The primary objective of this was to evaluate the safety of single doses of the drug in patients with UC flaring on stable doses of standard therapy. Patients were off anti-TNF therapy for at least 8 weeks prior to the study. Cohorts of patients were given a single infusion of the drug at doses of 0.3, 1.0, 3.0, or 10 mg/kg and were followed for at least 70 days post-infusion. A clinical response was defined as UCDAI decrease by ≥3 points at day 29 compared to baseline. Patients who responded were allowed to receive up to three additional infusions at the time of relapse. Peripheral blood mononuclear cells and colon biopsy specimens were studied for expression of CXCL10 and CXCL10-induced proteins. Three patients in the 1.0 mg/kg and two patients in the 3.0 mg/kg cohorts had clinical responses; however, one patient in the 1.0 mg/kg cohort also was started on concomitant immunomodulator therapy 2 months prior to MDX-1100 administration. Two of three responding patients who relapsed after 50, 85, and 93 days, respectively, and who had then been given additional MDX-1100 doses responded to re-treatment. One patient in the 3.0 mg/kg cohort was admitted to the hospital for anemia and worsening UC requiring a colectomy, but otherwise the drug was well tolerated.

Mayer and colleagues in 2014 published data from an 8-week phase II, double-blind, multicenter, randomized study in patients with active UC [57]. Patients with moderately to severely active UC were given either BMS-936557 (10 mg/kg) or placebo intravenously every other week. The primary endpoint was the rate of clinical response at day 57 and secondary endpoints were clinical remission and mucosal healing rates. Fifty-five patients received the drug and 54 patients received placebo. Primary and secondary endpoints were not met. However, what was found was that with higher steady-state trough levels of BMS-936557 (108–235 µg/ml), there was an increased clinical response (87.5 % vs. 37 % $P < 0.001$) and histological improvement (73 % vs. 41 % $P = 0.004$) compared to placebo. Infections occurred in 12.7 % of BMS-936557-treated patients and 5.8 % of placebo-treated patients. Two patients (or 3.6 %) discontinued due to adverse events.

Therefore, BMS-936557 appears promising at higher drug levels. Further dose-response studies are needed at this time.

## SB-656933

In humans, CXCR2 mediates neutrophil chemotaxis in response to tissue injury and many types of infections. Targeting the interaction of CXCR2 and its various ligands can potentially provide a potential mechanism to ameliorate neutrophil chemotaxis to sites of injury and thus inflammation.

SB-656933 is a novel and selective CXCR2 antagonist in the development for the treatment of CF and COPD [56, 65–67]. Polymorphonuclear migration to inflamed colonic tissue is a predominant feature of active UC. In preclinical models of colitis, SB-656933 has been shown to reduce polymorphonuclear neutrophil accumulation in the colon.

A 7 day open-label phase II study was underway evaluating the pharmacodynamics of daily dose of SB-656933 in patients with ulcerative colitis [68]. Primary outcome measures included changes from baseline to after 1 and 7 days in 99mTc-HMPAO-labeled leukocyte single-photon emission computed tomography (SPECT) scintigraphic activity scores (SAS). Secondary outcome measures included the safety and tolerability of the drug, amount of medicine in the blood, changes in fecal calprotectin levels, and induced CD11b levels in the blood. However, this study was terminated, and SB-656933 is no longer being developed for the treatment of UC.

## Abatacept

T cells play a role in the pathogenesis of UC. T-cell activity requires co-stimulatory signaling through CD28 (on T lymphocytes) and CD80 or CD86 (on antigen-presenting cells). T-lymphocyte antigen 4 is cytotoxic and induced on the T-cell surface 24–48 h after activation. This activates the CD28-mediated co-stimulation of T cells and prevents CD28 from binding to CD80 or CD86.

Abatacept is a recombinant fusion protein comprising a fragment of the Fc domain of human IgG1 and the extracellular domain of human cytotoxic T-lymphocyte antigen 4. This product competes with CD28 for CD80 and CD86 binding to block the interaction between CD80/CD86 and CD28 preventing the activation of T cells.

Abatacept is dosed intravenously every 2–4 weeks and has been shown to be effective for rheumatoid arthritis and juvenile idiopathic arthritis. In animal models of colitis, this has been shown to reduce inflammation.

By contrast, Amezcu a-Guerra and colleagues reported a case of a patient with severe rheumatoid arthritis who developed ulcerative colitis while being treated with CTLA-4Ig [69]. The patient had seropositive RA refractory to treatment with 20 mg/week methotrexate (MTX), 1.5 g/day sulfasalazine (SSZ), 400 mg/day hydroxychloroquine, and 100 mg/day azathioprine. The patient was in a CTLA-4Ig (10 mg/kg intravenously monthly) and methotrexate clinical trials. All other disease-modifying drugs were discontinued. The patient showed major clinical and serological responses with treatment. Fifteen months into treatment, the patient developed GI symptoms of diarrhea, rectal bleeding, crampy abdominal pain, tenesmus, and weight loss, and as a result, CTLA-4Ig and methotrexate were discontinued. After a thorough workup, the diagnosis of UC was made, and the patient was placed on mesalamine therapy with a good response. Eventually, the dose was reduced and the drug discontinued over the subsequent 3 months. Four months after stopping CTLA-4Ig, the patient remained asymptomatic for UC.

In placebo-controlled trials by Sandborn et al., abatacept was evaluated for the efficacy and safety as induction and maintenance therapy in adults with active moderate to severe CD and UC [70]. Patients were randomized to the drug at 30, 10, or 3 mg/kg or placebo and dosed at weeks 0, 2, 4, and 8. One hundred thirty-one patients with UC who responded to the drug at week 12 in induction trials were randomized to abatacept 10 mg/kg or placebo every 4 weeks through week 52. In UC patients during the induction phase, 21.4 %, 19.0 %, and 20.3 % of patients receiving abatacept 30, 10, and 3 mg/kg achieved a clinical response at week 12 vs. 29.5 % receiving placebo ($P=.124$, $P=.043$, and $P=.158$, respectively). In the maintenance portion of the trial, 12.5 % vs. 14.1 % of patients receiving abatacept vs. placebo were in remission at week 52. Safety was comparable between the groups. In this study, abatacept was not found to be efficacious for the treatment of moderate to severe UC.

## Fecal Microbiota Transplantation (FMT)

Fecal transplantation has attracted immense interest in the past several years and has been shown to be the most effective therapy for relapsing clostridium difficile infection. With advances in the understanding of the gastrointestinal microbiota in terms of structure and function, fecal transplantation is being investigated in other conditions where dysbiosis may occur such as in UC (Fig. 17.4).

A study was performed in children and young adults with UC recently and published by Kunde and colleagues in 2013 [71]. Ten children between the ages of 7 and 21 with mild to moderate UC received freshly prepared fecal enemas daily for 5 days. Data was collected during the fecal transplant and then weekly for 4 weeks afterward. No serious adverse events were noted. Mild (cramping, fullness, flatulence, bloating, diarrhea, blood in stool) to moderate (fever) adverse events were seen and were self-limiting. One patient could not retain the fecal enemas, and the average enema volume that was able to be tolerated by the remaining patients was 165 ml/day. After the transplant, 78 % [7] showed clinical response within 1 week, 67 % [6] maintained clinical response at 1 month, and 33 % [3] achieved clinical remission at 1 week after the fecal transplant. Median PUCAI improved after transplant compared with baseline with a ($P=0.03$).

A systematic review which included 17 studies and 41 patients with either UC or Crohn's disease who underwent a FMT demonstrated that 76 % had a reduction or complete resolution in symptoms, 76 % had cessation of all IBD medications, 63 % were in "prolonged remission" of previously active disease [72, 73].

In a publication by Harrell in 2012, 86 % of patients previously refractory to IBD medications became responsive to the meds after FMT [73, 74].

Damman and colleagues compiled the data of three publications which involved nine patients with refractory IBD. Eight patients had UC, and 1 patient had Crohn's disease. These patients were treated with fecal enemas, and all patients were in remission between 3 months and 13 years [75].

An ongoing phase II randomized, double-blind, controlled trial led by Paul Moayyedi and Christine Lee at McMaster University and St. Joseph's Hamilton Healthcare is evaluating fecal biotherapy (compared to placebo) in the form of weekly enemas (from healthy unrelated donors) for 6 weeks and its efficacy in the treatment of adults with active UC [76]. The primary outcome studied is remission of UC and mucosal healing. The secondary outcomes evaluated are endoscopic and clinical remission and improvement of symptoms.

There is a phase II randomized, double-blind, controlled study (FOCUS) of the efficacy and safety of FMT in the treatment and induction of remission in adults with mild to moderately active UC (>3 months duration excluding isolated proctitis <5 cm) that is being led by researchers at the University of New South Wales between September 2013 and 2016 [77]. Patients will either get a FMT infusion (from healthy screened donors) or a placebo (saline and glycerol) infusion. The primary outcome measured is clinical remission at 8 weeks as measured by Mayo subscores. The secondary outcomes measured will be endoscopic and clinical remission (Mayo subscores and UCEIS), clinical response (Mayo subscores), endoscopic healing (UCEIS), treatment failure rate (Mayo subscores), quality of life (IBDQ), and safety and tolerability (adverse event data) in the 8-week study period.

Several other clinical trials are currently in progress throughout the United States as on the clinicaltrials.gov website (including the University of Chicago) and other countries evaluating FMT in pediatric and adult patients with IBD [78].

Although fecal transplantation seems promising, there have been studies that have demonstrated otherwise. De Leon and colleagues in 2013 reported a patient with UC that had been quiescent for more than 20 years who developed a flare of UC after fecal microbiota transplantation [79]. The patient's colitis was under control without any maintenance medications prior to the fecal transplant and, after flaring, was treated with a short-term increase in his usual low prednisone dose for his panhypopituitarism in addition to

**Fig. 17.4** Fecal microbiota transplantation. Created from data taken from Brandt, LJ and Aroniadis OC. An overview of fecal microbiota transplantation: techniques, indications, and outcomes. Gastrointestinal Endoscopy 2013; 78(2): 240–249 [73]

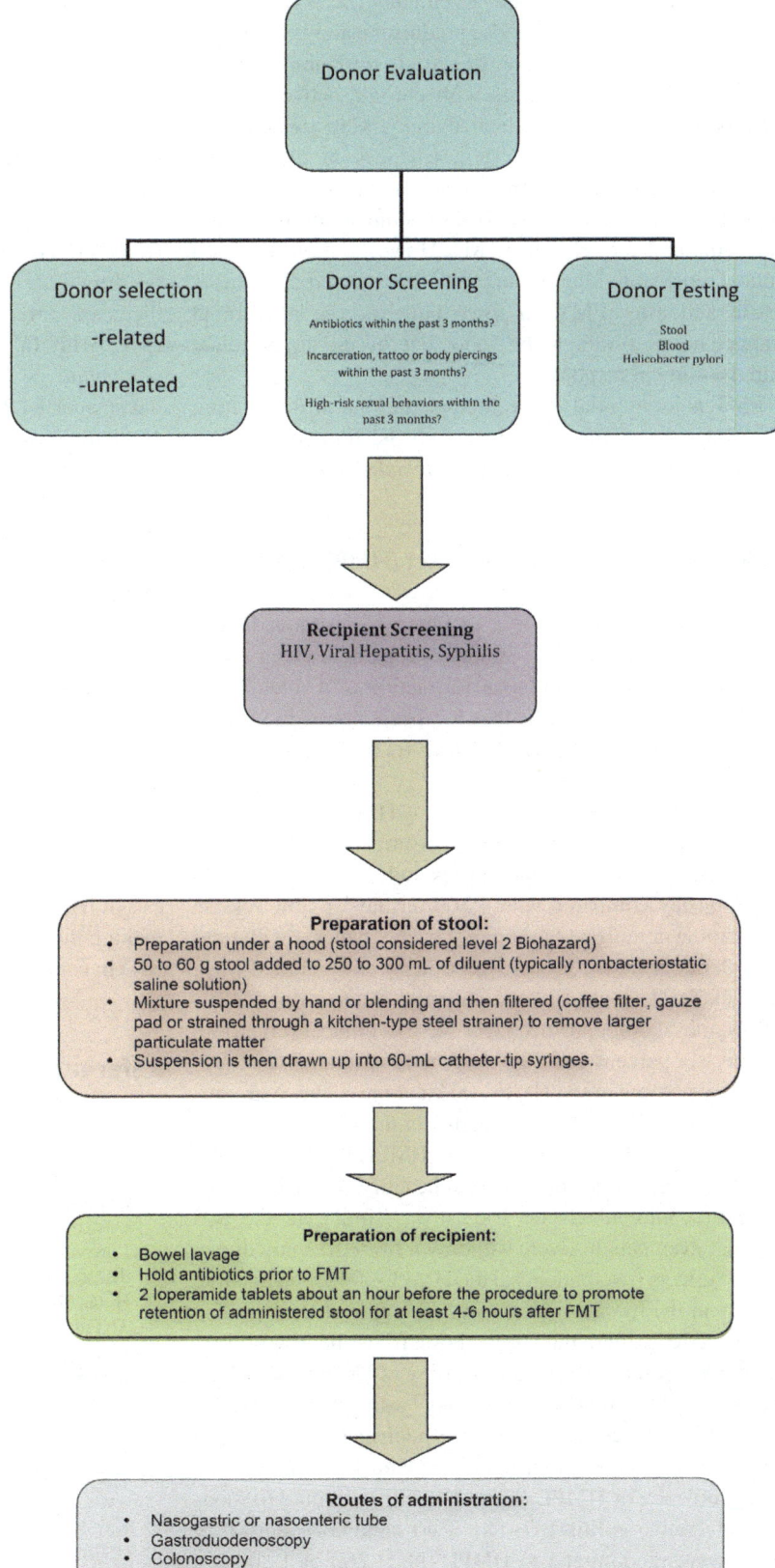

oral and topical mesalamine. Eventually, he was weaned back down to his usual low-dose prednisone and kept on oral mesalamine for maintenance. In a study by Kump and colleagues in 2013, six patients with chronic active UC not responsive to standard medical therapy were treated with FMT through colonoscopy [80]. Changes in the colonic microbiota were assessed from mucosal and stool samples. All patients experienced short-term clinical improvement within the first 2 weeks after FMT. However, none achieved clinical remission. Microbiota evaluation showed differences before and after FMT. In three patients, the microbiota changed to one similar to the donor, but this did not correlate with the clinical response.

FMT is a potential future therapeutic option for treating UC. However, at this time, based on the limited evidence available, FMT cannot yet be recommended at this time.

### *Androgmphis paniculata* Extract (HMPL-004)

*Androgmphis paniculata* is a member of the plant family Acanthaceae and has been an herbal remedy used in Asian countries like China and India. Extraction of *A. paniculata* leads to a mixture of herbs that has been shown in vitro to have inhibitory activity against TNF-α, IL-1β, and NF-Kb [81–84].

A phase I study was performed using HMPL-004 in China [85]. Then, Tang and colleagues performed a randomized, double-blind, 8-week parallel group study using HMPL-004 1,200 mg/day compared with 4,500 mg/day of slow release mesalamine granules. One hundred twenty patients with mild to moderately active ulcerative colitis were included [86]. At week 8, 21 % vs. 16 % of patients treated with HMPL-004 vs. mesalamine, respectively were in clinical remission. Seventy-six percent and 82 % had more than a 25 % reduction in symptoms in the HMPL-004 and mesalamine groups, respectively. 15/53 (28 % of patients in the intention-to-treat population) vs. 13/55 (24 %) in the HMPL-004 vs. mesalamine treatment groups had mucosal healing. The incidence of the most common adverse events was similar in the two groups. Seven patients were withdrawn from the study due to adverse effects (two patients in the HMPL-004 group and five patients in the mesalamine group). Two patients had serious adverse effects, and they were both from the HMPL-004 group. One of the SAEs was worsening of UC requiring hospitalization. The other was pregnancy (with a normal birth).

Sandborn and colleagues in 2013 published results from a randomized, double-blind, placebo-controlled trial evaluating the efficacy of HMPL-004 in patients with mild to moderate ulcerative colitis [87, 88]. Two hundred twenty-four adults were randomized to HMPL-004 1,200 or 1,800 mg daily or placebo for 8 weeks. Fifty-two percent (78 of 148) of patients receiving *A. paniculata* were in clinical response at week 8 as compared with 40 % (30 of 75) receiving placebo ($P=0.092$). A dose response for *A. paniculata* was demonstrated. Forty-five percent (*A. paniculata* 1,200 mg daily) vs. 40 % (placebo) were in clinical response at week 8 ($P=0.5924$). Sixty percent of patients receiving *A. paniculata* 1,800 mg daily vs. 40 % receiving placebo were in clinical response at week 8 ($P=0.0183$). Thirty-six percent vs. 25 % (drug vs. placebo) were in clinical remission at week 8 ($P=0.1173$). The rates of clinical remission for both doses of the drug were not significantly greater than placebo, although there was a trend toward significance for the 1,800 mg dose, $P=0.1011$. In all, 44 % vs. 33 % of patients receiving *A. paniculata* vs. placebo, respectively, achieved mucosal healing at week 8 ($P=0.1309$). The rate of mucosal healing for the 1,800 mg dose was significantly greater than placebo, but this was not true for the 1,200 mg group; therefore a dose response was seen. The incidence of adverse events was generally similar through week 8 although a mostly mild and reversible rash occurred in 8 % of patients receiving *A. paniculata* (compared to 1 % of patients receiving placebo).

### Conclusion

There are currently many agents in the pipeline for the treatment of ulcerative colitis that influence the disease course through either established or new mechanisms, and some of these treatments will be coming to market in the next decade. Also, with obtaining further information about the pathogenesis of IBD, many more therapeutic options will be developed, making this an exciting time in respect to the management of IBD in general.

### References

1. Simponi prescribing information: http://www.simponi.com/shared/product/simponi/prescribing-information.pdf.
2. Sandborn WJ, et al. Subcutaneous golimumab maintains clinical response in patients with moderate-to severe ulcerative colitis. Gastroenterology. 2014;146(1):96–109.
3. Lowenberg M, D'Haens G. Novel targets for inflammatory bowel disease therapeutics. Curr Gastroenterol Rep. 2013;13(2):311.
4. Hutas G. Golimumab, a fully human monoclonal antibody against TNFalpha. Curr Opin Mol Ther. 2008;10(4):393–406.
5. Perrier C, Rutgeerts P. New drug therapies on the horizon for IBD. Dig Dis. 2013;30 Suppl 1:100–5.
6. Smith K. IBD: golimumab shows promise in treatment of active ulcerative colitis. Nat Rev Gastroenterol Hepatol. 2013;10(7):386.
7. Danese S. IBD: golimumab in ulcerative colitis: a 'menage a trois' of drugs. Nat Rev Gastroenterol Hepatol. 2013;10(9):511–2.
8. www.fda.gov
9. Kay J, Smolen JS. Biosimilars to treat inflammatory arthritis: the challenge of proving identify. Ann Rheum Dis. 2013;72:1589–93.
10. Rietdijk ST, D'Haens GR. Recent developments in the treatment of inflammatory bowel disease. J Dig Dis. 2013;14(6):282–7.

11. Ghoreschi K, Laurence A, O'Shea J. Janus kinases in immune cell signaling. Immunol Rev. 2009;228:273–87.

12. Ghoreschi K, Jesson MI, Lee JL, et al. Modulation of innate and adaptive immune responses by tofacitinib (CP-690,550). J Immunol. 2011;186:4234–43.

13. Sandborn WJ, Ghosh S, Panes J, Vranic I, Su C, Rousell S, Niezychowski W. Study A3921063 Investigators. Tofacitinib, an oral Janus kinase inhibitor, in active ulcerative colitis. N Engl J Med. 2012;367(7):616–24.

14. A study of oral CP-690,550 as a maintenance therapy for ulcerative colitis (OCTAVE). ClinicalTrials.gov Identifier: NCT01458574.

15. West K. CP-690550, a JAK3 inhibitor as an immunosuppressant for the treatment of rheumatoid arthritis, transplant rejection, psoriasis and other immune-mediated disorders. Curr Opin Investig Drugs. 2009;10(5):491–504.

16. Kam JC, Szefler SJ, Surs W, Sher ER, Leung DY. Combination IL-2 and IL-4 reduces glucocorticoid receptor-binding affinity and T cell response to glucocor- ticoids. J Immunol. 1993;151: 3460–6.

17. Vuitton L, Koch S, Peyrin-Biroulet L. Janus kinase inhibition with tofacitinib: changing the face of inflammatory bowel disease treatment. Curr Drug Targets. 2013;14(12):1385–91.

18. Coskun M, Salem M, Pedersen J, Nielsen OH. Involvement of JAK/STAT signaling in the pathogenesis of inflammatory bowel disease. Pharmacol Res. 2013;76C:1–8.

19. Creed TJ, Norman MR, Probert CS, Harvey RF, Shaw IS, Smithson J, Anderson J, Moorghen M, Gupta J, Shepherd NA, Dayan CM, Hearing SD. Basiliximab (anti-CD25) in combination with steroids may be an effective new treatment for steroid-resistant ulcerative colitis. Aliment Pharmacol Ther. 2003;18(1):65–75.

20. Creed TJ, Probert CS, Norman MN, Moorghen M, Shepherd NA, Hearing SD, Dayan CM, BASBUC INVESTIGATORS. Basiliximab for the treatment of steroid-resistant ulcerative colitis: further experience in moderate and severe disease. Aliment Pharmacol Ther. 2006;23(10):1435–42.

21. Sands BE, Sandborn WJ, Creed TJ, Dayan CM, Dhanda AD, Van Assche GA, Greguš M, Sood A, Choudhuri G, Stempien MJ, Levitt D, Probert CS. Basiliximab does not increase efficacy of corticosteroids in patients with steroid-refractory ulcerative colitis. Gastroenterology. 2012;143(2):356–64.e1.

22. McLean LP, Shea-Donohue T, Cross R. Vedolizumab for the treatment of ulcerative colitis and Crohn's disease. Immunotherapy. 2012;4(9):883–98.

23. Feagan B, Macdonald J, Greenberg G, et al. An ascending dose of a humanized alpha 4 beta 7 antibody in ulcerative colitis (UC). Gastroenterology. 2000;118(4):A874.

24. Feagan BG, Greenberg GR, Wild G, Fedorak RN, Paré P, McDonald JW, Dubé R, Cohen A, Steinhart AH, Landau S, Aguzzi RA, Fox IH, Vandervoort MK. Treatment of ulcerative colitis with a humanized antibody to the alpha4beta7 integrin. N Engl J Med. 2005; 352(24):2499–507.

25. Parikh A, Leach T, Wyant T, Scholz C, Sankoh S, Mould DR, Ponich T, Fox I, Feagan BG. Vedolizumab for the treatment of active ulcerative colitis: a randomized controlled phase 2 dose-ranging study. Inflamm Bowel Dis. 2012;18(8):1470–9.

26. Tilg H, Kaser A. Vedolizumab, a humanized mAb against the $\alpha 4\beta 7$ integrin for the potential treatment of ulcerative colitis and Crohn's disease. Curr Opin Investig Drugs. 2010;11(11):1295–304.

27. Parikh A, Leach T, Xu J, Feagan B. P235. Long-term clinical experience with vedolizumab (VDZ) in patients with mild to moderate ulcerative colitis (UC). J Crohns Colitis. 2012;6(Suppl 1):S10328.

28. Feagan B, Rutgeerts P, Sands J, et al. 943b Induction therapy for ulcerative colitis: results of GEMINI I, a randomised placebo-controlled, double-blind, multicentre phase 3 trial. Gastroenterology. 2012;142(5):S160–1.

29. Rutgeerts P. Vedolizumab induction therapy for ulcerative colitis: results of GEMINI I, a randomized, placebo-controlled, double-blind, multicentre phase 3 trial. Gut. 2012;2012 Suppl 3:A65.

30. Rutgeerts P. Vedolizumab maintenance therapy for ulcerative colitis (uc): results of GEMINI I, a randomized, placebo-controlled, double-blind, multicenter phase 3 trial. Gut. 2012;61(Supp 3):A65.

31. Feagan BG, Rutgeerts P, Sands BE, Hanauer S, Colombel JF, Sandborn WJ, Van Assche G, Axler J, Kim HJ, Danese S, Fox I, Milch C, Sankoh S, Wyant T, Xu J, Parikh A. Vedolizumab as induction and maintenance therapy for ulcerative colitis. N Engl J Med. 2013;369:699–710.

32. Parikh A, Fox I, Leach T, Xu J, Scholz C, Patella M, Feagan BG. Long-term clinical experience with vedolizumab in patients with inflammatory bowel disease. Inflamm Bowel Dis. 2013; 19(8):1691–9.

33. Thomas S, Baumgart DC. Targeting leukocyte migration and adhesion in Crohns disease and ulcerative colitis. Inflammopharmacology. 2012;20(1):1–18.

34. Gledhill T, Bodger K. New and emerging treatments for ulcerative colitis: a focus on vedolizumab. Biologics. 2013;7:123–30.

35. Lobaton T, Vermeire S, Van Assche G, Rutgeerts P. Review article: anti-adhesion therapies for inflammatory bowel disease. Aliment Pharmacol Ther. 2014;39:579–94.

36. Vermeire S, Ghosh S, Panes J, et al. The mucosal addressin cell adhesion molecule antibody PF-00547,659 in ulcerative colitis: a randomised study. Gut. 2011;60:1068–75.

37. Pan WJ, Hsu H, Rees WA, Lear SP, Lee F, Foltz IN, Rathanaswami P, Manchulenko K, Chan BM, Zhang M, Xia XZ, Patel SK, Prince PJ, Doherty DR, Sheckler CM, Reynhardt KO, Krill CD, Harder BJ, Wisler JA, Brandvig JL, Lynch JL, Anderson AA, Wienkers LC, Borie DC. Pharmacology of AMG 181, a human anti-$\alpha 4$ $\beta 7$ antibody that specifically alters trafficking of gut-homing T cells. Br J Pharmacol. 2013;169(1):51–68.

38. Pan WJ, Sullivan B, Reese W. Clinical pharmacology and safety of AMG 181 a human anti-a4b7 antibody for treating inflammatory bowel diseases. 21st United European Gastroenterology Week (UEGWEEK2013). Contribution P914.

39. Pan WJ, Radford-Smith G, Andrews J, et al. Safety, pharmacology, and effect of AMG 181, a human antia4b7 antibody, in subjects with mild to moderate ulcerative colitis. 21st United European Gastroenterology Week (UEGWEEK2013) 2013, contribution OP264; 2013.

40. http://www.fiercebiotech.com/story/astrazeneca-amgen-crohns-drug-runs-phii-logistical-snafu/2013-10-16#ixzz2vLPnVf6C

41. ClinicalTrials.gov. Study to evaluate safety, tolerability, pharmacokinetics and pharmacodynamics of AMG 181; 2013.

42. ClinicalTrials.gov. A Phase 1, randomized, double-blind, placebo controlled, ascending single dose study to evaluate the safety, tolerability, pharmacokinetics and pharmacodynamics of AMG 181 in healthy subjects and subjects with mild to moderate ulcerative colitis; 2013.

43. ClinicalTrials.gov. AMG 181 Phase 2 study in subjects with moderate to severe ulcerative colitis. NCT016 94485.

44. http://www.ajinomoto seiyaku.co.jp/newsrelease/2013/1106e.pdf

45. Rutgeerts PJ, Fedorak RN, Hommes DW, Sturm A, Baumgan DC, Bressler B, Schreiber S, Mansfield JC, Williams M, Keir ME, Arian BS, Luca D, O'Byrne S. A phase I study of rHuMab Beta7 in moderate to severe ulcerative colitis (UC). Gastroenterology. 2011;140: S125.

46. Rutgeerts PJ, et al. A randomised phase I study of etrolizumab (rhuMAb $\beta 7$) in moderate to severe ulcerative colitis. Gut. 2013;62:1122–30.

47. Vermeire S, O'Bryne S, Williams M, Mansfield J. Differentiation between etrolizumab (Rhumab Beta7) and placebo in the eucalyptus phase II randomized double-blind placebo-controlled induction

study to evaluate efficacy and safety in patients with refractory moderate-to-severely active ulcerative colitis. Gastroenterology. 2013;144(5):S-36.

48. Gewirtz AT, Sitaraman S. Alicaforsen isis pharmaceuticals. Curr Opin Investig Drugs. 2001;2(10):1401–6.

49. Miner P, Wedel M, Bane B, Bradley J. An enema formulation of alicaforsen, an antisense inhibitor of intercellular adhesion molecule-1, in the treatment of chronic, unremitting pouchitis. Aliment Pharmacol Ther. 2004;19(3):281–6.

50. van Deventer SJ, Tami JA, Wedel MK. A randomised, controlled, double blind, escalating dose study of alicaforsen enema in active ulcerative colitis. Gut. 2004;53(11):1646–51.

51. Miner Jr PB, Geary RS, Matson J, Chuang E, Xia S, Baker BF, Wedel MK. Bioavailability and therapeutic activity of alicaforsen (ISIS 2302) administered as a rectal retention enema to subjects with active ulcerative colitis. Aliment Pharmacol Ther. 2006;23(10):1427–34.

52. Miner Jr PB, Wedel MK, Xia S, Baker BF. Safety and efficacy of two dose formulations of alicaforsen enema compared with mesalazine enema for treatment of mild to moderate left-sided ulcerative colitis: a randomized, double-blind, active-controlled trial. Aliment Pharmacol Ther. 2006;23(10):1403–13.

53. van Deventer SJ, Wedel MK, Baker BF, Xia S, Chuang E, Miner Jr PB. A phase II dose ranging, double-blind, placebo-controlled study of alicaforsen enema in subjects with acute exacerbation of mild to moderate left-sided ulcerative colitis. Aliment Pharmacol Ther. 2006;23(10):1415–25.

54. Vegter S, Tolley K, Wilson Waterworth T, Jones H, Jones S, Jewell D. Meta-analysis using individual patient data: efficacy and durability of topical alicaforsen for the treatment of active ulcerative colitis. Aliment Pharmacol Ther. 2013;38(3):284–93.

55. Barish CF. Alicaforsen therapy in inflammatory bowel disease. Expert Opin Biol Ther. 2005;5(10):1387–91.

56. Chapman RW, Phillips JE, Hipkin RW, Curran AK, Lundell D, Fine JS. CXCR2 antagonists for the treatment of pulmonary disease. Pharmacol Ther. 2009;121:55–68.

57. Mayer L, Sandborn WJ, Stepanov Y, Geboes K, Hardi R, Yellin M, Tao X, Xu LA, Salter-Cid L, Gujrathi S, Aranda R, Luo AY. Anti-IP-10 antibody (BMS-936557) for ulcerative colitis: a phase II randomised study. Gut. 2014;63(3):442–50.

58. Kuhne M, Preston B, Wallace S, Chen S, Vasudevan G, Witte A, Cardarelli P. MDX-1100, a fully human anti-CXCL10 (IP-10) antibody, is a high affinity, neutralizing antibody that has entered Phase I clinical trials for the treatment of Ulcerative Colitis (UC). J Immunol. 2007;178:131.20.

59. Uguccioni M, Gionchetti P, Robbiani DF, et al. Increased expression of IP-10, IL-8, MCP-1, and MCP-3 in ulcerative colitis. Am J Pathol. 1999;155:331–6.

60. Witte A, Kuhne MR, Preston BT, et al. W1170 CXCL10 expression and biological activities in inflammatory bowel disease. Gastroenterology. 2008;134:A-648.

61. Soejima K, Rollins BJ. A functional IFN-g-inducible protein-10/CXCL10-specific receptor expressed by epithelial and endothelial cells that is neither CXCR3 nor glycosaminoglycan. J Immunol. 2001;167:6576–82.

62. Sasaki S, Yoneyama H, Suzuki K, et al. Blockade of CXCL10 protects mice from acute colitis and enhances crypt cell survival. Eur J Immunol. 2002;32:3197–205.

63. Singh UP, Singh S, Taub DD, et al. Inhibition of IFN-gamma-inducible protein-10 abrogates colitis in IL-10–/–mice. J Immunol. 2003;171:1401–6.

64. Hyun JG, Lee G, Brown JB, et al. Anti-interferon-inducible chemokine, CXCL10, reduces colitis by impairing T helper-1 induction and recruitment in mice. Inflamm Bowel Dis. 2005;11:799–805.

65. Hardi R, Mayer L, Targan SR, et al. A phase 1 open-label, single-dose, dose-escalation study of MDX-1100, a high-affinity, neutralizing, fully human Igg1 (kappa) anti-CXCL10 (Ip10) monoclonal antibody, in ulcerative colitis. Gastroenterology. 2008;134:A-99–100.

66. Mayer L, Sandborn WJ, Stepanov Y, et al. A randomized placebo-controlled trial of MDX-1100, an anti-IP-10 antibody, for moderately-to-severely active ulcerative colitis. Oral presentation at DDW (abstract 711a) 2010.

67. Lazaar AL, Sweeney LE, MacDonald AJ, Alexis NE, Chen C, Tal-Singer R. SB-656933, a novel CXCR2 selective antagonist, inhibits ex vivo neutrophil activation and ozone-induced airway inflammation in humans. Br J Clin Pharmacol. 2011;72(2):282–93.

68. ClinicalTrials.gov. Study to EVALUATE THE PHARMACODYNAMICS of SB-656933 in patients with ulcerative colitis. ClinicalTrials.gov Identifier:NCT00748410.

69. Amezcua-Guerra LM, et al. Ulcerative colitis during CTLA-4Ig therapy in a patient with rheumatoid arthritis. Gut. 2006;55(7):1059–60.

70. Sandborn WJ, Colombel JF, Sands BE, Rutgeerts P, Targan SR, Panaccione R, Bressler B, Geboes K, Schreiber S, Aranda R, Gujrathi S, Luo A, Peng Y, Salter-Cid L, Hanauer SB. Abatacept for Crohn's disease and ulcerative colitis. Gastroenterology. 2012;143(1):62–9.

71. Kunde S, Pham A, Bonczyk S, Crumb T, Duba M, Conrad Jr H, Cloney D, Kugathasan S. Safety, tolerability, and clinical response after fecal transplantation in children and young adults with ulcerative colitis. J Pediatr Gastroenterol Nutr. 2013;56(6):597–601.

72. Anderson JL, Edney RJ, Whelan K. Systematic review: faecal microbiota transplantation in the management of inflammatory bowel disease. Aliment Pharmacol Ther. 2012;36:503–16.

73. Brandt LJ, Aroniadis OC. An overview of fecal microbiota transplantation: techniques, indications, and outcomes. Gastrointest Endosc. 2013;78(2):240–9.

74. Harrell L, Wang Y, Antonopoulos D, et al. Standard colonic lavage alters the natural state of mucosal-associated microbiota in the human colon. PLoS One. 2012;7:e32545.

75. Damman CJ, Miller SI, Surawicz CM, Zisman TL. The microbiome and inflammatory bowel disease: is there a therapeutic role for fecal microbiota transplantation? Am J Gastroenterol. 2012;107(10):1452–9.

76. Fecal biotherapy for the induction of remission in active ulcerative colitis. ClinicalTrials.gov Identifier: NCT01545908.

77. Faecal microbiota transplantation in ulcerative colitis (FOCUS). ClinicalTrials.gov Identifier: NCT01896635.

78. http://www.clinicaltrials.gov/ct2/results?term=fecal+transplant+and+ibd

79. De Leon LM, Watson JB, Kelly CR. Transient flare of ulcerative colitis after fecal microbiota transplantation for recurrent clostridium difficile infection. Clin Gastroenterol Hepatol. 2013;11(8):1036–8.

80. Kump PK, et al. Alteration of intestinal dysbiosis by fecal microbiota transplantation does not induce remission in patients with chronic active ulcerative colitis. Inflamm Bowel Dis. 2013;19:2155–65.

81. Paramsothy S, Agrawal G. Fecal microbiota transplantation: indications, methods, evidence, and future directions. Curr Gastroenterol Rep. 2013;15(8):337.

82. Chao WW, Kuo YH, Lin BF. Anti-inflammatory activity of new compounds from Andrographis paniculata by NF-kappaB transactivation inhibition. J Agric Food Chem. 2010;58:2505–12.

83. Parichatikanond W, Suthisisang C, Dhepakson P, et al. Study of anti-inflammatory activities of the pure compounds from Andrographis paniculata (burm.f.) Nees and their effects on gene expression. Int Immunopharmacol. 2010;10:1361–73.

84. Abu-Ghefreh AA, Canatan H, Ezeamuzie CI. In vitro and in vivo anti-inflammatory effects of andrographolide. Int Immunopharmacol. 2009;9:313–8.

85. Zhu HF. Clinical and experimental studies on minor prescription of bupleurum Chinese (Xiao Chaihu Tang) for ulcerative colitis. Zhonggo Gagchangbing Za Zhi. 2003;23:19–21.

86. Tang T, Targan SR, Li ZS, Xu C, Byers VS, Sandborn WJ. Randomised clinical trial: herbal extract HMPL-004 in active ulcerative colitis—a double-blind comparison with sustained release mesalazine. Aliment Pharmacol Ther. 2011;33:194–202.

87. Sandborn WJ, Targan SR, Byers VS, Rutty DA, Mu H, Zhang X, Tang T. *Andrographis paniculata* extract (HMPL-004) for active ulcerative colitis. Am J Gastroenterol. 2013;108:90–8.

88. Thomas S, Baumgart DC. Targeting leukocyte migration and adhesion in Crohn's disease and ulcerative colitis. Inflammopharmacology. 2012;20:1–18.

# Probiotics, Prebiotics, and Antibiotics for Ulcerative Colitis

# 18

Frank I. Scott and Faten N. Aberra

**Keywords**

Probiotics • Prebiotics • Antibiotics • Ulcerative colitis

The role of bacteria and antibiotics in the pathophysiology and treatment of ulcerative colitis has been postulated for over 60 years [1–3]. The first case reports of the use of antibiotics to treat inflammatory bowel disease (IBD) were published in the 1940s. Multiple studies since then have demonstrated a role for antibiotics in the treatment of perianal Crohn's disease (CD) and complications of IBD such as peritonitis, abscesses, and bacterial overgrowth [4–6]. The role for antibiotics in the treatment of ulcerative colitis (UC) has not been as clearly delineated.

Dysbiosis and microbiome alterations in the intestinal tract have been appreciated in several diseases, both within the gastrointestinal tract and beyond. The development of early bacterial populations in newborns can be modified by the delivery method at birth and antibiotic exposure, and these changes in bacterial composition may be long lasting [7–9]. Such modifications appear to have a significant impact on the early stages of postnatal immunologic development, potentially predisposing individuals to the development of autoimmune diseases such as type I diabetes, food allergies, and asthma [10–12].

Microbial composition has been demonstrated to play a significant role in IBD and other chronic diseases. Murine studies have demonstrated that mice raised in a germfree environment, i.e., lacking enteric flora, do not develop colitis despite a genetic predisposition to do so. These mice only develop colitis once specific commensal bacteria have been introduced [13, 14]. In humans with colitis, alterations in the location and concentration of intraluminal bacteria in relation to areas of inflammation have been appreciated [15, 16]. Modifications in microbial composition of the enteric microbiome have been demonstrated in several studies of humans with IBD, with increases in *Bacteroides, Escherichia coli,* and *Clostridium* species, as well as downregulation of *Bifidobacterium* and *Lactobacillus* species [4, 15, 17, 18]. There is a growing evidence demonstrating that these changes in flora may not only differ between different patients and phenotypes of IBD but also may differ significantly in local regions of the bowel in a single patient due to the presence or lack of inflammation in that specific region of the intestine [19, 20]. The composition of the gut microbiome may also have far-reaching implications, with studies suggesting a link between intestinal bacteria and the risk of type I diabetes mellitus, cardiovascular disease, and eczema [21, 22].

Given the growing body of evidence suggesting an effect of dysbiosis of the gut microbiome in IBD and other chronic medical conditions, medical therapy aimed at modulating these bacterial populations may have a significant impact on the resultant disease. Downregulating potentially deleterious organisms while upregulating beneficial strains could affect the degree of inflammation and alter the course of disease. This chapter will explore the current evidence that exists for therapies designed to directly modulate the gut flora in ulcerative colitis (UC), focusing on three classes of such treatment: (1) probiotics, which consist of live bacterial agents used to modify the composition of enteric flora; (2) prebiotics, or oligosaccharides and other compounds designed to affect

F.I. Scott, M.D., M.S.C.E.
Division of Gastroenterology, Department of Medicine, University of Pennsylvania Health System, Perelman School of Medicine at the University of Pennsylvania, 9 Penn Tower, 1 Convention Ave, Philadelphia, PA 19104, USA
e-mail: frankis@mail.med.upenn.edu

F.N. Aberra, M.D., M.S.C.E. (✉)
Division of Gastroenterology, Department of Medicine, Hospital of the University of Pennsylvania, Perelman School of Medicine at the University of Pennsylvania, 9 Penn Tower, 1 Convention Ave, Philadelphia, PA 19104, USA
e-mail: faten.aberra@uphs.upenn.edu

G.R. Lichtenstein (ed.), *Medical Therapy of Ulcerative Colitis,*
DOI 10.1007/978-1-4939-1677-1_18, © Springer Science+Business Media New York 2014

the growth of particular bacteria within the gut; and (3) antibiotics, or targeted pharmaceutical agents given to either limit the growth or kill specific bacteria.

## Probiotics

The hypothesis that specific strains of bacteria could be used to modulate the behavior of other bacteria and provide benefit to the host organism is often attributed to Elie Metchnikoff. In 1907, he proposed that the prolonged life spans of Bulgarians were due to lactic acid and other compounds produced by *Bacillus* species and other bacteria they consumed in sour milk on a daily basis, citing that these compounds inhibited other bacteria from producing toxins capable of producing "intestinal putrefaction" [23–25]. Despite these observations and those made by several other physicians and scientists of the potential beneficial effect of certain strains of bacteria, it was not until 1965 that the word "probiotic" was first used. This term was first used to describe certain products produced by one strain of bacteria in culture that would promote the growth of another strain of bacteria [26]. This definition has been refined several times since its inception to incorporate the concept that these compounds should consist of living bacteria, with the most widely accepted definition currently being "live microorganisms, which when consumed in adequate amounts, confer a health effect on the host" [27–29].

A number of commensal bacteria have been assessed as potential probiotics. While the initial commentary of prominent luminaries such as Metchnikoff and Tissier promoted the development of many compounds claimed to be probiotics, it has only been over the past 20 years that researchers have attempted to define and purify specific strains of bacteria and test the efficacy of these agents experimentally [24]. The majority of probiotic species used today are lactic-acid-producing strains such as *Lactobacillus* species, *Bifidobacteria* species, *Enterococcus*, *Lactococcus*, *Leuconostoc mesenteroides*, *Pediococcus acidilactici*, *Sporolactobacillus inulinus*, and *Streptococcus thermophilus*. Additionally, *Escherichia coli* Nissle 1917 and *Saccharomyces boulardii*, a yeast, have also been used as probiotics.

In addition to the individual strains noted above, there have been several studies looking at combinations of several bacteria, with the most studied combination being VSL#3. VSL#3 consists of 8 bacterial strains, including *L. plantarum*, *L. casei*, *L.acidophilus*, *L. bulgaricus*, *B. infantis*, *B. longum*, *B. breve*, and *Streptococcus thermophilus* [30].

## Probiotic Mechanisms of Action

There are a number of potential mechanisms of action for probiotic bacteria, and different strains have been shown to use different combinations of mechanisms. It is likely that each strain or combination of strains has multiple effects on the epithelial barrier, host immune system, and other bacterial populations within the gut.

Probiotics have been shown to have significant effects on the composition of a host's microbiome. These commensal organisms are capable of inhibiting the growth of or killing pathogenic bacteria via the production of antimicrobial peptides known as bacteriocins [31]. Both *Lactobacillus* and *Bifidobacteria* species have demonstrated direct effects against *Salmonella typhimurium* via this mechanism [32, 33]. Furthermore, as probiotic commensal populations expand, they can compete with pathogenic strains for various epithelial and mucin binding sites, preventing detrimental local mucosal surface colonization by more harmful, invasive bacteria while promoting the growth of beneficial strains [34, 35]. *Lactobacillus* species have been shown to increase the biodiversity of not only other *Lactobacilli* strains in patients with UC but also increase *Bifidobacteria* strains in neonates 5 days after birth when given to mothers prior to birth [36, 37]. VSL#3 has been shown to increase biodiversity in a DSS-based murine model, independent of its effects on mucosal inflammation or mucin production. This probiotic has also been shown to increase bacterial biodiversity while decreasing fungal biodiversity in patients with UC [38, 39]. It remains unclear whether these modulations in microbiome composition consistently translate into clinically meaningful changes, however [40].

Another potential mechanism of action of probiotic bacteria is direct modification of mucosal immunity via promoting barrier formation, upregulating defensin production, stimulating IgA production, and modulating local cytokine production. Both *Lactobacillus* and VSL#3 have been shown to promote mucous secretion, which functions as a protective layer against bacterial infiltration [41, 42]. *Lactobacillus*, *E. coli* Nissle, and VSL#3 are capable of upregulating genes responsible for defensin production [43–45]. These small peptides have direct antibacterial properties.

Several strains of commensal bacteria have exhibited the ability to directly modulate cytokine production. One study of patients with UC treated with 5-aminosalicylate (5-ASA) and *Lactobacillus* versus 5-ASA alone showed that 6 weeks of probiotic treatment reduced levels of IL-6, TNF-α, NF-κB, and leukocyte recruitment compared to controls [46]. *Bifidobacterium* has demonstrated similar effects in UC, reducing TNF-α, IL-8, and NF-κB+ mononuclear cells in colonic biopsies of inflamed mucosa [47].

## Probiotics in Ulcerative Colitis

Given the multitude of potential modulatory effects that probiotics have demonstrated in vitro and in murine models, there have been several recent studies ascertaining the clinical effects of these bacteria in patients with IBD.

The most extensive research has been done in pouchitis, but there is an expanding literature on the use of these agents in UC as well. Several studies have assessed different probiotic formulations, as well as different doses for these products.

Several agents have been assessed for their ability to induce remission in active UC. VSL#3, one of the more extensively studied probiotics in UC, has demonstrated the potential to induce remission and when used in combination with balsalazide was superior compared to balsalazide or mesalazine alone [48, 49]. In 2009, Sood et al. assessed the efficacy of VSL#3 in inducing remission in patients with mild to moderately active UC in a randomized, placebo-controlled trial [50]. Seventy-seven patients were randomized to the treatment arm, receiving 3,600 billion colony forming units (CFU) per day, compared to placebo. At 12 weeks, 42.9 % of the patients receiving VSL#3 were in remission, compared to 15.4 % of placebo-receiving patients ($P<0.001$). 32.5 % of patients in the treatment arm had a UCDAI decrease >50 %, compared to 10 % in the placebo arm. This study did have significant loss to follow-up, and the placebo arm had more patients on azathioprine which may indicate increased severity of disease in the placebo group [51]. In 2010, Tursi et al. conducted a randomized, placebo-controlled trial, using VSL#3 3600 billion CFU per day in 2 divided doses, with a primary end point of reduction of UCDAI >50 % at 8 weeks [52]. 57.7 % (41/71) of the patients in the treatment arm met this primary end point, compared to 39.7 % (29/73) in the placebo group ($p=0.031$). Induction of remission at 8 weeks was also assessed, though there was no significant difference between groups for this end point (43.7 % vs. 31.5 %, $p=0.132$).

Several studies have also examined the role of *Bifidobacterium* and other probiotics in inducing remission. Kato et al. examined the efficacy of *Bifidobacteria* in the induction of remission in 20 patients with mild to moderately active UC, randomizing them to a *Bifidobacteria*-fermented milk preparation versus placebo. Significant clinical improvement occurred in both the treatment group and placebo group, though significant endoscopic improvement occurred only in the treatment arm [53]. Furrie et al. also examined the efficacy of *Bifidobacteria* in combination with a prebiotic compared to placebo in 18 patients with active UC for 1 month. While reductions in sigmoidoscopic scores were appreciated in the treatment arm, they were not statistically significant [54]. A newer agent, BIO-THREE, which contains *Streptococcus faecalis*, *Clostridium butyricum*, and *Bacillus mesentericus*, was recently assessed in a small case series of 20 UC patients, demonstrating induction of remission in 9 of 20 patients and improvement in UCDAI in an additional 2 of 20 patients [55]. While promising, this agent will need further evaluation in prospective, randomized, placebo-controlled studies.

There have also been multiple systematic reviews of studies of probiotics for induction of remission. A Cochrane analysis in 2007 showed no evidence that probiotics were superior to ASA compounds or placebo for induction of remission. This pooled analysis was conducted prior to the Tursi and Sood studies, however [56]. A recent meta-analysis by Sang et al., published in 2010, assessed 13 randomized controlled trials involving several different preparations of probiotics, including *E. coli* Nissle, *Bifidobacterium*, *Lactobacillus* GG, VSL#3, and a combination product containing both *Bifidobacterium* and a prebiotic oligosaccharide called synbiotic [57]. The authors found no significant improvement in remission rate (OR 1.35, 95 % CI 0.98–1.85), though there was significant heterogeneity. The authors then performed an analysis stratified by probiotic, and neither *E. coli*, *Bifidobacterium*, nor VSL#3 demonstrated statistically significant improvement. However, This analysis also did not include the most recent study of VSL#3 by Tursi et al. The authors concluded that there was no significant benefit for using probiotics in inducing remission.

There have also been several studies assessing probiotics for the maintenance of remission as well. Kruis et al. examined the efficacy of *E. coli* Nissile 1917 for maintenance of remission compared to mesalazine and found them to have equivalent efficacy [58]. Kruis later assessed *E. coli* Nissile 1917 versus mesalazine in a larger randomized controlled trial of 327 patients with UC over 12 months. At the end of the study period, intention to treat analysis demonstrated that 45.1 % of patients receiving *E. coli* relapsed, compared to 37.0 % in the mesalazine group, with significant equivalence between the two groups [59]. Rembacken also examined the ability of *E. coli* to maintain remission in those who had successfully entered remission on prior *E. coli* therapy versus those who had entered remission on mesalazine. The probiotic preparation maintained remission in 67 % of patients, compared to 73 % who maintained remission with mesalazine [60]. These results were not significantly different. *Lactobacillus* GG has also been assessed in comparison to 5-ASA in prevention of relapse, without significant difference between groups [61]. *Bifidobacterium* was also assessed for maintenance of remission in two small studies published in 2004, with both studies demonstrating potential benefit for these agents [62, 63]. Given the small sample size, further research regarding this agent is required.

A recent systematic review has attempted to synthesize these results for maintenance of remission. Sang et al. assessed eight randomized controlled trials involving several different probiotics [57]. The authors found no significant improvement in prevention of relapse (OR 0.69, 95 % CI 0.47–1.01). Yet as with the induction trials, there was profound heterogeneity in both of these analyses. When assessing only placebo-controlled studies, there was a significant benefit of probiotic therapy in maintaining remission, with a remission ratio of 0.25 (95 % CI 0.12–0.51); there was no significant heterogeneity in this subgroup. Non-placebo-controlled trials did not demonstrate statistically significant benefit. Overall, the authors concluded that probiotics potentially provide benefit in the maintenance of remission. The degree of heterogeneity and variety of methods, agents, controls, and study duration in this meta-analysis make interpretation difficult.

In summary, with growing information on the impact of intestinal flora in disease activity and laboratory data demonstrating the beneficial effects of several specific strains of commensal bacteria, probiotics represent a potential adjunct to the current armamentarium in IBD. The data on efficacy of inducing and maintaining remission in UC has been mixed, although several recent placebo-controlled trials of VSL#3 have demonstrated benefit. A meta-analysis for induction of remission, which does not include two of the most recent trials and includes a heterogenous pool of 11 studies, has not confirmed these results. However, Another meta-analysis for maintenance of remission did appreciate a benefit when isolating only placebo-controlled trials. Further randomized controlled trials are still needed to confirm the efficacy of various probiotic preparations such as VSL#3 and *Bifidobacterium* in ulcerative colitis. Table 18.1 lists the probiotic clinical trials for induction and maintenance of remission in ulcerative colitis.

## Probiotics in Pouchitis

There have been several studies assessing the efficacy of probiotics in pouchitis. Pouchitis occurs in up to 45 % of patients after proctocolectomy and is thought to be secondary to alterations of the luminal flora in the pouch [64]. This hypothesized pathophysiology has made pouchitis an attractive candidate for probiotic therapy. In 2000, Gionchetti et al. published a randomized, double-blind, placebo-controlled trial assessing VSL#3 at 900 billion CFUs twice daily in the maintenance of remission of pouchitis in UC [30]. Forty patients in clinical and endoscopic remission were enrolled in the trial and followed for 9 months. Fifteen percent of patients (3 of 20) in the VSL#3 arm and 100 % (20/20) of the placebo arm relapsed. Gionchetti also demonstrated that the same dose of VSL#3 was capable of preventing onset of pouchitis after surgery in 2003 [65]. In 2004, Mimura et al. were able to demonstrate that a once daily dose of 600 billion CFUs of VSL#3 maintained remission in 85 % of pouchitis patients, compared to 5 % in the placebo arm [66]. A meta-analysis published in 2007 assessed 5 randomized controlled trials of probiotics in pouchitis. This study demonstrated an overall OR of 0.04 (95 % CI 0.0–0.14, $p < 0.0001$). There was significant heterogeneity between trials and variability in probiotics used, with one trial using *Lactobacillus rhamnosus* GG, while the other four used VSL#3 [67].

## Prebiotics and Synbiotics

The term "prebiotic" was coined by Glenn R. Gibson and Marcel B. Roberfroid in 1995 as "nondigestible food ingredients that beneficially affect the host by selectively stimulating the growth and/or activity of one or a limited number of bacterial species already resident in the colon, and thus attempt to improve host health" [68, 69]. This definition was refined in 2007 by Roberfroid to "a selectively fermented ingredient that allows specific changes, both in the composition and/or activity in the gastrointestinal microflora that confers benefits upon host well-being and health" [70]. Combining a prebiotic and probiotic in the same preparation is considered a "synbiotic" [69]. Such combinations are thought to enhance colonization, survival, and function of the probiotic species.

Prebiotics typically consist of oligosaccharides and polysaccharides that cannot be digested by the human host but can be digested by specific bacteria in the gut, providing them with a selective advantage. To be considered a prebiotic, a compound must be completely resistant to the host digestive tract, including gastric acid, host hydrolytic enzymes, and direct absorption. The compound must then be fermentable by host bacteria, resulting in stimulation of specific commensal bacteria. Two compounds that have been extensively researched and meet these criteria are inulin and trans-galactooligosaccharides (TOS) [70]. The bacterial "targets" of these agents are typically the same bacteria delivered in common probiotic formulation. When added to both pure strains of colonic flora and cultured human feces, inulin has been shown to selectively promote the growth of *Bifidobacterium* and may even inhibit the growth of other species such as *C. perfringens* and *E. coli* in mixed culture [71]. Furthermore, the end products of fermentation of these sugars include short chain fatty acids (SCFAs), which are an energy source of colonic enterocytes [69].

Research into the effects of both prebiotics and synbiotics in human disease, particularly with regard to disorders of the gastrointestinal tract, has begun. Inulin, oligofructose, and TOS have been assessed in the management of constipation, which is thought to be secondary to dysbiosis. A review by Macfarlane published in 2007 assessed 7 trials of various types and doses of prebiotics, with only two demonstrating a statistically significant improvement in stool output [72]. Further research has demonstrated a potential role for fructooligosaccharides (FOS) in a placebo-controlled, randomized trial, though results did not reach statistical significance [73]. Additional research demonstrated potential improvement in some symptoms in IBS with administration of TOS as well, though further research is required [74].

**Table 18.1** Probiotic clinical trials for induction of remission and maintenance of remission in ulcerative colitis

| Author | Ref. | Maintenance or induction of remission | Probiotic | Comparator | Study duration | UC population | Primary clinical outcome | Results Treatment arm | Results Control arm(s) | |
|---|---|---|---|---|---|---|---|---|---|---|
| Tursi et al. | [49] | Induction of remission | VSL#3 + balsalazide | Balsalazide or mesalazine | 8 weeks | Mild to moderate | Clinical remission | 24/30 (80 %) | Group 1: 21/30(70 %) Group 2: 16/30 (53.3 %) | P<0.02 |
| Rembacken | [60] | Induction of remission | E. coli Nissile 1917 | Mesalazine | 12 weeks | Mild to severe | Clinical remission | 39/57 (68 %) | 44/59(75 %) | P=0.0508 (for equivalence) |
| Tursi et al. | [52] | Induction of remission | VSL#3 | Placebo | 8 weeks | Mild to moderate | Reduction of UCDA >50 % | 41/71 (57.7 %) | 29/73 (39.7 %) | P=0.010 |
| Kato et al. | [53] | Induction of remission | Bifidobacterium-fermented milk preparation | Placebo | 12 weeks | Mild to moderate | Reduction in CAI by >3 pts | 7/10 (70 %) | 3/9 (33 %) | NR[a] |
| Furrie et al. | [54] | Induction of remission | Bifidobacterium longum+fructooligosaccharide/inulin mix | Placebo | 1 month | Mild to severe active (median SCCAI 5.6 2–13) | Reduction in CAI Endoscopic score reduction | 5/9 (56 %) xx (%) | 3/9 (33 %) xx (%) | NR[a] |
| Sood et al. | [50] | Induction of remission | VSL#3 | Placebo | 12 weeks | Mild to moderate | Reduction in UCDAI >50 % | 25/77 (32.5 %) | 7/70 (10 %) | P=0.001 |
| Kruis et al. | [58] | Maintenance of remission | E. coli Nissile 1917 | Mesalazine | 12 weeks | Remission | Maintenance of remission | 8/50 (16.0 %)[b] | 6/53 (11.3 %)[b] | NS[c] |
| Kruis et al. | [59] | Maintenance of remission | E. coli Nissile 1917 | Mesalazine | 12 months | Remission | Maintenance of remission | 73/162 (45.1 %)[b] | 61/165 (37.0 %)[b] | P=0.0013[d] |
| Rembacken | [60] | Maintenance of remission | E. coli Nissile 1917 | Mesalazine | 12 months | Remission | Maintenance of remission | 11/44 (25 %)[b] | 10/39 (26 %)[b] | NR[a] |
| Zocco et al. | [61] | Maintenance of remission | Lactobacillus GG (LGG) + mesalazine and LGG monotherapy | Mesalazine | 12 months | Remission | Maintenance of remission | LGG+mesalazine: 10/62 (16.1 %)[b] LGG alone: 10/65 (15.4 %)[b] | 12/60 (20 %)[b] | P=0.77 |
| Cui et al. | [62] | Maintenance of remission | Bifidobacterium | Placebo | 2 months | Remission | Maintenance of remission | 3/15 (20 %)[b] | 14/15 (93.3 %)[b] | P<0.01 |
| Ishakawa et al. | [63] | Maintenance of remission | Bifidobacterium-fermented milk preparation | Placebo | 12 months | Remission | Maintenance of remission | 3/11 (27.3 %) | 9/10 (90 %) | P=0.0184 |

[a]NR—statistical significance not reported in publication
[b]Relapse rate reported
[c]NS—not statistically significant
[d]Significance represents a test of statistical equivalence

With regard to ulcerative colitis, there have been several animal models suggesting efficacy, but there is limited human data. The effects of a wide range of agents, including FOS, inulin, lactulose, or combinations thereof, have demonstrated efficacy in increasing the quantity of *Bifidobacterium* and *Lactobacillus* species in several animal models of colitis, as well as modulating inflammatory markers [72, 75–79]. Controlled trials in humans are limited, however. Furrie et al. conducted a small randomized, placebo-controlled trial in 18 patients of a 1-month course of a synbiotic containing *Bifidobacterium longum* and a combination of inulin and oligofructose [54]. Patients were assessed before and after therapy via clinical index, endoscopic score, and several immunologic markers such as defensin excretion, TNF-α, IL-1α, and IL-10. After therapy with the synbiotic, all patients had a significant reduction in defensins, TNF-α, and IL-1α. There was also a 42-fold increase in concentration of *Bifidobacterium* on mucosal biopsies, determined via rRNA, after therapy. Histologically, there was also reduced inflammation in those in the treatment arm as well as reduced clinical symptoms. Statistical significance was not reported for these outcomes, however. Fujimori et al. conducted a 3-armed trial of a synbiotic (*Bifidobacterium* and psyllium) versus probiotic alone versus prebiotic alone in 120 patients with mild UC or in remission for 4 weeks [80]. Only the synbiotic group appreciated an improvement in IBDQ, a validated questionnaire of IBD symptoms and quality of life.

In summary, prebiotics and synbiotics represent a new method of modifying the microbiome, promoting the growth of potentially beneficial commensal and probiotic strains. There is a small but growing body of literature of the effect of these oligosaccharides on microbiome composition and their ability to modulate inflammation. There are also several small, randomized controlled trials, but much more research is needed to assess the efficacy of these agents.

## Antibiotics

As previously noted, the first publications of antibacterial agents being used to treat IBD were published in the 1940s [1–3]. However, the role of antibiotics in the pathogenesis and treatment of IBD has become considerably more complex since these early studies. Recent research has demonstrated that antibiotic exposure has been shown to have a significant and long-lasting effect on microbiome composition in neonates and infants [81, 82]. Amoxicillin can markedly reduce *Lactobacillus* species in the gut after administration, and this has been shown to have a significant effect on developmental gene expression in enterocytes [83]. Antibiotic-related dysbiosis has also been shown to create a permissive environment for several invasive, pathogenic strains of bacteria, including *Clostridium difficile*,

*Clostridium perfringens*, *Salmonella* species, and *E. coli* O157:H7 [84–86]. Promotion of these species may exacerbate IBD-related inflammation.

There is intriguing new data that suggests antibiotic exposure may increase the risk of later developing IBD. Margolis et al. performed a retrospective study in The Health Improvement Network database in the UK, assessing 94,487 patients with acne for exposure to tetracycline antibiotics. Tetracyclines are frequently used in the treatment of acne, and this class includes drugs such as minocycline, tetracycline, oxytetracycline, and doxycycline. The authors detected an increased risk of developing IBD with exposure to any of these antibiotics, with a hazard ratio (HR) of 1.39 (95 % CI 1.02–1.90). When stratified by IBD subtype and antibiotic, tetracycline/oxytetracycline remained associated with an increased risk of CD, while no antibiotics maintained significance for UC [87]. Further epidemiologic and animal-based research is needed to explore this potential relationship between antibiotic exposure and risk for developing IBD.

Once IBD has developed, antibiotic exposure may actually have a protective effect. A recent population-based cohort study using the General Practice Research Database (GPRD) in the UK assessed this effect [88]. The authors studied 1,205 patients with CD and 2,230 patients with UC, with a median of approximately 4 years' follow-up time for each group. In this cohort, exposure to antibiotics was associated with an overall reduced risk of disease flare for CD, with an OR of 0.78 (95 % CI 0.64–0.96), but this association was not present for UC. This protective effect was strongest with more recent exposure, suggesting that the acute changes in the microbiome may be responsible.

## Antibiotics in the Management of Ulcerative Colitis

There have been a multitude of studies looking at the role of antibiotics in the treatment of IBD. The two most commonly used classes of antibiotics are the fluoroquinolones, such as ciprofloxacin and levofloxacin, and the nitroimidazoles, including metronidazole. The combination of these two classes of antibiotics provides broad-spectrum coverage against most enteric bacteria, with the fluoroquinolone providing coverage against gram-negative and gram-positive aerobes and metronidazole covering gram-negative and gram-positive anaerobes [4]. Both classes are typically well tolerated, although fluoroquinolones can cause nausea, vomiting, abdominal pain, diarrhea, lightheadedness, photosensitivity, and an increased risk of tendon rupture. Side effects due to metronidazole include dysgeusia, resulting in a metallic taste. It has also been associated with nausea, vomiting, diarrhea, abdominal cramping, and a disulfiram-like reaction when combined with alcohol. Another common, though more serious, complication of metronidazole is peripheral neuropathy. The risk of this side effect appears to increase with prolonged exposure and increasing dose. It typically resolves upon cessation of the drug but may persist. A newer agent that has been assessed in several recent trials is rifaximin. This nonabsorbable rifamycin derivative is a nonabsorbable antibiotic with broad-spectrum coverage against gram-positive and gram-negative aerobes and anaerobes and is also well tolerated.

There appears to be an established role for antibiotic therapy in pouchitis. A small, randomized controlled trial by Madden et al. examined the benefit of metronidazole versus placebo in pouchitis in 1994. The authors appreciated a statistically significant decrease in the number of bowel movements, but no significant endoscopic or histological changes [89]. Another study compared metronidazole and budesonide enemas for a total of 6 weeks in active pouchitis, and a clinical improvement was appreciated in both groups, but there was no difference between the two groups [90]. Shen et al. performed a randomized trial in 2001 comparing ciprofloxacin to metronidazole, demonstrating a greater reduction in Pouchitis Disease Activity Index (PDAI) in the ciprofloxacin group. Ciprofloxacin was also better tolerated, with 33 % of patients experiencing adverse effects in the metronidazole group [91]. Another study looking at flora changes related to pouchitis suggested that more complete eradication of pathogenic *C. perfringens* and *E. coli* strains with ciprofloxacin may be responsible for the observed improvement in efficacy compared to metronidazole [92]. Mimura et al. also performed an open-label trial assessing the efficacy of combining both metronidazole and ciprofloxacin for refractory pouchitis [93]. Eighty-two percent (44 of 36) of their patients entered remission, with a significant decrease in median PDAI from 12 to 3 after therapy. The therapy was well tolerated. Rifaximin has also been assessed in open-label trials, either alone or in combination with other antibiotics [4, 94]. A recent case series demonstrated a reduction in PCDAI in 16 of 18 patients, with 6 patients entering remission. However, in a recent small, randomized, double-blind, placebo-controlled trial by Isaacs et al., rifaximin provided no benefit over placebo [95]. Based on this evidence, the American College of Gastroenterology currently recommends either metronidazole or ciprofloxacin for the treatment of pouchitis [96].

The data are less clear regarding the potential benefit of antibiotics in inducing remission in UC. As is the case with pouchitis, multiple antibiotics and combinations of antibiotics have been assessed for efficacy in active UC, with most studies focusing on ciprofloxacin or combination therapy. A number of other agents, such as tobramycin, oral vancomycin, or rifaximin, have been assessed, with mixed results. With regard to ciprofloxacin, there have been several

placebo-controlled trials. In 1997, Mantzaris et al. performed a randomized, placebo-controlled trial of a 2-week course of oral ciprofloxacin versus placebo in 70 patients with mild to moderately active UC in addition to 5-ASA and prednisolone [97]. No significant difference in response was appreciated between groups. Mantzaris also conducted a study in 55 patients with severe UC, examining the effects of IV ciprofloxacin versus placebo in addition to IV steroids and parenteral nutrition. IV ciprofloxacin provided no additional benefit [98]. In one of the few positive studies, Turunen et al. assessed 6 months of ciprofloxacin versus placebo in conjunction with 5-ASA and steroids for maintenance of remission of subjects with moderate to severe active UC. At 6 months, 79 % of patients in the ciprofloxacin group had maintained an initial response, compared to 56 % in the placebo group ($p = 0.02$) [99].

Several other antibiotic-based therapies have been assessed in randomized controlled trials of induction of remission in UC. Burke et al. performed a randomized controlled trial of oral tobramycin versus placebo in mild to severely active UC, in conjunction with steroid therapy, with 31 of 42 (74 %) patients achieving complete symptomatic remission compared to 18 of 42 (43 %) in the placebo arm ($p = 0.008$) [100]. Several combinations of antibiotics have been assessed as well. Mantzaris et al. assessed the combination of IV metronidazole and tobramycin versus placebo, along with parenteral nutrition and steroids, in 39 patients with acute severe UC. Sixty-three percent in the treatment arm and 65 % in the placebo arm noted significant improvement [101]. Rifaximin was assessed by Gionchetti et al. in a small placebo-controlled trial. Rifaximin 400 mg twice daily demonstrated significant decreases in clinical activity, with 9 of 14 patients receiving rifaximin demonstrating benefit compared to 5 of 12 receiving placebo [102].

Recent studies of antibiotic therapy have considered targeting specific organisms. In 2005, Okhusa et al. published a randomized controlled trial of a regimen specifically targeting *Fusobacterium varium*, containing amoxicillin, tetracycline, and metronidazole (ATM) versus placebo for 2 weeks in 20 patients with mild to moderately active UC [103]. At 3–5 months, the authors appreciated a statistically significant reduction in endoscopic score, but not histology or symptom index, in the treatment group. At 12–14 months after therapy, there were significant reductions in endoscopic score, symptom index, and histological grading. The same group performed a placebo-controlled, randomized trial of 2 weeks of oral ATM in 206 patients with mild to severe chronic relapsing UC [104]. The authors appreciated a greater clinical and endoscopic response at 3 months in the treatment group compared to placebo, though remission rates were not significantly different. Interestingly, this 2-week course of antibiotics improved clinical, endoscopic, and remission rates at 12 months in the treatment arm compared to placebo.

**Table 18.2** Antibiotic clinical trials for induction and maintenance of remission in ulcerative colitis

| Author | Ref. | Indication | Antibiotic | Comparator | Study duration | UC population | Primary clinical outcome | Results Treatment arm | Control arm | |
|---|---|---|---|---|---|---|---|---|---|---|
| Mantzaris et al. | [97] | Induction of remission | Ciprofloxacin (PO) | Placebo | 14 days | Mild to moderate | <3 bowel movements without blood per day | 24/34 (70.5 %) | 26/36 (72 %) | NS[a] |
| Mantzaris et al. | [98] | Induction of remission | Ciprofloxacin (IV) | Placebo | 10 days | Severe | <3 bowel movements without blood per day | 23/29 (79.3 %) | 20/26 (77 %) | NS[a] |
| Turunen et al. | [99] | Induction of remission | Ciprofloxacin (PO) | Placebo | 6 months | Moderate to severe | Treatment failure[b] | 8/38 (21.1 %) | 20/45 (44 %) | P=0.02 |
| Burke et al. | [100] | Induction of remission | Tobramycin (PO) | Placebo | 7 days | Active | Clinical remission | 31/42 (74 %) | 18/42 (43 %) | P=0.008 |
| Mantzaris et al. | [101] | Induction of remission | Metronidazole (IV)+Tobramycin (IV) | Placebo | 10 days | Severe | <3 bowel movements without blood per day | 12/19 (63.2 %) | 13/20 (65 %) | NS[a] |
| Gionchetti et al. | [102] | Induction of remission | Rifaximin | Placebo | 10 days | Moderate to severe | Improvement in CAI | 9/14 (64.3 %) | 5/14 (41.7 %) | NS[a] |
| Ohkusa et al. | [103] | Induction of remission | Amoxicillin (PO)+ tetracycline (PO)+ metronidazole (PO) | Placebo | 12–14 months | Mild to moderate | Decrease in median Lichtiger score | Median decrease in Lichtiger score from 3 (2–10) to 2 (1–5) (10 patients) | Median increase in Licthiger score from 3 (2–9) to 4 (3–8) (10 patients) | P=0.004 |
| Ohkusa et al. | [104] | Induction of remission | Amoxicillin (PO)+ tetracycline (PO)+ metronidazole (PO) | Placebo | 3 months | Mild to severe | Clinical Response (decrease in Mayo score >3) | 47/105 (44.8 %) | 23/101 (22.8 %) | P=0.0011 |
| Lobo et al. | [107] | Maintenance of remission | Tobramycin (PO) | Placebo | 12 and 24 months | Remission | Relapse with >3 stools per day with bleeding | 40 % @ 12 months[c] 20 % @ 24 months[c] | 24 % @ 12 months[c] 12 % @ 24 months[c] | NS[a] @ 12 months and 24 months |

[a]NS—not statistically significant
[b]Treatment failure was defined as a colonoscopic finding of moderate to severe activity in at least two segments of the colon after failure to respond to the treatment regimen
[c]Results reported in failure-free survival rates from Kaplan Meier analysis, i.e., continued remission rates

While such targeted approaches are compelling, further research is required to ascertain the exact effects such broad-spectrum therapies are having on the microbiome and clinical outcomes of UC patients.

There have also been several meta-analyses of the efficacy of antibiotics in UC. Rahimi et al. published a meta-analysis including ten randomized, placebo-controlled trials of antibiotics in addition to steroids for induction of remission in active UC [105]. Disease severity was not reported. Antibiotics assessed included vancomycin, metronidazole, tobramycin, ciprofloxacin, rifaximin. Two studies of the studies in the meta-analysis evaluated combinations of antibiotics for treatment of UC. Overall, there did appear to be a statistically significant benefit for antibiotic use in active UC, with an OR of 2.14 (95 % CI 1.48–3.09), without significant heterogeneity or detected publication bias. Khan et al. performed another meta-analysis in 2011, examining 9 trials including 662 patients for induction of remission of active UC. Of note, 7 of these trials were also included in the meta-analysis conducted by Rahimi et al. Those studies that commented on UC disease severity were typically moderate to severe. In this study, an overall benefit for antibiotic therapy was appreciated as well, with an Odds RatioR of not being in remission of 0.64 (95 % CI 0.43–0.96). They did detect moderate heterogeneity as well as possible publication bias. Of note, the authors rigorously reviewed the quality of these studies as well and found that only one of the 7 trials included for UC had a low risk of bias [106].

There is currently limited data regarding the role of antibiotics in the maintenance of remission in UC. Lobo et al.

performed a long-term follow-up of active UC patients who had received tobramycin and entered remission. In this trial, antibiotics were only given for a single 1-week period during the induction of the remission phase [107]. When examining those who were in remission, there was no significant difference between groups regarding relapse rates at 1 and 2 years. The previously mentioned trial by Turunen et al. which examined the benefits of ciprofloxacin for 6 months in active UC also reported the rates of relapse in those that responded from 6 months to 1 year after cessation of study medication, demonstrating similar failure rates in the treatment arm (9 of 30, 30 %) as in the placebo arm (7 of 25, 28 %) [99]. Both of these trials demonstrate failure rates after antibiotic cessation, however; a paucity of data regarding continued therapy may represent wariness in using long-term antibiotic therapy.

In summary, there is ample evidence demonstrating that antibiotic therapy has a significant impact on the microbiome of the intestinal track. Furthermore, there is a growing body of literature suggesting that antibiotic exposure may have an effect on the risk of developing IBD, and once diagnosed with IBD, antibiotic exposure may significantly impact the course of disease. It also appears that there is benefit to antibiotic therapy for treatment of IBD-related complications and for pouchitis. However, there is currently mixed evidence with regard to the efficacy of antibiotic therapy for the treatment of UC. There is considerable variation in efficacy in treatment based on the specific antibiotic, number of antibiotics used, and duration of treatment. Based on these data, more research is required before antibiotic therapy can be formally recommended for the management of ulcerative colitis in the absence of peritonitis, abscess, or toxic megacolon. Table 18.2 shows antibiotic clinical trials for induction and maintenance of remission in UC.

## Summary

There is growing evidence that dysbiosis plays a significant role in the pathogenesis of ulcerative colitis. As such, efforts to modify the composition of a patient's microbiome represent an attractive adjunct to the current therapeutic options in UC. In this chapter we explored the evidence for several different classes of agents designed to alter the microbial composition of a patient's enteric flora. Probiotics, which are living organisms ingested by a patient, can introduce commensal organisms into a patient's GI tract. Several different agents exist in this class, and there appears to be evidence of possible benefit in UC. Prebiotics promote the growth of beneficial commensal bacteria. The effects of these agents require significantly more research before specific recommendations can be made. Antibiotics are pharmaceutical agents designed to kill or halt the growth of existing bacteria and have a long history of efficacy in treating intraperitoneal complications of CD and UC. There is conflicting data supporting their use in UC. As such, they are not currently used in UC, except empirically in the setting of severe, fulminant colitis.

## References

1. Marks JA, Wright LT, Strax S. Treatment of chronic non-specific ulcerative colitis with aureomycin; a preliminary report. Am J Med. 1949;7(2):180–90.
2. Streicher MH. Oral administration of penicillin in chronic ulcerative colitis; a clinical, chemical and bacteriologic evaluation. JAMA. 1947;134(4):339–41.
3. Streicher MH, Pittard V. Clinical and bacteriologic evaluation of oral tyrothricin in chronic ulcerative colitis; preliminary report. Proc Annu Meet Cent Soc Clin Res U S. 1946;19:72.
4. Perencevich M, Burakoff R. Use of antibiotics in the treatment of inflammatory bowel disease. Inflamm Bowel Dis. 2006;12(7): 651–64.
5. Isaacs KL, Sartor RB. Treatment of inflammatory bowel disease with antibiotics. Gastroenterol Clin North Am. 2004;33(2): 335–45. x.
6. Sartor RB. Therapeutic manipulation of the enteric microflora in inflammatory bowel diseases: antibiotics, probiotics, and prebiotics. Gastroenterology. 2004;126(6):1620–33.
7. Dominguez-Bello MG, Costello EK, Contreras M, Magris M, Hidalgo G, Fierer N, et al. Delivery mode shapes the acquisition and structure of the initial microbiota across multiple body habitats in newborns. Proc Natl Acad Sci U S A. 2010;107(26):11971–5.
8. Biasucci G, Benenati B, Morelli L, Bessi E, Boehm G. Cesarean delivery may affect the early biodiversity of intestinal bacteria. J Nutr. 2008;138(9):1796S–800.
9. Salminen S, Gibson GR, McCartney AL, Isolauri E. Influence of mode of delivery on gut microbiota composition in seven year old children. Gut. 2004;53(9):1388–9.
10. Bjorksten B. Effects of intestinal microflora and the environment on the development of asthma and allergy. Springer Semin Immunopathol. 2004;25(3–4):257–70.
11. Negele K, Heinrich J, Borte M, von Berg A, Schaaf B, Lehmann I, et al. Mode of delivery and development of atopic disease during the first 2 years of life. Pediatr Allergy Immunol. 2004;15(1): 48–54.
12. Eggesbo M, Botten G, Stigum H, Nafstad P, Magnus P. Is delivery by cesarean section a risk factor for food allergy? J Allergy Clin Immunol. 2003;112(2):420–6.
13. Rath HC, Herfarth HH, Ikeda JS, Grenther WB, Hamm Jr TE, Balish E, et al. Normal luminal bacteria, especially Bacteroides species, mediate chronic colitis, gastritis, and arthritis in HLA-B27/human beta2 microglobulin transgenic rats. J Clin Invest. 1996;98(4):945–53.
14. Dianda L, Hanby AM, Wright NA, Sebesteny A, Hayday AC, Owen MJ. T cell receptor-alpha beta-deficient mice fail to develop colitis in the absence of a microbial environment. Am J Pathol. 1997;150(1):91–7.
15. Swidsinski A, Ladhoff A, Pernthaler A, Swidsinski S, Loening-Baucke V, Ortner M, et al. Mucosal flora in inflammatory bowel disease. Gastroenterology. 2002;122(1):44–54.
16. Tamboli CP, Neut C, Desreumaux P, Colombel JF. Dysbiosis in inflammatory bowel disease. Gut. 2004;53(1):1–4.
17. Scanlan PD, Shanahan F, O'Mahony C, Marchesi JR. Culture-independent analyses of temporal variation of the dominant fecal microbiota and targeted bacterial subgroups in Crohn's disease. J Clin Microbiol. 2006;44(11):3980–8.

18. Darfeuille-Michaud A, Boudeau J, Bulois P, Neut C, Glasser AL, Barnich N, et al. High prevalence of adherent-invasive Escherichia coli associated with ileal mucosa in Crohn's disease. Gastroenterology. 2004;127(2):412–21.

19. Frank DN, Robertson CE, Hamm CM, Kpadeh Z, Zhang T, Chen H, et al. Disease phenotype and genotype are associated with shifts in intestinal-associated microbiota in inflammatory bowel diseases. Inflamm Bowel Dis. 2011;17(1):179–84.

20. Walker AW, Sanderson JD, Churcher C, Parkes GC, Hudspith BN, Rayment N, et al. High-throughput clone library analysis of the mucosa-associated microbiota reveals dysbiosis and differences between inflamed and non-inflamed regions of the intestine in inflammatory bowel disease. BMC Microbiol. 2011;11:7.

21. Wen L, Ley RE, Volchkov PY, Stranges PB, Avanesyan L, Stonebraker AC, et al. Innate immunity and intestinal microbiota in the development of Type 1 diabetes. Nature. 2008;455(7216):1109–13.

22. Wang Z, Klipfell E, Bennett BJ, Koeth R, Levison BS, Dugar B, et al. Gut flora metabolism of phosphatidylcholine promotes cardiovascular disease. Nature. 2011;472(7341):57–63.

23. Sherman M. Perinatal profiles: Élie Metchnikoff: probiotic pioneer. NeoRev. 2011;12:495–7.

24. Joint FAO/WHO Expert Consultation on Evaluation of Health and Nutritional Properties of Probiotics in Food Including Powder Milk with Live Lactic Acid Bacteria. 2001.

25. Metchnikoff E. Lactic acid as inhibiting intestinal putrefaction. In: Chalmers Mitchell P, editor. The prolongation of life: optimistic studies. London: W. Heinemann; 1907. p. 161–83.

26. Lilly DM, Stillwell RH. Probiotics: growth-promoting factors produced by microorganisms. Science. 1965;147:747–8.

27. Fuller R. Probiotics in man and animals. J Appl Bacteriol. 1989;66(5):365–78.

28. Havenaar R, Huis in't Veld J. Probiotics: a general view. In: Wood B, editor. The lactic acid bacteria, vol 1: the lactic acid bacteria in health and disease. New York, NY: Chapman & Hall; 1992. p. 209–24.

29. Guarner F, Schaafsma G. Probiotics. Int J Food Microbiol. 1998;39:237–8.

30. Gionchetti P, Rizzello F, Venturi A, Brigidi P, Matteuzzi D, Bazzocchi G, et al. Oral bacteriotherapy as maintenance treatment in patients with chronic pouchitis: a double-blind, placebo-controlled trial. Gastroenterology. 2000;119(2):305–9.

31. Ohland CL, Macnaughton WK. Probiotic bacteria and intestinal epithelial barrier function. Am J Physiol Gastrointest Liver Physiol. 2010;298(6):G807–19.

32. Fayol-Messaoudi D, Berger CN, Coconnier-Polter MH, Lievin-Le Moal V, Servin AL. pH-, Lactic acid-, and non-lactic acid-dependent activities of probiotic Lactobacilli against Salmonella enterica Serovar Typhimurium. Appl Environ Microbiol. 2005;71(10):6008–13.

33. Lievin V, Peiffer I, Hudault S, Rochat F, Brassart D, Neeser JR, et al. Bifidobacterium strains from resident infant human gastrointestinal microflora exert antimicrobial activity. Gut. 2000;47(5):646–52.

34. Johnson-Henry KC, Donato KA, Shen-Tu G, Gordanpour M, Sherman PM. Lactobacillus rhamnosus strain GG prevents enterohemorrhagic Escherichia coli O157:H7-induced changes in epithelial barrier function. Infect Immun. 2008;76(4):1340–8.

35. Lee YK, Puong KY, Ouwehand AC, Salminen S. Displacement of bacterial pathogens from mucus and Caco-2 cell surface by lactobacilli. J Med Microbiol. 2003;52(Pt 10):925–30.

36. Fuentes S, Egert M, Jimenez-Valera M, Ramos-Cormenzana A, Ruiz-Bravo A, Smidt H, et al. Administration of Lactobacillus casei and Lactobacillus plantarum affects the diversity of murine intestinal lactobacilli, but not the overall bacterial community structure. Res Microbiol. 2008;159(4):237–43.

37. Gueimonde M, Sakata S, Kalliomaki M, Isolauri E, Benno Y, Salminen S. Effect of maternal consumption of lactobacillus GG on transfer and establishment of fecal bifidobacterial microbiota in neonates. J Pediatr Gastroenterol Nutr. 2006;42(2):166–70.

38. Gaudier E, Michel C, Segain JP, Cherbut C, Hoebler C. The VSL#3 probiotic mixture modifies microflora but does not heal chronic dextran-sodium sulfate-induced colitis or reinforce the mucus barrier in mice. J Nutr. 2005;135(12):2753–61.

39. Kuhbacher T, Ott SJ, Helwig U, Mimura T, Rizzello F, Kleessen B, et al. Bacterial and fungal microbiota in relation to probiotic therapy (VSL#3) in pouchitis. Gut. 2006;55(6):833–41.

40. Reiff C, Kelly D. Inflammatory bowel disease, gut bacteria and probiotic therapy. Int J Med Microbiol. 2010;300(1):25–33.

41. Mack DR, Ahrne S, Hyde L, Wei S, Hollingsworth MA. Extracellular MUC3 mucin secretion follows adherence of Lactobacillus strains to intestinal epithelial cells in vitro. Gut. 2003;52(6):827–33.

42. Caballero-Franco C, Keller K, De Simone C, Chadee K. The VSL#3 probiotic formula induces mucin gene expression and secretion in colonic epithelial cells. Am J Physiol Gastrointest Liver Physiol. 2007;292(1):G315–22.

43. Mondel M, Schroeder BO, Zimmermann K, Huber H, Nuding S, Beisner J, et al. Probiotic E. coli treatment mediates antimicrobial human beta-defensin synthesis and fecal excretion in humans. Mucosal Immunol. 2009;2(2):166–72.

44. Schlee M, Harder J, Koten B, Stange EF, Wehkamp J, Fellermann K. Probiotic lactobacilli and VSL#3 induce enterocyte beta-defensin 2. Clin Exp Immunol. 2008;151(3):528–35.

45. Schlee M, Wehkamp J, Altenhoefer A, Oelschlaeger TA, Stange EF, Fellermann K. Induction of human beta-defensin 2 by the probiotic Escherichia coli Nissle 1917 is mediated through flagellin. Infect Immun. 2007;75(5):2399–407.

46. Hegazy SK, El-Bedewy MM. Effect of probiotics on pro-inflammatory cytokines and NF-kappaB activation in ulcerative colitis. World J Gastroenterol. 2010;16(33):4145–51.

47. Bai AP, Ouyang Q, Xiao XR, Li SF. Probiotics modulate inflammatory cytokine secretion from inflamed mucosa in active ulcerative colitis. Int J Clin Pract. 2006;60(3):284–8.

48. Bibiloni R, Fedorak RN, Tannock GW, Madsen KL, Gionchetti P, Campieri M, et al. VSL#3 probiotic-mixture induces remission in patients with active ulcerative colitis. Am J Gastroenterol. 2005;100(7):1539–46.

49. Tursi A, Brandimarte G, Giorgetti GM, Forti G, Modeo ME, Gigliobianco A. Low-dose balsalazide plus a high-potency probiotic preparation is more effective than balsalazide alone or mesalazine in the treatment of acute mild-to-moderate ulcerative colitis. Med Sci Monit. 2004;10(11):I126–31.

50. Sood A, Midha V, Makharia GK, Ahuja V, Singal D, Goswami P, et al. The probiotic preparation, VSL#3 induces remission in patients with mild-to-moderately active ulcerative colitis. Clin Gastroenterol Hepatol. 2009;7(11):1202–9. 9 e1.

51. Shah SB. Probiotics for ulcerative colitis … Are the good bugs back? Gastroenterology. 2010;139(3):1054–6. discussion 6.

52. Tursi A, Brandimarte G, Papa A, Giglio A, Elisei W, Giorgetti GM, et al. Treatment of relapsing mild-to-moderate ulcerative colitis with the probiotic VSL#3 as adjunctive to a standard pharmaceutical treatment: a double-blind, randomized, placebo-controlled study. Am J Gastroenterol. 2010;105(10):2218–27.

53. Kato K, Mizuno S, Umesaki Y, Ishii Y, Sugitani M, Imaoka A, et al. Randomized placebo-controlled trial assessing the effect of bifidobacteria-fermented milk on active ulcerative colitis. Aliment Pharmacol Ther. 2004;20(10):1133–41.

54. Furrie E, Macfarlane S, Kennedy A, Cummings JH, Walsh SV, O'Neil DA, et al. Synbiotic therapy (Bifidobacterium longum/Synergy 1) initiates resolution of inflammation in patients with

active ulcerative colitis: a randomised controlled pilot trial. Gut. 2005;54(2):242–9.

55. Tsuda Y, Yoshimatsu Y, Aoki H, Nakamura K, Irie M, Fukuda K, et al. Clinical effectiveness of probiotics therapy (BIO-THREE) in patients with ulcerative colitis refractory to conventional therapy. Scand J Gastroenterol. 2007;42(11):1306–11.

56. Mallon P, McKay D, Kirk S, Gardiner K. Probiotics for induction of remission in ulcerative colitis. Cochrane Database Syst Rev. 2007;4, CD005573.

57. Sang LX, Chang B, Zhang WL, Wu XM, Li XH, Jiang M. Remission induction and maintenance effect of probiotics on ulcerative colitis: a meta-analysis. World J Gastroenterol. 2010;16(15):1908–15.

58. Kruis W, Schutz E, Fric P, Fixa B, Judmaier G, Stolte M. Double-blind comparison of an oral Escherichia coli preparation and mesalazine in maintaining remission of ulcerative colitis. Aliment Pharmacol Ther. 1997;11(5):853–8.

59. Kruis W, Fric P, Pokrotnieks J, Lukas M, Fixa B, Kascak M, et al. Maintaining remission of ulcerative colitis with the probiotic Escherichia coli Nissle 1917 is as effective as with standard mesalazine. Gut. 2004;53(11):1617–23.

60. Rembacken BJ, Snelling AM, Hawkey PM, Chalmers DM, Axon AT. Non-pathogenic Escherichia coli versus mesalazine for the treatment of ulcerative colitis: a randomised trial. Lancet. 1999;354(9179):635–9.

61. Zocco MA, dal Verme LZ, Cremonini F, Piscaglia AC, Nista EC, Candelli M, et al. Efficacy of Lactobacillus GG in maintaining remission of ulcerative colitis. Aliment Pharmacol Ther. 2006;23(11):1567–74.

62. Cui HH, Chen CL, Wang JD, Yang YJ, Cun Y, Wu JB, et al. Effects of probiotic on intestinal mucosa of patients with ulcerative colitis. World J Gastroenterol. 2004;10(10):1521–5.

63. Ishikawa H, Akedo I, Umesaki Y, Tanaka R, Imaoka A, Otani T. Randomized controlled trial of the effect of bifidobacteria-fermented milk on ulcerative colitis. J Am Coll Nutr. 2003;22(1):56–63.

64. Wu H, Shen B. Pouchitis and pouch dysfunction. Gastroenterol Clin North Am. 2009;38(4):651–68.

65. Gionchetti P, Rizzello F, Helwig U, Venturi A, Lammers KM, Brigidi P, et al. Prophylaxis of pouchitis onset with probiotic therapy: a double-blind, placebo-controlled trial. Gastroenterology. 2003;124(5):1202–9.

66. Mimura T, Rizzello F, Helwig U, Poggioli G, Schreiber S, Talbot IC, et al. Once daily high dose probiotic therapy (VSL#3) for maintaining remission in recurrent or refractory pouchitis. Gut. 2004;53(1):108–14.

67. Elahi B, Nikfar S, Derakhshani S, Vafaie M, Abdollahi M. On the benefit of probiotics in the management of pouchitis in patients underwent ileal pouch anal anastomosis: a meta-analysis of controlled clinical trials. Dig Dis Sci. 2008;53(5):1278–84.

68. Preidis GA, Versalovic J. Targeting the human microbiome with antibiotics, probiotics, and prebiotics: gastroenterology enters the metagenomics era. Gastroenterology. 2009;136(6):2015–31.

69. Gibson GR, Roberfroid MB. Dietary modulation of the human colonic microbiota: introducing the concept of prebiotics. J Nutr. 1995;125(6):1401–12.

70. Roberfroid M. Prebiotics: the concept revisited. J Nutr. 2007;137(3 Suppl 2):830S–7.

71. Wang X, Gibson GR. Effects of the in vitro fermentation of oligofructose and inulin by bacteria growing in the human large intestine. J Appl Bacteriol. 1993;75(4):373–80.

72. Macfarlane S, Macfarlane GT, Cummings JH. Review article: prebiotics in the gastrointestinal tract. Aliment Pharmacol Ther. 2006;24(5):701–14.

73. Cummings JH, Christie S, Cole TJ. A study of fructo oligosaccharides in the prevention of travellers' diarrhoea. Aliment Pharmacol Ther. 2001;15(8):1139–45.

74. Silk DB, Davis A, Vulevic J, Tzortzis G, Gibson GR. Clinical trial: the effects of a trans-galactooligosaccharide prebiotic on faecal microbiota and symptoms in irritable bowel syndrome. Aliment Pharmacol Ther. 2009;29(5):508–18.

75. Cherbut C, Michel C, Lecannu G. The prebiotic characteristics of fructooligosaccharides are necessary for reduction of TNBS-induced colitis in rats. J Nutr. 2003;133(1):21–7.

76. Moreau NM, Martin LJ, Toquet CS, Laboisse CL, Nguyen PG, Siliart BS, et al. Restoration of the integrity of rat caeco-colonic mucosa by resistant starch, but not by fructo-oligosaccharides, in dextran sulfate sodium-induced experimental colitis. Br J Nutr. 2003;90(1):75–85.

77. Rumi G, Tsubouchi R, Okayama M, Kato S, Mozsik G, Takeuchi K. Protective effect of lactulose on dextran sulfate sodium-induced colonic inflammation in rats. Dig Dis Sci. 2004;49(9):1466–72.

78. Camuesco D, Peran L, Comalada M, Nieto A, Di Stasi LC, Rodriguez-Cabezas ME, et al. Preventative effects of lactulose in the trinitrobenzenesulphonic acid model of rat colitis. Inflamm Bowel Dis. 2005;11(3):265–71.

79. Videla S, Vilaseca J, Antolin M, Garcia-Lafuente A, Guarner F, Crespo E, et al. Dietary inulin improves distal colitis induced by dextran sodium sulfate in the rat. Am J Gastroenterol. 2001;96(5):1486–93.

80. Fujimori S, Gudis K, Mitsui K, Seo T, Yonezawa M, Tanaka S, et al. A randomized controlled trial on the efficacy of synbiotic versus probiotic or prebiotic treatment to improve the quality of life in patients with ulcerative colitis. Nutrition. 2009;25(5):520–5.

81. Palmer C, Bik EM, DiGiulio DB, Relman DA, Brown PO. Development of the human infant intestinal microbiota. PLoS Biol. 2007;5(7):e177.

82. De La Cochetiere MF, Durand T, Lalande V, Petit JC, Potel G, Beaugerie L. Effect of antibiotic therapy on human fecal microbiota and the relation to the development of Clostridium difficile. Microb Ecol. 2008;56(3):395–402.

83. Schumann A, Nutten S, Donnicola D, Comelli EM, Mansourian R, Cherbut C, et al. Neonatal antibiotic treatment alters gastrointestinal tract developmental gene expression and intestinal barrier transcriptome. Physiol Genomics. 2005;23(2):235–45.

84. Bartlett JG. Clinical practice. Antibiotic-associated diarrhea. N Engl J Med. 2002;346(5):334–9.

85. Sekirov I, Tam NM, Jogova M, Robertson ML, Li Y, Lupp C, et al. Antibiotic-induced perturbations of the intestinal microbiota alter host susceptibility to enteric infection. Infect Immun. 2008;76(10):4726–36.

86. Wong CS, Jelacic S, Habeeb RL, Watkins SL, Tarr PI. The risk of the hemolytic-uremic syndrome after antibiotic treatment of Escherichia coli O157:H7 infections. N Engl J Med. 2000;342(26):1930–6.

87. Margolis DJ, Fanelli M, Hoffstad O, Lewis JD. Potential association between the oral tetracycline class of antimicrobials used to treat acne and inflammatory bowel disease. Am J Gastroenterol. 2010;105(12):2610–6.

88. Aberra FN, Brensinger CM, Bilker WB, Lichtenstein GR, Lewis JD. Antibiotic use and the risk of flare of inflammatory bowel disease. Clin Gastroenterol Hepatol. 2005;3(5):459–65.

89. Madden MV, McIntyre AS, Nicholls RJ. Double-blind crossover trial of metronidazole versus placebo in chronic unremitting pouchitis. Dig Dis Sci. 1994;39(6):1193–6.

90. Sambuelli A, Boerr L, Negreira S, Gil A, Camartino G, Huernos S, et al. Budesonide enema in pouchitis–a double-blind, double-dummy, controlled trial. Aliment Pharmacol Ther. 2002;16(1):27–34.

91. Shen B, Achkar JP, Lashner BA, Ormsby AH, Remzi FH, Brzezinski A, et al. A randomized clinical trial of ciprofloxacin and metronidazole to treat acute pouchitis. Inflamm Bowel Dis. 2001;7(4):301–5.

92. Gosselink MP, Schouten WR, van Lieshout LM, Hop WC, Laman JD, Ruseler-van Embden JG. Eradication of pathogenic bacteria and restoration of normal pouch flora: comparison of metronidazole and ciprofloxacin in the treatment of pouchitis. Dis Colon Rectum. 2004;47(9):1519–25.

93. Mimura T, Rizzello F, Helwig U, Poggioli G, Schreiber S, Talbot IC, et al. Four-week open-label trial of metronidazole and ciprofloxacin for the treatment of recurrent or refractory pouchitis. Aliment Pharmacol Ther. 2002;16(5):909–17.

94. Gionchetti P, Rizzello F, Venturi A, Ugolini F, Rossi M, Brigidi P, et al. Antibiotic combination therapy in patients with chronic, treatment-resistant pouchitis. Aliment Pharmacol Ther. 1999; 13(6):713–8.

95. Isaacs KL, Sandler RS, Abreu M, Picco MF, Hanauer SB, Bickston SJ, et al. Rifaximin for the treatment of active pouchitis: a randomized, double-blind, placebo-controlled pilot study. Inflamm Bowel Dis. 2007;13(10):1250–5.

96. Kornbluth A, Sachar DB. Ulcerative colitis practice guidelines in adults: American College Of Gastroenterology, Practice Parameters Committee. Am J Gastroenterol. 2010;105(3): 501–23. quiz 24.

97. Mantzaris GJ, Archavlis E, Christoforidis P, Kourtessas D, Amberiadis P, Florakis N, et al. A prospective randomized controlled trial of oral ciprofloxacin in acute ulcerative colitis. Am J Gastroenterol. 1997;92(3):454–6.

98. Mantzaris GJ, Petraki K, Archavlis E, Amberiadis P, Kourtessas D, Christidou A, et al. A prospective randomized controlled trial of intravenous ciprofloxacin as an adjunct to corticosteroids in acute, severe ulcerative colitis. Scand J Gastroenterol. 2001;36(9): 971–4.

99. Turunen UM, Farkkila MA, Hakala K, Seppala K, Sivonen A, Ogren M, et al. Long-term treatment of ulcerative colitis with ciprofloxacin: a prospective, double-blind, placebo-controlled study. Gastroenterology. 1998;115(5):1072–8.

100. Burke DA, Axon AT, Clayden SA, Dixon MF, Johnston D, Lacey RW. The efficacy of tobramycin in the treatment of ulcerative colitis. Aliment Pharmacol Ther. 1990;4(2):123–9.

101. Mantzaris GJ, Hatzis A, Kontogiannis P, Triadaphyllou G. Intravenous tobramycin and metronidazole as an adjunct to corticosteroids in acute, severe ulcerative colitis. Am J Gastroenterol. 1994;89(1):43–6.

102. Gionchetti P, Rizzello F, Ferrieri A, Venturi A, Brignola C, Ferretti M, et al. Rifaximin in patients with moderate or severe ulcerative colitis refractory to steroid-treatment: a double-blind, placebo-controlled trial. Dig Dis Sci. 1999;44(6):1220–1.

103. Ohkusa T, Nomura T, Terai T, Miwa H, Kobayashi O, Hojo M, et al. Effectiveness of antibiotic combination therapy in patients with active ulcerative colitis: a randomized, controlled pilot trial with long-term follow-up. Scand J Gastroenterol. 2005; 40(11):1334–42.

104. Ohkusa T, Kato K, Terao S, Chiba T, Mabe K, Murakami K, et al. Newly developed antibiotic combination therapy for ulcerative colitis: a double-blind placebo-controlled multicenter trial. Am J Gastroenterol. 2010;105(8):1820–9.

105. Rahimi R, Nikfar S, Rezaie A, Abdollahi M. A meta-analysis of antibiotic therapy for active ulcerative colitis. Dig Dis Sci. 2007;52(11):2920–5.

106. Khan KJ, Ullman TA, Ford AC, Abreu MT, Abadir A, Marshall JK, et al. Antibiotic therapy in inflammatory bowel disease: a systematic review and meta-analysis. Am J Gastroenterol. 2011; 106(4):661–73.

107. Lobo AJ, Burke DA, Sobala GM, Axon AT. Oral tobramycin in ulcerative colitis: effect on maintenance of remission. Aliment Pharmacol Ther. 1993;7(2):155–8.

# Novel Nonbiologic Therapies for Ulcerative Colitis

Pascal Juillerat and Joshua R. Korzenik

**Keywords**

Nonbiologic therapy • Ulcerative colitis • Heparin • Nicotine • Rosiglitazone • N-Acetylcysteine • Natural compounds • Aloe vera • Curcumin • Short-chain fatty acids • Bowman-Birk inhibitor

## Introduction

An extensive array of compounds has been studied for the treatment of UC. The most frequently used nonbiologic drugs for the oral and intravenous treatment of ulcerative colitis include 5-aminosalicylate (5-ASA) drugs (mesalamine and derivatives), sulfasalazine, and other azo-bonded molecules of 5-ASA, steroids, calcineurin inhibitors (cyclosporine, tacrolimus, and sirolimus), thiopurines (azathioprine, 6-mercaptopurine), and methotrexate, which are already presented in other sections of this book and are thus not considered in this chapter. The therapies presented in this section should be considered as potential alternatives, mostly for mild-to-moderate ulcerative colitis (UC). They are substances mostly used without FDA indications, such as heparin, nicotine, rosiglitazone, and N-acetylcysteine as well as "natural" compounds suggested to have anti-inflammatory or reparative properties, such as aloe vera, curcumin, short-chain fatty acids, and Bowman-Birk inhibitor.

The best evidence supportive of a potential clinical benefit for these kinds of therapies is mainly derived from uncontrolled open-label studies and is suggested for induction of remission and, rarely, maintenance of UC in remission. Few of the substances have yet been tested in randomized controlled trials (RCTs) and several that have been studied in RCTs did not prove to be of therapeutic benefit (such as omega-3 *fatty acid* and leukocytapheresis). This chapter aims to provide a practical guide to alternative treatments, including complementary medicine and nutritional measures, for UC patients (in particular, for those with mild-to-moderate UC on a stable dose of aminosalicylates or other conventional therapies who are seeking medications other than thiopurines and anti-TNF agents). Many agents in this diverse assortment of potential therapies appear promising and of interest for further study but the supportive evidence is inadequate to date.

Many patients seen in an ambulatory setting (60–85 % of all cases) have UC confined to the more distal part of the colon; this chapter is consequently dichotomized to systemic (oral and intravenous) and rectally administered treatments for this distally located manifestation of the disease [proctitis (suppositories), left-sided (foams)]. The latter, more cumbersome for the patient, is mainly used for induction of remission for a short period of time (tapered over a 1-month period) and is proposed less as a maintenance treatment.

## Oral and Intravenously Administered Therapies

### Nicotine

The development of inflammatory bowel disease (IBD) is the consequence of an inappropriate inflammatory response to intestinal microbes in a genetically susceptible host.

P. Juillerat, M.D., M.Sc. (✉)
Departement of gastroenterology, Clinic for Visceral Surgery and Medicine, Inselspital, Bern University Hospital, Bern, Switzerland
e-mail: pascal.juillerat@insel.ch

J.R. Korzenik, M.D.
Department of Gastroenterology, BWH Crohn's and Colitis Center, Brigham and Women's Hospital, 850 Boylston Street, Chestnut Hill, Boston, MA 02647, USA
e-mail: jkorzenik@partners.org

Several environmental factors, such as cigarette smoking, have been shown to play a significant role in the pathogenesis of IBD. Although cigarette smoking is known to be deleterious to most patients and may be associated with the development of lung cancer, atherosclerotic vascular disease, other kinds of cancers, and chronic obstructive pulmonary disease, it is now well accepted that ulcerative colitis primarily occurs in nonsmokers and former smokers. Additionally cigarette smoking exerts a universal protective effect against a patient developing ulcerative colitis [1]. Every clinician knows the history of a patient whom first manifestation of UC appears a couple of months after smoking cessation. Tobacco's protective role in the development and course of UC has been showed in epidemiologic studies [2] and therefore suggested a potential therapeutic role for nicotine, its principle ingredient. A Cochrane review by McGrath et al. concluded that transdermal nicotine administration is superior to placebo (odds ratio (OR) 2.56, 95 % confidence interval (CI) 1.02–6.45) for induction of remission in patients with UC but equal to standard medical therapy (OR 0.77, 95 % CI 0.37–1.60) [2, 3]. This study retrieved 5 RCTs, among them two double-blinded versus placebo. However, nicotine patch users were significantly more likely (OR 5.82, 95 % CI 1.66–20.47) to experience adverse side effects (i.e., light-headedness, tremor, nausea, vomiting, and contact dermatitis), and nicotine may have less of an effect in improving endoscopic appearance. Thus, nicotine remains of limited use in the therapy of UC, while its use in ex-smokers, refractory to conventional treatment, may be debatable. Some experts still suggest a potential interest in the use of nicotine patches for patients who presented initially after smoking cessation and who may at some point be likely to restart smoking in order to control their disease.

Rectal administration was thought to be better tolerated than patches [3]. Two uncontrolled pilot studies which produced clinical improvement in 54–71 % of 32 patients unresponsive to first-line therapy justified the need for an RCT. Unfortunately, this placebo-controlled trial demonstrated no significant benefit with daily 6 mg nicotine enemas. Clinical remission after 6 weeks was achieved in 14 of 52 (27 %) patients on active treatment and 14 of 43 (33 %) on placebo [4]. Part of the explanation for this failure may be the low dose of nicotine obtained with enema compared to the patch or cigarettes, the likelihood of a systemic rather than a local effect of nicotine, and a high proportion of treatment refractory patients.

## Phosphatidylcholine

The use of phosphatidylcholine (PC) originates from a concept of the potential pathogenesis of an UC flare, which is the impairment in the mucosal barrier linked to a decrease of PC in colonic mucus. PC is reduced by about 70 % in the mucus of the rectal mucosa in UC patients, independently of the state of inflammation [4, 5]. Supplementation of PC to increase mucosal PC could possibly prevent flares by augmenting the mucosal protection and reducing mucosal inflammation triggered by luminal bacteria antigens. A delayed-released oral PC preparation ($4 \times 0.5$ g daily) was randomized versus placebo by Stremmel et al. in 60 active UC patients over 3 months with a resulting 53 % of clinical remission (vs. 10 % placebo, $p < 0.001$) [6]. The same investigators treated 60 active steroid-dependent UC patients to either delayed-released PC or to placebo. Steroid withdrawal, with a concomitant achievement of remission or clinical response, was achieved in half of the 30 treated patients (vs. 10 % placebo, $p = 0.002$) [7]. Finally, a dose-finding study illustrated that a plateau of efficacy was obtained at around 3–4 g daily. The only adverse events reported were mild bloating (40 % independently of the dosage) and nausea (33 %, almost only in the higher-dose group) [8]. Moreover, endoscopic and histological healing also seemed to improve with PC treatment. Although PC has been demonstrated to reduce strictures and inflammation in experimental colitis studies, these three RCTs also suggest a possible influence on the causality itself, which adds to its interest as an emerging therapy. Larger studies are necessary to confirm the safety as well as short- and long-term benefit of this treatment in moderately active UC. This product is available commercially in North America under the brand name PhosChol® though not in a delayed-release formulation.

## Trichuris suis Ova

The use of Trichuris suis ova (or pig whipworm eggs) by Weinstock et al. as a therapy for treating inflammatory bowel disease (IBD) is based on the concept that a helminth infection induces a persistent immune alteration, though the precise mechanism remains uncertain. The host develops a Th2 immune response which paradoxically seems to prevent the development of other Th2 diseases (e.g., asthma), though other immunologic effects have been suggested [9]. Helminths promote the production of immunomodulatory molecules such as IL-10 [10], transforming growth factor β (beta), and prostaglandin E2, which could possibly have a protective effect. Moreover, in countries with a high rate of helminth colonization, the incidence of IBD is lower [11]. Weinstock et al. studied the impact of the ingestion of a dose of 2,500 Trichuris suis eggs in a sport drink with charcoal in 54 active ulcerative colitis patients versus placebo for 12 weeks. In an intention-to-treat analysis, they demonstrated a decrease in disease activity in 13 of 30 patients (43.3 %) with ova treatment compared to 4 of 24 patients (16.7 %) receiving placebo ($p = 0.04$) [12]. However, there was no statistical difference between the two groups in achieving remission. No side effects or complications were described.

According to Dr. Summers, the lead investigator of this trial, many patients were treated effectively well beyond the study periods, some for more than 3 years. This agent thus appears to be effective not only in treating active disease but also in maintaining remission [13] and has already been commercialized for online purchase by a German company, Ovamed GmbH. However, additional studies are needed to further optimize and ensure safety of helminth therapy for UC. Based on this publication from a single center, *Trichuris suis* ova therapy provides insufficient evidence and power to be recommended for the use in UC patients by the ECCO (European Crohn's and Colitis Organization) consensus [14].

Currently a large prospective, randomized placebo-controlled trial is ongoing evaluating the efficacy of *Trichuris suis* in patients with left-sided ulcerative colitis (ClinicalTrials.gov Identifier: NCT01953354). The study is a prospective, randomized, double-blind, placebo-controlled phase II clinical study of *Trichuris suis* ova treatment in left-sided ulcerative colitis, and it is also evaluating its effects on the mucosal immune state and the microbiota.

## Heparin and Parnaparin Sodium

There is evidence that IBD patients are at a higher risk of thromboembolism than the general population [15, 16]. Moreover, heparin-based anticoagulation is recommended during flares of the disease. A broader vascular hypothesis has been proposed that UC results from a dysfunction of endothelial cells and heparin has been proposed to counteract several potential pathophysiologic aspects, such as the development of microthrombi which may also play a role in the pathogenesis of UC [17]. Given the increased risk of thrombosis in patients with UC and reports suggesting an improvement in UC symptoms while on anticoagulant therapy, this led to randomized controlled studies of heparin and low-molecular-weight heparin in active UC. However, an increased risk of rectal bleeding due to anticoagulant therapy would need to be considered as a potential complication of treatment and balanced against any therapeutic benefit. In this situation, some improvement was observed which has been attributed to the in vitro-established anti-inflammatory properties of heparin. A Cochrane review performed by Chande et al. which evaluated the efficacy of unfractionated and low-molecular-weight heparin for remission induction in UC showed no benefit over placebo for any outcomes [18]. Higher expectations have recently been suggested by a newly developed oral colon-release form of low-molecular-weight heparin called parnaparin (*CB-01-05 MMX®*). A multicenter double-blind RCT conducted by Celasco et al. evaluated the efficacy and safety of an 8-week oral daily administration of 210 mg of parnaparin sodium in 114 mild-to-moderate left-sided UC patients treated with stable doses of aminosalicylates [19]. Clinical remission was achieved in 83.6 % of the active drug group and in 63.3 % of the comparator group ($p=0.011$). Notably, this effect was already visible and significant at week 4 (59.0 % vs. 38.9 %, $p=0.028$). Parnaparin had an acceptable safety profile and was not associated with bleeding complications. On the contrary, rectal bleeding was more frequently absent in the parnaparin group (75.4 % vs. 55.0 % in the placebo group; $p=0.018$). The mucosal friability also recovered better, but this was not accompanied by a significant difference in the histological healing rate. Endoscopic evaluation at week 8 may be too early to be able to estimate the maximal effect; however, mucosal healing has become an important standard in the evaluation of the efficacy of new IBD drugs. Further RCTs with longer follow-up periods and including patients with pancolitis are warranted to better identify the role of oral delayed-released heparin in UC [20].

## Ridogrel

Ridogrel, a combined thromboxane synthase inhibitor and receptor antagonist, is used to prevent thromboembolic events and as an adjunctive agent to thrombolytic therapy in acute myocardial infarction. As thromboxanes are produced in excess in the inflamed intestinal mucosa of IBD patients, the effect of low-dose (5 mg daily or less) ridogrel on active UC has been investigated over 12 weeks in one placebo-controlled trial ($n=439$) and one randomized trial ($n=445$) versus mesalazine 2.4 g [21]. Both trials failed to show any significant difference in primary outcome, the proportion of subjects in clinical remission, and there was a complete lack of dose response. A previous study using high-dose ridogrel (300 mg twice daily) demonstrated the same efficacy as mesalazine in clinical and endoscopic improvement [22]. The effective dose of ridogrel for the treatment of UC thus remains unknown.

Ridogrel was used as an enema in an open-label pilot trial in 11 UC patients. Five of 9 (56 %) patients responded clinically to the treatment, but this was inconsistently associated with the endoscopic and histological inflammation scores [23]. Auwerda et al. measured reduced mucosal thromboxane levels in all patients, but the other inflammatory cytokines, IL-6 and TNF, were unchanged. This preliminary study has indicated some efficacy, but as yet no further studies have been undertaken.

### *N*-Acetyl Cysteine

In the context of chronic inflammation, IBD patients often show a depletion in antioxidants such as ascorbate, β (beta)-carotene, α (alpha)-tocopherol, and glutathione [24]. The goal of combining *N*-acetyl-L-cysteine with 5-ASA was thus to restore the level of the very potent antioxidant glutathione.

Guijarro et al. recently published a pilot RCT in 37 mild-to-moderate UC patients with a 4-week treatment period. Twelve of 19 patients (63 %) in the combination treatment group experienced remission compared to 9 of 18 patients (50 %) on mesalamine monotherapy (odds ratios 1.71; 95 % CI: 0.46 to 6.36; $p = 0.19$; number needed to treat 7.7) [25]. However, the dose (0.8 g/d) of oral N-acetyl-L-cysteine was probably insufficient as no increase in serum glutathione levels occurred. This study also suggests a local beneficial effect related to a significant downregulation of chemokines such as MCP-1 and IL-8 which activate the recruitment of neutrophils and monocytes to the inflamed mucosa.

## Rosiglitazone

Recently, thiazolidinediones (glitazones)-PPAR-gamma (peroxisome proliferator-activated receptors gamma) agonists have been implicated to effectively control the inflammatory processes of the gastrointestinal tract. Three subtypes of peroxisome proliferator-activated receptors (PPARs) were identified in humans, i.e., alpha, beta (also called d or NUC-1), and gamma. They belong to the superfamily of nuclear steroid hormone receptors, which act as the transcription factors regulating the expression of genes [26–33]. PPARs-g are characterized by the widest spectrum of action and are present in many organs. Rosiglitazone (Avandia™, a member of the thiazolidinedione class used as an oral agent for diabetes mellitus) binds PPAR-gamma receptors which attenuate inflammatory cytokine production by inhibition of NF-kappaB [34] and induction of a TH2 response. Preclinical data have shown efficacy in murine colitis [35]. After a successful open-label study in 15 mild-to-moderate UC patients refractory to 5-ASA [36], Lewis et al. conducted a multicenter placebo double-blind RCT in similar patients [37]. A hundred and five individuals were enrolled in a 12-week therapy trial of either oral rosiglitazone 4 mg twice daily or placebo. The active drug was significantly superior to placebo for induction of clinical response (44 % vs. 23 %, $p = 0.04$) and clinical remission (17 % vs. 2 %, $p = 0.01$); however, endoscopic remission was uncommon in either group. Serious adverse events were rare. As anticipated, edema and weight gain were higher in the rosiglitazone group. However, based on the recent reporting concerning an increased risk of myocardial infarction [38], these drugs are now restricted to diabetic patients already being treated with these medicines and those whose blood sugar cannot be controlled with other antidiabetic medicines. Whether other agents in this class may be of equal benefit in UC remains unstudied.

Pedersen et al. assessed the clinical effectiveness of rosiglitazone enema (4 mg) in 14 patients with distal ulcerative colitis in an RCT versus mesalamine (1 g) on a nightly basis for 14 days. All 14 patients randomized in both groups achieved a similar clinical response (3-point decrease in the Mayo score) and endoscopic improvement. As expected, there was an in vivo increased expression of PPARγ(gamma)-activated genes. As mentioned in the section on systemic treatment, concerns have been raised about an increased risk of myocardial infarction when using this substance and it is currently only used in a limited fashion.

## Aloe Vera

Aloe vera is a perennial succulent plant belonging to the lily family which has been used medicinally for over 5,000 years. Its extract demonstrated some superiority over placebo in a trial in UC by Langmead et al. [39]. Forty-four patients with mild-to-moderate colitis were randomized to receive either oral aloe vera *liquid* or placebo for 4 weeks. Fourteen of the thirty UC patients (47 %) who ingested 100 ml of aloe vera twice daily showed clinical improvement compared to 2 of 14 (14 %) of those receiving placebo. Overall 30 % of the patients had clinical, endoscopic, and histological remission. These results failed, however, to reach statistical significance. Further evaluation of the therapeutic potential of aloe vera is thus needed. In view of the fact that it is a safe and well-tolerated treatment, many IBD patients may be willing to try it or may have used it already in conjunction with their conventional IBD medications.

## Curcumin (Turmeric)

Recently, curcumin, an active ingredient of turmeric (*Curcuma longa*), an Indian herb, which has been used in Indian Ayurvedic system for the treatment for inflammatory conditions, has been an area investigated subsequent to its recognized anti-inflammatory properties. In experimental models, curcumin has been shown to prevent trinitrobenzene sulfonic acid (TNBS)- [40] and dextran sodium sulfate (DSS)-induced colitis [41, 42]. Turmeric, also known as Indian saffron, is a plant belonging to the ginger family. It contains curcumin (chemically known as diferuloylmethane), a yellow pigment which has demonstrated anti-inflammatory and antioxidant properties. Similarly to sulfasalazine curcumin seems to be effective in reducing inducible nitric oxide synthase (iNOS) and nuclear factor kappa B (NF-kappaB) [43]. Recently, an RCT for the prevention of relapse in quiescent UC was carried out in 8 centers in Japan [44]. During a 6-month follow-up period, 2 of the 43 UC patients (4.7 %) who received curcumin as maintenance treatment (1 g twice daily) had a relapse compared to 8 of 39 patients (20.5 %) in the placebo group. The authors concluded that curcumin seems to be a promising and safe medication for maintaining remission in patients with ulcerative colitis but cautioned that further studies need to be conducted to reinforce these findings. Various doses have been studied for adults for a variety of treatments [45]: cut root, 1.5–3 g per day; dried, powdered root, 1–3 g per day; standardized powder (curcumin), 400–600 mg, 3 times per day; fluid extract (1:1) 30–90 drops a day; and tincture (1:2), 15–30 drops, 4 times per day, but an optimal dose in UC is uncertain. In 2011, Moss et al. reported one case of clinical and endoscopic remission in a female patient with left-sided UC who was refractory to 5-ASA, who needed multiple courses of steroids, and who refused other immunosuppressants [46].

Recently, a randomized, double-blind, single-center pilot trial was conducted in patients with mild-to-moderate active ulcerative colitis (with <25 cm of disease involvement). Forty-five patients were randomized to receive NCB-02 (standardized curcumin preparation) enema plus oral 5-ASA or placebo enema plus oral 5-ASA. The primary endpoint was disease response, defined as reduction in Ulcerative Colitis Diseases Activity Index by 3 points at 8 weeks, and secondary endpoints were improvement in endoscopic activity and disease remission at 8 weeks.

When assessed by intention-to-treat analysis, the response to active therapy with curcumin was seen in 56.5 % compared to 36.4 % ($p=0.175$) in the placebo group. At week 8, clinical remission was observed in 43.4 % of patients in curcumin-treated patients compared to 22.7 % in placebo group ($p=0.14$) and improvement on endoscopy in 52.2 % of patients in curcumin-treated patients compared to 36.4 % of patients in placebo group ($p=0.29$). When the study was analyzed by the per protocol analysis, there were beneficial outcomes in the curcumin group, in terms of clinical response (92.9 % vs. 50 %, $p=0.01$), clinical remission (71.4 % vs. 31.3 %, $p=0.03$), and improvement on endoscopy (85.7 % vs. 50 %, $p=0.04$). The authors thus note there is some evidence supporting the use of curcumin and further controlled trials are merited.

## Boswellia serrata

The plant *Boswellia serrata* is found mainly in India, but it is also grows in the northeastern coast of Africa and in the Middle East. Extract from the bark contains chemical constituents including alkaloids, phenols, saponins, tannins, terpenoids, and pentacyclic triterpenes. These compounds have been widely used in traditional Indian medicine. The extract of *Boswellia serrata* is used in the treatment of diseases with inflammatory characteristics such as rheumatoid arthritis, osteoarthritis, and intestinal diseases because these compounds have been shown to inhibit leukotrienes (LT). Leukotrienes are involved in the initiation and maintenance of inflammation, and inhibiting LT can effectively prevent the oxidation of lipids and release of inflammatory cytokines.

Resin extracts of *Boswellia serrata* (H15, indish incense), known from traditional Ayurvedic medicine, decrease leukotriene synthesis in vitro and blunt leucocytes recruitment by inhibiting the upregulation of P-selectin on endothelial cells in the inflamed colonic microvasculature [47]. Gupta et al. studied H15, a chloroform/methanol extract of *Boswellia serrata* gum resin (350 mg thrice daily for 6 weeks) for the treatment of mild-to-moderate UC [48]. The substance studied has a comparative effect to sulfasalazine, used as a control. As this trial was nonrandomized and included only a few patients, a larger RCT has been expected. Such a trial has been performed in Crohn's disease for maintenance of remission and was prematurely terminated due to a lack of demonstrable efficacy as an active treatment according to an independent interim analysis [49]. It is worth noting that *Boswellia serrata* extract is already taken by almost 40 % of IBD patients as complementary medicine in Germany [50] but not recommended by consensus guidelines [14].

## Bowman-Birk Inhibitor

The Bowman-Birk inhibitor (BBI) is a soybean-derived protease inhibitor. Inhibitors of the BBI family are present in all legumes. BBI concentrate (BBIC) is a soy extract enriched in BBI. Bowman-Birk inhibitor concentrate is a naturally occurring human proteases that has been demonstrated to have potential anti-inflammatory and chemopreventive properties [47]. The compact structure of this protein makes it resistant to the acidic conditions and proteolytic enzymes of the gastrointestinal tract and therefore a significant proportion reaches the colon in an intact form. A randomized, double-blind, placebo-controlled trial was performed by Lichtenstein et al. in 28 active ulcerative colitis patients [51]. Results only showed a beneficial trend for clinical improvement and remission. Bowman-Birk inhibitor was associated with no serious adverse events. A report on the successful use of another protease inhibitor in two UC patients was published in 1993 [52].

## Omega-3 Fatty Acids (Fish Oil)

Omega-3 fatty acids are incorporated into the wall of inflammatory cells, thus lowering the concentration of arachidonic acid (C20:4, n−6). By reducing the amount of arachidonic acid, omega-3 reduces the production of leukotriene B4 (which serves as a chemoattractant to polymorphonuclear leukocytes), thromboxane A2, prostaglandin E2, interleukin-1, interleukin-6, and tumor necrosis factor. Additionally, it has been shown to scavenge free radicals. Food and in particularly fish oil supplements rich in omega-3 fatty acids and eicosapentaenoic acid have been suggested to have anti-inflammatory properties by inhibiting 5-lipoxygenase and other enzymes involved in arachidonate metabolism of leukotriene [53]. Several studies including RCTs and meta-analyses failed to demonstrate any benefit of fish oil in the induction and maintenance of remission in UC [54, 55]. The pooled results of a recent Cochrane review showed a relative risk of 1.02 (95 % CI 0.51–2.03, $p=0.96$) for a new flare. The authors of the reviews evaluated the available studies on omega-3 as too small, heterogenous, and with a suggestive publication bias which did not permit the drawing of definitive conclusions [54, 55].

## Herbal Medicines, Other Complementary and Alternative Medicines

Over 30 % of the population of the Western world now uses some form of complementary and alternative medicine [56]. The single most commonly used modality in most surveys is herbal therapy. An excellent review paper by Langmead and Rampton also reported curcumin and *Boswellia* as potential complementary and alternative medicines for UC but also suggested taking a closer look at wheat grass juice and some specific Chinese herbs.

## Wheat Grass Juice

Wheat grass juice was investigated in a double-blind, RCT conducted in Israel [57]. Twenty-three patients with active distal UC were allocated to receive 100 cc of wheat grass juice or placebo. No side effects were reported and the intake of wheat grass juice was associated with significant improvement in terms of rectal bleeding and disease activity index ($p=0.031$).

## HMPL-004

*Andrographis paniculata* is a medicinal plant that has been used to treat inflammatory diseases in Asian countries. *Andrographis paniculata* extracts have been recently shown to have anti-inflammatory, antiviral, and antitumor properties. Several bioactive components have been identified in *Andrographis paniculata* including diterpenes, lactones, and flavonoids. Andrographolide, a diterpenoid lactone and the main bioactive component of *Andrographis paniculata*, has been demonstrated to possess strong anti-inflammatory activity via the inhibition of nuclear factor kappa B (NF-kB) signaling, suppression of the production of inducible nitric oxide synthase (iNOS), and reactive oxygen species. Recent animal studies have demonstrated that HMPL-004 inhibits the development of chronic colitis by affecting early T-cell

proliferation, differentiation, and TH1/TH17 responses in a T-cell-driven model of colitis, presenting a unique mechanism of action [58].

Two phase IIb RCTs using other herbal extracts have recently been published; they involved only Chinese centers and compared the efficacy and safety of herbal active drugs contained in a colonic-released capsule to mesalamine in mild-to-moderate UC. The first RCT tested a specific extract of *Andrographis paniculata* (*Acanthaceae* family) called HMPL-004 which has anti-inflammatory properties [59]. HMPL-004 has the capability to inhibit several cellular targets, resulting in the suppression of NF-κB and of several different cytokines, exerting an overall anti-inflammatory effect. After 8 weeks of treatment, 21 % of patients treated with HMPL-004 and 16 % of patients treated with mesalamine were in remission. In both groups, 36 % of the subjects could also be defined as being in partial remission. The endoscopic remission was 28 % and 24 %, respectively. A rare adverse event observed was urticaria. The authors concluded that this herbal extract could serve as a substitute induction therapy in those patients with a suboptimal response to mesalazine. There are, however, no data to date on its efficacy for maintenance. The second RCT used composite sophora colon-soluble capsules containing multiple Chinese herbs [60]. After an 8-week treatment, the total clinical efficacy rate in the two groups was very high, 92 % for the active drug and 83 for placebo, and the authors claimed at least an equivalence to conventional therapies. However, without further confirmation of safety, some preparations used in alternative medicine and their interactions with conventional drugs are unknown and thus they remain not recommended by consensus guidelines [14].

## Acupuncture and Moxibustion

Acupuncture and moxibustion are traditional Oriental medicine techniques which work through stimulation of acupuncture points. Acupuncture uses needles, whereas moxibustion requires the application of heat generated by burning herbal preparations directly or indirectly on the skin. The presumed mechanism of action of these local stimulations is through the autonomic nervous system which closely interact with the enteric nervous system and the hypothalamic-pituitary-adrenal axis. Thus, the expression of proinflammatory cytokines can be inhibited, as demonstrated in animal models of UC [61]. A meta-analysis of moxibustion for UC based on five RCTs of low methodological quality in 407 patients has been published [62]. The pooled effect was slightly favorable in terms of response rate compared to mostly sulfasalazine (risk ratio 1.24, 95 % CI 1.11–1.38; $p<0.0001$). However, current evidence is insufficient to show that moxibustion is an effective treatment for UC. The authors highlighted that the risk of bias was high and thus more rigorous studies are warranted. An RCT single-blinded trial (29 patients) performed in Germany compared acupuncture and moxibustion to a sham procedure over 5 weeks [63]. A decrease in disease activity was significantly higher in the acupuncture group. The secondary endpoints .such as quality of life, general well-being, and serum markers of inflammation did not show any difference. The authors concluded that both techniques seemed useful for mild-to-moderate UC. According to the European Crohn's and Colitis Organization, there is insufficient evidence for the use of acupuncture of UC [14].

## Psychological Interventions

Several studies in North America have demonstrated a much higher rate of major depression among IBD patients [64]. According to a Cochrane review which evaluated twelve eligible studies covering a wide range of psychological intervention in IBD, there is no evidence for efficacy in adult patients [65]. In adolescents, psychological interventions may be beneficial, but evidence is limited. The authors suggest that the need for psychological interventions may be better identified in specific vulnerable subgroups. This meta-analysis also demonstrated no benefit in directly measured disease activity or quality of life. Nevertheless, UC patients with long-term perceived life stress (in the previous 2 years) were found to be at increased risk of exacerbation over the following 8 months [66]. Attention to psychosocial factors and the appropriate use of psychosocial intervention could potentially improve the care of IBD patients.

## Diet

As consumption of refined sugar and certain carbohydrates have been suggested to be associated with IBD onset or relapse, a specific carbohydrate diet™ (SCD) was described by Elaine Gottschalk in her book called "Breaking the Vicious Cycle" [67]. While considerable anecdotal reports and emails in patient online communities support a role for this approach, the SCD has not been subjected to any scientific scrutiny. Other diet interventions have been suggested through identification of potential dietary risk factors for UC flares. In their study published in the journal Gut, Jowett et al. speculate that the high sulfur or sulfate content of nutrients increases the risk of relapse in a group of UC patients in remission for 1 year [68]. Using a food frequency questionnaire, they identified a higher likelihood of relapse in those consuming meat, particularly red and processed meat, protein, and alcohol (OR from 2.7 to 3.2). Another English group confirmed the effect of a high level of sulfite as a culprit and developed a list of deleterious and beneficial foods

based on a novel statistical method which associated endoscopic activity and food (the food sigmoidoscopy score) [69]. A reduced sulfur diet has not been studied in UC. Finally, a review of retrospective and prospective studies on food consumption and onset of IBD described an association between high intakes of total fat, polyunsaturated fatty acids, omega-6 fatty acids, and meat and the development of UC, whereas high vegetable intake was consistently associated with a decreased risk of UC [70]. Prebiotics (*short-chain carbohydrates*) and probiotics are described in detail in another section of this book.

## Additional Potential Therapies

In this section, promising drugs for the systemic treatment of ulcerative colitis at different preclinical development stages are described below with emphasis on the most convincing published results of the phase II/III trials. These substances are currently not available on the market and therefore cannot be prescribed off-label.

## Leukocytapheresis

Numerous open-label studies have demonstrated the superiority of granulocyte/monocyte apheresis over placebo or noninferiority when compared to steroids. Leukocytapheresis (LCAP) using a Cellsorba E column (Asahi Kasei Medical Co., Ltd., Tokyo, Japan), which is filled with nonwoven polyester fiber, is a blood purification therapy that exerts anti-inflammatory effects by removing activated leukocytes or platelets from the peripheral blood through an extracorporeal circulation [71–74]. An open-label multicenter randomized control study showed that LCAP with low-dose corticosteroids (26.9 mg/day on average) in the treatment of active UC had significantly higher efficacy (29/39, 74 %) than high-dose corticosteroids (47.9 mg/day on average; 14/37, 38 %) and had significantly lower (24 %) incidence of adverse events than high-dose steroid treatment (68 %).

A recent large multicenter RCT was conducted in the United States, Japan, and Europe (companion study) in 215 UC patients and demonstrated that granulocyte/monocyte apheresis was no more effective than sham apheresis for the induction of clinical remission and response in patients with moderate-to-severe UC [75]. More recently, another open-label randomized study compared two frequencies of leukocytapheresis administration (biweekly vs. standard weekly) and claimed that intensive treatment significantly increases effectiveness and reduces time to remission. Despite the relative safety of this intervention, its time-consuming and expensive nature would require a strong level of evidence of efficacy before its role in UC therapy could be reconsidered.

## Tetomilast

Tetomilast (OPC-6535) is a thiazole compound that belongs to the family of the phosphodiesterase-4 (PDE4) inhibitors. PDE4 is implicated in the breakdown of 3, 5′-adenosine cyclic monophosphate (cAMP) and is ubiquitously expressed in inflammatory cells. Consequently, selective PDE4 inhibitors have broad-spectrum anti-inflammatory effects such as inhibition of cell trafficking, cytokine, and chemokine release from inflammatory cells. In a phase II RCT, 186 patients with mild-to-moderate UC received oral tetomilast 25 mg, 50 mg, or placebo once daily for 8 weeks. In the intent-to-treat analysis, clinical improvement was 52 %, 39 %, and 35 %, respectively, which was not statistically significant. The remission rate was also higher in the tetomilast groups (16 %, 21 %, and 7 %, respectively) but also failed to reach statistical significance. Moreover, a high dropout rate was observed in the higher-dose group due to adverse events such as nausea/vomiting (32 % of the patients) but also fatigue, dizziness, and headache. The post hoc analysis suggests the efficacy of tetomilast was only significant in patients with objective criteria for inflammation. The phase III development (FACTS II and CORE study—in combination with 5-ASA) for ulcerative colitis, performed in North America, Europe, and Australia, has now been completed [76, 77].

## Janus Kinase (JAK) Inhibitor: Tofacitinib

The oral Janus kinase inhibitor tofacitinib (CS-690 550) showed good efficacy in moderate-to-severe UC according to a phase II multicenter double-blind trial [78]. The Janus kinase (JAK) family of intracellular, nonreceptor protein tyrosine kinases, which includes JAK1, JAK2, JAK3, and tyrosine kinase 2, transduce signals from multiple types I and II cytokine receptors. Upon receptor activation, JAKs phosphorylate signal transducer and activator of transcription proteins that translocate to the nucleus and regulate the expression of numerous genes. This drives additional participation in the inflammatory response. They were initially named "just another kinase" 1 and 2 (because they were just 2 of a large number of discoveries in a polymerase chain reaction-based screen of kinases). They were ultimately called "Janus kinase" as 1 domain exhibits the kinase activity, whereas the other negatively regulates the kinase activity of the first. Tofacitinib (CP-690,550), formerly known as CP-690, 550 and tasocitinib, is a selective oral inhibitor of JAK1 and JAK3 and, to a lesser extent, JAK2.

A total of 194 patients with moderate-to-severe active UC were randomized to receive twice daily tofacitinib at doses of 0.5, 3, 10, and 15 mg and placebo. Clinical benefit was suggested by the finding of response rates at 8 weeks in 32 %, 48 %, 61 %, 78 %, and 42 % of patients in each group, respectively [79]. Clinical and endoscopic remission showed significantly higher rates in the high-dose group (15 mg) compared to placebo (41 % vs. 10 % and 27 % vs. 2 %, respectively). No increase in adverse events associated with tofacitinib was observed, except for a dose-dependent rise in levels of low-density lipoprotein and triglyceride, which returned to baseline levels during the washout phase.

## RDP58

RDP58 (delmitide acetate) is a novel anti-inflammatory d-amino acid decapeptide that inhibits synthesis of proinflammatory cytokines (TNF-alpha, IFN-gamma, IL-12, and IL-2). By targeting the TRAF6/IRAK4/MyD88 protein complex, it inhibits phosphorylation of p38 and JNK and therefore AP1 and NF-kappaB activation. At a dosage of 200 and 300 mg, it was demonstrated to be safe and effective in the treatment of mild-to-moderate UC [80]. After 4 weeks of treatment and 4 weeks of observation, success rates (disease score ≤3) were 71 % and 72 %, respectively, versus 43 % for placebo ($p=0.016$). Histological, but not endoscopic, scores improved significantly ($p=0.002$) versus placebo. To date, approximately 400 patients and volunteers have been exposed to RDP58, with a good perceived safety profile. A phase III is awaited for this attractive molecule based on its mode of action.

## Exogenous Alkaline Phosphatase

In UC patients the mucosal surface of the colon wall is characterized by intermittent lesions and hyperpermeability caused by chronic inflammation. The alkaline phosphatase functions as resistance to bacterial and endotoxin transmigration but is also reduced secondary to the damage of the intestinal mucosa. The expected beneficial effect of alkaline phosphatase is then in the reduction of the amount of active luminal bacterial lipopolysaccharide which would diminish its ability to induce intestinal inflammation through the leaky inflamed intestinal mucosa. The safety and efficacy of exogenous alkaline phosphatase was evaluated in an open-label trial conducted in the Czech Republic and Italy [81]. Twenty-one hospitalized patients with moderate-to-severe disease (Mayo score 6–11) received 30,000 units of the enzyme administered daily via a naso-duodenal tube for a week. At day 21, 48 % (10/21) of patients showed clinical response, while 19 % (4/21) were in clinical remission and 33 % (7/21) did not respond. Clinical response and remission were associated with a decrease in C-reactive protein and stool calprotectin levels. This enteral administration of alkaline phosphatase was well tolerated, but there is a need for an acid-resistant oral form of this enzyme in order to be able to evaluate further its role in the therapeutic arsenal of UC.

## Vidofludimus Sc12267 (4SC-101)

The oral immunosuppressant vidofludimus (SC12267, 4SC-101) inhibits the dihydroorotate dehydrogenase, which is a key enzyme in pyrimidine biosynthesis and interleukin-17 (IL-17) release. There is an increased number of Il-17 producing cells, such as CD4 T helper 17 (Th17) and CD8+ T cells, in the lamina propria of UC patients and the IL-23/Th17 axis has been newly described as central to the pathogenesis of IBD [82]. This compound has been evaluated as a remission maintenance agent in steroid-dependent IBD patients after steroid weaning in an open-label phase IIa study in Germany, Bulgaria, and Romania [83]. Twelve UC patients were included and receive the treatment. After 12 weeks of a daily intake of vidofludimus 35 mg, remission was maintained in half of the UC patients without need for corticosteroids. One patient relapsed and five patients could not be weaned off the steroids but were maintained in remission. No serious adverse events were observed. An RCT is now planned.

## Additional Phase II Trials

To our knowledge, some interesting molecules are currently or have recently been studied in phase II trials [84] but results are incomplete at this point: Triolex® (HE-3286), a novel synthetic derivative of the steroid, β-AET (5-androstene-3β, 7β, 17β-triol). It has a broad-based anti-inflammatory activity (modulation of NF-kappaB pathway) but less adverse events such as immune suppression and bone loss as it does not interact with any of the steroid-binding nuclear hormone receptors [85]; a substance P antagonist (SR140333) on neurokinin receptor 1which interferes with the actions of this neuropeptide on inflammation sites and improves colitis in experimental models of colitis [86]; dersalazine sodium, a novel oral formulation, combining, through an azo bond, one molecule of 5-ASA with UR12715, a potent platelet-activating factor antagonist which induces anti-TNF-alpha effects and IL-17 downregulation [87]; and, finally, cannabidiol, a safe and non-psychotropic ingredient of the marijuana plant, because cannabinoid receptor activity promotes the reconstitution of injured colonic epithelium. It has also been recently demonstrated that cannabinoids accelerate wound closure during colitis and might have an inhibitory effect on the release of proinflammatory cytokines modulator of the gut neuro-immune axis [88].

Cannabidiol (CBD) is an interesting compound because of its ability to control reactive gliosis in the CNS, without any unwanted psychotropic effects. CBD targets enteric reactive gliosis and counteracts the inflammatory environment induced by LPS in mice and in human colonic cultures derived from UC patients. These actions lead to a reduction of intestinal damage mediated by PPAR-gamma receptor pathway. Our results therefore indicate that CBD indeed unravels a new therapeutic strategy to treat inflammatory bowel diseases [88].

## Other Rectally Administered Drugs for the Topical Treatment of Distal Colitis/Proctitis

### Tacrolimus (FK506)

Tacrolimus is a macrolide obtained from *Streptomyces tsukubaensis* that has similar but stronger immunosuppressive effects than cyclosporine. Both belong to the family of the calcineurin inhibitors which decrease T-cell proliferation without interfering with DNA synthesis but through diminished IL-2 and interferon-gamma production, for instance [89]. Two recent open-label pilot studies have started to investigate the efficacy of rectal tacrolimus in resistant distal colitis. In Australia, 8 patients with moderate-to-severe UC (5 proctitis, 2 left-sided, 1 extensive UC) received 4 weeks of topical tacrolimus [90]. At week 8, 75 % of the patients achieved clinical remission and most of them could taper or stop oral corticosteroids. In the Netherlands, van der Woude et al. have also reported the use of topical tacrolimus in 19 patients with resistant distal IBD colitis (12 proctitis (suppositories), 7 left-sided extension (enemas). Clinical and histological improvement was observed in 83 % and 67 % of the patients treated with suppositories and 60 % and 40 % of the enema group, respectively. In both studies, tacrolimus remained at a low serum level not usually associated with either toxicity or side effects [91]. As these studies performed in difficult-to-treat patients demonstrate promising results, further randomized placebo-controlled trials are warranted. It is worth noting that Pimecrolimus® cream is available on the market but is too frequently associated with a burning sensation on rectal application. Specific preparations were specially prepared for these studies and would require a compounding pharmacy to recreate formulations based on the original articles' description.

### Cyclosporine

Cyclosporine, the other anticalcineurin inhibitor, came into use as enema more than 10 years ago. Sandborn et al. performed an RCT versus placebo of cyclosporine enemas of 350 mg in 40 left-sided ulcerative colitis patients with or without concomitant therapy with oral steroids and 5-ASA (4 arms) [92]. At 4 weeks, the number of patients showing clinical improvement in the two comparison groups was similar (8 for cyclosporine and 9 in the placebo group). Blood cyclosporine levels were detectable in only two patients and no toxicity was noted. This negative finding may be related to the concentration of the medication on the mucosal surface. To our knowledge, the use of cyclosporine suppositories has not to date been investigated.

## Arsenic (Acetarsol)

The precise mechanism of action of acetarsol in proctitis is unknown. However, the rationale evocated to justify the initial trial done in St. Mark's Hospital was an antiprotozoal effect. This study on idiopathic colitis included 44 patients randomized to prednisolone suppositories or acetarsol suppositories 250 mg (containing 68 mg of 3-acetamido-4-hydroxyphenylarsonic acid) two suppositories nightly for 3 weeks [93]. The formulation used an organic arsenic, which is by far less toxic than the inorganic forms. Among the 20 patients who received the acetarsol, 18 showed clinical and 19 endoscopic improvement, whereas 17 of the 20 patients on prednisolone improved. One patient presented with jaundice in the acetarsol arm and stopped the treatment. Only one single small prospective open-label study has been reported using the same formulation of organic arsenic, given twice daily for 4 weeks [94]. In nine out of the ten treated patients with intractable proctitis, the symptoms and endoscopic signs of proctitis resolved within 2 weeks. Arsenic was absorbed systemically from the suppositories in the presence of active mucosal inflammation, but the level dropped rapidly after acetarsol was withdrawn. Minimal clinical side effects were reported, except for one transient thrombocytosis. To our knowledge, no further studies have been published since on the use of this agent in distal colitis.

## Probiotic Enemas, *Escherichia coli Nissle* 1917

As an altered microbial composition (dysbiosis) and function is probably involved in the pathogenesis of IBD through the microbiota-host interaction [95], prebiotics-, probiotics-, and antibiotics-based therapies have stimulated interest. These therapies are therefore also described in detail in another section of this book. Probiotics are containing numerous varieties of nonpathogenic bacteria. Their postulated beneficial role would be to directly exclude other microorganisms from the epithelial surface, including pathogens, due to competition for the adhesion sites and to interact with the intestinal epithelium to improve its function [96]. However, we choose to mention *E. coli Nissle 1917* which

has been studied in more detail as an oral preparation. Matthes et al. recently evaluated rectally administered *E. coli Nissle 1917* for acute distal UC. Ninety patients were randomly allocated to three different dosages (40 ml, 20 ml, 10 ml of probiotic enema (Mutaflor®)) or placebo. The intention-to-treat analysis was negative. However, patients did achieve remission according to a dose-related manner in the per-patient analysis: 53 % in the 40 ml group, 44 % in 20 ml, 27 % in 10 ml, and 185 in the placebo group ($p=0.0446$). Time to remission was also reduced with *E. coli Nissle* and the endoscopy results were favorable. Many patients in the trial were on concomitant oral therapy; *E. coli Nissle* 40 ml enema is a potential adjunctive, well-tolerated, treatment option.

## Fecal Bacteriotherapy

Fecal bacteriotherapy using fecal enemas for distal colitis was attempted by Borody et al. [97]. The rational idea behind it was to restore a normal balance in the colonic bacterial flora using feces from healthy donors (usually relatives) who were previously tested for numerous pathogens (*C. difficile* and other conventional enteropathogens and viral hepatitis). Their anecdotal report mentioned six patients who received fecal saline enemas (200–300 ml) administered within 10 min of preparation on a daily basis for 5 days and described symptom improvement after 1 week of follow-up and remission in all patients after 4 months without other UC medications. They also assessed remission maintained from 1 to 13 years in this very specific group of patients. However, concerns linked to the risks associated with fecal transplantation. However, IBD patients are probably more ready than caregivers to assume the risk and acceptability of this treatment [98]. A recent study was done representing the only placebo-controlled trial to date to treat patients with active ulcerative colitis with fecal enemas from nonrelated patients and did not demonstrate benefit for FMT as primary treatment in patients with active ulcerative colitis (who did not have *C. difficile* infection) [99].

## Lidocaine

Initial studies in the 1990s showed a low risk of systemic adverse effects with local anesthetic gels used for their potential anti-inflammatory properties [100]. The conceivable mode of action is through the blockage of hyperactive nervous reflex (possibly secondary to inflammation) which could reduce the release of neuropeptides and additional influence on inflammatory cell functions (such as adhesion, phagocytosis, lysis) [101]. A consecutive series of 100 patients with all forms of ulcerative colitis with a good response (83 %) to topical 2 % lignocaine gel (400 mg twice daily) within 6–34 weeks of treatment was reported at the time [101]. The relapse rate was high within the next 2 years after therapy, in particular for limited colitis. Finally, an RCT in 19 UC patients was unable to identify a change in the level of eicosanoids and neurotransmitters after the administration of topical ropivacaine [101]. The use of continuous intravenous administration of lidocaine, initially indicated for severe abdominal pain, to induce improvement in a patient with refractory panulcerative colitis was reported [102].

## Epidermal Growth Factor

Epidermal growth factor (EGF) is a mitogenic peptide produced by the salivary glands, which physiologically acts to maintain integrity of the oro-esophageal and gastric tissue by stimulating cellular proliferation, differentiation, and survival. However, circulating levels of EGF are low and not readily available to other parts of gastrointestinal mucosa. The objectives of this local therapy would be to propagate the abovementioned beneficial effects to the colonic mucosa and therefore improve healing of mucosal injuries and then preserve its integrity and barrier function. The efficacy of EGF enemas in left-sided ulcerative colitis has been assessed in a small RCT versus placebo involving 24 patients. After 2 weeks of treatment with daily enemas of 5 mcg of EGF in 100 ml of an inert carrier, all patients improved. Remission (defined by a St. Mark score ≤4 a non-stringent criteria) was achieved in 83 % of them compared to 8 % (one patient) in the control group. Endoscopic and histological assessments were also significantly better in the EGF than the placebo group and were maintained throughout the entire follow-up (12 weeks) [103]. These impressive results are the sole ones published till now on the use of EGF for UC. One possible explanation for lack of further studies to date is the concern over the carcinogenic potential of EGF therapy in patients already at high risk of developing colorectal cancer.

## Bismuth

Bismuth has been used for the treatment of gastric ulcer disease for over 100 years, and nowadays bismuth salicylate (Pepto-Bismol) is still used in *Helicobacter pylori* eradication and as over-the-counter antidiarrheal medication for nonsyndromic episodic diarrhea in both children and adults for its well-known antibacterial properties. In addition, its salicylate moiety and maybe bismuth as well could have anti-inflammatory properties. A multicenter randomized trial by Pullan et al. compared bismuth citrate enema to 5-ASA enema in 68 UC patient with distal colitis over a 4-week treatment period [104]. Clinical remission was observed in 18/32 (56 %) 5-ASA-treated and 12/31 (39 %) bismuth-treated patients ($p=0.16$), with an endoscopic remission in 20/32 (63 %) 5-ASA-treated and 15/31 (48 %) bismuth-treated patients ($p=0.26$). There were statistical differences between the groups: the 5-ASA-treated patients had less severe symptoms at inclusion and also experienced less bleeding at week 4. The authors conclude that bismuth enema could be a good alternative to 5-ASA enema in intolerant patients. Unfortunately, this study was not powered to confirm noninferiority of bismuth versus 5-ASA enemas. Moreover, only half of the recommended dose for gastric pathology was used (450 mg bismuth citrate, equivalent to 216 mg of metallic bismuth). Its potential antibacterial properties make it an interesting compound for future development.

## Rebamipide

Rebamipide (2-(4-chlorobenzoylamino)-3-(2-(1H)-quinolinon-4-yl)-propionic acid) is used in Japan as antiulcer agent. It was demonstrated not only to enhance epithelial restitution by increasing the expression of growth factors and endogenous prostaglandin but also to inhibit proinflammatory cytokines (such as tumor necrosis factor-alpha) and to suppress in vitro neutrophile functions [105, 106]. The first open-label study performed by Miyata et al. included 11 patients with steroid-resistant/dependent proctitis or proctosigmoiditis. Nine out of 11 patients (82 %) achieved clinical remission after 12 weeks of twice-daily rectal administration of 150 mg of rebamipide [107]. Seven patients continued on long-term treatment (80 days) with a similar success rate. Since then, two other open-label Japanese studies increased the total treated to 42 patients [108, 109] but no RCTs have been reported.

## Ecabet Sodium

Ecabet sodium is derived from pine resin and has been also initially used for gastritis and gastric ulcer; it was demonstrated to stimulate endogenous prostaglandins, the capsaicin-sensitive sensory nerves, nitric oxide, and the mucin metabolic pathway. The ability to provide a barrier to a mucosal antigen has also been suggested for ecabet sodium. This substance was tested as an enema in two small open-label cohorts of patients with ulcerative colitis. In the original study, 6 of 7 patients with limited distal colitis achieved clinical, endoscopic, and histological remission after 2 weeks [110]. In the most recent study performed entirely in 5 patients with more extensive colitis, two subjects almost achieved remission, one with a successful treatment of pouchitis, whereas two others with deep ulcers experience treatment failure [111]. To our knowledge, no further studies have been published.

## D-Alpha Tocopherol (Vitamin E)

Vitamin E is a lipophilic antioxidant which protects membrane lipids from peroxidation. A high production of reactive oxygen species has been demonstrated in the colonic mucosa of patients with IBD, and therefore, inhibition of lipid peroxidation and scavenging of oxygen free radicals are good strategies in order to prevent mucosal damage during the inflammation process in UC. Mirbagheri et al. performed an open-label series in 14 mild-to-moderate active UC patients [112]. All the patients received d-alpha tocopherol enema (8,000 U/days), the dominant isomer of vitamin E in the serum, for 12 weeks in addition to their oral therapy (5-ASA and/or thiopurines). All patients showed clinical response with a significant decrease in the value of the biological markers and 9 (64 %) achieved remission. These pilot results look promising and a larger trial is needed.

## SCFA, Butyrate and Sucralfate

Short-chain fatty acids, such as butyrate, are important energy source for colonic cells to help them maintain their homeostasis especially in the inflammatory state. In addition, the inflamed colonic mucosa seems to have a diminished capacity to oxidize butyrate maybe associated with TNF-alpha production [113]. It was also postulated that these compounds may play a role in colonic inflammation, whereas sucralfate protects ulcerated mucosa of further damages by local adherence. Very promising open studies have suggested that these compounds are effective treatments for active distal UC. However, for each of these substances, at least two RCTs involving more than 50 patients have now showed no therapeutic value by these drugs in the treatment of ulcerative colitis [14, 114, 115]. The daily oral administration of delayed-release tablets of butyrate has been explored and resulted in inconsistent data. The results were similar for enemas and the conclusion was that oral or rectal short-chain fatty acid was not an effective treatment for UC [116]. Interestingly, newly available tablets combining butyrate with mesalazine showed promising results in an open-label study. The treatment offered (mesalazine 800 mg + butyrate 0.3 g + inulin, thrice daily) to the 216 patients included in this multicenter Italian study was able to reduce disease activity, symptoms, and inflammation of the mucosa [117]. A blinded study is needed to confirm these results.

## Conclusion

Further understanding of the pathogenesis of ulcerative colitis has generated interesting new hypotheses and led to novel systemic and topical therapies. Many of them are nonbiologic, such as nicotine, helminths, probiotics, heparin, ridogrel, lidocaine, phosphatidylcholine, curcumin, aloe vera, and other herbal medicine used for their antioxidant and anti-inflammatory properties. Some small molecules which target cytokine receptors and inflammatory pathways are also emerging from promising phase II trials. However, not all these drugs have been subject to controlled studies and their current evidence of effectiveness and safety should be interpreted with caution. Ultimately, a shared decision between the patient and the clinician, including costs, availability, and weighting of risks and benefits, should lead to the initiation of these alternative drugs into the conventional management of ulcerative colitis.

**Acknowledgements** We gratefully acknowledge the contribution of Susan Giddons for editorial assistance. This study was supported by the Swiss National Science Foundation (SNF): grant N° PBLAP3-124341.

## References

1. Bastida G, Beltrán B. Ulcerative colitis in smokers, non-smokers and ex-smokers. World J Gastroenterol. 2011;17(22):2740–7.
2. Cosnes J. Tobacco and IBD: relevance in the understanding of disease mechanisms and clinical practice. Best Pract Res Clin Gastroenterol. 2004;18:481–96.
3. McGrath J, McDonald JWD, MacDonald JK. Transdermal nicotine for induction of remission in ulcerative colitis (systematic review). Cochrane Database Syst Rev. 2009(4):CD004722.
4. Ingram JR, Thomas GAO, Rhodes J, et al. A randomized trial of nicotine enemas for active ulcerative colitis. Clin Gastroenterol Hepatol. 2005;3:1107–14.
5. Braun A, Treede I, Gotthardt D, et al. Alterations of phospholipid concentration and species composition of the intestinal mucus barrier in ulcerative colitis: a clue to pathogenesis. Inflamm Bowel Dis. 2009;15:1705–20.
6. Stremmel W, Merle U, Zahn A, Autschbach F, Hinz U, Ehehalt R. Retarded release phosphatidylcholine benefits patients with chronic active ulcerative colitis. Gut. 2005;54:966–71.
7. Stremmel W, Ehehalt R, Autschbach F, Karner M. Phosphatidylcholine for steroid-refractory chronic ulcerative colitis: a randomized trial. Ann Intern Med. 2007;147:603–10.
8. Stremmel W, Braun A, Hanemann A, Ehehalt R, Autschbach F, Karner M. Delayed release phosphatidylcholine in chronic-active ulcerative colitis: a randomized, double-blinded, dose finding study. J Clin Gastroenterol. 2010;44:e101–7.
9. Weinstock JV, Elliott DE. Helminths and the IBD hygiene hypothesis. Inflamm Bowel Dis. 2009;15:128–33.
10. Schnoeller C, Rausch S, Pillai S, et al. A helminth immunomodulator reduces allergic and inflammatory responses by induction of IL-10-producing macrophages. J Immunol. 2008;180:4265–72.
11. Elliott DE, Urban JJ, Argo CK, Weinstock JV. Does the failure to acquire helminthic parasites predispose to Crohn's disease? FASEB J. 2000;14:1848–55.
12. Summers RW, Elliott DE, Urban Jr JF, Thompson RA, Weinstock JV. Trichuris suis therapy for active ulcerative colitis: a randomized controlled trial. Gastroenterology. 2005;128:825–32.
13. Summers RW. Novel and future medical management of inflammatory bowel disease. Surg Clin North Am. 2007;87:727–41.

14. Biancone L, Michetti P, Travis S, et al. European evidence-based Consensus on the management of ulcerative colitis: special situations. J Crohn's Colitis. 2008;2:63–92.

15. Bernstein CN, Blanchard JF, Houston DS, et al. The incidence of deep venous thrombosis and pulmonary embolism among patients with inflammatory bowel disease: a population-based cohort study. Thromb Haemost. 2001;85:430–4.

16. Kappelman MD, Horvath-Puho E, Sandler RS, et al. Thromboembolic risk among Danish children and adults with inflammatory bowel diseases: a population-based nationwide study. Gut. 2011;60:937–43.

17. Korzenik JR. IBD: a vascular disorder? the case for heparin therapy. Inflamm Bowel Dis. 1997;3:87–94.

18. Chande N, McDonald WDJ, MacDonald JK, Wang JJ. Unfractionated or low-molecular weight heparin for induction of remission in ulcerative colitis (systematic review). Cochrane Database Syst Rev 2010(10):CD006774.

19. Celasco G, Papa A, Jones R, et al. Clinical trial: oral colon-release parnaparin sodium tablets (CB-01-05 MMX) for active left-sided ulcerative colitis. Aliment Pharm Ther. 2010;31:375–86.

20. Baumgart DC. Extended colonic release low-molecular weight heparin (LMWH) not ready for use in ulcerative colitis. Evid Based Med. 2011;16:71–2.

21. Tytgat GN, Van Nueten L, Van De Velde I, Joslyn A, Hanauer SB. Efficacy and safety of oral ridogrel in the treatment of ulcerative colitis: two multicentre, randomized, double-blind studies. Aliment Pharmacol Ther. 2002;16:87–99.

22. Skandalis N, Rotenberg A, Meuwissen S, deGroot GH, Ouwendijk RJT, Tan TG. Ridogrel for the treatment of mild to moderate ulcerative colitis. Gastroenterology. 1996;110:A1016.

23. Auwerda JJ, Zijlstra FJ, Tak CJ, van den Ingh HF, Wilson JH, Ouwendijk RJ. Ridogrel enemas in distal ulcerative colitis. Eur J Gastroenterol Hepatol. 2001;13:397–400.

24. Sido B, Hack V, Hochlehnert A, Lipps H, Herfarth C, Droge W. Impairment of intestinal glutathione synthesis in patients with inflammatory bowel disease. Gut. 1998;42:485–92.

25. Guijarro LG, Mate J, Gisbert JP, et al. N-acetyl-L-cysteine combined with mesalamine in the treatment of ulcerative colitis: randomized, placebo-controlled pilot study. World J Gastroenterol. 2008;14:2851–7.

26. Celinski K, Dworzanski T, Korolczuk A, et al. Effects of peroxisome proliferator-activated receptors-gamma ligands on dextran sodium sulphate-induced colitis in rats. J Physiol Pharmacol. 2011;62:347–56.

27. Celinski K, Madro A, Prozorow-Krol B, et al. Rosiglitazone, a peroxisome proliferator-activated receptor gamma (PPAR- g)-specific agonist, as a modulator in experimental acute pancreatitis. Med Sci Monit. 2009;15:21–9.

28. Celinski K, Dworzanski T, Prozorow-Krol B, Korolczuk A. The role of PPAR-g receptors in gastrointestinal inflammation diseases. Gastroenterol Pol. 2009;16:51–6.

29. Andersen V, Christensen J, Ernst A, et al. Polymorphisms in NF-kB, PXR, LXR, PPARg and risk of inflammatory bowel disease. World J Gastroenterol. 2011;17:197–206.

30. Hontecillas R, Horne WT, Climent M, et al. Immunoregulatory mechanisms of macrophage PPAR-g in mice with experimental inflammatory bowel disease. Mucosal Immunol. 2011;4:304–13.

31. Saraf N, Sharma PK, Mondal SC, Garg VK, Singh AK. Role of PPARg2 transcription factor in thiazolidinedione-induced insulin sensitization. J Pharm Pharmacol. 2012;64:161–71.

32. Xiang GQ, Tang SS, Jiang LY, et al. PPARg agonist pioglitazone improves scopolamine-induced memory impairment in mice. J Pharm Pharmacol. 2012;64:589–96.

33. Ma JJ, Zhang T, Fang N, Zou Y, Gong QH, Yu LM, Chen DX. Establishment of a cell-based drug screening model for identifying agonists of human peroxisome proliferator activated receptor gamma (PPARg). J Pharm Pharmacol. 2012;64:719–26.

34. Rossi A, Kapahi P, Natoli G, et al. Anti-inflammatory cyclopentenone prostaglandins are direct inhibitors of IkappaB kinase. Nature. 2000;403:103–8.

35. Saubermann LJ, Nakajima A, Wada K, et al. Peroxisome proliferator-activated receptor gamma agonist ligands stimulate a Th2 cytokine response and prevent acute colitis. Inflamm Bowel Dis. 2002;8:330–9.

36. Lewis JD, Lichtenstein GR, Stein RB, et al. An open-label trial of the PPAR-gamma ligand rosiglitazone for active ulcerative colitis. Am J Gastroenterol. 2001;96:3323–8.

37. Lewis JD, Lichtenstein GR, Deren JJ, et al. Rosiglitazone for active ulcerative colitis: a randomized placebo-controlled trial. Gastroenterology. 2008;134:688–95.

38. Wertz DA, Chang CL, Sarawate CA, Willey VJ, Cziraky MJ, Bohn RL. Risk of cardiovascular events and all-cause mortality in patients treated with thiazolidinediones in a managed-care population. Circ Cardiovasc Qual Outcomes. 2010;3:538–45.

39. Langmead L, Feakins RM, Goldthorpe S, et al. Randomized, double-blind, placebo-controlled trial of oral aloe vera gel for active ulcerative colitis. Aliment Pharmacol Ther. 2004;19:739–47.

40. Sugimoto K, Hanai H, Tozawa K, Aoshi T, Uchijima M, Nagata T, et al. Curcumin prevents and ameliorates trinitrobenzene sulfonic acid induced colitis in mice. Gastroenterology. 2002;123:1912–22.

41. Deguchi Y, Andoh A, Inatomi O, Yagi Y, Bamba S, Araki Y, et al. Curcumin prevents the development of dextran sulfate Sodium (DSS)-induced experimental colitis. Dig Dis Sci. 2007;52:2993–8.

42. Arafa HM, Hemeida RA, El-Bahrawy AI, Hamada FM. Prophylactic role of curcumin in dextran sulfate sodium(DSS)-induced ulcerative colitis murine model. Food Chem Toxicol. 2009;47:1311–7.

43. Venkataranganna MV, Rafiq M, Gopumadhavan S, Peer G, Babu UV, Mitra SK. NCB-02 (standardized Curcumin preparation) protects dinitrochlorobenzene-induced colitis through down-regulation of NFkappa-B and iNOS. World J Gastroenterol. 2007;13:1103–7.

44. Hanai H, Iida T, Takeuchi K, et al. Curcumin maintenance therapy for ulcerative colitis: randomized, multicenter, double-blind, placebo-controlled trial. Clin Gastroenterol Hepatol. 2006;4:1502–6.

45. University of Maryland Medical center. http://www.umm.edu/altmed/articles/turmeric-000277.htm (2012). Accessed 14 October 2014.

46. Lahiff C, Moss AC. Curcumin for clinical and endoscopic remission in ulcerative colitis. Inflamm Bowel Dis. 2011;17(7):E66.

47. Anthoni C, Laukoetter MG, Rijcken E, et al. Mechanisms underlying the anti-inflammatory actions of boswellic acid derivatives in experimental colitis. Am J Physiol Gastrointest Liver Physiol. 2006;290:G1131–7.

48. Gupta I, Parihar A, Malhotra P, et al. Effects of Boswellia serrata gum resin in patients with ulcerative colitis. Eur J Med Res. 1997;2:37–43.

49. Holtmeier W, Zeuzem S, Preiss J, et al. Randomized, placebo-controlled, double-blind trial of Boswellia serrata in maintaining remission of Crohn's disease: good safety profile but lack of efficacy. Inflamm Bowel Dis. 2011;17:573–82.

50. Hilsden RJ, Verhoef MJ, Rasmussen H, Porcino A, DeBruyn JC. Use of complementary and alternative medicine by patients with inflammatory bowel disease. Inflamm Bowel Dis. 2011;17:655–62.

51. Lichtenstein GR, Deren JJ, Katz S, Lewis JD, Kennedy AR, Ware JH. Bowman-Birk inhibitor concentrate: a novel therapeutic agent

for patients with active ulcerative colitis. Dig Dis Sci. 2008; 53:175–80.

52. Senda S, Fujiyama Y, Bamba T, Hosoda S. Treatment of ulcerative colitis with camostat mesilate, a serine protease inhibitor. Intern Med. 1993;32:350–4.

53. Almallah YZ, El-Tahir A, Heys SD, Richardson S, Eremin O. Distal proctocolitis and n-3 polyunsaturated fatty acids: the mechanism(s) of natural cytotoxicity inhibition. Eur J Clin Invest. 2000;30:58–65.

54. Turner D, Steinhart AH, Griffiths AM. Omega 3 fatty acids (fish oil) for maintenance of remission in ulcerative colitis. Cochrane Database of Systematic Reviews 2007, Issue 3. Art. No.: CD006443. DOI:10.1002/14651858.CD006443.pub2.

55. De Ley M, de Vos R, Hommes DW, Stokkers PC. Fish oil for induction of remission in ulcerative colitis. Cochrane Database of Systematic Reviews 2007, Issue 4. Art. No.: CD005986. DOI:10.1002/14651858.CD005986.pub2.

56. Quattropani C, Ausfeld B, Straumann A, Heer P, Seibold F. Complementary alternative medicine in patients with inflammatory bowel disease: use and attitudes. Scand J Gastroenterol. 2003;38:277–82.

57. Ben-Arye E, Goldin E, Wengrower D, Stamper A, Kohn R, Berry E. Wheat grass juice in the treatment of active distal ulcerative colitis: a randomized double-blind placebo-controlled trial. Scand J Gastroenterol. 2002;37:444–9.

58. Michelsen KS, Wong MH, Ko B, Lisa BS, Thomas BS, Deepti D, Targan SR. HMPL-004 (Andrographis paniculata extract) prevents development of murine colitis by inhibiting T-cell proliferation and TH1/TH17 responses. Inflamm Bowel Dis. 2013;19:151–64.

59. Tang T, Targan SR, Li ZS, Xu C, Byers VS, Sandborn WJ. Randomised clinical trial: herbal extract HMPL-004 in active ulcerative colitis – a double-blind comparison with sustained release mesalazine. Aliment Pharm Ther. 2011;33:194–202.

60. Tong ZQ, Yang B, Chen B-Y, Zhao M-L. A multi-center, randomized, single-blind, controlled clinical study on the efficacy of composite sophora colon-soluble capsules in treating ulcerative colitis. Chin J Integr Med. 2010;16:486–92.

61. Wu HG, Zhou LB, Pan YY, et al. Study of the mechanisms of acupuncture and moxibustion treatment for ulcerative colitis rats in view of the gene expression of cytokines. World J Gastroenterol. 1999;5:515–7.

62. Lee DH, Kim JI, Lee MS, Choi TY, Choi SM, Ernst E. Moxibustion for ulcerative colitis: a systematic review and meta-analysis. BMC Gastroenterol. 2010;10:36.

63. Joos S, Wildau N, Kohnen R, et al. Acupuncture and moxibustion in the treatment of ulcerative colitis: a randomized controlled study. Scand J Gastroenterol. 2006;41:1056–63.

64. Walker JR, Ediger JP, Graff LA, et al. The Manitoba IBD cohort study: a population-based study of the prevalence of lifetime and 12-month anxiety and mood disorders. Am J Gastroenterol. 2008;103:1989–97.

65. Timmer A, Preiss JC, Motschall E, Rucker G, Jantschek G, Moser G. Psychological interventions for treatment of inflammatory bowel disease. Cochrane Database Syst Rev. 2011(2):CD006913.

66. Levenstein S, Prantera C, Varvo V, et al. Stress and exacerbation in ulcerative colitis: a prospective study of patients enrolled in remission. Am J Gastroenterol. 2000;95:1213–20.

67. Breaking the Vicious Cycle. http://www.breakingtheviciouscycle.info and http://www.scdiet.org/ (2011). Accessed 14 July 2011.

68. Jowett SL, Seal CJ, Pearce MS, et al. Influence of dietary factors on the clinical course of ulcerative colitis: a prospective cohort study. Gut. 2004;53:1479–84.

69. Magee EA, Edmond LM, Tasker SM, Kong SC, Curno R, Cummings JH. Associations between diet and disease activity in ulcerative colitis patients using a novel method of data analysis. Nutr J. 2005;4:7.

70. Hou JK, Abraham B, El-Serag H. Dietary intake and risk of developing inflammatory bowel disease: a systematic review of the literature. Am J Gastroenterol. 2011;106(4):563–73.

71. Hibi T, Sakuraba A. Is there a role for apheresis in gastrointestinal disorders? Nat Clin Pract Gastroenterol Hepatol. 2005;2:200–1.

72. Sawada K, Ohnishi K, Fukui S, Yamada K, Yamamura M, Amano K, et al. Leukocytapheresis therapy, performed with leukocyte removal filter, for inflammatory bowel disease. J Gastroenterol. 1995;30:322–9.

73. Sandborn WJ. Preliminary data on the use of apheresis in inflammatory bowel disease. Inflamm Bowel Dis. 2006;12:S15–21.

74. Emmrich J, Petermann S, Nowak D, Beutner I, Brock P. Klingelin the management of hospitalized patients with steroid refractory ulcerative colitis. Inflamm Bowel Dis. 2012;18:803–8.

75. Sands BE, Sandborn WJ, Feagan B, et al. A randomized, double-blind, sham-controlled study of granulocyte/monocyte apheresis for active ulcerative colitis. Gastroenterology. 2008;135:400–9.

76. Francis S, Conti M, Houslay M. Phosphodiesterases as drug targets. Berlin: Springer; 2011.

77. Keshavarzian A, Mutlu E, Guzman JP, Forsyth C, Banan A. Phosphodiesterase 4 inhibitors and inflammatory bowel disease: emerging therapies in inflammatory bowel disease. Expert Opin Investig Drugs. 2007;16:1489–506.

78. Sandborn WJ, Ghosh S, Panes J, et al. Tofacitinib, an oral janus kinase inhibitor, in active ulcerative colitis. N Engl J Med. 2012;367:616–24.

79. Sandborn WJ, Ghosh S, Panes J, Study A3921063 Investigators. Tofacitinib, an oral Janus kinase inhibitor, in active ulcerative colitis. N Engl J Med. 2012;367:616–24.

80. Travis S, Yap LM, Hawkey C, et al. RDP58 is a novel and potentially effective oral therapy for ulcerative colitis. Inflamm Bowel Dis. 2005;11:713–9.

81. Lukas M, Drastich P, Konecny M, et al. Exogenous alkaline phosphatase for the treatment of patients with moderate to severe ulcerative colitis. Inflamm Bowel Dis. 2010;16:1180–6.

82. Xavier RJ, Podolsky DK. Unravelling the pathogenesis of inflammatory bowel disease. Nature. 2007;448:427–34.

83. Herrlinger K, Diculescu M, Fellermann K, et al. Efficacy, safety, and tolerability of vidofludimus in patients with inflammatory bowel disease: the entrance study. Gastroenterology. 2011;140:S588–9.

84. Clinical trials registry, National Institute of Health, United States of America. www.clinicaltrial.gov (2011). Accessed 26 July 2011.

85. Ahlem C, Auci D, Mangano K, et al. HE3286: a novel synthetic steroid as an oral treatment for autoimmune disease. Ann N Y Acad Sci. 2009;1173:781–90.

86. Di Sebastiano P, Grossi L, Di Mola FF, et al. SR140333, a substance P receptor antagonist, influences morphological and motor changes in rat experimental colitis. Dig Dis Sci. 1999;44:439–44.

87. Camuesco D, Rodríguez-Cabezas ME, Garrido-Mesa N, et al. The intestinal anti-inflammatory effect of dersalazine sodium is related to a down-regulation in IL-17 production in experimental models of rodent colitis. Br J Pharmacol. 2012;165:729–40.

88. De Filippis D, Esposito G, Cirillo C, et al. Cannabidiol reduces intestinal inflammation through the control of neuroimmune axis. PLoS One. 2011;6:e28159.

89. van Dieren JM, Kuipers EJ, Samsom JN, Nieuwenhuis EE, van der Woude CJ. Revisiting the immunomodulators tacrolimus, methotrexate, and mycophenolate mofetil: their mechanisms of action and role in the treatment of IBD. Inflamm Bowel Dis. 2006;12:311–27.

90. Lawrance IC, Copeland TS. Rectal tacrolimus in the treatment of resistant ulcerative proctitis. Aliment Pharmacol Ther. 2008;28:1214–20.

91. van Dieren JM, van Bodegraven AA, Kuipers EJ, et al. Local application of tacrolimus in distal colitis: feasible and safe. Inflamm Bowel Dis. 2009;15:193–8.

92. Sandborn WJ, Tremaine WJ, Schroeder KW, et al. A placebo-controlled trial of cyclosporine enemas for mildly to moderately active left-sided ulcerative colitis. Gastroenterology. 1994;106:1429–35.

93. Connell AM, Lennard-Jones JE, Misiewicz JJ, Baron JH, Jones FA. Comparison of acetarsol and prednisolone-21-phosphate suppositories in the treatment of idiopathic proctitis. Lancet. 1965;1:238.

94. Forbes A, Britton TC, House IM, Gazzard BG. Safety and efficacy of acetarsol suppositories in unresponsive proctitis. Aliment Pharmacol Ther. 1989;3:553–6.

95. Sartor RB. Microbial influences in inflammatory bowel diseases. Gastroenterology. 2008;134:577–94.

96. Sans M. Probiotics for inflammatory bowel disease: a critical appraisal. Dig Dis. 2009;27:111–4.

97. Borody TJ, Warren EF, Leis S, Surace R, Ashman O. Treatment of ulcerative colitis using fecal bacteriotherapy. J Clin Gastroenterol. 2003;37:42–7.

98. Kahn SA, Gorawara-Bhat R, Rubin DT. Fecal bacteriotherapy for ulcerative colitis: patients are ready, are we? Inflamm Bowel Dis. 2012;18:676–84.

99. Moayyedi P et al. A randomized, placebo-controlled trial of fecal microbiota therapy in active ulcerative colitis. Gastroenterology. 2014;146(5):Suppl 1-abstract no. 929c.

100. Arlander E, Ost A, Stahlberg D, Lofberg R. Ropivacaine gel in active distal ulcerative colitis and proctitis – a pharmacokinetic and exploratory clinical study. Aliment Pharmacol Ther. 1996;10:73–81.

101. Björck S, Dahlstrom A, Ahlman H. Treatment of distal colitis with local anaesthetic agents. Pharmacol Toxicol. 2002;90:173–80.

102. Hillingso JG, Kjeldsen J, Schmidt PT, et al. Effects of topical ropivacaine on eicosanoids and neurotransmitters in the rectum of patients with distal ulcerative colitis. Scand J Gastroenterol. 2002;37:325–9.

103. Yokoyama Y, Onishi S. Systemic lidocaine and mexiletine for the treatment of a patient with total ulcerative colitis. Gut. 2005;54:441.

104. Travis SP, Higgins PD, Orchard T, et al. Review article: defining remission in ulcerative colitis. Aliment Pharmacol Ther. 2011;34:113–24.

105. Pullan RD, Ganesh S, Mani V, et al. Comparison of bismuth citrate and 5-aminosalicylic acid enemas in distal ulcerative colitis: a controlled trial. Gut. 1993;34:676–9.

106. Genta RM. Review article: the role of rebamipide in the management of inflammatory disease of the gastrointestinal tract. Aliment Pharm Ther. 2003;18:8–13.

107. Miyata M, Kasugai K, Ishikawa T, Kakumu S, Onishi M, Mori T. Rebamipide enemas-new effective treatment for patients with corticosteroid dependent or resistant ulcerative colitis. Dig Dis Sci. 2005;50 Suppl 1:S119–23.

108. Furuta R, Ando T, Watanabe O, et al. Rebamipide enema therapy as a treatment for patients with active distal ulcerative colitis. J Gastroenterol Hepatol. 2007;22:261–7.

109. Makiyama K, Takeshima F, Hamamoto T. Efficacy of rebamipide enemas in active distal ulcerative colitis and proctitis: a prospective study report. Dig Dis Sci. 2005;50:2323–9.

110. Kono T, Nomura M, Kasai S, Kohgo Y. Effect of ecabet sodium enema on mildly to moderately active ulcerative proctosigmoiditis: an open-label study. Am J Gastroenterol. 2001;96:793–7.

111. Iizuka M, Itou H, Konno S, et al. Efficacy of ecabet sodium enema on steroid resistant or steroid dependent ulcerative colitis. Gut. 2006;55:1523.

112. Mirbagheri S-A, Nezami B-G, Assa S, Hajimahmoodi M. Rectal administration of d-alpha tocopherol for active ulcerative colitis: a preliminary report. World J Gastroenterol. 2008;14:5990–5.

113. Nancey S, Moussata D, Graber I, Claudel S, Saurin JC, Flourie B. Tumor necrosis factor alpha reduces butyrate oxidation in vitro in human colonic mucosa: a link from inflammatory process to mucosal damage? Inflamm Bowel Dis. 2005;11:559–66.

114. Breuer RI, Soergel KH, Lashner BA, et al. Short chain fatty acid rectal irrigation for left-sided ulcerative colitis: a randomised, placebo controlled trial. Gut. 1997;40:485–91.

115. Steinhart AH, Hiruki T, Brzezinski A, Baker JP. Treatment of left-sided ulcerative colitis with butyrate enemas: a controlled trial. Aliment Pharmacol Ther. 1996;10:729–36.

116. Schoultz I, Soderholm JD, McKay DM. Is metabolic stress a common denominator in inflammatory bowel disease? Inflamm Bowel Dis. 2011;17(9):2008–18.

117. Assisi RF, Group GS. Combined butyric acid/mesalazine treatment in ulcerative colitis with mild-moderate activity. Results of a multicentre pilot study. Minerva Gastroenterol Dietol. 2008;54:231–8.

# Disease Modifiers in the Management of Ulcerative Colitis

Adam M. Berg and Francis A. Farraye

**Keywords**

Disease modifiers • Ulcerative colitis • Crohn's disease

## Introduction

Although an individual's susceptibility to develop inflammatory bowel disease (IBD) appears to be genetically determined, the actual development of the disease is largely influenced by environmental factors. In developed countries IBD emerged during the middle of the twentieth century, initially in the form of ulcerative colitis (UC), but over the past several decades, Crohn's disease (CD) has become the predominant form of IBD. Interestingly, in parts of the world where IBD was rare, epidemiologic studies have demonstrated the emergence of UC [1–3]. These data support the role of environmental influence on the development of IBD. Additionally, epidemiologic studies show an increased risk of IBD with immigration from a country with low IBD prevalence to high prevalence regions [4].

While important advances have been made in our understanding of the genetics, pathogenesis, diagnosis, and medical management of patients with IBD, our emphasis on environmental modifiers, health maintenance, and lifestyle factors that can affect the course, complications, and severity of the disease has not been nearly as significant. Several modifiable factors have been identified and are becoming increasingly relevant for physicians and patients alike. This chapter summarizes the available evidence surrounding the influence of disease modifiers on the natural history and course of UC, specifically prenatal and early childhood factors, medications, infections, appendectomy, and lifestyle influences.

A.M. Berg, M.D. • F.A. Farraye, M.D., M.Sc. (✉)
Section of Gastroenterology, Boston Medical Center,
Boston University School of Medicine, 85 East Concord Street,
7th Floor, Boston, MA 02118, USA
e-mail: adam2berg@gmail.com; francis.farraye@bmc.org

## Prenatal and Early Childhood

The first year of life is considered a crucial period for immune system maturation and development of immune tolerance. Childhood living conditions including socioeconomic status, hygiene, birth order, family size, urban living, and breastfeeding all may have an influence on UC development.

## Hygiene Hypothesis

Hygiene, especially early in life, appears to have an impact on the bacterial colonization of the gut and other infectious exposures that determine the development of the immune system [5]. Although in early reports, high socioeconomic status was postulated as a risk factor for UC [6, 7], subsequent studies have not confirmed this observation [8, 9]. These contradictory results may be explained by the reduction or disappearance of differences in living conditions between socioeconomic groups following the Second World War. The "hygiene hypothesis" which was initially formulated as an explanation for allergies [10] has been extended to autoimmune diseases including diabetes and inflammatory diseases including IBD [11]. It focuses on improved sanitation during the twentieth century leading to decreased exposure to enteric organisms in childhood and an inappropriate immunologic response to antigen exposure such as a gastrointestinal infection later in life [11]. This theory however is incompletely supported in the literature [12, 13].

Proxy markers of improved sanitation and decreased environmental exposures early in life that have been used as evidence to support the hygiene hypothesis include *Helicobacter pylori* infection, family size, birth order, sibship, urban living, and pet exposures [12–14].

G.R. Lichtenstein (ed.), *Medical Therapy of Ulcerative Colitis*,
DOI 10.1007/978-1-4939-1677-1_20, © Springer Science+Business Media New York 2014

There is conflicting data regarding urban environments and the risk of UC with some observational studies showing an increase risk [15, 16], whereas others found no such relationship [17, 18]. Some studies found exposure to farm animals was protective in the development of UC [19]. Use of toothpaste in Western societies has also been implicated as a possible risk factor for IBD [20]. In an isolated report, exposure to soft toys during childhood was found to be protective against the development of IBD [21]. This finding has not been validated or reproduced in other studies [22].

In summary, these reports suggest that strict attention to hygiene and a lack of environmental exposures during infancy and as a young child might prevent the development of tolerance to many bacteria commonly found in the environment and predispose the individual to active immune-mediated events if the exposure occurs later in life. Although interesting from an epidemiologic perspective, these findings are unlikely to lead to any specific recommendations to prevent IBD.

## Breastfeeding

Breastfeeding has an impact on both the immune system and bacterial colonization of the gut, and therefore, possible effects on the development of IBD are intriguing. However, the evidence for a possible inverse association between breastfeeding and IBD remains controversial. Although several studies suggested a protective effect of breastfeeding against the development of IBD, with a possible association between the duration of breastfeeding [23–28], in some studies, the association did not reach statistical significance and in others was not apparent at all [8, 29–31]. In general, the association appears to be stronger for CD than for UC. A meta-analysis that included seven studies suggested a protective effect of breastfeeding in developing early-onset IBD (OR, 0.69; 95 % CI, 0.51–0.94; $P=0.02$), but the composite data was limited by statistical flaws, methodological deficiencies, and recall bias of the primary data [32].

Early weaning has also been implicated as a risk factor for UC [30]. While the notion that early weaning has an impact on both the immune system and bacterial colonization of the gut is appealing, a case-control study did not confirm an association between early formula feeding and IBD [8]. It is thus possible that in studies showing a positive association, early weaning may be a surrogate marker for higher socioeconomic status. In general, breastfeeding studies are complicated by long recall intervals and the potential for introduction of recall bias; therefore, the evidence is controversial at best, and no firm conclusions can be made. Nonetheless, some authors recommend that as breastfeeding may be a possible protective factor for the development of IBD, any data that lends itself to increasing breastfeeding rates will also benefit the general population [32].

## Medications (See Table 20.1)

### Antibiotics

An increased use of antibiotics after the Second World War coincided with the increased incidence of IBD and has led some investigators to speculate that antibiotic use may cause IBD [33]. A possible mechanism includes "dysbiosis," which is the disruption of gut microflora that leads to an imbalance between protective and pathogenic bacteria [34]. Early evidence supporting antibiotics culpability showed an approximately threefold increase in antibiotic usage in IBD patients, but these data were retrospective and may have been influenced by recall and indication bias (i.e., patients receiving antibiotics for insidious symptoms not yet diagnosed as IBD) [16, 29, 35]. A case-control, population-based study in Manitoba using documented antibiotic exposure has shown a threefold increase in antibiotic use in childhood IBD patients compared to controls [36]. However, given the observational methodology of these studies, causation could not be established, and though some studies identified specific offending antibiotics (penicillin and extended-spectrum penicillin) [37], small sample sizes limit generalization. These results may indicate reverse causality and that infection more than the antibiotic use may actually cause IBD (see "Infections" section below). In addition, the prevalence of antibiotic use varies significantly between countries and does not appear to correlate well with the incidence of IBD [22]. Although there is no definitive causation between early antibiotic use and IBD, liberal use of antibiotics in childhood should be avoided with special attention to doxycycline for acne [38], penicillin, or extended penicillin [37].

**Table 20.1** Medications and the risk of inflammatory bowel disease

| Antibiotics | • No definitive cause between early use and IBD |
| | • Most studied include tetracyclines, penicillin |
| Oral contraceptives | • Weak association with CD that increases with length of exposure |
| | • Risk reverts to nonexposed population upon cessation |
| NSAIDs | • Possible association between NSAID use and exacerbation of IBD |
| | • Caution with all NSAIDs including COX-2 inhibitors |
| | • Short-term COX-2 inhibitors may not cause UC exacerbation |

*NSAIDs* nonsteroidal anti-inflammatory drugs, *IBD* inflammatory bowel disease, *CD* Crohn's disease, *UC* ulcerative colitis

## Probiotics

A possible mechanism leading to IBD as discussed above is dysbiosis, which leads to an imbalance of protective and pathogenic bacteria. Probiotics and prebiotics are thought to reestablish equilibrium. Probiotics are live, nonpathogenic microbial food ingredients, usually of the genus *Bifidobacterium* or *Lactobacillus*, that alter the enteric flora and have been associated with beneficial effects. Some non-invasive coliforms and nonbacterial organisms such as *Saccharomyces boulardii* are also categorized as probiotics [39]. Prebiotics are selectively fermented short-chain fatty acids including fructo-oligosaccharides and galacto-oligosaccharides [40], and together prebiotics and probiotics are termed synbiotics. Given their ability to prevent the overgrowth of potentially pathogenic organisms and stimulate the intestinal immune defense system [41], synbiotics are being increasingly used as an adjuvant or alternative therapy for IBD [42]. In two controlled studies, a nonpathogenic strain of *Escherichia coli* was as effective as a 5-ASA preparation in maintaining remission in patients with UC [43, 44]. Probiotic combinations have the strongest evidence in the treatment of chronic pouchitis, reducing the relapse rates when compared to placebo [45, 46], and in the primary prevention of pouchitis postsurgery [47], though not all studies were favorable [48]. The use of probiotics and prebiotics in IBD is discussed elsewhere in this book.

## Oral Contraceptives

Since the 1970s, several case reports as well as case-control and cohort studies have described an increased risk of IBD in women who use oral contraceptives (OCPs) [49–51]. Although cohort studies including more than 80,000 women reported increases in IBD risk ranging from 40 % to three-fold, the results were not statistically significant, especially after adjusting for cigarette smoking [50–53]. Other case-control studies have also suggested an association between OCP use and IBD, especially CD [54, 55]. The risk appears to be higher among longtime users [54, 56, 57] and among users of high-dose estrogen preparations [54].

In a meta-analysis of two cohort studies and seven case-control studies from 1995, the pooled OR for UC among OCP users was 1.29, but did not reach statistical significance (95 % CI: 0.9–1.8) [58]. A more recent meta-analysis from 1983 to 2007 that included a total of 75,815 patients (14 studies, with 36,797 exposed to OCP and 39,018 nonexposed women) showed that the pooled relative risk (RR) for UC in women currently taking the OCP was 1.53 (CI 1.21–1.94, $P=0.001$) and 1.28 (CI 1.06–1.54, $P=0.011$), adjusted for smoking. With cessation of smoking, the RR for UC did not change, but was no longer statistically significant [59].

In summary, available evidence supports a weak association between OCP use and IBD that increases with length of exposure, but with cessation of OCP, the risk reverts to that on the nonexposed population. The thrombogenic potential of OCPs, leading to multifocal gastrointestinal infarctions mediated by chronic mesenteric vasculitis, similar to those of smoking, is the proposed mechanism underlying the effect of OCPs [53, 60]. No recommendations can be made regarding the use of OCPs and the risk of developing IBD.

## Nonsteroidal Anti-inflammatory Drugs (NSAIDs)

NSAIDs are one of the most commonly used medications worldwide and have been implicated as a cause of flares secondary to an inhibitory effect on prostaglandins and through uncoupling mitochondrial oxidative phosphorylation [61]. The association between NSAIDs and IBD flares has not been clearly established, though several studies have examined this relationship [62–68]. In the United States, more than 70 million NSAID prescriptions and 30 billion over-the-counter preparations are sold every year [69]. Although NSAID use has typically been associated with the development of gastroduodenal injury, evidence implicating these agents in inducing and exacerbating damage in the distal gastrointestinal tract is also mounting. Colonic injury ranging from colitis resembling inflammatory bowel disease to colonic perforation and bleeding has been described [65, 70, 71].

More than 80 % of patients with IBD interviewed in one study reported use of NSAIDs within the previous month, and approximately one-third of these patients thought that there was an association between their IBD symptoms and NSAID use. In contrast, only 2 % of the IBS population used as a control group reported worsening symptoms following NSAID use [64, 66]. Most studies are case series or case reports and have reported an association between NSAIDs and IBD, though given the methodological shortcomings, causality cannot be established [62, 63, 67, 68]. For example, in new cases of IBD, there was a significant self-reported exposure to NSAIDs/salicylates within 3 months prior to presentation when compared to sex-matched community controls (OR = 9.1, 95 % CI:4.5–21.9) [68]. Some studies did not find a relationship between NSAIDs and IBD activity though these had significant limitations [64–66].

The exact mechanism by which NSAIDs can lead to exacerbations of IBD is not fully understood, though some speculate that small bowel mitochondrial dysfunction and colonic effects of prostaglandin are central. The key enzyme in the inhibition of colonic prostaglandin (PG) synthesis is cyclooxygenase (COX), which exists in two isoforms, COX-1, the constitutive enzyme involved in maintaining mucosal integrity in the GI tract, and COX-2, an inducible enzyme that is expressed at sites of inflammation [72]. COX-2 expression is significantly increased in the colonic mucosa of patients with active IBD when compared to inactive disease or healthy controls [73]. COX-2 appears to have a beneficial effect in healing experimental colitis, and in theory, COX-2 inhibition might impair colitis healing [72]. Alternatively, NSAIDs uncouple mitochondrial oxidative phosphorylation and reduce ATP levels, which can lead to increased permeability because of dysfunction at the mucosal tight junctions [74].

Because of the evidence suggesting that COX-2-specific inhibitors are less toxic to the gastrointestinal tract than traditional NSAIDs, patients and physicians have hoped that selective inhibition of COX-2 would result in anti-inflammatory and analgesic effects without exacerbating IBD. However, cases of IBD flares associated with the use of COX-2 inhibitors have been reported in the literature [75–77]. In a series of 33 patients with IBD who were prescribed with celecoxib or rofecoxib, 39 % experienced exacerbation of their disease [78]. A multicenter, randomized, double-blinded, placebo-controlled trial that enrolled 222 subjects with UC in remission found that rates of UC exacerbation were similar between groups who were taking 200 mg of celecoxib or placebo [67]. The general expert consensus is that the use of COX-2-specific inhibitors in patients with IBD should be viewed with the same caution as the use of traditional NSAIDs [79, 80].

There is no simple solution for patients who require NSAIDs and have significant IBD activity. When patients are using NSAIDs to control the pain from IBD-related arthritis, the intestinal disease should be treated aggressively hoping that the severity of the arthritis will decrease as the intestinal inflammatory activity resolves. Non-NSAID analgesics can be prescribed in the interim to control joint pain. Non-NSAID analgesics and local measures can be used for the treatment of trauma-related pain and inflammation in patients with IBD. If these fail, a short course of NSAIDs or COX-2-selective inhibitors may be prescribed with close monitoring of symptoms and side effects.

## Lifestyle Factors

Smoking is the best-described environmental factor affecting IBD. The overall effects of smoking on UC are summarized in Table 20.2. Other modifiable factors such as diet, exercise, and stress are less supported and are summarized in Table 20.3.

**Table 20.2** Effects of smoking and smoking cessation on inflammatory bowel disease

|  | Crohn's disease | Ulcerative colitis |
|---|---|---|
| Smoking | • Increased prevalence | • Decreased prevalence |
|  | • Negative effect on course | • "Protective effect" |
|  |   • More relapses |   • Less flares |
|  |   • Increased complications |   • ? Reduced hospitalizations |
|  |   • More surgeries |   • ? Reduced colectomy rates |
|  | • Increased need for use of immunomodulators | • Reduced incidence of pouchitis |
| Smoking cessation | • Decreased risk of relapse and postoperative recurrence | • Increased disease activity |
|  | • Decreased risk for steroids and immunomodulators | • Increased need for hospitalization, steroids, and immunomodulators |
|  |  | • ? Increased need for colectomy |

**Table 20.3** Role of lifestyle on ulcerative colitis

| Exercise | • May decrease the incidence |
|---|---|
|  | • Possible reduction in incidence of colon cancer |
|  | • Improvement in quality of life |
|  | • No association with reduction in flares or activity |
| Diet | • Refined sugars may increase risk |
|  | • Increased protein and fat may increase risk |
|  | • Red/processed meat, protein, and alcohol were associated with relapse |
|  | • High intake of dietary fiber, fruit, or vegetables may be protective against the development of IBD |
| Stress | • Depression, anxiety, IBS prevalent in IBD |
|  | • No clear evidence that stress causes IBD |
|  | • Increases use of medical services |
|  | • Improved social support can improve health outcomes |
|  | • Treatment of depression/anxiety may decrease relapse or severity |

*IBD* inflammatory bowel disease

## Smoking

Smoking is the best characterized of the environmental factors that can affect the severity and natural history of IBD, though the relationship between smoking and IBD is complex. Smoking has been recognized as a risk factor for IBD for over 25 years, where cigarettes were associated with an increased prevalence of CD, while nonsmoking was associated with the development of UC [81–83]. There is also strong evidence suggesting that smoking cigarettes has a negative effect on the course of CD and that smoking cigarettes may improve the disease severity or have a "protective" effect in some patients with UC [84].

## Smoking and Ulcerative Colitis

Ulcerative colitis is predominately a disease of nonsmokers or former smokers. The incidence of UC in the Mormon community where smoking is discouraged is fivefold higher than the general population [85, 86]. Lifetime nonsmokers are almost three times more likely to have UC than current smokers [87]. Several meta-analyses as well as observational and case-control studies have confirmed that the relative risk of developing ulcerative colitis is reduced in smokers when compared to people who have never smoked and to individuals who have quit smoking [88–90]. A meta-analysis that included a total of 245 articles found an association between former smoking and UC (OR, 1.79; 95 % CI, 1.37–2.34) and that current smoking had a protective effect on the development of UC when compared with controls (OR, 0.58; 95 % CI, 0.45–0.75) [90]. Furthermore, approximately two-thirds of former smokers with UC develop the disease after quitting smoking with a particularly high incidence in the first few years [91–93]. Smokers have also been noted to have a reduced incidence of conditions such as primary sclerosing cholangitis (PSC), with or without associated IBD [94–96] and pouchitis [97]. The protective effect against PSC suggests a systemic effect rather than a local effect on the colon [53].

Smoking also appears to have an effect on the clinical course of UC. A significant proportion of patients report that their colitis improves while smoking ~20 cigarettes daily. Similarly, smokers with UC report fewer bowel complaints than their nonsmoking counterparts [98]. Several studies have reported lower hospitalization rates in smokers with UC, higher colectomy rates in ex-smokers who quit smoking before the onset of their colitis [99], reduced rates of clinical relapse in patients who began smoking after diagnosis [100], and reduced incidence of pouchitis in smokers following proctocolectomy [97]. Conversely, smoking cessation is usually followed by a statistically significant increase in disease severity, hospitalization rate, and need for major medical therapy, when compared to continuing smoking [101].

The effects of passive smoking on the development or the course of UC are less clear. Early studies suggested that prenatal passive smoking or exposure during early childhood may offer protection against developing UC as in active smoking [102, 103]. Meta-analyses that included 13 studies did not find a positive relationship between UC and prenatal smoke exposure (OR 1.11, 95 % CI 0.63–1.97) or childhood passive smoke exposure (OR 1.01, CI 0.85–1.20) [104]. However, the small sample size prevented definitive conclusions. A follow-up survey and retrospective review that included 675 IBD patients (56 % CD and 44 % UC) found that UC patients who were passive smokers developed more pouchitis (100 % versus 44 %; $P<0.038$) and backwash ileitis (16 % versus 4 %; $P<0.023$) than nonpassive smokers, but passive smoking did not alter the need for medication, surgery, or hospitalizations [105].

## Pathogenesis of Smoking in IBD

Despite these well-described associations, the mechanism by which cigarette smoking affects UC and CD in opposite ways is not fully understood. In addition to nicotine, tobacco smoke contains hundreds of substances including free radicals and carbon monoxide (CO) [106]. Several effects of nicotine are likely contributors to the role of smoking as a disease modifier in IBD. Nicotine modifies the thickness of the mucus and abolishes the synthesis of inflammatory cytokines in the colonic mucosa in animal models [33, 55]. In humans, nicotine is known to decrease the production of mucosal eicosanoids and some cytokines such as IL-2, IL-8, and TNF-α [106–108]. Nicotine also reduces smooth muscle tone and contractile activity as a result of NO release, changes in the microcirculation, and transient ischemia [9, 109]. Cigarette smoke, in turn, increases lipid peroxidation and modifies the mucosal immune response [110]. Smoking increases carbon monoxide concentrations, which might amplify the impairment in vasodilation capacity in chronically inflamed microvessels, resulting in ischemia and perpetuating ulceration and fibrosis [106, 111].

Patient-related factors have also been found to play a role in the type and magnitude of the effects of smoking in IBD. The effects of nicotine on IBD appear to be dose related with significant changes seen with 15 or more cigarettes per day. Women appear to be more susceptible than men to the harmful effect of smoking on CD, and as seen in patients with UC, the protective effect of nicotine is more efficient in the distal intestine [106].

## Smoking and IBD in Clinical Practice

Although most evidence supports a beneficial effect of cigarette smoking on the course of UC, these patients should not be encouraged to smoke and should, as any other smoker, receive education about the health risks of nicotine use. Patients with UC should be educated about the relationship between smoking and their disease and should be allowed to make their own decision based on the available data.

## Diet

Various dietary exposures have been proposed as causative factors in IBD. Based on population and immigration studies, and considering the increase in the incidence of UC in countries like Japan and South Korea during the 1990s, a Westernized diet has been implicated in the development of IBD [22, 112–114]. Studies examining associations between diet and disease are difficult to perform because of recall bias and the possibility that the diet was modified before a formal diagnosis of IBD as a result of chronic gastrointestinal symptoms. Early dietary studies were poorly conducted and fraught with methodological deficiencies, making it impossible to draw any meaningful conclusion [115]. Refined sugar, fast foods, margarine, and dairy products, while vegetables, fruits, fish, and dietary fiber, have been investigated.

## Refined Sugar

Consumption of refined sugar has been found to be associated with IBD in several retrospective case-control studies [116, 117]. Trials that have aimed to minimize difficulties with dietary recall bias by studying patients diagnosed within 1 year have shown contradictory results, with some [117–119] but not all studies showing an association [116, 120, 121]. Because smoking is positively associated with sugar consumption, the interpretation of data derived from dietary studies is complicated. When analyzed separately, sugar intake and smoking have been shown to be independent risk factors; however, combined exposure did not result in a further increased risk [122, 123].

## Protein and Fat

A positive association has been demonstrated for both UC and CD with protein and fat consumption, although the results are inconsistent, and the studies may also be affected by methodological problems [113, 119, 124]. In a prospective study [125], dietary factors such as a high intake of red and processed meat, protein, and alcohol were associated with an increased likelihood of relapse in patients with UC.

## Fruits and Vegetables

High intake of dietary fiber, fruit, or vegetables may be protective against the development of IBD, but results vary among studies [113, 119, 126]. It is unclear whether this finding is the result of decreased fiber intake in response to symptoms of stricturing CD [53].

## Fast Food and Cola Drinks

Both fast food and cola drinks have been implicated as risk factors for UC and CD [21, 126]. Many more foods have been implicated in the development or worsening of IBD, including margarine [127], dairy products [128], baker's yeast [129, 130], coffee [126, 131], alcohol [131, 132], cornflakes [133, 134], and curry [135], among others. Lactase or other enzymatic deficiencies secondary to extensive mucosal involvement may be involved in specific food intolerance in patients with CD. In general, none of these associations has been irrefutably proven, and no firm clinical recommendations can be made in this regard.

## Other Foods and Food Allergies

Food allergies, food additives, and spices such as curry may play a role in the development of IBD. Food allergies may play a role in the pathogenesis of IBD because dietary antigens may act as immunoregulators [136, 137]. Small studies have shown that patients with CD demonstrate a stronger response to food antigens than healthy individuals [137]. The success of treatment with elemental or exclusion diets would support food allergy as a biological pathway in patients with CD. Similarly, food additives present in modern urban diets may be involved in immune reactions both locally and systemically and have been proposed as an etiological factor in IBD, especially CD [138, 139].

The low incidence of IBD in populations with high consumption of curried and highly spiced food is intriguing. It has been postulated that curcumin, a major component of curry, has antioxidant and anti-inflammatory activity, acting as a protective factor against the development of IBD [135]. Overall, the retrospective nature of diet-related studies makes any definitive conclusions difficult, but a well-balanced diet rich in fruits and vegetables and low in refined sugars would be generally recommended.

## Exercise

Sedentary and physically less demanding occupations have been associated with a higher incidence of IBD, though the data is limited and weak [140–143]. Exercise, in contrast, has been associated with improvements in quality of life, but not activity index scores, in patients with UC [144].

While GI symptoms such as nausea, heartburn, diarrhea, and occasionally GI bleeding are common during intense sports [145–148], physical activity has also been associated with long-term benefits in the GI tract, especially a consistent reduction in colon cancer risk, which, although documented in non-IBD patients, may also extend to individuals with IBD [149, 150].

Although the preventive effect of exercise remains inconclusive, it seems clear that physical activity is not harmful for patients with IBD. Another important reason to recommend regular physical activity is that IBD patients, especially those on chronic steroids, are at risk for osteoporosis and osteopenia [150, 151]. A low-impact exercise program can potentially increase bone density in these patients [152]. Exercise may also alleviate stress and allow people to deal with stressful events more effectively, increasing the sense of general well-being and quality of life [153]. Physical activity should be recommended, keeping in mind that there is limited data regarding exactly how much exercise is appropriate [79].

## Stress

Accumulating evidence suggests that stress appears to play a significant role in increasing disease activity and frequency of relapses, as well as the use of medical services in patients with IBD [80, 154–160]. Factors such as potential disability caused by the symptoms of IBD and the uncertainty regarding disease outcomes can produce significant stress in patients living with IBD, and this needs to be addressed by the clinician caring for IBD patients [154]. Although many patients and family members are convinced that stress is an essential factor in the onset and course of IBD, it has been difficult to correlate the development of disease with any psychological issues or disease exacerbations with stressful life events [161]. Many studies report that anxiety and depression are more prevalent in patients with IBD [162–164] and that stress [165] and adverse life events [166, 167] can trigger relapses. However, not all agree as one study found no evidence of an association between psychological stress, as measured by the death of a child, and the onset of IBD [168].

Strategies that improve social support, including local groups where individuals can share their experiences, may have a favorable impact on psychological distress and ultimately improve health outcomes in patients with IBD [158]. Additionally, diagnosis and treatment of concomitant mood disorders can have a positive impact on patient's outcomes. A retrospective study found that there was less relapse and steroid use among 14 ulcerative colitis and 15 Crohn's disease patients who were started on an antidepressant for a concomitant mood disorder compared to that of controls matched for age, sex, disease type, and medication over a 1-year period [169]. The possibility of concurrent irritable bowel syndrome (IBS)-related symptoms and their relation to stressful events should also be recognized to minimize the use of potent anti-inflammatory or disease-modifying therapies in the absence of a documented inflammatory component. Overall empathy, understanding, positive regard, and psychological support improve the patient-physician relationship and lead to better quality of life for the patients [170].

## Infections

IBD appears to result from the interaction of three essential cofactors: host susceptibility, enteric microflora, and mucosal immunity. Therefore, it has been proposed that intestinal bacteria may play a role in triggering and perpetuating chronic bowel inflammation. In susceptible individuals, a breakdown in the regulatory constraints of the mucosal immune response to enteric bacteria may result in the development of IBD [39]. Non-enteric systemic infections have

**Table 20.4** Infectious agents possibly linked to the occurrence of inflammatory bowel disease

*Bacterial*
- *Mycobacterium paratuberculosis*
- *Listeria*
- Pharyngitis and otitis
- *Helicobacter pylori*

*Viral*
- Unspecified childhood gastroenteritis
- Measles and measles vaccination
- Mumps
- Influenza
- Varicella

*Parasites*
- Helminthic parasites

also been proposed as causing a flare of IBD by releasing cytokines. The role of infections in the development and during the course of IBD is summarized in Table 20.4.

### *Mycobacterium avium* subspecies *paratuberculosis* (MAP)

*M. paratuberculosis* (MAP), a subspecies of *M. Avium*, is known to cause Johne's disease, a granulomatous enterocolitis that resembles Crohn's disease, in sheep and cattle and has been widely studied for its possible role in the development of IBD, particularly CD, though there is some data for UC. DNA from that organism has been detected in blood of 50 % (14/28) of patients with Crohn's disease, 22 % (2/9) with ulcerative colitis, and none (0/15) in individuals without inflammatory bowel disease [171]. Fecal samples have also detected MAP DNA in UC patients [172]. Although the hypothesis involving mycobacteria in the pathogenesis of IBD is intriguing, the theory has not been proven, and antimycobacterial therapy cannot be recommended in the management of affected patients [53].

### *Listeria monocytogenes*

Early reports suggested that *Listeria monocytogenes* may have the potential to cause IBD [173, 174]. Recently, this theory has lost strength when studies utilizing tissue culture and PCR have not found the bacteria in biopsy specimens from IBD patients [175].

### Enteric *Salmonella* or *Campylobacter* Infection

Following infectious gastroenteritis, in a population-based cohort of 43,013 subjects, the risk of IBD increased 2.4 times over a 3.5-year follow-up with the greatest risk during the first year. The estimated incidence rate of IBD was 68.4 per 100,000 person-years after an episode of gastroenteritis and 29.7 per 100,000 person-years in the control cohort [176]. In a Danish population-based cohort, comparing patients with *Salmonella* or *Campylobacter* exposure to unexposed controls found an HR of 2.9 for developing IBD during a 7.5-year follow-up [177]. However, a large population-based study including 6.9 million people had examined temporal risk patterns following a positive or negative test and concluded that the increased occurrence of IBD following detection of these enteric organisms was likely from detection bias and not causality [178].

### Helicobacter pylori

*H. pylori* is acquired early in life and has a negative association with CD [179] and UC. This suggests a possible protective effect from developing IBD perhaps through an *H. pylori*-mediated alternation in T-cell gene expression [180]. In a cohort of 1,061 patients with IBD and 64,451 controls, *H. pylori* was inversely associated with CD (0.48, CI 0.27–0.79) and UC (0.59, CI 0.39–0.84) compared to controls [181]. Another study found that the adjusted OR for UC was 0.59 (95 % CI 0.39–0.84) and *H. pylori*-negative gastritis was positively associated with UC 2.25 (95 % CI 1.31–3.60) [181].

### Mumps/Measles Infection or Mumps/Measles Vaccination

In the 1950s, an association between exposure to mumps or measles and the development with IBD was described, but the data supporting this relationship is controversial. A chronic granulomatous vasculitis of the mesenteric endothelium has been postulated as the mechanism to explain the onset of IBD [182].

Several studies have found an association between early infection and development of IBD. Data from the Mayo Clinic suggested that there was a trend towards IBD in a retrospective, survey-based study that included 1,164 subjects with measles prior to age 5. However, this study was limited by a 57 % rate of questionnaire completion, recall bias, and retrospective design [183]. In a British cohort study, mumps infection before age 2 years was found to be a risk for UC (odds ratio, 25.12; 95 % confidence interval, 6.35–99.36) [184]. No significant relationship between measles infection or vaccination at a young age and subsequent IBD was found in this cohort. An increased incidence of IBD following concurrent epidemics of mumps and measles has also been reported in other parts of the world [185, 186]. Other studies however have found no such relationship, including measles

vaccinations and CD, measles epidemics and development of IBD, or perinatal measles and an IBD diagnosis [187–189].

Similarly, the use of attenuated live measles vaccine was implicated as a possible cause of CD when the prevalence of the disease in a group of people who received the vaccine was two to three times higher than in the group that did not. However, the findings from population, as well as microbiologic studies, do not support the relationship between viral infections or MMR vaccinations and IBD [190–193]. Several studies showed no significant differences in the titers of serum anti-mumps IgG in IBD patients when compared to healthy controls [194–196]. Similarly, studies using amplification techniques found no evidence of mumps viral genome in intestinal mucosa or peripheral lymphocytes of patients with IBD [197–199]. In general, the available evidence does not support the theory that measles or mumps infection or vaccination leads to IBD.

### Other Infections

Childhood infections have also been postulated as a potential factor associated with the development of IBD. In a population study, patients with CD were more likely to report an increased frequency of childhood infections in general (OR 4.67, 95 % CI 2.65–8.23) and pharyngitis specifically (OR 2.14, 95 % CI 1.30–3.51) than healthy counterparts. Treatment with antibiotics for both otitis media (OR 2.07, 95 % CI 1.03–4.14) and pharyngitis (OR 2.14, 95 % CI 1.20–3.84) was also more common in the group with CD. Patients with UC also reported an excess of infections in general (odds ratio 2.37, 95 % CI 1.19–4.71), but not an excess of specific infections or treatments with antibiotics. Persons who reported an increased frequency of infections tended to have an earlier onset of CD (*P* < 0.0001) and ulcerative colitis (*P* = 0.04) [16].

Several studies have reported a higher frequency of gastroenteritis or diarrheal illness during infancy among future IBD patients [9, 24, 30, 178]. As noted earlier, recall or detection bias may affect the validity of the conclusions obtained from these studies.

An adhesive strain of *E. coli* has been implicated in the pathogenesis of UC [200]. Many other agents including *Clostridium*, *Pseudomonas*, *Mycoplasma*, *Cytomegalovirus*, herpes, and rotaviruses have been considered but not proven to have a role in IBD [201].

Reduced immunologic exposure to helminthic parasites has also been proposed as a potential factor to explain the increased incidence of CD in industrialized societies when compared to developing countries [39]. Colonization with pathogenically attenuated helminths has been used to switch the mucosal cytokine profile in patients with CD. In a small open-label trial, the administration of porcine whipworm eggs was safe and resulted in the improvement of CDAI scores for both CD and UC [202].

In summary, although the bulk of the evidence does not suggest that IBD is an infectious or a self-antigen-specific autoimmune disease, recent findings suggest that mucosal damage might be initiated and driven by common, ubiquitous microbial agents derived from the normal bacterial flora in the intestinal lumen [203].

## Appendectomy/Appendicitis

Appendectomy has been consistently found to be protective against the development of UC [29, 179, 204–207]. A meta-analysis of 17 case-control studies including more than 3,600 cases and over 4,600 controls showed that appendectomy was associated with a 69 % reduction in the subsequent risk of UC [53, 208]. The results of cohort studies have been less consistent, with two large series producing conflicting results. A Swedish inpatient registry of 212,963 patients with more than 5 million person-years of follow-up showed that patients who underwent appendectomy for appendicitis and mesenteric lymphadenitis had a 25 % reduction of the risk of developing UC. The protective effect was only seen if the appendectomy was performed before the age of 20 years. Appendectomy for noninflammatory conditions such as non-specific abdominal pain did not appear to confer protection against UC [209]. In another large cohort from Denmark, 154,000 patients who had undergone appendectomy were followed for over 1 million person-years. Although the cohort was found to be 13 % less likely to be diagnosed with UC than previously documented national averages, the difference was not statistically significant [209]. Despite these somewhat conflicting results, most evidence from case-control and cohort studies suggest that appendectomy is a protective factor against UC [53].

The influence of appendicitis and appendectomy on UC is not limited to the onset of the disease. Appendectomy also appears to influence the clinical course of UC. When compared to patients with UC and an intact appendix, patients who have undergone appendectomy and develop UC are diagnosed at an older age [210, 211], develop less recurrent symptoms [210], require colectomy less frequently [206, 212], and require less immunosuppressive therapy to control the disease [206]. The effect of appendectomy on the clinical course of patients with known UC is limited to case reports and small case series and results are conflicting [53].

The mechanism by which appendectomy protects against UC is unknown. The appendix is part of the mucosa-associated lymphoid tissue system and is involved in B-lymphocyte-mediated immune responses and extrathymic T lymphocytes. A T-cell receptor alpha chain knockout mouse model of colitis showed that inflammation was suppressed in animals that underwent appendectomies [213]. Because of its role as a reservoir for enteric bacteria, removal of the appendix may influence the mucosal immune system and the antigenic exposure in the bowel lumen [201].

## Summary

The role of certain environmental and lifestyle factors on the onset, severity, and course of IBD is significant. Patient education and, when possible, modifications of these risk factors should be an integral part of the care provided to patients with IBD. Smoking is the best studied of the disease modifiers in IBD, and smoking cessation should be encouraged for all IBD patients. Although achieving long-term smoking cessation is difficult, IBD patients, including those with UC, should be encouraged to quit smoking. The benefits of smoking cessation outweigh the risk of aggravating UC, and providers caring for these patients should be prepared to adjust the medical regimen to mitigate the adverse effects of nicotine discontinuation. While appendectomy appears to be protective against UC, the chronic use of both traditional NSAIDs and selective COX-2 inhibitors appears to exert a negative effect on the onset and course of IBD. Breastfeeding may offer some protection from IBD and given its other beneficial attributes should be encouraged. The influence of other factors such as diet, childhood infections, socioeconomic factors, psychological stress, and oral contraceptives is less clear, and specific recommendations cannot be generalized at this time for our patients.

## References

1. Bernstein CN. New insights into IBD epidemiology: are there any lessons for treatment? Dig Dis. 2010;28:406–10.
2. Zheng JJ, Zhu XS, Huangfu Z, Gao ZX, Guo ZR, Wang Z. Crohn's disease in mainland China: a systematic analysis of 50 years of research. Chin J Dig Dis. 2005;6:175–81.
3. Desai HG, Gupte PA. Increasing incidence of Crohn's disease in India: is it related to improved sanitation? Indian J Gastroenterol. 2005;24:23–4.
4. Pinsk V, Lemberg DA, Grewal K, Barker CC, Schreiber RA, Jacobson K. Inflammatory bowel disease in the South Asian pediatric population of British Columbia. Am J Gastroenterol. 2007;102:1077–83.
5. Ekbom A. The epidemiology of IBD: a lot of data but little knowledge. How shall we proceed? Inflamm Bowel Dis. 2004;10 Suppl 1:S32–4.
6. Acheson ED, Nefzger MD. Ulcerative colitis in the United States Army in 1944. Epidemiology: comparisons between patients and controls. Gastroenterology. 1963;44:7–19.
7. Sonnenberg A. Disability from inflammatory bowel disease among employees in West Germany. Gut. 1989;30:367–70.
8. Ekbom A, Adami HO, Helmick CG, Jonzon A, Zack MM. Perinatal risk factors for inflammatory bowel disease: a case-control study. Am J Epidemiol. 1990;132:1111–9.

9. Whorwell PJ, Holdstock G, Whorwell GM, Wright R. Bottle feeding, early gastroenteritis, and inflammatory bowel disease. Br Med J. 1979;1:382.

10. Strachan DP. Hay fever, hygiene, and household size. BMJ. 1989;299:1259–60.

11. Okada H, Kuhn C, Feillet H, Bach JF. The 'hygiene hypothesis' for autoimmune and allergic diseases: an update. Clin Exp Immunol. 2010;160:1–9.

12. Lashner BA, Loftus Jr EV. True or false? The hygiene hypothesis for Crohn's disease. Am J Gastroenterol. 2006;101:1003–4.

13. Amre DK, Lambrette P, Law L, et al. Investigating the hygiene hypothesis as a risk factor in pediatric onset Crohn's disease: a case-control study. Am J Gastroenterol. 2006;101:1005–11.

14. Bernstein CN, Rawsthorne P, Cheang M, Blanchard JF. A population-based case control study of potential risk factors for IBD. Am J Gastroenterol. 2006;101:993–1002.

15. Klement E, Lysy J, Hoshen M, Avitan M, Goldin E, Israeli E. Childhood hygiene is associated with the risk for inflammatory bowel disease: a population-based study. Am J Gastroenterol. 2008;103:1775–82.

16. Wurzelmann JI, Lyles CM, Sandler RS. Childhood infections and the risk of inflammatory bowel disease. Dig Dis Sci. 1994;39:555–60.

17. Bernstein CN, Blanchard JF, Rawsthorne P, Wajda A. Epidemiology of Crohn's disease and ulcerative colitis in a central Canadian province: a population-based study. Am J Epidemiol. 1999;149:916–24.

18. Malekzadeh F, Alberti C, Nouraei M, et al. Crohn's disease and early exposure to domestic refrigeration. PLoS One. 2009;4:e4288.

19. Radon K, Windstetter D, Poluda AL, Mueller B, von Mutius E, Koletzko S. Contact with farm animals in early life and juvenile inflammatory bowel disease: a case-control study. Pediatrics. 2007;120:354–61.

20. Sullivan SN. Hypothesis revisited: toothpaste and the cause of Crohn's disease. Lancet. 1990;336:1096–7.

21. Russel MG, Engels LG, Muris JW, et al. Modern life' in the epidemiology of inflammatory bowel disease: a case-control study with special emphasis on nutritional factors. Eur J Gastroenterol Hepatol. 1998;10:243–9.

22. Ekbom A, Montgomery SM. Environmental risk factors (excluding tobacco and microorganisms): critical analysis of old and new hypotheses. Best Pract Res Clin Gastroenterol. 2004;18:497–508.

23. Bergstrand O, Hellers G. Breast-feeding during infancy in patients who later develop Crohn's disease. Scand J Gastroenterol. 1983;18:903–6.

24. Koletzko S, Sherman P, Corey M, Griffiths A, Smith C. Role of infant feeding practices in development of Crohn's disease in childhood. BMJ. 1989;298:1617–8.

25. Rigas A, Rigas B, Glassman M, et al. Breast-feeding and maternal smoking in the etiology of Crohn's disease and ulcerative colitis in childhood. Ann Epidemiol. 1993;3:387–92.

26. Gruber M, Marshall JR, Zielezny M, Lance P. A case-control study to examine the influence of maternal perinatal behaviors on the incidence of Crohn's disease. Gastroenterol Nurs. 1996;19:53–9.

27. Thompson NP, Montgomery SM, Wadsworth ME, Pounder RE, Wakefield AJ. Early determinants of inflammatory bowel disease: use of two national longitudinal birth cohorts. Eur J Gastroenterol Hepatol. 2000;12:25–30.

28. Gearry RB, Richardson AK, Frampton CM, Dodgshun AJ, Barclay ML. Population-based cases control study of inflammatory bowel disease risk factors. J Gastroenterol Hepatol. 2010;25:325–33.

29. Gilat T, Hacohen D, Lilos P, Langman MJ. Childhood factors in ulcerative colitis and Crohn's disease. An international cooperative study. Scand J Gastroenterol. 1987;22:1009–24.

30. Koletzko S, Griffiths A, Corey M, Smith C, Sherman P. Infant feeding practices and ulcerative colitis in childhood. BMJ. 1991;302:1580–1.

31. Thompson NP, Pounder RE, Wakefield AJ. Perinatal and childhood risk factors for inflammatory bowel disease: a case-control study. Eur J Gastroenterol Hepatol. 1995;7:385–90.

32. Barclay AR, Russell RK, Wilson ML, Gilmour WH, Satsangi J, Wilson DC. Systematic review: the role of breastfeeding in the development of pediatric inflammatory bowel disease. J Pediatr. 2009;155:421–6.

33. Demling L. Is Crohn's disease caused by antibiotics? Hepatogastroenterology. 1994;41:549–51.

34. De Vroey B, De Cassan C, Gower-Rousseau C, Colombel JF. Editorial: antibiotics earlier, IBD later? Am J Gastroenterol. 2010;105:2693–6.

35. Hildebrand H, Malmborg P, Askling J, Ekbom A, Montgomery SM. Early-life exposures associated with antibiotic use and risk of subsequent Crohn's disease. Scand J Gastroenterol. 2008;43:961–6.

36. Shaw SY, Blanchard JF, Bernstein CN. Association between the use of antibiotics in the first year of life and pediatric inflammatory bowel disease. Am J Gastroenterol. 2010;105:2687–92.

37. Hviid A, Svanstrom H, Frisch M. Antibiotic use and inflammatory bowel diseases in childhood. Gut. 2011;60:49–54.

38. Rosh JR. Does "Bug Juice" give kids IBD? Inflamm Bowel Dis. 2011;17:1822–3.

39. Shanahan F. Inflammatory bowel disease: immunodiagnostics, immunotherapeutics, and ecotherapeutics. Gastroenterology. 2001;120:622–35.

40. Gibson GR, Roberfroid MB. Dietary modulation of the human colonic microbiota: introducing the concept of prebiotics. J Nutr. 1995;125:1401–12.

41. Bengmark S. Colonic food: pre- and probiotics. Am J Gastroenterol. 2000;95:S5–7.

42. Hedin C, Whelan K, Lindsay JO. Evidence for the use of probiotics and prebiotics in inflammatory bowel disease: a review of clinical trials. Proc Nutr Soc. 2007;66:307–15.

43. Kruis W, Schulz T, Fric P, et al. Double blind comparison of an oral *Eschericia coli* preparation and mesalazine in maintaining remission of ulcerative colitis. Aliment Pharmacol Ther. 1997;11:853–8.

44. Rembacken BJ, Snelling AM, Hawkey PM, et al. Non-pathogenic *Escherichia coli* versus mesalazine for the treatment of ulcerative colitis: a randomized trial. Lancet. 1999;354:635–9.

45. Gionchetti P, Rizzello F, Venturi A, Campieri M. Probiotics in infective diarrhoea and inflammatory bowel diseases. J Gastroenterol Hepatol. 2000;15:489–93.

46. Mimura T, Rizzello F, Helwig U, et al. Once daily high dose probiotic therapy (VSL#3) for maintaining remission in recurrent or refractory pouchitis. Gut. 2004;53:108–14.

47. Gionchetti P, Rizzello F, Helwig U, et al. Prophylaxis of pouchitis onset with probiotic therapy: a double-blind, placebo-controlled trial. Gastroenterology. 2003;124:1202–9.

48. Shen B, Brzezinski A, Fazio VW, et al. Maintenance therapy with a probiotic in antibiotic-dependent pouchitis: experience in clinical practice. Aliment Pharmacol Ther. 2005;22:721–8.

49. Rhodes JM, Cockel R, Allan RN, Hawker PC, Dawson J, Elias E. Colonic Crohn's disease and use of oral contraception. Br Med J (Clin Res Ed). 1984;288:595–6.

50. Ramcharan S, Pellegrin FA, Ray RM, Hsu JP. The Walnut Creek Contraceptive Drug Study. A prospective study of the side effects of oral contraceptives. Volume III, an interim report: a comparison of disease occurrence leading to hospitalization or death in users and nonusers of oral contraceptives. J Reprod Med. 1980;25:345–72.

51. Logan RF, Kay CR. Oral contraception, smoking and inflammatory bowel disease—findings in the Royal College of General

Practitioners Oral Contraception Study. Int J Epidemiol. 1989;18:105–7.

52. Vessey M, Jewell D, Smith A, Yeates D, McPherson K. Chronic inflammatory bowel disease, cigarette smoking, and use of oral contraceptives: findings in a large cohort study of women of child-bearing age. Br Med J (Clin Res Ed). 1986;292:1101–3.

53. Loftus Jr EV. Clinical epidemiology of inflammatory bowel disease: incidence, prevalence, and environmental influences. Gastroenterology. 2004;126:1504–17.

54. Boyko EJ, Theis MK, Vaughan TL, Nicol-Blades B. Increased risk of inflammatory bowel disease associated with oral contraceptive use. Am J Epidemiol. 1994;140:268–78.

55. Corrao G, Tragnone A, Caprilli R, et al. Risk of inflammatory bowel disease attributable to smoking, oral contraception and breastfeeding in Italy: a nationwide case-control study. Cooperative Investigators of the Italian Group for the Study of the Colon and the Rectum (GISC). Int J Epidemiol. 1998;27:397–404.

56. Lesko SM, Kaufman DW, Rosenberg L, et al. Evidence for an increased risk of Crohn's disease in oral contraceptive users. Gastroenterology. 1985;89:1046–9.

57. Katschinski B, Fingerle D, Scherbaum B, Goebell H. Oral contraceptive use and cigarette smoking in Crohn's disease. Dig Dis Sci. 1993;38:1596–600.

58. Godet PG, May GR, Sutherland LR. Meta-analysis of the role of oral contraceptive agents in inflammatory bowel disease. Gut. 1995;37:668–73.

59. Cornish JA, Tan E, Simillis C, Clark SK, Teare J, Tekkis PP. The risk of oral contraceptives in the etiology of inflammatory bowel disease: a meta-analysis. Am J Gastroenterol. 2008;103:2394–400.

60. Wakefield AJ, Sawyerr AM, Hudson M, Dhillon AP, Pounder RE. Smoking, the oral contraceptive pill, and Crohn's disease. Dig Dis Sci. 1991;36:1147–50.

61. Somasundaram S, Sigthorsson G, Simpson RJ, et al. Uncoupling of intestinal mitochondrial oxidative phosphorylation and inhibition of cyclooxygenase are required for the development of NSAID-enteropathy in the rat. Aliment Pharmacol Ther. 2000; 14:639–50.

62. Tanner AR, Raghunath AS. Colonic inflammation and nonsteroidal anti-inflammatory drug administration. An assessment of the frequency of the problem. Digestion. 1988;41:116–20.

63. Evans JM, McMahon AD, Murray FE, McDevitt DG, MacDonald TM. Non-steroidal anti-inflammatory drugs are associated with emergency admission to hospital for colitis due to inflammatory bowel disease. Gut. 1997;40:619–22.

64. Bonner GF, Walczak M, Kitchen L, Bayona M. Tolerance of non-steroidal antiinflammatory drugs in patients with inflammatory bowel disease. Am J Gastroenterol. 2000;95:1946–8.

65. Gibson GR, Whitacre EB, Ricotti CA. Colitis induced by nonsteroidal anti-inflammatory drugs. Report of four cases and review of the literature. Arch Intern Med. 1992;152:625–32.

66. Felder JB, Korelitz BI, Rajapakse R, Schwarz S, Horatagis AP, Gleim G. Effects of nonsteroidal antiinflammatory drugs on inflammatory bowel disease: a case-control study. Am J Gastroenterol. 2000;95:1949–54.

67. Sandborn WJ, Stenson WF, Brynskov J, et al. Safety of celecoxib in patients with ulcerative colitis in remission: a randomized, placebo-controlled, pilot study. Clin Gastroenterol Hepatol. 2006;4:203–11.

68. Gleeson MH, Davis AJ. Non-steroidal anti-inflammatory drugs, aspirin and newly diagnosed colitis: a case-control study. Aliment Pharmacol Ther. 2003;17:817–25.

69. Wolfe MM, Lichtenstein DR, Singh G. Gastrointestinal toxicity of nonsteroidal antiinflamatory drugs. N Engl J Med. 1999; 340:1888–99.

70. Katsinelos P, Christodoulou K, Pilpilidis I, et al. Colopathy associated with the systemic use of nonsteroidal antiinflammatory medications. An underestimated entity. Hepatogastroenterology. 2002;49:345–8.

71. Oren R, Ligumsky M. Indomethacin-induced colonic ulceration and bleeding. Ann Pharmacother. 1994;28:883–5.

72. Wallace JL. Nonsteroidal anti-inflammatory drugs and gastroenteropathy: the second hundred years. Gastroenterology. 1997;112:1000–16.

73. Hendel J, Nielsen OH. Expression of cyclooxygenase-2 mRNA in active inflammatory bowel disease. Am J Gastroenterol. 1997; 92:1170–3.

74. Mahmud T, Scott DL, Bjarnason I. A unifying hypothesis for the mechanism of NSAID related gastrointestinal toxicity. Ann Rheum Dis. 1996;55:211–3.

75. Bonner GF. Exacerbation of inflammatory bowel disease associated with use of celecoxib. Am J Gastroenterol. 2001;96:1306–8.

76. Goh J, Wight D, Parkes M, Middleton SJ, Hunter JO. Rofecoxib and cytomegalovirus in acute flare-up of ulcerative colitis: coprecipitants or coincidence? Am J Gastroenterol. 2002;97:1061–2.

77. Gornet JM, Hassani Z, Modiglian R, Lemann M. Exacerbation of Crohn's colitis with severe colonic hemorrhage in a patient on rofecoxib. Am J Gastroenterol. 2002;97:3209–10.

78. Matuk R, Crawford J, Abreu M, Targan S, Vasiliauskas E, Papadakis K. The spectrum of gastrointestinal toxicity and effect on disease activity of selective COX-2 inhibitors in patients with inflammatory bowel disease. Inflamm Bowel Dis. 2004; 10:352–6.

79. Oviedo J, Farraye FA. Self-care for the inflammatory bowel disease patient: what can the professional recommend? Semin Gastrointest Dis. 2001;12:223–36.

80. Singh S, Graff LA, Bernstein CN. Do NSAIDs, antibiotics, infections, or stress trigger flares in IBD? Am J Gastroenterol. 2009; 104:1298–313. quiz 314.

81. Harries AD, Baird A, Rhodes J. Non-smoking: a feature of ulcerative colitis. Br Med J. 1982;284:706.

82. Somerville KW, Logan RF, Edmond M, Langman MJ. Smoking and Crohn's disease. Br Med J (Clin Res Ed). 1984;289:954–6.

83. Logan RF, Edmond M, Somerville KW, Langman MJ. Smoking and ulcerative colitis. Br Med J (Clin Res Ed). 1984;288:751–3.

84. Sutherland LR, Ramcharan S, Bryant H, Fick G. Effect of cigarette smoking on recurrence of Crohn's disease. Gastroenterology. 1990;98:1123–8.

85. Penny WJ, Penny E, Mayberry JF, et al. Mormons, smoking and ulcerative colitis. Lancet. 1983;1315.

86. Penny WJ, Penny E, Mayberry JF, et al. Prevalence of inflammatory bowel disease amongst mormons in Britain and Ireland. Soc Sci Med. 1985;21:287–90.

87. Calkins BM. A meta-analysis of the role of smoking in inflammatory bowel disease. Dig Dis Sci. 1989;34:1841–54.

88. Gareth AO, Thomas BS, Rhodes J, Green JT. Inflammatory bowel disease and smoking—a review. Am J Gastroenterol. 1998;93: 144–9.

89. Reif S, Lavy A, Keter D, et al. Lack of association between smoking and Crohn's disease but the usual association with ulcerative colitis in Jewish patients in Israel: a multicenter study. Am J Gastroenterol. 2000;95:474–8.

90. Mahid SS, Minor KS, Soto RE, Hornung CA, Galandiuk S. Smoking and inflammatory bowel disease: a meta-analysis. Mayo Clin Proc. 2006;81:1462–71.

91. Motley RJ, Rhodes J, Ford GA, et al. Time relationship between cessation of smoking and onset of ulcerative colitis. Digestion. 1987;37:125–7.

92. Boyko EJ, Koepsell TD, Perera DR, et al. Risk of ulcerative colitis among former and current cigarette smokers. N Engl J Med. 1987;316:707–10.

93. Lindberg E, Tysk C, Anderson K, et al. Smoking and inflammatory bowel disease. A case-control study. Gut. 1988;29:352–7.

94. Loftus Jr EV, Sandborn WJ, Tremaine WJ, et al. Primary sclerosing cholangitis is associated with nonsmoking: a case-control study. Gastroenterology. 1996;110:1496–502.

95. van Erpecum KJ, Smits SJ, van de Meeberg PC, et al. Risk of primary sclerosing cholangitis is associated with nonsmoking behavior. Gastroenterology. 1996;110:1503–6.

96. Mitchell SA, Thyssen M, Orchard TR, Jewell DP, Fleming KA, Chapman RW. Cigarette smoking, appendectomy, and tonsillectomy as risk factors for the development of primary sclerosing cholangitis: a case control study. Gut. 2002;51:567–73.

97. Merrett MN, Mortensen N, Kettlewell M, Jewell DO. Smoking may prevent pouchitis in patients with restorative proctocolectomy for ulcerative colitis. Gut. 1996;38:362–4.

98. Russel MG, Nieman FH, Bergers JM, Stockbrugger RW. Cigarette smoking and quality of life in patients with inflammatory bowel disease. South Limburg IBD Study Group. Eur J Gastroenterol Hepatol. 1996;8:1075–81.

99. Boyko EJ, Perera DR, Koepsell TD, et al. Effects of cigarette smoking on the clinical course of ulcerative colitis. Scand J Gastroenterol. 1988;23:1147–52.

100. Fraga XF, Vergara M, Medina C, Casellas F, Bermejo B, Malagelada JR. Effects of smoking on the presentation and clinical course of inflammatory bowel disease. Eur J Gastroenterol Hepatol. 1997;9:683–7.

101. Beaugerie L, Massot N, Carbonnel F, et al. Impact of cessation of smoking on the course of ulcerative colitis. Am J Gastroenterol. 2001;96:2113–6.

102. Lashner BA, Shaheen NJ, Hanauer SB, et al. Passive smoking is associated with an increased risk of developing inflammatory bowel disease in children. Am J Gastroenterol. 1993;88:356–9.

103. Sandler RS, Sandler DP, McDonnell CW, Wurzelmann JI. Childhood exposure to environmental tobacco smoke and the risk of ulcerative colitis. Am J Epidemiol. 1992;135:603–8.

104. Jones DT, Osterman MT, Bewtra M, Lewis JD. Passive smoking and inflammatory bowel disease: a meta-analysis. Am J Gastroenterol. 2008;103:2382–93.

105. van der Heide F, Dijkstra A, Weersma RK, et al. Effects of active and passive smoking on disease course of Crohn's disease and ulcerative colitis. Inflamm Bowel Dis. 2009;15:1199–207.

106. Cosnes J. Tobacco and IBD: relevance in the understanding of disease mechanisms and clinical practice. Best Pract Res Clin Gastroenterol. 2004;18:481–96.

107. Motley RJ, Rhodes J, Williams G, et al. Smoking, eicosanoids and ulcerative colitis. J Pharm Pharmacol. 1990;42:288–9.

108. Madretsma S, Wolters LM, van Dijk JP, et al. In-vivo effect of nicotine on cytokine production by human non-adherent mononuclear cells. Eur J Gastroenterol Hepatol. 1996;8:1017–20.

109. Gent AE, Hellier MD, Grace RH, Swarbrick ET, Coggon D. Inflammatory bowel disease and domestic hygiene in infancy. Lancet. 1994;343:766–7.

110. Euler DE, Dave SJ, Guo H. Effect of cigarette smoking on pentane excretion in alveolar breath. Clin Chem. 1996;42:303–8.

111. Hatoum OA, Binion DG, Otterson MF, Gutterman DD. Acquired microvascular dysfunction in inflammatory bowel disease: loss of nitric oxide-mediated vasodilation. Gastroenterology. 2003;125:58–69.

112. Probert CS, Jayanthi V, Pinder D, Wicks AC, Mayberry JF. Epidemiological study of ulcerative proctocolitis in Indian migrants and the indigenous population of Leicestershire. Gut. 1992;33:687–93.

113. Shoda R, Matsueda K, Yamato S, Umeda N. Epidemiologic analysis of Crohn disease in Japan: increased dietary intake of n-6 polyunsaturated fatty acids and animal protein relates to the increased incidence of Crohn disease in Japan. Am J Clin Nutr. 1996;63:741–5.

114. Yang SK, Hong WS, Min YI, et al. Incidence and prevalence of ulcerative colitis in the Songpa-Kangdong District, Seoul, Korea, 1986-1997. J Gastroenterol Hepatol. 2000;15:1037–42.

115. Persson PG, Ahlbom A, Hellers G. Crohn's disease and ulcerative colitis. A review of dietary studies with emphasis on methodologic aspects. Scand J Gastroenterol. 1987;22:385–9.

116. Jarnerot G, Jarnmark I, Nilsson K. Consumption of refined sugar by patients with Crohn's disease, ulcerative colitis, or irritable bowel syndrome. Scand J Gastroenterol. 1983;18:999–1002.

117. Mayberry JF, Rhodes J, Allan R, et al. Diet in Crohn's disease two studies of current and previous habits in newly diagnosed patients. Dig Dis Sci. 1981;26:444–8.

118. Tragnone A, Valpiani D, Miglio F, et al. Dietary habits as risk factors for inflammatory bowel disease. Eur J Gastroenterol Hepatol. 1995;7:47–51.

119. Reif S, Klein I, Lubin F, Farbstein M, Hallak A, Gilat T. Pre-illness dietary factors in inflammatory bowel disease. Gut. 1997;40:754–60.

120. Brauer PM, Gee MI, Grace M, Thomson AB. Diet of women with Crohn's and other gastrointestinal diseases. J Am Diet Assoc. 1983;82:659–64.

121. Andersen V, Olsen A, Carbonnel F, Tjonneland A, Vogel U. Diet and risk of inflammatory bowel disease. Dig Liver Dis. 2012;44:185–94.

122. Katschinski B, Logan RF, Edmond M, Langman MJ. Smoking and sugar intake are separate but interactive risk factors in Crohn's disease. Gut. 1988;29:1202–6.

123. Thornton JR, Emmett PM, Heaton KW. Smoking, sugar, and inflammatory bowel disease. Br Med J (Clin Res Ed). 1985; 290:1786–7.

124. Geerling BJ, Dagnelie PC, Badart-Smook A, Russel MG, Stockbrugger RW, Brummer RJ. Diet as a risk factor for the development of ulcerative colitis. Am J Gastroenterol. 2000;95: 1008–13.

125. Jowett SL, Seal CJ, Pearce MS, et al. Influence of dietary factors on the clinical course of ulcerative colitis: a prospective cohort study. Gut. 2004;53:1479–84.

126. Persson PG, Ahlbom A, Hellers G. Diet and inflammatory bowel disease: a case-control study. Epidemiology. 1992;3:47–52.

127. Sonnenberg A. Geographic and temporal variations of sugar and margarine consumption in relation to Crohn's disease. Digestion. 1988;41:161–71.

128. Millar D, Ford J, Sanderson J, et al. IS900 PCR to detect Mycobacterium paratuberculosis in retail supplies of whole pasteurized cows' milk in England and Wales. Appl Environ Microbiol. 1996;62:3446–52.

129. Main J, McKenzie H, Yeaman GR, et al. Antibody to Saccharomyces cerevisiae (bakers' yeast) in Crohn's disease. BMJ. 1988;297:1105–6.

130. Barclay GR, McKenzie H, Pennington J, Parratt D, Pennington CR. The effect of dietary yeast on the activity of stable chronic Crohn's disease. Scand J Gastroenterol. 1992;27:196–200.

131. Boyko EJ, Perera DR, Koepsell TD, Keane EM, Inui TS. Coffee and alcohol use and the risk of ulcerative colitis. Am J Gastroenterol. 1989;84:530–4.

132. Hendriksen C, Binder V. Social prognosis in patients with ulcerative colitis. Br Med J. 1980;281:581–3.

133. James AH. Breakfast and Crohn's disease. Br Med J. 1977; 1:943–5.

134. Mayberry JF, Rhodes J, Newcombe RG. Breakfast and dietary aspects of Crohn's disease. Br Med J. 1978;2:1401.

135. Ukil A, Maity S, Karmakar S, Datta N, Vedasiromoni JR, Das PK. Curcumin, the major component of food flavour turmeric, reduces mucosal injury in trinitrobenzene sulphonic acid-induced colitis. Br J Pharmacol. 2003;139:209–18.

136. Suchner U, Kuhn KS, Furst P. The scientific basis of immunonutrition. Proc Nutr Soc. 2000;59:553–63.

137. Van Den Bogaerde J, Cahill J, Emmanuel AV, et al. Gut mucosal response to food antigens in Crohn's disease. Aliment Pharmacol Ther. 2002;16:1903–15.

138. Lomer MC, Thompson RP, Powell JJ. Fine and ultrafine particles of the diet: influence on the mucosal immune response and association with Crohn's disease. Proc Nutr Soc. 2002;61:123–30.

139. Lomer MC, Harvey RS, Evans SM, Thompson RP, Powell JJ. Efficacy and tolerability of a low microparticle diet in a double blind, randomized, pilot study in Crohn's disease. Eur J Gastroenterol Hepatol. 2001;13:101–6.

140. Narula N, Fedorak RN. Exercise and inflammatory bowel disease. Can J Gastroenterol. 2008;22:497–504.

141. Sonnenberg A. Occupational distribution of inflammatory bowel disease among German employees. Gut. 1990;31:1037–40.

142. Persson PG, Leijonmarck CE, Bernell O, Hellers G, Ahlbom A. Risk indicators for inflammatory bowel disease. Int J Epidemiol. 1993;22:268–72.

143. Klein I, Reif S, Farbstein H, Halak A, Gilat T. Preillness non dietary factors and habits in inflammatory bowel disease. Ital J Gastroenterol Hepatol. 1998;30:247–51.

144. Elsenbruch S, Langhorst J, Popkirowa K, et al. Effects of mind-body therapy on quality of life and neuroendocrine and cellular immune functions in patients with ulcerative colitis. Psychother Psychosom. 2005;74:277–87.

145. Oktedalen O, Lunde OC, Opstad PK, et al. Changes in the gastrointestinal mucosa after long-distance running. Scand J Gastroenterol. 1992;27:270–4.

146. Peters HP, Bos M, Seebregts L, et al. Gastrointestinal symptoms in long-distance runners, cyclists and triathletes: prevalence, medication, and etiology. Am J Gastroenterol. 1999;94:1570–81.

147. Peters HP, Zweers M, Backx FJ, et al. Gastrointestinal symptoms during long-distance walking. Med Sci Sports Exerc. 1999;31:767–73.

148. Lucas W, Schroy PC. Reversible ischemic colitis in a high endurance athlete. Am J Gastroenterol. 1998;93:2231–4.

149. Oliveria SA, Christos PJ. The epidemiology of physical activity and cancer. Ann N Y Acad Sci. 1997;833:79–90.

150. Peters HP, De Vries WR, Vanberge-Henegouwen GP, Akkermans LM. Potential benefits and hazards of physical activity and exercise on the gastrointestinal tract. Gut. 2001;48:435–9.

151. Robinson RJ, al-Azzawi F, Iqbal SJ, et al. Osteoporosis and determinants of bone density in patients with Crohn's disease. Dig Dis Sci. 1998;43:2500–6.

152. Robinson RJ, Krzywicki T, Almond L, et al. Effect of a low-impact exercise program on bone mineral density in Crohn's disease: a randomized controlled trial. Gastroenterology. 1998;115:36–41.

153. Loudon CP, Corroll V, Butcher J, Rawsthorne P, Bernstein CN. The effects of physical exercise on patients with Crohn's disease. Am J Gastroenterol. 1999;94:697–703.

154. Drossman DA, Leserman J, Mitchell M, et al. Health status and healthcare use in persons with inflammatory bowel disease. A national sample. Dig Dis Sci. 1991;36:1746–55.

155. Porcelli P, Zaka S, Centonze S, Sisto G. Psychological distress and levels of disease activity in inflammatory bowel disease. Ital J Gastroenterol. 1994;26:111–5.

156. Porcelli P, Leoci C, Guerra V. A prospective study of the relationship between disease activity and psychologic distress in patients with inflammatory bowel disease. Scand J Gastroenterol. 1996;31:792–6.

157. North CS, Alpers DH, Helzer JE, et al. Do life events or depression exacerbate inflammatory bowel disease? A prospective study. Ann Intern Med. 1991;114:381–6.

158. Sewitch MJ, Abrahamowicz M, Bitton A, et al. Psychological distress, social support, and disease activity in patients with inflammatory bowel disease. Am J Gastroenterol. 2001;96:1470–9.

159. Rampton DS. The influence of stress on the development and severity of immune-mediated diseases. J Rheumatol Suppl. 2011;88:43–7.

160. Bernstein CN, Singh S, Graff LA, Walker JR, Miller N, Cheang M. A prospective population-based study of triggers of symptomatic flares in IBD. Am J Gastroenterol. 2010;105:1994–2002.

161. Hanauer SB, Sandborn WJ, et al. Management of Crohn's disease in adults. Am J Gastroenterol. 2001;96:635–43.

162. Addolorato G, Capristo E, Stefanini GF, Gasbarrini G. Inflammatory bowel disease: a study of the association between anxiety and depression, physical morbidity, and nutritional status. Scand J Gastroenterol. 1997;32:1013–21.

163. Kovacs Z, Kovacs F. Depressive and anxiety symptoms, dysfunctional attitudes and social aspects in irritable bowel syndrome and inflammatory bowel disease. Int J Psychiatry Med. 2007;37:245–55.

164. Kurina LM, Goldacre MJ, Yeates D, Gill LE. Depression and anxiety in people with inflammatory bowel disease. J Epidemiol Community Health. 2001;55:716–20.

165. Levenstein S, Prantera C, Varvo V, et al. Stress and exacerbation in ulcerative colitis: a prospective study of patients enrolled in remission. Am J Gastroenterol. 2000;95:1213–20.

166. Duffy LC, Zielezny MA, Marshall JR, et al. Relevance of major stress events as an indicator of disease activity prevalence in inflammatory bowel disease. Behav Med. 1991;17:101–10.

167. Bitton A, Sewitch MJ, Peppercorn MA, et al. Psychosocial determinants of relapse in ulcerative colitis: a longitudinal study. Am J Gastroenterol. 2003;98:2203–8.

168. Li J, Norgard B, Precht DH, Olsen J. Psychological stress and inflammatory bowel disease: a follow-up study in parents who lost a child in Denmark. Am J Gastroenterol. 2004;99:1129–33.

169. Goodhand JR, Greig FI, Koodun Y, et al. Do antidepressants influence the disease course in inflammatory bowel disease? A retrospective case-matched observational study. Inflamm Bowel Dis. 2012;18:1232–9.

170. Moser G, Drossman DA. Managing patients' concerns. In: Bayless TM, Hanauer SB, editors. Advanced therapy of inflammatory bowel disease. London: BC Decker Inc; 2001. p. 527–9.

171. Naser SA, Ghobrial G, Romero C, Valentine JF. Culture of Mycobacterium avium subspecies paratuberculosis from the blood of patients with Crohn's disease. Lancet. 2004;364:1039–44.

172. Tuci A, Tonon F, Castellani L, et al. Fecal detection of Mycobacterium avium paratuberculosis using the IS900 DNA sequence in Crohn's disease and ulcerative colitis patients and healthy subjects. Dig Dis Sci. 2011;56:2957–62.

173. Van Kruiningen HJ, Colombel JF, Cartun RW, et al. An in-depth study of Crohn's disease in two French families. Gastroenterology. 1993;104:351–60.

174. Liu Y, van Kruiningen HJ, West AB, Cartun RW, Cortot A, Colombel JF. Immunocytochemical evidence of Listeria, Escherichia coli, and Streptococcus antigens in Crohn's disease. Gastroenterology. 1995;108:1396–404.

175. Swidsinski A, Ladhoff A, Pernthaler A, et al. Mucosal flora in inflammatory bowel disease. Gastroenterology. 2002;122:44–54.

176. Garcia Rodriguez LA, Ruigomez A, Panes J. Acute gastroenteritis is followed by an increased risk of inflammatory bowel disease. Gastroenterology. 2006;130:1588–94.

177. Gradel KO, Nielsen HL, Schonheyder HC, Ejlertsen T, Kristensen B, Nielsen H. Increased short- and long-term risk of inflammatory bowel disease after salmonella or campylobacter gastroenteritis. Gastroenterology. 2009;137:495–501.

178. Jess T, Simonsen J, Nielsen NM, et al. Enteric Salmonella or Campylobacter infections and the risk of inflammatory bowel disease. Gut. 2010;60:318–24.

179. Feeney MA, Murphy F, Clegg AJ, Trebble TM, Sharer NM, Snook JA. A case-control study of childhood environmental risk factors for the development of inflammatory bowel disease. Eur J Gastroenterol Hepatol. 2002;14:529–34.

180. Luther J, Dave M, Higgins PD, Kao JY. Association between Helicobacter pylori infection and inflammatory bowel disease: a meta-analysis and systematic review of the literature. Inflamm Bowel Dis. 2010;16:1077–84.

181. Sonnenberg A, Genta RM. Low prevalence of Helicobacter pylori infection among patients with inflammatory bowel disease. Aliment Pharmacol Ther. 2012;35:469–76.

182. Wakefield AJ, Ekbom A, Dhillon AP, Pittilo RM, Pounder RE. Crohn's disease: pathogenesis and persistent measles virus infection. Gastroenterology. 1995;108:911–6.

183. Pardi DS, Tremaine WJ, Sandborn WJ, et al. Early measles virus infection is associated with the development of inflammatory bowel disease. Am J Gastroenterol. 2000;95:1480–5.

184. Montgomery SM, Morris DL, Pounder RE, Wakefield AJ. Paramyxovirus infections in childhood and subsequent inflammatory bowel disease. Gastroenterology. 1999;116:796–803.

185. Montgomery SM, Bjornsson S, Johannsson JH, Thjodleifsson B, Pounder RE, Wakefield AJ. Concurrent measles and mumps epidemics in Iceland are a risk factor for later inflammatory bowel disease. Gut. 1998;42:A41.

186. Lavy A, Broide E, Reif S, et al. Measles is more prevalent in Crohn's disease patients. A multicentre Israeli study. Dig Liver Dis. 2001;33:472–6.

187. Nielsen LL, Nielsen NM, Melbye M, Sodermann M, Jacobsen M, Aaby P. Exposure to measles in utero and Crohn's disease: Danish register study. BMJ. 1998;316:196–7.

188. Pardi DS, Tremaine WJ, Sandborn WJ, Loftus Jr EV, Poland GA, Melton III LJ. Perinatal exposure to measles virus is not associated with the development of inflammatory bowel disease. Inflamm Bowel Dis. 1999;5:104–6.

189. Haslam N, Mayberry JF, Hawthorne AB, Newcombe RG, Holmes GK, Probert CS. Measles, month of birth, and Crohn's disease. Gut. 2000;47:801–3.

190. Anonymous. Case control study finds no link between measles vaccine and inflammatory bowel disease. Commun Dis Rep CDR Wkly 1997;7:339.

191. Feeney M, Ciegg A, Winwood P, Snook J. A case-control study of measles vaccination and inflammatory bowel disease. The East Dorset Gastroenterology Group. Lancet. 1997;350:764–6.

192. Morris DL, Montgomery SM, Thompson NP, Ebrahim S, Pounder RE, Wakefield AJ. Measles vaccination and inflammatory bowel disease: a national British Cohort Study. Am J Gastroenterol. 2000;95:3507–12.

193. Davis RL, Kramarz P, Bohlke K, et al. Measles-mumps-rubella and other measles-containing vaccines do not increase the risk for inflammatory bowel disease: a case-control study from the Vaccine Safety Datalink project. Arch Pediatr Adolesc Med. 2001;155:354–9.

194. Iizuka M, Saito H, Yukawa M, et al. No evidence of persistent mumps virus infection in inflammatory bowel disease. Gut. 2001;48:637–41.

195. Peltola H, Patja A, Leinikki P, Valle M, Davidkin I, Paunio M. No evidence for measles, mumps, and rubella vaccine-associated inflammatory bowel disease or autism in a 14-year prospective study. Lancet. 1998;351:1327–8.

196. Bernstein CN, Rawsthorne P, Blanchard JF. Population-based case-control study of measles, mumps, and rubella and inflammatory bowel disease. Inflamm Bowel Dis. 2007;13:759–62.

197. Haga Y, Funakoshi O, Kuroe K, et al. Absence of measles viral genomic sequence in intestinal tissues from Crohn's disease by nested polymerase chain reaction. Gut. 1996;38:211–5.

198. Afzal MA, Armitage E, Begley J, et al. Absence of detectable measles virus genome sequence in inflammatory bowel disease tissues and peripheral blood lymphocytes. J Med Virol. 1998;55:243–9.

199. Folwaczny C, Jager G, Schnettler D, Wiebecke B, Loeschke K. Search for mumps virus genome in intestinal biopsy specimens of patients with IBD. Gastroenterology. 1999;117:1253–5.

200. Burke DA, Axon AT. Adhesive Escherichia coli in inflammatory bowel disease and infective diarrhoea. BMJ. 1988;297:102–4.

201. Howlett M, Gibson P. Environmental influences on IBD. IBD Monitor. 2004;5:74–83.

202. Summers RW, Elliott DE, Qadir K, Urban Jr JF, Thompson R, Weinstock JV. Trichuris suis seems to be safe and possibly effective in the treatment of inflammatory bowel disease. Am J Gastroenterol. 2003;98:2034–41.

203. Merger M, Croitoru K. Infections in the immunopathogenesis of chronic inflammatory bowel disease. Semin Immunol. 1998; 10:69–78.

204. Rutgeerts P, D'Haens G, Hiele M, Geboes K, Vantrappen G. Appendectomy protects against ulcerative colitis. Gastroenterology. 1994;106:1251–3.

205. Duggan AE, Usmani I, Neal KR, Logan RF. Appendicectomy, childhood hygiene, Helicobacter pylori status, and risk of inflammatory bowel disease: a case control study. Gut. 1998; 43:494–8.

206. Radford-Smith GL, Edwards JE, Purdie DM, et al. Protective role of appendicectomy on onset and severity of ulcerative colitis and Crohn's disease. Gut. 2002;51:808–13.

207. Gardenbroek TJ, Eshuis EJ, Ponsioen CI, Ubbink DT, D'Haens GR, Bemelman WA. The effect of appendectomy on the course of ulcerative colitis: a systematic review. Colorectal Dis. 2012; 14:545–53.

208. Koutroubakis IE, Vlachonikolis IG, Kouroumalis EA. Role of appendicitis and appendectomy in the pathogenesis of ulcerative colitis: a critical review. Inflamm Bowel Dis. 2002;8:277–86.

209. Andersson RE, Olaison G, Tysk C, Ekbom A. Appendectomy and protection against ulcerative colitis. N Engl J Med. 2001; 344:808–14.

210. Naganuma M, Iizuka B, Torii A, et al. Appendectomy protects against the development of ulcerative colitis and reduces its recurrence: results of a multicenter case-controlled study in Japan. Am J Gastroenterol. 2001;96:1123–6.

211. Selby WS, Griffin S, Abraham N, Solomon MJ. Appendectomy protects against the development of ulcerative colitis but does not affect its course. Am J Gastroenterol. 2002;97:2834–8.

212. Cosnes J, Carbonnel F, Beaugerie L, Blain A, Reijasse D, Gendre JP. Effects of appendicectomy on the course of ulcerative colitis. Gut. 2002;51:803–7.

213. Mombaerts P, Mizoguchi E, Grusby MJ, Glimcher LH, Bhan AK, Tonegawa S. Spontaneous development of inflammatory bowel disease in T cell receptor mutant mice. Cell. 1993;75:274–82.

Robert Burakoff and Jonathon S. Levine

**Keywords**

Proctitis • Ulcerative colitis • 5-ASA • Suppository • Infliximab • Rectum • Sigmoidoscopy

Ulcerative proctitis (UP) is defined as disease limited to the rectum or the first 15–20 cm from the anal verge. This is to be distinguished from ulcerative proctosigmoiditis, which involves both the rectum and sigmoid colon, or left-sided ulcerative colitis, which begins in the rectum and extends as far as the splenic flexure. One distinguishing principal in ulcerative proctitis is that the rectum is intensely inflamed, whereas in left-sided ulcerative colitis, the rectum may appear relatively spared and inflammation may be concentrated in the sigmoid or descending colon. The principals of treatment for extensive ulcerative colitis and proctitis are the same with the notable difference that the limited extent of disease in ulcerative proctitis allows for more intensive use of rectally administered therapy. The natural course of ulcerative proctitis is unknown but does not appear to increase the risk for colorectal cancer [1].

## 5-ASA Therapies

5-ASA therapy remains the mainstay of treatment for ulcerative proctitis. Both oral and topical therapies are commonly employed. A meta-analysis of controlled trials indicates that topical mesalamine is superior to oral mesalamine in achieving clinical improvement in patients with mild to moderate disease [2–4].

R. Burakoff, M.D., M.P.H. (✉)
Department of Gastroenterology, Brigham and Women's Hospital, 45 Franics St., Boston, MA 02458, USA
e-mail: rburakoff@partners.org

J.S. Levine, M.D.
Gastroenterology, Harvard Medical School,
45 Franics St., Boston, MA 02458, USA
e-mail: jslevine@partners.org

5-ASA suppositories are the first-line treatment for both induction and maintenance of mild to moderate UP. Scintigraphic studies have demonstrated this formulation allows effective delivery of the drug to the rectum [5, 6]. Suppositories generally reach the upper rectum (at about 15–20 cm). Enemas are also commonly used as alternative means of topical therapy; however, they are more effective for ulcerative proctosigmoiditis and left-sided colitis as the inflamed rectum physiologically moves them to the more proximal colon, and so they concentrate proximal to the inflamed segment. Although the total dose of suppositories is lower, a 1,000 mg suppository will deliver a higher concentrated dose to the rectum than a 4 g mesalamine enema. Patients often find enemas cosmetically more difficult to administer, and the choice of topical therapy often depends on patient preference.

Mesalamine is currently the only available 5-ASA medication in suppository form. Suppositories are generally administered in a dose of 500 mg twice daily or as a single 1,000 mg suppository given at bedtime. A recent multicenter randomized study comparing efficacy of BID versus nightly dosing showed comparable efficacy in both inducing and maintaining remission [7–9]. Patients who achieve adequate remission are often able to be maintained on therapy given every other or every third night. Only a small percentage of patients are able to discontinue therapy completely, with 47–86 % relapsing within 1 year of discontinuing therapy [4, 7].

Oral 5-ASA therapy is less effective at inducing or maintaining remission in UP as compared to proctosigmoiditis or left-sided ulcerative colitis. The lower efficacy of oral preparations may be due to proximal colonic stasis causing the medication to concentrate above the rectum [8]. Despite a lower response rate, oral 5-ASA therapy is commonly used for treatment and is beneficial in inducing and maintaining

G.R. Lichtenstein (ed.), *Medical Therapy of Ulcerative Colitis*,
DOI 10.1007/978-1-4939-1677-1_21, © Springer Science+Business Media New York 2014

**Table 21.1** 5-ASA therapies

| Medication | |
| --- | --- |
| Mesalamine DR (Asacol, Asacol HD) | 800 mg DR, 1–2 tabs TID |
| Mesalamine ER (Apriso, currently only approved for maintenance) | 0.375 g ER, 4 tabs QAM |
| Mesalamine ER (Pentasa) | 250/500 mg ER, 1,000 mg QID |
| Mesalamine DR (Lialda) | 1.2 g DR, 2–4 tabs/day |
| Sulfasalazine | 500 mg tabs, 1 tab QID |
| Balsalazide | 750 mg tabs, 3 tabs PO TID |
| Olsalazine | 250 mg, 2 tabs PO BID |
| Mesalamine enema (Rowasa, sulfite-free formulation available) | One 4 g enema QHS |
| Mesalamine suppositories (Canasa) | 1,000 mg supp PR QHS |

remission [10]. Oral aminosalicylates include sulfasalazine, olsalazine, mesalamine, and balsalazide. Dosing recommendations for sulfasalazine are 4–6 g per day in divided doses [11], for olasalzine 250 mg to 2 g daily, and balsalazide 750 mg up to 6.75 g daily. Multiple delayed release formulations have been developed over the past 15 years with the goal of minimizing pill burden; these include Pentasa (500 mg tablets up to 4 g daily), Asacol HD (800 mg tablets up to 6 tablets daily), Apriso (375 mg up to 6 tablets daily), and Lialda (1.2 g up to 4 tablets daily (see Table 21.1)). They generally exert their effects within 2–4 weeks of the onset of therapy [12]. Oral 5-ASA agents are generally well tolerated, but uncommon side effects include alopecia, nausea, and paradoxical diarrhea. The occurence of nephrotoxicity is rare but is a known potential adverse effect [13]. It occurs most frequently during the first year of treatment but can occur at later points. There does not appear to be a dose effect relationship. It is recommended that serum creatinine and a urinalysis should be measured prior to initiating therapy and monitored yearly thereafter.

It needs to be emphasized that patients seem to achieve maximum benefit and an earlier response using a combination of oral and topical therapy, generally with an oral dose of 2.4–4 mg of mesalamine [11].

## Steroids

Therapies with hydrocortisone enemas or foam are effective for inducing remission [2, 10, 14, 15]. Suppository foam reaches approximately 15–20 cm from the anal verge and enemas often as far as the splenic flexure [2, 3, 16–22]. They have not been shown to be effective in maintaining remission [3]. Due to difficulty retaining liquid enemas, particularly at times when the patient is in an acute flair, 10 % hydrocortisone foam is well recognized to be often better tolerated. The author's general approach has been to use hydrocortisone foam for 2 weeks nightly and then attempt converting to either oral, topical, or dual mesalamine. Depending on the severity of patient's symptoms and time of remission, the foam can be alternated nightly with mesalamine for a short

period of time also. Patient's refractory to this should use a combination of oral and topical mesalamine therapy. Other formulations beside hydrocortisone include Prednisolone 21-phosphate and beclomethasone dipropionate. These are both available as suppositories and enemas although are less commonly available in the USA.

Budesonide is a steroid which undergoes rapid first pass hepatic metabolism resulting in less systemic absorption of the medication. It is used orally for the treatment of right-sided colonic and ileal disease for patients with Crohn's disease. It is available in enema form. The recommended dose of 2 mg is not available yet in the United States but seems to be as effective as hydrocortisone with less systemic side effects [2, 16, 17]. Recently, oral Budesonide MMX gained regulatory approval for ulcerative colitis.

Rarely, systemic corticosteroids are required for the treatment of UP. This should be reserved for patients who are failing maximal topical therapy as well as maximum dose oral mesalamine. Inflamed rectal mucosa shows relatively poor absorption of oral steroid formulations. Given this fact and the well-known high rate of systemic side effects, oral corticosteroids are generally a temporizing measure to a more definitive therapy with either an immunomodulator or biologic agent.

## Immunomodulator Therapy

Azathioprine (AZA) and 6-mercaptopurine (6-MP) are immunomodulator medications used in the treatment of both Crohn's disease and ulcerative colitis. Small studies have shown benefit of 6-MP for ulcerative proctosigmoiditis. Love et al. [23] reported improvement in 63 % of patients with steroid refractory disease while on doses of 25–150 mg/day. About 1/3 of these patients developed a relapse while on 6-MP, but remission was restored in 88 % with a short course of steroids and continued 6-MP use. Their primary role in ulcerative colitis and ulcerative proctitis is as steroid-sparing agents rather than as primary therapy to induce remission. It needs to be emphasized that no specific studies have shown a beneficial effect of 6-MP in the use of ulcerative proctitis (as opposed to the studies noted above looking at ulcerative proctosigmoiditis).

Methotrexate is often used to induce remission in patients with Crohn's disease or Crohn's colitis, but no controlled data supports the use of methotrexate in patients with ulcerative colitis.

## Steroid and Immunomodulator Refractory Disease

Infliximab is a chimeric anti-TNF-alpha antibody that has been demonstrated in large randomized placebo-controlled trials to be effective for the treatment of moderate to severe ulcerative colitis [24]. More recently, a fully human monoclonal antibody that binds TNF-alpha, Adalimumab, has been approved for induction and maintenance of remission in patients with moderate to severe ulcerative colitis. Infliximab has not been evaluated in large studies on ulcerative proctitis patients: however, several small studies have shown efficacy. Out of 13 patients treated with infliximab at 5 mg/kg for refractory ulcerative proctitis at 6 referral centers between 2005 and 2009, 9/13 (69 %) had a complete response, 2/13 (15 %) had a partial response, and 2/13 (15 %) were primary nonresponders [25, 26]. This suggests a role for infliximab for patient's refractory to other agents. Adalimumab has not been studied specifically for ulcerative proctitis. Case reports have described the use of topically administered infliximab for patient's refractory to systemic therapy, but no controlled studies have been performed [27].

Recent studies have looked at the use of oral tacrolimus for treatment of ulcerative colitis (although not specifically in ulcerative proctitis) [28]. Tacrolimus is a potent immunosuppressant in the FK506 family of agents often used for immunosuppression in the setting of organ transplant. Oral tacrolimus is associated with numerous side effects including hypertension, hematologic abnormalities, renal impairment, and increase in skin cancers. Topical tacrolimus is effective in numerous inflammatory conditions, and several studies have showed efficacy in ulcerative proctitis resistant to other therapies. In one study, 19 patients with ulcerative proctitis were treated for 4 weeks with a daily 2–4 mg enema or a 2 mg suppository [29]. 13/19 patients showed clinical and histologic improvement of disease activity after 4 weeks of treatment. More importantly, blood trough levels were followed and were too low to induce systemic immune suppression, and patients had minimal side effects. Cyclosporine has a similar mechanism of action to tacrolimus but is not available topically and has not specifically been studied for ulcerative proctitis.

## Other Therapies

Several experimental therapies have been tried for ulcerative proctitis although none have been approved by the FDA. In a case report, granulocyte, macrophage, and monocyte apheresis was effective, and the patient was able to be bridged to azathioprine [29]. Antibiotics have shown poor efficacy in the treatment of ulcerative colitis generally. Nicotine enemas [30, 31] have not proven effective. Limited data on the use of short-chain fatty acid enemas in combination with oral 5-ASA agents [32] have shown modest benefits but are not readily available. A small prospective study showed a modestly good effect in the use of arsenic suppositories 250 mg twice daily for 4 weeks with minimal side effects [33]. Probiotics are an area of active interest for ulcerative colitis although no studies have shown beneficial effects.

Recently regulatory approval for vedolizumab was introduced in the United States for refractory ulcerative colitis and Crohn's disease. Though this agent has not been formally assessed in patients with ulcerative colitis limited to proctitis, the perception is that this agent is effective in patients with all disease distributions.

## Conclusion

Ulcerative proctitis can be a challenging condition for both physicians and patients to treat. The pathophysiology of inflammation confined to the rectum makes effective drug delivery a unique challenge in UP. The mainstay of treatment remains 5-ASA therapy (see Fig. 21.1). Combination therapy with oral and topical treatment is most effective, followed by topical therapy alone and lastly oral therapy alone.

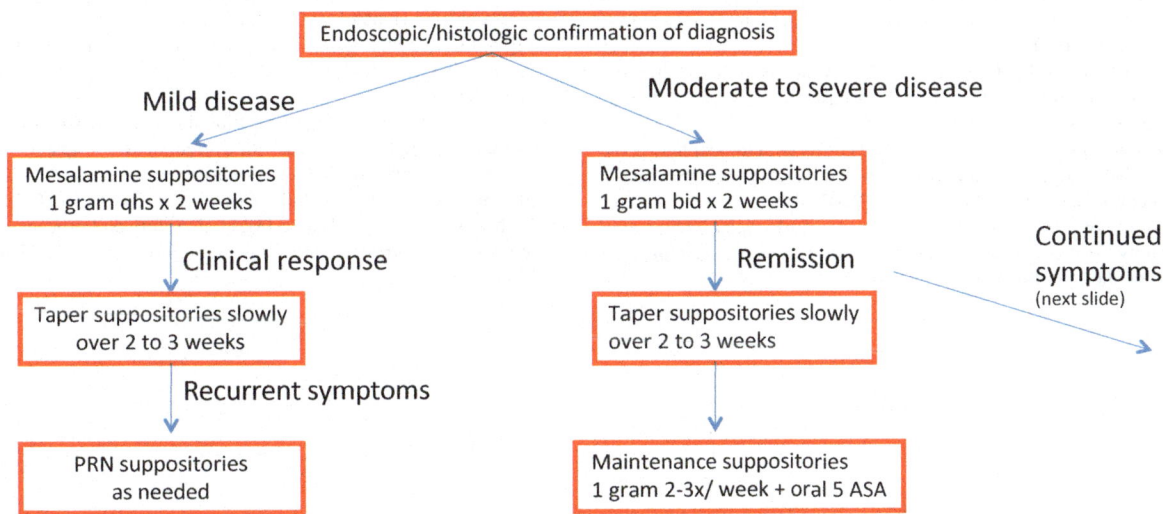

**Fig. 21.1** Medical management of ulcerative proctitis

Patients who are steroid refractory are now often managed with infliximab, adalimumab, or golimumab although multiple other experimental approaches have been shown to be efficacious. Vedolizumab, although not formally tested in patients with ulcerative proctitis, is likely effective in this patient population.

# References

1. Eaden JA, Abrams KR, Mayberry JF. The risk of colorectal cancer in ulcerative colitis: a meta-analysis. Gut. 2001;48:526–35.
2. Kornbluth A, Sachar DB. Ulcerative colitis practice guidelines in adults: American College of Gastroenterology, Practice Parameters Committee. AMJ Gastroenterol. 2010;105:501–23.
3. Cohen RD, Woseth DM, Thisted RA, et al. A meta-analysis and overview of the literature on treatment options for left-sided ulcerative colitis and ulcerative proctitis. Am J Gastroenterol. 2009; 95:1263–76.
4. Regueiro M, Loftus Jr EV, Steinhart AH, et al. Medical management of left-sided ulcerative colitis and ulcerative proctitis: summary statement. Inflamm Bowel Dis. 2006;12:972–8.
5. Wilding IR, Kenyon CJ, Chauhan S, et al. Colonic spreading of a non-chlorofluorocarbon mesalazine rectal foam enema in patients with quiescent ulcerative colitis. Aliment Pharmacol Ther. 1995; 9:161–6.
6. Van Bodegraven AA, Bower RO, Lourens J, et al. Distribution of mesalazine enemas in active and quiescent ulcerative colitis. Aliment Pharmacol Ther. 1996;10:327–32.
7. Banerjee S, Peppercorn MA. Inflammatory bowel disease: medical therapy for specific clinical presentations. Gastroenterol Clin North Am. 2002;31:185–202.
8. Gionchetti P, Rizzello F, Morselli C, et al. Review article: aminosalicylates for distal colitis. Aliment Pharmacol Ther. 2006;24 suppl 3:41–4.
9. Lamet M. A multicenter, randomized study to evaluate the efficacy and safety of mesalamine suppositories 1 g at bedtime and 500 mg twice daily in patients with active mild-to-moderate ulcerative proctitis. Dig Dis Sci. 2011;56:513–22.
10. Sutherland LR. Topical treatment of ulcerative colitis. Med Clin North Am. 1990;74:119–31.
11. Baron JH, Connell AM, Lennard-Jones JE, et al. Sulphasalazine and salicylazosulphadimidine in ulcerative colitis. Lancet. 1962;1: 1094–6.
12. Sutherland L, Macdonald JK. Oral 5-aminosalicylic acid for induction of remission in ulcerative colitis. Cochrane Database Syst Rev. 2006; CD000543
13. Gilbert JP, Lonzalez-Lama Y, Mate J. 5-Aminosalicylates and renal function in inflammatory bowel disease: a systematic review. Inflamm Bowel Dis. 2007;13:629–38.
14. Watkinson G. Treatment of ulcerative colitis with topical hydrocortisone hemisuccinate sodium; a controlled trial employing restricted sequential analysis. Br Med J. 1958;2:1077–82.
15. Truelove SC, Hambling MH. Treatment of ulcerative colitis with local hydrocortisone hemisuccinate sodium; a report on a controlled therapeutic trial. Br Med J. 1958;2:1072–7.
16. Hanauer SB, Robinson M, Pruitt R, et al. Budesonide enema for the treatment of active, distal ulcerative colitis and proctitis: a dose-ranging study. US Budesonide Enema Study Group. Gastroenterology. 1998;115:525–32.
17. Budesonide enema in distal ulcerative colitis. A randomized dose–response trial with prednisolone enema as positive control. The Danish Budesonide Study Group. Scand J Gastroenterol 1991;26:1225–30.
18. Lofberg R, Danielsson A, Suhr O, et al. Oral budesonide vs. prednisolone in patients with active extensive and left-sided ulcerative colitis. Gastroenterology. 1996;110:1713–8.
19. Farthing MJ, Rutland MD, Clark ML. Retrograde spread of hydrocortisone containing foam given intrarectally in ulcerative colitis. Br Med J. 1979;2:822–4.
20. Jay M, Digenis GA, Foster TS, et al. Retrograde spreading of hydrocortisone enema in inflammatory bowel disease. Dig Dis Sci. 1986;31:139–44.
21. Chapman NJ, Brown ML, Phillips SF, et al. Distribution of mesalamine enemas in patients with active distal ulcerative colitis. Mayo Clin Proc. 1992;67:245–8.
22. Williams CN, Haber G, Aquino JA. Double-blind, placebo-controlled evaluation of 5-ASA suppositories in active distal proctitis and measurement of extent of spread using 99mTc-labeled 5-ASA suppositories. Dig Dis Sci. 1987;32(12 Suppl):71S–5.
23. Love MA, Rubin PH, Chapman ML, Present DH. 6-merecaptopurine is effective in intractable proctosigmoiditis. Gastroenterology. 1995;100:A832.
24. Rutgeerts P, Sandborn WJ, Feagan BG, et al. Infliximab for induction and maintenance therapy for ulcerative colitis. N Engl J Med. 2005;353:2462–76.
25. Sandborn W, Assche G, Reinisch W, et al. Adalimumab induces and maintains clinical remission in patient with moderate-to severe ulcerative colitis. Gastroenterology. 2011;142:257–65.
26. Bouguen G, Roblin X, Bourreille A, et al. Infliximab for refractory ulcerative proctitis. Aliment Pharmacol Ther. 2010;31:1178–85.
27. Molnar T, Farkas K, Nagy F. Topically administered infliximab can work in ulcerative proctitis despite the ineffectiveness of intravenous induction therapy. AJG. 2009;104:1857. Letters to the editor.
28. Ogata H, Matsui T, Nakamure M, et al. A randomized dose finding study of oral tacrolimus (FK506) therapy in refractory ulcerative colitis. Gut. 2006;55:1255–62.
29. Van Dieren JM, Van Bodegraven AA, Kuipers EJ. Local application of tacrolimus in distal colitis: feasible and safe. Inflamm Bowel Dis. 2009;15(2):193–8.
30. Premchand P, Takeuchi K, Bjarnason I. Granulocyte, macrophage, monocyte apheresis for refractory ulcerative proctitis. Eur J Gastroenterol Hepatol. 2004;16(9):943–5.
31. Ingram JR, Thomas GA, Rhodes J, et al. A randomized trial of nicotine enemas for active ulcerative colitis. Clin Gastroenterol Hepatol. 2005;3:1107–14.
32. Vernia P, Monteleone G, Grandinetti G, et al. Combined oral sodium butyrate and mesalazine treatment compared to oral mesalazine alone in ulcerative colitis: randomized, double-blind, placebo-controlled pilot study. Dig Dis Sci. 2000;45:976–81.
33. Forbes A, Britton TC, House IM, et al. Safety and efficacy of acetarsol suppositories in unresponsive proctitis. Aliment Pharmacol Ther. 1989;3:553–6.

# Treatment of Distal/Left-Sided Ulcerative Colitis

**22**

Jason M. Swoger and Miguel D. Regueiro

**Keywords**

Distal ulcerative colitis • Left-sided ulcerative colitis • Topical therapy • 5-ASA • Maintenance therapy • Long-term use • Rectal administration • Oral formulation

## Abbreviations

| | |
|---|---|
| 5-ASA | 5-Aminosalicylic acid |
| ACTH | Adrenocorticotropic hormone |
| BDP | Beclomethasone dipropionate |
| DAI | Disease activity index |
| IPAA | Ileal pouch-anal anastomosis |
| L-UC | Left-sided ulcerative colitis |
| POR | Pooled odds ratio |
| UC | Ulcerative colitis |

## Introduction

Ulcerative colitis (UC) has an incidence of 8–12/100,000 people per year, and there are approximately 500,000 individuals in the United States affected by this condition [1, 2]. The distribution of ulcerative colitis always involves the rectum and spreads proximally, in a continuous manner, to involve a part or all of the colon. At the time of diagnosis, up to 80 % of patients will present with left-sided colitis (L-UC), defined as a disease distribution that does not extend proximally to the splenic flexure [3, 4]. Early and aggressive intervention is paramount, and this may lessen the risk of disease progression over time, though this has not been proven in studies [5]. As with ulcerative colitis in general, the goals of therapy for L-UC are the induction and maintenance of remission [1, 3, 6]. The mainstay of the treatment of L-UC is rectally administered topical therapy, which has been proven in multiple studies to rapidly induce both symptomatic improvement and remission. Most patients will require long-term maintenance therapy, and rectal 5-aminosalicylic acid (5-ASA) therapy has been shown to be effective in this regard. However, maintenance therapy may be complicated by compliance factors inherent in the use of long-term rectally administered therapy, and patients often prefer oral formulations for maintenance therapy.

This chapter will discuss treatment approaches to L-UC, not including ulcerative proctitis; the treatment of which is detailed elsewhere. The first section will focus on the treatment of active L-UC, reviewing the evidence-based data on topical 5-ASA, topical corticosteroids, oral 5-ASA, and oral corticosteroids. Data will be presented comparing each medication to placebo, as well as to the alternate medications. A treatment algorithm for active L-UC is presented.

J.M. Swoger, M.D., M.P.H. (✉) • M.D. Regueiro, M.D.
Department of Gastroenterology, Hepatology, and Nutrition,
University of Pittsburgh Medical Center,
200 Lothrop Street, C-Wing, Mezzanine Level, Pittsburg,
PA 15213, USA
e-mail: swogerjm@upmc.edu; mdr7@pitt.edu

G.R. Lichtenstein (ed.), *Medical Therapy of Ulcerative Colitis*,
DOI 10.1007/978-1-4939-1677-1_22, © Springer Science+Business Media New York 2014

The treatment of 5-ASA nonresponse, a challenging patient population, is also discussed. Subsequently, maintenance therapy of L-UC is discussed, again reviewing the evidence-based data for each available medication. A table describing options for the maintenance therapy of L-UC is presented. There is some debate in the medical literature regarding the terminology used for rectally administered enema/suspension therapy. For the purpose of this review, "rectally administered" therapy and "topical" therapy will be used interchangeably.

## Treatment of Active Left-Sided Ulcerative Colitis

### Topical 5-ASA Therapy

The most effective therapy for L-UC is topical 5-ASA, which is recommended as a first-line agent in treatment guidelines both in the United States and Europe [1, 6]. Advantages of rectal therapy include direct delivery of the medication to the site of inflammation, superior efficacy, and decreased systemic absorption compared to oral formulations, which may limit potential toxicities [3, 7]. Although 5-ASA topical therapy has well-established efficacy, other considerations, including tolerability and patient acceptance, may impact their usage and reduce compliance. Additionally, rectal compliance is diminished in the presence of active inflammation, and enema preparations may be more difficult to retain. Another limitation of enema therapy is that the most distal part of the rectum may remain untreated, as the majority of the enema is distributed in the descending and sigmoid colons [3]. Symptomatic improvement with rectally administered 5-ASA products can be expected in as early as 2–4 weeks [8]. If there is no symptomatic improvement after this time period, alternative therapies should be considered.

### Rectal 5-ASA vs. Placebo

Multiple studies have demonstrated the superiority of rectal 5-ASA therapy compared to placebo, and several meta-analyses have supported these findings [7, 9, 10]. Cohen et al. performed a meta-analysis to compare treatment options for L-UC [9]. Two trials compared 2 g 5-ASA enemas to placebo and found a significant benefit for the 5-ASA enemas in terms of both clinical improvement and clinical remission, at 2 and 4 weeks of therapy [11, 12]. In the meta-analysis, enema therapies had a 37–47 % advantage over placebo, depending on dose, at 2-, 4-, and 6-week end points. In contrast, the advantages over placebo for oral 5-ASA formulations (olsalazine or 4 g mesalamine) were only 17–25 % [9].

Marshall and Irvine reported an initial meta-analysis for L-UC, which found topical 5-ASA to be superior for the treatment of active diseases, compared to placebo, for symptomatic improvement and remission and endoscopic and histologic end points [7]. Seven trials were included in this meta-analysis, with each of the individual studies showing topical 5-ASA to be significantly superior to placebo for the induction of clinical remission. When combining the results in the meta-analysis, the authors reported a pooled odds ratio (POR) of 7.71 (4.84–12.30) for symptomatic remission, 6.55 (4.15–10.36) for endoscopic remission, and 6.91 (3.82–12.50) for histologic remission, all in favor of topical 5-ASA.

The same authors reported a Cochrane systematic review of rectal 5-ASA therapy for the induction of remission of L-UC, which included ten studies comparing rectal 5-ASA and placebo [10]. As with the prior meta-analysis, each individual study found topical therapy to be significantly superior to placebo for all end points, including symptomatic, endoscopic, and histologic improvement and remission. When analyzing the individual data, the authors reported a POR for symptomatic improvement and remission of 8.87 (5.30–14.83) and 8.30 (4.28–16.12) in favor of topical 5-ASA therapy. Similarly, for the end points of endoscopic improvement and remission, PORs in favor of topical mesalamine therapy were 11.18 (5.99–20.88) and 5.31 (3.15–8.92), respectively. Based on the results of these meta-analyses and the significant odds ratios reported in the individual studies, topical 5-ASA therapy has been proven to be superior to placebo for the treatment of active left-sided UC.

### Topical Corticosteroid Therapy

Topical corticosteroid therapy is effective for the induction of remission of L-UC [13]. Available formulations include a hydrocortisone enema (100 mg), which delivers medication to the level of the splenic flexure [1]. In addition, there is hydrocortisone foam (10 %) available, which delivers medication to the rectosigmoid colon and can be used in patients with proctosigmoiditis [1]. Though not available in the United States, several studies have evaluated budesonide enemas for the treatment of L-UC. Budesonide is rapidly metabolized by the liver and is not associated with as many systemic side effects as hydrocortisone. Beclomethasone dipropionate (BDP) is another second-generation corticosteroid, with limited absorption and a high hepatic first-pass metabolism.

The newer corticosteroid formulations may have efficacy similar to traditional corticosteroids, such as hydrocortisone, but are associated with fewer side effects, due to more limited absorption. Budesonide enemas have been shown to be as effective as hydrocortisone enemas but are associated with significantly fewer side effects. Three studies have compared the different formulations of rectal corticosteroids, most often comparing either budesonide or BDP to hydrocortisone, with no differences being found in any of the studies [14–16]. In a meta-analysis, rectal hydrocortisone was found to be similar to rectal budesonide for both improvement and remission end points [17]. These results suggest that rapidly metabolized corticosteroids are as effective as conventional corticosteroids, as well as rectal 5-ASA formulations.

## Rectal Corticosteroids vs. Placebo

Several studies have found rectal corticosteroid therapy to be superior to placebo for the induction of remission of L-UC. These studies have also been systematically reviewed in two meta-analyses [9, 17]. Significant improvement in symptomatic, endoscopic, and histologic remission, compared to placebo, has been found for hydrocortisone enemas as well as the second-generation corticosteroids, budesonide, and BDP.

In the Cohen et al. meta-analysis, hydrocortisone and budesonide enemas had an advantage over placebo of 32 % and 56 %, respectively [9]. Marshall and Irvine performed a meta-analysis of rectal corticosteroids, compared to other treatments of L-UC [17]. Among the pooled studies, symptomatic improvement rates with rectal corticosteroids were 73–77 %, with remission rates of 45 %. Endoscopic improvement rates were 66–69 %, with endoscopic remission seen in 31–34 % of subjects. When compared to placebo, rectal corticosteroids showed superiority, with a pooled odds ratio of 0.21 (0.07–0.71) for symptomatic improvement and a POR of 0.27 (0.10–0.77) for endoscopic improvement. This translates into rectal steroids being 4–5 times more likely to lead to symptomatic and endoscopic improvements than placebo. Similar results were found when the end points were symptomatic and endoscopic remission. This meta-analysis also included studies of BDP and budesonide enemas.

A study of 233 patients with L-UC and proctitis showed that a 2 g budesonide enema was significantly more effective than placebo for the induction of remission (19 % vs. 4 %, $p \leq 0.05$) [18]. Furthermore, 90 % of patients had normal adrenocorticotropic hormone (ACTH) levels at the end of the 6-week treatment period. Lindgren et al. studied once vs. twice daily dosing of budesonide enemas and found no difference in remission rates at 8 weeks [19]. In addition, there was significantly less impairment of adrenal function in the once-daily group (32 % vs. 4.8 %, $p = 0.001$). There was no increase in efficacy with a 4 g enema compared to a 2 g enema, but the higher dose was associated with more cortisol suppression.

## Rectal 5-ASA vs. Rectal Corticosteroids

Several clinical trials have found rectal 5-ASA medications to be superior to rectal corticosteroids for the induction of symptomatic, endoscopic, and histologic remission. An early trial of 123 patients with mild-to-moderate L-UC randomized patients to receive 5-ASA or prednisolone enemas [10]. After 2 weeks, improvement rates were similar, but remission rates were significantly better in the 5-ASA group (51 % vs. 31 %, $p < 0.05$). 5-ASA was found to be an acceptable alternative to rectal corticosteroids. Bianchi Porro et al. compared 1 g 5-ASA enemas to 100 mg hydrocortisone enemas, in a randomized trial of 52 patients [20]. In the 5-ASA group, clinical, endoscopic, and histologic improvement was seen in 89, 74, and 56 %, compared to 70, 56, and 60 % in the corticosteroid group, making rectal 5-ASA a safe and alternative treatment for L-UC.

Lee et al. compared 5-ASA foam to prednisolone foam in 295 patients with L-UC [21]. Clinical remission was achieved in 52 % of 5-ASA patients, compared to 31 % of prednisolone patients ($p < 0.001$), though there was no significant difference in endoscopic or histologic remission. Finally, in a trial of 18 patients who had not responded to hydrocortisone enemas, Friedman et al. compared 5-ASA enemas to continued hydrocortisone enema therapy [22]. Clinical, endoscopic, and histologic improvement rates were significantly better for the 5-ASA patients than those patients who continued hydrocortisone enemas. Patients who received hydrocortisone enemas and did not respond were then switched over to open-label 5-ASA enemas, with four of six demonstrating clinical improvement. Thus, 5-ASA enemas were effective in patients with L-UC who did not previously responded to hydrocortisone enemas.

In addition to the traditional rectal corticosteroid formulations, studies have compared the second-generation, topically active corticosteroids to mesalamine enemas for the treatment of active L-UC. In a study of 99 patients with L-UC, BDP (3 mg) enema and foam were compared to 5-ASA (2 g) enema and foam [23]. Response rates at weeks 4 and 8 were comparable between these medications, and though remission rates were numerically higher in the 5-ASA group (52 % vs. 36 %), these did not reach statistical significance. Gionchetti et al. compared BDP enemas (3 g daily) to 5-ASA enemas (1 g daily) in 217 patients, with a 6-week end point [24]. Rates of clinical improvement and remission were 49 and 25 % for the 5-ASA group, compared to 37 and 30 % for the BDP group, which were not statistically significant. Both treatments improved disease activity and were well tolerated, and the authors concluded equivalence between the two treatments. A meta-analysis specifically pooled four trials comparing rectal BDP and 5-ASA. 5-ASA therapy led to an improvement/remission in 69.9 % of patients, compared to 65.3 % for BDP ($p = $NS), suggesting equal efficacy between these medications for the treatment of active L-UC [25].

Rectal budesonide therapy has also been studied in active L-UC. Lemann et al., in a study of 97 patients, found a statistically significantly higher clinical remission rate for rectal

5-ASA (1 g daily) compared to a budesonide enema (2.3 mg daily), at a 4-week end point (60 % vs. 38 %, $p=0.03$) [26]. Clinical improvement rates, as well as endoscopic and histologic improvement and remission rates, were similar between the two groups, but the study may have been underpowered to prove equivalence. A smaller study of 62 patients, by Lamers et al., did not find a difference in rates of clinical, endoscopic, or histologic remission between topical 5-ASA and budesonide [27]. These results suggest that rapidly metabolized corticosteroids may be as effective as conventional corticosteroids, as well as rectal 5-ASA, for the treatment of active L-UC.

An early meta-analysis, published in 1997, included seven trials comparing rectal corticosteroid to rectal 5-ASA therapy [17]. Different dosages and formulations of the medications among the individual studies make comparisons somewhat difficult. There were no differences noted between the therapies in terms of symptomatic or endoscopic improvement, though histologic improvement was found to be superior with 5-ASA therapy. However, for the more stringent end points of remission, the authors found rectal 5-ASA therapy to be superior to rectal corticosteroid therapy for symptomatic (POR 2.42, 1.72–3.41), endoscopic (POR 1.89, 1.29–2.76), and histologic remissions (POR 2.03, 1.28–3.20).

The Cohen et al. meta-analysis reported data on trials comparing rectal 5-ASA to rectal corticosteroids [9]. In their analysis of trials that passed their quality assessment, robust results comparing topical 5-ASA and corticosteroid enemas were not reported. When all 67 studies on the treatment of active diseases were reported, remission rates for topical 5-ASA therapies were higher than those in studies of topical corticosteroid therapies, at both 6- and 8-week end points. Clinical improvement rates were similar between these therapies at 2- and 4-week end points, though there was an advantage in one study for 5-ASA enema compared to prednisolone enema at a 6-week end point. In general, the symptomatic improvement and remission rates for 5-ASA enemas were 10–20 % higher than those for corticosteroid enemas and oral 5-ASA.

Finally, Marshall et al. updated their prior meta-analyses with a Cochrane systematic review, published in 2010, which included 11 studies comparing rectal 5-ASA and corticosteroids [10]. For the outcome of symptomatic improvement, only one of nine studies showed a statistically significant difference between therapies, in favor of rectal 5-ASA. However, when the studies were pooled, with a total of 937 patients included, the authors found a POR of 1.56 (1.15–2.11) in favor of rectal 5-ASA therapy. Similarly, for symptomatic remission, only two of the six studies included showed a significant difference on an individual basis, both of which were in favor of rectal 5-ASA. When the studies were combined, 942 patients were included, and the POR was 1.65 (1.11–2.45)

in favor of rectal 5-ASA therapy. There were also trends noted for other end points, including endoscopic and histologic improvement and remission, in favor of rectal 5-ASA.

Based on the results described above, demonstrating both superior efficacy and a more favorable side-effect profile compared to conventional corticosteroids, rectal 5-ASA therapy should be the first-line treatment of L-UC. In addition, as will be discussed subsequently, rectal corticosteroids are not effective for the maintenance of remission of distal UC, which makes topical mesalamine a better option for long-term treatment. Rectal corticosteroids should be reserved for patients who do not respond to or cannot tolerate topical 5-ASA formulations.

## Rectal 5-ASA vs. Oral 5-ASA

Few randomized trials have compared rectal 5-ASA to oral 5-ASA formulations for the treatment of active L-UC. Kam et al. randomized 37 patients to receive daily 5-ASA enema (4 g) vs. sulfasalazine 1,000 mg, given four times daily [28]. At week 6, clinical global improvement scores were improved in 85 % of patients in the enema group compared to 77 % in the sulfasalazine group ($p=0.02$). In addition, significantly more patients in the sulfasalazine group experienced adverse events ($p=0.02$). There was no difference between the groups in the disease activity index (DAI), though topical 5-ASA was found to have a more rapid onset and improved tolerability. In this study, improvement with rectal therapy occurred rapidly and was noticeable within 2 weeks. This trend has been noted in additional studies, as Sutherland et al. reported that cessation of rectal bleeding with topical 5-ASA therapy occurred in as little as 3 days (median 8 days), which is shorter than the time reported for oral 5-ASA therapies [8, 29]. At week 3, cessation of rectal bleeding was seen in 60 % of 5-ASA group, compared to 15.1 % of placebo.

More recently, oral MMX mesalamine was compared with 5-ASA enemas in patients with L-UC [30]. At week 4, more patients in the topical therapy group had experienced clinical response (68.4 % vs. 57.5 %). However, at week 8, clinical response was seen in 60 % of MMX patients compared to 50 % of 5-ASA enema patients (CI for difference, −12.0 to +32.0). There were no significant differences in clinical response noted at either week 4 or week 8, and the authors concluded that the treatments were comparable. There was also no difference between endoscopic and histologic remissions. Not surprisingly, compliance was significantly greater in the oral MMX-mesalamine group. Similarly, Safdi et al. did not find an efficacy difference between topical and oral therapies for L-UC but did find combination therapy to be superior, which will be discussed further in the following section [31].

An initial meta-analysis comparing rectal and oral formulations of 5-ASA was reported by Marshall and Irvine, in 2000, with a POR for symptomatic remission and improvement of 4.1 (1.4–10.9) and 6.3 (2.7–14.5), respectively, in favor of topical therapy [7]. This was despite only one individual trial, which studied suppository therapy for ulcerative proctitis, showing a positive result [32]. A more recent update of this meta-analysis, which included an additional study showing a nonsignificant superiority of oral therapy, made the meta-analysis findings nonsignificant (POR 2.25, 0.53–9.54) [10]. However, the additional study has been criticized for having a high dropout rate in the topical therapy group and using an 8-week primary end point, as opposed to the 4-week end point used in other studies [30].

Cohen et al. also reported a meta-analysis of rectal therapy for L-UC, including comparisons of rectal and oral 5-ASA [9]. For the end point of clinical improvement, enema therapies were superior at the 2-week time point to oral therapies at all time points studied, again demonstrating the rapid onset of topical therapy. In addition, compared to the oral 5-ASA compounds, 5-ASA enemas demonstrated higher clinical improvement rates. In general, the symptomatic improvement and remission rates for 5-ASA enemas were 10–20 % higher than those reported for the oral 5-ASA formulations.

## Combination Therapy

As detailed above, oral or topical therapy with either 5-ASA formulations or corticosteroids has been found to be effective for the induction of remission in L-UC. Additional studies have examined whether combination therapies lead to even greater efficacy.

Mulder et al. compared BDP enemas (3 mg daily) to 5-ASA enemas (2 g daily) in 60 patients with L-UC, limited to the distal 20 cm of the colon [33]. One treatment arm in this study received a combination enema, containing both medications. At a 4-week end point, there was no difference in clinical improvement scores between the monotherapy groups. However, the group receiving combination therapy was found to have significantly higher clinical improvement scores compared to either monotherapy group. The clinical and endoscopic improvement rates in the combination therapy group were 100 %, compared to 70–75 % in the rectal 5-ASA and corticosteroid monotherapy groups. For all end points, including clinical, endoscopic, and histologic improvement, combination therapy was statistically significantly better than either monotherapy alone.

Safdi et al., in a study of 60 patients with L-UC, found the combination of oral and topical therapy to be superior to either therapy alone, for both disease activity improvement and cessation of rectal bleeding [31]. Patients received 4 g 5-ASA enemas daily, along with at least 2.4 g of oral 5-ASA daily. Cessation of rectal bleeding occurred in 89 % of the combination therapy group, compared to 69 % in rectal therapy group and 46 % in oral monotherapy group. The average time to cessation of rectal bleeding was 11.9 days in the combination therapy group, compared to approximately 25 days in either monotherapy group. Each monotherapy group achieved similar reductions in the DAI, but combination therapy was found to achieve a superior reduction.

Studies in patients with more extensive UC (proximal to the splenic flexure) have also shown combination oral and topical 5-ASA therapy to be superior to either treatment alone. Marteau et al. compared oral 5-ASA (4 g divided twice daily) plus placebo to oral 5-ASA plus a 5-ASA enema (1 g daily) [34]. Remission rates were similar at 4 weeks among the groups, achieved in 34 % of the monotherapy group and 44 % of the combination therapy group ($p = 0.31$). However, at 8 weeks, 64 % of the combination group achieved remission compared to 43 % of the monotherapy group ($p = 0.0008$). Additionally, symptomatic improvement end points at weeks 4 and 8 were superior in the combination therapy group, with differences in response rates at each time point of 18–27 %. Finally, Rizzello et al. randomized 119 patients with either extensive or L-UC to receive oral 5-ASA alone or oral 5-ASA in addition to oral BDP [35]. At the 4-week end point, combination therapy was associated with significantly higher rates of remission and significantly lower DAI scores.

Thus, combination therapy with rectal 5-ASA and corticosteroids, or with oral and rectal 5-ASA, is more effective than monotherapy regimens and should be considered in patients who do not respond to either 5-ASA rectal or oral monotherapy.

## Rectal 5-ASA Dosing

Multiple studies of 5-ASA enemas for left-sided UC have used different medication doses making trials somewhat difficult to compare. Campieri et al. compared different doses of 5-ASA enemas to evaluate for a possible dose–response effect. No difference was found between enemas containing 1, 2, or 4 g of mesalamine daily [11]. These results were confirmed in both a larger study, of 287 patients, by Hanauer et al. and a meta-analysis that found 1 g-daily enemas to be as effective as 4 g-daily enemas for the induction of remission [9, 36]. These studies suggest that response to rectal 5-ASA therapy is more dependent on the duration of therapy than on dosage for the induction of remission. One hypothesis to explain the superiority of combination therapy suggests that this approach may lead to a more homogeneous drug distribution, suggesting that geographic coverage, not dose, may be the most significant factor in gaining response [10].

## Rectal 5-ASA Formulations

Several studies have evaluated alternative delivery methods for rectal therapies, including liquid enemas, foams, and gels. As of the writing of this chapter, in the United States, 5-ASA is available only in a 4 g liquid enema form, and corticosteroids are available in both enema and foam formulations. Gionchetti et al. compared 5-ASA gel and foam enemas in 103 patients with L-UC [37]. At 4 weeks, clinical, endoscopic, and histologic remission rates were similar between the groups, and DAI scores showed significant improvements in both groups. While there was no difference in efficacy or safety between the groups, the gel enema was better tolerated. In a study of 375 patients with L-UC, comparing 5-ASA foam and liquid enemas, clinical remission rates again were similar, and the trial showed the non-inferiority of the foam preparation at 2 and 4 weeks [38]. Finally, Malchow et al. compared 5-ASA foam and liquid enemas, finding no difference in efficacy, though quality of life scores were higher in the foam group [39].

In summary, multiple studies have found similar results when comparing different rectal 5-ASA formulations, in that they seem to have equivalent efficacy [40]. However, in general, foam preparations are preferred compared to liquid enemas, even if they contain a larger volume of medication [10].

## Oral 5-ASA Therapy

The different oral 5-ASA preparations have been shown to be effective in the treatment of ulcerative colitis, though few studies have specifically focused on patients with L-UC [1, 6]. These agents can be used for patients who either do not tolerate or do not respond to topical therapy.

Though efficacious, sulfasalazine is often associated with side effects, including headache, nausea, and rash, thus making non-sulfa-based 5-ASA preparations preferred [1]. The newer 5-ASA formulations are effective in 50–75 % of patients, are better tolerated, and do not have dose-related side effects [1, 13, 14]. Oral mesalamine (2.4–4.8 g daily) and balsalazide (6.75 g) are effective therapies for mild-to-moderate L-UC [1, 6]. One study suggested that, in patients with active L-UC, more patients experienced remission at 4 weeks with balsalazide compared to mesalamine [3]. However, in general, it is thought that all oral 5-ASA medications are equally effective in the treatment of L-UC, with cost and compliance issues often directing therapy with specific medications [41, 42]. Some studies have suggested an improved efficacy with a 4.8 g compared to a 2.4 g daily dose in patients with moderately active UC, though other studies have not been able to demonstrate a significant dose–response relationship [43, 44]. In patients who are refractory to initial oral 5-ASA therapy, rectal therapy should be introduced, as this may lead to improved efficacy.

## Oral Nonabsorbed Corticosteroids

Finally, a colonic release form of oral budesonide (MMX) has recently been studied in active left-sided UC [45]. Budesonide MMX demonstrated a significant reduction in the colitis activity index, while placebo did not. Improvement was rapid (50 % at 4 weeks), and there were no effects on cortisol levels or the pituitary-adrenal axis.

## 5-ASA Nonresponse

For patients who do not respond to either topical or oral 5-ASA, topical corticosteroids, or a combination therapy regimen, the treatment of L-UC parallels that of moderate-to-severe extensive colitis, which is discussed in more detail elsewhere. No studies involving the additional medication classes, including oral corticosteroids, immunomodulators (azathioprine or 6-mercaptopurine), or infliximab, have specifically evaluated patients with L-UC. These patients may be among the most difficult to treat, as evidence-based treatment recommendations in this specific patient population are lacking. It is the authors' opinion that the use of immunomodulators and/or biologic agents is warranted, and, in nonresponders, surgery is indicated.

Prior to labeling a patient as a treatment failure and escalating to more aggressive therapy, alternative explanations for the lack of response should be sought. Alternate diagnoses that may explain refractory disease include infection, medication effects (nonsteroidal anti-inflammatory drugs and antibiotics), medication noncompliance, irritable bowel syndrome, Crohn's disease, and, rarely, malignancy [46]. Common infections that should be excluded include *Clostridium difficile*, *Salmonella*, *Shigella*, *Campylobacter jejuni*, cytomegalovirus, and parasitic infections.

A minority of patients may experience a worsening of their colitis symptoms when mesalamine medications are initiated, due to a hypersensitivity to this class of medications. 5-ASA hypersensitivity is indistinguishable from a flare of acute colitis, almost always recurs with rechallenge, and patients experience rapid improvement with cessation of the offending medication [46].

Oral corticosteroids (40–60 mg/day prednisone) should be initiated in patients who do not respond to the above therapies or those with severe L-UC [1, 6]. Oral corticosteroid therapy is a well-established treatment for active UC and is effective in up to 75 % of patients. Prednisone therapy is usually initiated at a dose of 40 mg/day, which is continued for 1–2 weeks, or until symptomatic improvement is noted. This medication is generally tapered by a dose of 5–10 mg every 1–2 weeks, with more rapid reductions in dosage having been associated with earlier relapse [6]. During a course of oral corticosteroid therapy, oral and rectal 5-ASA medications may be continued, with the aim of maintaining long-term remission with these medications. If patients do not respond to a course of oral corticosteroids, intravenous corticosteroids are indicated [1, 6]. If patients require inpatient admission for intravenous corticosteroid therapy, 5-ASA products may be discontinued in order to avoid any possible contribution of 5-ASA hypersensitivity to the refractory symptoms.

For nonresponders to 3–5 days of intravenous corticosteroid therapy, cyclosporine and infliximab have been found to be effective treatments [47–49]. However, long-term usage of cyclosporine is limited by significant drug toxicities, and cyclosporine is often used as a bridge to an alternate maintenance therapy, such as azathioprine or 6-mercaptopurine. No studies have evaluated the efficacy of cyclosporine specifically in patients with L-UC. More recently, multiple controlled and uncontrolled studies have demonstrated the effectiveness of infliximab in patients with moderate-to-severe UC, and up to 56 % of the patients in these trials had L-UC [50–53]. However, in one of the larger randomized controlled trials of infliximab for UC, the rate of steroid-free remission at week 30 was only 21 % [50]. Infliximab is a treatment option in patients with steroid-refractory L-UC and can be continued as a maintenance therapy should patients experience clinical improvement, though long-term data in UC is sparse.

Laharie et al. compared cyclosporine to infliximab in patients with severe acute UC, refractory to 5 days of IV corticosteroids. Neither response rates, colectomy rates (day 98), nor adverse events significantly differed among patients receiving cyclosporine or infliximab rescue therapy. However, the a priori assumptions of the trial were for a 60 % failure rate in the infliximab group and a 30 % failure rate in the cyclosporine group, which may have affected study power [54].

Patients with severe disease, unresponsive to intravenous steroids, cyclosporine, or infliximab, should be considered for total proctocolectomy with ileal pouch-anal anastomosis (IPAA). Surgery for L-UC is less common than that for patients with extensive UC, with approximately 10–35 % of colectomies being performed in patients with L-UC [55]. Again, the treatment of severe colitis, as well as alternate medications (immunomodulators, cyclosporine, biologics), is discussed in more detail elsewhere.

Key points highlighting the evidence-based data for the treatment of active L-UC discussed above are detailed in Table 22.1.

## Treatment Recommendations for Active Left-Sided UC (Fig. 22.1)

Based on multiple clinical trials, as well as several meta-analyses, rectal 5-ASA should be the first-line therapy for L-UC. Enemas should be administered on a daily basis, in doses of 1–4 g. If patients achieve adequate clinical response,

**Table 22.1** Key points: treatment of active left-sided ulcerative colitis

- Rectally administered 5-ASA is the most effective therapy for active L-UC and can be continued as a maintenance therapy
- Topical corticosteroids are more effective than placebo for active L-UC but inferior to topical 5-ASA
- Newer topical corticosteroids (BDP, budesonide) are as effective as hydrocortisone, with fewer systemic side effects
- Rectal 5-ASA therapy is likely superior to oral 5-ASA therapy for active L-UC
- Combination rectal and oral 5-ASA therapy is superior to either agent alone
- A dose–response relationship has not been found with 5-ASA enema therapy
- 5-ASA nonresponders require oral corticosteroid therapy and are subsequently treated similarly to patients with severe extensive UC

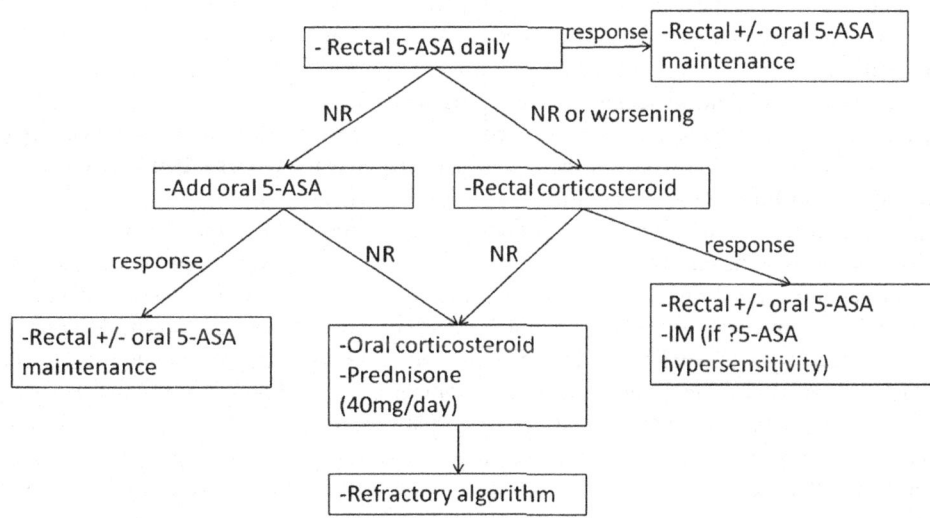

**Fig. 22.1** Treatment recommendations for active left-sided ulcerative colitis. *NR* nonresponse

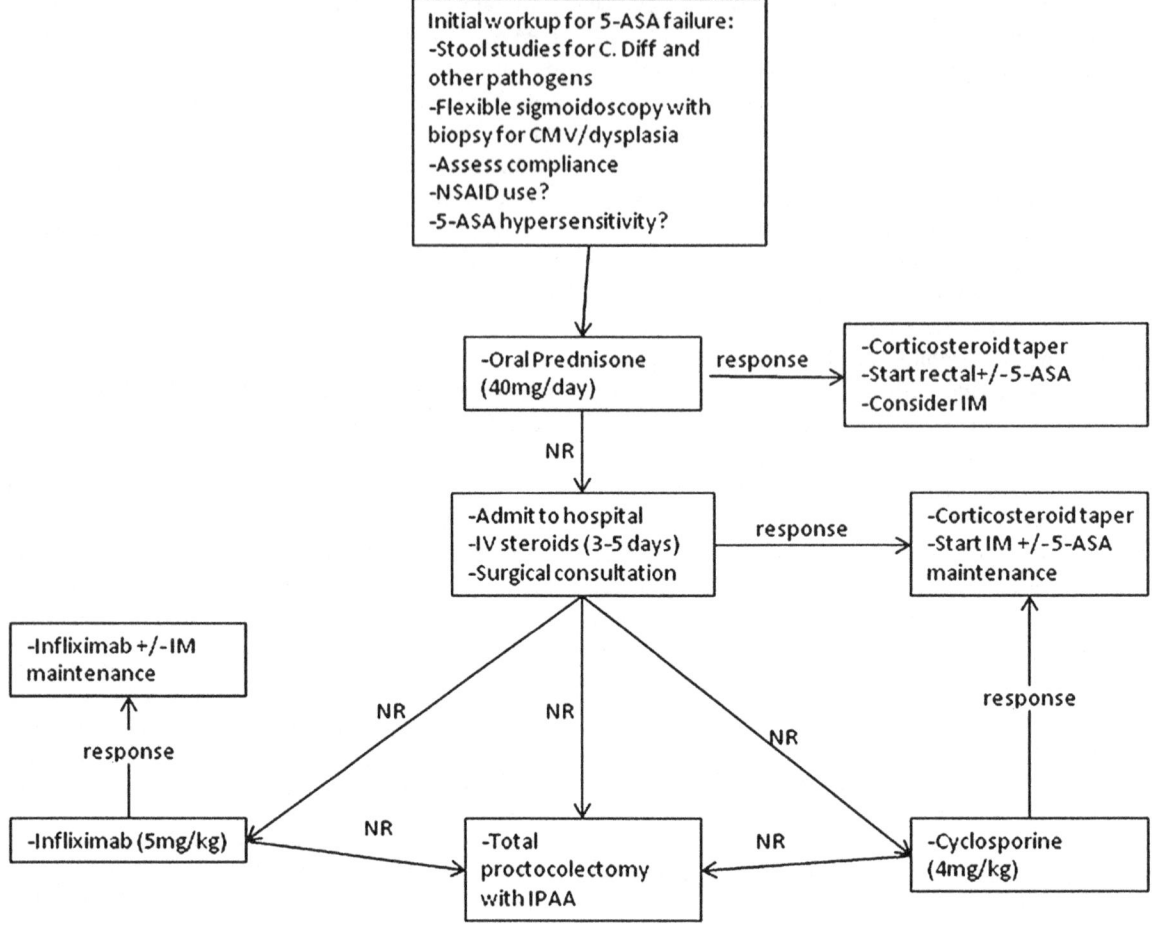

**Fig. 22.2** Steroid-refractory disease warrants hospital admission for further evaluation with stool studies, endoscopy with biopsies, and intravenous corticosteroid therapy. *NR* nonresponse, *NSAIDs* nonsteroidal anti-inflammatory drugs, *mg* milligrams, *IM* immunomodulation (azathioprine/6-MP), *IV* intravenous, *IPAA* ileal pouch-anal anastomosis

enemas may be continued for maintenance therapy, which will be discussed in the following sections. If patients do not demonstrate clinical improvement with rectal 5-ASA therapy, an oral 5-ASA medication may be added, in a dose of 2.4–4.8 g daily. In addition, switching to hydrocortisone enemas, at a dose of 100 mg daily, may be considered in rectal 5-ASA nonresponders after 2–4 weeks of therapy. If patients have a worsening of symptoms upon initiation of rectal 5-ASA therapy, these medications should be discontinued and corticosteroid enemas initiated.

In patients who do not respond to monotherapy with a rectal 5-ASA or corticosteroid, or an oral 5-ASA, combination therapy with an oral and rectal 5-ASA may lead to improved outcomes. However, patients who remain refractory to 5-ASA therapy and/or rectal corticosteroids should receive systemic corticosteroids. As detailed above, steroid-refractory disease warrants hospital admission for further

evaluation with stool studies, endoscopy with biopsies, and intravenous corticosteroid therapy (Fig. 22.2). Further therapy of severe L-UC parallels that of severe extensive UC.

## Maintenance Therapy for Left-Sided Ulcerative Colitis

In general, patients with ulcerative colitis, including L-UC, require long-term maintenance therapy following the induction of remission. All patients with L-UC are at risk for disease relapse. In addition to decreasing the risk of symptomatic relapse, maintenance therapy may also decrease the likelihood of proximal disease progression (though this has not been proven in an evidence-based fashion), as well as the development of colorectal cancer [5]. The lowest effective dose of the medication that induced remission is generally continued as a maintenance therapy, excluding corticosteroids, which are not effective medications for the maintenance of remission [1].

## 5-ASA Therapy

Both topical and oral 5-ASA medications have been shown to be effective for the maintenance of remission of L-UC [1, 6]. Often, topical 5-ASA therapy can be tapered during maintenance therapy. Studies have found that mesalamine enemas can maintain remission if used on an every other day or every third day schedule [1]. In a meta-analysis, 5-ASA enemas (4 g) had maintenance of remission rates of 78 %, slightly decreasing to 72 % for every other night dosing, and 65 % for every third night dosing, with no statistical difference being found between dosing intervals [9, 13]. The main difficulty with this approach is patient acceptance of long-term rectally administered therapy. In addition, topical 5-ASA at a dose of as low as 1 g daily has been shown to be effective as a maintenance therapy [6]. Additional studies have demonstrated 1-year remission rates of 52–92 %, with no differences being found between 2 and 4 g doses of rectal 5-ASA, which parallels findings from the induction studies [40].

In general, a dose of 2.4 g/day of oral 5-ASA has been shown to be effective for maintenance therapy. Maintenance rates ranged from 60 to 92 % for the various oral formulations, with no apparent dose response [9]. However, if patients require corticosteroids or higher doses of 5-ASA to induce remission, it is the authors' opinion that they may benefit from higher maintenance doses. If patients required combination therapy to induce remission, both medications should be continued during the maintenance phase.

Finally, studies have compared rectal and oral 5-ASA formulations for the maintenance of remission of L-UC. Mantzaris et al. compared every third night 5-ASA enemas to 1.5 g/day oral 5-ASA (thrice daily divided dosing) [56]. At 2 years, remission was maintained in 75 % of the patients in the enema group, compared to only 32 % of the oral 5-ASA group ($p < 0.001$). Topical 5-ASA maintenance therapy was found to be more efficacious than oral 5-ASA therapy, up to a 24-month end point, in a meta-analysis [7]. This meta-analysis included 3 studies comparing rectal and oral 5-ASA for the maintenance of remission of L-UC, with durations of therapy from 6 to 24 months. The POR for the maintenance of remission was 2.3 (1.1–4.8) in favor of topical therapy.

Finally, combination maintenance therapy utilizing rectal and oral 5-ASA formulations has been evaluated. D'Albasio et al. randomized 60 patients to receive either 4 g 5-ASA enema for the first 7 days each month or sulfasalazine (2 g daily) [57]. At a 2-year end point, there was no difference in relapse rate between the two groups. The same authors then randomized 72 patients to receive 1.6 g daily oral 5-ASA combined with twice weekly 5-ASA enemas (4 g) or oral 5-ASA plus a placebo enema [58]. The 1-year relapse rate in the combination therapy group was significantly less than in the monotherapy group (39 % vs. 69 %, $p < 0.036$).

For the maintenance of remission of L-UC, rectal 5-ASA therapy is superior to placebo and at least as efficacious as oral 5-ASA. In addition, oral and rectal combination maintenance therapy may be superior to either therapy alone.

## Corticosteroid Therapy

Multiple studies have shown corticosteroids to be an ineffective maintenance therapy for the maintenance of remission of UC [1, 6, 13]. In addition, these medications are associated with multiple well-described side effects, including hospitalization and mortality [59]. A randomized trial of oral corticosteroid maintenance therapy compared to placebo, for a treatment duration of 6 months, did not find any difference in remission rates, with approximately 40 % of each group being in remission [60]. Lindgren et al.'s study of different dosages of budesonide enemas included a maintenance phase to determine relapse rates [19]. By week 24, 40–50 % of patients in the corticosteroid enema group had experienced disease relapse, depending on dosing strategy. Clinical guidelines recommend against the use of corticosteroids for maintenance therapy in patients with UC, and the use of these medications should be limited due to their significant side effects and lack of efficacy [1, 6, 46].

## 5-ASA Nonresponse

For patients who cannot maintain remission with 5-ASA medications alone, either topical or oral, or who have corticosteroid-dependent disease, treatment should be escalated to an immunomodulator or biologic agent [1, 13]. As discussed above, corticosteroids are not effective for the maintenance of remission, and steroid-sparing medications are indicated for patients with moderate-to-severe disease that requires systemic corticosteroids to achieve remission.

Though there is not extensive data to support the effectiveness of immunomodulators for the treatment of active UC, these medications may be effective steroid-sparing maintenance medications [13, 61, 62]. Thiopurine therapy has been found to be superior to placebo in the maintenance of remission of UC, though there have been no comparative studies specifically evaluating these medications specifically in patients with L-UC [55, 62]. Studies have demonstrated the maintenance of remission rates for immunomodulators of approximately 65 % over 1 year, for UC [13]. In steroid-dependent UC patients, azathioprine was found to lead to higher rates of clinical and endoscopic remissions, as well as steroid cessation, compared to patients randomized to receive oral 5-ASA. However, at least four double-blind, randomized, placebo-controlled studies did not demonstrate benefit of azathioprine therapy compared to placebo in patients with steroid-dependent UC [13]. Finally, infliximab can be used for the maintenance of remission of L-UC, though there are few studies with follow-up past 52 weeks [1]. However, some guidelines do not recommend infliximab maintenance therapy for UC due to low corticosteroid-free remission rates after 1 year [6].

## Treatment Recommendations for the Maintenance of Remission of Left-Sided UC (Table 22.2)

Treatment options for the maintenance of remission of L-UC depend on the medication that was able to successfully induce remission. If remission was induced by a rectal or oral 5-ASA, these medications can be continued indefinitely, either as monotherapy or in combination. If compliance with rectal therapy is problematic, enema dosing for maintenance therapy can be recommended on an every other or every third night schedule. If topical corticosteroids were used to induce remission, therapy should be switched to a rectal and/or oral 5-ASA. If patients experience disease relapse on 5-ASA maintenance therapy, they should be treated as recommended in the induction of remission algorithm (Fig. 22.1). With disease relapse, special attention should be given to assessing for alternative causes of symptoms, including infection, noncompliance, etc.

**Table 22.2** Treatment algorithm for the maintenance of remission in patients with left-sided ulcerative colitis

| Induction medication | Maintenance medication options |
| --- | --- |
| 5-ASA (oral and/or rectal) | Rectal 5-ASA (every 2–3 days) |
| | Oral 5-ASA |
| | Combination rectal + oral 5-ASA |
| Rectal corticosteroid | Rectal 5-ASA (every 2–3 days) |
| | Oral 5-ASA |
| | Combination rectal + oral 5-ASA |
| Oral corticosteroid | Rectal ± oral 5-ASA |
| | IM (AZA/6-MP) |
| IV corticosteroid | Rectal ± oral 5-ASA (less likely) |
| | IM (AZA/6-MP) |
| | Infliximab ± IM |
| Cyclosporine | IM (AZA/6-MP) |
| | ?5-ASA |
| Infliximab | Infliximab ± IM (AZA/6-MP) |
| | ?5-ASA |

AZA = azathioprine, 6-MP = 6-mercaptopurine, IM = immunomodulator

Patients who require either oral or especially intravenous corticosteroids to achieve remission often require immunomodulator or biologic agents in order to maintain remission. However, it is worthwhile attempting treatment with maximum 5-ASA therapy prior to escalating therapy to an immunomodulator. In these cases, oral 5-ASA should be given in a dose of 4.8 g daily, and patients should also receive concomitant topical 5-ASA therapy. If patients relapse following an attempt at 5-ASA therapy and require an additional oral corticosteroid course, immunomodulators should be initiated and continued long term. Further treatment recommendations in these cases parallel those for extensive UC.

## Conclusions

Treatment strategies for L-UC differ from those for more extensive UC, in that topical therapies are able to deliver medication directly to the site of inflammation. Multiple studies have found rectal 5-ASA formulations to be superior to conventional corticosteroid enemas for the induction of remission. Additionally, rectal 5-ASA is more effective than oral 5-ASA, making rectal 5-ASA formulations the first-line treatment for patients with L-UC. These medications have also demonstrated efficacy in the maintenance of remission of L-UC.

While rectal corticosteroids can be considered in 5-ASA treatment failures, they are not effective for the maintenance of remission of L-UC. Oral 5-ASA may be more accepted by patients than rectal therapies, due to ease of administration, and has been found to be effective for both the induction and maintenance of remission in L-UC. Several studies have suggested that a combination therapy strategy, utilizing both rectal and oral 5-ASA, is more effective than monotherapy with either formulation [4, 31, 58].

The treatment of L-UC in patients who do not respond to either oral or rectal 5-ASA therapy or rectal steroids mirrors that of more extensive UC. Patients may require oral or intravenous corticosteroids to induce remission. Options for steroid-refractory patients include intravenous cyclosporine, infliximab, or surgery. If remission is achieved, immunomodulators or infliximab may be utilized for the maintenance of steroid-free remission. However, no studies have specifically evaluated these medications in patients with L-UC, and recommendations are based on the treatment guidelines for extensive UC.

## References

1. Kornbluth A, Sachar DB. Ulcerative colitis practice guidelines in adults: American College Of Gastroenterology. Practice Parameters Committee. Am J Gastroenterol. 2010;105(3):501–23. quiz 524.
2. Loftus Jr EV, Silverstein MD, Sandborn WJ, Tremaine WJ, Harmsen WS, Zinsmeister AR. Ulcerative colitis in Olmsted

County, Minnesota, 1940-1993: incidence, prevalence, and survival. Gut. 2000;46(3):336–43.

3. Nilsson A. Optimizing management of distal ulcerative colitis. Scand J Gastroenterol. 2006;41(5):511–23.

4. Loftus Jr EV. Clinical epidemiology of inflammatory bowel disease: incidence, prevalence, and environmental influences. Gastroenterology. 2004;126(6):1504–17.

5. Pica R, Paoluzi OA, Iacopini F, et al. Oral mesalazine (5-ASA) treatment may protect against proximal extension of mucosal inflammation in ulcerative proctitis. Inflamm Bowel Dis. 2004; 10(6):731–6.

6. Mowat C, Cole A, Windsor A, et al. Guidelines for the management of inflammatory bowel disease in adults. Gut. 2011;60(5): 571–607.

7. Marshall JK, Irvine EJ. Putting rectal 5-aminosalicylic acid in its place: the role in distal ulcerative colitis. Am J Gastroenterol. 2000;85(7):1628–36.

8. Sutherland LR, Martin F, Greer S, et al. 5-Aminosalicylic acid enema in the treatment of distal ulcerative colitis, proctosigmoiditis, and proctitis. Gastroenterology. 1987;92(6):1894–8.

9. Cohen RD, Woseth DM, Thisted RA, Hanauer SB. A meta-analysis and overview of the literature on treatment options for left-sided ulcerative colitis and ulcerative proctitis. Am J Gastroenterol. 2000;95(5):1263–76.

10. Marshall JK, Thabane M, Steinhart AH, Newman JR, Anand A, Irvine EJ. Rectal 5-aminosalicylic acid for induction of remission in ulcerative colitis. Cochrane Database Syst Rev. 2010;(1): CD004115.

11. Campieri M, Gionchetti P, Belluzzi A, et al. Optimum dosage of 5-aminosalicylic acid as rectal enemas in patients with active ulcerative colitis. Gut. 1991;32(8):929–31.

12. Campieri M, Gionchetti P, Belluzzi A. Sucralfate, 5-aminosalicylic acid, and placebo enemas in the treatment of distal ulcerative colitis. Eur J Gastroenterol Hepatol. 1991;3:41–4.

13. Regueiro M, Loftus Jr EV, Steinhart AH, Cohen RD. Medical management of left-sided ulcerative colitis and ulcerative proctitis: critical evaluation of therapeutic trials. Inflamm Bowel Dis. 2006;12(10):979–94.

14. Bar-Meir S, Fidder HH, Faszczyk M, et al. Budesonide foam vs. hydrocortisone acetate foam in the treatment of active ulcerative proctosigmoiditis. Dis Colon Rectum. 2003;46(7): 929–36.

15. Campieri M, Cottone M, Miglio F, et al. Beclomethasone dipropionate enemas versus prednisolone sodium phosphate enemas in the treatment of distal ulcerative colitis. Aliment Pharmacol Ther. 1998;12(4):361–6.

16. Hammond A, Andus T, Gierend M, Ecker KW, Scholmerich J, Herfarth H. Controlled, open, randomized multicenter trial comparing the effects of treatment on quality of life, safety and efficacy of budesonide foam and betamethasone enemas in patients with active distal ulcerative colitis. Hepatogastroenterology. 2004;51(59): 1345–9.

17. Marshall JK, Irvine EJ. Rectal corticosteroids versus alternative treatments in ulcerative colitis: a meta-analysis. Gut. 1997;40(6): 775–81.

18. Hanauer SB, Robinson M, Pruitt R, et al. Budesonide enema for the treatment of active, distal ulcerative colitis and proctitis: a dose-ranging study. U.S. Budesonide enema study group. Gastroenterology. 1998;115(3):525–32.

19. Lindgren S, Lofberg R, Bergholm L, et al. Effect of budesonide enema on remission and relapse rate in distal ulcerative colitis and proctitis. Scand J Gastroenterol. 2002;37(6):705–10.

20. Bianchi Porro G, Ardizzone S, Petrillo M, Fasoli A, Molteni P, Imbesi V. Low Pentasa dosage versus hydrocortisone in the topical treatment of active ulcerative colitis: a randomized, double-blind study. Am J Gastroenterol. 1995;90(5):736–9.

21. Lee FI, Jewell DP, Mani V, et al. A randomised trial comparing mesalazine and prednisolone foam enemas in patients with acute distal ulcerative colitis. Gut. 1996;38(2):229–33.

22. Friedman LS, Richter JM, Kirkham SE, DeMonaco HJ, May RJ. 5-Aminosalicylic acid enemas in refractory distal ulcerative colitis: a randomized, controlled trial. Am J Gastroenterol. 1986; 81(6):412–8.

23. Biancone L, Gionchetti P, Blanco Gdel V, et al. Beclomethasone dipropionate versus mesalazine in distal ulcerative colitis: a multicenter, randomized, double-blind study. Dig Liver Dis. 2007; 39(4):329–37.

24. Gionchetti P, D'Arienzo A, Rizzello F, et al. Topical treatment of distal active ulcerative colitis with beclomethasone dipropionate or mesalamine: a single-blind randomized controlled trial. J Clin Gastroenterol. 2005;39(4):291–7.

25. Manguso F, Balzano A. Meta-analysis: the efficacy of rectal beclomethasone dipropionate vs. 5-aminosalicylic acid in mild to moderate distal ulcerative colitis. Aliment Pharmacol Ther. 2007; 26(1):21–9.

26. Lemann M, Galian A, Rutgeerts P, et al. Comparison of budesonide and 5-aminosalicylic acid enemas in active distal ulcerative colitis. Aliment Pharmacol Ther. 1995;9(5):557–62.

27. Lamers CB, Wagtmans MJ, van der Sluys VA, van Hogezand RA, Griffioen G. Budesonide in inflammatory bowel disease. Neth J Med. 1996;48(2):60–3.

28. Kam L, Cohen H, Dooley C, Rubin P, Orchard J. A comparison of mesalamine suspension enema and oral sulfasalazine for treatment of active distal ulcerative colitis in adults. Am J Gastroenterol. 1996;91(7):1338–42.

29. Sandborn WJ, Hanauer S, Lichtenstein GR, Safdi M, Edeline M, Scott HM. Early symptomatic response and mucosal healing with mesalazine rectal suspension therapy in active distal ulcerative colitis - additional results from two controlled studies. Aliment Pharmacol Ther. 2011;34(7):747–56.

30. Prantera C, Viscido A, Biancone L, Francavilla A, Giglio L, Campieri M. A new oral delivery system for 5-ASA: preliminary clinical findings for MMx. Inflamm Bowel Dis. 2005;11(5):421–7.

31. Safdi M, DeMicco M, Sninsky C, et al. A double-blind comparison of oral versus rectal mesalamine versus combination therapy in the treatment of distal ulcerative colitis. Am J Gastroenterol. 1997; 92(10):1867–71.

32. Gionchetti P, Rizzello F, Venturi A, et al. Comparison of mesalazine suppositories in proctitis and distal proctosigmoiditis. Aliment Pharmacol Ther. 1997;11(6):1053–7.

33. Mulder CJ, Fockens P, Meijer JW, van der Heide H, Wiltink EH, Tytgat GN. Beclomethasone dipropionate (3 mg) versus 5-aminosalicylic acid (2 g) versus the combination of both (3 mg/2 g) as retention enemas in active ulcerative proctitis. Eur J Gastroenterol Hepatol. 1996;8(6):549–53.

34. Marteau P, Probert CS, Lindgren S, et al. Combined oral and enema treatment with Pentasa (mesalazine) is superior to oral therapy alone in patients with extensive mild/moderate active ulcerative colitis: a randomised, double blind, placebo controlled study. Gut. 2005;54(7):960–5.

35. Rizzello F, Gionchetti P, D'Arienzo A, et al. Oral beclomethasone dipropionate in the treatment of active ulcerative colitis: a double-blind placebo-controlled study. Aliment Pharmacol Ther. 2002; 16(6):1109–16.

36. Hanauer SB. Dose-ranging study of mesalamine (PENTASA) enemas in the treatment of acute ulcerative proctosigmoiditis: results of a multicentered placebo-controlled trial. The U.S. PENTASA Enema Study Group. Inflamm Bowel Dis. 1998;4(2):79–83.

37. Gionchetti P, Ardizzone S, Benvenuti ME, et al. A new mesalazine gel enema in the treatment of left-sided ulcerative colitis: a randomized controlled multicentre trial. Aliment Pharmacol Ther. 1999; 13(3):381–8.

38. Cortot A, Maetz D, Degoutte E, et al. Mesalamine foam enema versus mesalamine liquid enema in active left-sided ulcerative colitis. Am J Gastroenterol. 2008;103(12):3106–14.

39. Malchow H, Gertz B. A new mesalazine foam enema (Claversal Foam) compared with a standard liquid enema in patients with active distal ulcerative colitis. Aliment Pharmacol Ther. 2002; 16(3):415–23.

40. Harris MS, Lichtenstein GR. Review article: delivery and efficacy of topical 5-aminosalicylic acid (mesalazine) therapy in the treatment of ulcerative colitis. Aliment Pharmacol Ther. 2011;33(9): 996–1009.

41. Haghighi DB, Lashner BA. Left-sided ulcerative colitis. Gastroenterol Clin North Am. 2004;33(2):271–84. ix.

42. James SL, Irving PM, Gearry RB, Gibson PR. Management of distal ulcerative colitis: frequently asked questions analysis. Intern Med J. 2008;38(2):114–9.

43. Brain O, Travis SP. Therapy of ulcerative colitis: state of the art. Curr Opin Gastroenterol. 2008;24(4):469–74.

44. Hanauer SB, Sandborn WJ, Kornbluth A, et al. Delayed-release oral mesalamine at 4.8 g/day (800 mg tablet) for the treatment of moderately active ulcerative colitis: the ASCEND II trial. Am J Gastroenterol. 2005;100(11):2478–85.

45. D'Haens GR, Kovacs A, Vergauwe P, et al. Clinical trial: preliminary efficacy and safety study of a new Budesonide-MMX(R) 9 mg extended-release tablets in patients with active left-sided ulcerative colitis. J Crohns Colitis. 2010;4(2):153–60.

46. Regueiro M, Loftus Jr EV, Steinhart AH, Cohen RD. Clinical guidelines for the medical management of left-sided ulcerative colitis and ulcerative proctitis: summary statement. Inflamm Bowel Dis. 2006;12(10):972–8.

47. Cohen RD, Stein R, Hanauer SB. Intravenous cyclosporin in ulcerative colitis: a five-year experience. Am J Gastroenterol. 1999; 94(6):1587–92.

48. Lichtiger S, Present DH, Kornbluth A, et al. Cyclosporine in severe ulcerative colitis refractory to steroid therapy. N Engl J Med. 1994;330(26):1841–5.

49. Campbell S, Travis S, Jewell D. Ciclosporin use in acute ulcerative colitis: a long-term experience. Eur J Gastroenterol Hepatol. 2005;17(1):79–84.

50. Rutgeerts P, Sandborn WJ, Feagan BG, et al. Infliximab for induction and maintenance therapy for ulcerative colitis. N Engl J Med. 2005;353(23):2462–76.

51. Kohn A, Daperno M, Armuzzi A, et al. Infliximab in severe ulcerative colitis: short-term results of different infusion regimens and long-term follow-up. Aliment Pharmacol Ther. 2007;26(5): 747–56.

52. Probert CS, Hearing SD, Schreiber S, et al. Infliximab in moderately severe glucocorticoid resistant ulcerative colitis: a randomised controlled trial. Gut. 2003;52(7):998–1002.

53. Jarnerot G, Hertervig E, Friis-Liby I, et al. Infliximab as rescue therapy in severe to moderately severe ulcerative colitis: a randomized, placebo-controlled study. Gastroenterology. 2005;128(7): 1805–11.

54. Laharie D, Bourreille A, Branche J, et al. Cyclosporin versus infliximab in severe acute ulcerative colitis refractory to intravenous steroids: a randomized trial. Gastroenterology. 2011;140(5):S112.

55. Koutroubakis IE. Recent advances in the management of distal ulcerative colitis. World J Gastrointest Pharmacol Ther. 2010; 1(2):43–50.

56. Mantzaris GJ, Hatzis A, Petraki K, Spiliadi C, Triantaphyllou G. Intermittent therapy with high-dose 5-aminosalicylic acid enemas maintains remission in ulcerative proctitis and proctosigmoiditis. Dis Colon Rectum. 1994;37(1):58–62.

57. d'Albasio G, Trallori G, Ghetti A, et al. Intermittent therapy with high-dose 5-aminosalicylic acid enemas for maintaining remission in ulcerative proctosigmoiditis. Dis Colon Rectum. 1990; 33(5):394–7.

58. d'Albasio G, Pacini F, Camarri E, et al. Combined therapy with 5-aminosalicylic acid tablets and enemas for maintaining remission in ulcerative colitis: a randomized double-blind study. Am J Gastroenterol. 1997;92(7):1143–7.

59. Lichtenstein GR, Feagan BG, Cohen RD, et al. Serious infections and mortality in association with therapies for Crohn's disease: TREAT registry. Clin Gastroenterol Hepatol. 2006;4(5):621–30.

60. Lennard-Jones JE, Misiewicz JJ, Connell AM, Baron JH, Jones FA. Prednisone as maintenance treatment for ulcerative colitis in remission. Lancet. 1965;1(7378):188–9.

61. Timmer A, McDonald JW, Macdonald JK. Azathioprine and 6-mercaptopurine for maintenance of remission in ulcerative colitis. Cochrane Database Syst Rev. 2007; (1):CD000478.

62. Gisbert JP, Linares PM, McNicholl AG, Mate J, Gomollon F. Meta-analysis: the efficacy of azathioprine and mercaptopurine in ulcerative colitis. Aliment Pharmacol Ther. 2009;30(2): 126–37.

Seamus J. Murphy and Asher Kornbluth

**Keywords**

Severe • Ulcerative colitis • Treatment • Assessment score • Investigation • Monitoring • Corticosteroids • Cyclosporine • 6-Mercaptopurine/azathioprine • Infliximab antibiotics • Parenteral nutrition • Surgery • Fulminant colitis • Toxic megacolon

## Definitions and Assessing Severity

Severe ulcerative colitis (UC) was first defined by Truelove and Witts in 1955 using six simple criteria without any requirement for a sigmoidoscopic examination—six or more stools per day with one of the following: large amounts of blood, fever >37.8 °C, tachycardia >90, ESR > 30 mm/h, and hemoglobin <10.5 g/dl. These criteria are easily measured and have stood the test of time over half a century [1]. The Mayo Clinic Index (with slight variations also known as the Sutherland Index or the UC Disease Activity Index) has become a frequently used scoring index in clinical trials and includes sigmoidoscopic appearance and the physician's global assessment. Another score known as the Modified Truelove-Witts Scoring Index, or the Lichtiger score, has been used most frequently in patients with intravenous (IV) corticosteroid-refractory UC. The Lichtiger score includes assessments for nocturnal bowel movements, incontinence, abdominal pain, cramping and tenderness, and the overall sense of "well-being." While all of these scores list the salient features defining disease activity, the term "severe

ulcerative colitis" as used in this chapter will refer to those patients with ongoing frequent bloody diarrhea with systemic signs and/or symptoms that significantly limit the patient's quality of life and who fail to improve with maximal outpatient therapies and require hospitalization for further management.

Toxic megacolon refers to patients with dilation of the colon of >6 cm diameter associated with severe systemic toxicity. It is important to recognize that patients may present with toxicity without colonic dilation and are still at graver risk than patients with severe colitis without toxicity. Fulminant colitis is defined as any colitis that, in addition to the features of severe colitis, becomes rapidly worse, usually manifesting as severe abdominal pain and continuous bleeding requiring multiple transfusions. Medical therapy is inappropriate in fulminant colitis, and colectomy is the only suitable treatment.

## Management: Investigations and Monitoring

The immediate goals of therapy are to reduce the signs and symptoms of the severe acute attack, allow the taper of corticosteroids, and initiate a strategy to achieve a long-term corticosteroid-free remission. The primary goal is *not* the avoidance of surgery. This is important to emphasize that the mortality from severe UC reduced dramatically from 24 to 7 % with the introduction of IV corticosteroids in the 1960s. Now the mortality in most units should be <1 %, and this reduction over the last 50 years is almost exclusively due to timely and expert surgical input. Close collaboration with a surgeon is therefore essential.

S.J. Murphy, F.R.C.P., Ph.D. (✉)
Department of Medicine, Daisy Hill Hospital,
5 Hospital Road, Newry, Co., Down, N. Ireland, UK
e-mail: seamus.murphy2@southerntrust.hscni.net

A. Kornbluth, M.D.
The Henry D. Janowitz Division of Gastroenterology,
The Icahn School of Medicine at Mount Sinai,
1751 York Ave., New York 10128, NY, USA
e-mail: asher.kornbluth@gmail.com

A sigmoidoscopy is done to assess disease severity and obtain biopsies to exclude a superimposed etiology, e.g., infection with *Clostridium difficile* (*C. difficile*) and cytomegalovirus (CMV). A full colonoscopy incurs the risk of perforation in these patients, so an unprepped sigmoidoscopy with minimal air insufflation is sufficient and yields the information required at that moment in time to correctly manage the patient.

The incidence of *C. difficile* in hospitalized patients with UC is rising dramatically and results in increased length of stay and morbidity and mortality [2]. The diagnosis is challenging because patients with severe UC may not have the usual risk factors of antibiotic exposure or recent hospitalization, pseudomembranes are generally not seen at sigmoidoscopy, and if stool toxin assays are relied upon, multiple stool specimens may be necessary before the infection is confirmed. The use of a polymerase chain reaction test for *C. difficile* significantly reduces false-negative results [3].

CMV superinfection may occur in severe colitis and should be considered in the patient who is not responding to maximal immunosuppressive therapy. The diagnosis can be confirmed with sigmoidoscopic biopsy and viral culture; treatment with ganciclovir may lead to clinical improvement. Evidence of CMV disease can be found in 30 % of cases of severe colitis and its exact role continues to be debated [4]. However, in the patient with fulminant colitis with continuing deterioration, colectomy should not be deferred while awaiting a possible response to treatment for CMV infection.

A plain abdominal film should be performed on admission. Not only will this detect a megacolon but also more subtle radiographic findings of increased small intestinal gas, which predicts a greater likelihood of failure of medical therapy [5]. Any complaints of increasing abdominal pain or distention, especially in a febrile patient, should prompt a CT scan of the abdomen and pelvis to detect subtle signs of colonic perforation, which may be first seen as air within the wall of the colon. The presence of these findings should be followed by emergent subtotal colectomy. In general, medications with anticholinergic or narcotic properties should be avoided because of the theoretical risk of reducing bowel tone and worsening colonic dilatation.

## Corticosteroids

IV corticosteroids have been the mainstay of treatment for acute severe colitis for over 50 years [1]. Patients are treated with IV hydrocortisone 100 mg three times daily or an equivalent dose of an alternative IV corticosteroid. There is no benefit to treatment with a higher daily dose of corticosteroids, which exposes the patient to a higher risk of side effects without increased rate of success. There is no benefit to continuous IV corticosteroid infusion compared to bolus dosing three times daily. Historically, almost half of patients with severe colitis did not respond to high-dose IV corticosteroids and required colectomy [6]. The colectomy rate for severe UC has remained consistent over the last 40 years [7].

More recently, it has been recognized that by day 3 of IV corticosteroids, there is a high rate of colectomy in those patients with continued bleeding and greater than six bowel movements daily, elevated CRP, or fevers [8, 9]. These patients, as well as patients who are not decisively improved by days 5–7, should be offered IV cyclosporine, infliximab, or surgery.

## Cyclosporine

IV cyclosporine is effective therapy in severe colitis. Multiple series have replicated the 80 % immediate response rate in hospitalized patients failing IV corticosteroids first demonstrated by Lichtiger et al. [10]. Van Assche and colleagues found no difference in efficacy when they compared IV cyclosporine 2–4 mg/kg [11]. It is thought that cyclosporine levels of approximately 200–400 µg/ml are therapeutic during the IV phase. The median time to response is 4 days [12], and predictive factors for failure to respond to cyclosporine include persistent fevers, tachycardia, elevated CRP, hypoalbuminemia, and deep colonic ulcerations [13].

Cyclosporine should only be used by clinicians experienced with its use and who have access to drug level monitoring. Contraindications to its use include active infection, uncontrolled hypertension, renal impairment, and unreliable patients since frequent physician visits are required following discharge from hospital. More common but less severe side effects include paresthesias, hypertension, hypertrichosis, headache, abnormal liver function tests, hyperkalemia, and gingival hyperplasia [14]. Renal function must be monitored closely and serum cholesterol and magnesium should be checked. Low levels of either increase the risk of neurotoxicity, including seizures. Patients with low levels of cholesterol (cholesterol < 120 mg/dl or 3 mmol/l) should be started on lower doses of cyclosporine (or avoid cyclosporine and use infliximab instead, see below), and cholesterol and cyclosporine levels should be monitored daily.

During intervals of triple immunosuppression with corticosteroids, cyclosporine, and thiopurine, we give patients prophylaxis against *Pneumocystis jiroveci* (*carinii*) with trimethoprim/sulfamethoxazole 960 mg daily. Serious infections during the IV cyclosporine phase may be due to the concomitant use of corticosteroids rather than the serum level of cyclosporine.

For transitioning to oral cyclosporine before hospital discharge, the IV dose the patient was receiving at the end of the IV phase is doubled and is given in two divided doses daily and generally aiming for trough oral cyclosporine levels of 100–250 μg/ml. In addition, treatment with a thiopurine (6-mercaptopurine or azathioprine) is continued or initiated, and the patient is started on a weekly corticosteroid taper. Failure to taper the prednisone and cyclosporine by 3–6 months is considered a failure. Patients who have already been treated unsuccessfully with an adequate course of a thiopurine prior to cyclosporine are less likely to maintain a long-term remission after the discontinuation of cyclosporine.

## 6-Mercaptopurine/Azathioprine

Multiple open-label series have demonstrated long-term success with initiating thiopurine therapy during the oral cyclosporine phase in those patients not previously exposed to thiopurines. However, the long-term success rate is lower in those patients who have previously failed adequate courses of thiopurine therapy [15, 16]. In the largest series to date, 83 % of 142 patients had an initial response to cyclosporine and avoided colectomy during hospitalization [16]. Of the 118 patients who responded, 41 (35 %) required a future colectomy. The rate of colectomy in those already taking azathioprine compared with those not previously exposed to azathioprine was 59 % vs. 31 %, respectively. Life-table analysis demonstrated that although only 33 % of patients required colectomy at 1 year, 88 % required colectomy at 7 years.

For patients who have a complete remission in response to cyclosporine and then have a relapse months or years later, a second course of IV cyclosporine followed by oral cyclosporine may be a successful strategy. In 32 patients who flared a mean of 24 months after their initial cyclosporine-induced remission, 44 % avoided colectomy at 3 years after the second course of cyclosporine [17]. Predictors of higher rate of colectomy in these patients were hypoalbuminemia and the presence of *C. difficile.*

## Infliximab

There are limited controlled trial data regarding the role of infliximab in patients with severe UC refractory to IV corticosteroids. In one double-blind series, 45 patients who were naïve to infliximab and refractory to IV corticosteroids, with either fulminant colitis at day 3 or severe colitis at days 6–8, were randomized to either a single dose of infliximab 5 mg/kg or placebo [18]. At day 90, 29 % of infliximab-treated patients with predefined *severe* colitis had undergone colectomy vs. 67 % of placebo-treated patients. In patients with *fulminant* colitis, 47 % of infliximab-treated patients underwent colectomy, compared to 69 % of placebo-treated patients. Long-term follow-up of these patients suggested a continued benefit from a single infusion of infliximab even

after 3 years [19] with lower colectomy rates in infliximab compared to placebo-treated patients (50 % and 76 %, respectively). However, most of the benefit of infliximab occurred in the first 3 months. In fact, five patients in the infliximab group required colectomy during the long-term follow-up period (i.e., after 3 months and before 3 years) compared to only two in the placebo group. It is possible that a single dose of infliximab may have simply delayed colectomy in the treated patients, leading to more infliximab-treated patients requiring colectomy later on. However, infliximab is rarely given as a single infusion, more commonly being given as three induction doses at 0, 2, and 6 weeks. A retrospective series of severe colitic patients treated with infliximab reported a 50 % colectomy rate at 5 years [20]. Forty percent of patients in this series had more than one infusion. The true long-term benefit of infliximab is unknown, and we think that any strategy involving infliximab will require maintenance infliximab treatment and/or thiopurine therapy.

## Infliximab or Cyclosporine as Rescue Therapy?

As discussed above, patients who have previously been intolerant of, or failed to respond to, thiopurine therapy should be offered infliximab preferentially since a large part of the cyclosporine strategy relies on transitioning to thiopurine so that cyclosporine can be stopped after 3–6 months. In contrast, infliximab can be continued as maintenance therapy in those patients who respond to it.

An open-label clinical (CYSIF) trial comparing cyclosporine with infliximab in corticosteroid-refractory severe UC found similar response rates and similar adverse event rates among 115 trial participants [21]. Treatment failure occurred in 60 % patients given cyclosporine and 54 % given infliximab ($p=0.52$), while 16 % of patients in the cyclosporine group and 25 % in the infliximab group had severe adverse events. There are no trial data to support the use of other anti-TNF agents (adalimumab and golimumab) in corticosteroid-refractory severe UC.

## Immediate and Delayed Sequential Use of Cyclosporine and Infliximab

The immediate sequential use of one of these drugs in the event of failure of the first drug has been studied. A series reported findings among 19 patients who were treated with cyclosporine followed by infliximab (ten patients) or infliximab followed by cyclosporine (nine patients), with either agent being used within 30 days of the other [22]. The 1-year remission rates were low in both groups at 40 % and 33 %, respectively.

Serious adverse events occurred in three patients (16 %), including one death due to septicemia. A Spanish group reported their experience among 47 patients treated with infliximab within 1 month of discontinuation of cyclosporine [23]. They reported an immediate colectomy rate of 30 % among this group of patients and one death from sepsis. The French GETAID group reported a colectomy-free survival of 61 % at 3 months and 41 % at 12 months among 86 patients [24]. There was wide variation in timing of the second drug after failure of the first (range 7–163 days). One death and nine infectious complications were reported. It may therefore be inadvisable to use cyclosporine and infliximab or vice versa within 1 month of each other given the limited long-term success and the potential for serious toxicity.

Delayed sequential use of infliximab (at least *1 month after* discontinuation of the other drug) appears to be a more acceptable strategy. In a small series among 11 patients, a corticosteroid-free remission occurred in over 64 % of these patients at 1 year and without any serious adverse events when these two drugs were used in this fashion [25]. Delayed use of cyclosporine after infliximab failure, on the other hand, only resulted in 25 % (two of eight patients) of patients achieving a steroid-free remission.

## Aminosalicylates

There are no studies to demonstrate that oral aminosalicylates are of clinical benefit in severe colitis, so we have a low threshold for stopping them if the patient has difficulty taking them, but they may be continued if the patient is eating and can tolerate them. Likewise, no controlled studies have confirmed any incremental benefit of rectal medications in this setting, but we still often prescribe them if they can be retained and tolerated, as they help the symptoms of urgency and incontinence, which many patients find distressing.

## Antibiotics

In the absence of any proven infection, controlled trials of antibiotics have demonstrated no therapeutic benefit from the use of oral vancomycin, intravenous metronidazole, or ciprofloxacin when added to IV corticosteroids. However, protocols outlining treatment regimens for severe colitis generally include broad-spectrum antibiotics for patients with signs of toxicity or with worsening symptoms despite maximal medical therapy [26]. Antibiotics should be initiated (with coverage for gram negative and anaerobic enteric infections) in the presence of fever or other signs of toxicity, but these may be stopped after 48 h if negative blood and stool culture results return.

## Parenteral Nutrition

Controlled studies showed no benefit from total parenteral nutrition (TPN) as a primary therapy for UC [27]. There is no evidence that maintaining oral nutrition is harmful, and it should be continued in patients who can tolerate it, with the exception of patients with colonic dilatation. However, TPN may be useful as a nutritional adjunct in patients with significant nutritional depletion. Those patients with limited expectations of restoring adequate nutritional status and especially in those patients who have a high likelihood of failure of medical therapy and requiring imminent surgery are started on TPN early in their hospital course.

## Venous Thromboembolism

This potentially lethal complication occurs approximately twice as frequently in hospitalized UC patients compared to hospitalized controls [28]. For this reason, prophylactic subcutaneous heparin is mandatory for all patients with severe colitis, and the presence of frequent rectal bleeding should not dissuade the clinician of this. Thrombotic events may occur in atypical locations, e.g., portal veins, upper extremities, at sites of IV cannulae, the central nervous system, and in both arterial and venous circulations. For the patient with a series of thrombotic or embolic events during a course of severe colitis, emergent colectomy may be potentially life-saving in preventing additional, potentially fatal thrombi.

## Fulminant Colitis and Toxic Megacolon

Patients with fulminant colitis or toxic megacolon should be treated as above; in addition they should be kept NPO, a nasogastric tube or small bowel decompression tube should be considered if a small bowel ileus is present, particularly in patients with vomiting, and the patients should be instructed to rotate frequently into the prone or knee-elbow [29] position to aid in evacuation of bowel gas. A baseline CT should be obtained and followed with daily abdominal x-rays. Broad-spectrum antibiotics are generally used empirically in these patients. The duration of medical treatment of megacolon is controversial; some experts advocate surgery within 72 h if no significant improvement is noted [30], while we may take a more watchful stance if no toxic symptoms are present. However, if there are any clinical, laboratory, or radiologic deterioration on medical therapy, we proceed to emergent subtotal colectomy.

## Surgery

Absolute indications for surgery are exsanguinating hemorrhage and frank or suspected perforation. Perforation occurs in 2–3 % of hospitalized UC patients at tertiary referral centers. It is essential to recognize that perforation can occur without being preceded by megacolon and that the initial signs can be masked by corticosteroid use. The surgical procedure of choice is a subtotal colectomy with either a rectosigmoid mucous fistula or Hartmann's closure. In experienced hands, a laparoscopic approach is not contraindicated if this can be carried out in an expedient fashion.

Patients should be informed of the various *future* operations available, i.e., total proctocolectomy with permanent ileostomy vs. the ileal pouch-anal anastomosis (IPAA) procedure. IPAA has become the most commonly performed operation for UC and is performed in 1, 2, or 3 stages, but in the patient undergoing urgent colectomy for acute severe colitis, the construction of the ileoanal pouch should always be deferred to a future date, when the patient has been tapered from corticosteroids and has been restored to good health.

## References

1. Truelove SC, Witts LJ. Cortisone in ulcerative colitis; final report on a therapeutic trial. Br Med J. 1955;2(4947):1041–8.
2. Issa M, Vijayapal A, Graham MB, et al. Impact of Clostridium difficile on inflammatory bowel disease. Clin Gastroenterol Hepatol. 2007;5(3):345–51.
3. Peterson LR, Manson RU, Paule SM, et al. Detection of toxigenic Clostridium difficile in stool samples by real-time polymerase chain reaction for the diagnosis of C. difficile associated diarrhea. Clin Infect Dis. 2007;45(9):1152–60.
4. Lawlor G, Moss AC. Cytomegalovirus in inflammatory bowel disease: pathogen or innocent bystander? Inflamm Bowel Dis. 2010;16(9):1620–7.
5. Caprilli R, Vernia P, Latella G, et al. Early recognition of toxic megacolon. J Clin Gastroenterol. 1987;9(2):160–4.
6. Gustavsson A, Halfvarson J, Magnuson A, et al. Long-term colectomy rate after intensive intravenous corticosteroid therapy for ulcerative colitis prior to the immunosuppressive treatment era. Am J Gastroenterol. 2007;102(11):2513–9.
7. Turner D, Walsh CM, Steinhart AH, et al. Response to corticosteroids in severe ulcerative colitis: a systematic review of the literature and a metaregression. Clin Gastroenterol Hepatol. 2007;5:103–10.
8. Ho GT, Mowat C, Goddard CJ, et al. Predicting the outcome of severe ulcerative colitis: development of a novel risk score to aid early selection of patients for second-line medical therapy or surgery. Aliment Pharmacol Ther. 2004;19(10):1079–87.
9. Seo M, Okada M, Yao T, et al. An index of disease activity in patients with ulcerative colitis. Am J Gastroenterol. 1992;87(8):971–6.
10. Lichtiger S, Present DH, Kornbluth A, et al. Cyclosporine in severe ulcerative colitis refractory to steroid therapy. N Engl J Med. 1994;330(26):1841–5.
11. Van Assche G, D'Haens G, Noman M, et al. Randomized, double-blind comparison of 4 mg/kg versus 2 mg/kg intravenous cyclosporine in severe ulcerative colitis. Gastroenterology. 2003;125(4):1025–31.
12. D'Haens G, Lemmens L, Geboes K, et al. Intravenous cyclosporine versus intravenous corticosteroids as single therapy for severe attacks of ulcerative colitis. Gastroenterology. 2001;120:1323–9.
13. Cacheux W, Seksik P, Lemann M, et al. Predictive factors of response to cyclosporine in steroid-refractory ulcerative colitis. Am J Gastroenterol. 2008;103(3):637–42.
14. Sternthal MB, Murphy SJ, George J, et al. Adverse events associated with the use of cyclosporine in patients with inflammatory bowel disease. Am J Gastroenterol. 2008;103(4):937–43.
15. Cohen RD, Stein R, Hanauer SB. Intravenous cyclosporin in ulcerative colitis: a five-year experience. Am J Gastroenterol. 1999;94(6):1587–92.
16. Moskovitz DN, Van Assche G, Maenhout B, et al. Incidence of colectomy during long-term follow-up after cyclosporine-induced remission of severe ulcerative colitis. Clin Gastroenterol Hepatol. 2006;4(6):760–5.
17. Sauk J, Present DH, Kornbluth A, et al. Outcomes after cyclosporine retreatment in hospitalized ulcerative colitis patients: a 7-year review from a single institution (abstract DDW). Gastroenterology. 2009;136:A-87.
18. Jarnerot G, Hertervig E, Friis-Liby I, et al. Infliximab as rescue therapy in severe to moderately severe ulcerative colitis: a randomized, placebo-controlled study. Gastroenterology. 2005;128(7):1805–11.
19. Gustavsson A, Järnerot G, Hertervig E, et al. Clinical trial: colectomy after rescue therapy in ulcerative colitis—3-year follow-up of the Swedish-Danish controlled infliximab study. Aliment Pharmacol Ther. 2010;32(8):984–9.
20. Lees CW, Heys D, Ho GT, et al. A retrospective analysis of the efficacy and safety of infliximab as rescue therapy in acute severe ulcerative colitis. Aliment Pharmacol Ther. 2007;26(3):411–9.
21. Laharie D, Bourreille A, Branche J, et al. Cyclosporine versus infliximab in patients with severe ulcerative colitis refractory to intravenous steroids: a parallel open label randomized controlled trial. Lancet. 2012;380(9857):1909–15.
22. Maser EA, Deconda D, Lichtiger S, et al. Cyclosporine and infliximab as rescue therapy for each other in patients with steroid refractory ulcerative colitis. Clin Gastroenterol Hepatol. 2008;6(10):1112–6.
23. Chaparro M, Burgueño P, Iglesias E, et al. Infliximab salvage therapy after failure of ciclosporin in corticosteroid-refractory ulcerative colitis: a multicentre study. Aliment Pharmacol Ther. 2012;35(2):275–83.
24. Leblanc S, Allez M, Seksik P, et al. Successive treatment with cyclosporine and infliximab in steroid-refractory ulcerative colitis. Am J Gastroenterol. 2011;106(4):771–7.
25. Katz J, Maser EA, Ullman T, et al. Cyclosporine and infliximab as delayed salvage therapy for each other in patients with steroid-refractory ulcerative colitis (abstract DDW). Gastroenterology 2009.
26. Truelove SC, Jewell DP. Intensive intravenous regimen for severe attacks of ulcerative colitis. Lancet. 1974;1(7866):1067–70.
27. Dickinson RJ, Ashton MG, Axon AT, et al. Controlled trial of intravenous hyperalimentation and total bowel rest as an adjunct to the routine therapy of acute colitis. Gastroenterology. 1980;79(6):1199–204.
28. Present DH, Wolfson D, Gelernt IM, et al. Medical decompression of toxic megacolon by "rolling". A new technique of decompression with favorable long-term follow-up. J Clin Gastroenterol. 1988;10(5):485–90.
29. Kappelman MD, Horvath-Puho E, Sandler RS, et al. Thromboembolic risk among Danish children and adults with inflammatory bowel diseases: a population-based nationwide study. Gut. 2011;60(7):937–43.
30. Truelove SC, Marks CG. Toxic megacolon. Part I: pathogenesis, diagnosis and treatment. Clin Gastroenterol. 1981;10(1):107–17.

# Pregnancy and Fertility in Ulcerative Colitis

Kim L. Isaacs

**Keywords**

Pregnancy • Fertility • Ulcerative colitis • Inheritance • Surgery • Medical therapy • Aminosalicylates • Corticosteroids • Azathioprine/6-mercaptopurine • Methotrexate • Cyclosporine/tacrolimus • Biologics • Breastfeeding • Ileoanal pouch

## Introduction

Ulcerative colitis is a disease that has its peak incidence during the second and third decades of life which are also the prime childbearing years for men and women. As a result, there are multiple concerns that patients have regarding the ability to get pregnant, the advisability of childbearing, disease activity during pregnancy, medication use during pregnancy, and the possibility of passing ulcerative colitis to their offspring. This chapter will review the current data available on these issues.

## Fertility

Fertility is the ability to conceive and become pregnant through normal sexual activity. Infertility is defined as a failure to conceive after a year of unprotected intercourse in women under the age of 35 [1]. The background rate of infertility in the noninflammatory bowel disease (IBD) population is approximately 14 % which accounts for one in seven couples. In women with ulcerative colitis, who have not had surgery, fertility rates are similar to the non-IBD population. Hudson and colleagues found in a Scottish ulcerative colitis population that there was a 13 % infertility rate

in a medically treated IBD population compared to 14 % in the control population [2]. There was a high rate of patients choosing not to conceive (21 %). In a US study, there was a 2–4 % incidence of involuntary childlessness or secondarily infertile women in both the UC and control groups and a 15–20 % rate of pregnancy that required more than 1 year of attempts to conceive [3]. Similarly to the Scottish study, there was a higher level of voluntary childlessness in patients with UC (21 %) compared to controls (14 %). Voluntary childlessness may be multifactorial including advice from health-care providers to avoid pregnancy, disease activity, fear of passing on ulcerative colitis to a child, and medication concerns.

Surgery does adversely affect fertility in patients with ulcerative colitis. In the Hudson study, there was a 30 % rate of infertility in the patients that had surgical therapy for ulcerative colitis [2]. In most cases, infertility was related to tubal factors including adhesions related to surgery. This study included a small number of patients in whom most of the surgical intervention was total abdominal colectomy with end ileostomy. In the 1980s, there was a transition of surgical therapy for ulcerative colitis to a restorative proctocolectomy (RPC) with ileal pouch-anal anastomosis (IPAA). Olsen and colleagues studied the fecundability of 290 women before and after RPC with IPAA compared to a non-IBD population. Fecundability is the ability to conceive per menstrual cycle with unprotected intercourse. In this study, the fecundability ratio dropped from 1.01 before surgery to 0.20 ($p < 0.001$) after surgery [4]. These findings have been confirmed in several meta-analyses which demonstrate that the average infertility rate after RPC with IPAA is in the range of 48–63 % [5, 6]. The risk of infertility after IPAA increases

K.L. Isaacs, M.D., Ph.D. (✉)
Department of Gastroenterology and Hepatology, University of North Carolina at Chapel Hill, CB3 7032, Room 7200 MBRB, Chapel Hill, NC 27599-7032, USA
e-mail: klisaacs@med.unc.edu

G.R. Lichtenstein (ed.), *Medical Therapy of Ulcerative Colitis*,
DOI 10.1007/978-1-4939-1677-1_24, © Springer Science+Business Media New York 2014

three- to fourfold as compared to the medically treated and control populations [5, 6]. The cause of the infertility is thought to be due to pelvic adhesions related to the surgery with one study showing abnormal tubal anatomy in 14 out of 21 patients studied with hysterosalpingography (HSG) after RPC [7]. Despite these findings, only a small percentage of patients experiencing infertility after RPC are referred for fertility treatments [8]. There is a small amount of evidence that an ileorectal anastomosis (IRA) may preserve female fertility in patients with ulcerative colitis who require surgery for management [9].

Male infertility in ulcerative colitis is less well studied. In one small study, 62 men with ulcerative colitis were compared to 140 controls with the mean number of pregnancies not statistically different in the two populations [10]. Fecundability was the same in the ulcerative colitis and control populations. Drugs may significantly affect semen quality and subsequently fertility in men with ulcerative colitis. Sulfasalazine causes oligospermia and leads to male infertility in patients treated with this for ulcerative colitis [11]. Other medications used for the treatment of ulcerative colitis may also affect sperm quality and will be discussed later in this chapter. In patients with Crohn's disease, disease activity and poor nutritional status are associated with abnormal semen quality. This likely can be extrapolated to patients with ulcerative colitis suggesting that patients whose disease is in remission are more likely to have healthy sperm and therapy improved chances at conception [12]. Men who undergo RPC with IPAA for ulcerative colitis may develop erectile dysfunction and retrograde ejaculation which may affect fertility [13]. However, at least one study demonstrated that male sexual function improved after IPAA [14].

## Inheritance

The etiology of inflammatory bowel disease is multifactorial with genetic predisposition playing a major role in the development of IBD. Genetic susceptibility appears to be associated with the interaction of gut commensal microbiota and the host [15]. Patients with IBD often are concerned about passing the disease to their children. This concern often plays a role in the decision to have children. There are now multiple studies looking at the role of gene variants in the development of inflammatory bowel disease [15].

If a single parent is affected with ulcerative colitis, the risks of their children developing UC are 2–15 times higher than in the general population [16]. This transmission risk is slightly less than if the parent had Crohn's disease. The absolute risk of developing IBD for a child with a single parent affected with ulcerative colitis ranges from 2.9 to 11 % [16]. If both parents are affected with inflammatory bowel disease, the risk to the child of developing IBD is 36 % over their lifetime [17]. Twin studies have also demonstrated increased genetic susceptibility for ulcerative colitis with monozygotic twins that were 49 % concordant (95 % CI 35.7, 63.3). The corresponding risk for dizygotic twins is not elevated for ulcerative colitis although it is elevated for twins with Crohn's disease [18]. There are some families that have multiple family members affected with IBD in which the genetic susceptibility/risk will be much higher for first-degree relatives of the proband. These risk factors should all be taken into consideration when counseling a patient on pregnancy issues.

Interestingly, there are several studies looking at the potential protective effect of maternal breastfeeding and the subsequent development of IBD in the newborn [12]. In a recent population-based study, breastfeeding greater than 3 months was associated with a 30 % reduced risk of developing ulcerative colitis or 0.71 (0.52–0.96) [19]. Other environmental factors were also identified that affected the development of ulcerative colitis. These included having a childhood vegetable garden as reducing the UC risk by 35 % or 0.65 (0.45–0.94) [19]. This is consistent with the findings that environmental manipulations can affect the genetic susceptibility to disease.

## Effect of Pregnancy on Disease Activity

One of the most important considerations during the family planning process is the activity of ulcerative colitis at the time of conception and during the pregnancy. Disease activity at the time of conception influences disease activity during the course of the pregnancy. If disease is in remission at the beginning of the pregnancy, it will stay in remission in approximately 2/3 of patients [20]. Relapse tends to occur in the first trimester and postpartum; however, this is in part dependent on disease activity at conception. In those patients with ulcerative colitis who have active disease at the onset of pregnancy, in only ¼ of the patients will the disease go into remission. Half of the patients will have continued disease activity or become worse during the pregnancy [20]. In their series of patients, Willoughby and Truelove found that those patients who had active disease at conception had disease that was less responsive to therapy [20]. In another study of 97 women with ulcerative colitis, with 173 pregnancies, the risk of UC flare was 34 % during pregnancy as compared to 32 % when not pregnant [21]. Discontinuation of medical therapy during the first trimester in hopes of decreasing drug exposure to the growing fetus often will lead to a flare in disease activity and should be discouraged.

There also have been reports of lower disease activity during pregnancy in patients with autoimmune disease. Kane and colleagues demonstrated that improvement of IBD symptoms during pregnancy was associated with disparity in HLA class II antigens between the mother and the fetus [22]. A total of 50 pregnancies in 38 patients were studied, of which 13 had ulcerative colitis.

Pregnancy may decrease the rate of relapse following the pregnancy. In a large European cohort, there was a reduction in the rate of relapse in patients with ulcerative colitis with a decrease of 0.34–0.18 flares per year ($p = 0.008$) [23].

## Effect of Disease on Pregnancy and Pregnancy Outcomes

The effect of ulcerative colitis on pregnancy outcome is in a large part related to disease activity at conception [21]. Several large population-based studies and a meta-analysis have reported that there is an increased risk of preterm delivery and low birth weight infants in patients with IBD [24, 25]. Most of these studies do not take into account disease activity in their analysis. In a nationwide Danish cohort study, Norgard et al. reported that the risk of preterm birth was increased in the children of women with ulcerative colitis [26]. This was most prominent when the first hospitalization for ulcerative colitis occurred during the pregnancy. There was not an increased risk of LBW infants in this cohort [26]. A recent large European, multicenter, prospective case-control study that included measures of active disease found that for ulcerative colitis patients older age and active disease were associated with low birth weight and older age and combination therapy were risk factors for preterm delivery [27]. There are several theories as to why preterm labor and low birth weight infant may be seen in patients with active disease. Maternal low-grade inflammation may lead to suboptimal placental development due to affects on the endothelium leading to vascular dysfunction [28]. Ernst and colleagues looked at CRP levels in 6016 women during pregnancy and found that women with elevated maternal CRP>25 mg/L as compared to a reference group with CRP levels than 5 mg/L had an increased incidence of fetal growth restriction and increased risks of preterm birth and small for gestational age (SGA) infants at birth [28]. Circulating proinflammatory cytokines have also been shown to lead to increased miscarriage rates and neonates who were SGA [29, 30]. These findings suggest that improved control of systemic inflammation may lead to better birth outcomes.

## Medical Therapy of Ulcerative Colitis During Pregnancy

Ulcerative colitis management goals during pregnancy are similar to those in the non-pregnant patient. It is even more important in the pregnant patient to control disease activity due to potential adverse effects of active disease on the growing fetus. With a few exceptions, most of the medications used in the non-pregnant UC patient can be used in the pregnant UC patient. In the next section, the medications used for ulcerative colitis in the context of pregnancy and breastfeeding will be reviewed.

## Aminosalicylates

Mesalamine compounds and sulfasalazine have been used extensively in pregnant patients with ulcerative colitis. These compounds do cross the placenta, and levels in the fetal circulation are similar to the levels in the maternal circulation [31]. Sulfasalazine use up to the time of delivery has not been associated with kernicterus or neonatal jaundice [31]. When used in pregnancy, there is no reported increase in congenital defects or in neonatal toxicity. Sulfasalazine is a folic acid antagonist, and folate supplementation is required during pregnancy to help prevent neural tube defects as well as cardiovascular, oral cleft, and urinary tract defects [32]. The Asacol HD mesalamine formulation has dibutyl phthalate (DBP) as an inactive ingredient in its enteric coating. DBP at high levels has been associated with external and skeletal malformations and male reproductive system effects in animals [33]. This is at a dose greater than 80 time the human dose and likely has no effect in terms of fetal exposure at the doses that are used for the treatment of ulcerative colitis.

Sulfasalazine adversely affects spermatogenesis in men leading to decreased sperm counts and motility. It should be discontinued at least 2 months prior to conception [34]. Mesalamine does not have the same effects on sperm and can be used in place of sulfasalazine.

*Pregnancy recommendation*: Human data suggests low risk; use folate supplements in patients on sulfasalazine [35].

*Men*: Avoid sulfasalazine in men who are trying to conceive; mesalamine has no effect on sperm.

## Corticosteroids

Prednisone and prednisolone are felt to pose a small amount of risk to the developing fetus. A population-based case-control study in 1999 and a meta-analysis in 2000 both suggested a possible causal association between cleft lip and palate and steroid use in the first trimester [36, 37]. In the meta-analysis, the increased risk of cleft lip/palate was 3.4-fold, which is consistent with animal studies [37]. These investigators also performed a case-control study in 184 exposed subjects which showed a 3.35-fold increase in cleft lip/palate (95 % CI 1.97–5.69). There were no significant differences in the rate of major birth defects in the case-control study.

*Pregnancy recommendation*: Human data suggests risk. Use when risk of disease outweighs risk of medication. Better after the first trimester [35].

## Azathioprine/6-Mercaptopurine

6-Mercaptopurine and its parent compound azathioprine are playing an increasing role in the maintenance of steroid-dependent ulcerative colitis. These agents do cross the placenta and trace amounts can be found in fetal blood [38]. These agents are teratogenic in animals but have not been shown to cause abnormalities when used in the first trimester in humans [35]. A large cohort study in IBD patients from France showed no increase in the risk of congenital abnormalities in thiopurine-exposed subjects [39]. There was increased incidence of low birth weight and prematurity that may be related to disease activity. In a kidney transplant population, maternal azathioprine use has been associated with neonatal leukopenia. The maternal leukocyte count at 32 weeks gestation was correlated with the cord blood leukocyte count [40]. In this study, there was less leukopenia and thrombocytopenia in the newborn if the azathioprine dose was halved in mothers who had a leukocyte count below 1 SD for normal pregnancy [41].

*Pregnancy recommendation*: Human data suggests risk in the third trimester; consider decreasing azathioprine/6-mercaptopurine dose at that time [35].

*Men*: Azathioprine/6MP does not affect sperm quality and can be used during conception [41].

## Methotrexate

Methotrexate is associated with a diverse group of congenital defects that collectively are known as the aminopterin-methotrexate syndrome. Defects include skeletal abnormalities, oxycephaly, low-set ears, long webbed fingers, and wide set eyes. Methotrexate is contraindicated during pregnancy and should not be initiated in childbearing women unless there is complete understanding of the need for contraception and avoidance of pregnancy.

*Pregnancy recommendation*: Contraindicated.

*Men*: Case reports of decreased sperm count, stop if there are contraception difficulties [42].

## Cyclosporine/Tacrolimus

Cyclosporine is not an animal teratogen, and in small numbers of patients, there is no evidence that it is teratogenic in humans. Growth retardation of the fetus has been seen in some pregnancies but it is thought to be due to the underlying disease process. It has been used in severe steroid-refractory ulcerative colitis during pregnancy with some success in small numbers of patients. Using cyclosporine in this population allowed the pregnancies to progress to term without the need for colectomy, which would be high risk to the fetus in this population [43].

*Pregnancy recommendation*: Limited human data; animal data suggests risk however in severe medically refractory colitis cyclosporine may be preferred to surgery [35, 43].

*Men*: Compatible [44].

## Biologics

Infliximab and adalimumab both have been used for therapy in aggressive ulcerative colitis. Exposure during pregnancy may be part of an ulcerative colitis maintenance regimen or as acute salvage therapy for the pregnant patient presenting with fulminant colitis [45]. These are both parenteral IgG1 molecules with little transfer through the placenta until approximately week 20. Babies born to mothers who are receiving infliximab during pregnancy will have detectable levels of the drug for up to 6 months after birth. Infants that have detectable infliximab in their blood after delivery do not appear to have an increased risk of infection, and studies have demonstrated a normal response to non-live vaccines [46]. The long-term potential adverse effects on the infant's immune system are not known. Vaccination of exposed infants with live viruses should be avoided for at least 6 months or until circulating infliximab levels are negative [46]. There is no clear role for holding therapy for 8 or more weeks prior to delivery to decrease fetal exposure to infliximab. Zelinkova and colleagues show that infants born to mothers who stopped infliximab 21–30 weeks prior to delivery still had therapeutic infliximab levels in cord blood and peripheral blood infliximab level two- to threefold higher than their mothers [47]. Certolizumab, as a PEGylated Fab' monoclonal antibody, is not actively passed through the placenta to the fetus and may not pose the same potential risks. The degree of passive transfer is thought to be low.

*Pregnancy recommendation*: Based on the small amount of data available, infliximab and adalimumab are compatible with pregnancy; avoid live virus vaccines in offspring for 6 months after delivery or when circulating infliximab levels are negative.

*Men*: Slight decrease in sperm motility and oval forms [48].

## Breastfeeding and Pregnancy

Breastfeeding has numerous benefits in the health of the neonate including the studies mentioned above that suggest that there may be a decreased risk of developing IBD in children

277

**Table 24.1** Medications used to maintain remission in ulcerative colitis compatible with breastfeeding

| Medication | FDA pregnancy category[a] | Pregnancy Recommendation | Breastfeeding Recommendation |
|---|---|---|---|
| *5-ASA* | | | |
| Sulfasalazine | B | Low risk, replace folate daily | Probably compatible, possible diarrhea |
| Mesalamine[a] | B | Low risk | Probably compatible, possible diarrhea |
| | C[a] | Asacol[a]—phthalate in coating AE in animals | |
| Olsalazine | C | Low risk | Probably compatible, possible diarrhea |
| Balsalazide | B | Low risk | Probably compatible, possible diarrhea |
| Corticosteroids | C | Low risk: possible increased risk of cleft palate, adrenal insufficiency, premature rupture of membranes | Compatible |
| *Antibiotics* | | | |
| Metronidazole | B | Low risk, possibly avoid 1st trimester | Potential toxicity with higher doses and longer duration |
| Quinolones | C | Avoid, potential damage to cartilage | Probably compatible in short courses |
| Amoxicillin/clavulanate | B | Low risk | Probably compatible |
| Cephalosporins | B | Low risk | Compatible |
| *Immunomodulators* | | | |
| 6MP/azathioprine | D | Low risk, animal teratogen, possible risk in third trimester | Probably compatible, discard breast milk for 4 h after dose |
| Methotrexate | X | Contraindicated, teratogenic to humans | Contraindicated, immunosuppression |
| Cyclosporine | C | Low risk | Potential toxicity, immunosuppression |
| Thalidomide | X | Contraindicated, teratogenic to humans | Contraindicated |
| *Biologics* | | | |
| Infliximab | B | Low risk, continue dosing through pregnancy | Probably compatible |
| Adalimumab | B | Low risk, continue dosing through pregnancy | Probably compatible |
| Certolizumab pegol | B | Low risk, continue dosing through pregnancy | Probably compatible |
| Natalizumab | C | Low risk | Probably compatible |

Adapted from: Briggs G, Freeman R, Yaffe S. Drugs in Pregnancy and Lactation: A Reference Guide to Fetal and Neonatal Risk. 9th edition ed. Philadelphia, Pennsylvania: Lippincott Williams & Wilkins; 2011 [35]; Kwan L, Mahadevan U. Inflammatory bowel disease and pregnancy: an update. *Expert Review of Clinical Immunology* 2010;*6*:643–657 [64]; Mahadevan U, Kane S. American Gastroenterological Association Institute Technical Review on the Use of Gastrointestinal Medications in Pregnancy. *Gastroenterology* 2006;*131*(1):283–311 [65]
[a]FDA pregnancy categories are given for historical reference; however, they are being phased out of routine usage for evaluation of medications during pregnancy

that have been breastfed [19, 49]. There are both medication concerns and concerns regarding a risk of flare in disease activity associated with breastfeeding. If patients discontinue IBD medication to breastfeed, there is a twofold risk of flare compared to patients who do not breastfeed (95 % CI 1.2–2.7); however, if medication discontinuation is corrected for, there is no increased risk of flare of disease [50]. In a Canadian population-based study, Moffatt and colleagues found that women with IBD were as likely to breastfeed as the general population. The risk of flare postpartum in those with ulcerative colitis who breastfed vs. those who did not breastfeed was 289.2 % vs. 44.4 % ($p = 0.44$) [49, 51].

There is a concern that if a mother is on medication while breastfeeding that there are potential adverse effects on the nursing infant if it is secreted in the breast milk. If at all possible, the medications used to treat ulcerative colitis should not be discontinued in order to breastfeed. Most of the medications that are used to maintain remission in

ulcerative colitis are compatible with breastfeeding (Table 24.1). The notable exceptions are cyclosporine, tacrolimus, and methotrexate.

## Aminosalicylates

This class of medication is felt to be compatible with breastfeeding with caution due to potential adverse effects on the fetus [35]. Small amounts of mesalamine are excreted into human milk as well as its metabolite, acetyl-5-aminosalicylate. The estimated daily intake of the neonate is felt to be negligible, and adverse events have not been seen [52]. Diarrhea has been reported in a nursing infant after the maternal exposure to rectal mesalamine [53]. Sulfasalazine is broken down to sulfapyridine and acetyl-5-aminosalicylate. Sulfapyridine is excreted in low levels into breast milk. The low doses that are seen do not increase the risk of kernicterus and that there is no significant displacement of bilirubin from albumin [31]. There is at least one report of bloody diarrhea associated with sulfasalazine use [54]. If diarrhea or bloody diarrhea develops in a breastfed infant on aminosalicylates, either the mother should stop breastfeeding or if clinically reasonable stop the drug.

## Corticosteroids

Very small amounts of prednisone and prednisolone are excreted into breast milk. In a study using radioactively labeled prednisolone in seven patients and examining the levels in breast milk, there was 0.14 % of the administered 5 mg dose found per liter of milk [55]. In a second study, doses of 10–80 mg/day lead to milk concentrations of 5–25 % of serum concentrations. It is estimated that the infant, at even high levels, receives <0.1 % of the dose, which is less than 10 % of the nursing infant's own endogenous cortisol production [56].

*Breastfeeding recommendation*: Compatible [35].

## Azathioprine/6-Mercaptopurine

There is only a small amount of human data available on maternal use of thiopurines during breastfeeding.

Christensen et al. studied the pharmacokinetics of azathioprine in eight patients—looking at milk and plasma levels after dose of azathioprine from 75 to 200 mg. They found that the highest concentration of azathioprine was seen in the milk with the first 4 h of dosing. Levels seen were very low, and on the basis of maximum concentrations measured, the infant received <0.008 mg/kg body weight over a 24-h period [57].

Angelberger and colleagues followed the babies of 11 mothers taking AZA (median 150 mg/day) for IBD during pregnancy and lactation and compared this group to 12 mothers on no immunosuppressants. Duration of breastfeeding was 6 months in the AZA group vs. 8 months in the non-AZA group [58]. The children were followed to median age of 3.3 years in the AZA group and 4.7 years in the non-exposed group. There were no differences in childhood infections between the AZA exposed and non-exposed groups. Common cold and conjunctivitis were more common in the non-AZA exposed group. This data suggests that exposure to AZA in utero and in breastfeeding does not increase the risk of infection in the neonates [58].

*Breastfeeding recommendations*: Probably compatible, discard milk 4 h after dosing [35].

## Methotrexate

Methotrexate is excreted in small amounts into breast milk. Methotrexate may accumulate in neonatal tissues. Breastfeeding is contraindicated for patients on methotrexate [35].

## Cyclosporine/Tacrolimus

Cyclosporine is excreted into breast milk. In one study, the infant's blood levels were as high as 78 % of the maternal trough concentrations. The estimated exposure is from 0.2 to 2.1 % of the mother's weight-adjusted dose [35].

*Breastfeeding recommendation*: Limited human data—potential toxicity due to detectable levels in the blood of neonates and subsequent immunosuppression [35].

## Biologics

Infliximab and certolizumab have not been detected in breast milk in patients who are receiving these agents for inflammatory bowel disease.

*Breastfeeding recommendation*: Limited human data—thought to be low risk and compatible with breastfeeding [59].

## Pregnancy and the Ileoanal Pouch

As discussed above, fertility is decreased in women who undergo a colectomy with IPAA for ulcerative colitis. There is less information available on pouch function in women who do become pregnant with an ileal pouch. Hahnloser and colleagues studied 232 pregnancies in 135 women, 1–16 years after IPAA for ulcerative colitis [60]. They found that daytime stool frequency 7 months after delivery was the same as in the pregravid state (5.4 vs. 5.4) but that at 68 months after delivery, there was a slight increase (5.4 vs. 6.4). In this group of women, there was an increase in occasional fecal incontinence, 21 % pregravid as compared to 36 % at the last post-pregnancy follow-up. Pregnancy did not increase the incidence of stricture formation, pouchitis, or obstruction [60]. In a review of all the available literature on pouch complications associated with pregnancy, Seligman et al. reported that stool frequency and incontinence was not significantly affected by pregnancy or mode of delivery [61]. Antepartum small bowel obstruction was reported in 8 out of 283 pregnancies reviewed [61]. These all resolved nonoperatively after delivery. Other complications seen in this review were postpartum SBO in 6.7 %, pouchitis in 1.8 %, and a perianal abscess in 1 patient [61]. Overall, the literature supports the fact that pregnancy in patients with ileal pouches is well tolerated.

## Labor and Delivery

There is an increased rate of Cesarean section as mode of delivery in patients with ulcerative colitis. Nguyen et al. reported a rate of 42 % compared to 30.9 % in a non-IBD population ($p=0.0002$) [62]. Lower Cesarean section rates of 13.8 % (all IBD) and 29 % (UC) have been reported in two large community-based practice studies [24, 63]. In general, the decision for a Cesarean section in patients with ulcerative colitis should be made for obstetric indications. Patients who have had a total abdominal colectomy with IPAA can have a successful vaginal delivery as it relates to pouch function [60]. The main delivery concern in this population relates to potential of damage to the anal sphincter. In a patient with borderline continence related to the IPAA, a tear or episiotomy that affects the sphincter may significantly worsen continence issues. The potential risks to the sphincter of vaginal delivery should be discussed with the patient, obstetrician, and surgeon as delivery decisions are being made [12].

## Summary

Patients with ulcerative colitis typically do quite well during pregnancy, and pregnancy should not be discouraged in this patient population. Fertility in the medically treated patient is no different than in the non-UC population but is affected by surgical therapy with IPAA. Ideally, patients should be in remission prior to conception and should continue to be optimally treated throughout their pregnancy. Compliance with medical regimen should be encouraged to avoid flares of disease which then may impact the pregnancy in terms of preterm delivery and low birth weight infants. Most medications used for the treatment of ulcerative colitis can be used safely during pregnancy. Delivery method should be based on obstetric indications. Collaborative management of the pregnant ulcerative colitis patient with the obstetrician, gastroenterologist, and surgeon (in IPAA patient) is recommended.

## References

1. Medicine Practice Committee of the American Society for Reproductive Medicine. Definitions of infertility and recurrent pregnancy loss. Fertil Steril. 2008;90 Suppl 5:60.

2. Hudson M, Flett G, Sinclair T, Brunt P, Templeton A, Mowat N. Fertility and pregnancy in inflammatory bowel disease. Int J Gynaecol Obstet. 1997;58(2):229–37.

3. Baird D, Narendranthan M, Sandler R. Increased risk of preterm birth for women with inflammatory bowel disease. Gastroenterology. 1990;99(4):987–94.

4. Olsen K, Juul S, Berndtsson I, Oresland T, Laurberg S. Ulcerative colitis: female fecundity before diagnosis, during disease and after surgery compared with a population sample. Gastroenterology. 2002;122(1):15–9.

5. Rajaratnam S, Eglinton T, Hider P, Fearnhead N. Impact of ileal pouch-anal anastomosis on female fertility: meta-analysis and systematic review. Int J Colorectal Dis. 2011;26(11):1365–74.

6. Waljee A, Waljee J, Morris A, Higgins P. Threefold increased risk of infertility: a meta-analysis of infertility after ileal pouch anal anastomosis in ulcerative colitis. Gut. 2006;55:1575–80.

7. Oresland T, Palmblad S, Ellstron M, Berndtsson I, Crona N, Hulten L. Gynaecological and sexual function related to anatomical changes in the female pelvis after restorative proctocolectomy. Int J Colorectal Dis. 1994;9:77–81.

8. Cornish JA, Tan E, Singh B, Bundock H, Mortensen N, Nicholls RJ, et al. Female infertility following restorative proctocolectomy. Colorectal Dis. 2011;13(10):e339–44.

9. Mortier P, Gambiez L, Karoui M, Cortot A, Paris J, Quandalle P, et al. Colectomy with ileorectal anastomosis preserves female fertility in ulcerative colitis. Gastroenterol Clin Biol. 2006;30(4):594–7.

10. Narendranthan M, Sandler R, Suchindran C, Savitz D. Male infertility in inflammatory bowel disease. J Clin Gastroenterol. 1989;11(4):403–6.

11. Riley S, Lecarpentier J, Mani V, Goodman M, Mandal B, Turnberg L. Sulphasalazine induced seminal abnormalities in ulcerative colitis: results of mesalazine substitution. Gut. 1987;28(8):1008–12.

12. Mahadevan U. Fertility and pregnancy in the patient with inflammatory bowel disease. Gut. 2006;55(8):1198–206.

13. Tiainen J, Matikainen M, Hiltunen K. Ileal J-pouch–anal anastomosis, sexual dysfunction, and fertility. Scand J Gastroenterol. 1999;34(2):185–8.

14. Gorgun E, Remzi F, Montague D, Connor J, O'Brien K, Loparo B, et al. Male sexual function improves after ileal pouch anal anastomosis. Colorectal Dis. 2005;7(6):545–50.

15. Sun L, Nava G, Stappenbeck M. Host genetic susceptibility, dysbiosis, and viral triggers in inflammatory bowel disease. Curr Opin Gastroenterol. 2011;27(4):321–7.

16. Russell R, Satsangi J. IBD: a family affair. Best Pract Res Clin Gastroenterol. 2006;18(3):525–39.

17. Bennett R, Rubin P, Present D. Frequency of inflammatory bowel disease in offspring of couples both presenting with inflammatory bowel disease. Gastroenterology. 1991;100(6):1638–43.

18. Bengtson M, Aamodt G, Vatn M, Harris J. Concordance for IBD among twins compared to ordinary siblings – a Norwegian population-based study. J Crohn Colitis. 2010;4(3):312–8.

19. Gearry R, Richardson A, Frampton C, Dodgshun A, Barclay M. Population-based cases control study of inflammatory bowel disease risk factors. J Gastroenterol Hepatol. 2010;25:325–33.

20. Willoughby C, Truelove S. Ulcerative colitis and pregnancy. Gut. 1980;21:469–74.

21. Nielsen O, Andreasson B, Bondesen S, Jarnum S. Pregnancy in ulcerative colitis. Scand J Gastroenterol. 1983;18(6):735–42.

22. Kane S, Kisiel J, Shih L, Hanauer S. HLA disparity determines disease activity through pregnancy in women with inflammatory bowel disease. Am J Gastroenterol. 2004;99:1523–6.

23. Riis L, Vind I, Politi P, Wolters F, Vermeire S, Tsianos E, et al. Does pregnancy change the disease course[quest] a study in a European cohort of patients with inflammatory bowel disease. Am J Gastroenterol. 2006;101(7):1539–45.

24. Dominitz JA, Young JCC, Boyko EJ. Outcomes of infants born to mothers with inflammatory bowel disease: a population-based cohort study. Am J Gastroenterol. 2002;97(3):641–8.

25. Cornish J, Tan E, Teare J, Teoh TG, Rai R, Clark SK, et al. A meta-analysis on the influence of inflammatory bowel disease on pregnancy. Gut. 2007;56(6):830–7.

26. Norgard B, Fonager K, Sorensen HT, Olsen J. Birth outcomes of women with ulcerative colitis: a nationwide Danish cohort study. Am J Gastroenterol. 2000;95(11):3165–70.

27. Bortoli A, Pedersen N, Duricova D, D'Inca R, Gionchetti P, Panelli MR, et al. Pregnancy outcome in inflammatory bowel disease: prospective European case–control ECCO-EpiCom study, 2003–2006. Aliment Pharmacol Ther. 2011;34(7):724–34.

28. Ernst G, de Jonge L, Hofman A, Lindemans J, Russcher H, Steegers E, et al. C-reactive protein levels in early pregnancy, fetal growth patterns, and the risk for neonatal complications: the generation R study. Am J Obstet Gynecol. 2011;205(2):132.e1–12.

29. Calleja-Aguis J, Muttukrishna S, Pizzey A, Jauniaux E. Pro- and antiinflammatory cytokines in threatened miscarriages. Am J Obstet Gynecol. 2011;205:e8–16.

30. Georgiou H, Thio Y, Russell C, Permezel M, Heng Y, Lee S, et al. Association between maternal serum sytokine profiles at 7–10 weeks' gestation and birthweight in small for gestational age infants. Am J Obstet Gynecol. 2011;204(415):e1–12.

31. Jarnerot G, Into-Malmberg M-B, Esbjorner E. Placental transfer of sulfasalazine and sulfapyridine and some of its metabolites. Scand J Gastroenterol. 1981;16:693–8.

32. Hernandez-Diaz S, Werler M, Walker A, Mitchell A. Folic acid antagonists during pregnancy and the risk of birth defects. N Eng J Med. 2000;343:1608–14.

33. Hernandez-Diaz S, Mitchell A, Kelley K, Calafat A, Hauser R. Medications as a potential source of exposure to phthalates in the US population. Environ Health Perspect. 2009;117:185–9.

34. Toovey S, Hudson E, Hendry W, Levi A. Sulphasalazine and male infertility; reversibility and possible mechanism. Gut. 1981;22:445–51.

35. Briggs G, Freeman R, Yaffe S. Drugs in pregnancy and lactation: a reference guide to fetal and neonatal risk. 9th ed. Philadelphia, PA: Lippincott Williams & Wilkins; 2011.

36. Carmichael S, Shaw G. Maternal corticosteroid use and risk of selected congenital anomalies. Am J Med Genet. 1999;86(3):242–4.

37. Park-Wyllie L, Mazzotta P, Pastuszak A, Moretti M, Beique L, Hunnisett L, et al. Birth defects after maternal exposure to corticosteroids: prospective cohort study and meta-analysis of epidemiological studies. Teratology. 2000;62:385–92.

38. Sarrikoski S, Seppala M. Immunosuppression during pregnancy. Transmission of azathioprine and its metabolites from mother to the fetus. Am J Obstet Gynecol. 1973;115:1100–6.

39. Coelho J, Beaugerie L, Colombel J, Hebuterne X, Lerebours E, Lemann M, et al. Pregnancy outcome in patients with inflammatory bowel disease treated with thiopurines: cohort from the CESAME study. Gut. 2011;60:198–203.

40. Davison J, Dellagrammatikas H, Parkin J. Maternal azathioprine therapy and depressed haemopoiesis in the babies of renal allograft patients. Br J Obstet Gynaecol. 1985;92:233–9.

41. Dejaco C, Mittermaier C, Reinisch W, Gasche C, Waldhoer T, Strohmer H, et al. Azathioprine treatment and male fertility in inflammatory bowel disease. Gastroenterology. 2001;121(5):1048–53.

42. Sussman A, Leonard J. Psoriasis, methotrexate and oligospermia. Arch Dermatol. 1980;116:215–7.

43. Branche J, Cortot A, Bourreille A, Coffin B, de Vos M, de Saussure P, et al. Cyclosporine treatment of steroid-refractory ulcerative colitis during pregnancy. Inflamm Bowel Dis. 2009;15(7):1044–8.

44. Haberman J, Karwa G, Greenstein S, Soberman R, Glicklich D, Tellis V, et al. Male fertility in cyclosporine-treated renal transplant patients. J Urol. 1991;145:294–6.

45. Aratari A, Margagnoni G, Koch M, Papi C. Intentional infliximab use during pregnancy for severe steroid-refractory ulcerative colitis. J Crohn Colitis. 2010;5:262.

46. Djokanovic N, Klieger-Grossman C, Pupco A, Koren G. Safety of infliximab use during pregnancy. Reprod Toxicol. 2011;32(1):93–7.

47. Zelinkova Z, de Haar C, de Ridder L, Pierik MJ, Kuipers EJ, Peppelenbosch MP, et al. High intra-uterine exposure to infliximab following maternal anti-TNF treatment during pregnancy. Aliment Pharmacol Ther. 2011;33(9):1053–8.

48. Mahadevan U, Terdiman JP, Aron J, Jacobsohn S, Turek P. Infliximab and semen quality in men with inflammatory bowel disease. Inflamm Bowel Dis. 2005;11(4):395–9.

49. Klement E, Cohen R, Boxman J, Joseph A, Reif S. Breastfeeding and risk of inflammatory bowel disease: a systematic review with meta-analysis. Am J Clin Nutr. 2004;80:1342–52.

50. Kane S, Lemieux N. The role of breastfeeding in postpartum disease activity in women with inflammatory bowel disease. Am J Gastroenterol. 2005;100:102–5.

51. Moffatt D, Ilnyckyi A, Bernstein C. A population-based study of breastfeeding in inflammatory bowel disease: initiation, duration, and effect on disease in the postpartum perio. Am J Gastroenterol. 2009;104:2517–23.

52. Klotz U, Harings-Kaim A. Negligible excretion of 5-aminosalicylic acid in breast milk. Lancet. 1993;342:618–9.

53. Nelis G. Diarrheoea due to 5-aminosalicylic acid in breast milk. Lancet. 1989;1:383.

54. Branski D, Kerem E, Gross-Kieselstein E, Hurvitz H, Litt R, Abrahamov A. Bloody diarrhea – a possible complication of sulfasalazine transferred through human breast milk. J Pediatr Gastroenterol Nutr. 1986;5:316–7.

55. McKenzie S, Selley J, Agnew J. Secretion of prednisone into breast milk. Arch Dis Child. 1975;50:894–6.

56. Ost L, Wettrell G, Bjorkhem I, Rane A. Prednisolone excretion in human milk. J Pediatr Gastroenterol Nutr. 1985;106:1008–11.

57. Christensen L, Dahlerup J, Nielsen M, Fallingborg J, Schmiegelow K. Azathioprine treatment during lactation. Aliment Pharmacol Ther. 2008;28:1209–13.

58. Angelberger SRW, Messerschmidt A, Miehsler W, Novacek G, Vogelsang H, Dejaco C. Long-term follow-up of babies exposed to azathioprine in utero and via breastfeeding. J Crohns Colitis. 2011;5(2):95–100.

59. Mahadevan U, Cucchiara S, Hyams J, Steinwurz F, Nuti F, Travis S, et al. The London position statement of the world congress of gastroenterology on biological therapy for IBD with the European Crohn's and Colitis Organisation: pregnancy and pediatrics. Am J Gastroenterol. 2011;106(2):214–23.

60. Hahnloser D, Pemberton JH, Wolff BG, Larson D, Harrington J, Farouk R, et al. Pregnancy and delivery before and after ileal pouch-anal anastomosis for inflammatory bowel disease: immediate and long-term consequences and outcomes. Dis Colon Rectum. 2004;47(7):1127–35. doi:10.1007/s10350-004-0569-0.

61. Seligman NS, Sbar W, Berghella V. Pouch function and gastrointestinal complications during pregnancy after ileal pouch-anal anastomosis. J Matern Fetal Neonatal Med. 2011;24(3):525–30.

62. Nguyen GC, Boudreau H, Harris ML, Maxwell CV. Outcomes of obstetric hospitalizations among women with inflammatory bowel disease in the United States. Clin Gastroenterol Hepatol. 2009;7(3):329–34.

63. Mahadevan U, Sandborn WJ, Li DK, Hakimian S, Kane S, Corley DA. Pregnancy outcomes in women with inflammatory bowel disease: a large community-based study from northern California. Gastroenterology. 2007;133(4):1106–12.

64. Kwan L, Mahadevan U. Inflammatory bowel disease and pregnancy: an update. Expert Rev Clin Immunol. 2010;6:643–57.

65. Mahadevan U, Kane S. American gastroenterological association institute technical review on the use of gastrointestinal medications in pregnancy. Gastroenterology. 2006;131(1):283–311.

# Pediatric Issues in Treating Ulcerative Colitis

Lindsey Albenberg, Robert N. Baldassano,
and Judith Kelsen

**Keywords**

Pediatrics • Ulcerative colitis • Approach • 5-ASA • Antibiotics • Probiotics • Corticosteroids • 6-Mercaptopurine (6-MP) • Azathioprine • Methotrexate • Biologics • Surgical care

## Overview

While the diagnosis of inflammatory bowel disease (IBD) can occur at any age, approximately 25 % of patients with inflammatory bowel disease will become symptomatic during childhood or adolescence [1]. Clinicians who care for pediatric patients with IBD are faced with certain challenges and responsibilities. Some of the distinct issues which must be addressed include growth, skeletal health, and psychosocial development. Such issues may affect the choice and the ultimate success of the therapy. In this chapter, we will focus on the treatment of ulcerative colitis (UC) in this unique patient population.

Worldwide, the incidence of IBD is increasing, particularly in industrialized countries. The increase in incidence seems to be most prominent for Crohn's disease (CD). The majority of studies in pediatric ulcerative colitis have demonstrated a relatively stable incidence. However, a retrospective epidemiological study evaluating the incidence of pediatric IBD between 1991 and 2002 in Texas also found an increased incidence of UC in patients less than 17 years of age [2]. In North America, the incidence of UC in patients 10–19 years of age is approximately 2 cases per 100,000 persons [3]. The pediatric literature suggests that the highest age-related incidence of UC occurs in patients greater than 10 years of age [2].

The presentation of ulcerative colitis in pediatric patients is similar to the presentation in adults. Children with UC often present with persistent symptoms of abdominal pain, diarrhea, and rectal bleeding. In pediatric UC, 83–95 % of patients present with rectal bleeding [4]. As compared to adults, children with UC are more likely to experience acute, severe symptoms at the time of diagnosis [5]. It is not uncommon for pediatric patients to require hospitalization during the initial presentation. Another unique feature of ulcerative colitis in children and adolescence is the effect of the disease on growth. While Crohn's disease is more likely to affect growth, long-standing and severe symptoms from ulcerative colitis may result in malnutrition. Linear growth may subsequently be impacted. The degree of growth failure will often influence treatment decisions.

In regard to diagnosis, a complete laboratory evaluation should be performed to evaluate for anemia, hypoalbuminemia, elevated inflammatory markers, and hepatic function abnormalities. In addition, imaging of the small bowel should be performed in order to differentiate Crohn's disease from UC as this can be challenging in the pediatric population. Colonoscopy with biopsy remains the most valuable procedure in the evaluation of a pediatric patient in whom the diagnosis of ulcerative colitis is suspected. A complete examination of the entire colon, as well as the terminal ileum, is necessary in order to determine the extent of the disease and to distinguish between Crohn's disease and UC.

The gross appearance of the colon and the histologic findings in ulcerative colitis are similar in children and adults. There are differences, however, in disease location. While isolated left-sided colitis is common in adults, most children with UC present with inflammation extending proximal to the

R.N. Baldassano, M.D. • J. Kelsen, M.D. • L. Albenberg, D.O. (✉)
Pediatrics, Division of Gastroenterology, Heptaology,
and Nutrition, The Children's Hospital of Philadelphia,
University of Pennsylvania, 7 NW 3400 Civic Center Blvd.,
Philadelphia, PA 19104, USA
e-mail: baldassano@email.chop.edu; kelsen@email.chop.edu;
albenbergl@ema.l.chop.edu

G.R. Lichtenstein (ed.), *Medical Therapy of Ulcerative Colitis*,
DOI 10.1007/978-1-4939-1677-1_25, © Springer Science+Business Media New York 2014

splenic flexure. A statewide epidemiological study in Wisconsin evaluating pediatric patients newly diagnosed with IBD found left-sided colitis in only 10 % of children with UC at the time of presentation. Conversely, 90 % of children newly diagnosed with UC presented with pancolitis [6]. As mentioned previously, pediatric patients with UC often present initially with acute, severe exacerbations, and this is likely related to the more extensive disease location frequently observed.

Most pediatric patients with UC can be treated on an outpatient basis. However, hospitalization is necessary in certain situations such as when maximal outpatient therapy is unsuccessful or when patients develop severe disease. There is, in fact, a greater risk of hospitalization in pediatric UC patients as compared to the adult population [7].

## Approach to Treatment

The general goals for managing UC in children are to eliminate symptoms of disease, improve quality of life, and avoid hospitalization and surgery. One of the primary aims is to promote and allow normal, unrestricted activity (i.e., attending school). Although clinical improvement is imperative, in order to increase the chance of lasting remission and decrease the potential for adverse effects of long-standing inflammation, it is important to attain mucosal healing. In terms of therapy, the most common approach in pediatric ulcerative colitis is the "step-up" approach, in which medications with the least toxicity are used early. Then, further therapies are added or replaced if the desired response is not achieved. Recently, a "top-down" approach has been utilized, in which patients with moderate to severe disease are treated more aggressively early [8]. Theoretically, this strategy may be appropriate for specific pediatric patients such as in patients who have pancolitis or who require hospitalization. However, to date, there is only one published study evaluating a top-down approach in the treatment of pediatric IBD [9].

There have been very few studies in pediatric patients evaluating the safety and efficacy of the different therapies used in ulcerative colitis. When making therapeutic decisions, the best available evidence is frequently limited to retrospective studies in children and adolescents and prospective studies performed in the adult population.

## 5-Aminosalicylate (5-ASA)

### Oral 5-ASA

Oral 5-ASA medications are commonly utilized as first-line therapy in the treatment of mild to moderately active ulcerative colitis. The exact mechanism through which the 5-ASA preparations decrease inflammation is unclear. They are thought to decrease inflammation through inhibition of cyclooxygenase and lipoxygenase, enzymes that are responsible for the production of inflammatory mediators. The 5-ASA medications are thought to act directly on the gastrointestinal mucosa. In other words, the effect is largely topical rather than systemic. Adult studies have clearly demonstrated a role for 5-ASA medications in both induction of remission and maintenance of remission in ulcerative colitis [10, 11].

To date, there have been two prospective, multicenter, randomized trials examining the efficacy of 5-ASA medications in children with active UC. In a study published by Ferry and colleagues, patients with mild to moderate disease were randomized to receive either 30 mg/kg/day of olsalazine or 60 mg/kg/day of sulfasalazine for induction of remission [12]. After 3 months, clinical improvement was seen in 39 % of patients treated with olsalazine versus 79 % of patients treated with sulfasalazine. It was hypothesized that olsalazine was less effective than sulfasalazine in this trial because of the small sample size and the relatively low dose of olsalazine studied. A more recent prospective, multicenter, randomized study demonstrated that in pediatric patients (ages 5–17) with mild to moderately active UC, balsalazide was well tolerated and improved clinical signs and symptoms of disease [13].

Similarly, there have been a small number of studies examining the pharmacokinetics of 5-ASA medications in the pediatric population. In general, the data in children is comparable to the data in adults [14]. In the available literature, a wide range of 5-ASA dosages have been used. The overall tendency in clinical practice is to recommend 80–100 mg/kg/day of mesalamine for induction therapy and 30–100 mg/kg/day of mesalamine for maintenance therapy. Mesalamine is used much more commonly in children than sulfasalazine due to lower side effect profile. In addition, mesalamine is available in pH-dependent (Asacol®) and time-release (Pentasa®) formulations which allow the drug to become active in different sites within the GI tract. Conversely, sulfasalazine preparations target the colon exclusively. Despite this, sulfasalazine is still occasionally prescribed for young children who cannot swallow pills because it is available in a liquid preparation.

The side effects and adverse events reported in children treated with 5-ASA medications are similar to those reported in adults. There are adverse events associated exclusively with sulfasalazine which are thought to be related to the sulfa component. These include hypersensitivity reactions and hemolytic anemia. In general, the side effects associated with mesalamine preparations are milder and include symptoms such as headache, abdominal pain, nausea, and vomiting. There have been case reports in children and adolescents describing more severe adverse events with mesalamine such as pancreatitis, hepatitis, nephritis, and pericarditis. There have also been reports of mesalamine intolerance mimicking exacerbation of colitis [15].

## Topical 5-ASA

Many symptoms of ulcerative colitis, such as urgency and tenesmus, are secondary to rectal disease or left-sided colitis. 5-ASA suppositories and enemas have been widely used worldwide in the treatment of adults with ulcerative colitis with good success. These preparations may be used alone or in combination with oral 5-ASAs. However, the efficacy and safety of mesalamine suppositories in pediatric patients have not been well studied until recently. A multicenter trial published by Heyman and colleagues found that once daily mesalamine (500 mg) suppositories were well tolerated and effective in treating mild to moderate ulcerative proctitis in children ages 5–17 [16]. In this study, ulcerative proctitis was diagnosed by biopsy at the time of study entry, and improvement was based on a clinical disease improvement index. Clinical response was achieved in more than 90 % of patients 3 weeks and 6 weeks following initiation of therapy. Limitations of this study included the open-label and uncontrolled study design.

## Combination 5-ASA Therapy

As mentioned previously, the majority of pediatric patients with ulcerative colitis present with disease which extends beyond the splenic flexure. However, there are patients who present with left-sided disease exclusively. In these patients, a common approach is treatment with a combination of oral and topical mesalamine. Combination therapy is also useful in patients who have symptoms suggestive of proctitis such as tenesmus, urgency, and frequency.

Compliance with a treatment regimen that includes per rectum medications can be difficult in pediatric patients. In fact, compliance with medications in pediatric patients, in general, is a frequently encountered problem. For example, treatment with 5-ASA medications involves multiple pills per day and also frequent dosing. Also, the pills themselves are large and can be difficult for a child to swallow. The literature suggests that pediatric patients with IBD miss up to 50 % of 5-ASA doses [17]. There are current research efforts directed toward identifying simpler methods of administration for 5-ASA medications. However, it is also essential for providers to assess adherence at each office visit and to recognize barriers to compliance.

## Antibiotics

In clinical practice, antibiotics are commonly used in the treatment of pediatric inflammatory bowel disease. Although no specific bacterial infection has been implicated in the pathogenesis of IBD, there is a growing body of evidence which supports a relationship between the gut microbiota and inflammation. Among humans, a significant amount of gut microbial diversity exists. However, the gut microbial composition in patients with IBD appears to be altered as compared to healthy controls [18]. In the treatment of IBD, it is thought that antibiotics produce a response by altering the composition of the gut flora [14]. An immunomodulatory effect has also been proposed [19].

Adult studies suggest a role for antibiotics, such as ciprofloxacin and metronidazole, in the treatment of perianal Crohn's disease, postoperative Crohn's disease, and pouchitis [20]. However, there is little evidence based on the current published literature supporting the use of antibiotics in the treatment of ulcerative colitis except in the case of pouchitis. Antibiotics are important in children presenting with fulminant ulcerative colitis and signs of toxicity such as fever, leukocytosis, bandemia, or peritoneal symptoms [21]. However, these medications should not be used routinely in less severely ill patients.

## Probiotics

Probiotics are defined as live microbial food products that have beneficial effects on the host. Probiotics have been suggested as potential treatments for numerous digestive disorders. However, the routine use of probiotics in such disorders remains controversial. A Cochrane review of randomized, controlled trials of probiotics in ulcerative colitis concluded that probiotics, when added to standard therapy, may add modest benefit in mild to moderately active UC [22]. Probiotics may have a more important role in treating patients with ulcerative colitis who have pouchitis. In a double-blind study in an adult population with pouchitis treated with VSL#3, 85 % of patients maintained remission of pouchitis for 1 year [23]. Another study suggested that probiotics may be effective in pouchitis as a preventative strategy [24]. In the treatment of children and adolescents with UC, the current notion is that probiotics may be a useful adjunctive treatment strategy. Further investigations are clearly needed in this area.

## Corticosteroids

Topical corticosteroids can be utilized in the treatment of pediatric patients with ulcerative colitis. Rectal steroid foams or suppositories can be used for proctitis, and steroid enemas can be used for proctocolitis and left-sided disease. Studies in adults have demonstrated benefit with short-term use. However, the literature suggests that corticosteroids administered per rectum are not sufficient to maintain remission [25].

Budesonide is a glucocorticoid which undergoes extensive first-pass metabolism in the liver and therefore has a lower incidence of systemic side effects. Studies have shown that enteric-coated budesonide has a role in the induction of remission in pediatric patients who have mild to moderately active Crohn's disease [26]. Budesonide MMX has been demonstrated in adult patients to induce remission in patients with active ulcerative colitis. Conversely, there are no studies which evaluate the efficacy of oral budesonide in children with ulcerative colitis. Studies in adults have suggested that oral enteric-coated budesonide is both less effective than mesalamine and is not superior to placebo in the induction of remission in patients with ulcerative colitis [27]. Treatment with oral enteric-coated budesonide in children who have ulcerative colitis is therefore not currently recommended. Oral enteric-coated budesonide is released in the upper GI tract which likely explains the lack of efficacy in ulcerative colitis when compared to Crohn's disease. Extended-release formulations such as budesonide MMX (multi-matrix) are now available and have been demonstrated to be effective in treating patients with ulcerative colitis—including patients who have left-sided disease [28–30].

In pediatric patients with ulcerative colitis, oral corticosteroids are commonly utilized to induce remission when the 5-ASA medications have failed. Inpatient admission for IV corticosteroids is sometimes required if the disease is severe or if oral corticosteroids are ineffective. Although valuable in controlling acute exacerbations of disease, the long-term use of systemic corticosteroids is undesirable due to the large number of adverse affects seen with this class of medications. Side effects which are frequently encountered include increased appetite, skin changes such as acne, cushingoid appearance, hypertension, increased blood glucose levels, and emotional lability. Also, the negative effects of corticosteroids on growth and bone health should always be considered [31].

The vast majority of pediatric patients with ulcerative colitis demonstrate response to corticosteroid treatment. However, maintenance of remission is difficult to achieve with this therapy alone. Population-based studies in adults suggest that in those patients, who require treatment with corticosteroids initially, very few maintain remission and corticosteroid dependence is a significant issue [32]. More recently, a similar result was found in pediatric patients. In a prospective study evaluating UC patients from the Pediatric Inflammatory Bowel Disease Research Collaborative, a cohort of patients from various referral centers in the USA, the majority of patients received systemic corticosteroids at the time of diagnosis, and most of these patients were considered corticosteroid responders. However, the rate of corticosteroid dependence in this cohort of pediatric patients was approximately 45 % [33]. In addition to the many side

**Table 25.1** Pediatric ulcerative colitis activity index [36]

| Item | Points |
| --- | --- |
| 1. Abdominal pain | |
| No pain | 0 |
| Pain can be ignored | 5 |
| Pain cannot be ignored | 10 |
| 2. Rectal bleeding | |
| None | 0 |
| Small amount only, in less than 50 % of stools | 10 |
| Small amount with most stools | 20 |
| Large amount (>50 % of the stool content) | 30 |
| 3. Stool consistency of most stools | |
| Formed | 0 |
| Partially formed | 5 |
| Completely unformed | 10 |
| 4. Number of stools per 24 h | |
| 0–2 | 0 |
| 3–5 | 5 |
| 6–8 | 10 |
| >8 | 15 |
| 5. Nocturnal stools (any episode causing wakening) | |
| No | 0 |
| Yes | 10 |
| 6. Activity level | |
| No limitation of activity | 0 |
| Occasional limitation of activity | 5 |
| Severe restricted activity | 10 |

Sum of PUCAI: 0–85

effects and the risk of dependence, it is clear that while corticosteroids may provide symptomatic relief, histological remission and mucosal healing occur uncommonly in pediatric patients with UC treated with corticosteroids [34].

To avoid complications of prolonged corticosteroid use, there are several indices used in the adult population to help predict which patients will fail to respond to corticosteroids early on in the course of therapy [35]. In these patients, second-line or "rescue" therapies can then be promptly instituted. Until recently, no such tool existed in pediatrics. In 2007, the Pediatric Ulcerative Colitis Activity Index (PUCAI) was developed (Table 25.1) [36]. The PUCAI uses noninvasive items such as degree of abdominal pain, amount of rectal bleeding, and the number of stools per 24 h to measure disease activity in pediatric UC. The PUCAI was initially validated by means of a prospective cohort of 48 pediatric patients with ulcerative colitis undergoing colonoscopy. The PUCAI correlated well with established indices including Beattie index (colonoscopic appearance), physician global assessment (PGA), and Mayo score [36]. The PUCAI was more recently prospectively evaluated in 215 children with UC. This study confirmed the validity of the PUCAI as a primary outcome measure in determining disease activity in pediatric UC. Furthermore, it correlated well with therapeutic decisions [37].

The PUCAI score is now used commonly to direct therapeutic decision-making in pediatric patients presenting with severe, acute ulcerative colitis. The literature supports the use of the PUCAI, calculated on day 3 and 5 of corticosteroid treatment, to predict response to corticosteroid therapy and to identify those patients who will require escalation of therapy [7]. For example, a PUCAI of greater than 45 on day 3 can be used to predict nonresponse to IV corticosteroids [5]. In addition, patients who have a calculated PUCAI of greater than 70 on day 5 of corticosteroids should be regarded as steroid-refractory, and rescue therapy with infliximab should be considered [5].

## 6-Mercaptopurine (6-MP) and Azathioprine

Immunomodulatory agents used in the treatment of children and adolescents with IBD include purine analogs that inhibit purine ribonucleotide synthesis and cell proliferation, 6-mercaptopurine (Purinethol) and azathioprine (Imuran). These agents are used in patients with UC who are steroid dependent or whose disease is refractory to steroid treatment. These medications generally require approximately 1–3 months to produce an effect and, therefore, are not used in acute exacerbations of the disease. Because of the delay in response, immunomodulators are frequently combined with corticosteroids initially.

The first controlled trial evaluating the efficacy of 6-MP in pediatric patients was published in 2000 [38]. Markowitz and colleagues hypothesized that 6-MP would reduce the need for corticosteroids in pediatric patients newly diagnosed with Crohn's disease. At the time of diagnosis, pediatric patients with disease activity scores in the moderate to severe range were randomized to receive a corticosteroid plus 6-MP or a corticosteroid plus placebo. Patients were followed for 18 months. The results suggested that children in the 6-MP group required corticosteroids for a shorter period of time and were able to remain off of corticosteroids for longer. The adverse effects seen with 6-MP were similar to those seen in adults and included pancreatitis, hepatitis, and bone marrow suppression. There were limitations to this study, however, including small sample size.

Recently, a cohort of pediatric patients with ulcerative colitis treated with a thiopurine was prospectively observed [39]. At 1 year following initiation of thiopurine therapy, 50 % of patients had achieved corticosteroid-free inactive disease. The study further demonstrated that the likelihood of avoiding rescue therapy with a biologic, calcineurin inhibitor, or colectomy was 73 % at 1 year. Treatment with a thiopurine also seemed to improve the likelihood of avoiding rescue therapy at 2 years (59 %). When these patients were followed further than 1 year, however, the results were less favorable.

In clinical practice, for the treatment of patients with UC, 6-MP and azathioprine are used interchangeably. The standard initial dose in pediatric patients is 1.0–1.5 mg/kg/day of 6-MP or 2.0–2.5 mg/kg/day of azathioprine. Dosing is also based on the thiopurine methyltransferase (TPMT) enzyme activity level. The TPMT enzyme activity is typically assessed prior to initiation of therapy in order to prevent toxicity. Some individuals either lack the TPMT enzyme or have low levels, which increases their risk of toxicity. The active 6-thioguanine (6-TGN) metabolites can also be followed in order to ensure that therapeutic levels of the medication are achieved. There is recent data to suggest that in very young patients with IBD (age 6 and younger), the standard per kilogram dose may not be adequate [40]. When these patients are closely monitored, dosage escalations are acceptable and are generally effective and well tolerated.

## Methotrexate

Methotrexate is an analog of folic acid and of aminopterin, a folic acid antagonist. The mechanism of action is through dihydrofolate reductase, the enzyme involved in the de novo synthesis pathway for purines and pyrimidines. The exact anti-inflammatory effect of low-dose methotrexate is unclear [41]. The treatment of juvenile idiopathic arthritis (JIA) with low-dose oral methotrexate is well established and is the source of the majority of the literature regarding the safety of low-dose methotrexate in pediatric patients. Methotrexate has also been used to maintain remission in children with IBD who are steroid dependent and fail to respond to or are unable to tolerate thiopurines [42]. Parenteral (SQ) administration seems to be more effective than oral administration in IBD patients. A potential benefit of methotrexate is that the onset of action is slightly more rapid than 6-MP or azathioprine.

There is limited data available for the use of methotrexate in ulcerative colitis, although there is more significant evidence for its use in Crohn's disease. There is only one double-blind, placebo-controlled study evaluating the efficacy of methotrexate in ulcerative colitis [43]. In this study, methotrexate was not found to be superior to placebo in the induction or maintenance of remission in UC patients. However, methotrexate was administered orally in this study. Additionally, lower dosing than what has been demonstrated to be effective in Crohn's disease was used.

In the treatment of pediatric UC, methotrexate seems to be well tolerated [44]. However, further studies are required in order to establish efficacy. Common side effects include nausea and anorexia. More serious adverse events such as hepatotoxicity, bone marrow suppression, hypersensitivity pneumonitis, and opportunistic infections are rare. Finally, methotrexate is a known teratogen, and as such, many clinicians will avoid its use in adolescent females.

## Biologics

Infliximab is a monoclonal antibody against tumor necrosis factor (TNF)-alpha, and it is the most commonly used biologic medication in the treatment of ulcerative colitis. Clinical trials in adults with UC have demonstrated a role for infliximab in the treatment of moderate to severe disease or corticosteroid-resistant disease [41]. Infliximab has also become especially valuable as rescue therapy in the treatment of acute, severe exacerbations. There is adult literature to suggest that infliximab is effective in preventing or delaying colectomy in UC patients with steroid-refractory disease [42]. However, the long-term efficacy of infliximab in the treatment of UC remains largely unknown.

Available pediatric data supports the use of infliximab in the treatment of moderate to severe ulcerative colitis. In fact, in 2011, the FDA approved infliximab to treat moderately to severely active UC in children older than 6 years of age who have had inadequate response to conventional therapy. The infliximab dosage used in pediatric patients is 5 mg/kg. Similar to the adult population, intravenous infusions are given at 0, 2, and 6 weeks for induction. Hyams and colleagues recently performed a multicenter, prospective, observational cohort study of 332 pediatric patients with UC [45]. In this study, 61 % of patients who had failed intravenous corticosteroids and had been prescribed infliximab as a second-line therapy avoided colectomy at 24 months. In addition, at 12 months and 24 months, 28 % and 21 % of patients were in remission and off corticosteroids, respectively.

As discussed previously, pediatric patients with ulcerative colitis often present with acute, severe disease, and in these situations, the treatment options are limited. Corticosteroids are considered to be first-line therapy in acute, severe exacerbations. However, as is the case in adults, approximately 1/3 of pediatric patients with severe UC will not have a complete response to corticosteroids. A recent multicenter, prospective, observational study was designed in order to evaluate outcomes in severe pediatric UC [7], in which pediatric patients hospitalized for severe UC were enrolled. The PUCAI, calculated on day 3 and 5 of IV corticosteroid treatment, was able to predict patients who would require rescue therapy. Of the patients who required rescue treatment with infliximab, 76 % responded and 52 % remained well 1 year following initiation of therapy.

Adalimumab, a fully humanized monoclonal anti-TNF, can be used in the treatment of ulcerative colitis. Generally, adalimumab is reserved for patients who either lose response or become intolerant to infliximab. The onset of action of adalimumab may be slower to demonstrate efficacy as compared to infliximab which would make it somewhat less suitable for the treatment of acute, severe exacerbations [46]. Recently, adalimumab was found to be effective in the induction of remission in adult patients with moderate to severe UC who had failed corticosteroids and/or other immunosuppressive medications [47]. There are currently no studies which examine the efficacy of adalimumab in the treatment of pediatric UC patients.

Golimumab is the most recently approved fully humanized monoclonal anti-TNF for the treatment of patients with ulcerative colitis. Golimumab is a human anti-TNF monoclonal antibody-binding soluble and transmembrane TNF-$\alpha$ (therefore, the binding of TNF to its receptors, with consequent activation of inflammation, is inhibited). It is administered subcutaneously. Since 2009, the therapy of golimumab has been approved for the treatment of autoimmune diseases, such as rheumatoid arthritis, psoriatic arthritis, and ankylosing spondylitis, in Europe. In 2013 this agent gained regulatory approval in the USA for the treatment of refractory ulcerative colitis.

There are no currently published trials that have evaluated golimumab in pediatric patients with ulcerative colitis; however, a recent trial was published that assessed the efficacy and safety of golimumab in polyarticular pediatric juvenile idiopathic arthritis patients (aged 2 to <18 years) with active arthritis despite methotrexate for ≥3 months. The results of this study demonstrated that JIA patients with active polyarticular disease demonstrated rapid response to golimumab [48].

## Other Immunosuppressive Medications

Cyclosporine is a potent inhibitor of the inflammatory cascade, and it has occasionally been used as salvage therapy in pediatric patients with UC who do not respond to corticosteroids. There have been several retrospective pediatric studies evaluating the efficacy of cyclosporine in severe UC. However, the cohorts have been small. No prospective studies have been performed in children. The available literature suggests that in the short term, cyclosporine can effectively induce remission and obviate the need for immediate surgical intervention [5]. However, multiple studies have shown that the use of cyclosporine as monotherapy in steroid-refractory UC patients is associated with high failure rates [49]. Currently, in pediatric patients, cyclosporine is rarely used. When cyclosporine is prescribed, it is prescribed in combination with an immunomodulator such as 6-MP or azathioprine. As a rule, cyclosporine is used exclusively as a bridging therapy to allow 6-MP or azathioprine to become therapeutic. Because cyclosporine is a potent immunosuppressive agent, infections which can mimic IBD exacerbations, such as CMV, must be ruled out prior to initiating therapy. Also, patients must be monitored closely for the side effects and adverse events associated with cyclosporine treatment. For example, cyclosporine is nephrotoxic and may cause irreversible renal insufficiency.

In some centers, tacrolimus has been utilized in pediatric patients with steroid-refractory colitis. A retrospective analysis of a single center's experience with tacrolimus in the treatment of steroid-refractory pediatric UC was recently published [50]. During the study period, 46 hospitalized patients were treated with tacrolimus. All but five patients responded to tacrolimus therapy, and response was defined as an improvement in the PUCAI score of more than 20 points. Most patients were able to be discharged from the hospital without undergoing colectomy. However, many patients experienced exacerbation of disease when transitioned to maintenance therapy, and 60 % still ultimately required colectomy. Tacrolimus may be valuable as a bridge to maintenance therapy in pediatric patients with steroid-refractory UC. There may also be a role for tacrolimus in the stabilization of acutely ill steroid-refractory UC patients prior to surgery [50]. However, further studies are necessary before routine use can be recommended.

## Surgical Care

At some point during the course of the illness, surgical removal of the colon may become a necessity for patients with ulcerative colitis. Because in UC the disease is limited to the colon, colectomy is considered a curative procedure. The most commonly performed procedure in children with UC is the ileal pouch-anal anastomosis (IPAA), which is performed in 2–3 stages. The rate of surgery in pediatric patients is higher than in the adult population. In pediatrics, 40 % of patients require colectomy 10 years after diagnosis [51]. This is compared to 5–20 % of adult patients who require colectomy 10 years after diagnosis [52]. In children, elective colectomy is considered when severe, medically refractory disease significantly interferes with growth

and nutrition, when symptoms prevent the patient from maintaining a normal lifestyle, or when dysplasia or malignancy is detected. Because of the potential toxicities of therapy, colectomy should be considered in patients who will require prolonged escalation of therapy in order to maintain remission. Apart from elective colectomy, a smaller percentage of pediatric patients will require acute surgical intervention because of fulminant colitis refractory to medical therapy.

Pediatric patients with Crohn's disease often present with isolated colonic involvement. Patients with Crohn's disease who undergo IPAA often have a poor outcome. Therefore, it is critical to distinguish the disease type (i.e., Crohn's disease versus UC) prior to surgical intervention. In a study performed in 151 pediatric patients with ulcerative colitis who underwent IPAA, 15 % were found to have Crohn's disease and had poor outcomes including pouchitis and pouch failure [53]. The risk of reclassification of inflammatory bowel disease, from ulcerative colitis to Crohn's disease, varies in the literature between 2 and 15 % [53–55]. Prior to recommending colectomy in a pediatric patient, imaging is often performed to exclude small bowel disease. In addition, IBD serology can be useful to help distinguish between Crohn's disease and ulcerative colitis. If despite the evaluation, the disease subtype remains unclear, a temporary diverting ileostomy can be considered. While this procedure is performed rarely, it is valuable in young patients with indeterminate colitis.

## Summary

Ulcerative colitis is common in the pediatric population. In children with UC, the therapeutic goal is to gain clinical and laboratory control of the disease with minimal adverse effects while permitting the patient to function as normally as possible. The "step-up" approach has been outlined here and is the most common therapeutic approach utilized; however, there are cases in which the "top-down" approach is appropriate. The treatment of pediatric patients with UC can be challenging, especially given the lack of pediatric literature describing the safety and efficacy of ulcerative colitis therapies. Clearly, further prospective randomized, controlled trials in pediatric patients are essential. In addition, as the fields of genomics, metagenomics, and the microbiome expand, novel treatments will undoubtedly be developed. The goal of patient-targeted therapy may also become more realistic. Table 25.2 lists commonly used medications in treating ulcerative colitis in pediatric patients.

**Table 25.2** Commonly used medications in treating ulcerative colitis in pediatric patients

| Medication | Available formulations | Pediatric dosage | Notes |
|---|---|---|---|
| *5-ASA* | | | |
| Mesalamine | | | |
| Asacol | Tablet 400 mg, 800 mg | 40–80 mg/kg/day PO in 3–4 divided doses | |
| Pentasa | Capsule 250 mg, 500 mg | 40–80 mg/kg/day PO in 3–4 divided doses | May open the capsule and sprinkle contents on food, but beads should not be crushed or chewed |
| Rowasa | Rectal suspension 4 g/60 mL | 4 g once nightly at bedtime | |
| Canasa | Rectal suppository 1,000 mg | ½–1 suppository once nightly at bedtime | |
| Balsalazide (Colazal) | Capsule 750 mg | 110–170 mg/kg/day in 3 divided doses | May open the capsule and sprinkle contents on food |
| *Immunomodulators* | | | |
| 6-Mercaptopurine (Purinethol) | Tablet 50 mg | 1.5–2.5 mg/kg/dose once nightly at bedtime | |
| Azathioprine (Imuran) | Tablet 50 mg | 1.5–3 mg/kg/dose once nightly at bedtime | |
| Methotrexate | Tablet 2.5 mg, 10 mg Injection 25 mg/mL | Oral or subcutaneous once weekly: 20–29 kg: 10 mg 30–39 kg: 15 mg 40–49 kg: 20 mg 50 kg or >25 mg | Supplement folic acid 1 mg/day PO |
| *Biologics* | | | |
| Infliximab (Remicade) | Powder for injection 100 mg | Induction: 5 mg/kg IV infused over 2 h at weeks 0, 2, and 6 weeks Maintenance: 5 mg/kg IV infused over 2 h every 8 weeks | |
| Adalimumab (Humira) | Injection solution (subcutaneous) 20 mg/0.4 mL prefilled syringe 40 mg/0.8 mL prefilled syringe or pen | Induction: <40 kg: 80 mg on day 1 followed by 40 mg 2 weeks later >40 kg: 160 mg on day 1 followed by 80 mg 2 weeks later Maintenance: <40 kg: 20 mg every other week >40 kg: 40 mg every other week | No studies in pediatric UC, dosing for pediatric CD shown |
| Golimumab (Simponi) | Subcutaneous solution: 50 mg/0.5 mL prefilled syringe or autoinjector 100 mg/mL prefilled syringe or autoinjector | <45 kg: Week 0: 90 mg/m$^2$ Week 2: 45 mg/m$^2$ Every 4 weeks: 45 mg/m$^2$ Consider adult dosing in children >45 kg | No studies demonstrating safety or efficacy in pediatric IBD, unpublished dosing shown |

# References

1. Kelsen J, Baldassano RN. Inflammatory bowel disease: the difference between children and adults. Inflamm Bowel Dis. 2008;14 Suppl 2:S9–11.
2. Malaty HM, et al. Rising incidence of inflammatory bowel disease among children: a 12-year study. J Pediatr Gastroenterol Nutr. 2010;50(1):27–31.
3. Benchimol EI, et al. Epidemiology of pediatric inflammatory bowel disease: a systematic review of international trends. Inflamm Bowel Dis. 2011;17(1):423–39.
4. Bousvaros A, et al. Differentiating ulcerative colitis from Crohn disease in children and young adults: report of a working group of the North American Society for Pediatric Gastroenterology, Hepatology, and Nutrition and the Crohn's and Colitis Foundation of America. J Pediatr Gastroenterol Nutr. 2007;44(5):653–74.

5. Turner D, Griffiths AM. Acute severe ulcerative colitis in children: a systematic review. Inflamm Bowel Dis. 2011;17(1):440–9.

6. Kugathasan S, et al. Epidemiologic and clinical characteristics of children with newly diagnosed inflammatory bowel disease in Wisconsin: a statewide population-based study. J Pediatr. 2003; 143(4):525–31.

7. Turner D, et al. Severe pediatric ulcerative colitis: a prospective multicenter study of outcomes and predictors of response. Gastroenterology. 2010;138(7):2282–91.

8. Rutgeerts P, et al. Infliximab for induction and maintenance therapy for ulcerative colitis. N Engl J Med. 2005;353(23):2462–76.

9. Kim MJ, et al. Infliximab therapy in children with Crohn's disease: a one-year evaluation of efficacy comparing 'top-down' and 'step-up' strategies. Acta Paediatr. 2011;100(3):451–5.

10. Sutherland L, Macdonald JK. Oral 5-aminosalicylic acid for maintenance of remission in ulcerative colitis. Cochrane Database Syst Rev. 2006; (2): CD000544.

11. Sutherland L, Macdonald JK. Oral 5-aminosalicylic acid for induction of remission in ulcerative colitis. Cochrane Database Syst Rev. 2006; (2): CD000543.

12. Ferry GD, et al. Olsalazine versus sulfasalazine in mild to moderate childhood ulcerative colitis: results of the Pediatric Gastroenterology Collaborative Research Group Clinical Trial. J Pediatr Gastroenterol Nutr. 1993;17(1):32–8.

13. Quiros JA, et al. Safety, efficacy, and pharmacokinetics of balsalazide in pediatric patients with mild-to-moderate active ulcerative colitis: results of a randomized, double-blind study. J Pediatr Gastroenterol Nutr. 2009;49(5):571–9.

14. Escher JC, et al. Treatment of inflammatory bowel disease in childhood: best available evidence. Inflamm Bowel Dis. 2003;9(1):34–58.

15. Iofel E, et al. Mesalamine intolerance mimics symptoms of active inflammatory bowel disease. J Pediatr Gastroenterol Nutr. 2002; 34(1):73–6.

16. Heyman MB, et al. Efficacy and safety of mesalamine suppositories for treatment of ulcerative proctitis in children and adolescents. Inflamm Bowel Dis. 2010;16(11):1931–9.

17. Ingerski LM, et al. Barriers to oral medication adherence for adolescents with inflammatory bowel disease. J Pediatr Psychol. 2010;35(6):683–91.

18. Frank DN, St. Amand A, Feldman RA, Boedeker EC, Harpaz N, Pace NR. Molecular-phylogenetic characterization of microbial community imbalances in human inflammatory bowel diseases. Proc Natl Acad Sci U S A. 2007;104:13780–5.

19. Sartor RB. Therapeutic manipulation of the enteric microflora in inflammatory bowel diseases: antibiotics, probiotics, and prebiotics. Gastroenterology. 2004;126(6):1620–33.

20. Perencevich M, Burakoff R. Use of antibiotics in the treatment of inflammatory bowel disease. Inflamm Bowel Dis. 2006;12(7): 651–64.

21. Thukral C, Travassos WJ, Peppercorn MA. The role of antibiotics in inflammatory bowel disease. Curr Treat Opt Gastroenterol. 2005;8(3):223–8.

22. Mallon P et al. Probiotics for induction of remission in ulcerative colitis. Cochrane Database Syst Rev. 2007; (4): CD005573.

23. Mimura T, et al. Once daily high dose probiotic therapy (VSL#3) for maintaining remission in recurrent or refractory pouchitis. Gut. 2004;53(1):108–14.

24. Gionchetti P, et al. Oral bacteriotherapy as maintenance treatment in patients with chronic pouchitis: a double-blind, placebo-controlled trial. Gastroenterology. 2000;119(2):305–9.

25. Lindgren S, et al. Effect of budesonide enema on remission and relapse rate in distal ulcerative colitis and proctitis. Scand J Gastroenterol. 2002;37(6):705–10.

26. Levine A, et al. Evaluation of oral budesonide for treatment of mild and moderate exacerbations of Crohn's disease in children. J Pediatr. 2002;140(1):75–80.

27. Sherlock ME et al. Oral budesonide for induction of remission in ulcerative colitis. Cochrane Database Syst Rev. 2010; (10): CD007698.

28. D'Haens GR, et al. Clinical trial: preliminary efficacy and safety study of a new Budesonide-MMX(R) 9 mg extended-release tablets in patients with active left-sided ulcerative colitis. J Crohns Colitis. 2010;4(2):153–60.

29. Sandborn WJ, Travis S, Moro L, et al. Once-daily budesonide MMX(R) extended-release tablets induce remission in patients with mild to moderate ulcerative colitis: results from the CORE I study. Gastroenterology. 2012;143:e1–2.

30. Travis SP, Danese S, Kupcinskas L, et al. Once-daily budesonide MMX in active, mild-to-moderate ulcerative colitis: results from the randomised CORE II study. Gut. 2014;63:433–41.

31. Leonard MB. Glucocorticoid-induced osteoporosis in children: impact of the underlying disease. Pediatrics. 2007;119 Suppl 2: S166–74.

32. Faubion Jr WA, et al. The natural history of corticosteroid therapy for inflammatory bowel disease: a population-based study. Gastroenterology. 2001;121(2):255–60.

33. Hyams J, et al. The natural history of corticosteroid therapy for ulcerative colitis in children. Clin Gastroenterol Hepatol. 2006;4(9):1118–23.

34. Beattie RM, et al. Endoscopic assessment of the colonic response to corticosteroids in children with ulcerative colitis. J Pediatr Gastroenterol Nutr. 1996;22(4):373–9.

35. Seo M, et al. Evaluation of the clinical course of acute attacks in patients with ulcerative colitis through the use of an activity index. J Gastroenterol. 2002;37(1):29–34.

36. Turner D, et al. Development, validation, and evaluation of a pediatric ulcerative colitis activity index: a prospective multicenter study. Gastroenterology. 2007;133(2):423–32.

37. Turner D, et al. Appraisal of the pediatric ulcerative colitis activity index (PUCAI). Inflamm Bowel Dis. 2009;15(8):1218–23.

38. Markowitz J, et al. A multicenter trial of 6-mercaptopurine and prednisone in children with newly diagnosed Crohn's disease. Gastroenterology. 2000;119(4):895–902.

39. Hyams JS, et al. Outcome following thiopurine use in children with ulcerative colitis: a prospective multicenter registry study. Am J Gastroenterol. 2011;106(5):981–7.

40. Grossman AB, et al. Increased dosing requirements for 6-mercaptopurine and azathioprine in inflammatory bowel disease patients six years and younger. Inflamm Bowel Dis. 2008;14(6): 750–5.

41. Rosenberg LN, Peppercorn MA. Efficacy and safety of drugs for ulcerative colitis. Expert Opin Drug Saf. 2010;9(4):573–92.

42. Ng SC, Kamm MA. Therapeutic strategies for the management of ulcerative colitis. Inflamm Bowel Dis. 2009;15(6):935–50.

43. Oren R, et al. Methotrexate in chronic active ulcerative colitis: a double-blind, randomized, Israeli multicenter trial. Gastroenterology. 1996;110(5):1416–21.

44. Willot S, Noble A, Deslandres C. Methotrexate in the treatment of inflammatory bowel disease: an 8-year retrospective study in a Canadian pediatric IBD center. Inflamm Bowel Dis. 2011;17:2521.

45. Hyams JS, et al. Outcome following infliximab therapy in children with ulcerative colitis. Am J Gastroenterol. 2010;105(6): 1430–6.

46. Reinisch W, et al. Adalimumab for induction of clinical remission in moderately to severely active ulcerative colitis: results of a randomised controlled trial. Gut. 2011;60(6):780–7.

47. Reinisch W, et al. Long-term infliximab maintenance therapy for ulcerative colitis: the ACT-1 and -2 extension studies. Inflamm Bowel Dis. 2011;18(2):201–11.

48. Brunner H, Ruperto N, Tzaribachev N, Horneff G, Wouters C, Panaviene V, Chasnyk V, Abud-Mendoza C, Cuttica R, Reiff A, Maldonado-Velázquez M, Rubio-Perez N, Alexeeva E, Joos R,

Keltsev V, Nasonov E, Kingsbury D, Bandeira M, Silverman E, Weller-Heinemann F, van Royen-Kerkhof A, Mendelsohn A, Kim L, Lovell D, Martini A. A148: a multi-center, double-blind, randomized-withdrawal trial of subcutaneous golimumab in pediatric patients with active polyarticular course juvenile idiopathic arthritis despite methotrexate therapy: week 48 results. Arthritis Rheumatol. 2014;66 Suppl 11:S191–2. doi:10.1002/art.38569.

49. Moskovitz DN, et al. Incidence of colectomy during long-term follow-up after cyclosporine-induced remission of severe ulcerative colitis. Clin Gastroenterol Hepatol. 2006;4(6):760–5.

50. Watson S, et al. Outcomes and adverse events in children and young adults undergoing tacrolimus therapy for steroid-refractory colitis. Inflamm Bowel Dis. 2011;17(1):22–9.

51. Shikhare G, Kugathasan S. Inflammatory bowel disease in children: current trends. J Gastroenterol. 2010;45(7):673–82.

52. Solberg IC, et al. Clinical course during the first 10 years of ulcerative colitis: results from a population-based inception cohort (IBSEN Study). Scand J Gastroenterol. 2009;44(4):431–40.

53. Alexander F, et al. Fate of the pouch in 151 pediatric patients after ileal pouch anal anastomosis. J Pediatr Surg. 2003;38(1):78–82.

54. Pakarinen MP, et al. Long-term outcomes of restorative proctocolectomy in children with ulcerative colitis. Pediatrics. 2009;123(5):1377–82.

55. Durno C, et al. Outcome after ileoanal anastomosis in pediatric patients with ulcerative colitis. J Pediatr Gastroenterol Nutr. 1998; 27(5):501–7.

# Chemoprevention in Ulcerative Colitis

Fernando Velayos

**Keywords**

Chemoprevention • Ulcerative colitis • Colorectal cancer • Familial adenomatous polyposis (FAP) • Hereditary nonpolyposis colorectal cancer (HNPCC)

## Background

Colorectal cancer (CRC) is a feared complication of chronic ulcerative colitis (UC). The cumulative probability of developing colorectal cancer (CRC) among persons with UC is significantly higher than in the general population [1]. UC is the third highest-risk condition for colorectal cancer after two genetic syndromes, familial adenomatous polyposis syndrome (FAP) and hereditary nonpolyposis colorectal cancer (HNPCC) [2]. Data from a comprehensive meta-analysis suggest that the probability of CRC in IBD is 2 % after 10 years of disease, 8 % after 20 years, and 18 % after 30 years [3, 4]. In comparison, the cumulative lifetime probability of developing CRC for the general population in the United States is approximately 5 % [3, 4].

Described in terms of relative risk, UC increases the risk of CRC five- to sixfold relative to the general population [1]. The risk of developing CRC increases as a greater proportion of the colon is involved by inflammation [1]. Interestingly, not all populations of IBD patients have an increased risk of CRC. In a Danish population-based cohort, the risk was 0.4 % after 10 years, 1.1 % after 20 years, and 2.1 % after 30 years of disease [5]. These probabilities are comparable to those of an American population-based cohort where the cumulative probability of developing CRC was 0 % at 5 years, 0.4 % at 15 years, and 2.0 % at 25 years after a CUC diagnosis [6]. Also

notable is that high-risk populations may be experiencing a reduction in cancer risk and mortality over time. A UK surveillance colonoscopy cohort reported a reduction in cancer risk over the past 30 years (1970–2000) and quantified the risk as a 2.5 % at 20 years, 7.6 % at 30 years, and 10.8 % after 40 years of disease [7]. A cohort in Sweden found a still elevated, but declining, trend in CRC incidence and mortality over a 35-year time period (1960–2004) [8].

It is not known why the risk of CRC is lower in certain populations than others or if the risk of CRC and mortality from CRC are declining in all populations. However, these promising data suggest that the risk of CRC in IBD is modifiable. Greater rates of proctocolectomy for medical treatment failures, better rates of surveillance colonoscopy with proctocolectomy for dysplasia, and finally greater use of potentially chemopreventive drugs used for IBD, vitamins, and other therapies used by UC patients could all be important factors that reduce the risk of CRC in a given population [9, 10].

To mitigate the risk of colorectal cancer, many patients and their physicians choose to follow a diagnostic program of *screening* and *surveillance* colonoscopy with a goal of detecting dysplasia and other early neoplastic lesions at a curable stage [11]. The rationale for undergoing surveillance colonoscopy is based on the premise that determining which patients are likely to progress to cancer in the near term can be reliably predicted by the presence or absence of histological dysplasia on colonoscopy. Surveillance colonoscopy is a *secondary prevention* strategy, whereby the risk of colorectal cancer is mitigated by either (1) identification and removal of dysplastic polypoid tissue or (2) detection of flat or subtle dysplasia followed by proctocolectomy. In other words, intervention occurs after dysplasia occurs.

F. Velayos, M.D., M.P.H. (✉)
Department of Gastroenterology, University of California, San Francisco, 2330 Post St., Suite 610, San Francisco, CA 94115, USA
e-mail: fernando.velayos@ucsf.edu

G.R. Lichtenstein (ed.), *Medical Therapy of Ulcerative Colitis*,
DOI 10.1007/978-1-4939-1677-1_26, © Springer Science+Business Media New York 2014

This strategy of secondary prevention is quite successful in colon cancer screening in the general population. However, dysplasia in inflammatory bowel disease is different. There is greater incidence of flat or subtle dysplasia that may be missed during colonoscopy, and important lesions can be obscured in the setting of inflammatory polyps [12, 13]. Thus instead of relying exclusively on secondary prevention (detecting and intervening after dysplasia has occurred), there has been significant interest in exploring strategies for primary prevention (intervening early to prevent the development of dysplasia in the first place). Chemoprevention is a primary prevention strategy.

The National Cancer Institute defines chemoprevention as the use of drugs, vitamins, or other agents to try to reduce the risk of or delay the development or recurrence of cancer. This chapter will review the relationship between drugs used to treat UC, vitamins, and other therapies used by UC patients and the risk of the development of colorectal cancer. This chapter will also review the most recent recommendations and guidelines from the American Gastroenterological Association with regard to chemoprevention.

## Medications Used to Treat UC

Chronic inflammation has a key role in the development of CRC in UC through years of repeated cycles of cellular damage and repair. Thus, it is logical that medications used to treat ulcerative colitis may reduce chronic inflammation and have important chemopreventive properties.

## 5-Aminosalicylates

There has been significant attention regarding the potential chemopreventive properties of 5-aminosalicylates. 5-aminosalicylates are among the oldest therapies used to treat ulcerative colitis. Sulfasalazine, composed of a sulfa moiety bonded to mesalamine, has been used in UC since the 1940s [14]. Modern mesalamine derivatives, which lack the sulfa moiety (contributes to GI side effects of sulfasalazine), have been available and approved by the US Food and Drug Administration (FDA) since the late 1980s after the first pivotal randomized control trials using these newer derivatives were published [15].

Interest in the chemopreventive properties of 5-ASA agents started in the mid-1990s, coincident with publications that aspirin and NSAIDs reduced the risk of colorectal cancer in the general population. In 1991, Thun et al. published an observational study showing regular aspirin users had an approximate 40 % reduction in fatal colon cancer [16]. In 1993, Greenberg et al. published an observational study showing that aspirin users had a 48 % reduction in adenomas [17].

A variety of clinical and experimental studies demonstrated that 5-aminosalicylates share several important antiinflammatory and anticancer properties with aspirin and nonsteroidal antiinflammatory medications (NSAIDs). These properties include increased apoptosis, decreased cell proliferation, reduced production of oxidative radicals such as prostaglandins and leukotrienes, and finally improved cellular repair [18].

The first major observational population-based study examining the association between 5-ASA use and cancer risk was published in 1994 by Pinczowski et al. [19]. The authors conducted a nested case-control study in a population of Swedish patients in the Uppsala region with ulcerative colitis treated between 1965 and 1983. They noted that those who used more than 3 months of continuous sulfasalazine had a 60 % reduction in the risk of colorectal cancer compared to those with less than 3 months. It was noted that most subjects used more than 3 months of continuous therapy or in fact were long-term and regular users with high rates of adherence to sulfasalazine [19].

In their study, Pinczowski et al. described the important next step to advance the 5-ASA hypothesis and wrote: "clinical trials should be initiated in patients with inactive ulcerative colitis to determine if continuous treatment with sulfasalazine… has an impact on dysplasia or malignant transformation" [19]. This statement is similar to that from Greenberg et al. the year prior regarding aspirin use in the general population and colorectal adenomas: "this study supports the hypothesis that aspirin has an anti-neoplastic effect in the large bowel. Nevertheless, the question of whether aspirin *should be used* to prevent large bowel tumors would be best answered by a randomized controlled clinical trial specifically designed to address this issue."

This historical perspective is relevant in that a randomized trial of aspirin to prevent colorectal adenomas in patients without IBD was published a decade later and showed a 39 % reduction in advanced neoplasia risk. For ulcerative colitis, no such trial has been conducted given complexities in design as well as sample size. Thus, the available data for 5-ASA chemoprevention and the 5-ASA hypothesis remains based on experimental and human observational studies, but not randomized trials. These observational studies are notable for a variety of clinical designs and quality, as well as heterogeneous population of patients.

A systematic synthesis of these early trials was published in a meta-analysis. The pooled data supported the hypothesis that 5-aminosalicylates reduce the risk of colorectal neoplasia in patients with ulcerative colitis [10]. A total of nine studies (three cohort, six case-control) containing 334 cases of colorectal cancer, 140 cases of dysplasia, and a total of 1,932 subjects were analyzed. Pooled analysis showed a protective association with regular 5-ASA therapy and a risk reduction of 49 %. This estimate is consistent with the range of risk reduction observed with aspirin and nonsteroidal use in the general population and colorectal neoplasia risk.

Since then, additional studies have been published showing heterogeneous results. An example of two recent large-scale studies includes a Canadian and a French study. The Canadian study included 8,744 subjects with IBD who are part of the population-based epidemiologic database in Manitoba. The authors found no difference in the incidence of CRC among 5-ASA users nor differences between cases and controls with regard to duration of prior 5-ASA use [20]. In contrast, a nested case-control study within the CESAME population-based cohort found a 54 % reduction in CRC risk among 5-ASA users [21]. As such, the 5-ASA hypothesis is unlikely to be definitively answered with further observational studies.

Thus the question is how to synthesize and apply seemingly conflicting data to patient care. We can summarize what is known and not known and make educated guesses based on this information. It is known that chronic inflammation of the colon causes DNA damage and is a risk factor for colorectal dysplasia in ulcerative colitis [18, 22]. It is known that 5-ASA is an effective maintenance therapy for ulcerative colitis and has in vitro and in vivo antineoplastic effects [18, 23]. It is not proven but likely that maintenance 5-ASA therapy manages remission in UC through the reduction of chronic inflammation. It is known that the question of whether 5-ASA *should be used* to prevent large bowel tumors would be best answered by a randomized controlled clinical trial specifically designed to address this issue, and this is unlikely to occur in the near future if at all.

We can analyze this experimental and clinical data to provide some reasonable conclusions and also refer to the most recent AGA evidence ratings on this topic. For those patients with an indication for maintenance 5-ASA therapy, it is reasonable to suggest that maintenance 5-ASA therapy may in fact have a secondary benefit of reducing the risk of long-term dysplasia and colorectal cancer. Patients should be aware that this does not eliminate the need for regular surveillance nor changes the recommended frequency of surveillance [11]. Whether patients on immunomodulators or anti-TNF therapy but not on a 5-ASA therapy should have such therapy added is not answered with the available data. The AGA evidence rating for 5-ASA as a chemopreventive agent in UC is B (moderate certainty that the magnitude of net benefits is moderate) [24].

## Immunomodulators

The class of immunomodulator agents includes azathioprine, its metabolite 6-mercaptopurine, and methotrexate. Given the lack of data for the use of methotrexate in ulcerative colitis, most immunomodulator use in UC and chemopreventive studies has assessed only azathioprine and 6-mercaptopurine.

Both azathioprine and 6-mercaptopurine do not have any obvious or inherent anticancer properties in colonocytes. The biologic effect appears to be on lymphocytes. Azathioprine and 6-mercaptopurine inhibit DNA and RNA synthesis and proliferation of lymphocytes. AZA and 6-MP have antineoplastic effects in certain leukemias. They have pro-neoplastic effects in certain lymphoproliferative tumors and are associated with a fourfold increased risk of non-Hodgkin's lymphoma in persons with inflammatory bowel disease [25].

There have been at least four studies that have examined the association between azathioprine or 6-MP use and colorectal cancer risk in ulcerative colitis. One study showed a threefold increased risk of cancer; however, this study included high-risk patients for colorectal cancer who had primary sclerosing cholangitis and whose indication for azathioprine or 6-MP was posttransplant immunosuppression [12]. Of the remaining studies, two studies (one unpublished [26], one published [27]) showed a 70 % reduction in colorectal cancer risk [22, 26], whereas one showed no effect [27].

Given the lack of experimental data showing a chemopreventive effect for immunomodulators, the mixed results from clinical data, and the elevated relative risk of lymphoma reported with AZA/6-MP, the AGA evidence rating for immunomodulator use as a chemopreventive agent in UC is I (no recommendation, insufficient evidence to recommend for or against) [24].

As with 5-ASA, how should the above data be synthesized and used clinically? Given that AZA/6-MP use has a specific role within the algorithm for management of ulcerative colitis, it appears reasonable to emphasize to patients that the same therapy that is maintaining the ulcerative colitis in remission is likely having a secondary benefit of reducing long-term colorectal cancer risk. It is important to again emphasize that the only recommended modality for reducing long-term colorectal cancer risk is screening and surveillance colonoscopy [11].

## Corticosteroids and Anti-TNF Therapy

Two other important drug classes used in the management of ulcerative colitis are oral corticosteroids and anti-TNF biologic therapy. Corticosteroids are effective for the short-term management of acute flares of ulcerative colitis. They are ineffective as long-term therapies, and most chemopreventive agents need to meet the requirement of safe use on a long-term basis. Known long-term side effects from steroids include but are not limited to osteopenia, osteoporosis, hypertension, as well as cataracts. Nearly 20 % of patients with ulcerative colitis who start oral corticosteroids become corticosteroid dependent, meaning that they cannot taper off of corticosteroids [28]. It is recommended that these patients transition onto immune modulator therapy or anti-TNF therapy in order to achieve a durable remission off of corticosteroids [29]. Thus, even if compelling data were available regarding a chemopreventive effect of corticosteroids, modern management of ulcerative colitis attempts to minimize long-term steroid use and steroid dependence [29]. The AGA evidence rating for corticosteroids for chemoprevention in UC is D (high certainty that the net magnitude of benefit is negative) [24].

Data are sparse with regard to the use of anti-TNF therapy and chemoprevention. The FDA approved anti-TNF therapy for UC in late 2006 after the publication of two pivotal randomized controlled trials [30]. Longer-term data will be necessary in order to specifically address the question regarding anti-TNF and chemoprevention. Accordingly, there is no evidence rating on the most recent AGA guidelines for anti-TNF therapy for chemoprevention [24].

## Vitamins

### Folic Acid

Folate is a water-soluble B vitamin that plays several important biologic roles, including carcinogenesis. Folate deficiency is associated with aberrant DNA synthesis and repair. There are folate-sensitive sites on genes important for carcinogenesis such as the p53 suppressor gene. Folate deficiency in inflammatory bowel disease can occur through a variety of mechanisms. These include intestinal losses, poor intake, as well as competitive absorption from sulfasalazine.

Given the consequences of folate deficiency, there has been significant interest in using folic acid supplementation as a chemopreventive agent in ulcerative colitis. At least four studies have assessed this relationship [12, 22, 31, 32]. Supplementation was assessed in a variety of ways. Some studies assessed the use of 0.4 mg per day, others 1 mg per day, and others any use of folic acid either as direct supplementation or in the form of a multivitamin. Although all showed a trend toward reduction in risk ranging anywhere from 15 to 62 %, all failed to show statistical significance likely due to small sample size.

To put these data in context, in patients without inflammatory bowel disease, observational studies have noted a reduction in colorectal cancer risk after prolonged use of folic acid supplementation. The Nurses' Health Study demonstrated no benefit in reduction in the first 4 years of use (RRR, 1.02), a nonsignificant risk reduction after 5–15 years of use (RR, 0.80–0.83), but a markedly lower risk after 15 years of use (RR, 0.25 (CI 0.13–0.51)) [33]. Given the potentially antineoplastic effects of folic acid supplementation in the large bowel, Cole et al. conducted a randomized controlled trial whereby subjects were randomly assigned to receive 1 mg a day of folic acid or placebo [34]. The primary end point, the occurrence of at least one colorectal adenoma, was no different among the groups (44.1 % for folic acid, 42.4 % for placebo). However, for secondary end points, subjects in the folic acid group tended to have slightly higher rates of advanced adenomas and were more likely to have more than three adenomas.

As with therapy used to treat UC, how should the above data be applied? Given the known association between folate deficiency and neoplasia risk and potential risk for folate deficiency in patients with UC, it is reasonable to screen for folate deficiency in patients with ulcerative colitis (especially those on sulfasalazine) and to supplement those who are deficient. Based on extrapolation of the trial by Cole et al., empiric supplementation of all patients is unlikely to significantly reduce colorectal cancer risk and may potentially increase the risk of advanced neoplasia or multiple foci of neoplasia. The AGA evidence rating for folic acid supplementation and multivitamin use for chemoprevention in UC is I (no recommendation, insufficient evidence to recommend for or against) [24].

## Drugs Other Than Those Used to Treat UC

### Ursodeoxycholic Acid

Another medication that has been studied as a potential chemopreventive agent is ursodeoxycholic acid. Secondary bile acids are carcinogenic to the colon and are increased in patients with cholestatic liver disease. Primary sclerosing cholangitis (PSC) is a chronic cholestatic liver disease characterized by fibrosing inflammation and destruction of intrahepatic bile ducts and is an important indication for liver transplantation. At least 70 % of cases of PSC are associated with IBD, mostly UC [35]. There are no effective therapies. A randomized controlled trial by Lindor et al. showed that ursodeoxycholic at a dose of 13–15 mg/kg/day showed biochemical improvement and trend toward improving time to progression, although this was not statistically significant [36]. Given the lack of effective therapies, these findings prompted investigation into the use of higher doses as a therapy for PSC, and this trial was recently published.

Ursodeoxycholic acid is an exogenous bile acid that reduces the concentration of toxic secondary bile acids in the colon and thus an attractive candidate as a chemopreventive agent in patients with PSC/UC, independent of any potential effects in the management of PSC. This is relevant in primary sclerosing cholangitis because the risk of dysplasia and colorectal cancer is significantly elevated [37]. As evidence, quite aggressive colonoscopic surveillance (every year and upon diagnosis of primary sclerosing cholangitis) is recommended [38].

Initial studies regarding the use ursodeoxycholic acid as a chemopreventive agent were quite promising. Two studies that demonstrated its use were associated with at least a significant 80 % reduced risk of CRC [39, 40], and a third demonstrated a nonsignificant 41 % reduced risk [41]. Among the favorable studies was a subgroup analysis published in 2003 of a prospective randomized trial by Lindor. Accordingly, the AGA evidence rating for ursodeoxycholic acid for chemoprevention in UC is A (high certainty that the magnitude of net benefit is substantial) [24].

Since publication of these guidelines, a new study has raised doubts regarding the use of high-dose ursodeoxycholic acid (28–30 mg/kg/day) for chemoprevention and for managing PSC patients in general. Lindor et al. published the follow-up clinical trial studying high-dose ursodeoxycholic acid in PSC with unexpected results. Patients in the high-dose ursodeoxycholic acid arm had a 2.3-fold greater rate of a negative primary end point (cirrhosis, varices, cholangiocarcinoma, liver transplantation, or death) and serious adverse events (63 % vs. 37 %) [35]. A subgroup analysis published in 2011 examining colon cancer risk also had unexpected results. Patients who received high-dose ursodeoxycholic acid had a 4.4-fold increased risk of neoplasia (dysplasia or cancer) compared to those receiving placebo (95 % CI 1.3–20.01, $p = 0.02$) [42]. In comparison, the subgroup analysis published in 2003 from the low-dose UDCA clinical trial showed a 74 % reduction in neoplasia risk [40].

A recently published subgroup analysis of a European RCT for high-dose UDA (defined as 17–23 mg/kg/day) did not show higher risk of colorectal neoplasia in the UDCA group, but definitely did not show a reduction in the incidence of neoplasia (13 % vs. 16 %) [43]. Thus, the question is how to weigh and clinically resolve this discrepancy regarding safety and efficacy with regard to low- and high-dose USDA and the elevated colorectal cancer risk in PSC/UC. Based on these data, the American Association for the Study of Liver Diseases (AASLD) in their most recent practice guidelines does not endorse the routine use of UDCA as chemoprevention for CRC in patients with PSC/UC and do not distinguish between high and low dose (evidence 1B: strength strong, quality moderate). It also recommends against the use of UDCA as medical therapy in PSC (evidence 1A: strength strong, quality high) [44].

## Statins

There is interest in assessing the potential role of statins not only as a chemoprotective agent in UC but also in the general population. Data in IBD are quite sparse. The AGA evidence rating for statin use for chemoprevention in UC is I (no recommendation, insufficient evidence to recommend for or against) [24].

## Conclusion

The concept of chemoprevention in IBD is attractive and needed and promising but as of yet unproven. There is a biologic rationale for several agents, yet the clinical evidence in many cases is mixed, with definitive clinical trials unlikely to be performed. Even so, several conclusions can be drawn based on extrapolation of the available data. With regard to drugs used to treat UC, long-term 5-ASA use and long-term maintenance of remission in UC are likely to yield a secondary benefit of chemoprevention. Given the association between chronic inflammation and neoplasia risk in UC, it may be that other agents used to treat UC may have a chemoprotective effect through long-term maintenance of remission. The data do not support using a specific drug exclusively for the purpose of chemoprevention. Chronic steroid use is not encouraged and not relevant in the discussion of chemoprevention. The known carcinogenic potential of folate deficiency demonstrated in experimental models alone does not provide sufficient biologic rationale to supplement all patients with UC based on the clinical data. However, UC patients have risk factors for folate deficiency, and thus it appears relevant and logical to screen and treat folate deficiency, especially in patients on sulfasalazine. At this time, the AASLD does not recommend UDCA to patients with PSC/UC for chemoprevention. At this time, the primary strategy for cancer prevention in UC is that of secondary prevention (regular surveillance colonoscopy). Surveillance guidelines should not be altered based on the use of presumptive chemopreventive agents [11].

## References

1. Ekbom A, Helmick C, Zack M, Adami HO. Ulcerative colitis and colorectal cancer. A population-based study. N Engl J Med. 1990;323(18):1228–33.
2. Clevers H. Colon cancer–understanding how NSAIDs work. N Engl J Med. 2006;354(7):761–3.
3. Eaden JA, Abrams KR, Mayberry JF. The risk of colorectal cancer in ulcerative colitis: a meta-analysis. Gut. 2001;48(4):526–35.
4. Canavan C, Abrams KR, Mayberry J. Meta-analysis: colorectal and small bowel cancer risk in patients with Crohn's disease. Aliment Pharmacol Ther. 2006;23(8):1097–104.
5. Winther KV, Jess T, Langholz E, Munkholm P, Binder V. Long-term risk of cancer in ulcerative colitis: a population-based cohort study from Copenhagen county. Clin Gastroenterol Hepatol. 2004; 2(12):1088–95.
6. Jess T, Loftus Jr EV, Velayos FS, et al. Risk of intestinal cancer in inflammatory bowel disease: a population-based study from Olmsted county Minnesota. Gastroenterology. 2006;130(4): 1039–46.
7. Rutter MD, Saunders BP, Wilkinson KH, et al. Thirty-year analysis of a colonoscopic surveillance program for neoplasia in ulcerative colitis. Gastroenterology. 2006;130(4):1030–8.

8. Soderlund S, Brandt L, Lapidus A, et al. Decreasing time-trends of colorectal cancer in a large cohort of patients with inflammatory bowel disease. Gastroenterology. 2009;136(5):1561–7. quiz 1818-1569.

9. Munkholm P. Review article: the incidence and prevalence of colorectal cancer in inflammatory bowel disease. Aliment Pharmacol Ther. 2003;18 Suppl 2:1–5.

10. Velayos FS, Terdiman JP, Walsh JM. Effect of 5-aminosalicylate use on colorectal cancer and dysplasia risk: a systematic review and metaanalysis of observational studies. Am J Gastroenterol. 2005;100(6):1345–53.

11. Itzkowitz SH, Present DH. Consensus conference: colorectal cancer screening and surveillance in inflammatory bowel disease. Inflamm Bowel Dis. 2005;11(3):314–21.

12. Velayos FS, Loftus Jr EV, Jess T, et al. Predictive and protective factors associated with colorectal cancer in ulcerative colitis: a case-control study. Gastroenterology. 2006;130(7):1941–9.

13. Rutter MD, Saunders BP, Wilkinson KH, et al. Cancer surveillance in longstanding ulcerative colitis: endoscopic appearances help predict cancer risk. Gut. 2004;53(12):1813–6.

14. Svartz M. The treatment of 124 cases of ulcerative colitis with salazopyrine and attempts of desensibilization in cases of hypersensitiveness to sulfa. Acta Med Scand. 1948;131 Suppl 206:465–72.

15. Schroeder KW, Tremaine WJ, Ilstrup DM. Coated oral 5-aminosalicylic acid therapy for mildly to moderately active ulcerative colitis. A randomized study. N Engl J Med. 1987; 317(26):1625–9.

16. Thun MJ, Namboodiri MM, Heath Jr CW. Aspirin use and reduced risk of fatal colon cancer. N Engl J Med. 1991;325(23):1593–6.

17. Greenberg ER, Baron JA, Freeman Jr DH, Mandel JS, Haile R. Reduced risk of large-bowel adenomas among aspirin users. The Polyp Prevention Study Group. J Natl Cancer Inst. 1993;85(11): 912–6.

18. Allgayer H. Review article: mechanisms of action of mesalazine in preventing colorectal carcinoma in inflammatory bowel disease. Aliment Pharmacol Ther. 2003;18 Suppl 2:10–4.

19. Pinczowski D, Ekbom A, Baron J, Yuen J, Adami HO. Risk factors for colorectal cancer in patients with ulcerative colitis: a case-control study. Gastroenterology. 1994;107(1):117–20.

20. Bernstein CN, Nugent Z, Blanchard JF. 5-aminosalicylate is not chemoprophylactic for colorectal cancer in IBD: a population based study. Am J Gastroenterol. 2011;106(4):731–6.

21. Carrat F, Seksik P, Bouvier A-M, et al. 255 Aminosalicylates, thiopurines and the risk of colorectal cancer in inflammatory bowel diseases: a case-control study nested in the CESAME cohort. Gastroenterology. 2010;138(5, Suppl 1):S-47.

22. Rutter M, Saunders B, Wilkinson K, et al. Severity of inflammation is a risk factor for colorectal neoplasia in ulcerative colitis. Gastroenterology. 2004;126(2):451–9.

23. Sutherland L, Macdonald JK. Oral 5-aminosalicylic acid for maintenance of remission in ulcerative colitis. Cochrane Database Syst Rev. 2006;2, CD000544.

24. Farraye FA, Odze RD, Eaden J, Itzkowitz SH. AGA medical position statement on the diagnosis and management of colorectal neoplasia in inflammatory bowel disease. Gastroenterology. 2010; 138(2):738–45.

25. Kandiel A, Fraser AG, Korelitz BI, Brensinger C, Lewis JD. Increased risk of lymphoma among inflammatory bowel disease patients treated with azathioprine and 6-mercaptopurine. Gut. 2005;54(8):1121–5.

26. Beaugerie L, Brousse N, Bouvier AM, et al. Excess risk of lymphoproliferative disorders (LPD) in inflammatory bowel diseases (IBD): interim results of the CESAME cohort. Gastroenterology. 2008;134(A):116–7.

27. Matula S, Croog V, Itzkowitz S, et al. Chemoprevention of colorectal neoplasia in ulcerative colitis: the effect of 6-mercaptopurine. Clin Gastroenterol Hepatol. 2005;3(10):1015–21.

28. Faubion Jr WA, Loftus Jr EV, Harmsen WS, Zinsmeister AR, Sandborn WJ. The natural history of corticosteroid therapy for inflammatory bowel disease: a population-based study. Gastroenterology. 2001;121(2):255–60.

29. Kornbluth A, Sachar DB. Ulcerative colitis practice guidelines in adults: American College Of Gastroenterology, Practice Parameters Committee. Am J Gastroenterol. 2010;105(3):501–23. quiz 524.

30. Rutgeerts P, Sandborn WJ, Feagan BG, et al. Infliximab for induction and maintenance therapy for ulcerative colitis. N Engl J Med. 2005;353(23):2462–76.

31. Lashner BA, Heidenreich PA, Su GL, Kane SV, Hanauer SB. Effect of folate supplementation on the incidence of dysplasia and cancer in chronic ulcerative colitis. A case-control study. Gastroenterology. 1989;97(2):255–9.

32. Lashner BA, Provencher KS, Seidner DL, Knesebeck A, Brzezinski A. The effect of folic acid supplementation on the risk for cancer or dysplasia in ulcerative colitis. Gastroenterology. 1997;112(1): 29–32.

33. Giovannucci E, Stampfer MJ, Colditz GA, et al. Multivitamin use, folate, and colon cancer in women in the Nurses' Health Study. Ann Intern Med. 1998;129(7):517–24.

34. Cole BF, Baron JA, Sandler RS, et al. Folic acid for the prevention of colorectal adenomas: a randomized clinical trial. JAMA. 2007;297(21):2351–9.

35. Lindor KD, Kowdley KV, Luketic VA, et al. High-dose ursodeoxycholic acid for the treatment of primary sclerosing cholangitis. Hepatology. 2009;50(3):808–14.

36. Lindor KD. Ursodiol for primary sclerosing cholangitis. Mayo Primary Sclerosing Cholangitis-Ursodeoxycholic Acid Study Group. N Engl J Med. 1997;336(10):691–5.

37. Soetikno RM, Lin OS, Heidenreich PA, Young HS, Blackstone MO. Increased risk of colorectal neoplasia in patients with primary sclerosing cholangitis and ulcerative colitis: a meta-analysis. Gastrointest Endosc. 2002;56(1):48–54.

38. Farraye FA, Odze RD, Eaden J, Itzkowitz SH. AGA technical review on the diagnosis and management of colorectal neoplasia in inflammatory bowel disease. Gastroenterology. 2010;138(2):746–74. 774 e741-744; quiz e712-743.

39. Tung BY, Emond MJ, Haggitt RC, et al. Ursodiol use is associated with lower prevalence of colonic neoplasia in patients with ulcerative colitis and primary sclerosing cholangitis. Ann Intern Med. 2001;134(2):89–95.

40. Pardi DS, Loftus Jr EV, Kremers WK, Keach J, Lindor KD. Ursodeoxycholic acid as a chemopreventive agent in patients with ulcerative colitis and primary sclerosing cholangitis. Gastroenterology. 2003;124(4):889–93.

41. Wolf JM, Rybicki LA, Lashner BA. The impact of ursodeoxycholic acid on cancer, dysplasia and mortality in ulcerative colitis patients with primary sclerosing cholangitis. Aliment Pharmacol Ther. 2005;22(9):783–8.

42. Eaton JE, Silveira MG, Pardi DS, et al. High-dose ursodeoxycholic acid is associated with the development of colorectal neoplasia in patients with ulcerative colitis and primary sclerosing cholangitis. Am J Gastroenterol. 2011;106(9):1638–45.

43. Lindstrom L, Boberg KM, Wikman O, et al. High dose ursodeoxycholic acid in primary sclerosing cholangitis does not prevent colorectal neoplasia. Aliment Pharmacol Ther. 2012; 35(4):451–7.

44. Chapman R, Fevery J, Kalloo A, et al. Diagnosis and management of primary sclerosing cholangitis. Hepatology. 2010;51(2): 660–78.

# Safety Considerations in the Medical Therapy of Ulcerative Colitis

Caroline Kerner, James D. Lewis, and Mark T. Osterman

**Keywords**

Safety • Medical therapy • Ulcerative colitis • Aminosalicylates • Infection • Malignancy • Renal injury • Steroids • Thiopurine analogues • Biologics • Cyclosporine • Death

Every day in the routine care of patients with ulcerative colitis, physicians are forced to consider the potential benefits and harms of a variety of medical therapies. There are numerous medications that have demonstrated efficacy for the treatment of ulcerative colitis, each of which has the potential to also cause unintended harm. Because most adverse events are reversible with early recognition and treatment, it is important for the practicing physician to be able to recognize and appropriately manage them.

This chapter will focus primarily on three categories of complications: infection, malignancy, and renal injury. In addition, we will comment briefly on the risk of mortality with medical therapy.

C. Kerner, M.D., M.S.C.E. (✉)
Division of Gastroenterology, Department of Medicine,
University of Pennsylvania, Pennsylvania Hospital,
230 West Washington Square, 4th Floor,
Philadelphia, PA 19106, USA
e-mail: caroline.kerner@uphs.upenn.edu

J.D. Lewis, M.D., M.S.C.E.
Department of Medicine, University of Pennsylvania,
720 Blockley Hall, 423 Guardian Drive, Philadelphia,
PA 19104, USA
e-mail: lewisjd@mail.med.upenn.edu

M.T. Osterman, M.D., M.S.C.E.
Division of Gastroenterology, Department of Medicine,
Pennsylvania Presbyterian Medical Center,
University of Pennsylvania, 218 Wright-Saunders Building,
51 N. 39th St., Philadelphia, PA 19104, USA
e-mail: mark.osterman@uphs.upenn.edu

## Aminosalicylates

### Infection

The mechanism of action of sulfasalazine and mesalamine is multifactorial and may to some extent cause immune suppression [1], impairment of white cell adhesion [2], and inhibition of cytokine production [3]. However, these medications are not known to increase infection risk. For example, a Mayo Clinic case-control study of inflammatory bowel disease (IBD) patients performed 1:2 matching of 100 cases of opportunistic infection (OI) to controls without OI [4]. Mesalamine use was not associated with opportunistic infection (OR 1, 95 % CI 0.6–1.6). Similarly, mesalamine use was not associated with an increased risk of herpes zoster among a cohort of patients with IBD in the United Kingdom [5]. The low infectious risk may be related to the low systemic availability of these medications.

### Malignancy

There is no known association between aminosalicylates and increased cancer risk. Rather, there is some evidence to support an association between mesalamine and decreased colorectal cancer risk [6, 7]. However, other studies have not found an association between mesalamine and decreased colorectal cancer risk [8–10]. Chronic colonic inflammation is associated with a higher risk of colorectal cancer [11], and the apparent benefit of mesalamine at reducing colorectal cancer incidence may be related to greater mucosal healing. At present, the use of mesalamine solely for the purpose of preventing colorectal cancer when other medications have completely healed the colonic mucosa is likely safe but of unclear benefit.

## Renal Injury

While renal disease in IBD is often thought to be caused by the medications used to treat it, IBD itself, irrespective of medication use, may be a risk factor for renal disease. A study of 1,529 patients (over half of whom were taking 5-ASA medications) reported a 2.2 % annual incidence of renal impairment and 0.9 % incidence of chronic kidney disease (CKD), the causes of which included prerenal damage, nephrolithiasis, nephroangiosclerosis, focal segmental glomerulosclerosis, and amyloidosis [12]. Unfortunately, this study lacked a non-IBD control group. However, in another study, IBD patients who were not treated with 5-ASA had a 50 % higher incidence of kidney injury than those receiving 5-ASA [13]. Other studies have shown that many IBD patients exhibit microalbuminuria, irrespective of 5-ASA use [14–17]. Chronic nephrolithiasis, an extraintestinal complication of IBD, can also cause CKD [18]. Finally, many IBD patients will experience at least transient elevations of serum creatinine due to disease flares during which diarrhea, inadequate oral intake of fluids, abdominal pain, nausea/vomiting, and fever often lead to dehydration.

Animal studies have shown that 5-ASA drugs may cause renal tubular injury [19, 20]. There have been at least 46 case reports of kidney injury, particularly interstitial nephritis and nephrotic syndrome, with the use of 5-ASA in IBD patients [21]. This is not surprising given the structural similarity of 5-ASA (5-aminosalicylic acid) to aspirin (acetylsalicylic acid). There is a wealth of data, both laboratory and clinical, demonstrating that aspirin and other nonsteroidal anti-inflammatory drugs (NSAIDs) can directly cause acute and chronic kidney injury, including ischemic renal insufficiency, interstitial nephritis, progressive hypertensive nephropathy, minimal change glomerulonephropathy, and papillary necrosis, some of which can be acute and chronic [22–25]. These toxic effects may be dose dependent (e.g., papillary necrosis) or idiosyncratic (e.g., interstitial nephritis). Combined data from the 46 case reports of renal disease (mostly interstitial nephritis) in IBD patients taking 5-ASA agents showed that renal injury may occur at widely various time points during 5-ASA therapy, from 1 month to 7 years of therapy, with 43 % having nephrotoxicity within 1 year of initiation of therapy [21].

Retrospective studies specifically examining the association of 5-ASA agents and kidney injury in IBD patients have reported conflicting results [13, 15, 16, 26–30]. One of the most rigorous of these studies, a nested case-control study using the General Practice Research Database (GPRD), observed an increased risk of kidney injury (defined as a combined endpoint of acute glomerulonephritis, nephritic

syndrome, chronic glomerulonephritis, other nephritis or nephropathy, or acute, chronic, or unspecified renal failure) with recent, but not current or past, 5-ASA use [13]. A review of over 30 studies, many of which were randomized clinical trials, of 5-ASA use in IBD published through 2005, in which serum creatinine or creatinine clearance was measured regularly showed rates of renal injury ranging from 0 to 6 % in these patients who were treated with 5-ASA for 1.5–48 months, thus representing highly variable estimates of risk [21]. Four recent randomized clinical trials of UC patients treated for up to 1 year with various dose and formulations of 5-ASA drugs have shown low levels of renal injury, from 0 to 0.2 %, but this duration of treatment is still relatively short [31–34].

Thus, the risk of kidney injury with the use of 5-ASA medications is unclear at the present time. For this reason, it is difficult to design guidelines for monitoring of serum creatinine levels in IBD patients receiving 5-ASA therapy. In an early report of renal injury among 16 patients treated with 5-ASA, serum creatinine levels were higher and recovery of renal function after withdrawal of 5-ASA was less common in those with more than 1 year of therapy [35]. This led the authors to recommend that "serum creatinine concentration should be measured each month for the first 3 months of treatment, 3-monthly for the remainder of the first year and annually thereafter. The use of concurrent immunosuppressive therapy may necessitate extension to the period of intensive monitoring." A subsequent study also demonstrated greater recovery of renal function when nephrotoxicity was diagnosed within 12 months of starting 5-ASA, but again was unable to provide definitive recommendations for timing of monitoring (or even whether 5-ASA use increases the risk of nephrotoxicity) [36]. Ultimately, there have been a wide range of recommendations due to a perception that the risk of renal toxicity may be quite low and the absence of evidence to define optimal screening intervals [37]. Current FDA-approved prescribing instructions for 5-ASA products include a nonspecific recommendation to measure creatinine before initiation of therapy and intermittently thereafter [38–40] [27–29]. The rationale is that: (1) there are no satisfactory urinary markers of early renal injury; (2) renal injury is often asymptomatic and when diagnosed at later stages may lead to irreversible damage and possibly end-stage renal disease; and (3) detection of early renal injury in these patients and subsequent early withdrawal of 5-ASA therapy may lead to recovery of renal function.

## Steroids

### Infection

Corticosteroids are effective in treating inflammation by inhibiting multiple inflammatory genes, but the broad inhibition of both innate and adaptive immune functions also increases susceptibility to infection [41]. The infectious risk of corticosteroids in IBD has been evaluated in multiple population-based and single-center studies.

In the Mayo Clinic case-control study referred to previously [4], corticosteroid use was associated with significantly increased odds of OI (OR 3.4, 95 % CI 1.8–6.2). In the multivariate analysis, the use of two or three immunosuppressive drugs was associated with markedly increased odds of OI (OR 14.5, 95 % CI 4.9–43). *Candida albicans* was the most common opportunistic infection in patients receiving only corticosteroids for immunosuppression.

A population-based cohort study in British Columbia subsequently examined the association between corticosteroid use and serious bacterial infections [42]. Serious infection was defined as bacteremia, pneumonia, osteomyelitis, pyelonephritis, meningitis, encephalitis, or endocarditis. Corticosteroid use was not associated with the composite outcome of serious bacterial infection (RR 1.22, 95 % CI 0.7–2.13), but was associated with an increased risk of *Clostridium difficile* colitis (RR 2.65, 95 % CI 1.53–4.57).

Steroids have also been shown to increase the risk of postoperative infections among patients with IBD. In a retrospective study of 159 patients with IBD undergoing elective bowel surgery, there was significantly increased odds of any (OR 3.69, 95 % CI 1.24–10.97) and major (OR 5.54, 95 % CI 1.12–27.26) postoperative infectious complications [43].

## Malignancy

Corticosteroids are used in some chemotherapy regimens because of their apoptotic effects in lymphoid cells and their ability to reduce symptoms from cancer-related complications. However, there are various mechanisms by which corticosteroids may play a role in oncogenesis, including inactivation of B and T lymphocytes, decreased expression of major histocompatibility class I antigen, and inhibition of immunosurveillance [44]. Several population-based studies have examined the association between corticosteroid use and malignancy, though these studies were not limited to patients with IBD.

A Danish population-based study compared observed and expected numbers of cases of non-Hodgkin's lymphoma and nonmelanoma skin cancers among 59,043 patients who were exposed to corticosteroids [45]. Patients exposed to other immunosuppressive drugs were excluded from the analysis. Patients who received 10–14 corticosteroid prescriptions had an increased risk of non-Hodgkin's lymphoma (SIR 2.68, 95 % CI 1.16–5.29). There was also a statistically significant association between having 15 or more corticosteroid prescriptions and squamous cell (SIR 2.45, 95 % CI 1.37–4.04) or basal cell (SIR 1.52, 95 % CI 1.09–2.07) skin cancers. Similarly, a case-control study in New Hampshire found that

after controlling for confounding by other skin cancer risk factors and excluding patients with organ transplant, there was an association between oral corticosteroid use and squamous cell carcinoma (OR 2.31, 95 % CI 1.27–4.18), but not basal cell carcinoma (OR 1.49, 95 % CI 0.90–2.47) [46].

However, the potential confounding by other immunosuppressant use and comorbidity raises the question of whether these associations were causal. Jensen et al. attempted to address this limitation in a 2009 population-based case-control study in North Jutland County, Denmark [47]. After adjusting for chronic diseases and other immunosuppressant use, there was a small statistically significant association between oral glucocorticoid use and basal cell carcinoma (IRR 1.15, 95 % CI 1.07–1.25) but not squamous cell carcinoma, malignant melanoma, or non-Hodgkin's lymphoma.

## Thiopurine Analogues

### Infection

There are multiple case reports and case series describing infectious complications in patients exposed to thiopurines. In 1989, Present et al. [48] described their 18-year experience with 6-MP in IBD and found 29 (7.4 %) cases of infectious complications among 396 patients. Only seven (1.8 %) of these cases were determined to be severe, and all infections resolved with treatment. "Hepatitis" was the most commonly reported infectious complication with a total of ten cases, though only one case each of hepatitis A and B were reported and all biochemical abnormalities resolved in the other cases. There were also eight cases of herpes zoster (including one severe encephalitis), five pneumonias, two liver abscesses, and one case each of disseminated cytomegalovirus, septic phlebitis, Q fever, and fever of unknown origin.

There are also case reports in the literature of serious or fatal Epstein-Barr virus (EBV) infections in adults exposed to azathioprine [49–54]. The patients were all men ages 19–33 years old with a diagnosis of Crohn's disease. In 2009, Hagel et al. reported a case of serious EBV infection in a 21-year-old woman with ulcerative colitis who was exposed to thiopurines [55].

The previously described Mayo Clinic case-control study also found that the OR for OI among azathioprine or 6-MP-exposed patients was 3.1 (95 % CI 1.7–5.5) [4] and thiopurine use was also associated with an increased risk of herpes zoster in the UK cohort [5]. However, other studies do not demonstrate an increased risk of serious infection among patients with IBD exposed to thiopurines. The Crohn's Therapy, Resource, Evaluation, and Assessment Tool (TREAT) registry, a prospective multicenter study of North

American patients with CD, found no increased risk of serious infection among patients exposed to immunomodulators (OR 0.78, 95 % CI .52–1.8) [56]. Immunomodulator use in this study included both azathioprine and methotrexate.

In the previously described retrospective study of the risk of postoperative complications in 159 patients with IBD undergoing elective bowel surgery, there were no increased odds of postoperative infection (OR 1.68, 95 % CI .65–4.27) or major infectious complications (OR 1.20, 95 % CI .37–3.94) among patients exposed to thiopurines preoperatively [43].

While the above studies mainly examined the risk of serious and opportunistic infections, Seksik et al. performed a prospective cohort study of 230 patients with IBD to determine the risk of less serious infections, including upper respiratory infections, herpes simplex virus cutaneous infections, and human papillomavirus warts [57]. When comparing azathioprine-exposed versus azathioprine-unexposed patients, there was a statistically significant increased risk of herpes simplex virus (HSV) flares (1.0±2.6 events per observation year vs. 0.2±0.8 events per observation year, $p=.04$) and HPV warts (17.2 vs. 3.3 %, $p=.004$) but not upper respiratory infections.

## Malignancy

### Lymphoproliferative Disorders

When assessing the risk of lymphoproliferative disorders among patients exposed to thiopurines, the first question to address is whether there is an increased risk of lymphoma among patients with IBD independent of immunosuppressive use [58]. The evidence based on multiple population-based studies suggests that the absolute risk of lymphoma in this population is similar to the general population [59–65].

A 2005 meta-analysis of 6 studies in IBD patients found a pooled relative risk of 4.18 (95 % CI 2.07–7.51) for the risk of lymphoma in thiopurine users compared with nonusers [66]. However, five of the included studies were single-center studies [67–71], and there was significant heterogeneity. The other study included in this meta-analysis used the United Kingdom's General Practice Research Database (GPRD) through 1997 and found that among 1,465 patients with IBD, there was no increased risk of lymphoma among patients treated with thiopurine analogues compared to patients who did not receive thiopurines (relative risk 1.27, 95 % CI 0.03–8.20) [63]. Of note, there was only one case of lymphoproliferative disease among the 1,465 patients, specifically Hodgkin's lymphoma in a patient with UC whose azathioprine exposure occurred 10 months prior to the lymphoma diagnosis.

A subsequent population-based study in 2010 also used the GPRD to perform a nested case-control study within a cohort of patients with IBD [72]. When defining azathioprine exposure as a dichotomous outcome of ever used versus never used, the OR for the association between azathioprine and lymphoma risk was significant at 3.22 (95 % CI 1.01–10.18). However, when azathioprine exposure was calculated as a prescription density (number of prescriptions per calendar year), there was no statistically significant association between azathioprine exposure and lymphoma risk (OR 1.37, 95 % CI 0.79–2.40). This study did not control for anti-TNF exposure, but anti-TNF medication became available only in the last few years of the study. In the Cancers Et Surrisque Associe aux Maladies inflammatoires intestinales En France (CESAME) cohort of 19,486 French patients with IBD enrolled between May 2004 and June 2005 with a median follow-up of 35 months, there were 23 new cases of lymphoproliferative disorder diagnosed (22 non-Hodgkin's lymphoproliferative disorder and 1 Hodgkin's lymphoma) [73]. There were no reported cases of hepatosplenic T-cell lymphoma (HSTCL). In multivariate analysis, the adjusted hazard ratio for the risk of lymphoproliferative disorders among thiopurine users compared with never users was 5.28 (95 % CI 2.01–13.9). In addition, standardized incidence ratios (SIRs) were calculated to compare the risk of lymphoproliferative disorders in patients exposed to thiopurines compared with the general population. They found that ongoing thiopurine use was associated with an increased risk (SIR 6.86, 95 % CI 3.84–11.31) of lymphoproliferative disorders, but patients who discontinued (SIR 1.44, 95 % CI .17–5.20) or were never exposed to thiopurines (SIR 1.43, 95 % CI .53–3.12) had risks similar to that of the general population.

A recent meta-analysis estimated the relative risk (RR) of lymphoma in patients with IBD exposed to thiopurines and compared RR values derived from population-based studies with those from referral center-based studies [74]. Also, they investigated whether active use increased risk compared with past use, and whether sex, age, or duration of use, affects risk of lymphoma. Overall, 18 studies (among 4,383 citations) met inclusion criteria. Overall, the SIR for lymphoma was 4.49 (95 % CI, 2.81–7.17), ranging from 2.43 (95 % CI, 1.50–3.92) in eight population studies to 9.16 (95 % CI, 5.03–16.7) in ten referral studies. Population studies demonstrated an increased risk among current users (SIR=5.71; 95 % CI, 3.72–10.1) but not former users (SIR=1.42; 95 % CI, 0.86–2.34). Level of risk became significant after 1 year of exposure. Men have a greater risk than women (RR=2.05; $P<.05$); both sexes were at increased risk for lymphoma (SIR for men=3.60; 95 % CI, 2.68–4.83 and SIR for women=1.76, 95 % CI, 1.08–2.87). Patients younger than 30 years had the highest RR (SIR=6.99; CI, 2.99–16.4); younger men had the highest risk. The absolute risk was highest in patients older than 50 years (1:377 cases per patient-years). The authors concluded that compared with studies from referral centers, population-based studies of IBD patients show a lower but significantly increased risk of lymphoma among patients taking thiopurines. The increased risk does not appear to persist after discontinuation of therapy. The risks of lymphoma and potential benefits of therapy should be considered for all patients.

There is also evidence suggesting a possible association between Epstein-Barr virus (EBV)-positive lymphoma and thiopurine use. In a 2002 study [74], 18 lymphoma cases were identified among all patients with IBD seen at the Mayo Clinic between 1985 and 2000. Of these 18 lymphomas, six occurred in thiopurine-exposed patients. Of the seven EBV-positive lymphomas, five (71 %) were treated with thiopurines. Of the 11 EBV-negative lymphomas, one (9 %) was exposed to thiopurines. In the CESAME cohort, 10/15 (67 %) cases of lymphoma were EBV positive among patients currently using thiopurines, whereas 2/8 (25 %) cases of lymphoma were EBV positive among patients who were not using thiopurines [73]. Similarly, in a study of 44 cases of lymphoma among 17,834 IBD cases identified in PALGA, the Dutch national registry of histo- and cytopathology, EBV status was assessed in 33 of the cases [75]. Thiopurine exposure was noted in 11/12 (92 %) EBV-positive lymphomas, compared with 4/21 (19 %) of EBV-negative lymphomas.

## Nonmelanoma Skin Cancer

Nonmelanoma skin cancer (NMSC) is comprised primarily of basal cell carcinoma and squamous cell carcinoma. Thiopurines are thought to increase the risk of NMSC through enhanced ultraviolet light tumorigenesis and perhaps immunosuppressive effects related to human papillomavirus infection [76]. Long et al. [77] examined this question in a large US database, in which each of 53,377 patients with IBD were matched with three non-IBD controls. The incidence of NMSC was higher in patients with IBD compared with controls, with an incidence of 7.33 per 1,000 patient-years of follow-up in IBD patients compared with 4.47 per 1,000 patient-years in controls and an incidence rate ratio of 1.64 (95 % CI 1.51–1.78). The authors also reported the results of a nested case-control study that found that thiopurine use within the previous 90 days was associated with an increased risk of NMSC with an adjusted odds ratio of 3.56 (95 % CI 2.81–4.50).

In the CESAME cohort, the crude incidence rates of NMSC ranged from 0.66 per 1,000 patient-years in current thiopurine users less than age 50 to 4.04 cases per 1,000 patient-years in current thiopurine users over the age of 65. There was an increased risk of NMSC in patients with ongoing thiopurine use (HR 5.9, 95 % CI 2.1–16.4) as well as previous thiopurine users (HR 3.9, 95 % CI 1.3–12.1) [78].

In contrast, a study using the University of Manitoba IBD Epidemiology Database found an increased risk of squamous cell carcinoma of the skin (HR 5.4, 95 % CI 2–14.56), but no increased risk of basal cell carcinoma (HR 1.12, 95 % CI 0.68–1.85) or NMSC overall (HR 1.31, 95 % CI 0.85–2.03) [79]. Furthermore, a study in a Dutch database of 2,887 patients with IBD and a follow-up of 18,663 person-years found no increased risk of NMSC among thiopurine users [80]. The incidence rate was 4.4 per 1,000 patient-years in thiopurine users compared with 4.7 per 1,000 person-years in nonusers, and a Cox proportional hazard regression analysis found no association between thiopurine use and NMSC risk after adjusting for confounders. They attributed their lower incidence of NMSC compared with the Long et al. study partly to a more strict definition of thiopurine exposure. Similarly, the nested case-control study of patients with IBD in the GPRD discussed earlier found no increased risk of nonmelanoma skin cancer among patients when comparing thiopurine-exposed to unexposed patients (OR 0.99, 95 % CI .35–2.81) [72].

Trying to put these discordant findings into context is challenging. NMSC is not routinely reported to many cancer databases and may not be routinely recorded in the electronic medical records or claims data. The CESAME and Manitoba studies were unique in that they used pathology reports to determine the cancer type and did not rely exclusively on claims data to identify NMSC. Geography may also be important since sun exposure is an important risk factor for NMSC. Thus, the lack of an association in the Dutch and British studies may reflect lower rates of sun exposure. Regardless, there is currently sufficient evidence that thiopurines may increase the risk of NMSC and that regular use of sunblock may reduce this risk. As such, sunblock should be widely recommended for patients treated with thiopurines and frequent dermatologic evaluations should be considered as well.

## Other Malignancies

Several single-center studies reporting their experience with long-term thiopurine treatment demonstrate no patterns of increased risk of other malignancies. A study from St. Mark's Hospital in London reported 31 cancer cases among 755 patients with IBD who were treated with azathioprine between 1962 and 1991. This incidence rate was not significantly higher than that in the general population (SIR 1.27). A New Zealand center performed a long-term follow-up of 2,204 patients with IBD, of which 626 had used azathioprine, and reported similar results with malignancies diagnosed in 4.5 % of azathioprine-exposed and 4.5 % of azathioprine-unexposed patients [69].

In the nested case-control study in GPRD discussed above, Armstrong et al. [72] identified 392 cancers among 15,471 patients with IBD. In addition to the lymphoma and NMSC discussed earlier, these malignancies included 36 breast cancers, 139 gastrointestinal malignancies and 38 lung cancers. After adjusting for age and smoking, azathioprine use was not associated with an increased risk of malignancy overall (OR 1.08, 95 % CI 0.78–1.51), breast (OR 0.47, 95 % CI .11–1.97), gastrointestinal (OR 0.68, 95 % CI .35–1.29), or lung (OR 0.96, 95 % CI 0.29–3.13) cancers.

## Biologics

### Infection

In a Mayo Clinic case series of 500 consecutive patients with CD treated with infliximab between the years 1998 and 2002, there were 48 infections, 41 (8.2 %) of which were thought to be related to infliximab use [81]. 20 of these infections were considered to be serious and included eight with sepsis (all fatal), 8 pneumonias (2 fatal), 6 viral infections, 2 abdominal abscesses requiring surgery, 1 cellulitis, and 1 histoplasmosis. However, the uncontrolled nature of these data prevented drawing strong conclusions on whether infliximab increased the risk of infection.

In a Mayo Clinic case-control study [4] evaluating risk factors for OI among patients with IBD, the univariate analysis detected an association between infliximab use and OI (OR 4.4, 95 % CI 1.2–17.1). The multivariate analysis demonstrated that the use of any immunosuppressive (corticosteroid, thiopurine, or infliximab) had an OR of 2.9 (95 % CI 1.5–5.3), but use of 2 or more immunosuppressants resulted in an OR of 14.5 (95 % CI 4.9–43). In the multivariable Cox proportional hazards regression model using the TREAT registry data, there was a statistically significant association between infliximab exposure in the prior 6 months and serious infection (HR 1.43, 95 % CI 1.11–1.84) [82].

However, there are other studies demonstrating no significant association between infliximab use and serious infection in patients with IBD. A population-based cohort in British Columbia found no association between infliximab use and serious bacterial infection including *Clostridium difficile* [42]. Using safety data from 21 randomized controlled trials of anti-TNF in the treatment of Crohn's disease, Peyrin-Biroulet performed a meta-analysis to assess risk of serious infection [83]. There was no significant difference in the frequency of serious infection in patients randomized to anti-TNF therapy versus placebo (2.09 vs. 2.13 %). There are several possible interpretations of these data. One possibility is that there is truly no increased risk of serious infections among patients treated with anti-TNF therapy for Crohn's disease. An alternate interpretation is that any increased risk of medication-related infection is counterbalanced by a reduction in disease-related infections, such as intra-abdominal abscess.

Despite mixed results from the population and registry data regarding the association between anti-TNF use and serious infections, case reports have demonstrated evidence of reactivation of latent tuberculosis (TB) among patients exposed to these medications. Infliximab was first approved by the FDA in 1998. By May 2001, 70 cases of tuberculosis infections had been reported among patients exposed to infliximab [84]. The publication of these findings led to the recommendation for screening for latent and active tuberculosis prior to starting anti-TNF therapy. The American College of Gastroenterology (ACG) recommends screening with a clinical history to assess TB risk factors, physical exam, intradermal purified protein derivative (PPD) tuberculin skin test (TST), and a chest x-ray prior to initiation of anti-TNF therapy [85]. However, because a high prevalence of anergy to the TST has been demonstrated among patients with IBD [86], the ACG guidelines suggest that physicians consider using the QuantiFERON-TB Gold assay in patients with previous BCG vaccination or who are using concomitant immunosuppressants.

There are also case reports of reactivation of chronic hepatitis B in patients with IBD receiving infliximab [87]. As a result, the ACG recommends vaccination for patients at risk for hepatitis B virus prior to initiation of anti-TNF therapy [85].

Case reports have also demonstrated the risk of infection with endemic fungal infection among patients receiving anti-TNF therapy, with *Histoplasma capsulatum* being the most commonly reported [88]. Furthermore, these infections often appear as disseminated disease. As a result, the FDA issued a black box warning in 2008 to increase awareness of the risk of endemic fungal infection among patients exposed to TNF-alpha inhibitor therapy [89].

There are extremely limited data comparing the risk of infection with different anti-TNF therapies. A recent cohort study among patients with rheumatoid arthritis identified a higher risk of serious infections among patients treated with infliximab compared to other anti-TNF therapies [90]. As more data on anti-TNF therapy for IBD becomes available, similar analyses will be warranted in this population.

## Malignancy

### Lymphoproliferative Disorders
It is difficult to estimate the risk of lymphoma from anti-TNF use in inflammatory bowel disease because of confounding factors, including concomitant immunosuppressive medication exposure and disease severity.

In the randomized controlled trials studying the use of infliximab, adalimumab, and certolizumab for induction and maintenance in both ulcerative colitis and Crohn's disease, there was only one reported case of lymphoma (Table 27.1).

**Table 27.1** Randomized controlled trials studying the use of infliximab, adalimumab, and certolizumab for induction and maintenance in both ulcerative colitis and Crohn's disease

| Study | Drug | Population | Number of patients | Follow-up (wks) | Number of lymphoma cases | Number of other malignancies |
|---|---|---|---|---|---|---|
| Targan [91] | IFX | CD (I) | 83 | 12 | 0 | 0 |
| Present [92] | IFX | Fistulizing CD (I) | 63 | N/R (at least 18) | 0 | 0 |
| Rutgeerts [93] | IFX | CD (M) | 73 | 48 | 1[a] | 0 |
| Hanauer [94] | IFX | CD (M) | 573 | 54 | 1[a] | 5[b] |
| Sands [95] | IFX | Fistulizing CD (M) | 282 | 54 | 0 | 2[c] |
| Rutgeerts [96] | IFX | UC (I, M) | 243 (ACT 1) | 54 (ACT 1) | 0 | 3 (ACT 1)[d] |
| | | | 241 (ACT 2) | 30 (ACT 2) | | 2 (ACT 2)[e] |
| Hanauer [97] | ADA | CD (I) | 225 | 4 | 0 | 0 |
| Colombel [98] | ADA | CD (M) | 517 | 56 | 0 | 1[f] |
| Sandborn [99] | ADA | CD (M) | 241 | 56 | 0 | 0 |
| Sandborn [100] | ADA | CD (I) | 159 | 4 | 0 | 0 |
| Colombel [101] | ADA | Fistulizing CD (I) | 70 | 56 | 0 | 0 |
| Reinisch [102] | ADA | UC (I) | 260 | 8 | 0 | 0 |
| Schreiber [103] | CTZ | CD (I) | 219 | 12 | 0 | 0 |
| Sandborn [104] | CTZ | CD (I) | 331 | 26 | 0 | 2[g] |
| Schreiber [105] | CTZ | CD (M) | 215 | 26 | 0 | 0 |
| Lichtenstein [106] | CTZ | CD (M) | 141 | 54 | 0 | 1[h] |
| Sandborn [107] | CTZ | CD (I) | 868 | 26 | 0 | 1[i] |
| Sandborn [108] | CTZ | CD (I) | 223 | 6 | 0 | 1[j] |

*ADA* adalimumab, *CD* Crohn's disease, *CTZ* certolizumab, *I* induction, *IFX* infliximab, *M* maintenance, *UC* ulcerative colitis
[a]Intravascular duodenal B-cell lymphoma in a 61-year-old man with a 30-year history of CD (same patient)
[b]Epithelial cell skin cancer, basal cell carcinoma, hypernephroma, breast, bladder
[c]Rectal
[d]Prostate cancer, basal cell carcinoma, colon dysplasia
[e]Basal cell carcinoma, rectal adenocarcinoma
[f]Breast
[g]Rectal, lung
[h]Small bowel carcinoma
[i]Squamous cell skin carcinoma
[j]Metastatic adenocarcinoma with history of breast cancer prior to treatment

Population-based cohort studies of anti-TNF-exposed patients reveal a mixed picture in terms of the lymphoma risk. In a Swedish population-based cohort study of Stockholm County patients with IBD exposed to infliximab between 1999 and 2001, there were three cases of lymphoma, all in patients with CD. Two cases were fatal. The incidence of lymphoma in the study population was 1.5 % compared with a 0.015 % incidence in the general Swedish population [109]. On the other hand, there were no reported cases of lymphoma in a population-based cohort of 651 Danish patients with IBD exposed to infliximab between 1999 and 2005 [110].

In the 6,273-patient TREAT registry, which included 3,420 patients exposed to infliximab, there was no significant difference in the rate of lymphoma in infliximab-exposed (0.05 per 100 patient-years) versus unexposed (0.06 per 100 patient-years) patients (RR 0.80, 95 % CI 0.31–2.07) [111].

As mentioned previously, it is difficult to assess the lymphoma risk attributed directly to anti-TNF use because of confounding by disease severity and present or past exposure to concomitant immunosuppressants. In the CESAME cohort, the risk for lymphoproliferative disorders was markedly increased among patients receiving ongoing combination therapy with a thiopurine analogue and anti-TNF therapy compared to the general population (SIR 10.2, 95 % CI 1.24–36.9) [73]. Another recent retrospective cohort study compared patients in the Kaiser Permanente IBD registry to the general Kaiser population. Of the patients exposed to thiopurine or anti-TNF therapy, only 3 % were exposed only to anti-TNF therapy, and 16 % were exposed to both medications. The SIRR among patients with current anti-TNF exposure (with or without thiopurine exposure) was 4.4 (95 % CI 3.4–5.4), while the SIRR for patients currently receiving both anti-TNF and thiopurines was 6.6 (95 % CI 4.4–8.8) [112]. These data suggest a possible further increased risk of lymphoma with combination thiopurine and anti-TNF therapy.

A recent study however is contradictory. Using The TREAT registry, a prospective, observational, multicenter long-term registry of 6,273 patients with Crohn's disease evaluated the clinical safety outcomes of various treatment regimens, including infliximab. Multivariate Cox regression analysis demonstrated that baseline age (hazard ratio (HR) = 1.59/10 years; $P < 0.001$), disease duration (HR = 1.64/10 years; $P = 0.012$), and smoking (HR = 1.38; $P = 0.045$) but neither immunosuppressive therapy alone (HR = 1.43; $P = 0.11$), infliximab therapy alone (HR = 0.59; $P = 0.16$), nor their combination (HR = 1.22, $P = 0.34$) was independently associated with the risk of malignancy. When compared with the general population, no significant increase in incidence was observed in any malignancy category. In an exposure-based analysis, the use of immunosuppressants alone (odds ratio = 4.19) or in combination with infliximab (3.33) seemed to be associated with a numerically, but not significantly, greater risk of malignancy than did treatment with infliximab alone (1.96) relative to treatment with neither. Thus, the authors noted that in the TREAT registry, age, disease duration, and smoking were independently associated with increased risk of malignancy. Although results for immunosuppressant use were equivocal, no significant association between malignancy and infliximab was observed.

## Hepatosplenic T-Cell Lymphoma

Hepatosplenic T-cell lymphoma (HSTCL) is a rare and aggressive peripheral T-cell lymphoma characterized by hepatomegaly, splenomegaly, and thrombocytopenia. The disease primarily affects young males, with a median age of diagnosis of 35 and a median survival time of 16 months despite consolidative or salvage high-dose chemotherapy [113]. A systematic review of published articles and abstracts, pharmaceutical company records, and the Medwatch Adverse Event Reporting System of the FDA identified 36 reported cases of hepatosplenic T-cell lymphoma in IBD patients [114]. The cases were predominantly male patients (80.5 %) with Crohn's disease (72 %). These patients were all exposed to thiopurines. Of the 30 cases with information on the timing of therapy, 93 % were exposed to thiopurines for at least 2 years prior to the diagnosis of HSTCL. Of the 36 cases, 20 patients (55.5 %) had received infliximab in combination with a thiopurine. Three of those 20 patients had received both infliximab and adalimumab prior to the diagnosis, and one patient had exposure to infliximab, adalimumab, and natalizumab. As a result of the above cases, the black box warning for azathioprine, 6-mercaptopurine, infliximab, and adalimumab all warn of an increased risk of malignancy and specifically reference the reports of HSTCL among patients exposed to these medications.

## Other Malignancies

Two large single centers found a low risk of non-lymphoma malignancies in patients exposed to infliximab. In the Mayo Clinic experience of 500 consecutive patients, there were 7

non-lymphoma malignancies reported, of which 2 (both lung cancers) were attributed to infliximab exposure [81]. A Belgian center followed 734 patients with IBD exposed to infliximab and 666 IBD patients unexposed to infliximab for a median of 58 months and found no difference in the risk of malignancy (OR 0.97, 95 % CI 0.56–1.65) [115].

Similarly, population-based cohorts have also reported low rates of malignancies. In the Swedish [109] population-based cohorts of infliximab-exposed patients with IBD discussed previously, there were no cases of non-lymphoma malignancies. In the Danish [110] population-based cohort, there were four cases of cancer (melanoma, ovarian, esophageal, and rectal), but 5.9 were expected, with an SIR of 0.7 (95 % CI 0.2–1.7).

While the above studies assessed the risk of malignancies overall, a previously discussed case-control study using an administrative database specifically assessed the risk of nonmelanoma skin cancers in patients with IBD [77]. After adjusting for other medication use, they found that adalimumab or infliximab use was associated with an increased risk of nonmelanoma skin cancer (OR 2.18, 95 % CI 1.07–4.46).

At least one meta-analysis of placebo-controlled trials of anti-TNF therapy for rheumatoid arthritis identified an increased risk of malignancy in the anti-TNF-treated patients [116]. However, other meta-analyses have not confirmed these findings, and no increased risk of cancer was observed in the placebo-controlled trials of anti-TNF therapies for Crohn's disease [83].

# Cyclosporine

## Infection

Infections have been reported in patients with IBD treated with cyclosporine (CsA). Since CsA is indicated in the treatment of severe UC [117], and patients who respond to intravenous CsA are then treated with outpatient oral therapy while initiating another immunosuppressive agent, the combination immunosuppression likely increases this risk of infection.

In the original randomized controlled trial assessing the efficacy of CsA for severe ulcerative colitis, 11 patients were followed until hospital discharge or colectomy, and no infections were reported [117]. However, in a larger chart review of 111 patients with IBD treated with CsA, 25 infections were reported in 23 (20 %) patients [118]. 16 (73 %) were mild infections, and 7 infections were determined to be serious. These included one case of *Pneumocystis jiroveci* (*carinii*) pneumonia and three cases of catheter-related sepsis. Another retrospective chart review was performed in 86 Belgian patients with IBD treated with CsA between 1992 and 2000 with a mean follow-up of 773 days [119]. Infections were reported in 16 (18.6 %) patients. Three (3.5 %) died of opportunistic infections (one case of *Pneumocystis jiroveci* pneumonia and two cases of *Aspergillus fumigatus* pneumonia). There were eight cases of catheter-related sepsis, and two cases of anal abscess. The several cases of *Pneumocystis jiroveci* reported in these case series are noteworthy as this is an uncommon complication of other medical therapies for ulcerative colitis. As such, routine prophylaxis against Pneumocystis pneumonia is often used for patients treated with CsA.

## Lymphoma

Estimating the risk of lymphoma associated with CsA use in IBD is limited by the small number of patients exposed to these drugs and confounding by concomitant immunosuppressive use.

The organ transplant literature provides the most information relating to CsA and lymphoma risk. The largest study that estimated lymphoma risk of CsA in an organ transplant population comes from the Collaborative Transplant Study database, an international database of solid organ transplant patients [120]. Among cadaver kidney transplant recipients, the relative risk of lymphoma was higher among patients exposed CsA compared with a normal population matched by age, sex, and geographic region, but this relative risk was not significantly different than the relative risk of lymphoma in kidney transplant patients treated with steroids and azathioprine (RR 12.7 vs. 14.3, *p*-value 0.91). A 1998 study examined the outcomes of different CsA doses by randomizing 231 patients 1-year post kidney transplant to normal- or low-dose CsA. After a 66-month follow-up period, four lymphoproliferative disorders were diagnosed, three of which occurred in the normal-dose group and one in the low-dose group [121]. In 1989, Cockburn and Krupp [122] detailed the malignancies including lymphoma or other lymphoproliferative disease reported to the Sandoz Drug Monitoring Center. There were 186 neoplasms among CsA recipients reported, and the largest percentage of malignancies reported were lymphomas or leukemia (29 %). They also reported the results of postmarketing surveillance of 4,040 renal transplant recipients who received at least one dose of CsA. These patients were followed for up to 7 years, and the lymphoma risk was estimated to be 28 times that of the normal population.

In the IBD literature, there are at least three cases of non-Hodgkin's lymphoma reported among CsA-exposed patients. In a retrospective study of 782 patients with IBD followed at St. James's Hospital in Dublin from 1990 to 1999, there were four cases of non-Hodgkin's lymphoma [71]. The patients were all exposed to immunosuppressants, and one of these patients had received 5 months of methotrexate followed by 12 months of CsA prior to a colectomy that revealed diffuse large B-cell lymphoma. A case of rectal diffuse large B-cell lymphoma was reported in a patient with UC and pyoderma gangrenosum treated with 4 years of CsA and low-dose prednisone [123]. Another patient with UC treated with exposure to prednisone, CsA, 6-mercaptopurine, and infliximab developed an EBV-positive non-Hodgkin's lymphoma of the ileal pouch [124].

## Other Malignancy

Skin cancer appears to be the most frequent malignancy other than lymphoproliferative disease reported among users of CsA. Again, this evidence comes largely from the dermatologic and transplant literature. Cockburn and Krupp [122] reported that of the 186 neoplasms reported by 1989 to the Sandoz Drug Monitoring Center for CsA, 58 (39 %) were skin cancers. Among these cases, Kaposi's sarcoma was the most commonly reported skin cancer (45 %), followed by basal cell (29 %) and squamous cell skin cancer (26 %). Cockburn [122] also studied the malignancies reported among 4,040 renal transplant patients who received CsA and were followed post transplant. They estimated the risk of skin cancer in this population to be seven times that of the normal population.

The major difference between CsA treatment for transplant recipients and patients with ulcerative colitis is the duration of therapy. While there is clear evidence of an increased risk of malignancy among transplant recipients, it is difficult to quantitatively translate this for patients with ulcerative colitis who typically receive less than 6 months of therapy. Nonetheless, because the risk of cancer appears to be correlated with the degree of immunosuppression, there is a rationale to try to minimize the period of time that patients are simultaneously treated with CsA, steroids, and thiopurines.

## Renal Injury

Nephrotoxicity due to CsA is well defined in the solid organ transplantation population, including kidney, liver, heart, and lung transplants [125–128]. CsA can cause both acute and chronic kidney injury [126–129]. CsA is thought to cause acute kidney injury (AKI) by reducing renal blood flow due to vasoconstriction of the afferent arteriole, thus leading to a decrease in the glomerular filtration rate and an increase in the serum creatinine. The vasoconstriction is thought to be mediated by a number of factors, including endothelin, thromboxane A2, inhibition of nitric oxide synthase, and activation of the sympathetic nervous system [130]. Fortunately, this form of nephrotoxicity is reversible and often appears to be associated with the dose of CsA used. CsA therapy can also lead to CKD by causing interstitial fibrosis and tubular nephropathy, which tends to develop after 6–12 months of therapy. It is thought that intrarenal activation of the renin-angiotensin system may play a role in the development of CsA-induced CKD [131]. Unfortunately, this form of nephrotoxicity is not reversible and constitutes the major limitation of the use of CsA in the transplantation population.

In contrast to the transplantation world, nephrotoxicity due to CsA in the IBD population is less well described. In IBD, CsA is used most often to induce remission in patients with severely active ulcerative colitis. In the acute setting, three randomized controlled trials of intravenous (IV) CsA for induction of remission in patients with severely active ulcerative colitis have been published [117, 132, 133]. The first study, by Lichtiger et al., in which 20 patients refractory to IV corticosteroids were treated with IV CsA or placebo, found that none of the patients had nephrotoxicity [117]. The second study, by D'Haens et al., comparing IV CsA to IV corticosteroids in 30 patients, reported a significant decrease in renal function, as measured by inulin clearance, after 8 days of CsA treatment; however, renal function returned to normal in these patients after CsA was discontinued [132]. Of note, patients treated with corticosteroids did not experience a reduction in renal function. The third study, by Van Assche et al., compared the efficacy of IV CsA at daily doses of 4 mg/kg versus 2 mg/kg in 73 patients and observed an increase in serum creatinine of 10 % or more in 18 % of patients treated with 4 mg/kg and 17 % of patients treated with 2 mg/kg; of note, no patient had a serum creatinine increase of 30 % or greater [133].

While these data in the acute setting are useful, patients treated with IV CsA for 7–14 days then remain on oral CsA typically at 8 mg/kg daily (with dose adjustment to maintain trough serum levels of 150–300 ng/mL) after hospital discharge for 3–9 months while bridging to thiopurine therapy and weaning corticosteroids. Long-term retrospective follow-up data of UC patients treated with CsA at tertiary care medical centers represent the best information we have to date regarding the nephrotoxicity of CsA in IBD patients. At least five such long-term outcome series have been published [118, 119, 134–136]. Cohen et al. found that none of the 42 patients followed for up to 5.5 years had renal toxicity [134]. Arts et al. reported that only 6 % of the 86 patients treated with CsA and followed for a mean of 2.1 years developed renal insufficiency, defined as an increase in serum creatinine of at least 20 %, most of which occurred during the IV phase [119]. In a study by Campbell et al., of the 76 patients followed for a median of 2.9 years, only one had to discontinue the use of CsA due to renal toxicity [135]. Moskovitz et al. retrospectively followed 142 patients for up to 7 years and observed that only 3.5 % developed renal toxicity [136].

Finally, Sternthal et al. found that of the 111 patients treated with CsA for a mean of 9.3 months, 5.4 % had to discontinue CsA due to major nephrotoxicity, defined as serum creatinine of $\geq 1.4$ mg/dL or an increase of at least 33 % from baseline not responding to dose adjustment, while 19 % developed minor nephrotoxicity, defined as above but with return to normal serum creatinine after dose adjustment [118]. Thus, overall the available data in the IV inpatient and oral outpatient setting indicate that the risk of major nephrotoxicity with CsA use is low and that minor nephrotoxicity, which may occur more frequently in the IV inpatient phase, is often reversible with dose adjustment. It is likely that the higher incidence of CsA-induced nephrotoxicity in the transplantation population compared to the IBD population is due to the long-term use of CsA in transplant recipients who remain on CsA for years, in contrast to the 3–9 months of CsA therapy for IBD patients.

Risk factors for CsA-induced nephrotoxicity in IBD patients are unknown. However, in renal transplantation patients, risk factors for the development of CsA-induced CKD include: the number of CsA-induced episodes of AKI, the number of unexplained episodes of AKI, CsA trough level, primary renal function, and the number of nephrotoxic drugs [137]. With respect to monitoring of serum creatinine in UC patients treated with CsA, no specific guidelines exist. During inpatient IV therapy, serum creatinine is generally measured at least every other day, while during outpatient long-term oral therapy, serum creatinine is often checked weekly for 1 month and at least monthly thereafter and also rechecked 1 week after each dose adjustment of CsA [118]. With respect to monitoring of CsA levels, these levels are generally checked at least every other day during the IV phase with a target level of 250–450 ng/ml, whereas they are usually checked weekly for 1 month and at least monthly thereafter and also rechecked 1 week after each dose adjustment of CsA during the oral phase with a target level of 150–300 ng/mL [117, 118, 133–135].

## Risk of Death with Medical Therapy

The prior discussion has focused on a variety of rare adverse events. However, the potential for patients to die as a result of these complications is one of the major reasons that both patients and physicians are cautious about using potent immunosuppressive therapies. This question is further complicated because colectomy represents a "pseudocure" for ulcerative colitis. In a recent study among patients hospitalized with ulcerative colitis in the United Kingdom, those who underwent an elective colectomy had a very low rate of perioperative mortality and subsequently had a life expectancy comparable to that of the general population [138]. Patients who underwent an emergency colectomy had a higher rate of perioperative mortality but also had a subsequent survival that was comparable to the general population. In contrast, those patients who were hospitalized for ulcerative colitis and received medical rather than surgical therapy had a progressive decline in relative survival compared to the general population. While this study did not examine the medical therapies that were employed after discharge from the hospital, another study of ulcerative colitis patients in the United Kingdom demonstrated that corticosteroid therapy, but not thiopurine therapy, was associated with an increased risk of death [139]. Interestingly, a study based in Kaiser Permanente Northern California found that in recent years there had been a trend to lower surgery rates and higher rates of long-term steroid use [140].

Interpretation of such data needs to consider the full therapeutic armamentarium available to patients with ulcerative colitis. Were steroids the only available therapy, their efficacy would almost certainly outweigh any potential complications of therapy. However, in the current era, prolonged steroid therapy is likely a sign of inadequately controlled disease, and it is this which likely leads to the increased mortality observed in the UK studies. Of note, there are very limited data on the risk of death with anti-TNF therapies for ulcerative colitis. A prior meta-analysis of placebo-controlled trials demonstrated no increased risk of mortality in patients with Crohn's disease who were treated with anti-TNF therapies [141]. It is likely that the same would apply to ulcerative colitis. However, the risks of anti-TNF therapy must be considered against the option of surgery and must also account for the possibility that ulcerative colitis surgical complications may be more common in patients who have recently been treated with anti-TNF therapies [142–145].

## Conclusions

The introduction of novel therapies has made the management of ulcerative colitis more complicated. At present, the benefit to harm profile of all currently available therapies for ulcerative colitis appears generally favorable with the exception of long-term steroids. We can anticipate that even more medical therapies will be approved in the coming years, further complicating treatment algorithms. Patients and physicians both hope that newly developed therapies will have clearly favorable balance of benefit to risk. Almost certainly, most of these new therapies will be associated with some unique adverse events, and over the course of several years, we will learn how to best optimize the use of the new therapies. As the choice of therapies becomes more complex, there will be greater need for clinicians to be able to personalize treatment regimens such that patients receive the therapy that maximizes the balance of potential benefits and harms.

## References

1. Macdermott RP, Schloemann SR, Bertovich MJ, Nash GS, Peters M, Stenson WF. Inhibition of antibody secretion by 5-aminosalicylic acid. Gastroenterology. 1989;96:442–8.
2. Rhodes JM, Bartholomew TC, Jewell DP. Inhibition of leukocyte motility by drugs used in ulcerative-colitis. Gut. 1981;22:642–7.
3. Bantel H, Berg C, Vieth M, Stolte M, Kruis W, Schulze-Osthoff K. Mesalazine inhibits activation of transcription factor NF-kappa B in inflamed mucosa of patients with ulcerative colitis. Am J Gastroenterol. 2000;95:3452–7.
4. Toruner M, Loftus Jr EV, Harmsen WS, et al. Risk factors for opportunistic infections in patients with inflammatory bowel disease. Gastroenterology. 2008;134:929–36.
5. Gupta G, Lautenbach E, Lewis JD. Incidence and risk factors for herpes zoster among patients with inflammatory bowel disease. Clin Gastroenterol Hepatol. 2006;4:1483–90.
6. Tang J, Sharif O, Pai C, Silverman AL. Mesalamine protects against colorectal cancer in inflammatory bowel disease. Dig Dis Sci. 2010;55:1696–703.
7. van Staa TP, Card T, Logan RF, Leufkens HGM. 5-aminosalicylate use and colorectal cancer risk in inflammatory bowel disease: a large epidemiological study. Gut. 2005;54:1573–8.
8. Bernstein CN, Blanchard JF, Metge C, Yogendran M. Does the use of 5-aminosalicylates in inflammatory bowel disease prevent the development of colorectal cancer? Am J Gastroenterol. 2003;98:2784–8.
9. Bernstein CN, Nugent Z, Blanchard JF. 5-Aminosalicylate is not chemoprophylactic for colorectal cancer in IBD: a population based study. Am J Gastroenterol. 2011;106:731–6.
10. Terdiman JP, Steinbuch M, Blumentals WA, Ullman TA, Rubin DT. 5-aminosalicylic acid therapy and the risk of colorectal cancer among patients with inflammatory bowel disease. Inflamm Bowel Dis. 2007;13:367–71.
11. Rutter M, Saunders B, Wilkinson K, et al. Severity of inflammation is a risk factor for colorectal neoplasia in ulcerative colitis. Gastroenterology. 2004;126:451–9.
12. Elseviers MM, D'Haens G, Lerebours E, et al. Renal impairment in patients with inflammatory bowel disease: association with aminosalicylate therapy? Clin Nephrol. 2004;61:83–9.
13. Van Staa TP, Travis S, Leufkens HG, Logan RF. 5-aminosalicylic acids and the risk of renal disease: a large British epidemiologic study. Gastroenterology. 2004;126:1733–9.
14. Mahmud N, Stinson J, O'Connell MA, et al. Microalbuminuria in inflammatory bowel disease. Gut. 1994;35:1599–604.
15. Kreisel W, Wolf LM, Grotz W, Grieshaber M. Renal tubular damage: an extraintestinal manifestation of chronic inflammatory bowel disease. Eur J Gastroenterol Hepatol. 1996;8:461–8.
16. Herrlinger KR, Noftz MK, Fellermann K, Schmidt K, Steinhoff J, Stange EF. Minimal renal dysfunction in inflammatory bowel disease is related to disease activity but not to 5-ASA use. Aliment Pharmacol Ther. 2001;15:363–9.
17. Poulou AC, Goumas KE, Dandakis DC, et al. Microproteinuria in patients with inflammatory bowel disease: is it associated with the disease activity or the treatment with 5-aminosalicylic acid? World J Gastroenterol. 2006;12:739–46.
18. Wrong O. Nephrocalcinosis. In: Davidson A, Cameron J, Grunfeld J, editors. Oxford textbook of clinical nephrology. Oxford, UK: Oxford University Press; 2005. p. 1375–96.
19. Calder IC, Funder CC, Green CR, Ham KN, Tange JD. Nephrotoxic lesions from 5-aminosalicylic acid. Br Med J. 1972;1:152–4.
20. Bilyard KG, Joseph EC, Metcalf R. Mesalazine: an overview of key preclinical studies. Scand J Gastroenterol Suppl. 1990;172:52–5.

21. Gisbert JP, Gonzalez-Lama Y, Mate J. 5-Aminosalicylates and renal function in inflammatory bowel disease: a systematic review. Inflamm Bowel Dis. 2007;13:629–38.

22. Blackshear JL, Davidman M, Stillman MT. Identification of risk for renal insufficiency from nonsteroidal anti-inflammatory drugs. Arch Intern Med. 1983;143:1130–4.

23. Kleinknecht D. Interstitial nephritis, the nephrotic syndrome, and chronic renal failure secondary to nonsteroidal anti-inflammatory drugs. Semin Nephrol. 1995;15:228–35.

24. Sandler DP, Burr FR, Weinberg CR. Nonsteroidal anti-inflammatory drugs and the risk for chronic renal disease. Ann Intern Med. 1991;115:165–72.

25. Segasothy M, Samad SA, Zulfigar A, Bennett WM. Chronic renal disease and papillary necrosis associated with the long-term use of nonsteroidal anti-inflammatory drugs as the sole or predominant analgesic. Am J Kidney Dis. 1994;24:17–24.

26. Riley SA, Lloyd DR, Mani V. Tests of renal function in patients with quiescent colitis: effects of drug treatment. Gut. 1992;33:1348–52.

27. Mahmud N, McDonald GS, Kelleher D, Weir DG. Microalbuminuria correlates with intestinal histopathological grading in patients with inflammatory bowel disease. Gut. 1996;38:99–103.

28. Schreiber S, Hamling J, Zehnter E, et al. Renal tubular dysfunction in patients with inflammatory bowel disease treated with aminosalicylate. Gut. 1997;40:761–6.

29. Birketvedt GS, Berg KJ, Fausa O, Florholmen J. Glomerular and tubular renal functions after long-term medication of sulphasalazine, olsalazine, and mesalazine in patients with ulcerative colitis. Inflamm Bowel Dis. 2000;6:275–9.

30. Fraser JS, Muller AF, Smith DJ, Newman DJ, Lamb EJ. Renal tubular injury is present in acute inflammatory bowel disease prior to the introduction of drug therapy. Aliment Pharmacol Ther. 2001;15:1131–7.

31. Kamm MA, Lichtenstein GR, Sandborn WJ, et al. Randomised trial of once- or twice-daily MMX mesalazine for maintenance of remission in ulcerative colitis. Gut. 2008;57:893–902.

32. Dignass AU, Bokemeyer B, Adamek H, et al. Mesalamine once daily is more effective than twice daily in patients with quiescent ulcerative colitis. Clin Gastroenterol Hepatol. 2009;7:762–9.

33. Sandborn WJ, Korzenik J, Lashner B, et al. Once-daily dosing of delayed-release oral mesalamine (400-mg tablet) is as effective as twice-daily dosing for maintenance of remission of ulcerative colitis. Gastroenterology. 2010;138:1286–96, 96 e1-3.

34. Kruis W, Jonaitis L, Pokrotnieks J, et al. Randomised clinical trial: a comparative dose-finding study of three arms of dual release mesalazine for maintaining remission in ulcerative colitis. Aliment Pharmacol Ther. 2011;33:313–22.

35. World MJ, Stevens PE, Ashton MA, Rainford DJ. Mesalazine-associated interstitial nephritis. Nephrol Dial Transplant. 1996;11:614–21.

36. Muller AF, Stevens PE, McIntyre AS, Ellison H, Logan RF. Experience of 5-aminosalicylate nephrotoxicity in the United Kingdom. Aliment Pharmacol Ther. 2005;21:1217–24.

37. Moscandrew M, Mahadevan U, Kane S. General health maintenance in IBD. Inflamm Bowel Dis. 2009;15:1399–409.

38. Shire US, Inc. Lialda Full Prescribing Information, 2014. Accessed October 2, 2014 at http://www.lialda.com/hcp/lialda-prescribing-information.aspx

39. Salix Pharmaceuticals, Inc. Apriso Prescribing Information, 2009. Accessed October 2, 2014 at http://www.salix.com/assets/pdf/prescribe_info/apriso-pi.pdf

40. Warner Chilcott, LLC. Asacol HD Prescribing Information, 2013. Accessed October 2, 2014 at http://pi.actavis.com/data_stream. asp?product_group=1875&p=pi&language=E

41. Barnes PJ. How corticosteroids control inflammation: quintiles prize lecture 2005. Br J Pharmacol. 2006;148:245–54.

42. Schneeweiss S, Korzenik J, Solomon DH, Canning C, Lee J, Bressler B. Infliximab and other immunomodulating drugs in patients with inflammatory bowel disease and the risk of serious bacterial infections. Aliment Pharmacol Ther. 2009;30:253–64.

43. Aberra FN, Lewis JD, Hass D, Rombeau JL, Osborne B, Lichtenstein GR. Corticosteroids and immunomodulators: postoperative infectious complication risk in inflammatory bowel disease patients. Gastroenterology. 2003;125:320–7.

44. Gutierrez-Dalmau A, Campistol JM. Immunosuppressive therapy and malignancy in organ transplant recipients: a systematic review. Drugs. 2007;67:1167–98.

45. Sorensen HT, Mellemkjaer L, Nielsen GL, Baron JA, Olsen JH, Karagas MR. Skin cancers and non-hodgkin lymphoma among users of systemic glucocorticoids: a population-based cohort study. J Natl Cancer Inst. 2004;96:709–11.

46. Karagas MR, Cushing Jr GL, Greenberg ER, Mott LA, Spencer SK, Nierenberg DW. Non-melanoma skin cancers and glucocorticoid therapy. Br J Cancer. 2001;85:683–6.

47. Jensen AO, Thomsen HF, Engebjerg MC, et al. Use of oral glucocorticoids and risk of skin cancer and non-Hodgkin's lymphoma: a population-based case-control study. Br J Cancer. 2009;100:200–5.

48. Present DH, Meltzer SJ, Krumholz MP, Wolke A, Korelitz BI. 6-Mercaptopurine in the management of inflammatory bowel disease: short- and long-term toxicity. Ann Intern Med. 1989;111:641–9.

49. Garrido Serrano A, Perez Martin F, Guerrero Igea FJ, Galbarro Munoz J, Palomo GS. Fatal infectious mononucleosis during azathioprine treatment in Crohn's disease. Gastroenterol Hepatol. 2000;23:7–8.

50. Posthuma EF, Westendorp RG, van der Sluys VA, Kluin-Nelemans JC, Kluin PM, Lamers CB. Fatal infectious mononucleosis: a severe complication in the treatment of Crohn's disease with azathioprine. Gut. 1995;36:311–3.

51. Angelucci E, Cesarini M, Caturelli E, Vernia P. EBV hepatitis in a young Crohn's disease patient on prolonged remission with azathioprine. Inflamm Bowel Dis. 2011;17:E1.

52. Bargallo A, Carrion S, Domenech E, et al. Infectious mononucleosis in patients with inflammatory bowel disease under treatment with azathioprine. Gastroenterol Hepatol. 2008;31:289–92.

53. N'Guyen Y, Andreoletti L, Patey M, et al. Fatal Epstein-Barr virus primo infection in a 25-year-old man treated with azathioprine for Crohn's disease. J Clin Microbiol. 2009;47:1252–4.

54. Moreira T, Lago P, Salgado M, Pimentel R. Epstein-Barr virus and parvovirus B19 coinfection in a Crohn's disease patient under azathioprine. Inflamm Bowel Dis. 2010;16:905–6.

55. Hagel S, Bruns T, Kantowski M, Fix P, Seidel T, Stallmach A. Cholestatic hepatitis, acute acalculous cholecystitis, and hemolytic anemia: primary Epstein-Barr virus infection under azathioprine. Inflamm Bowel Dis. 2009;15:1613–6.

56. Lichtenstein GR, Feagan BG, Cohen RD, et al. Serious infections and mortality in association with therapies for Crohn's disease: TREAT registry. Clin Gastroenterol Hepatol. 2006;4:621–30.

57. Seksik P, Cosnes J, Sokol H, Nion-Larmurier I, Gendre JP, Beaugerie L. Incidence of benign upper respiratory tract infections, HSV and HPV cutaneous infections in inflammatory bowel disease patients treated with azathioprine. Aliment Pharmacol Ther. 2009;29:1106–13.

58. Bewtra M, Lewis JD. Safety profile of IBD: lymphoma risks. Med Clin North Am. 2010;94:93–113.

59. Ekbom A, Helmick C, Zack M, Adami HO. Extracolonic malignancies in inflammatory bowel disease. Cancer. 1991;67:2015–9.

60. Karlen P, Lofberg R, Brostrom O, Leijonmarck CE, Hellers G, Persson PG. Increased risk of cancer in ulcerative colitis: a

population-based cohort study. Am J Gastroenterol. 1999;94: 1047–52.

61. Loftus Jr EV, Tremaine WJ, Habermann TM, Harmsen WS, Zinsmeister AR, Sandborn WJ. Risk of lymphoma in inflammatory bowel disease. Am J Gastroenterol. 2000;95:2308–12.

62. Bernstein CN, Blanchard JF, Kliewer E, Wajda A. Cancer risk in patients with inflammatory bowel disease: a population-based study. Cancer. 2001;91:854–62.

63. Lewis JD, Bilker WB, Brensinger C, Deren JJ, Vaughn DJ, Strom BL. Inflammatory bowel disease is not associated with an increased risk of lymphoma. Gastroenterology. 2001;121: 1080–7.

64. Winther KV, Jess T, Langholz E, Munkholm P, Binder V. Long-term risk of cancer in ulcerative colitis: a population-based cohort study from Copenhagen county. Clin Gastroenterol Hepatol. 2004;2:1088–95.

65. Askling J, Brandt L, Lapidus A, et al. Risk of haematopoietic cancer in patients with inflammatory bowel disease. Gut. 2005;54: 617–22.

66. Kandiel A, Fraser AG, Korelitz BI, Brensinger C, Lewis JD. Increased risk of lymphoma among inflammatory bowel disease patients treated with azathioprine and 6-mercaptopurine. Gut. 2005;54:1121–5.

67. Connell WR, Kamm MA, Dickson M, Balkwill AM, Ritchie JK, Lennard-Jones JE. Long-term neoplasia risk after azathioprine treatment in inflammatory bowel disease. Lancet. 1994; 343:1249–52.

68. Korelitz BI, Mirsky FJ, Fleisher MR, Warman JI, Wisch N, Gleim GW. Malignant neoplasms subsequent to treatment of inflammatory bowel disease with 6-mercaptopurine. Am J Gastroenterol. 1999;94:3248–53.

69. Fraser AG, Orchard TR, Robinson EM, Jewell DP. Long-term risk of malignancy after treatment of inflammatory bowel disease with azathioprine. Aliment Pharmacol Ther. 2002;16:1225–32.

70. Kinlen LJ. Incidence of cancer in rheumatoid arthritis and other disorders after immunosuppressive treatment. Am J Med. 1985;78:44–9.

71. Farrell RJ, Ang Y, Kileen P, et al. Increased incidence of non-Hodgkin's lymphoma in inflammatory bowel disease patients on immunosuppressive therapy but overall risk is low. Gut. 2000;47: 514–9.

72. Armstrong RG, West J, Card TR. Risk of cancer in inflammatory bowel disease treated with azathioprine: a UK population-based case-control study. Am J Gastroenterol. 2010;105:1604–9.

73. Beaugerie L, Brousse N, Bouvier AM, et al. Lymphoproliferative disorders in patients receiving thiopurines for inflammatory bowel disease: a prospective observational cohort study. Lancet. 2009;374:1617–25.

74. Dayharsh GA, Loftus Jr EV, Sandborn WJ, et al. Epstein-Barr virus-positive lymphoma in patients with inflammatory bowel disease treated with azathioprine or 6-mercaptopurine. Gastroenterology. 2002;122:72–7.

75. Vos ACW, Bakkal N, Minnee RC, et al. Risk of malignant lymphoma in patients with inflammatory bowel diseases: a Dutch nationwide study. Inflamm Bowel Dis. 2011;17(9):1837–45.

76. Maddox JS, Soltani K. Risk of nonmelanoma skin cancer with azathioprine use. Inflamm Bowel Dis. 2008;14:1425–31.

77. Long MD, Herfarth HH, Pipkin CA, Porter CQ, Sandler RS, Kappelman MD. Increased risk for non-melanoma skin cancer in patients with inflammatory bowel disease. Clin Gastroenterol Hepatol. 2010;8:268–74.

78. Peyrin-Biroulet L, Khosrotehrani K, Carrat F, et al. Increased risk for nonmelanoma skin cancers in patients who receive thiopurines for inflammatory bowel disease. Gastroenterology. 2011;141: 1621–28 e1-5.

79. Singh H, Nugent Z, Demers AA, Bernstein CN. Increased risk of nonmelanoma skin cancers among individuals with inflammatory bowel disease. Gastroenterology. 2011;141:1612–20.

80. van Schaik FD, van Oijen MG, Smeets HM, van der Heijden GJ, Siersema PD, Oldenburg B. Risk of nonmelanoma skin cancer in patients with inflammatory bowel disease who use thiopurines is not increased. Clin Gastroenterol Hepatol. 2011;9:449–50.

81. Colombel JF, Loftus Jr EV, Tremaine WJ, et al. The safety profile of infliximab in patients with Crohn's disease: the Mayo clinic experience in 500 patients. Gastroenterology. 2004;126:19–31.

82. Lichtenstein GR, Cohen RD, Feagan BG, et al. Safety of infliximab and other Crohn's disease therapies: TREAT registry data with a mean of 5 years of follow-up. Gastroenterology. 2011;140: S-773.

83. Peyrin-Biroulet L, Deltenre P, de Suray N, Branche J, Sandborn WJ, Colombel JF. Efficacy and safety of tumor necrosis factor antagonists in Crohn's disease: meta-analysis of placebo-controlled trials. Clin Gastroenterol Hepatol. 2008;6:644–53.

84. Keane J, Gershon S, Wise RP, et al. Tuberculosis associated with infliximab, a tumor necrosis factor alpha-neutralizing agent. N Engl J Med. 2001;345:1098–104.

85. Kornbluth A, Sachar DB. Ulcerative colitis practice guidelines in adults: American College of Gastroenterology, Practice Parameters Committee. Am J Gastroenterol. 2010;105:501–23. quiz 24.

86. Mow WS, Abreu-Martin MT, Papadakis KA, Pitchon HE, Targan SR, Vasiliauskas EA. High incidence of anergy in inflammatory bowel disease patients limits the usefulness of PPD screening before infliximab therapy. Clin Gastroenterol Hepatol. 2004;2: 309–13.

87. Esteve M, Saro C, Gonzalez-Huix F, Suarez F, Forne M, Viver JM. Chronic hepatitis B reactivation following infliximab therapy in Crohn's disease patients: need for primary prophylaxis. Gut. 2004;53:1363–5.

88. Smith JA, Kauffman CA. Endemic fungal infections in patients receiving tumour necrosis factor-alpha inhibitor therapy. Drugs. 2009;69:1403–15.

89. FDA Safety Alerts for Human Medical Products. Tumor necrosis factor-alpha blockers (TNF blockers), Cimzia (certolizumab pegol), Enbrel (etanercept), Humira (adalimumab), and Remicade (infliximab) Sept 2008. http://www.fda.gov/Safety/MedWatch/SafetyInformation/SafetyAlertsforHumanMedicalProducts/ucm163195.htm (2008). Accessed 2 Dec, 2011.

90. Grijalva CG, Chen L, Delzell E, et al. Initiation of tumor necrosis factor-alpha antagonists and the risk of hospitalization for infection in patients with autoimmune diseases. JAMA. 2011;306:2331–9.

91. Targan SR, Hanauer SB, van Deventer SJ, et al. A short-term study of chimeric monoclonal antibody cA2 to tumor necrosis factor alpha for Crohn's disease. Crohn's Disease cA2 Study Group. N Engl J Med. 1997;337:1029–35.

92. Present DH, Rutgeerts P, Targan S, et al. Infliximab for the treatment of fistulas in patients with Crohn's disease. N Engl J Med. 1999;340:1398–405.

93. Rutgeerts P, D'Haens G, Targan S, et al. Efficacy and safety of retreatment with anti-tumor necrosis factor antibody (infliximab) to maintain remission in Crohn's disease. Gastroenterology. 1999;117:761–9.

94. Hanauer SB, Feagan BG, Lichtenstein GR, et al. Maintenance infliximab for Crohn's disease: the ACCENT I randomised trial. Lancet. 2002;359:1541–9.

95. Sands BE, Anderson FH, Bernstein CN, et al. Infliximab maintenance therapy for fistulizing Crohn's disease. N Engl J Med. 2004;350:876–85.

96. Rutgeerts P, Sandborn WJ, Feagan BG, et al. Infliximab for induction and maintenance therapy for ulcerative colitis. N Engl J Med. 2005;353:2462–76.

97. Hanauer SB, Sandborn WJ, Rutgeerts P, et al. Human anti-tumor necrosis factor monoclonal antibody (adalimumab) in Crohn's disease: the CLASSIC-I trial. Gastroenterology. 2006;130: 323–33. quiz 591.

98. Colombel JF, Sandborn WJ, Rutgeerts P, et al. Adalimumab for maintenance of clinical response and remission in patients with Crohn's disease: the CHARM trial. Gastroenterology. 2007;132: 52–65.

99. Sandborn WJ, Hanauer SB, Rutgeerts P, et al. Adalimumab for maintenance treatment of Crohn's disease: results of the CLASSIC II trial. Gut. 2007;56:1232–9.

100. Sandborn WJ, Rutgeerts P, Enns R, et al. Adalimumab induction therapy for Crohn disease previously treated with infliximab: a randomized trial. Ann Intern Med. 2007;146:829–38.

101. Colombel JF, Schwartz DA, Sandborn WJ, et al. Adalimumab for the treatment of fistulas in patients with Crohn's disease. Gut. 2009;58:940–8.

102. Reinisch W, Sandborn WJ, Hommes DW, et al. Adalimumab for induction of clinical remission in moderately to severely active ulcerative colitis: results of a randomised controlled trial. Gut. 2011;60:780–7.

103. Schreiber S, Rutgeerts P, Fedorak RN, et al. A randomized, placebo-controlled trial of certolizumab pegol (CDP870) for treatment of Crohn's disease. Gastroenterology. 2005;129:807–18.

104. Sandborn WJ, Feagan BG, Stoinov S, et al. Certolizumab pegol for the treatment of Crohn's disease. N Engl J Med. 2007;357: 228–38.

105. Schreiber S, Khaliq-Kareemi M, Lawrance IC, et al. Maintenance therapy with certolizumab pegol for Crohn's disease. N Engl J Med. 2007;357:239–50.

106. Lichtenstein GR, Thomsen OO, Schreiber S, et al. Continuous therapy with certolizumab pegol maintains remission of patients with Crohn's disease for up to 18 months. Clin Gastroenterol Hepatol. 2010;8:600–9.

107. Sandborn WJ, Abreu MT, D'Haens G, et al. Certolizumab pegol in patients with moderate to severe Crohn's disease and secondary failure to infliximab. Clin Gastroenterol Hepatol. 2010;8:688–95 e2.

108. Sandborn WJ, Schreiber S, Feagan BG, et al. Certolizumab pegol for active Crohn's disease: a placebo-controlled, randomized trial. Clin Gastroenterol Hepatol. 2011;9:670–8 e3.

109. Ljung T, Karlen P, Schmidt D, et al. Infliximab in inflammatory bowel disease: clinical outcome in a population based cohort from Stockholm County. Gut. 2004;53:849–53.

110. Caspersen S, Elkjaer M, Riis L, et al. Infliximab for inflammatory bowel disease in Denmark 1999-2005: clinical outcome and follow-up evaluation of malignancy and mortality. Clin Gastroenterol Hepatol. 2008;6:1212–7. quiz 176.

111. Lichtenstein GR, Cohen RD, Feagan BG et al. Safety of Infliximab and other Crohn's disease therapies: Treat™ registry data with a mean of 5 years of follow-up. Gastroenterology. 2011;140:S773.

112. Herrinton LJ, Liu L, Weng X, Lewis JD, Hutfless S, Allison JE. Role of thiopurine and Anti-TNF therapy in lymphoma in inflammatory bowel disease. Am J Gastroenterol. 2011;106:2146–53.

113. Belhadj K, Reyes F, Farcet JP, et al. Hepatosplenic gammadelta T-cell lymphoma is a rare clinicopathologic entity with poor outcome: report on a series of 21 patients. Blood. 2003;102:4261–9.

114. Kotlyar DS, Osterman MT, Diamond RH, et al. A systematic review of factors that contribute to hepatosplenic T-cell lymphoma in patients with inflammatory bowel disease. Clin Gastroenterol Hepatol. 2011;9:36–41 e1.

115. Fidder H, Schnitzler F, Ferrante M, et al. Long-term safety of infliximab for the treatment of inflammatory bowel disease: a single-centre cohort study. Gut. 2009;58:501–8.

116. Bongartz T, Sutton AJ, Sweeting MJ, Buchan I, Matteson EL, Montori V. Anti-TNF antibody therapy in rheumatoid arthritis and the risk of serious infections and malignancies: systematic review and meta-analysis of rare harmful effects in randomized controlled trials. JAMA. 2006;295:2275–85.

117. Lichtiger S, Present DH, Kornbluth A, et al. Cyclosporine in severe ulcerative colitis refractory to steroid therapy. N Engl J Med. 1994;330:1841–5.

118. Sternthal MB, Murphy SJ, George J, Kornbluth A, Lichtiger S, Present DH. Adverse events associated with the use of cyclosporine in patients with inflammatory bowel disease. Am J Gastroenterol. 2008;103:937–43.

119. Arts J, D'Haens G, Zeegers M, et al. Long-term outcome of treatment with intravenous cyclosporin in patients with severe ulcerative colitis. Inflamm Bowel Dis. 2004;10:73–8.

120. Opelz G, Dohler B. Lymphomas after solid organ transplantation: a collaborative transplant study report. Am J Transplant. 2004;4:222–30.

121. Dantal J, Hourmant M, Cantarovich D, et al. Effect of long-term immunosuppression in kidney-graft recipients on cancer incidence: randomised comparison of two cyclosporin regimens. Lancet. 1998;351:623–8.

122. Cockburn IT, Krupp P. The risk of neoplasms in patients treated with cyclosporine A. J Autoimmun. 1989;2:723–31.

123. Shibahara T, Miyazaki K, Sato D, et al. Rectal malignant lymphoma complicating ulcerative colitis treated with long-term cyclosporine A. J Gastroenterol Hepatol. 2006;21:336–8.

124. Schwartz LK, Kim MK, Coleman M, Lichtiger S, Chadburn A, Scherl E. Case report: lymphoma arising in an ileal pouch anal anastomosis after immunomodulatory therapy for inflammatory bowel disease. Clin Gastroenterol Hepatol. 2006;4:1030–4.

125. de Mattos AM, Olyaei AJ, Bennett WM. Nephrotoxicity of immunosuppressive drugs: long-term consequences and challenges for the future. Am J Kidney Dis. 2000;35:333–46.

126. Porayko MK, Textor SC, Krom RA, et al. Nephrotoxic effects of primary immunosuppression with FK-506 and cyclosporine regimens after liver transplantation. Mayo Clin Proc. 1994;69: 105–11.

127. Bertani T, Ferrazzi P, Schieppati A, et al. Nature and extent of glomerular injury induced by cyclosporine in heart transplant patients. Kidney Int. 1991;40:243–50.

128. Zaltzman JS, Pei Y, Maurer J, Patterson A, Cattran DC. Cyclosporine nephrotoxicity in lung transplant recipients. Transplantation. 1992;54:875–8.

129. Kopp JB, Klotman PE. Cellular and molecular mechanisms of cyclosporin nephrotoxicity. J Am Soc Nephrol. 1990;1:162–79.

130. Bennett WM, DeMattos A, Meyer MM, Andoh T, Barry JM. Chronic cyclosporine nephropathy: the Achilles' heel of immunosuppressive therapy. Kidney Int. 1996;50:1089–100.

131. Shang MH, Yuan WJ, Zhang SJ, Fan Y, Zhang Z. Intrarenal activation of renin angiotensin system in the development of cyclosporine A induced chronic nephrotoxicity. Chin Med J (Engl). 2008;121:983–8.

132. D'Haens G, Lemmens L, Geboes K, et al. Intravenous cyclosporine versus intravenous corticosteroids as single therapy for severe attacks of ulcerative colitis. Gastroenterology. 2001;120:1323–9.

133. Van Assche G, D'Haens G, Noman M, et al. Randomized, double-blind comparison of 4 mg/kg versus 2 mg/kg intravenous cyclosporine in severe ulcerative colitis. Gastroenterology. 2003;125: 1025–31.

134. Cohen RD, Stein R, Hanauer SB. Intravenous cyclosporin in ulcerative colitis: a five-year experience. Am J Gastroenterol. 1999;94:1587–92.

135. Campbell S, Travis S, Jewell D. Ciclosporin use in acute ulcerative colitis: a long-term experience. Eur J Gastroenterol Hepatol. 2005;17:79–84.

136. Moskovitz DN, Van Assche G, Maenhout B, et al. Incidence of colectomy during long-term follow-up after cyclosporine-induced

remission of severe ulcerative colitis. Clin Gastroenterol Hepatol. 2006;4:760–5.

137. Mihatsch MJ, Steiner K, Abeywickrama KH, Landmann J, Thiel G. Risk factors for the development of chronic cyclosporine-nephrotoxicity. Clin Nephrol. 1988;29:165–75.

138. Roberts SE, Williams JG, Yeates D, Goldacre MJ. Mortality in patients with and without colectomy admitted to hospital for ulcerative colitis and Crohn's disease: record linkage studies. BMJ. 2007;335:1033.

139. Lewis JD, Gelfand JM, Troxel AB, et al. Immunosuppressant medications and mortality in inflammatory bowel disease. Am J Gastroenterol. 2008;103:1428–35. quiz 36.

140. Herrinton LJ, Liu L, Fireman B, et al. Time trends in therapies and outcomes for adult inflammatory bowel disease, Northern California, 1998-2005. Gastroenterology. 2009;137:502–11.

141. Casal M, Leao C. Utilization of acetic acid and other short-chain monocarboxylic acids in the yeasts Torulaspora delbrueckii and Saccharomyces cerevisiae: transport and its regulation. Folia Microbiol (Praha). 1994;39:512–3.

142. Gainsbury ML, Chu DI, Howard LA, et al. Preoperative infliximab is not associated with an increased risk of short-term postoperative complications after restorative proctocolectomy and ileal pouch-anal anastomosis. J Gastrointest Surg. 2011;15: 397–403.

143. Ferrante M, D'Hoore A, Vermeire S, et al. Corticosteroids but not infliximab increase short-term postoperative infectious complications in patients with ulcerative colitis. Inflamm Bowel Dis. 2009;15:1062–70.

144. Mor IJ, Vogel JD, da Luz MA, Shen B, Hammel J, Remzi FH. Infliximab in ulcerative colitis is associated with an increased risk of postoperative complications after restorative proctocolectomy. Dis Colon Rectum. 2008;51:1202–7. discussion 7-10.

145. Selvasekar CR, Cima RR, Larson DW, et al. Effect of infliximab on short-term complications in patients undergoing operation for chronic ulcerative colitis. J Am Coll Surg. 2007;204:956–62. discussion 62-3.

# Management of Steroid-Dependent and Steroid-Refractory Ulcerative Colitis

Keely R. Parisian and Bret A. Lashner

**Keywords**

Management • Steroid-dependent ulcerative colitis • Steroid-refractory ulcerative colitis • Corticosteroids

## Background

Corticosteroids remain an effective therapy for inducing remission in patients with ulcerative colitis (UC); however, they have not been shown to be effective for the maintenance of remission [1]. Response to corticosteroids has been defined as the clinical improvement within 30 days of treatment with high-dose oral corticosteroids (40–60 mg prednisone or equivalent) or clinical improvement within 7–10 days of treatment with high-dose intravenous corticosteroids [2]. Patients with inflammatory bowel disease (IBD) who initially respond to corticosteroids but then relapse with tapering corticosteroids or shortly after discontinuation and require reintroduction of corticosteroids to maintain control of symptoms have been defined as steroid dependent. Patients who fail to respond to corticosteroids within this time frame have been defined as steroid refractory (Table 28.1) [2]. In a population-based cohort study, Faubion et al. assessed a 1-year outcome in 358 patients with IBD after the first course of oral corticosteroids [3]. They showed that after 1 year, 49 % of UC patients treated with oral prednisone maintained remission [95 % confidence interval (CI), 36–62 %], 22 %

K.R. Parisian, M.D. (✉)
Gastroenterology Group of Rochester, 919 Westfall Road, Suit 100, Rochester, NY 14618, USA
e-mail: keelyparisian@gmail.com

B.A. Lashner, M.D.
Department of Gastroenterology and Hepatology, Digestive Disease Institute, Cleveland Clinic, 9500 Euclid Avenue/A30, Cleveland, OH 44195, USA
e-mail: Lashneb@ccf.org

were corticosteroid dependent (95 % CI, 13–34 %), and 29 % underwent colectomy (95 % CI, 18–40 %).

The risks of long-term corticosteroid therapy including osteoporosis, pathological fractures, cataract, metabolic changes, acne, striae, hirsutism, psychological disturbance, and infection outweigh their benefits in some patients. Management of steroid-dependent and steroid-refractory UC may include stepped-up medical treatment or surgery. At any time, approximately 20–34 % of patients with UC have chronic active disease requiring several courses of corticosteroids to achieve remission [1, 3]. This chapter will discuss the management of steroid-dependent UC followed by the management of steroid-refractory UC.

## Management of Steroid-Dependent UC

Immunosuppression with thiopurines is a mainstay in managing steroid-dependent UC. Thiopurine therapy, although more widely used in steroid-dependent Crohn's disease (CD), may be useful for patients with steroid-dependent as well as steroid-refractory UC. Ardizzone et al. randomized 72 patients with steroid-dependent UC to receive azathioprine (AZA) 2 mg/kg daily or oral 5-aminosalicylic acid (5-ASA) 3.2 g daily for a 6-month follow-up period [4]. Steroid dependence was defined as a requirement for steroid therapy ≥10 mg daily during the preceding 6 months, with at least two attempts to discontinue the medication. They found that significantly more patients in the AZA than in the 5-ASA group had clinical and endoscopic remission and discontinued steroid therapy (53 vs. 21 %, $P = 0.003$).

More recently, a cohort study of 42 patients with steroid-dependent UC initiated on AZA therapy with a steroid taper

G.R. Lichtenstein (ed.), *Medical Therapy of Ulcerative Colitis*,
DOI 10.1007/978-1-4939-1677-1_28, © Springer Science+Business Media New York 2014

**Table 28.1** Definitions of corticosteroid-dependent ulcerative colitis [1, 24]

| Therapeutic outcome | Definition |
|---|---|
| Response to corticosteroids | Clinical improvement after treatment with high-dose oral steroids (40–60 mg prednisone or equivalent) within 30 days or clinical improvement after treatment with high-dose intravenous steroids within 7–10 days |
| Corticosteroid refractory (steroid refractory) | Patients who fail to respond in the time frame described above |
| Corticosteroid dependent (steroid dependent) | Patients who initially respond to corticosteroids but then relapse during tapering or shortly after drug discontinuation of corticosteroids and require reintroduction of corticosteroid therapy to maintain symptom control |

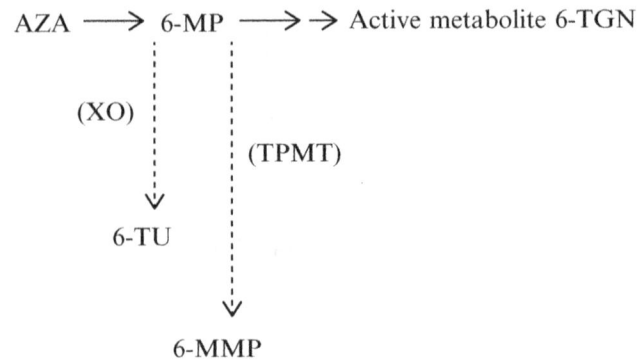

**Fig. 28.1** Metabolism of azathioprine

showed the proportion of patients remaining in steroid-free remission at 12, 24, and 36 months was 55, 52, and 45 %, respectively [5]. AZA was dosed at 50 mg daily for the first 15 days followed by a target dose of 2–3 mg/kg daily. Steroid-dependent UC was defined as the inability to successfully reduce steroids below the equivalent of prednisone 10 mg daily within 3 months of starting steroids, relapse within 3 months of stopping steroids, or symptoms only controlled by continued use of steroids requiring a daily oral dose of 15–25 mg of prednisone for at least 6 months.

In light of these and several other studies, the American College of Gastroenterology (ACG) and the American Gastroenterological Association (AGA) recommend that patients with corticosteroid-dependent inflammatory bowel disease (IBD) be treated with AZA 2–3 mg/kg daily or 6-mercaptopurine (6-MP) 1.0–1.5 mg/kg daily in an attempt to lower or eliminate corticosteroid use (grade A) [6, 7].

The metabolites of AZA and 6-MP may influence the management of patients with IBD. AZA is nonenzymatically converted to 6-MP, which may be activated through several enzymatic steps to the active metabolites, 6-thioguanine nucleotides (6-TGN). 6-MP may also be metabolized to 6-methylmercaptopurine (6-MMP) by the enzyme thiopurine methyltransferase (TPMT) and to 6-thiouric acid (6-TU) by the enzyme xanthine oxidase. Both 6-MMP and 6-TU are inactive metabolites. (Please see Fig. 28.1.) TPMT activity may be both genetically determined and inducible, and a deficiency of this enzyme may lead to myelosuppression.

The toxicity induced by AZA and 6-MP in patients with IBD includes bone marrow suppression in 10 % of patients (secondary to elevated 6-TGN levels) [5], pancreatitis in 3.3 % of patients, allergic reactions in 2 % of patients, drug hepatitis in 0.3 % of patients (secondary to elevated 6-MMP levels), infection in 7.4 % of patients, and neoplasm in 3.1 %

of patients [8]. Routine monitoring of complete blood count with differential weekly for 4 weeks, biweekly for 4 weeks, and then every 1–2 months for the duration of treatment is suggested [9]. The ACG and AGA recommend measuring liver function tests periodically and assessing TPMT genotype or phenotype before initiation of therapy with AZA or 6-MP to detect individuals with low enzyme activity who may be at risk for myelosuppression [6, 7]. Roblin et al. performed a cross-sectional worldwide survey and showed that the use of TMPT phenotype and genotype testing was performed in only 43 and 30 % of responding gastroenterologists, respectively [10].

Dubinsky et al. showed that clinical response was highly correlated with 6-TGN levels ($P < 0.0001$) in pediatric patients with IBD. Further, they showed that the frequency of therapeutic response increased at 6-TGN levels >235 pmol/8 × 10 [8] erythrocytes ($P < 0.001$) [11]. Other studies have found that 6-MP dose is weakly associated with 6-TGN levels [12, 13]. As a result of the discrepancy in data, a controlled study to evaluate the utility of these tests is needed before recommendations for clinical use can be instituted. Thiopurine testing may play a role in assessing nonadherence or to explain therapeutic failure in patients taking AZA or 6-MP.

The antimetabolite methotrexate (MTX) is widely used in certain autoimmune diseases such as rheumatoid arthritis and psoriasis. A pilot study by Kozarek et al. in 1989 showed that 25 mg/week intramuscular injection of MTX for 12 weeks resulted in a significant reduction in prednisone dosage in patients with refractory UC or CD [14]. The chronic UC activity index decreased from 13.3 to 6.3 ($P = 0.007$); however, no patient with UC showed complete histological or endoscopic remission. This early study also addressed the side effects of MTX, including nausea and diarrhea, liver function test increase, leukopenia, brittle nails, and hypersensitivity pneumonitis.

Baron et al. in 1993 evaluated the efficacy and safety of oral MTX 15 mg daily in patients with refractory IBD for

18 weeks [15]. Refractory IBD was defined as a chronic active disease that lasts for more than 6 months and the failure to respond to steroids or the requirement of 20 mg/day of prednisone or more with disease flare when the dose was tapered. Ten of the 11 UC patients included were previously unsuccessfully treated with ASA or 6-MP. UC patients treated with low-dose MTX showed a statistically significant decrease in daily prednisone dose from 26.3 to 12.7 mg ($P < 0.001$) and a decrease in sigmoidoscopic score (graded on a scale of 0–15 based on mucopus, friability, vascular pattern, granularity, and erythema) from 10.9 to 8.0 ($P < 0.003$). Mild side effects including mouth ulcers, alopecia, insomnia, facial flushing, nausea and vomiting, and transient decrease in night vision were reported. This pilot study supports the previous study by Kozarek et al. concluding that low-dose oral MTX is reasonably safe as a steroid-sparing agent in patients with refractory IBD.

Oren et al. randomized 67 patients with active UC to receive oral MTX 12.5 mg weekly or placebo for 9 months [16]. Disease chronicity was defined as the requirement of steroid therapy for at least 4 of the preceding 12 months. At each visit the Mayo Clinic score was calculated, and a sigmoidoscopy was performed every 3 months. There was no significant difference in achieving remission and complete steroid withdrawal between patients assigned to MTX and patients assigned to placebo (47 vs. 49 %, $P = 0.87$).

In a non-placebo-controlled study, Paoluzi et al. treated steroid-dependent UC patients with oral AZA 2 mg/kg followed by intramuscular MTX 12.5 mg/week if intolerant or not responding to AZA [17]. Disease activity was monitored monthly and colonoscopy with histology performed at 3 months, 6 months, and then every 6 months thereafter. In the short-term treatment, achieving complete remission and demonstrating improvement on AZA was similar to MTX (69 vs. 60 %, 20 vs. 40 %, respectively). Of the patients who achieved complete remission in the short-term treatment, 12 of 22 patients taking AZA and all 6 patients taking MTX remained in remission at the end of long-term treatment (54 % vs. 100 %, $P < 0.05$). This study confirms the beneficial role of AZA in refractory UC and shows that MTX may be effective in those unresponsive or intolerant to AZA. A limitation to this study is the small study population.

It is important to mention that the dose of MTX used to treat patients with CD successfully (25 mg IM weekly) has not been tried in patients with UC. The use of lower-dose MTX has shown some promise in the studies discussed and may be of potential benefit in patients with UC. Although evidence supports the use of MTX for induction and remission with corticosteroid withdrawal in active CD, the ACG and AGA state that there is insufficient evidence to support the use of MTX in patients with active UC [6, 7].

Mycophenolate mofetil (MMF) is another drug that shows potential in steroid-dependent UC. Similar to MTX, MMF reduces the production of interferon gamma by T cells. MMF is traditionally used to prevent graft rejection in organ transplant patients. An early trial randomized patients with CD to receive AZA (2.5 mg/kg) plus 50 mg prednisolone orally versus MMF (15 mg/kg) plus 50 mg prednisolone orally [18]. Corticosteroid dosage was titrated weekly to a maintenance dose of prednisolone 5 mg daily. This study showed that treatment of patients with a Crohn's disease activity index (CDAI) greater than 300 with MMF plus corticosteroids had a greater decrease in CDAI score during the first month of treatment compared to patients in the AZA plus corticosteroid treatment arm. Over 6 months this resulted in a greater number of MMF-treated patients entering remission. Additionally, this study showed that there were no severe adverse events in either group. Two patients in the MMF-treated group developed drug exanthema and vomiting.

Shortly after, Orth et al. carried out a prospective study to compare MMF versus AZA in patients with chronic active UC [19]. In a similar fashion, they randomized 24 patients with UC to MMF (20 mg/kg) plus prednisolone orally or AZA (2 mg/kg) plus prednisolone orally. They found that the number of patients not requiring steroids was higher in the AZA plus prednisolone group than in the MMF plus prednisolone group. Further, there were no severe adverse events reported in the AZA plus prednisolone group but two severe adverse events observed in the MMF plus prednisolone group (recurrent upper airway infections in one patient and bacterial meningitis in another patient). The authors conclude that AZA plus prednisolone appears to be more effective and more safe compared to MMF plus prednisolone in patients with UC. This trial employed dosages lower than those typically used in renal transplantation and may explain why diarrhea, hematological toxicity, primary neutropenia, or thrombocytopenia was not seen. A later study showed adverse events that include malaise, irritability, depression, joint pain, skin rash, pancreatitis, alopecia, diarrhea, and abnormal liver function tests [20]. As a result of conflicting data, the ACG and the AGA do not recommend the use of MMF in patients with steroid-dependent UC [6, 7]. If a patient has a contraindication to AZA, then MMF may be a reasonable alternative; however, further studies are essential to evaluate the effects of MMF in active UC.

The immunosuppressant tacrolimus is a calcineurin inhibitor currently approved for the prophylaxis of organ rejection in patients receiving allogeneic liver or kidney transplants. Tacrolimus may also inhibit interleukin 2 (IL-2) and therefore play a role in the pathogenesis of IBD. A retrospective study in 2006 observed 53 patients with steroid-refractory or steroid-dependent IBD [21]. The study included

40 patients with UC, 11 patients with CD, and 2 patients with pouchitis. Patients had previously failed or not tolerated therapy with 5-ASA, AZA, MTX, infliximab, cyclosporine, MMF, and budesonide in the UC group. In those patients with UC, 57 % had pancolitis, 30 % had left-sided colitis, 10 % had other parts of their colon affected, and 2.5 % had proctitis. Tacrolimus was administered orally at an initial dose of 0.1 mg/kg per day in two divided doses with goal serum trough levels of 4–8 ng/mL. At 39 months, 27 of 40 patients (67.5 %) in the UC group were in remission, 2 of 40 patients (5 %) did not respond, and 2 of 40 patients (5 %) withdrew. A reduction or discontinuation of prednisolone was achieved in 33 of 36 UC patients (91.7 %) receiving prednisolone. It is important to note that 77 % of all IBD patients included in the study were receiving concomitant AZA. Nine of 40 UC patients (22.5 %) underwent colectomy for intractable bleeding, premalignant or malignant polyps, intractable paresthesias, or the desire of the patient to have surgery rather than continue immunosuppression. Colectomy-free survival in UC patients was 56.5 % at 43 months. There were no reported side effects in 75 % of all IBD patients included. They did have opportunistic infections in 3 % of patients, increase in creatinine in 7.5 % of patients, hyperkalemia in 1.9 % of patients, hypertension in 1.9 % of patients, and tremor or paresthesias in 9.4 % of patients. The authors conclude that tacrolimus appears safe and effective in refractory IBD.

In a prospective randomized controlled trial, patients with active refractory UC were assigned to tacrolimus with a high trough concentration (10–15 ng/ml), low trough concentration (5–10 ng/ml), or placebo [22]. Patients were permitted to continue 5-ASA drugs or steroids during the study as long as the dosage was not adjusted; however, AZA or 6-MP concomitant use was prohibited. An improvement in the disease activity index (DAI) score was observed in 68.4 % of patients in the high trough concentration group compared to 10 % in the placebo group at week 2 ($P < 0.001$). Clinical remission was observed in 4 of 20 patients (20 %) of the high trough concentration group, 2 of 19 patients (10.5 %) of the low trough concentration group, and 1 of 17 patients (5.9 %) in the placebo group at week 2. Mucosal healing was achieved in 15 of 19 patients (78.9 %) in the high trough concentration group, 8 of 18 patients (44.4 %) in the low trough concentration group, and 2 of 16 patients (12.5 %) in the placebo group at week 2. In an open-label extension, 55.2 % of patients receiving tacrolimus therapy showed an improvement in the DAI score at week 10. The mean dose of prednisolone was reduced at week 10. Reported adverse events in this trial included: finger tremor, headache, serious viral gastroenteritis, decreases in serum magnesium, and increases in serum creatinine. This study concluded that oral tacrolimus, with optimal target trough concentration of 10–15 ng/ml, appears to be efficacious and

**Table 28.2** Medical therapy for steroid-dependent UC

| Medical therapy | Adverse events | References |
|---|---|---|
| Thiopurines | Bone marrow suppression (elevated 6-TGN levels) | Chebli et al. [5] |
| AZA | Infection | Kornbluth et al. [6] |
| 6-MP | Pancreatitis | Lichtenstein et al. [7] |
| | Neoplasm | Present et al. [8] |
| | Allergic reactions | |
| | Drug hepatitis (elevated 6-MMP levels) | |
| MTX[a] | Neutrophilic dermatitis (Sweet's syndrome) | Baron et al. [15] |
| | Dermatitis | Oren et al. [16] |
| | Leukopenia | Paoluzi et al. [17] |
| | Headache | |
| | Mouth ulcers | |
| | Ulceration of nasal mucosa | |
| | Alopecia | |
| | Insomnia | |
| | Facial flushing | |
| | Nausea, vomiting | |
| | Transient decreased night vision | |
| MMF[a] | Diarrhea | Neurath et al. [18] |
| | Neutropenia | Orth et al. [19] |
| | Thrombocytopenia | Palaniappan et al. [20] |
| | Hematological toxicity | |
| | Nausea, vomiting | |
| | Elevated liver function tests | |
| | Malaise | |
| | Behavioral changes | |
| | Depression | |
| | Joint pain | |
| | Skin rash | |
| | Pancreatitis | |
| | Alopecia | |
| Tacrolimus[a] | Opportunistic infections | Baumgart et al. [21] |
| | Viral gastroenteritis | Ogata et al. [22] |
| | Increase in creatinine | |
| | Hyperkalemia | |
| | Hypomagnesemia | |
| | Hypertension | |
| | Headache | |
| | Hand tremor | |
| | Paresthesias | |

[a]The ACG and AGA do not recommend this therapy. There is insufficient evidence to support the use of these medications for steroid-dependent UC. However, if there is a contraindication to AZA, these medical therapies may be reasonable alternatives

safe as therapy in refractory UC. As a result of few data, the ACG and the AGA do not recommend tacrolimus at this time for the management of steroid-dependent or steroid-refractory UC (Table 28.2) [6, 7].

## Management of Steroid-Refractory UC

The medical management of steroid-refractory UC may overlap with the therapy used to manage steroid-dependent UC. In general, intravenous (IV) corticosteroids, cyclosporine, infliximab, and surgery are the mainstay of the therapy for steroid-refractory UC (Table 28.3).

In an editorial comparing oral versus intravenous steroids to define refractory UC, Chiorean reminds us that corticosteroids remain the first-line treatment of choice for patients with moderate to severe flares of UC despite little evidence-based data to support the optimal dose and delivery [23]. One may speculate that IV steroids have superior efficacy over oral steroids in patients with UC secondary to impaired absorption in the setting of an inflamed colon. The landmark study by Truelove and Jewell in 1974 treated 49 patients with severe UC with a regimen to include IV steroids for 5 days [24]. They define severe UC as having six or more bloody bowel movements daily, fever, tachycardia, anemia, and elevated erythrocyte sedimentation rate (ESR). Remission after 5 days was shown in 36 of 49 patients (73 %) treated with IV steroids. Of the 36 patients in remission at day 5, 33 remained in remission for 6 weeks. Based on this study and the fact that gastroenterologists have treated UC with steroids for more than 50 years, Chiorean suggests that IV steroids may define refractory disease.

Still, we include IV steroids in this section as there is not a definitive definition for steroid-refractory UC. In addition, the ACG and AGA recommend hospitalization for parenteral corticosteroids in patients failing to respond to oral corticosteroids or for patients with severe UC (grade A) [6, 7]. It is important to monitor for infection, glucose intolerance, and metabolic abnormalities while treating with IV steroids. There should be a plan for a specific duration and a specific tapering regimen of steroids at the initiation of therapy due to the toxicity associated with the use of corticosteroids.

Cyclosporine was first discovered and used in organ transplantation in the 1970s. Like tacrolimus, cyclosporine competitively binds to and inhibits calcineurin, leading to the suppression of signaling pathways that play a role in the pathogenesis of IBD. In 1990, Lichtiger and Present showed that IV cyclosporine is an effective treatment for patients with severe active UC who have not responded to steroids [25]. Reported adverse effects were hypertrichosis, paresthesias, resting tremor, gingival hyperplasia, transient hypertension, and nephrotoxicity.

In a landmark randomized placebo-controlled trial, 20 patients with severe active UC who had not clinically improved after at least 7 days of IV corticosteroid therapy received either IV cyclosporine (4 mg/kg/day) for up to 14 days or placebo [26]. All patients received 100 mg of IV hydrocortisone every 8 h and hydrocortisone enemas nightly if the drug could be retained. Oral sulfasalazine, mesalamine, olsalazine, or mesalamine enemas were continued, however, not initiated during the study. Serum cyclosporine concentrations of 100–400 ng/ml by radioimmunoassay with a monoclonal antibody or concentrations of 400–800 ng/ml by radioimmunoassay with a polyclonal antibody were considered therapeutic. Nine of 11 patients (82 %) in the IV cyclosporine group had an improvement in the clinical activity score within a mean of 7 days as compared to 0 of 9 patients in the placebo group (P<0.001). Five patients in the placebo group went on to receive open-label IV cyclosporine after the study period with a decrease in their mean clinical activity score from 11 to 7 within a mean time of 7 days. A total of nine patients in the trial responded to IV cyclosporine and were subsequently treated with oral cyclosporine 8 mg/kg/day. Four of nine patients went to colectomy. Documented adverse effects were similar to the pilot study

**Table 28.3** Medical therapy for steroid-refractory UC

| Medical therapy | Adverse events | References |
| --- | --- | --- |
| IV corticosteroids | Osteoporosis | Kornbluth et al. (ACG practice guidelines) [6] |
| | Pathological fractures | |
| | Glaucoma | |
| | Cataracts | |
| | Metabolic changes | |
| | Acne | |
| | Striae | |
| | Hirsutism | |
| | Psychological disturbance | |
| | Infection | |
| | Gastroduodenal mucosal injury | |
| Cyclosporine | Hypertrichosis | Lichtiger et al. [25] |
| | Paresthesias | Van Assche et al. [27] |
| | Resting tremor | |
| | Gingival hyperplasia | |
| | Transient hypertension | |
| | Nephrotoxicity | |
| | Seizures | |
| Infliximab | Abdominal pain | Rutgeerts et al. [28] |
| | Infusion reactions | Jarnerot et al. [29] |
| | Upper respiratory tract infection | |
| | Pharyngitis | |
| | Sinusitis | |
| | Oral candidiasis | |
| | Pain | |
| | Rash | |
| | Arthralgia | |
| | Anemia | |
| | Fatigue | |
| | Tuberculosis | |
| | Varicella-zoster virus | |

with the addition of seizures. This trial was terminated early due to the overwhelming beneficial effect of cyclosporine.

The coadministration of maintenance agents such as AZA or 6-MP after induction with IV cyclosporine has been documented as a therapy that may avoid colectomy. In addition, triple therapy with oral prednisone, oral cyclosporine, and an oral purine analogue with subsequent tapering of the corticosteroid and cyclosporine may lead to long-term maintenance. As such, the AGA recommends IV cyclosporine at 2–4 mg/kg/day or colectomy in patients with severe UC who have failed to respond to 7–10 days of oral or parenteral corticosteroids (grade B) [7]. Further, they recommend IV cyclosporine as an effective means of avoiding surgery in patients with severe corticosteroid-refractory UC (grade A) [7]. This, however, is based upon the data from 2006 prior to the widespread use of infliximab in patients with severe UC.

Van Assche et al. published findings of patients with severe UC randomized to a high-dose cyclosporine group (4 mg/kg) or low-dose cyclosporine group (2 mg/kg) for 8 days [27]. At day 8, all responding patients were switched to 8 mg/kg oral cyclosporine. Concomitant medications allowed included IV corticosteroids if given prior to enrollment and at a stable dose (oral corticosteroids were converted to IV corticosteroids), AZA or 6-MP if started 3 months prior, oral and rectal 5-ASA, and antibiotics. The primary end point clinical response was achieved by 32 of 38 patients (84 %) in the high-dose group and 30 of 35 patients (85 %) in the low-dose group. The median time to response was 4 days in both groups, and the short-term colectomy rates were similar in both groups. The authors conclude that there is no difference between 4 mg/kg and 2 mg/kg IV cyclosporine. Adverse effects of cyclosporine were seen in both groups and included tremor or paresthesia, hypertension, an increase in serum creatinine, fever, headache, and diabetes mellitus.

Infliximab, a tumor necrosis factor-alpha chimeric monoclonal antibody, is approved by the FDA for use in UC, CD, rheumatoid arthritis, ankylosing spondylitis, psoriatic arthritis, and plaque psoriasis. The Active Ulcerative Colitis Trials 1 and 2 (ACT 1 and ACT 2) are two large randomized control trials that evaluated infliximab versus placebo for induction and maintenance therapy for corticosteroid-refractory UC.

In ACT 1, patients were treated with infliximab at weeks 0, 2, and 6 and then every 8 weeks through week 46; patients in ACT 2 were treated at weeks 0, 2, and 6 and then every 8 weeks through week 22 [28]. Patients were randomly assigned to receive IV infliximab 5 mg/kg, IV infliximab 10 mg/kg, or placebo at each treatment session. In both studies, patients continued their treatment with corticosteroids alone or in combination with immunomodulators or 5-ASA. After week 8, corticosteroids were tapered until discontinuation.

In ACT 1 and ACT 2 at week 8, clinical response rates in patients in the infliximab 5 mg/kg group and infliximab 10 mg/kg group were significantly greater as compared to patients in the placebo group [infliximab 5 mg/kg group (69 %) vs. placebo group (37 %), P<0.001, and infliximab 10 mg/kg group (62 %) vs. placebo group (37 %), P<0.001, in ACT 1 and infliximab 5 mg/kg group (65 %) vs. placebo group (29 %), P<0.001, and infliximab 10 mg/kg group (69 %) vs. placebo group (29 %), P<0.001, in ACT 2]; clinical remission rates in patients in the infliximab 5 mg/kg group and infliximab 10 mg/kg group were significantly higher as compared to patients in the placebo group [infliximab 5 mg/kg group (39 %) vs. placebo group (15 %), P<0.001, and infliximab 10 mg/kg group (32 %) vs. placebo group (15 %), P=0.002, in ACT 1 and infliximab 5 mg/kg group (34 %) vs. placebo group (6 %), P<0.001, and infliximab 10 mg/kg group (28 %) vs. placebo group (6 %), P<0.001, in ACT 2]; and mucosal healing rates in patients in the infliximab 5 mg/kg group and infliximab 10 mg/kg group were significantly higher as compared to the patients in the placebo group [infliximab 5 mg/kg group (62 %) vs. placebo group (34 %), P<0.001, and infliximab 10 mg/kg group (59 %) vs. placebo group (34 %), P<0.001, in ACT 1 and infliximab 5 mg/kg group (60 %) vs. placebo group (31 %), P<0.001, and infliximab 10 mg/kg group (62 %) vs. placebo (31 %), P<0.001, in ACT 2]. In ACT 2 at week 30, clinical response rates in patients in the infliximab 5 mg/kg group and infliximab 10 mg/kg group were significantly greater than the placebo group (47 %, 60 %, and 26 %, respectively; both P values <0.001); clinical remission rates in patients in the infliximab 5 mg/kg group and infliximab 10 mg/kg group were significantly higher than the placebo group [infliximab 5 mg/kg group (26 %) vs. placebo group (11 %), P=0.003; infliximab 10 mg/kg group (36 %) vs. placebo (11 %), P<0.001]; and mucosal healing rates in the infliximab 5 mg/kg group and infliximab 10 mg/kg group were significantly greater than the placebo group [infliximab 5 mg/kg group (46 %) vs. placebo group (30 %), P=0.009; infliximab 10 mg/kg group (57 %) vs. placebo group (30 %), P<0.001]. In ACT 1 at week 54, patients in the infliximab 5 mg/kg group and infliximab 10 mg/kg group showed greater clinical response, clinical remission, and mucosal healing rates as compared to the placebo group (P<0.001 in all comparisons). Additionally, the proportion of patients who had discontinued corticosteroids at week 30 in both studies and at week 54 in ACT 1 was higher in the infliximab groups than in the placebo groups.

The proportion of patients reporting any adverse event in ACT 1 and ACT 2 was similar among the three groups. Adverse events occurring in ≥10 % of patients in the infliximab groups included: abdominal pain, nausea, upper respiratory tract infections, pharyngitis, sinusitis, pain, rash, arthralgia, headache, fever, anemia, and fatigue. Other adverse events occurring in a smaller percentage of patients in the infliximab groups included: fungal dermatitis, pneumonia, varicella-zoster virus infection, herpes zoster, and abscess. One patient in the infliximab 10 mg/kg group developed tuberculosis. It is concluded that the risks of infliximab use must be weighed against the risks of the alternative, which is colectomy and the creation of an ileoanal pouch. Physicians and patients must be diligent in monitoring for signs and symptoms of infection.

Jarnerot et al. published a paper comparing infliximab to placebo as rescue therapy in severe to moderately severe UC [29]. Patients were treated with betamethasone 4 mg IV twice daily on day 0 and then randomized to receive infliximab (4–5 mg/kg) or placebo on day 3 if they met the index criteria for fulminant UC (based on the fulminant colitis index ≥8) or on day 5, 6, or 7 if they fulfilled the criteria for a severe or moderately severe attack of UC not responding to IV corticosteroids (based on the Seo index >150). The primary end point was colectomy. Significantly more patients in the placebo group (14 of 21) than in the infliximab group (7 of 24) had colectomy ($P=0.017$). Of the patients with fulminant UC, 69 % of patients in the placebo group and 47 % of patients in the infliximab group had a colectomy. In patients with less severe UC, 63 % of patients in the placebo group and no patients in the infliximab group had a colectomy ($P=0.009$). Side effects included central venous line septicemia, arthralgias, upper respiratory tract infections, exanthema, nausea, vomiting, abnormal liver function tests, oral candidiasis, and pruritus during infusion. The authors conclude that infliximab 4–5 mg/kg is an effective and safe rescue therapy in patients with acute severe or moderately severe UC not responding to conventional corticosteroids.

A recent prospective randomized trial compared cyclosporine to infliximab in steroid-resistant acute severe UC [30]. Steroid-resistant severe UC was defined as a Lichtiger score >10 after at least 5 days of IV methylprednisolone ≥0.8 mg/kg/day. Patients were randomized to either intravenous cyclosporine (2 mg/kg/day for 1 week and then transitioned to oral dosing) or infliximab (5 mg/kg at weeks 0, 2, and 6). Patients with clinical response at day 7 (Lichtiger score <10 with a decrease of at least three points compared to the baseline) were started on AZA 2.5 mg/kg/day, and steroids were decreased. Treatment failure was 60 % in the cyclosporine group and 54 % in the infliximab group ($P=0.49$). Response rates at day 7 in the cyclosporine group and infliximab group were 84 and 86 %, respectively ($P=0.76$). Colectomy was performed in ten patients treated with cyclosporine and 13 patients treated with infliximab. The authors conclude that cyclosporine is not more effective than infliximab to achieve short-term remission and avoid urgent colectomy in patients with steroid-resistant acute severe UC.

Finally, failure to obtain remission with the use of the abovementioned medical therapy for steroid-resistant UC may lead to colectomy. Unlike medical therapy, surgical therapy provides a definitive treatment for UC. Sandborn et al. extracted data to include the incidence of colectomy from ACT 1 and ACT 2 in 2009. The cumulative incidence of colectomy through 54 weeks in patients with UC was 10 and 17 % for the infliximab group and placebo group, respectively ($P=0.02$) [31]. Complications following colectomy with ileoanal pouch include the risk for pouchitis, pouch failure, female infertility, and nocturnal fecal incontinence. Certainly, quality of life and functional outcome will be important to the patient with UC. Therefore, the risks and benefits of surgery as well as timing must be weighed by both the gastroenterologist and patient.

In conclusion, steroid-dependent UC is best medically managed with thiopurines; however, if UC is unresponsive or intolerant to thiopurines, it may be managed with methotrexate, MMF, or tacrolimus. Steroid-resistant UC may be managed with IV corticosteroids, cyclosporine, infliximab, or colectomy. The risks and benefits of therapy in each individual case must be thoroughly appraised by both the gastroenterologist and the patient.

## References

1. Porro GB, Cassinotti A, Ferrara E, Maconi G, et al. Review article: the management of steroid dependency in ulcerative colitis. Aliment Pharmacol Ther. 2007;26:779–94.
2. Munkholm P, Langholz E, Davidsen M, Binder V. Frequency of glucocorticoid resistance and dependency in Crohn's disease. Gut. 1994;35:360–2.
3. Faubion WA, Loftus EV, Harmsen WS, Zinsmeister AR, et al. The natural history of corticosteroid therapy for inflammatory bowel disease: a population-based study. Gastroenterology. 2001;121:255–60.
4. Ardizzone S, Maconi G, Russo A, Imbesi V, Colombo E, Porro GB. Randomised controlled trial of azathioprine and 5-aminosalicylic acid for treatment of steroid dependent ulcerative colitis. Gut. 2006;55:47–53.
5. Chebli LA, Chaves LD, Pimentel FF, Guerra DM, Barros RM, Gaburri PD, Zanini A, Chebli JM. Azathioprine maintains long-term steroid-free remission through 3 years in patients with steroid-dependent ulcerative colitis. Inflamm Bowel Dis. 2010;16:613–9.
6. Kornbluth A, Sachar DB, The Practice Parameters Committee of the American College of Gastroenterology. Ulcerative colitis practice guidelines in adults: American College of Gastroenterology, Practice Parameters Committee. Am J Gastroenterol. 2010;105:501–23.
7. Lichtenstein GR, Abreu MT, Cohen R, Tremaine W, et al. American Gastroenterological Association Institute technical review on corticosteroids, immunomodulators, and infliximab in inflammatory bowel disease. Gastroenterology. 2006;130(3):940–87.
8. Present DH, Meltzer SJ, Krumholz MP, Wolke A, Korelitz BI. 6-Mercaptopurine in the management of inflammatory bowel disease: short- and long-term toxicity. Ann Intern Med. 1989;111:641–9.

9. Sandborn WJ. A review of immune modifier therapy for inflammatory bowel disease: azathioprine, 6-mercaptopurine, cyclosporine, and methotrexate. Am J Gastreoenterol. 1996;91:423–33.

10. Roblin X, Oussalah A, Chevaux JB, Sparrow M, Peyrin-Biroulet L. Use of thiopurine testing in the management of inflammatory bowel disease in clinical practice: a worldwide survey of experts. Inflamm Bowel Dis. 2011;17(12):2480–7.

11. Dubinsky MC, Lamothe S, Yang HY, Targan SR, Sinnett D, Theoret Y, Seidman EG. Pharmacogenomics and metabolite measurement for 6-mercaptopurine therapy in inflammatory bowel disease. Gastroenterology. 2000;118:705–13.

12. Lowry PW, Franklin CL, Weaver AL, Pike MG, Mays DC, Tremaine WJ, Lipsky JJ, Sandborn WJ. Measurement of thiopurine methyltransferase activity and azathioprine metabolites in patients with inflammatory bowel disease. Gut. 2001;49:665–70.

13. Morales A, Salquti S, Miao CL, Lewis JD. Relationship between 6-mercaptopurine dose and 6-thioguanine nucleotide levels in patients with inflammatory bowel disease. Inflamm Bowel Dis. 2007;13:380–5.

14. Kozarek RA, Patterson DJ, Gelfand MD, Botoman VA, Ball TJ, Wilske JR. Methotrexate indices for clinical and histological remission in patients with refractory inflammatory bowel disease. Ann Intern Med. 1989;110:352–6.

15. Baron TH, Truss CD, Elson CO. Low-dose oral methotrexate in refractory inflammatory bowel disease. Dig Dis Sci. 1993;38:1851–6.

16. Oren R, Arber N, Odes S, Moshkowitz M, Keter D, Pomeranz I, Ron Y, Reisfeld I, Broide E, Lavy A, Fich A, Eliakim R, Patz J, Bardan E, Villa Y, Gilat T. Methotrexate in chronic active ulcerative colitis: a double-blind, randomized, Israeli multicenter trial. Gastroenterology. 1996;110:1416–21.

17. Paoluzi OA, Pica R, Marcheggiano A, Crispino P, Iacopini F, Iannoni C, Rivera M, Paoluzi P. Azathioprine or methotrexate in the treatment of patients with steroid- ependent or steroid-resistant ulcerative colitis: results of an open-label study on efficacy and tolerability in inducing and maintaining remission. Alliment Pharmacol Ther. 2002;16:1751–9.

18. Neurath MF, Wanitschke R, Peters M, Krummenauer F, Meyer Zum Buschenfelde KH, Schlaak JF. Randomized trial of mycophenolate mofetil versus azathioprine for treatment of chronic active crohn's disease. Gut. 1999;44:625–8.

19. Orth T, Peters M, Schlaak JF, Krummenauer F, Wanitschke R, Mayet WJ, Galle PR, Neurath MF. Mycophenolate mofetil versus azathioprine in patients with chronic active ulcerative colitis: a 12-month pilot study. Am J Gastroenterol. 2000;95:1201–7.

20. Palaniappan S, Ford AC, Greer D, Everett SM, et al. Mycophenolate mofetil therapy for refractory inflammatory bowel disease. Inflamm Bowel Dis. 2007;13:1488–92.

21. Baumgart DC, Pintoffl JP, Strum A, Wiedenmann B, Dignass AU. Tacrolimus is safe and effective in patients with severe steroid-refractory or steroid-dependent inflammatory bowel disease – a long-term follow up. Am J Gastroenterol. 2006;101:1048–56.

22. Ogata H, Matsui T, Nakamura M, Lida M, Takazoe M, Suzuki Y, Hibi T. A randomised dose finding study of oral tacrolimus (FK506) therapy in refractory ulcerative colitis. Gut. 2006;55:1255–62.

23. Chiorean MV. Oral versus intravenous steroids to define refractory ulcerative colitis. Inflamm Bowel Dis. 2011;17(12):2503–4.

24. Truelove SC, Jewell DP. Intensive intravenous regimen for severe attacks of ulcerative colitis. Lancet. 1974;1:1067–70.

25. Lichtiger S, Present DH. Preliminary report: cyclosporine in treatment of severe active ulcerative colitis. Lancet. 1990;335:16–9.

26. Lichtiger S, Present DH, Kornbluth A, Gelernt I, Bauer J, Galler G, Michelassi F, Hanauer S. Cyclosporine in severe ulcerative colitis refractory to steroid therapy. N Engl J Med. 1994;330:1841–5.

27. Van Assche G, D'Haens G, Noman M, Vermeire S, Hiele M, Asnong K, Arts J, D'Hoore A, Penninckx F, Rutgeerts P. Randomized, double-blind comparison of 4 mg/kg versus 2 mg/kg intravenous cyclosporine in severe ulcerative colitis. Gastroenterology. 2003;125:1025–31.

28. Rutgeerts P, Sandborn WJ, Feagan BG, Reinisch W, Olson A, Johanns J, Travers S, Rachmilewitz D, Hanauer SB, Lichtenstein GR, de Villiers WJS, Present D, Sands BE, Colombel JF. Infliximab for induction and maintenance therapy for ulcerative colitis. N Engl J Med. 2005;353:2462–76.

29. Jarnerot G, Hertervig E, Friis-Liby I, Blomquist L, Karlen P, Granno C, Vilien M, Strom M, Danielsson A, Verbaan H, Hellstrom PM, Magnuson A, Curman B. Infliximab as rescue therapy in severe to moderately severe ulcerative colitis: a randomized, placebo-controlled study. Gastroenterology. 2005;128:1805–11.

30. Laharie D, Bourreille A, Branche J, Allez M, et al. Cyclosporin versus infliximab in severe acute ulcerative colitis refractory to intravenous steroids: a randomized trial. Presentation given on 10 May 2010 at Digestive Disease Week, Chicago (2010).

31. Sandborn WJ, Rutgeerts P, Feagan BG, Reinisch W, Olson A, Johanns J, Lu J, Horgan K, Rachmilewitz D, Hanauer SB, Lichtenstein GR, De Villiers WJS, Present D, Sands BE, Colombel JF. Colectomy rate comparison after treatment of ulcerative colitis with placebo or infliximab. Gastroenterology. 2009;137:1250–60.

# Medical Therapy in the Preoperative and Postoperative Patient

Caroline Kerner

**Keywords**

Medical therapy • Preoperative • Postoperative • Ulcerative colitis • Immunosuppression medication • Risk of colectomy • Ileostomy • Aminosalicylates • Glucocorticoids • Azathioprine and 6-mercaptopurine • Biologic agents • Cyclosporine • Venous thromboembolism (VTE) prophylaxis • Pain management

## Introduction

Medical therapy in ulcerative colitis (UC) often includes the use of immunosuppressant medications including prednisone, thiopurine analogues, biologic medications or cyclosporine. While patients with UC are being treated with medical therapy, the need for surgery may arise. The surgery may be related to a complication of the UC, or may be a non-intestinal surgery that is unrelated to the UC diagnosis. This chapter will cover medical management in patients with ulcerative colitis (UC) in the preoperative and postoperative settings.

The 10-year cumulative risk of colectomy in patients with UC is 8.7 %, with a 20 % risk in patients with extensive ulcerative colitis [1]. Indications for surgery in UC include refractory disease, cancer or dysplasia, or emergencies including perforation, massive hemorrhage or megacolon. The surgical options in these patients include subtotal or total colectomy with ileostomy in emergency situations, versus total proctocolectomy with ileal pouch-anal anastomosis (IPAA) as a one, two or three-stage procedure.

Early complications of UC-related surgeries can include anastomotic leak, wound dehiscence, pelvic sepsis, intra-abdominal abscess, small bowel obstruction, prolonged ileus and sepsis. Late complications can include fistulae (peri-

anal, enterocutaneous), anastomotic stricture and pouch dysfunction. Risk factors for surgical morbidity for any surgery include diabetes, obesity, cigarette smoking, malnutrition, preoperative disease severity and prolonged surgery. There is some evidence that surgical technique and expertise also influence the risk of postoperative morbidity and mortality. Laparoscopic surgery in inflammatory bowel disease (IBD) has been shown to demonstrate no increased complication rates compared with open surgery, as well as a decrease in postoperative length of stay [2]. In addition, postoperative mortality following colectomy for UC is lower in hospitals which perform the highest volume of these operations [3].

There is a paucity of data regarding the frequency of and complications related to non-intestinal surgeries among patients with UC and those with IBD in general. Furthermore, there are no consensus statements from either gastroenterological or rheumatologic societies regarding the perioperative management of immunosuppressives in either setting. In this chapter we will present the data available to help guide the decisions regarding medical therapy in the preoperative and postoperative patient. In addition, we will discuss perioperative pain management and venous thromboembolism prophylaxis in the patient with UC.

## Aminosalicylates

5-Aminosalicylic acid (5-ASA) medication is the first-line therapy for UC. There are at least 46 case reports in the literature of renal disease—mainly interstitial nephritis—associated with the use of 5-ASA medications. Combined

C. Kerner, M.D., M.S.C.E. (✉)
Division of Gastroenterology, Department of Medicine,
Perelman School of Medicine of the University of Pennsylvania,
Pennsylvania Hospital, 230 West Washington Square, 4th Floor,
Philadelphia, PA 19106, USA
e-mail: caroline.kerner@uphs.upenn.edu

G.R. Lichtenstein (ed.), *Medical Therapy of Ulcerative Colitis*,
DOI 10.1007/978-1-4939-1677-1_29, © Springer Science+Business Media New York 2014

data from the 46 case reports showed that renal injury may occur at widely various time points during 5-ASA therapy, from 1 month to 7 years of therapy, with 43 % having nephrotoxicity within 1 year of initiation of therapy [4]. These medications have a half-life of 6–10 h. There are no studies examining the perioperative risk of 5-ASA medications.

It is reasonable to discontinue 5-ASA medications 2 days before surgery and to resume the medications as soon as the patient is clinically stable post-operatively, particularly in patients who are at increased risk for acute kidney injury in the perioperative setting. Risk factors for acute kidney injury in the perioperative setting include age >65, preoperative kidney disease, diabetes, peripheral vascular disease, congestive heart failure, chronic obstructive pulmonary disease and obesity. Patients who undergo total proctocolectomy for ulcerative colitis will not need to resume 5-ASA medications postoperatively.

## Glucocorticoids

Glucocorticoids are commonly used in UC for induction of remission and treatment of flares. However, long-term use is not recommended because of the risks of infection, osteoporosis, glucose intolerance and glaucoma, among others. Indications for colectomy in patients with UC include steroid-dependent or steroid-refractory disease, and thus patients undergoing surgery may have been exposed to either long-term corticosteroid use, or high-dose short-term corticosteroid use. The other clinical scenario that may be encountered is a UC patient who is steroid-dependent who requires a surgery for a condition unrelated to the IBD.

A main concern of perioperative corticosteroid use is the risk of post-infectious complications including infection and poor wound healing. In animal studies, glucocorticoids have been demonstrated to decrease TGF-beta and IGF-1 levels in wound fluid and hydroxyproline content in tissue, which can result in impaired wound healing [5]. The TREAT (The Crohn's Therapy, Resource, Evaluation, and Assessment Tool) registry data has demonstrated an association between corticosteroid use and increased risk for infection (HR 1.57, 95 % CI 1.17–2.10) [6]. In both pediatric and adult patients undergoing colectomy for UC, steroids have been associated with an increased risk of postoperative complications including infection [7–10]. The association between preoperative corticosteroid use and postoperative infection was also found in a retrospective study of 159 patients with IBD undergoing elective bowel surgery [11]. Thus, in the case of elective surgery, corticosteroids should be tapered to the lowest dose possible prior to surgery and should be tapered completely if possible.

The physiologic stress of surgery activates the hypothalamic-pituitary-adrenal (HPA) axis, resulting in increased corticotrophin (ACTH) and cortisol secretion. Patients with UC who are treated with corticosteroids may have a suppressed HPA axis. They are therefore at risk of adrenal insufficiency and shock if they do not produce adequate ACTH and cortisol levels during the intraoperative and postoperative period [12]. There is, however, conflicting evidence about whether perioperative supplementary corticosteroids are needed. A recent systematic review of the literature determined that the evidence is not sufficient to either support or refute the need for perioperative supplementary corticosteroids in patients maintained on corticosteroid therapy [13].

As a result of the inconclusive literature and the theoretical risk of potentially life-threatening adrenal insufficiency and shock in the postoperative setting amongst patients maintained on chronic glucocorticoids, most experts generally recommend considering glucocorticoid supplementation. The decision about whether additional glucocorticoids are needed depends on the preoperative glucocorticoid dose and duration of therapy, whether there is a known preoperative diagnosis of adrenal insufficiency, as well as the degree of physiologic stress expected from the surgery [12]. Patients with UC and ongoing corticosteroid use must also be monitored carefully in the perioperative setting for hyperglycemia.

## Azathioprine and 6-Mercaptopurine

Azathioprine is a pro-drug of 6-mercaptopurine, which is converted by hypoxanthine-guanine-phosphoribosyltransferase to the active metabolite 6-thioguanine (6-TG) nucleotides. The 6-TG nucleotides have both cytotoxic and immunosuppressive effects via inhibition of RNA and DNA synthesis, and T and B cell proliferation [14]. These effects are beneficial in reducing disease activity in IBD, but also may in theory decrease healing in the setting of surgery. However, a recent experimental study in rats demonstrated no effect of azathioprine on the strength of intestinal anastomoses [15].

The evidence does not suggest an increased risk of postoperative complications amongst patients with UC undergoing IPAA. In a retrospective study of patients with UC who underwent proctocolectomy with IPAA at the University of California at San Francisco between 1997 and 1999, azathioprine and 6-mercaptopurine were not associated with an increased risk of complications at 30 days or at 6 months [9]. Similarly, a retrospective study at the Cleveland Clinic in Florida demonstrated no increased risk of postoperative complications among patients with UC undergoing total proctocolectomy with IPAA [16].

Studies including patients with Crohn's disease similarly do not demonstrate increased risk for postoperative complications after bowel surgery. Aberra et al. [11] performed a retrospective cohort study of 159 patients with IBD who underwent elective bowel surgery, of which 52 patients were receiving azathioprine or 6-mercaptopurine either alone or with corticosteroids. The adjusted odds ratios for any infectious complication and major infectious complications were 1.68 (05 % CI 0.65–4.27), and 1.20 (95 % CI 0.37–3.94). A systematic review in 2006 similarly concluded that preoperative immunomodulator use was not associated with an increased rate of postoperative complications amongst patients with IBD undergoing abdominal surgery [17].

There is a paucity of data examining the perioperative risks of azathioprine and 6-mercaptopurine in other disease and in surgeries unrelated to IBD. These medications have a short half-life, but are predominantly renally cleared and thus could accumulate in the setting of acute kidney injury in the perioperative setting. Furthermore, thiopurines can cause nausea and vomiting when taken on an empty stomach. Thus, it is reasonable to hold thiopurines 2 days before surgery and to resume the medication 3 days after surgery, once the patient is clinically stable and has resumed oral intake. In the setting of total proctocolectomy for ulcerative colitis, azathioprine and 6-mercaptopurine are not resumed postoperatively.

## Biologic Agents

The biologic agents that are FDA-approved for the treatment of UC include infliximab and adalimumab. These drugs are tumor necrosis factor α inhibitors (anti-TNF). Adverse effects reported in association with the use of these medications include lymphoma, infection (including reactivation of tuberculosis or Hepatitis B, opportunistic infections, pneumonia), lymphoma, worsening of congestive heart failure, demyelinating disease, lupus-like syndrome, induction of auto-antibodies and hypersensitivity reactions [18].

There are a multitude of studies examining the risk of postoperative complications associated with perioperative anti-TNF use among patients with UC. These include a small single-center study [19] including 29 infliximab-exposed and 52 non-infliximab controls with UC undergoing IPAA in which multivariable regression models revealed that infliximab was not associated with postoperative complications (OR 0.78, $p=0.67$). The largest and only population-based study to date included 199 patients with UC in the Danish National Health Registry who underwent colectomy, and found no difference in postoperative complications (including fever, infection, anastomotic leak, death) among patients exposed to biologics [20]. Another recent large single-center retrospective case-control study of 473 abdominal surgeries among IBD patients (both UC and Crohn's disease) in which 195 were exposed to biologics found no difference in postoperative complications between the biologic-exposed versus unexposed patients [21]. A subgroup analysis of patients undergoing subtotal colectomy similarly showed no increased rates of postoperative complications among the patients exposed to biologics. Finally, a 2012 meta-analysis of 13 studies including 2,933 patients undergoing abdominal surgery for UC concluded that preoperative infliximab does not increase the risk of early postoperative total complications (OR 1.09, 95 % CI 0.87–1.37), infectious complications (OR 1.10, 95 % CI 0.51–2.38) or non-infectious complications (OR 1.10, 95 % CI 0.76–1.59) [22].

In summary, the evidence is more supportive of a lack of increased risk of postoperative complications among UC patients exposed to infliximab. At the same time, it must be noted that no studies have examined the risk of IBD flare on postoperative outcomes in the setting of discontinuing medications preoperatively. In the case of colectomy for ulcerative colitis, surgery should not be delayed because of recent anti-TNF use. Since colectomy is curative in the case of UC, anti-TNF medications do not need to be resumed postoperatively.

In the case of non-intestinal surgery, there is less data to guide the clinical decision and it must be made on a case-by-case basis in conjunction with the surgeon. If the patient is at low risk for disease flare with discontinuation of anti-TNF therapy and the surgical procedure is considered high risk in terms of infectious complications, the dose could be held for one cycle before the surgery and resumed as soon as the patient is clinically stable post-operatively. However, the risk of postoperative complications must be weighed against the risk of disease flare.

## Cyclosporine

Cyclosporine is a calcineurin inhibitor given intravenously as a second-line therapy in severe steroid-refractory UC. Drug levels must be monitored closely, and patients who respond are then switched to oral cyclosporine while initiating a steroid-sparing therapy such as azathioprine or 6-mercaptopurine.

Adverse events associated with the use of cyclosporine include nephrotoxicity, seizures, anaphylaxis, paresthesias, hypomagnesaemia, hyperkalemia, hypertension, hypertrichosis, headache and infection [23]. In a case series of 86 patients treated with cyclosporine for severe UC, 3 (3.5 %) died from opportunistic infection including pneumocystic jirovecii pneumonia and aspergillus fumigatus pneumonia [24]. Thus, we recommend considering prophylaxis with trimethoprim-sulfamethoxazole in these patients.

Based on case series data, preoperative cyclosporine use has not resulted in higher than expected postoperative complication rates. In 1995, Fleshner et al. [25] found that in 14 patients requiring urgent colectomy and ileostomy for UC after failing cyclosporine, there were no postoperative deaths. The 57 % complication rate included three cases of ileus and two of deep venous thrombosis. There was one wound infection, and one partial dehiscence of a rectal stump. A later series of 25 patients who underwent procto-colectomy after failing cyclosporine found no postoperative deaths, and a 36 % rate of early complications. However, all patients were able to retain their pouch. The largest series published to date is a British study of 80 patients with severe ulcerative colitis, of which 29 % received cyclosporine, found that the patients with major postoperative complications had a significantly longer duration of time between admission and medical therapy (mean 8 days versus 5 days, $p = 0.036$) [26]. However, treatment with cyclosporine was not associated with an increased risk of postoperative complications.

One study compared the postoperative risk of preoperative cyclosporine and steroids compared to preoperative steroids alone in patients undergoing emergency colectomy for severe UC and found no increased risk of perioperative complications in the cyclosporine group (24 % steroids alone versus 15.8 % steroids and cyclosporine) [27].

Based on the available data, we do not recommend delaying colectomy in patients exposed to cyclosporine preoperatively. In patients receiving cyclosporine who require non-IBD-related surgery, we suggest delaying elective surgery if possible until the cyclosporine is discontinued and the patient is tolerating steroid-sparing therapy. However, if surgery is urgently needed in a patient taking cyclosporine, the available data do not support the need to discontinue the drug prior to surgery.

## Venous Thromboembolism (VTE) Prophylaxis

Patients with inflammatory bowel disease have an increased risk of venous thromboembolism (VTE) compared with controls (HR 3.4, 95 % CI 2.7-4.3), and this risk is increased during flare states (HR 8.4, 95 % CI 5.5–12.8) [28]. A retrospective analysis using a national surgical database found that VTE was more common among patients with IBD compared to controls (OR 2.03, 95 % CI 1.52–2.70), and that nonintestinal surgical cases had a higher rate of DVT or PE (OR 4.45, CI 1.72–11.49) compared with intestinal surgeries [29].

Several studies have examined risk factors for VTE in patients with IBD who are undergoing surgery. Laparoscopic surgery has been associated with a decreased risk for venous thromboembolism compared with open surgery [30, 31]. However, causality has not been established, as patients selected for laparoscopic surgery may otherwise be at lower risk for venous thromboembolism. A study [32] of 10,431

colorectal surgeries amongst patients with IBD in the American College of Surgeons National Surgical Quality Improvement 2004–2010 database found that venous thromboembolic events occurred in 1.4 % of patients with CD and 3.3 % of patients with UC. Risk factors for postoperative venous thromboembolic events included bleeding disorder, steroid use, anesthesia time, emergency surgery, hematocrit <37 %, malnutrition and functional status. Some of these risk factors are modifiable and could be optimized in patients who are planning to undergo surgery.

Based on the available data, prophylaxis for VTE is recommended in all hospitalized patients with UC, including those undergoing surgery [33–35]. The options include low molecular weight heparin at a dose of 5,000 international units every 8 h or enoxaparin 40 mg every 24 h, though patients with weights less than 50 kg may need dose reduction. Flare of disease with hematochezia is not a contraindication to VTE prophylaxis with anticoagulation. However, prospective studies are needed to demonstrate the efficacy of VTE prophylaxis among patients with UC.

## Pain Management

We suggest avoiding non-steroidal anti-inflammatory medications (NSAIDs) because of the potential association with disease flare in UC. Narcotic pain medications are associated with increased risk of mortality and serious infection in patients with IBD based on TREAT registry data [6]. Narcotics are also thought to increase the risk for toxic megacolon in patients with UC flares. A recent retrospective review found no increased risk of colectomy in patients exposed to narcotics, but prospective studies are needed to confirm this finding [36]. Acetaminophen and tramadol may be reasonable options to treat pain in this patient population. However, narcotics may be needed, particularly to treat postoperative pain. In that case, the dose and frequency should be minimized, and the patient should be monitored closely for prevention or early detection of toxic megacolon and infection.

Tables 29.1 and 29.2 show the stress-dose corticosteroid dosing in the perioperative setting and perioperative medication management, respectively.

## Conclusion

This chapter provides suggestions about management of medical therapy in the preoperative and postoperative patient with ulcerative colitis. However, there is limited published literature available regarding the perioperative use of these medications. As a result, no formal guidelines have been

**Table 29.1** Stress-dose corticosteroid dosing in the perioperative setting

| | Minor surgical stress (hernia repair) | Moderate surgical stress (cholecystectomy, colectomy) | Major surgical stress (cardiac surgery, hepatobiliary surgery) |
|---|---|---|---|
| No HPA axis suppression:<br>• <5 mg prednisone or equivalent/day, any duration<br>• <3 weeks of glucocorticoid use, any dose | Continue usual daily glucocorticoid dose | Continue usual daily glucocorticoid dose | Continue usual daily glucocorticoid dose |
| HPA axis suppression<br>• >20 mg prednisone or equivalent for ≥3 weeks<br>• Cushingoid<br>• Positive ACTH stimulation test | Continue usual daily glucocorticoid dose | Hydrocortisone 50 mg IV (induction),then 25 mg IV every 8 h for 24–48 h, then resume normal dose | Hydrocortisone 100 mg IV (induction), then 50 mg IV every 8 h for 48–72 h, then resume normal dose |
| Uncertain HPA axis suppression<br>• 5–20 mg prednisone or equipvalent for ≥3 weeks<br>• ≥5 mg of prednisone or equivalent for ≥3 weeks in the last year | Continue usual daily glucocorticoid dose | Perform ACTH stimulation test<br>• If suppressed, give hydrocortisone 50 mg IV (induction), then 25 mg IV every 8 h for 24–48 h, then resume normal dose<br>• Otherwise continue usual daily glucocorticoid dose | Perform ACTH stimulation test<br>• If suppressed, give hydrocortisone 100 mg IV (induction), then 50 mg IV every 8 h for 48–72 h, then resume normal dose<br>• Otherwise continue usual daily glucocorticoid dose |

HPA=hypothalamus-pituitary-adrenal, IV=intravenous, induction=prior to induction of anesthesia, ACTH=adrenocorticotropic hormone. Adapted from Schiff RL et al., *Med Clin North Am* [12]

**Table 29.2** Perioperative medication management in ulcerative colitis

| Drug | Colectomy/IPAA (level of evidence) | Other surgery (level of evidence) |
|---|---|---|
| 5-Aminosalicylates | Discontinue 2 days before surgery; do not resume postoperatively (C) | Hold 2 days before surgery; resume 3 days postoperatively or when creatinine is stable (C) |
| Glucocorticoids | Minimize dose preoperatively; administer stress-dose steroids if indicated (see Table 29.2); taper postoperatively (B) | Minimize dose preoperatively; administer stress-dose steroids if indicated (B) |
| Azathioprine or 6-MP | No need to postpone surgery; hold 2 days prior to elective surgery if possible; do not resume postoperatively (unless indicated for a non-IBD diagnosis) (B,C) | No need to postpone surgery; hold 2 days prior to elective surgery if possible; resume 3 days after surgery when eating and when creatinine is stable (B,C) |
| Biologics | No need to postpone surgery; continue prior to colectomy if needed; do not resume postoperatively (unless indicated for a non-IBD diagnosis) (B) | Discuss with surgeon; if high risk for disease flare with discontinuation of biologic, continue biologic and monitor closely postoperatively (B) |
| Cyclosporine | No need to postpone surgery; do not resume postoperatively; watch for opportunistic infections (B,C) | Delay elective surgery until cyclosporine therapy completed if possible; if surgery is urgent, continue cyclosporine, watch for opportunistic infections and consider trimethoprim-sulfamethoxazole prophylaxis (B,C) |

*IPAA* ileal pouch-anal anastomosis, *6-MP* 6-mercaptopurine, *Pre* preoperatively, *Post* postoperatively

published by the major gastroenterological or rheumatologic societies. Prospective data from high-quality studies are needed in order to inform the decision regarding the perioperative use of immunosuppressant medications. In the meantime, the decision regarding the use of 5-ASA and immunosuppressant therapy in the perioperative setting must be individualized for each patient and should involve a discussion between the gastroenterologist and the surgeon.

# References

1. Hoie O, Wolters FL, Riis L, et al. Low colectomy rates in ulcerative colitis in an unselected European cohort followed for 10 years. Gastroenterology. 2007;132:507–15.
2. Ananthakrishnan AN, McGinley EL, Saeian K, Binion DG. Laparoscopic resection for inflammatory bowel disease: outcomes from a nationwide sample. J Gastrointest Surg. 2010;14: 58–65.

3. Kaplan GG, McCarthy EP, Ayanian JZ, Korzenik J, Hodin R, Sands BE. Impact of hospital volume on postoperative morbidity and mortality following a colectomy for ulcerative colitis. Gastroenterology. 2008;134:680–7.

4. Gisbert JP, Gonzalez-Lama Y, Mate J. 5-Aminosalicylates and renal function in inflammatory bowel disease: a systematic review. Inflamm Bowel Dis. 2007;13:629–38.

5. Wicke C, Halliday B, Allen D, et al. Effects of steroids and retinoids on wound healing. Arch Surg. 2000;135:1265–70.

6. Lichtenstein GR, Feagan BG, Cohen RD, et al. Serious infection and mortality in patients with Crohn's disease: more than 5 years of follow-up in the TREAT registry. Am J Gastroenterol. 2012; 107:1409–22.

7. Miki C, Ohmori Y, Yoshiyama S, et al. Factors predicting postoperative infectious complications and early induction of inflammatory mediators in ulcerative colitis patients. World J Surg. 2007;31:522–9. discussion 30–1.

8. Markel TA, Lou DC, Pfefferkorn M, et al. Steroids and poor nutrition are associated with infectious wound complications in children undergoing first stage procedures for ulcerative colitis. Surgery. 2008;144:540–5. discussion 5–7.

9. Mahadevan U, Loftus Jr EV, Tremaine WJ, et al. Azathioprine or 6-mercaptopurine before colectomy for ulcerative colitis is not associated with increased postoperative complications. Inflamm Bowel Dis. 2002;8:311–6.

10. Subramanian V, Saxena S, Kang JY, Pollok RC. Preoperative steroid use and risk of postoperative complications in patients with inflammatory bowel disease undergoing abdominal surgery. Am J Gastroenterol. 2008;103:2373–81.

11. Aberra FN, Lewis JD, Hass D, Rombeau JL, Osborne B, Lichtenstein GR. Corticosteroids and immunomodulators: postoperative infectious complication risk in inflammatory bowel disease patients. Gastroenterology. 2003;125:320–7.

12. Schiff RL, Welsh GA. Perioperative evaluation and management of the patient with endocrine dysfunction. Med Clin North Am. 2003;87:175–92.

13. Yong SL, Coulthard P, Wrzosek A. Supplemental perioperative steroids for surgical patients with adrenal insufficiency. Cochrane Database Syst Rev. 2012;12, CD005367.

14. Sandborn WJ. A review of immune modifier therapy for inflammatory bowel disease: azathioprine, 6-mercaptopurine, cyclosporine, and methotrexate. Am J Gastroenterol. 1996;91:423–33.

15. Stolzenburg T, Ljungmann K, Christensen H. The effect of azathioprine on anastomotic healing: an experimental study in rats. Dis Colon Rectum. 2007;50:2203–8.

16. Zmora O, Khaikin M, Pishori T, et al. Should ileoanal pouch surgery be staged for patients with mucosal ulcerative colitis on immunosuppressives? Int J Colorectal Dis. 2007;22:289–92.

17. Subramanian V, Pollok RC, Kang JY, Kumar D. Systematic review of postoperative complications in patients with inflammatory bowel disease treated with immunomodulators. Br J Surg. 2006;93:793–9.

18. Scheinfeld N. A comprehensive review and evaluation of the side effects of the tumor necrosis factor alpha blockers etanercept, infliximab and adalimumab. J Dermatolog Treat. 2004;15:280–94.

19. Gainsbury ML, Chu DI, Howard LA, et al. Preoperative infliximab is not associated with an increased risk of short-term postoperative complications after restorative proctocolectomy and ileal pouch-anal anastomosis. J Gastrointest Surg. 2011;15:397–403.

20. Norgard BM, Nielsen J, Qvist N, Gradel KO, de Muckadell OB, Kjeldsen J. Pre-operative use of anti-TNF-alpha agents and the risk of post-operative complications in patients with ulcerative colitis—a nationwide cohort study. Aliment Pharmacol Ther. 2012;35: 1301–9.

21. Waterman M, Xu W, Dinani A, et al. Preoperative biological therapy and short-term outcomes of abdominal surgery in patients with inflammatory bowel disease. Gut. 2013;62:387–94.

22. Yang Z, Wu Q, Wang F, Wu K, Fan D. Meta-analysis: effect of preoperative infliximab use on early postoperative complications in patients with ulcerative colitis undergoing abdominal surgery. Aliment Pharmacol Ther. 2012;36:922–8.

23. Sternthal MB, Murphy SJ, George J, Kornbluth A, Lichtiger S, Present DH. Adverse events associated with the use of cyclosporine in patients with inflammatory bowel disease. Am J Gastroenterol. 2008;103:937–43.

24. Arts J, D'Haens G, Zeegers M, et al. Long-term outcome of treatment with intravenous cyclosporin in patients with severe ulcerative colitis. Inflamm Bowel Dis. 2004;10:73–8.

25. Fleshner PR, Michelassi F, Rubin M, Hanauer SB, Plevy SE, Targan SR. Morbidity of subtotal colectomy in patients with severe ulcerative colitis unresponsive to cyclosporin. Dis Colon Rectum. 1995;38:1241–5.

26. Randall J, Singh B, Warren BF, Travis SP, Mortensen NJ, George BD. Delayed surgery for acute severe colitis is associated with increased risk of postoperative complications. Br J Surg. 2010; 97:404–9.

27. Hyde GM, Jewell DP, Kettlewell MG, Mortensen NJ. Cyclosporin for severe ulcerative colitis does not increase the rate of perioperative complications. Dis Colon Rectum. 2001;44:1436–40.

28. Grainge MJ, West J, Card TR. Venous thromboembolism during active disease and remission in inflammatory bowel disease: a cohort study. Lancet. 2010;375:657–63.

29. Merrill A, Millham F. Increased risk of postoperative deep vein thrombosis and pulmonary embolism in patients with inflammatory bowel disease: a study of National Surgical Quality Improvement Program patients. Arch Surg. 2012;147:120–4.

30. Shapiro R, Vogel JD, Kiran RP. Risk of postoperative venous thromboembolism after laparoscopic and open colorectal surgery: an additional benefit of the minimally invasive approach? Dis Colon Rectum. 2011;54:1496–502.

31. Nguyen NT, Hinojosa MW, Fayad C, et al. Laparoscopic surgery is associated with a lower incidence of venous thromboembolism compared with open surgery. Ann Surg. 2007;246:1021–7.

32. Wallaert JB, De Martino RR, Marsicovetere PS, et al. Venous thromboembolism after surgery for inflammatory bowel disease: are there modifiable risk factors? Data from ACS NSQIP. Dis Colon Rectum. 2012;55:1138–44.

33. Murthy SK, Nguyen GC. Venous thromboembolism in inflammatory bowel disease: an epidemiological review. Am J Gastroenterol. 2011;106:713–8.

34. Nguyen GC, Sam J. Rising prevalence of venous thromboembolism and its impact on mortality among hospitalized inflammatory bowel disease patients. Am J Gastroenterol. 2008;103:2272–80.

35. Gould MK, Garcia DA, Wren SM, et al. Prevention of VTE in non-orthopedic surgical patients: antithrombotic therapy and prevention of thrombosis, 9th ed: American College of Chest Physicians Evidence-Based Clinical Practice Guidelines. Chest. 2012;141: e227S–77.

36. Lian L, Fazio VW, Hammel J, Shen B. Impact of narcotic use on the requirement for colectomy in inpatients with ulcerative colitis. Dis Colon Rectum. 2010;53:1295–300.

# Medication Adherence in Ulcerative Colitis

Sunanda V. Kane

**Keywords**

Medication adherence • Ulcerative colitis • Maintenance medications • Non-adherence in management of ulcerative colitis • Optimize adherence

## Introduction

While literature on other chronic diseases such as coronary artery disease, congestive heart failure, and diabetes has tried to address the issue of medication non-adherence and its effect on disease outcomes, the impact of medication adherence on specific inflammatory bowel disease (IBD) outcomes has just recently become of interest. The published literature of the efficacy of IBD maintenance medications underestimates the extent of the problem, as patients often conceal their failure to take medications as directed once outside of controlled clinical trial environments. The remainder of this chapter will discuss the state of knowledge regarding the issues surrounding non-adherence in the management of ulcerative colitis (UC).

## Current Data on Non-adherence

### Non-adherence to Medications

Multiple studies have demonstrated the efficacy of aminosalicylates as first line therapy to induce and maintain remission in UC [1–5]. These well-designed multi-center trials have used pill count and patient inquiry to assess adherence, with rates ranging from 70 to >95 %. Based upon

community-based follow-up studies in other chronic illnesses, the percentage of long-term adherence tends to be much lower, about 40–50 % [6]. This wide variance across studies can be explained by (1) a study's definition of adherence, (2) the degree to which the investigators were proactive in adherence measures, and (3) patient population. Particularly after remission has been established, patients may not believe (or understand) the importance of continuing on maintenance therapy. Many patients openly admit they do not take their medications as prescribed; medication-taking probably makes patients more uncomfortably aware of their chronic illness status, they have a fear of long-term side effects from medications, and they question the need for medication in the setting of quiescent disease.

Patient adherence is defined as the extent to which an individual's behavior coincides with medical or health advice [7]. The term "adherence" replaces "compliance", the latter a term that conveys a paternalistic concept of medical care and patient obedience to the physician's authority (Table 30.1). Despite research attempting to profile non-adherent patients, there are no characteristics consistently linked to non-adherence. This is not surprising, given that patient non-adherence varies between and within individuals as well as across time, recommended behaviors, and diseases.

The issue of adherence was first introduced several decades ago, in several published studies addressing long-term sulfasalazine use in UC. Das and colleagues defined its metabolism in patients with ulcerative colitis, during both the active and quiescent phases of the disease. They subsequently studied the relationship between clinical status and serum concentrations of sulfasalazine and its metabolites [8]. Levels of total sulphapyridine (SP) were demonstrated to be different in slow versus rapid acetylators, and that a serum

S.V. Kane, M.D., M.S.P.H. (✉)
Division of Gastroenterology and Hepatology,
Department of Medicine, Mayo Clinic,
200 First Street SW, Rochester, MN 55905, USA
e-mail: kane.sunanda@mayo.edu

G.R. Lichtenstein (ed.), *Medical Therapy of Ulcerative Colitis*,
DOI 10.1007/978-1-4939-1677-1_30, © Springer Science+Business Media New York 2014

**Table 30.1** Definitions of the key terms commonly used to describe the concept of non-adherence [8]

*Compliance* is defined as "the extent to which the patient's behavior matches the prescriber's recommendations".

*Adherence* is defined as "the extent to which the patient's behavior matches agreed recommendations from the prescriber".

*Concordance* is a relatively new concept, predominantly applied outside the US, defined as a two-way relationship between patient and physician, where treatment decisions are discussed and the treatment of choice is the one most acceptable to both parties.

*Persistence* is defined as the continued adherence over time to the prescribed medication.

concentration of 20–50 μg/ml appeared to coincide with clinical improvement in the absence of side effects. One year follow up on 64 outpatients revealed that of the 43 patients with quiescent disease, 32 had total SP levels above 20 μg/ml remained in remission [9]. Ten of 21 with active disease had levels below 20 μg/ml and remained symptomatic. The correlation between "therapeutic" levels and disease activity suggested that adherence was associated with an improved outcome, and that following metabolite levels may be a method to monitor patient adherence.

In a second study, Van Hees et al. measured urine levels of acetylated sulfasalazine as a marker for adherence in 51 patients 1–6 months after hospital discharge and in 171 outpatients over several years [10]. The authors found that non-adherence, as defined by undetectable urine levels, in the months after hospital discharge approximated 40 %. In the cohort of outpatients followed on maintenance doses of sulfasalazine, 12 % had undetectable urine levels at 6-month follow up.

In a study by a group of Italian psychiatrists treating IBD patients, Nigro et al. examined the effect of psychiatric disorders on adherence with medications [11]. They found a correlation between duration of disease and adherence but an inverse relationship between disease severity and the presence of significant psychiatric disorders with regular medication consumption. Their recommendation was preventive liaison interventions for these patients to improve disease outcomes.

In an attempt to understand the possible effect of adherence on disease outcome, Riley and colleagues included adherence as a potential factor leading to disease relapse in patients with quiescent UC [12]. Medication adherence was determined by pill count and direct patient inquiry. After 48 weeks, there was no difference in adherence rates between the patients who relapsed versus those who remained in remission. However, the total adherence for both groups was >95 % throughout the study, making the interpretation of these findings difficult.

Farup et al., in their trial of mesalazine (European term for mesalamine) versus hydrocortisone foam enemas,

incorporated the issue of tolerability, ease and adherence into the data collection [13]. In this 4-week trial, patients were asked to mark on a 100 mm visual analog scale an assessment of their medication regimen with regard to ease of administration and practicality. Adherence, as measured by the return of unused bottles, was >80 % at 2 weeks in both groups, then dropped to 73 % for the foam patients but remained >90 % for the mesalazine group. The authors suggested that the better outcome in the mesalazine group was in part due to convenience and simplicity and thus better adherence to that treatment regimen.

Riley and colleagues, in another subsequent prospective study, studied 98 outpatients with IBD prescribed maintenance delayed-release mesalazine [14]. Adherence was studied by both direct inquiry and by analysis of urine samples for the presence of 5-aminosalicylic acid (ASA) and *N*-acetyl 5-ASA. Demographic variables, disease and treatment related factors, quality of life, psychiatric morbidity and aspects of the doctor patient relationship were all assessed as possible determinants of adherence. Self-reporting revealed non-adherence (taking less than 80 % of the prescribed dose) in 42 patients (43 %). Logistic regression revealed three times daily dosing (OR 3.1 (95 % CI 1.8–8.4)), full-time employment (OR 2.7 (1.8–8.9)) and depression (Hospital Anxiety and Depression rating scale >7) (OR 10.5 (1.8–79)) were the only independent predictors of non-adherence. Urinary drug measurements revealed 12 patients with no detectable 5-ASA or *N*-acetyl 5-ASA. Of interest, self-reporting correctly identified 66 % of patients judged to be non-adherent on the basis of urinary drug measurements but only 2 of the 12 patients with undetectable drug levels admitted to complete non-adherence.

In a published prevalence survey, Kane and colleagues found the overall adherence rate with a maintenance dose of Asacol to be only 40 % [15]. Adherence was measured by pharmacy refill data rather than patient inquiry or pill count. The median amount of medication dispensed per patient was 71 % (range 8–130 %) of the prescribed regimen over a 6-month period. Noncompliant patients were more likely to be male (67 % vs. 52 %, $p < 0.05$), single (68 % vs. 53 %, $p = 0.04$) and to have disease limited to the left side of the colon vs. pancolitis (83 % vs. 51 %, $p < 0.01$). Sixty-eight percent of patients who took >4 prescription medications were found to be noncompliant versus only 40 % of those patients taking fewer medications ($p = 0.05$). Age, occupation, a family history of IBD, length of remission or quality-of-life score was not associated with nonadherence. Logistic regression identified that a history of >4 prescriptions (OR 2.5 (1.4–5.7)) and male gender (OR 2.06 (1.17–4.88)) increased the risk of nonadherence. Two statistically significant variables that were protective against nonadherence were endoscopy within the past 24 months (OR 0.96 (0.93–0.99)) and being married (OR 0.46 (0.39–0.57)).

In a recent systematic review, Jackson et al. noted that the number of daily doses is not consistently related to non-adherence, and none of the significant relationships that have been observed relate to once daily dosing compared to twice daily [16]. Although there remains much discussion regarding the optimum dosage of 5-ASA, it would be important to keep in mind the patient's preferences and not assume that a once daily formulation is "better" than one taken twice a day. What does seem apparent that even for active disease no 5-ASA has to be dosed more than twice a day [17].

## Non-adherence with Non-medication Related Treatment and Therapies

Patient adherence rates with surveillance colonoscopy are not well documented. In the only study that directly addressed this issue, Woolrich et al. reported on 7 patients of their cohort of 121 that were found to have cancer [18]. In two of these patients, previous colonoscopy had found dysplasia in the setting of quiescent disease, and neither of these patients were adherent with recommendations for close follow up colonoscopy or colectomy. It was the conclusion of the authors that quiescent disease was a risk factor for non-adherence with physician recommendations.

## Adherence and Outcomes

What data do we have that would compel a patient to continue taking medication in the setting of well-being? A prospective 2-year follow up on a cohort of patients with quiescent UC was done to help answer this question [19]. Patients in remission were enrolled and then stratified by adherence based on the previous 6-month pharmacy refill data. At 6 months, 12 patients (12 %) had clinical recurrence of disease symptoms, all of whom were noncompliant with medication. At 12 months, 19 of 86 patients had recurrent disease, 13 (68 %) of whom were noncompliant. Multiple Cox proportional hazards model revealed that patients not compliant with medication had more than fivefold greater risk of recurrence than the compliant patients (hazard ratio 5.47, 95 % confidence interval 2.26–13.22, $p < 0.001$). As part of the study, non-adherent patients were asked why they were not taking their medications [20]. The majority stated that they simply forgot one of their doses. Fewer than 10 % of patients complained of side effects and cost.

There are now several studies that suggest that documented medication consumption is protective for colon cancer, which is an important concern for the long-term natural history of UC. Moody et al. studied 168 patients with UC diagnosed between 1972 and 1981 and correlated sulfasalazine non-adherence with risk of colorectal cancer [21]. A patient was classified as non-compliant if there was clear evidence in the medical record of medications not taken, or upon the advice of a physician medication was discontinued. Their crude colectomy rate was 23 % in 10 years with a 3 % rate in those patients on maintenance sulfasalazine, and 31 % in patients either non-compliant or off all medications. Since the authors found a colectomy rate and cancer incidence similar to previously published series, they concluded that medications were beneficial in reducing cancer risk. In a second retrospective case control study, Pinczowski found that a record of at least a 3-month history of therapy with sulfasalazine had a protective effect for colon cancer [22]. There was a 62 % reduction in risk with any history of therapy in the 102 patients studied. It is difficult to interpret this finding however, as documentation of dose and duration of therapy for each patient was imprecise. More recently, a published meta-analysis suggests that the risk reduction for dysplasia and colorectal cancer is significant [23].

Eaden and colleagues found in a case-control study that mesalamine at a dose of 1.2 g/day or greater reduced colorectal cancer risk by 91 % in patients with UC compared to no treatment [24]. There was also a protective effect of >2 visits to the physician per year, but the same was not found for the number of surveillance colonoscopies. More data on mesalamine comes from investigators at Mount Sinai Medical Center in New York who followed patients whose colon biopsies were indeterminant for dysplasia [25]. Those patients on 2 g or more of 5-ASA per day did not progress to definite dysplasia, suggesting that any chemoprotective effect occurs early in the cancer progression pathway. Rubin and colleagues studied the University of Chicago experience with all forms of 5-ASA in ulcerative colitis patients [26]. The use of at least 1.2 g daily of a 5-ASA carried a 76 % relative risk reduction for the development of colorectal cancer, when controlled for disease extent, duration and folic acid use. In contrast, IBD patients on 5-ASA agents followed in Canada did not appear to have the same protective effect [27].

There have also been recently published data on the effects of non-adherence on health care costs. Kane et al. demonstrated that those UC patients without an active prescription cost 30 % more in hospital and outpatient costs than patients who were taking medication [28]. In addition, those taking less than 80 % of medication were also associated with higher health costs. Yen et al. performed a cost effectiveness study and showed that over a year period adherence with 5-ASA was associated with a higher health care quality of life than those who were not [29].

## Methods to Optimize Adherence

Optimizing adherence is most effective when open lines of communication characterize the relationship between physician and patient (Table 30.2). Allowing the patient the time to voice his concerns and questions is the first step in effective

**Table 30.2** Methods to enhance patient compliance

- Communication regarding medication concerns
- Education about necessity of medications long term
- Simplification of patient regimens as much as possible
- Provision of patient autonomy and self-management

education. Open-ended questions during a patient visit can be time consuming, but setting an appropriate tone so as not to overestimate the patient's level of education is paramount in establishing a good relationship. One study from the psychology literature featuring IBD patients revealed that, when asked, their greatest concern was the uncertain nature of their disease [30]. In addition, patients expressed a significant concern about the effect of medications on their disease. In another more recent study, patients were asked what were the most important attributes to therapy [31]. While 76 of the 100 patients surveyed said that convenience was important, 95 of them stated that the most important attribute should be the ability to provide consistent relief from symptoms.

It has been suggested that physicians may overestimate patient comprehension in regard to instructions and education. Martin and colleagues showed that of IBD patients polled, 62 % of ulcerative colitis patients felt ill informed about their disease [32]. While 86 % of patients responding knew of the increased risk of cancer, only 44 % know that it was possible to screen for dysplasia and possible prevention of invasive cancer. Other literature also suggests that non-adherence is linked to patient non-comprehension [33]. Another study yet to be published in full form reported that in a GI outpatient clinic that 15 % of patients did not know how their medication worked, 22 % felt dissatisfied with their medications, primarily from unexpected side effects, and 12 % admitted they do not tell their physician all the medications that they take [34].

A new model of patient adherence has been proposed in which effective patient-physician dialog is central to promoting patient adherence [35]. This theoretical framework is in part supported by findings that higher patient physician discordance has been associated with unfavorable health outcomes as well as with decreased patient satisfaction, a variable that is related to poorer adherence. In a study of 153 patients, the non-adherence rate for IBD medications within 2 weeks of a clinic visit was 41 % [36]. Eighty-one percent of these patients were found to have "non-intentional" non-adherent behavior, i.e. forgetfulness or carelessness in taking medication. Intentional non-adherence was found to be associated with patients who were considered "non-distressed" by psychosocial measurements but showed high discordance with their physician in terms of disease activity. The clinical implications of these findings suggest that the therapeutic relationship can influence adherence just as much as individual clinical and psychosocial characteristics.

Closely linked to this is the concept of health literacy. Patients may not fully understand their condition or the purpose of their medication, so an element of patient education could be included in consultations [37]. There are a number of sources of information and support available throughout the wider healthcare system. In particular, it may be beneficial to direct patients to relevant patient groups, which can provide valuable information and support. A well-informed patient may be better equipped to make reasoned, logical decisions regarding their treatment. Additionally, patient education could help to reinforce the necessity of maintenance therapy. For example, patients should be reminded of the evidence that there is a far higher risk of relapse if they do not adhere to their medication. In addition, it may be beneficial to discuss the potential chemoprotective effects of 5-ASA.

Simplifying patient regimens can be an effective way to increase adherence. A pilot feasibility trial assessed short-term outcomes in patients on once daily mesalamine compared to a conventional (twice or three times daily) regimen for maintenance of ulcerative colitis [38]. Secondary aims included overall medication consumption rates and patient satisfaction. Twenty-two patients were randomized, and followed for 6 months. The number of clinical relapses after 6 months was similar in the once daily and conventional dosing groups. While there was no statistically significant difference in 6-month adherence rates between the two groups, there was a numerical advantage for overall consumption with a once daily regimen and patients in the once daily group were on the whole more satisfied with their regimen as compared to the conventional dosing patients. Since that time, two large trials have been published that have documented the efficacy of once daily therapy [39, 40].

Patient autonomy is also a means to enhance adherence with medications. Realizing the potential difficulties for long term adherence with sulfasalazine, Dickinson et al. studied continuous versus "on demand" sulfasalazine in 28 patients with quiescent ulcerative colitis [41]. Of the 18 patients in the "on demand" group, directed to take 3 g of sulfasalazine per day starting within 24 h of symptom recurrence, seven relapsed within the study period, four within the first 2 months of the trial. Three of the ten patients randomized to the continuous group relapsed. Adherence was measured by serum sulfapyridine levels every 4 months for 1 year or until relapse, and was reported as adequate for patients in either group. The authors concluded that because there was no difference in relapse rates between the two groups, and that by serologic testing sulfapyridine levels were therapeutic, that an "on demand" regimen may be as efficacious as continuous therapy. These results were published as preliminary, and unfortunately no larger studies have been published to date that corroborate these results.

This patient-centered, self-management approach offers the opportunity to improve outcomes through patient education

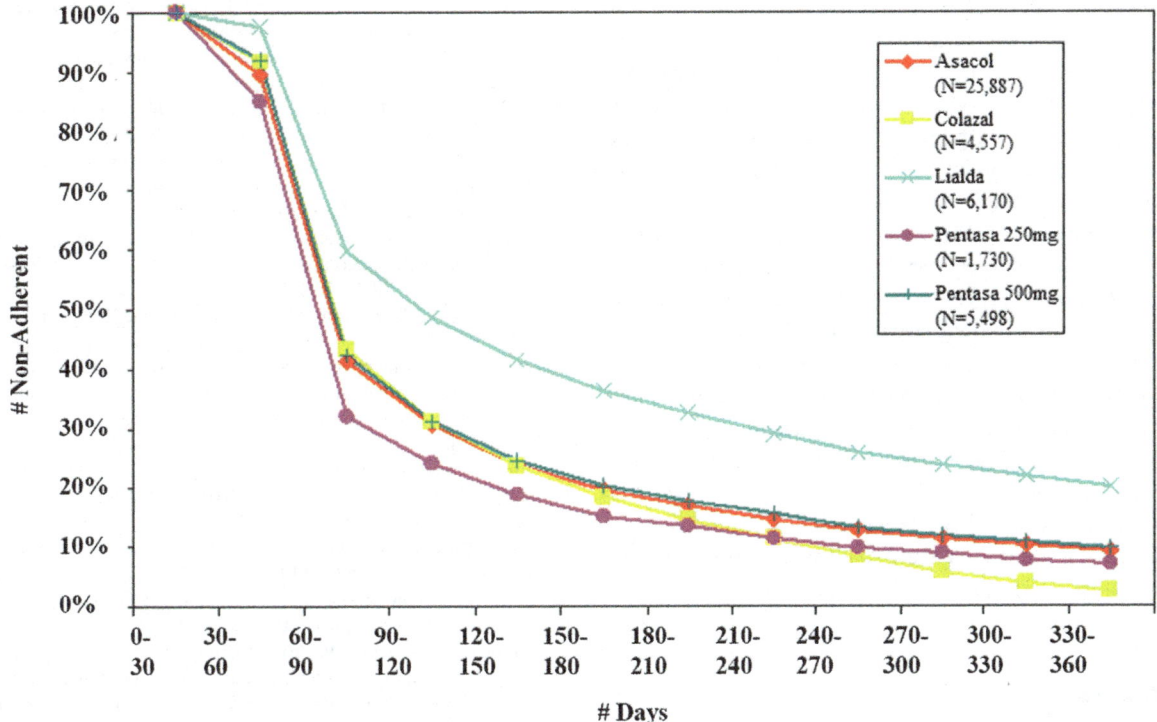

**Fig. 30.1** 5-ASA persistency over 12 months. Adapted from Kane S, Sumner M, Solomon D, Jenkins M. Persistency with Mesalamine Therapy: Long term Results in Patients Persistent with Therapy at Onset. Am J Gastroenterol 2009; 104 (Suppl 3)A 1269 [44]

and empowerment. In a British study, 203 patients with UC were randomized to either routine treatment by a specialist or patient-centered self-management in the primary care setting [42]. Patient training included a written algorithm for treatment and a 15–30 min training session. In the self-management group, relapses were treated significantly more rapidly than in the conventional group (14.8 h vs. 49.6 h, $p<0.01$), had fewer office visits (0.9/year vs. 2.9/year, $p<0.01$), and the length of the flares that did occur was shorter.

Evidence suggests that adherence varies with time, with patients often becoming less adherent with increasing duration of treatment. Maintaining adherence for extended periods of time is defined as persistence. A study investigating the prescription refill data from more than 3,500 UC patients over a 2-year period demonstrated that there is a marked decrease in adherence over time, with 57 % of patients adherent at 3 months, but only 55 % of those patients were still adherent after 12 months [43]. Another similar study in a larger group of patients over 12 months including Lialda® prescriptions demonstrates the same trend over time (Fig. 30.1) [44]. This suggests that patients may need some reinforcement of the importance of their medication at certain time points. This is the premise behind a concept which could be termed "interval empathy", whereby patients are contacted at certain times when the risk of non-adherence is judged to be greater [45]. For example, after 3 months, a

patient is likely to be in remission but may be at increased risk of non-adherence. The patient could be contacted to reinforce the message that continuing with their treatment is beneficial to their health. This could also give patients an opportunity to voice any new concerns that may have arisen since their last consultation. Various approaches are being piloted, with doctors or specialist nurses contacting patients by means such as telephone, text message or email.

The use of validated tools to help clinicians screen for those patients who are non-adherent has become of interest recently. Trindade et al. demonstrated that the use of the Morisky Medication Adherence Rating Scale was able to predict in a population of patients with inflammatory bowel disease those at high risk for non-adherence [46]. A follow up study performed by Kane and colleagues showed that patient scores could indeed correlate with non-adherence ($p=0.006$), but when stratified by class of therapy, it was only immunomodulators that this correlation was seen ($r=0.26$, $p=0.02$) [47].

## Conclusions

Medication non-adherence is prevalent in chronic illnesses, and ulcerative colitis is no exception. The problem is still not well-understood since it is difficult to predict who and when non-adherence becomes a clinically important issue. As discussed above, there is emerging data to show the long-term benefits of adherence, and then risks of non-adherence, with medications or other physician recommendations. Through physician and patient education, the clinical relevance of adherence can be emphasized and in the long-term disease outcomes will be improved.

Whilst predictive tools to identify patients at risk of non-adherence are likely to be very useful, it is still important to monitor adherence between consultations and identify, at the earliest opportunity, those patients who slip through the net and do still become non-adherent. One approach that could be developed in the future might be the adoption of a more integrated approach, whereby pharmacies and primary care could coordinate with secondary care clinicians to identify signs that a patient is not adhering to their medication. This may assist clinicians who, when encountering relapsing patients, may wish to take steps to ensure that the prescribed regimen is being adhered to before starting a new course of therapy.

# References

1. An oral preparation of mesalamine as long-term maintenance therapy for ulcerative colitis. A randomized, placebo-controlled trial. The Mesalamine Study Group. Ann Intern Med 1996;124: 204–11.
2. Ardizzone S, Petrillo M, Molteni P, et al. Coated oral 5-aminosalicylic acid (Claversal) is equivalent to sulfasalazine for remission maintenance in ulcerative colitis. A double-blind study. J Clin Gastroenterol. 1995;21:287–9.
3. Fockens P, Mulder CJ, Tytgat GN, et al. Comparison of the efficacy and safety of 1.5 compared with 3.0 g oral slow-release mesalazine (Pentasa) in the maintenance treatment of ulcerative colitis. Dutch Pentasa Study Group. Eur J Gastroenterol Hepatol. 1995;7: 1025–30.
4. Green JR, Gibson JA, Kerr GD, et al. Maintenance of remission of ulcerative colitis: a comparison between balsalazide 3 g daily and mesalazine 1.2 g daily over 12 months. ABACUS Investigator group. Aliment Pharmacol Ther. 1998;12:1207–16.
5. Miner P, Hanauer S, Robinson M, et al. Safety and efficacy of controlled-release mesalamine for maintenance of remission in ulcerative colitis. Pentasa UC Maintenance Study Group. Dig Dis Sci. 1995;40:296–304.
6. Miller NH. Compliance with treatment regimens in chronic asymptomatic diseases. Am J Med. 1997;102(2A):43–9.
7. Haynes RB. Determinants of compliance: the disease and the mechanisms of treatment. In: Haynes RB, Taynor DW, Sackett DL, editors. Compliance in health care. Baltimore: Johns Hopkins University Press; 1979.
8. Das K, Estwood MA, McManus JPA, et al. The metabolism of salicylazaosulphapyridine in ulcerative colitis. Gut. 1973;14:631–41.
9. Cowan GO, Das KM, Eastwood MA. Further studies of sulphasalazine metabolism in the treatment of ulcerative colitis. Br Med J. 1977;2(6094):1057–9.
10. van Hees PA, van Tongeren JH. Compliance to therapy in patients on a maintenance dose of sulfasalazine. J Clin Gastroenterol. 1982; 4:333–6.
11. Nigro G, Angelini G, Grosso SB, et al. Psychiatric predictors of noncompliance in inflammatory bowel disease. Psychiatry and compliance. J Clin Gastroenterol. 2001;32:66–8.
12. Riley S, Mani V, Goddman MJ, et al. Why do patients with ulcerative colitis relapse? Gut. 1990;31:179–83.
13. Farup PG, Hovde O, Halvorsen FA, et al. Mesalazine suppositories versus hydrocortisone foam in patients with distal ulcerative colitis. A comparison of the efficacy and practicality of two topical treatment regimens. Scand J Gastroenterol. 1995;30(2):164–70.
14. Shale MJ, Riley SA. Studies of compliance with delayed-release mesalazine therapy in patients with inflammatory bowel disease. Aliment Pharmacol Ther. 2003;18(2):191–8.
15. Kane SV, Aikens J, Hanauer SB. Medication regimens are associated with non-adherence in quiescent ulcerative colitis. Am J Gastroenterol. 2002;97(9):S770.
16. Jackson CA, Clathworthy J, Robinson A, Horne R. Factors associated with non-adherence to oral medication for inflammatory bowel disease: a systematic review. Am J Gastroenterol. 2010;105(3):525–39.
17. Kane S. Does treatment schedule matter? Once daily versus divided doses of 5-ASAs. Dig Dis. 2010;28(3):478–82.
18. Woolrich AJ, DeSilva MD, Korelitz BI. Surveillance in the routine management of ulcerative colitis: the predictive value of low-grade dysplasia. Gastroenterology. 1992;103(2):431–8.
19. Kane SV, Aikens J, Huo D, et al. Medication adherence is associated with improved outcomes in patients with quiescent ulcerative colitis. Am J Med. 2003;113:39–42.
20. Kane SV. Medication adherence and the physician-patient relationship. Am J Gastroenterol. 2002;97(7):1853.
21. Moody GA, Jayanthi V, Probert CS, et al. Long-term therapy with sulphasalazine protects against colorectal cancer in ulcerative colitis: a retrospective study of colorectal cancer risk and compliance with treatment in Leicestershire. Eur J Gastroenterol Hepatol. 1996;8:1179–83.
22. Pinczowski D, Ekbom A, Baron J, et al. Risk factors for colorectal cancer in patients with ulcerative colitis: a case-control study. Gastroenterology. 1994;107:117–20.
23. Velayos FS, Terdiman JP, Walsh JM. Effect of 5-aminosalicylate use on colorectal cancer and dysplasia risk: a systematic review and metaanalysis of observational studies. Am J Gastroenterol. 2005;100(6):1345–53.
24. Eaden J, Abrams K, Ekbom A, et al. Colorectal cancer prevention in ulcerative colitis: a case-control study. Aliment Pharmacol Ther. 2000;14:145–53.
25. Ullman T, Croog V, Itzkowitz S, et al. Preventing neoplastic progression in ulcerative colitis: role of mesalamine. Gastroenterology. 2003;124(4):S1662.
26. Rubin DT, LoSavio A, Yadron N, Huo D, Hanauer SB. Aminosalicylate therapy in the prevention of dysplasia and colorectal cancer in ulcerative colitis. Clin Gastroenterol Hepatol. 2006;4(11):1346–50.
27. Bernstein CN, Nugent Z, Blanchard JF. 5-Aminosalicylate is not chemoprophylactic for colorectal cancer in IBD: a population based study. Am J Gastroenterol. 2011;106(4):731–6.
28. Kane S, Shaya F. Medication non-adherence is associated with increased medical health care costs. Dig Dis Sci. 2008;53(4):1020–4.
29. Yen EF, Kane SV, Ladabaum U. Cost-effectiveness of 5-aminosalicylic acid therapy for maintenance of remission in ulcerative colitis. Am J Gastroenterol. 2008;103:3094–105.
30. Drossman DA, Leserman K, Li Z, et al. The rating form of IBD patient concerns. A new measure of health status. Psychosom Med. 1991;53:701–12.
31. Gray JR, Leung E, Scales J. Treatment of ulcerative colitis from the patient's perspective: a survey of preferences and satisfaction with therapy. Aliment Pharmacol Ther. 2009;29(1):1114–20.
32. Martin A, Leone L, Fries W, et al. What do patients want to know about their inflammatory bowel disease. Ital J Gastroenterol. 1992;24(8):477–80.
33. Levy R, Feld AD. Increasing patient adherence to gastroenterology treatment and prevention regimens. Am J Gastroenterols. 1999;94:1733–42.

34. Kane SV, Dang J. Medication taking behavior in a gastroenterology clinic: a disconnect between patient behavior and physician knowledge. Gastroenterology. 2004;126(4):A605.

35. Nobel LM. Doctor-patient communication and adherence to treatment. In: Myers LB, Midence K, editors. Adherence to treatment in medical conditions. New York: Harwood Academic Publishers; 1998. p. 51–82.

36. Sewitch MJ, Abrahamowicz M, Barkun A, et al. Patient nonadherence to medication in inflammatory bowel disease. Am J Gastroenterol. 2003;98(7):1535–44.

37. Wolf MS, Davis TC, Bass PF, et al. Improving prescription drug warnings to promote patient comprehension. Arch Intern Med. 2011;170(1):50–6.

38. Kane SV, Huo D, Magnanti K. A pilot feasibility trial of once daily vs. conventional dosing of mesalamine for treatment of ulcerative colitis. Clin Gastroenterol Hepatol. 2003;1:170–3.

39. Dignass AU, Bokemeyer B, Adamek H, et al. Mesalamine once daily is more effective than twice daily in patients with quiescent ulcerative colitis. Clin Gastroenterol Hepatol. 2009;7(7):762–9.

40. Sandborn WJ, Korzenik J, Lashner B, et al. Once daily dosing of delayed-release oral mesalamine (400 mg tablet) for maintenance of remission of ulcerative colitis: the QDIEM trial. Gastroenterology. 2010;138:1286–96.

41. Dickinson RJ, King A, Wight DG, et al. Is continuous sulfasalazine necessary in the management of patients with ulcerative colitis? Results of a preliminary study. Dis Colon Rectum. 1985;28:929–30.

42. Robinson A, Thompson DG, Wilkin D, et al. Guided self-management and patient-directed follow-up of ulcerative colitis: a randomized trial. Lancet. 2001;358(9268):976–81.

43. Kane SV, Accortt NA, Magowan S, Brixner D. Predictors of persistence with 5-aminosalicylic acid therapy for ulcerative colitis. Aliment Pharmacol Ther. 2009;29(8):855–62.

44. Kane S, Sumner M, Solomon D, Jenkins M. Persistency with mesalamine therapy: long term results in patients persistent with therapy at onset. Am J Gastroenterol. 2009;104 Suppl 3:A 1269.

45. Dl R, Ja H, Kern DE, et al. Improving physicians' interviewing skills and reducing patients' emotional distress. A randomized controlled trial. Arch Intern Med. 1995;155(17):1877–84.

46. Trindade AJ, Ehrlich A, Kornbluth A, Ullman TA. Are your patients taking their medicine? Validation of a new adherence scale in patients with inflammatory bowel disease and comparison with physician perception of adherence. Inflamm Bowel Dis. 2011;17(2):599–604.

47. Kane SV, Loftus EV, Sandborn WJ, et al. Limited clinical utility of a self-administered tool for predicting medication adherence behavior in IBD. Gastroenterology. 2011;139(Suppl):Sa1303 (Abstract).

# The Role of Telemedicine for Management of Ulcerative Colitis

Sandra M. Quezada and Raymond K. Cross

**Keywords**

Telemedicine • Ulcerative colitis • Management • Medical therapy

## Introduction

Inflammatory bowel disease (IBD) comprised of ulcerative colitis (UC), and Crohn's disease (CD) is a chronic idiopathic intestinal disorder that afflicts more than one million people in the United States [1]. Its impact on quality of life is profound and results in a substantial economic burden [2, 3]. Effective therapies are available to induce and maintain symptom remission; however, there are multiple barriers to successful patient outcomes. Such barriers include but are not limited to poor adherence to medical therapy [4–8], limited patient education [9], inadequate patient monitoring, limited access to care, and medication side effects [10, 11].

Diseases like IBD are associated with a high-risk of medication nonadherence because of the unpredictable disease course with long periods of low activity in between flares of disease. Only 40–60 % of patients with quiescent UC are adherent to aminosalicylate (5-ASA) therapy [7, 8, 12, 13]. Nonadherence to therapy is not trivial because nonadherent patients are five times more likely to have disease exacerbations [6], and direct health-care costs are increased in nonadherent patients [14]. The reasons for nonadherence vary. Sewitch et al. found that most instances of nonadherence in IBD were unintentional with 31 % of patients simply forgetting to take medicines. Variables positively associated with unintentional nonadherence include younger age, less active disease, new patient status, no prescription for steroids,

and lower patient-physician discordance [8]. Patient miscomprehension is another important factor leading to nonadherence since 62 % of patients with IBD perceive that they are misinformed about their illness [15]. Miscomprehension can be linked to nonadherence when patients do not understand why they are taking medications or when they are surprised by unexpected side effects [5, 16].

Despite the fact that effective therapies exist to treat IBD, all current medications have potential side effects [17] that can result in cessation of therapy, decrease adherence with therapy [5], and worsen symptoms [11]. Improved detection of side effects and better patient education regarding side effects may improve outcomes. Improved monitoring of IBD symptoms is another potential mechanism to improve outcomes. Currently, patients with IBD are seen at scheduled intervals. Because exacerbations of bowel symptoms are sporadic, scheduled office visits are often discordant with disease flares. In addition, when patients develop recurrent symptoms, long delays may ensue before office visits are scheduled.

Self-management could be implemented to encourage patient self-monitoring and earlier initiation of treatment. Robinson successfully implemented a self-care plan in patients with UC. In this study, UC patients treated successfully with steroids during a hospitalization were randomized to usual care (scheduled clinical visits after hospital discharge) or to self-management for 1 year. Participants in the self-management group received individualized, written action plans without clinical follow-up. Relapses in the self-management group were treated earlier and were shorter in duration, and utilization of health-care resources was decreased [18]. Similarly, self-care plans implemented in UC patients in the United Kingdom decreased hospitalization rates, sustained quality of life, and increased coping

S.M. Quezada, M.D., M.S. • R.K. Cross, M.D., M.S. (✉)
Division of Gastroenterology and Hepatology,
Department of Medicine, University of Maryland,
100 North Greene Street, Lower Level, Baltimore, MD 21093, USA
e-mail: rcross@medicine.umaryland.edu

G.R. Lichtenstein (ed.), *Medical Therapy of Ulcerative Colitis*,
DOI 10.1007/978-1-4939-1677-1_31, © Springer Science+Business Media New York 2014

without increasing the number of outpatient visits or increasing patient anxiety [19]. Neither of these studies utilized telemedicine to administer action plans.

## Telemedicine in Chronic Disease and Inflammatory Bowel Disease

Telemedicine is a candidate intervention that can help practitioners follow current clinical guidelines, prompt patients to adhere to medications, help providers educate patients, assist providers in monitoring patients, increase patient and provider interactions, help providers and patients initiate therapy earlier, and help patients adhere to self-care plans (see Fig. 31.1).

Although not routinely applied to chronic gastrointestinal illnesses such as UC, telemedicine has been applied to chronic conditions similar to UC, and patients' acceptance of telemedicine systems is high [20–26]. IBD shares many similarities to these other chronic illnesses in that patients have long-term symptoms, experience frequent recurrence of symptoms, and require ongoing medical therapy to control symptoms and prevent relapses. A home telemanagement system similar to that described below was well accepted by patients with asthma [21], resulted in greater adherence with self-action plans [27], improved quality of life and patient knowledge, and decreased urgent care visits [28]. In a follow-up study by Finkelstein et al, significant improvements were noted in asthma symptoms, self-administered spirometry, adherence to action plans, and decreased use of quick-relief inhalers [28]. Likewise, a large randomized trial from a different center demonstrated that Internet-based monitoring reduced asthma symptoms and improved lung function and quality of life compared to specialist or general practitioner monitoring [29]. In diabetes, several studies

demonstrated reduced glycosylated hemoglobin with the use of telemedicine [30–35]. Telemedicine was shown to improve quality of life and to decrease hospitalizations and length of stay, emergency room visits, and office visits [36, 37]. Moreover, even studies that showed no improvement in glycosylated hemoglobin showed that telemedicine results in equivalent outcomes with decreased clinical visits [38]. A recent systematic review summarizes the effect of telemedicine interventions in patients with diabetes. Overall, telemedicine interventions decrease glycosylated hemoglobin and complications of disease [39]. In congestive heart failure, telemedicine improved clinical outcomes and quality of life [40, 41]. Further, telemedicine interventions decreased utilization of health-care resources [40, 42]. Roth and colleagues showed that telemedicine decreased hospitalizations by 66 %, and Benatar et al. demonstrated decreased hospitalization costs in the telemedicine group [40, 42].

Pilot testing of telemedicine in IBD has demonstrated that it is feasible to use and that patient acceptance is excellent [43–45]. One pilot study assessed the acceptance of a home telemanagement system for IBD (IBD HAT) in ten patients with IBD. IBD HAT was comprised of three components: a patient home unit, a decision support server, and a web-based clinician portal. The patient home unit included an electronic weight scale connected to a laptop computer via a serial port for self-testing [44].

The laptop computer contained a symptom diary, side effect inventory, adherence check, and assessment of body weight. Patients answered questions directly using the laptop; weight was assessed after audio prompts from the laptop. Individualized patient data was entered into the secure web portal; information collected included contact information, medication prescriptions, IBD HAT testing schedules, and disease history. Clinicians used the web portal to customize medication and side effect profiles for each patient. Furthermore, a clinical alert system was customized for each patient based on responses to the symptom diary, medication side effect questions, self-reported adherence, and body weight. Figure 31.2 demonstrates the flow of data communication in this telemedicine system. Once self-testing was completed, patients received an IBD-related educational prompt in the format of a "tip of the day"; the following week, patients were asked a question about the tip. Patients could not advance in the educational curriculum unless they answered the question correctly. The results of self-testing were submitted telephonically and were available for review immediately thereafter on the secure web server [44].

IBD HAT was tested on ten adult patients with IBD. Participants underwent a single 45-min training session during which they were taught how to use the equipment. They then completed self-testing without supervision. All participants reported that self-testing was not complicated

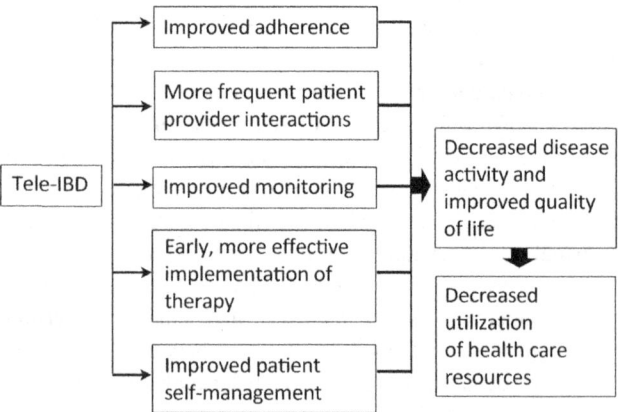

**Fig. 31.1** Theoretical model for improved outcomes with the use of telemedicine [Tele-inflammatory bowel disease (IBD)] in patients with IBD

**Fig. 31.2** Model of the home telemanagement system for patients with inflammatory bowel disease

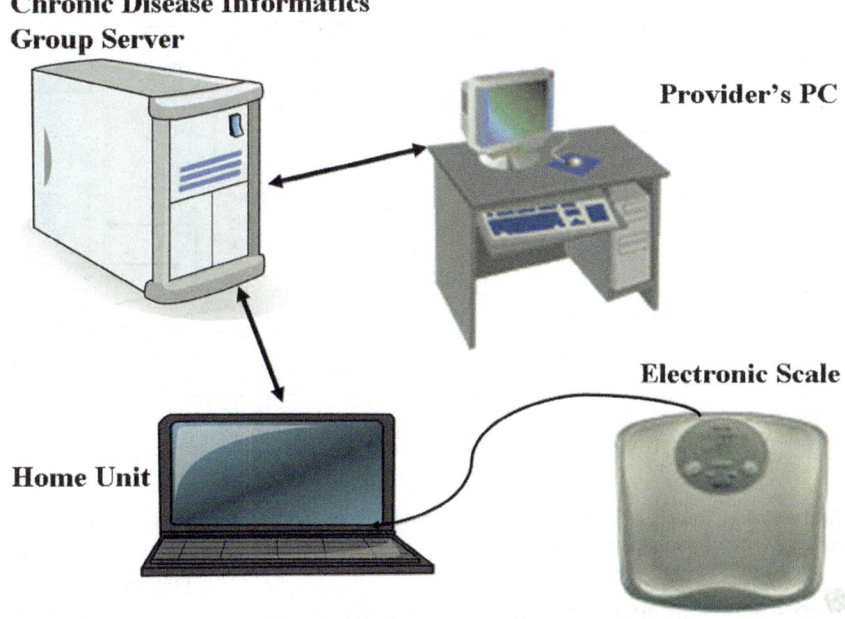

and that the symptom diary and side effect questions were easy to answer. Participants felt that self-testing took very little time and that they could adhere to self-testing at least three times per week. Most patients thought IBD HAT would make them feel safer, and 80 % would agree to use the system in the future [44].

Based on the positive pretesting results, a 6-month open-label trial to assess the feasibility and patient acceptance of IBD HAT in patients with IBD was performed. Thirty-four patients were enrolled. Each participant received an initial 45-min instruction session at their home during which they were taught how to operate the equipment. After this initial training session, the participants were asked to complete weekly self-testing sessions over a 6-month period. During the study period, participants continued to receive standard IBD care in addition to the weekly HAT sessions. Twenty-five participants successfully completed the 6-month study. Fifteen participants had CD, nine had UC, and one had indeterminate colitis. Over the study period, 89 % of participants were adherent with weekly self-testing. Attitudes toward IBD HAT were also very good; 95 % of participants said that self-testing was not complicated. Ninety percent of patients reported that use of the weight scale was not difficult, and 100 % reported use of the computer was not difficult. Similarly, 90 % reported that answering the symptom diary and medication side effect questions were not difficult. Participants reported that self-testing took very little time and did not interrupt their usual activities. Seventy percent of patients felt safer using the system. Mean self-reported adherence with IBD medications was 90 % throughout the

study. Clinical disease activity, disease-specific quality of life, and patient knowledge improved after using IBD HAT for 6 months compared to baseline [45].

## Home Automated Telemanagement for Ulcerative Colitis (UC HAT)

Several modifications to the IBD HAT system were made to make it specific for patients with UC (UC HAT). First, the symptom diary and alert criteria were changed to make them specific to patients with UC. The UC symptom diary consisted of 14 questions, which assessed overall well-being, functional status, bowel symptoms, systemic symptoms, and extraintestinal manifestations of UC. Subscores were generated for questions that dealt with overall well-being, number of liquid stools per day, nocturnal awakening, and amount of visible blood in bowel movements. Total and subscore thresholds were individualized for each participant to increase or decrease sensitivity. Second, self-care or action plans were added to the system (see Fig. 31.3). Based on scores generated from the UC symptom diary, participants received self-action or action plans in one of three categories: (1) green zone, for patients with no to mild symptoms; (2) yellow zone, for patients with moderate symptoms (Table 31.1); or (3) red zone, for patients with severe symptoms. Each severity zone lists several actions that providers can choose for participants to initiate as part of their self-management plan. These action plans could also be modified by the provider on the web portal as needed. Third, an electronic

**Fig. 31.3** Information flow in Tele-inflammatory bowel disease (IBD)

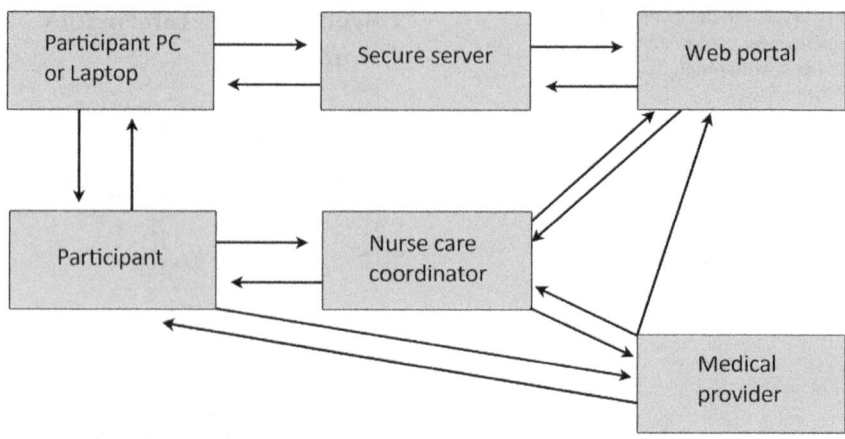

**Table 31.1** Example of self-care or action plan delivered by the UC HAT system for participants in the yellow zone

| Yellow zone | Symptoms | Actions |
|---|---|---|
| Moderate symptoms | Overall health poor | Continue your current meds; it can take a few weeks to take effect |
| | 4–6 BMs/day | Take one Canasa suppository nightly |
| | 1–3 nocturnal awakenings | Take one Rowasa enema nightly |
| | More than trace blood in stool | Double the dose of oral aminosalicylate |
| | | Start prednisone 20 or 40 mg daily |
| | | Call your nurse or physician to Schedule infliximab |
| | | Call your nurse or physician |

*BM* bowel movements

messaging system (automated and free text) was developed for participants to communicate to the research team [46].

The feasibility and acceptance of UC HAT were assessed in ten patients with UC. Pretesting yielded similar results in the UC population compared to the overall IBD population. All participants felt that using the computer and self-testing system was not complicated, and nine of the ten participants reported no difficulty in using the weight scale or in answering the symptom diary and side effect questions. Seven participants reported that they would feel safer using UC HAT, and eight felt it was important that the IBD center physicians monitored their results [46].

In a follow-up controlled trial, forty-seven patients with UC were randomized to receive either UC HAT (25 participants) or best available care (22 participants). Participants in the UC HAT group underwent self-testing weekly. Participants in the best available care group underwent routine and as needed clinic and telephone follow-up, received educational fact sheets about IBD, and received self-action plans without reinforcement. Disease activity

was measured by the Seo Index [47], and disease-related quality of life was measured by the Inflammatory Bowel Disease Questionnaire (IBDQ) [48].

At baseline, 27 % of participants in the best available care group used immune suppressants compared to 56 % in the UC HAT group ($p = 0.05$). Further, IBDQ scores at baseline were lower in UC HAT participants compared to the best available care group. During the trial, 8 participants withdrew in the UC HAT arm compared to 1 in the best available care arm. There was no difference in disease activity scores or remission rates between the treatment groups at 4, 8, and 12 months. After adjustment for baseline quality of life, disease activity scores decreased 12 points from baseline in the UC HAT arm ($p = 0.08$) compared to 1 point in the best available care arm ($p = 0.84$). IBDQ scores increased in the UC HAT arm and remained stable in the best available care arm, though these differences were not significant at any time point after baseline. However, after the adjustment for baseline disease knowledge, UC HAT participants were noted to have a 16-point improvement in quality of life scores at 12 months from baseline compared to the best available care group ($p = 0.04$) (see Fig. 31.4). Adherence was low in both groups at baseline but improved in both groups over 12 months; no significant differences in adherence were noted between the two groups [48].

These results suggest that telemedicine may decrease disease activity and increase disease-specific quality of life in patients with UC. This seems to occur despite the finding that self-reported adherence did not improve in the UC HAT group. The negative findings in the intention to treat analysis were likely affected by the high attrition rate in the UC HAT arm, which calls into question the utility of UC HAT for long-term use. It is possible that a different telemedicine system, such as a web-based unit, would decrease attrition rates in future trials and improve outcomes. Furthermore, future studies are warranted to identify what if any factor in the UC HAT system is associated with improved outcomes.

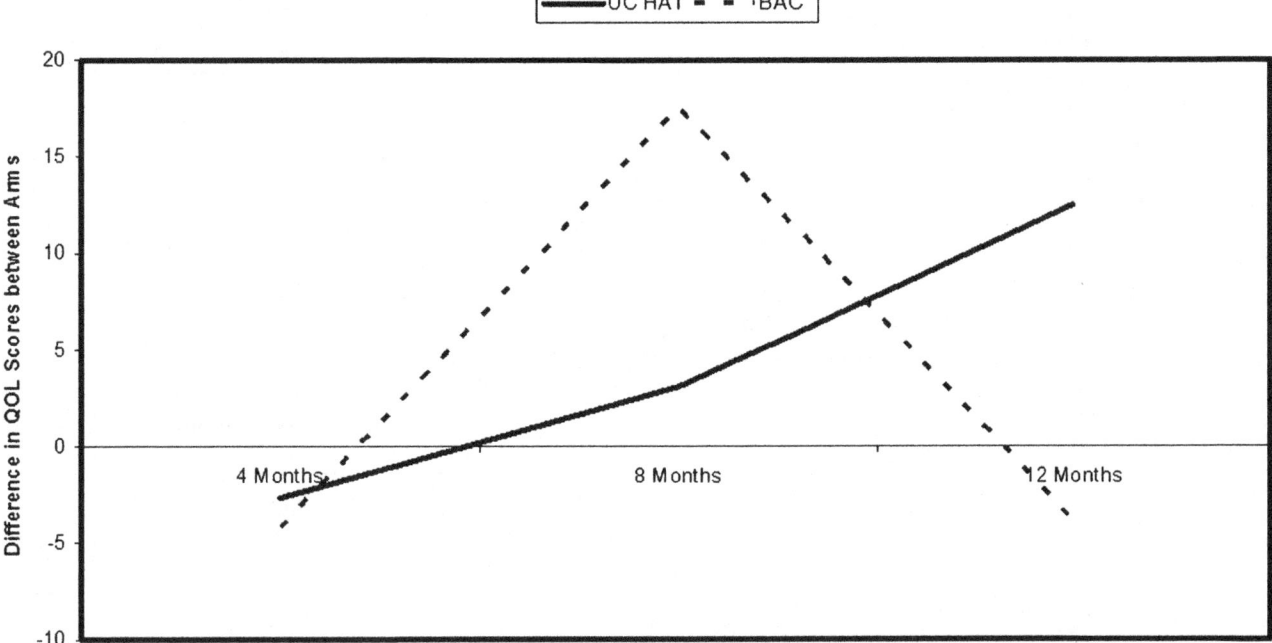

**Fig. 31.4** Differences in disease-specific quality of life scores from baseline between UC HAT and BAC groups at 12 months [48]. Reprinted from Cross RK, Cheevers N, Rustgi A, Langenberg P, Finkelstein J. Randomized, controlled trial of home telemanagement in patients with ulcerative colitis (UC HAT). Inflamm Bowel Dis. 2012 Jun;18(6):1018–25., with permission from Wiley

## Constant Care for Ulcerative Colitis

Researchers from Denmark developed a web-based telemedicine system for patients with UC called "Constant Care" (http://www.constant-care.dk). Construction of the 24-h Constant Care website began in 2001 and was created to be available in Danish and English. Using this system, doctors were able to prescribe 5-ASA and topical steroid medications electronically based on patient symptoms, to monitor patients longitudinally, and to provide patient education [49].

Prior to using the website, all participants in the web group and their relatives were given educational training with a 1.5-h slide presentation on IBD etiology, pathology, anatomy, medical and surgical treatments, disease course, adherence, nutrition, mortality risk, colorectal cancer chemoprevention, pregnancy, and breastfeeding. Participants and family members also underwent a 1.5-h training session in using the Constant Care website. Guidelines for indications on when to call the provider included having greater than six stools per day, daily rectal bleeding, rectal bleeding occurring between relapses, fever >37.5 °C, heart rate >90 beats per minute, severe abdominal pain, symptoms persisting more than 11 days despite escalation of therapy, unexplained weight loss, and/or for any doubts or questions regarding the study. Disease-specific quality of life was measured on the website with the Short Inflammatory Bowel Disease Questionnaire (SIBDQ) [50], and the Simple Clinical Colitis Activity Index (SCCAI) [51] was used to assess disease activity [49].

Ten participants with UC and five of their relatives participated in the validation study of Constant Care. All participants in the validation group felt capable of self-initiating treatment after the educational training. Eight of ten participants expected to see an improvement in quality of life, quality of the treatment, and knowledge of their disease after the educational training session [49].

Subsequently, a randomized controlled trial in Denmark and Ireland was conducted to assess the impact of the Constant Care website compared to standard care. Patients with mild-to-moderate UC were randomly assigned to either Constant Care with disease-specific education and self-treatment or a control group that received standard care for 12 months. Outcomes of interest included feasibility of the Constant Care web system and its influence on participants' medication adherence, UC knowledge, quality of life, safety, and health-care costs. Exclusion criteria included use of infliximab and immunosuppressant therapy, narcotic dependence, previous IBD surgery or likelihood of surgery during the study period, 2 or more flares per year requiring high-dose steroid therapy, pregnancy, and breastfeeding [52].

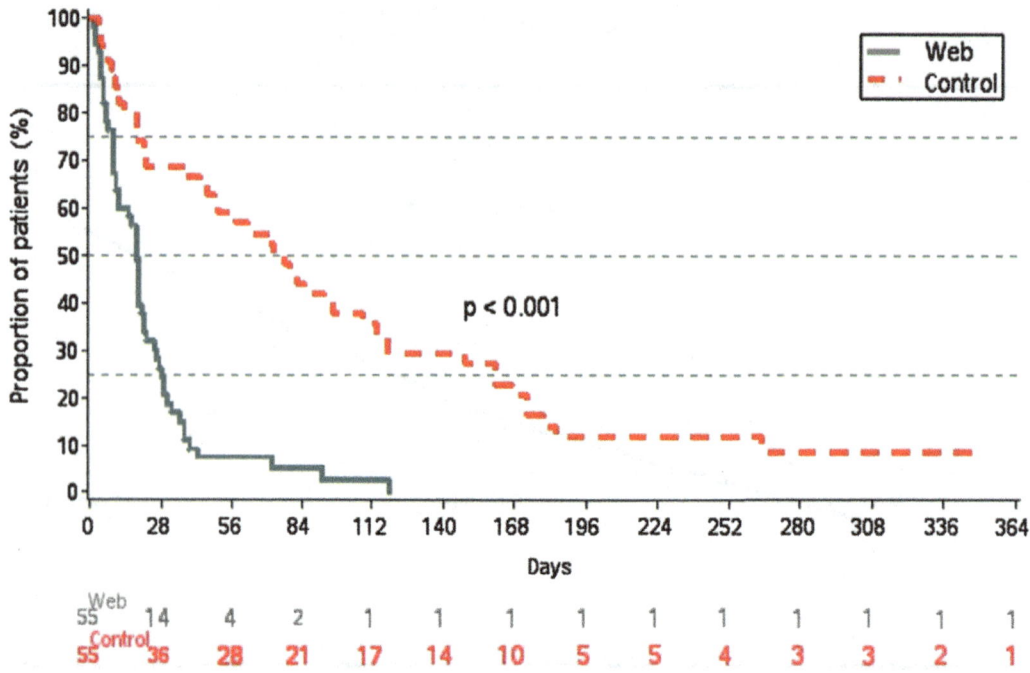

**Fig. 31.5** Time (days) from the first relapse to remission in web and control patients during 1 year of follow-up [52]. Reproduced from Elkjaer M, Shuhaibar M, Burisch J, Bailey Y, Scherfig H, Laugesen B, et al. E-health empowers patients with ulcerative colitis: a randomised controlled trial of the web-guided "Constant-care" approach. Gut. 2010 Dec;59(12):1652–61, with permission from BMJ Publishing Group Ltd

Symptoms were categorized as follows: quiescent-to-mild symptoms appeared as a green traffic light, moderate symptoms appeared as a yellow light, and highly active symptoms appeared as a red light. During symptom flare, participants were instructed to log onto the system daily to complete the SCCAI until their symptoms entered the green zone. Entry frequency was then reduced to once weekly until 4 weeks after the initial relapse. The SIBDQ was to be completed at the beginning and end of each relapse. Once in remission, participants were to log into the system once monthly until the next relapse occurred. If symptoms were entered such as rectal bleeding, three or more bowel movements per day, or nighttime bowel movements, the system recommended initiation of 4 g daily or more of 5-ASA for a total of 28 days. Participants were given the option to extend this treatment period by an additional 28 days if remission into the green zone was not achieved. Participants could also choose additional topical 5-ASA treatment and prednisolone, based on previous maximal extent of disease and participants' prior treatment experience [52].

All participants were to have study visits at baseline, 6 months, and 12 months. During each of these visits, participants were asked to complete a series of questionnaires, including the SCCAI, SIBDQ, Crohn's Colitis Knowledge Score (CCKNOW) [53], SF-36 [54], Hospital Anxiety and Depression Scale [55], and Compliance Questionnaire. The Compliance Questionnaire included 5 questions on the following topics: ease of access to prescription, ability of relapse recognition, following the medical doctor's advice, ability to self-initiate acute treatment, and adherence to 5-ASA treatment [52].

In total, 333 adult participants were randomized. Of these, 263 (79 %) participants completed the 12-month follow-up visit. In the Danish arm of the study, there were no differences in 5-ASA adherence between the web and control participants (68 % vs. 69 % respectively refilled at least 80 % of their medication). However, the web group demonstrated significantly higher adherence to four weeks of acute treatment compared to controls (73 % vs. 42 %, $p=0.003$). There were significantly greater improvements among web group participants in IBD knowledge, disease-specific quality of life ($p=0.04$), general health ($p=0.009$), vitality ($p=0.03$), and emotional ($p<0.0001$) and social functioning ($p=0.002$) as compared with the control group. Half of all participants experienced at least one flare of symptoms during the study period, with no difference in flare rates between the groups. However, relapses were significantly shorter in the web group compared to the control group (median 18 days vs. 77 days, $p<0.0001$) (see Fig. 31.5). Furthermore, at the time of relapse, 100 % of web participants initiated therapy with high-dose oral 5-ASA compared to 10 % of controls. There was otherwise no difference between the groups in disease activity scores as measured by the SCCAI or in the rate of hospitalizations [52].

UC-related acute visits were higher in the control group compared to the web group (107 visits vs. 21 visits, $p < 0.0001$). There were also fewer routine visits in the web group. Conversely, there were a significantly higher number of emails (86) and phone calls (21) from web participants than from controls (seven emails and 17 phone calls) and greater 5-ASA use in the web group [52].

Similarly, medication adherence to four weeks of treatment was significantly greater in the web group compared to controls (73 % vs. 29 %, $p = 0.03$) in the Irish arm of the study. The web group also demonstrated improved mental health ($p = 0.01$), physical functioning ($p = 0.03$), and social functioning ($p = 0.02$) compared to controls. However, there were no differences between study groups in terms of IBD knowledge or disease-specific quality of life. Thirty-nine percent of web participants experienced a relapse compared to 24 % of controls; however, these were shorter than the relapses experienced by controls (median 30 days vs. 70 days, $p < 0.03$). Interestingly, only 15 % of web participants initiated high-dose oral 5-ASA at the time of relapse compared to 10 % of controls. Routine visits were decreased in web participants relative to controls; however, acute care visits were identical between the two groups [52].

This study demonstrated that a web-based treatment strategy such as Constant Care can improve short-term adherence, improve quality of life, shorten relapses, and decrease utilization of some health-care resources.

## Conclusion

In summary, use of telemedicine appears to be feasible and well accepted by patients with UC. In addition, available studies have demonstrated improvements in clinical outcomes. The quasi-experimental study by Cross et al. reported decreased disease activity, improved quality of life, and increased knowledge after use of IBD HAT for 6 months [45]. Similarly, both randomized controlled trials of telemedicine for UC showed improvements in disease activity as measured by disease activity indices or length of flares and improvements in quality of life. Despite improvements in disease activity, adherence was not better in the telemedicine arms in either study, except for adherence with acute treatment in the Constant Care study [48, 52]. Quality of life improved in the telemedicine arms of both studies, and utilization of some health-care resources was less in the telemedicine group in the European study [48, 52]. For example, routine visits and acute care visits were decreased in web participants; however, email and phone calls increased, and use of 5-ASA increased in the telemedicine group resulting in a net increase in costs [52]. Use of telemedicine systems in the UC population seems feasible; however, attrition rates range from as low as 8 % to as high as 32 % in the telemedicine arms [45, 48, 52].

This raises concerns about long-term adherence to telemedicine systems. Larger studies are needed to explore subgroups that might particularly benefit from telemedicine, specifically patients with decreased access to care, a history of nonadherence, poor social support, more severe disease (moderate-to-severe UC), patients with active disease versus disease in remission, and patients initiating new drug therapy. Also, the financial impact of telemedicine on UC care, positive or negative, needs to be explored.

In UC, use of telemedicine is feasible and well accepted, can improve access to care, and can increase a patients' sense of empowerment. Technology will continue to advance in quality and ease of use and will likely incorporate the use of handheld devices in the future. This progress should result in the increased use of telemedicine as a treatment alternative or as an adjunctive component to disease management in UC.

## References

1. Loftus CG, Loftus EV, Jr., Harmsen WS, Zinsmeister AR, Tremaine WJ, Melton LJ, 3rd, et al. Update on the incidence and prevalence of Crohn's disease and ulcerative colitis in Olmsted County, Minnesota, 1940–2000. Inflamm Bowel Dis. 2006 Dec 19.
2. Guthrie E, Jackson J, Shaffer J, Thompson D, Tomenson B, Creed F. Psychological disorder and severity of inflammatory bowel disease predict health-related quality of life in ulcerative colitis and Crohn's disease. Am J Gastroenterol. 2002;97(8):1994–9.
3. Kappelman MD, Rifas-Shiman SL, Porter C, Ollendorf DA, Sandler RS, Galanko JA, et al. Direct health care costs of Crohn's disease and ulcerative colitis in US children and adults. Gastroenterology. 2008;135(6):1907–13.
4. Kane S. Patient compliance and outcomes. Inflamm Bowel Dis. 1999;5(2):134–7.
5. Kane S, Dang J. Medication taking behavior in a gastroenterology clinic: a disconnect between patient behavior and physician knowledge. Gastroenterology. 2004;126(4):A605.
6. Kane S, Huo D, Aikens J, Hanauer S. Medication nonadherence and the outcomes of patients with quiescent ulcerative colitis. Am J Med. 2003;114(1):39–43.
7. Kane SV, Cohen RD, Aikens JE, Hanauer SB. Prevalence of nonadherence with maintenance mesalamine in quiescent ulcerative colitis. Am J Gastroenterol. 2001;96(10):2929–33.
8. Sewitch MJ, Abrahamowicz M, Barkun A, Bitton A, Wild GE, Cohen A, et al. Patient nonadherence to medication in inflammatory bowel disease. Am J Gastroenterol. 2003;98(7):1535–44.
9. Quan H, Present JW, Sutherland LR. Evaluation of educational programs in inflammatory bowel disease. Inflamm Bowel Dis. 2003;9(6):356–62.
10. Cross RK, Lapshin O, Finkelstein J. Patient subjective assessment of drug side effects in inflammatory bowel disease. J Clin Gastroenterol. 2008;24.
11. Cross RK, Wilson KT, Binion DG. Polypharmacy and Crohn's disease. Aliment Pharmacol Ther. 2005;21(10):1211–6.
12. Bernal I, Domenech E, Garcia-Planella E, Marin L, Manosa M, Navarro M, et al. Medication-taking behavior in a cohort of patients with inflammatory bowel disease. Dig Dis Sci. 2006;51(12):2165–9.
13. D'Inca R, Bertomoro P, Mazzocco K, Vettorato MG, Rumiati R, Sturniolo GC. Risk factors for non-adherence to medication in

inflammatory bowel disease patients. Aliment Pharmacol Ther. 2008;27(2):166–72.

14. Shaya F, El Khoury AC, Wong W, Whitelaw N, Whitelaw G, Joseph RE, Cohen RD. Persistence with pharmacotherapy for gastrointestinal disease: associated costs of health care. P&T. 2006;31(11):657–65.

15. Martin A, Leone L, Castagliuolo I, Di Mario F, Naccarato R. What do patients want to know about their inflammatory bowel disease? Ital J Gastroenterol. 1992;24(9):477–80.

16. Levy RL, Feld AD. Increasing patient adherence to gastroenterology treatment and prevention regimens. Am J Gastroenterol. 1999;94(7):1733–42.

17. Navarro F, Hanauer SB. Treatment of inflammatory bowel disease: safety and tolerability issues. Am J Gastroenterol. 2003;98(12 Suppl):S18–23.

18. Robinson A, Thompson DG, Wilkin D, Roberts C. Guided self-management and patient-directed follow-up of ulcerative colitis: a randomised trial. Lancet. 2001;358(9286):976–81.

19. Kennedy AP, Nelson E, Reeves D, Richardson G, Roberts C, Robinson A, et al. A randomised controlled trial to assess the effectiveness and cost of a patient orientated self management approach to chronic inflammatory bowel disease. Gut. 2004;53(11):1639–45.

20. Farzanfar R, Finkelstein J, Friedman RH. Testing the usability of two automated home-based patient management systems. J Med Syst. 2004;28(2):143–53.

21. Finkelstein J, Hripcsak G, Cabrera MR. Patients' acceptance of Internet-based home asthma telemonitoring. Proc AMIA Symp. 1998;336–40.

22. Finkelstein J, Feldman J, Safi C, Mitchell P, Khare R, editors. The feasibility and patient acceptance of computer-assisted asthma education in Emergency Department setting. Proceedings of the Academic Emergency Medicine 2003 Annual Meeting. Academic Emergency Medicine; 2003.

23. Finkelstein J, Cabrera MR, Hripcsak G. Internet-based home asthma telemonitoring: can patients handle the technology? Chest. 2000;117(1):148–55.

24. Finkelstein J, Khare, R, Ansell, J. Feasibility and patient's acceptance of home automated telemanagement of oral anticoagulation therapy. AMIA Annu Symp Proc. 2003:230–4.

25. Finkelstein J, Arora M, Joshi A, editor. Home automated telemanagement in hypertension. Proceedings of the IEEE 17th symposium on computer-based medical systems. Bethesda, MD; 2004.

26. Finkelstein J, Friedman RH. Potential role of telecommunication technologies in the management of chronic health conditions. Dis Manage Health Outcomes. 2000;8(2):57–63.

27. Finkelstein J, O'Connor G, Friedman RH. Development and implementation of the home asthma telemonitoring (HAT) system to facilitate asthma self-care. Medinfo. 2001;10(Pt 1):810–4.

28. Joshi A, Amelung P, Arora M, Finkelstein J. Clinical impact of home automated telemanagement in asthma. AMIA Annu Symp Proc. 2005:1000.

29. Rasmussen LM, Phanareth K, Nolte H, Backer V. Internet-based monitoring of asthma: a long-term, randomized clinical study of 300 asthmatic subjects. J Allergy Clin Immunol. 2005;115(6):1137–42.

30. Hee-Sung K. Impact of Web-based nurse's education on glycosylated haemoglobin in type 2 diabetic patients. J Clin Nurs. 2007;16(7):1361–6.

31. Montori VM, Helgemoe PK, Guyatt GH, Dean DS, Leung TW, Smith SA, et al. Telecare for patients with type 1 diabetes and inadequate glycemic control: a randomized controlled trial and meta-analysis. Diabetes Care. 2004;27(5):1088–94.

32. Shea S, Weinstock RS, Starren J, Teresi J, Palmas W, Field L, et al. A randomized trial comparing telemedicine case management with usual care in older, ethnically diverse, medically underserved patients with diabetes mellitus. J Am Med Inform Assoc. 2006;13(1):40–51.

33. Dang S, Ma F, Nedd N, Florez H, Aguilar E, Roos BA. Care coordination and telemedicine improves glycaemic control in ethnically diverse veterans with diabetes. J Telemed Telecare. 2007;13(5):263–7.

34. Quinn CC, Clough SS, Minor JM, Lender D, Okafor MC, Gruber-Baldini A. WellDoc mobile diabetes management randomized controlled trial: change in clinical and behavioral outcomes and patient and physician satisfaction. Diabetes Technol Ther. 2008;10(3):160–8.

35. Quinn CC, Gruber-Baldini AL, Shardell M, Weed K, Clough SS, Peeples M, et al. Mobile diabetes intervention study: testing a personalized treatment/behavioral communication intervention for blood glucose control. Contemp Clin Trials. 2009;30(4):334–46.

36. Barnett TE, Chumbler NR, Vogel WB, Beyth RJ, Qin H, Kobb R. The effectiveness of a care coordination home telehealth program for veterans with diabetes mellitus: a 2-year follow-up. Am J Manag Care. 2006;12(8):467–74.

37. Chumbler NR, Neugaard B, Kobb R, Ryan P, Qin H, Joo Y. Evaluation of a care coordination/home-telehealth program for veterans with diabetes: health services utilization and health-related quality of life. Eval Health Prof. 2005;28(4):464–78.

38. Howells L, Wilson AC, Skinner TC, Newton R, Morris AD, Greene SA. A randomized control trial of the effect of negotiated telephone support on glycaemic control in young people with Type 1 diabetes. Diabet Med. 2002;19(8):643–8.

39. Jaana M, Pare G. Home telemonitoring of patients with diabetes: a systematic assessment of observed effects. J Eval Clin Pract. 2007;13(2):242–53.

40. Roth A, Kajiloti I, Elkayam I, Sander J, Kehati M, Golovner M. Telecardiology for patients with chronic heart failure: the "SHL" experience in Israel. Int J Cardiol. 2004;97(1):49–55.

41. Schofield RS, Kline SE, Schmalfuss CM, Carver HM, Aranda Jr JM, Pauly DF, et al. Early outcomes of a care coordination-enhanced telehome care program for elderly veterans with chronic heart failure. Telemed J E Health. 2005;11(1):20–7.

42. Benatar D, Bondmass M, Ghitelman J, Avitall B. Outcomes of chronic heart failure. Arch Intern Med. 2003;163(3):347–52.

43. Castro HK, Cross RK, Finkelstein J. Using a home automated telemanagement (HAT) system: experiences and perceptions of patients with inflammatory bowel disease. AMIA Annu Symp Proc. 2006;872.

44. Cross RK, Arora M, Finkelstein J. Acceptance of telemanagement is high in patients with inflammatory bowel disease. J Clin Gastroenterol. 2006;40(3):200–8.

45. Cross RK, Finkelstein J. Feasibility and acceptance of a home telemanagement system in patients with inflammatory bowel disease: a 6-month pilot study. Dig Dis Sci. 2007;52(2):357–64.

46. Cross RK, Cheevers N, Finkelstein J. Home telemanagement for patients with ulcerative colitis (UC HAT). Dig Dis Sci. 2009;54(11):2463–72.

47. Seo M, Okada M, Yao T, Ueki M, Arima S, Okumura M. An index of disease activity in patients with ulcerative colitis. Am J Gastroenterol. 1992;87(8):971–6.

48. Cross RK, Cheevers N, Rustgi A, Langenberg P, Finkelstein J. Randomized, controlled trial of home telemanagement in patients with ulcerative colitis (UC HAT). Inflamm Bowel Dis. 2012;18(6):1018–25.

49. Elkjaer M, Burisch J, Avnstrom S, Lynge E, Munkholm P. Development of a Web-based concept for patients with ulcerative colitis and 5-aminosalicylic acid treatment. Eur J Gastroenterol Hepatol. 2010;22(6):695–704.

50. Irvine EJ, Zhou Q, Thompson AK. The short inflammatory bowel disease questionnaire: a quality of life instrument for community

physicians managing inflammatory bowel disease. CCRPT Investigators. Canadian Crohn's Relapse Prevention Trial. Am J Gastroenterol. 1996;91(8):1571–8.

51. Walmsley RS, Ayres RC, Pounder RE, Allan RN. A simple clinical colitis activity index. Gut. 1998;43(1):29–32.

52. Elkjaer M, Shuhaibar M, Burisch J, Bailey Y, Scherfig H, Laugesen B, et al. E-health empowers patients with ulcerative colitis: a randomised controlled trial of the web-guided "Constant-care" approach. Gut. 2010;59(12):1652–61.

53. Eaden JA, Abrams K, Mayberry JF. The Crohn's and colitis knowledge score: a test for measuring patient knowledge in inflammatory bowel disease. Am J Gastroenterol. 1999;94(12):3560–6.

54. Ware Jr JE, Sherbourne CD. The MOS 36-item short-form health survey (SF-36). I. Conceptual framework and item selection. Med Care. 1992;30(6):473–83.

55. Bjelland I, Dahl AA, Haug TT, Neckelmann D. The validity of the hospital anxiety and depression scale. An updated literature review. J Psychosom Res. 2002;52(2):69–77.

# Assessment of Disease Activity in Ulcerative Colitis

**32**

Rebecca Palmer, Alissa Walsh, and Simon Travis

**Keywords**

Ulcerative colitis • Remission • Mucosal healing

## Introduction

Management of ulcerative colitis (UC) is guided by the anatomical distribution of disease, severity of symptoms, response to medical therapy and ability of the patient to tolerate treatment. In its most severe form, acute ulcerative colitis can carry major morbidity and can be fatal. Disease severity indices help guide clinical decisions regarding appropriate initial treatment and are particularly helpful for patients who fail to show adequate response to first-line therapy but are also essential for evaluating therapeutic response and defining outcomes in clinical trials [1]. Indeed, severity indices were all developed for use in clinical trials, although almost none have been formally validated and none have had responsiveness defined in clinical practice.

Indices measure a "snapshot" of activity, but responsiveness has been assumed, rather than tested. This matters, because there are several steps in defining the properties of an index (see below). Initial validation of the index determines the intrinsic reliability (degree of intra- and interobserver variation, as well as interaction between descriptors) of the index. Thresholds for active disease (perhaps divided into mild/moderate/severe) and remission need to be set and tested, before responsiveness (the ability to detect change in disease activity) is determined. It is inherently improbable that patients relapse or respond to treatment in a linear fashion: indeed, clinical practice proves otherwise, since patients can relapse suddenly and severely or have a saltatory pattern of improvement in symptoms. Unfortunately, out of almost a dozen disease activity indices in UC [1], only the Pediatric Ulcerative Colitis Activity Index (PUCAI) [2] has formally been validated for symptom severity. Other measures for evaluating disease activity include endoscopy, quality of life and histopathology. Fortunately there are validated instruments for all these measures (unlike indices of symptoms), notably the Ulcerative Colitis Endoscopic Index of Severity (UCEIS) [3], Geboes Histopathology Index [4] and Inflammatory Bowel Disease Questionnaire (IBDQ) [5]. Nevertheless, with the exception of the PUCAI, uncertainty remains over their predictive value and their responsiveness in practice. Even a universal definition of remission has not been agreed for clinical trials or practice [6].

Although disparity between clinical, endoscopic and histological assessments of disease activity in ulcerative colitis (UC) has been recognised since 1956 [7], there has been little systematic study of the relationship. Comparisons between measures of disease activity in UC show relatively poor correlation between the different measures, but this should be expected: were any one measure to match another, then one of the two would be irrelevant.

Consequently, there are many challenges with the formal evaluation of disease activity in UC, but the problems are further compounded by confusing terminology, different names or abbreviations for the same index and the tendency to use composite indices that combine symptoms with endoscopy and quality of life. Subjective terms (Physician's Global Assessment) are introduced as a fudge factor to

R. Palmer, M.R.C.P. • S. Travis, D.Phil., F.R.C.P. (✉)
Translational Gastroenterology Unit, John Radcliffe Hospital, Oxford OX3 9DU, UK
e-mail: rebeccapalmer@doctors.org; simon.travis@ndm.ox.ac.uk

A. Walsh, F.R.A.C.P.
Gastroenterology Unit, St. Vincent's Hospital, Sydney, NSW, Australia
e-mail: alissa.walsh@gmail.com

G.R. Lichtenstein (ed.), *Medical Therapy of Ulcerative Colitis*,
DOI 10.1007/978-1-4939-1677-1_32, © Springer Science+Business Media New York 2014

345

**Table 32.1** List of disease activity indices for UC, with common synonyms and abbreviations

| Type of index | Index main name | aka[a] | Abbreviation | Reference |
|---|---|---|---|---|
| Symptoms | Partial Mayo score | | | [13] |
| | Simple clinical colitis activity index | | SCCAI | [14] |
| | Modified Truelove and Witts index | Lichtiger score | MTWSI | [15] |
| | Ulcerative colitis clinical score | | UCCS | [16] |
| | Paediatric ulcerative colitis activity index | | PUCAI | [2] |
| | Beattie paediatric UC index | | | [17] |
| Symptoms and endoscopy | Mayo Clinic score | Disease activity index; Mayo score | DAI | [18] |
| | Sutherland index | Ulcerative colitis disease activity index | UCDAI | [19] |
| | Powell-Tuck index | St Mark's score | PTI | [20] |
| | Rachmilewitz index | Clinical activity index | CAI | [21] |
| Symptoms and biomarkers[b] | Seo index | Activity index | Seo | [22] |
| | Truelove and Witts index | | T&W | [23] |
| | Montréal classification | | | [24] |
| Endoscopy[c] | Baron score | | Baron | [16, 25] |
| | Modified Mayo Clinic endoscopy subscore | Mayo endoscopy score | | [18] |
| | Rachmilewitz endoscopy subscore | | | [21] |
| | Endoscopy activity index | | EAI | [26] |
| | Ulcerative colitis endoscopic index of severity | | UCEIS | [3] |
| Histopathology | Geboes | | | [4] |
| | Riley | | | [27] |
| | Saverymuttu | | | [28] |
| | Truelove and Richards histology index | | | [7] |
| Quality of life | Inflammatory bowel disease questionnaire | | IBDQ | [5] |
| | Short inflammatory bowel disease questionnaire | | SIBDQ | [29] |
| | UK inflammatory bowel disease questionnaire | | UKIBDQ | [30] |
| | Rating form of IBD patient concerns | | | [31] |

[a]*aka* also known as
[b]Biomarkers: haemoglobin, albumin or erythrocyte sedimentation rate
[c]Only the most common endoscopic indices are included (see Table 32.3)

allow an overall impression, because of limitations in the sensitivity of objective measures of assessment to distinguish between mild and moderately active disease. It is therefore hardly surprising that people are confused about relative drug efficacy or outcomes in clinical trials, since the activity index, endpoints and measures of response or remission may all differ between trials [1]. The development of an index of disease activity should follow a multistep process of descriptor (item) generation, reduction, grading and weighting [8–10]. The final product, the clinical index, is then evaluated to define cut-off scores that correspond to clinically important disease states covering the spectrum from remission to severe disease activity. Once the instrument has been developed, it must be evaluated for its psychometric properties including validity, reliability, responsiveness and feasibility [5, 11, 12].

In an attempt to reduce confusion in terminology, the word "index" refers to an instrument for assessing disease activity; "descriptor" refers to an item within that index with the level of severity often allocated on a Likert scale. The word "level" (as in the level of a Likert scale) is used to refer to the severity graded for an item. The word "score," so often used as a synonym for index, is best used to describe the overall measure provided by an index. Common usage has often confused these terms, but they will be used as consistently as possible in this chapter. To reduce confusion in the names of indices, synonyms and abbreviations, common names and abbreviations for indices used in UC are summarised (Table 32.1) [13–31].

**Table 32.2** Commonly used index scores for defining remission, mild, moderate or severe activity[a]

| Index | Remission[b] | Mild | Moderate | Severe | Other |
|---|---|---|---|---|---|
| Simple clinical colitis activity index | ≤2 | 3–5 | 6–9 | ≥10 | <3 Validated for remission and ≥5 for active disease |
| Modified Truelove and Witts index | ≤3 | 4–6 | 7–11 | ≥12 | |
| Ulcerative colitis clinical score | ≤1 | 2–4 | 5–9 | ≥10 | |
| PUCAI | ≤10 | | | | Predictive |
| Mayo Clinic score | ≤2 | 3–5 | 6–10 | ≥11 | |
| Sutherland index | ≤2 | 3–5 | 6–8 | ≥9 | |
| Powell-Tuck index | ≤3 | 4–10 if endoscopy ≤1 | 4–10 if endoscopy ≥2 | ≥11 | |
| Rachmilewitz index | ≤2 | ≤8 | >8 | | |
| Seo index | <108 | 120–<150 | 150–220 | >220 | |
| Truelove and Witts index | No definition | <4 Bloody tools/day, no systemic features | In between | ≥6 Bloody stools/day, with $P$ >90 bpm, or $T$ >37.8 °C, or Hb <10.5 g/dL, or ESR >30 mm/h | |

[a]Thresholds vary between clinical trials; see prospective comparison of indices [33]; some clinical trials continue to use inappropriate definitions of remission, especially those using a Rachmilewitz score ≤4 [6, 33]

[b]Criteria are more complex than indicated, since they may be contingent on subscores for rectal bleeding, stool frequency, endoscopy or change from the initial score [1, 33]

## Evaluating Symptomatic Activity

In clinical practice we conventionally assess patients' symptoms, but often this is done without using activity indices to guide management, perhaps with the exception of Truelove and Witts' criteria to define acute severe colitis [32]. Many indices have arbitrarily assigned quantitative scores for improvement and lack rigorous design or evaluation but have been used in clinical trials [33]. Indices tend to have been designed for particular disease severities or purpose (such as the MTWSI for hospitalised patients with severe colitis, in contrast to the Mayo Clinic score for outpatients with mild or moderately active disease). Therefore, if applied to patients with a different pattern of disease, activity may be over- or underestimated, which causes further confusion when interpreting outcome data.

*Partial Mayo Score.* Six indices evaluate symptoms independently of endoscopic scoring or biochemical markers (Table 32.1). The Partial Mayo score evolved from the need to evaluate patients in clinical trials during the interval between endoscopies [34]. Although readily criticised because it is an unvalidated derivation of an unvalidated index, it serves a purpose when examining the speed of symptom relief or trends in response. When compared with other noninvasive indices, it performed well for discriminating remission from active disease and responsiveness [33] but depends on a Physician's Global Assessment (PGA).

*Simple Clinical Colitis Activity Index.* The Simple Clinical Colitis Activity Index [14] was based on the Powell-Tuck Index, modified to exclude sigmoidoscopic assessment but to include nocturnal bowel movements and urgency of defecation. Urgency is a symptom of vital importance to patients, but neglected by other indices. The general well-being score was based on the Harvey-Bradshaw Index for Crohn's disease [35]. The index was derived from a study of 57 patients with variable disease extent and severity. It included hospitalised patients. Scores range from 0 to 19 points, with generally applied thresholds shown in Table 32.2. It has been compared prospectively with the Partial Mayo score, Lichtiger (MTWSI), PUCAI, Rachmilewitz (CAI) and Seo indices in 86 adult patients [33]. Along with the PUCAI, it performed best of all noninvasive indices for validity, reliability, responsiveness and feasibility. Since it does not include a PGA, it can readily be completed by patients.

*Modified Truelove and Witts Severity Index.* The MTWSI (Lichtiger Index) was introduced during a pilot study of cyclosporine for acute severe colitis in 1990 [15]. It is important to remember that like its progenitor (Truelove & Witts' Index), the focus was on patients with severe colitis and it may be less responsive or reliable for patients with less severe disease. The MTWSI has a score of 0–21 and comprises eight descriptors: number of daily stools, nocturnal stools, visible blood in stools, faecal incontinence, abdominal pain/cramping, general well-being and need for antidiarrhoeal agents. The authors arbitrarily defined "response" as a

50 % decrease in baseline score, and remission was subsequently defined as a score ≤3 [36] although this does not necessarily mean absence of symptoms. Although neither the score, thresholds nor response has been validated, it quantitates activity which the original Truelove & Witts' Index fails to do, so it may yet be the most suitable index for trials on hospitalised patients with acute severe UC [37].

*Ulcerative Colitis Clinical Score.* The Ulcerative Colitis Clinical Score was designed for a placebo-controlled trial of an α(alpha)4β(beta)7 integrin antagonist for UC [16]. The UCCS is a modification of the Mayo Clinic score excluding endoscopy, so it is very similar to the Partial Mayo score. It comprises four descriptors: stool frequency, rectal bleeding, patient's functional status and PGA. By including patient's functional status in the index, it differs from the Partial Mayo score (which comprises the three other descriptors, even though functional status is separately scored). Although remission (score 0 or 1, as long as the endoscopy score was 0–1 on a modified Baron grading defined in the paper) and response (improvement by ≥3 points) were described, neither the score nor these thresholds have been validated. Nevertheless, it disarticulated symptom scoring from endoscopy, even though it recognised interdependence in the PGA. The Partial Mayo score has largely superseded the UCCS for clinical trials, since the full Mayo Clinic score is currently (2012) the most widely used index in trial design.

*Pediatric Ulcerative Colitis Activity Index.* The PUCAI was devised by paediatric gastroenterologists to provide a noninvasive instrument to assess disease activity in children in whom repeated endoscopy is less acceptable to patients and parents [2]. It comprises six descriptors with different levels, creating a total score ranging from 0 to 85: abdominal pain, rectal bleeding, average stool consistency, number of stool in 24 h, nocturnal stools and activity level. The PUCAI was rigorously developed using descriptor generation by a group of 36 experts and descriptor weighting by stepwise multiple regression analysis of prospectively collected data from 157 paediatric UC patients. Validation was assessed on a separate prospective cohort of 48 children with UC undergoing colonoscopy. Responsiveness was evaluated at follow-up visits in 75 children. It has predictive value for children admitted with acute severe colitis, for whom it has become the standard of care for evaluating activity and decision-making (see below). The PUCAI has also been shown to be valid, reliable and responsive in adults [33]. This may permit less frequent endoscopic assessment for patients with UC both in clinical practice and clinical trials [33].

Beattie and colleagues developed a disease activity instrument for children in a study published in 1996 [17]. This index generated a numerical score from 0 to 10 with four descriptors: stool frequency, rectal bleeding, abdominal pain and rectal prolapse. It has been evaluated in adults but did not perform as well as the PUCAI (which supersedes it in children) or the SCCAI [33].

## Composite Clinical and Endoscopic Indices

Several disease activity instruments combine clinical symptoms, endoscopy and quality of life descriptors into a composite index. This is superficially appealing, because the physician in clinical practice considers all aspects and makes a judgement. Nevertheless, the subjectivity of that judgement creates concern for consistency, and validating a composite index creates particular difficulty, where interaction between descriptors has to be evaluated. It is easier to separately validate the symptomatic, endoscopic, quality of life and (if appropriate) histological components. Indeed, since independent indices have been validated for all aspects bar symptoms, a composite index appears to swim against the tide. On the other hand, the archetypal composite index, the Mayo Clinic score, is the index most widely used in clinical trials. This has an inherent value, since it allows the efficacy of different trials to be compared, assuming the same endpoints and definitions of response [38, 39]. Nevertheless, not many gastroenterologists routinely use the Mayo Clinic score in clinical practice.

*Mayo Clinic Score.* The Disease Activity Index (DAI) was first described in 1987 for a placebo-controlled trial of mesalamine for active UC [18]. There are four descriptors: stool frequency, rectal bleeding, findings at proctosigmoidoscopy and PGA. The stool frequency score is not an absolute number, but relative to "normal" for that subject, which may itself introduce variation between observers that has yet to be quantified. Symptoms are assessed over 3 days: some clinical trialists take the average of symptom scores, others the worst score in the 3 days preceding the visit. Scores range from 0 to 12 points. The physician has access to the patient's functional assessment as a measure of general well-being when determining the PGA, but the patient's functional assessment is not used to calculate the score. Definitions of remission and improvement depend on descriptor subscores. Complete resolution is defined as a DAI of 0 (normal stool frequency, no rectal bleeding, normal proctosigmoidoscopy and a PGA of 0). Response has been defined as improvement in the PGA and at least one other item subscore and no worsening in any other descriptor subscore, although definitions of response vary [1]. A more liberal definition of remission (≤2) has been recognised by the FDA for registration trials of infliximab in the treatment of UC [34]. A trial endpoint is more easily reached with a lower threshold (i.e. a higher score) for remission. This is apparent from the ACT

(Active Ulcerative Colitis Trials [ACT] I and II) of infliximab for patients with UC refractory to standard therapy. The definition of remission was a DAI ≤2, with no individual subscore >1 [34]. When this definition was applied to a population of patients without treatment-refractory disease in a retrospective analysis of two large trials of mesalazine [40, 41], the remission rate for 2.4 g mesalazine increased from 22 % (according to the original trial definition) to 50 % [42]. The Mayo Clinic score is the activity index for UC against which others have to be compared; at present (2012) the advantages of common usage outweigh its inherent disadvantages.

*Sutherland Index.* The UC Disease Activity Index (UCDAI) was originally used in a placebo-controlled trial of mesalamine enemas for the treatment of distal UC [19]. This is a notably different patient population to the MTWSI (above). It is a simplified composite index, quite similar to the Mayo Clinic score, incorporating four descriptors: stool frequency relative to normal, rectal bleeding, endoscopic mucosal appearance and the PGA. Scores range from 0 to 12 points. Subsequent studies defined remission as a DAI of 1, with a score of 0 for rectal bleeding and 0 for stool frequency and at least a 1 point reduction from baseline in sigmoidoscopy score with friability moved from a score of 1 to two within the sigmoidoscopy score making a more stringent definition of remission [1]. The Sutherland Index has not been formally validated. The relative simplicity of the index provides a means of reducing the impact of physician and patient subjectivity in disease scoring. The index has been adopted in large clinical studies [43, 44]. Of particular note, a score <2.5 points has been shown to correlate with patient-defined remission [45], indicating that sigmoidoscopy contributes little to the definition of remission in clinical practice.

*Powell-Tuck Index.* The PTI was originally developed at St Mark's Hospital, London, when comparing dosing schedules of oral prednisolone for the treatment of active UC [20]. The index scores from 0 to 20 points and includes ten descriptors: general well-being, abdominal pain, bowel frequency, stool consistency, bleeding, nausea/vomiting, anorexia, abdominal tenderness, extra-intestinal manifestations and fever. Later studies used a variation of the PTI which added an extra two possible points by including a sigmoidoscopy assessment score. Remission was defined as a score of 0 and improvement as a decrease in the baseline score 2 or more points. Neither the PTI nor the definitions of remission or improvement have been validated, but the index was the basis for developing the SCCAI (above). The relative complexity reflects the lack of validation, which would have identified redundant descriptors. It is unlikely to have a role in future clinical trials and is impracticable for everyday practice.

*Rachmilewitz Index.* The Clinical Activity Index (CAI) was originally used in a controlled trial of coated mesalamine compared to sulfasalazine for the treatment of active UC. This index generates a score from 0 to 29 points based on seven descriptors: number of stools weekly, presence of blood, investigators global assessment of symptomatic state, abdominal pain/cramps, temperature, extra-intestinal manifestations and laboratory findings (ESR and haemoglobin). It continues to be used in some clinical trials [46]. Like many indices, the CAI considers an "investigator's global assessment" to be an essential component. This, however, introduces a layer of subjectivity, depending on the amount and quality of time spent with the patient. Similarly, the endoscopic element of the CAI depends on the subjective assessment of mucosal properties, including friability. Its main weakness is that clinical remission has come to be defined as any score less than that used to define disease activity (CAI score >4). By this measure, a score ≤4 points includes a level of symptoms that cannot conceivably be used to define remission: this might mean, for instance, that a patient with 36–60 stools/week (score 2) and a little blood in the stools (score 2, total=4) met the criteria for "remission"! It fails to recognise the simple fact that there is a "grey area" in scoring systems between the level used to define remission and the threshold used for defining disease activity. In the prospective comparison of different disease activity indices, a score ≤2 best reflected remission [33].

## Composite Symptom and Biomarker Indices

*Seo Index.* The Activity Index (a term best avoided, since it is so readily confused with CAI, DAI or UCDAI) was devised using multivariate regression analysis, similar to that used to develop the Crohn's Disease Activity Index (CDAI) [22]. 18 clinical, laboratory and sigmoidoscopy variables were initially derived from prospective data collected from 72 patients during 85 clinical events. The Seo needs a calculator: $60 \times$ blood in the stool + $13 \times$ bowel movements + $0.5 \times$ ESR − $4 \times$ haemoglobin (in g/dL) − $15 \times$ albumin + 200. When correlated against the MTWSI as a standard, subjects in remission had a mean Seo of $100 \pm 11$: 90 % those with mild disease had scores <150; 83 % those with moderate activity had scores between 150 and 220 and those with severe disease on average scored above 220. The definition of remission was therefore set at 120, but a prospective comparison has shown that a score of 108 is more appropriate [33]. This comparison, however, showed that the Seo failed one of the four fundamental psychometric criteria for indices: that of feasibility. It also performed less well than others with regard to discriminative ability, test-retest reliability and responsiveness. Nevertheless, a subsequent study in patients with moderate to severe UC suggested that the Seo Index might have predictive value:

following 2 weeks treatment with intravenous corticosteroids, 65 % of subjects with a score >180 underwent colectomy [47], and following infliximab treatment, the index predicted response to therapy or need for colectomy [48]. Indices such as the Seo use multiple biomarkers and may yet identify patients who meet the "regulatory definition" of remission, without the need for endoscopy (i.e. patients with no more than grade I or II on a modified Baron endoscopic score), and the absence of visible blood are identified using a cut-off score of <120 [45]. The associations are relatively weak (around 60 %) and the index is too complex to use in practice.

*Truelove and Witts.* The first instrument to assess disease activity in UC was devised in 1955 by Truelove and Witts in the first clinical trial in gastroenterology, evaluating cortisone treatment for UC [23]. This index has five descriptors: bloody stool frequency, temperature, heart rate, haemoglobin and erythrocyte sedimentation rate (ESR). The original instrument provided definitions for mild and severe UC, with all cases in-between classified as moderate. This apparent lack of precision is off-set by the objective criteria for defining (acute) severe colitis, which are widely used to define a course of action (hospital admission for intravenous therapy, in 27/32 trials of steroids for UC) [49] and which predict outcome [50]. Its principal disadvantage is that it does not generate a quantitative activity score, which makes it unsuitable for assessing outcomes in clinical trials. Instead, ambiguous terms for evaluating response were originally proposed ("improved," "no change" or "worse"), which have no place in clinical trials today [1]. On the other hand, the T&W Index is the most amenable for daily clinical practice by defining acute severe colitis and continues to be used as an entry or exclusion criteria for clinical trials (e.g. CONSTRUCT ISRCTN22663589) and is almost universally recommended by national or international guidelines for the management of acute severe colitis [51–53].

*Montréal Classification.* The Montréal Classification was developed by an international working group for the World Congress of Gastoenterology in 2006 [54]. It incorporates both extent of disease, divided into proctitis (distal to the rectosigmoid junction=E1), left sided (distal to the splenic flexure=E2) and pancolitis (proximal to splenic flexure=E2) and severity. The severity scores are based on the Truelove and Witts Index, with S0=remission [54]. Mild activity (S1) was defined as 4 or fewer bloody stools/day without signs of systemic toxicity and with a normal ESR. Moderate activity (S2) was defined as more than 4 bloody stools/day, with minimal systemic toxicity. Severe colitis was defined in the classical T&W description, with 6 or more bloody stools/day with a pulse >90 bpm, temperature >37.8 °C, haemoglobin <10.5 g/dL or ESR >30 mm/h. The index is pragmatic and

was meant to be applied in clinical practice, especially with regard to large clinical studies (such as those involving genetics or disease databases), but although responsiveness has never formally been tested, it appears too insensitive for use in clinical trials—other than as a threshold for defining acute severe colitis.

## Evaluating Endoscopic Activity

Endoscopic indices evolved from the Baron score, initially developed for rigid proctoscopy in ambulatory patients with mild to moderate disease, which rated mucosal bleeding and friability [25]. Subsequent endoscopic indices were of increasing complexity and incorporated the presence of ulcers, mucopus, granularity or light scattering in addition to bleeding and friability [18, 19, 54, 55]. Such modifications were intended to improve the capture of disease activity, but they invariably increased the subjectivity of the scoring system.

In clinical practice, endoscopic assessment of disease activity is used to confirm diagnosis and assess disease activity. Endoscopic confirmation of disease improvement is uncommon in clinical practice if the patient's symptoms have resolved. In the context of clinical trials, endoscopic assessment has a key role for measuring outcome, because it is intended to be independent of symptom score. The newly introduced term of "mucosal healing" has shown that where treatment achieves this within 8 weeks, this correlates with a lower colectomy rate over the succeeding 12 months ($p=0.0004$) and steroid-free remission ($p<0.0001$) [56]. In composite indices its relative weighting varies. The FDA currently uses two measures for defining remission: endoscopic mucosal healing and rectal bleeding. Although considerable efforts have been made to derive a patient symptom score that negates the need for endoscopy [45] and the endoscopic component of some, symptom scores (such as the UCDAI) have been calculated to contribute only 2.5 % of the total score [45]. There has been renewed interest in endoscopy with the advent of a validated endoscopic scoring system [3]. Efforts have been made to compare indices, which have resulted in another activity index that shows good interobserver agreement ((kappa)$\kappa=0.65$–$0.79$ between 4 expert endoscopists) but has not followed the criteria for index development (Table 32.3) [57].

*Ulcerative Colitis Endoscopic Index of Severity.* The UCEIS (Table 32.4) was developed because there was wide interobserver variation in endoscopic assessment [3]. There was only 76 % agreement for "severe" and 27 % agreement for "normal" endoscopic mucosal appearances between 10 experienced investigators and a central reader. 30 different investigators then rated 25/60 different videos for 10

**Table 32.3** Endoscopic indices of disease activity in UC: activity thresholds

| Endoscopic index | Remission | Mild | Moderate | Severe |
|---|---|---|---|---|
| Truelove and Witts [23] | Ambiguous terms without definitions have not been widely utilised for endoscopic assessment | | | |
| Matts' endoscopic grading [58] | Normal | Mild granularity of the mucosa, with mild contact bleeding | Marked granularity and oedema of mucosa, contact bleeding, and spontaneous bleeding | Severe ulceration of mucosa with haemorrhage |
| Baron score [25] | Normal: Matt mucosa, ramifying vascular pattern clearly visible throughout, no spontaneous bleeding, no bleeding to light touch (0) | Abnormal but not haemorrhagic: appearances between (0) and (2) | Moderately haemorrhagic: bleeding to light touch, but no spontaneous bleeding seen ahead of instrument on initial inspection (2) | Severely haemorrhagic: spontaneous bleeding seen ahead of instrument at initial inspection and bleeds to light touch (3) |
| Modified Baron [16] | Normal mucosa (0) | Granular mucosa with abnormal vascular pattern (1) | Friable mucosa (2) | Micro-ulceration of mucosa with spontaneous bleeding (3)    Denuded mucosa (4) |
| Powell-Tuck sigmoidoscopic assessment [20] | Non-haemorrhagic (0) | | Friable (1) | Spontaneous bleeding (2) |
| Blackstone index [59] | Distorted or absent mucosal vascular pattern = 1 Granularity = 2 | Continuous or focal erythema = 3 Friability (touch bleeding) = 4 | Mucopurulent exudate (mucopus) = 5 Single or multiple ulcers (<5 mm), fewer than 10 per 10-cm Segment = 6 | Large ulcers (>5 mm); more than 10 per 10-cm segment = 7 Spontaneous bleeding = 8 |
| Rachmilewitz Endoscopic Index [21] | Granulation scattering reflected light: No = 0 Yes = 2 | Vascular Pattern: Normal = 0 Faded/disturbed = 1 Completely absent = 2 | Vulnerability of mucosa: None = 0 Slightly increased (contact bleeding) = 2 Greatly increased (spontaneous bleeding) = 4 | Mucosal damage (mucous, fibrin, exudates, erosions, ulcer): None = 0 Slight = 2 Pronounced = 4 |
| Mayo Clinic flexible proctoscopy assessment [18] | Normal or inactive disease | Mild disease (erythema, decreased vascular pattern, mild friability) | Moderate disease (marked erythema, absent vascular pattern, friability, erosions) | Severe disease (spontaneous bleeding, ulceration) |
| Modified Mayo Clinic proctoscopy score [60] | Normal | Erythema, decreased vascular pattern and minimal granularity | Marked erythema, friability, granularity, absent vascular pattern, bleeding with minimal trauma and no ulcerations | Ulceration and spontaneous bleeding |
| Sutherland mucosal appearance assessment [19] | Normal | Mild friability | Moderate friability | Exudation, spontaneous haemorrhage |
| Endoscopic activity index [26] | Scale 0–16, describing size and depth of ulcers, redness, bleeding, mucosal oedema and mucous exudates with a higher score indicating the more severe condition | | | |
| Modified 6-point activity index | Scale 1–6, describing vascular pattern, erythema, oedema, friability, erosions and ulcers of different size or number | | | |
| Ulcerative Colitis Endoscopic Index of Severity (UCEIS) [3, 61] | Scale 0–8, based on three descriptors: vascular pattern (three levels); mucosal bleeding (4 levels) and erosions and ulcers (4 levels), giving a range 0–8 that covers normal endoscopy to the most severe UC seen by independent investigators (accounts for 94 % of variance between observers, $R^2 = 0.94$) | | | |

descriptors and assessed overall severity on a 0–100 visual analogue scale. Kappa statistics tested inter- and intra-observer variability for each descriptor. Kappa statistics ranged from 0.34–0.65 to 0.30–0.45 within and between observers for the ten descriptors. Different models to predict the overall assessment of severity as judged by a visual analogue scale were developed using general linear mixed regression. The final model incorporated just three

**Table 32.4** The Ulcerative Colitis Endoscopic Index of Severity (UCEIS) [3, 61]

| Descriptor (score most severe lesions) | Likert scale anchor points | Definition |
|---|---|---|
| Vascular pattern | Normal (0) | Normal vascular pattern with arborisation of capillaries clearly defined or with blurring or patchy loss of capillary margins |
| | Patchy obliteration (1) | Patchy obliteration of vascular pattern |
| | Obliterated (2) | Complete obliteration of vascular pattern |
| Bleeding | None (0) | No visible blood |
| | Mucosal (1) | Some spots or streaks of coagulated blood on the surface of the mucosa ahead of the scope, which can be washed away |
| | Luminal mild (2) | Some free liquid blood in the lumen |
| | Luminal moderate or severe (3) | Frank blood in the lumen ahead of endoscope or visible oozing from mucosa after washing intraluminal blood or visible oozing from a haemorrhagic mucosa |
| Erosions and ulcers | None (0) | Normal mucosa, no visible erosions or ulcers |
| | Erosions (1) | Tiny (≤5 mm) defects in the mucosa, of a white or yellow colour with a flat edge |
| | Superficial ulcer (2) | Larger (>5 mm) defects in the mucosa, which are discrete fibrin-covered ulcers when compared to erosions but remain superficial |
| | Deep ulcer (3) | Deeper excavated defects in the mucosa, with a slightly raised edge |

Copyright Warner Chilcott Pharmaceuticals (index is freely available for use)

descriptors, each with precise definitions (Table 32.4). A third validation phase used another 25 different investigators from North America and Europe, who assessed in a randomly selected subset of 28/60 videos, including two duplicated videos to assess test-retest reliability. Intra-observer Kappa values were 0.82, 0.72 and 0.78 for vascular pattern, bleeding and erosions and ulcers descriptors and interobserver Kappa values were 0.83, 0.56, and 0.77, respectively. The correlation between UCEIS and overall severity evaluation was 0.94 ($p < 0.0001$) [59–61].

The UCEIS dispensed with the term "mucosal friability," because the model including friability as a descriptor did not perform significantly better than one including bleeding and the term friability always needs explanation, while bleeding is well understood. In practical terms, the most severely affected part of the mucosa is scored. There are, however, still limitations: thresholds for remission, mild, moderate and severe disease have yet to be set. The extent to which full colonoscopy may influence the score compared to the flexible sigmoidoscopy upon which it was based has only started to be evaluated [62]. How knowledge of symptoms influences the score also needs further evaluation, while the UCEIS also needs formal evaluation compared to the Mayo Clinic endoscopy subscore. All this is work in progress. Nevertheless, the UCEIS is simple enough to use in clinical practice and should achieve its goal of reducing variation in endoscopic assessment of activity between observers.

## Histological Assessment

Histological assessment of activity in UC is important not just to confirm the diagnosis, but once this is established, to confirm that symptoms are due to active disease rather than some other cause. Normal rectal mucosal biopsies effectively exclude active ulcerative colitis as a cause of symptoms. Although normal histopathology does not exclude a diagnosis of ulcerative colitis since the mucosa may return to normal during remission, it is completely at odds with the presence of active disease. A biopsy serves as an independent arbiter of activity, since there is appreciable interobserver variation in assessing endoscopy, even among experienced observers [3]. It may also have prognostic value since patients with persistent microscopic inflammation are more likely to relapse [27, 63]. In a study of 91 patients followed up for a median 29 months, clinical, endoscopic and histological measures of disease activity agreed in 53/91 (58 %, 28/53 remission, 25/53 active disease), indicating moderate agreement ($k = 0.44$) [64]. The strongest predictor of steroid-free remission over the following 2.5 years was the concordance of all three measures of remission (HR 0.20; 95 % CI 0.08–0.47, $p < 0.001$). Histological remission was the only measure associated with lower hospitalisation rates (HR 0.27; 95 % CI 0.07–0.99, $p = 0.048$), with a trend to lower colectomy rates (HR 0.15; 95 % CI 0.02–1.28, $p = 0.08$) in this small sample.

Currently no single histopathology index meets all needs, but the Geboes Index has been validated and tested for reproducibility. It has 6 descriptors: architectural disturbance, chronic inflammatory infiltrate, lamina propria inflammatory infiltrate, epithelial neutrophils, crypt destruction and erosion or ulceration [4]. Its main advantage is validation that shows that it reliably discriminates active from inactive disease. Its principal disadvantage from a clinical trial's perspective is that it was designed for use in clinical practice and a cumulative numerical score was consciously avoided. Hence it does not readily lend itself to evaluating histological response. The Riley Index also has 6 parameters which include presence of crypt abscesses and mucin depletion [27]. Its main value is its potential for predicting relapse: in 82 people with clinically quiescent UC, 52 % relapsed if they had an acute inflammatory infiltrate of neutrophils on rectal biopsy, whereas in the absence of such an infiltrate only 25 % relapsed ($p=0.02$).

Use of a pictorial scale to convey precise definitions improves interobserver agreement [4]. There are several other histopathology indices (Table 32.1). That of Truelove and Richards [7] is simple and has been correlated with endoscopy and also with long-term outcome [64]. Matts' histopathology grading is popular in Japan [57, 58] but is rarely used in the West now that the Geboes Index has been validated. That described by Saverymuttu [28] is also simple and has been compared with an independent measure of disease activity (indium 111-labelled granulocyte scanning). It has been used in recent clinical trials to confirm disease activity at entry and for evaluating improvement in response to treatment [65]. Detailed appraisals of histopathology for evaluating UC have been published [66].

## Evaluating Quality of Life

When consulting with patients, we are very familiar with establishing the pattern of symptoms but are not always so good at recognising how they impact on the patient's daily life. It is important to recognise that aims of medical therapy for the patient may differ from that of the physician. For example, the patient is likely to be most concerned with resolution of symptoms and few side effects, compared to the physician's focus, which may be on endoscopic mucosal healing for predicting the future course of disease. Assessment of quality of life is inevitably subjective and therefore can be difficult to interpret. Interested readers are referred to recent reviews [67, 68].

Formal assessment of quality of life in clinical practice has been limited but has gained much greater importance in clinical trial design over the last 20 years. It has been recommended that that the inflammatory bowel disease questionnaire (IBDQ) [5] and short form-36 (SF-36) [69] are used routinely as a secondary outcome measure in prospective randomised controlled trials of medical treatment in UC to be sure that quality of life has improved [1]. Most studies use a combination of generic and disease-specific health-related quality of life (HRQOL) instruments. One of the most commonly used generic instruments is the SF-36 which has been validated in several clinical conditions including UC, in several languages and countries including the USA and UK. It is composed of 8 health concept subscores covering physical, social, emotional and mental health [69]. The EuroQol or EQ-5D is another example of a generic HRQOL instrument which has been used in trials in many diseases in many countries [70]. It was designed to be self-administered and well suited to postal surveys. It is relatively simple with five domains, mobility, self-care, usual activities, pain/discomfort and anxiety/depression, and has the advantage of taking only a few minutes to complete. It has become the standard for assessment used by institutions such as the National Institute for Health and Clinical Excellence (NICE) in the UK.

Disease-specific instruments for UC include the IBDQ which has been validated in Canada and the USA and in different languages [5, 30]. The IBDQ uses 32 items in four subcategories, bowel, systemic, social and emotional, and can be either self-administered or interviewer-administered. A self-administered version and a shortened version of the IBDQ have also been validated [29]. More recently, an anglicised version the UK-IBDQ [30] has been validated in the UK and is currently being used as the primary outcome measure, with EQ-5D as secondary outcome measure, in a nationwide UK clinical trial evaluating infliximab versus cyclosporine for steroid-refractory acute severe colitis [71]. The rating form for IBD patient concerns [31, 72] is no longer used in clinical trials, or in practice, with the advent of the IBDQ.

When interpreting clinical trials, HRQOL instruments are usually the outcome of most relevance to patients, even if quality of life tracks disease activity evaluated by other indices. Physicians generally underestimate the impact of UC in patients who appear to be leading a normal life [73]. Patient global self-assessment of disease activity correlates poorly with objective measures of disease activity [74] and is worse than the Physician's Global Assessment, illustrating the importance of a patient-rated HRQOL scale when evaluating treatment effect. Traditional indices often ignore symptoms which matter to patients and highlighted by focus groups [73]. Other outcomes that may matter greatly to patients but are not directly measured by indices commonly used in therapeutic trials for UC include, for example, the number of hospitalisations, number of work days missed due to symptoms or even the colectomy rate. The reason is not hard to discern: clinical trials generally last 12 months at most, which is a brief period in the course of a disease that lasts a life time. It is therefore easier to show a therapeutic effect on symptom or endoscopy scores than it is on relatively uncommon outcomes that may matter more to patients. Surgeons have been better than physicians in evaluating the impact of their (surgical) treatment on the quality of life for patients with UC [74].

## Predictive Indices

The need for colectomy requires careful judgement. While early colectomy may be unnecessary, delayed colectomy may have significant morbidity and can be fatal. Therefore it is important to consider the factors that help predict those who are likely to fail medical therapy and require rescue therapy or indicate the need for timely surgery [73]. It is worth noting that these are all slightly different outcomes. It should also be remembered that current indices relate to the failure of steroid therapy and do not necessarily translate to failure of other therapies or infection complicating colitis. Factors which may predict the need for colectomy can be broadly divided into clinical, laboratory, radiological, endoscopic and genetic. Many have focussed on steroid failure, but some prospective studies also included patients treated with ciclosporin or infliximab [32, 75–77]. Most predictive indices are composites, combining two or more factors. To be clinically useful, an index must be easy to remember, simple to apply and reliable. Validation of indices for acute severe colitis is needed to avoid surgical decisions based on clinical impression, rather than objective assessment.

*Clinical markers* can help predict the risk of colectomy, and therefore objective clinical parameters can help with management decisions. They generally depend on the objective measures of stool frequency, pulse or temperature. A stool frequency >12/day on day 2 was associated with 55 % colectomy in a retrospective study of 189 admissions in 166 patients [78], while a frequency >8/day on day 3 of intensive treatment predicted colectomy in 85 % ($p < 0.001$) on that admission in a prospective analysis of 51 admissions [32]. Stool frequency has been validated in 128 children: in the only prospective study yet to compare different indices, the number of daily stools on day 3 (closely followed by amount of blood in the stool) was the main factor identified in multivariate analysis associated with lack of response to intravenous steroids [77]. The value of this Pediatric Ulcerative Colitis Activity Index (PUCAI) [2] to facilitate the decision about "rescue" therapy has been demonstrated [78, 79]. The question of what counts as a "stool" is not trivial. There is no standardisation, and it is generally regarded as an evacuation (be it blood, liquid or solid stool) that is counted as a bowel movement by the nursing staff. This is inevitably imprecise. Other clinical factors have been considered, including disease extent, duration, previous therapy (steroids, thiopurines), number of previous attacks and even gender, but all arise from retrospective analysis of admission outcome and none are in widespread use. Disease activity is independent of disease duration and age in prospective studies, even if old age is associated with mortality.

*Truelove and Witts' Criteria on Admission.* Clinical criteria on admission also help predict outcome, rather than after 3 days' treatment. Recent data suggest that the number of Truelove and Witts' criteria [23] on admission is associated with colectomy [50] The more of these criteria in addition to a bloody stool frequency of ≥6/day, the more severe the systemic inflammatory response, and it is not surprising that the biological severity of an attack of colitis predicts colectomy. In a retrospective study of 294 episodes of colitis in 186 patients, the risk of colectomy was 9 % (11/129) if patients had one additional criterion, compared to 31 % (29/94) if two additional criteria were present and 48 % (34/71) if three or more additional criteria were present ($p = 1.4 \times 10^{-5}$; OR 4.35, 95 % CI 2.20–8.56 one criterion vs. two or more). Therefore, simply counting the number of additional criteria on admission helps identify those patients at higher risk of colectomy.

*Laboratory criteria* are objective parameters which help measure the inflammatory response. Biochemical markers include C-reactive protein (CRP) and albumin, among others [6]. Although the ESR was one of the original Truelove and Witts' criteria, it has not been shown to be of predictive value in prospective studies. In the prospective OSCI study (Outcome of Steroid Therapy in Colitis Individuals) [77] to evaluate short-term corticosteroid response rates in 128 children hospitalised with acute severe colitis, the significant predictors at day 3 were nocturnal diarrhoea (OR 3.4, 95 % CI 1.9–6.1), number of daily stools (OR 2.7, 95 % CI 1.7–4.3), amount of blood in stool (OR 4.2, 95 % CI 2.0–8.9) and CRP (OR 1.3, 95 % CI 1.1–1.6). The faecal calprotectin differed ($p = 0.039$) but was not significant by odds' ratio. Confirmation in different patient groups provides reassurance that the CRP is a useful objective marker of predictive value for steroid failure. This resonates with clinical practice, because CRP is commonly measured and stool frequency can simply be monitored in patients with acute severe colitis. There is some evidence that the rate of change in CRP during intensive treatment predicts response [73], but this has not yet been quantified in a clinically useful tool. Albumin is a marker of inflammation, and low levels in acute severe colitis should raise concern as this has been associated with colectomy in retrospective case series: 42 % with an albumin <30 g/L at the end of the first day came to colectomy in the early series of 189 admissions from St Mark's [80]. In a large series from Edinburgh, sensitivity was increased by combining albumin with clinical (stool frequency) and radiological data. However, multivariate analysis in prospective case series has not identified albumin as an independent marker of colectomy [32, 77, 81]. Faecal calprotectin is a marker of intestinal inflammation but so far has been less successful at predicting colectomy than the combination of stool frequency and CRP: this also holds true for other faecal markers [73].

*Endoscopy* is useful for helping to predict remission and the risk of colectomy. Data from a subsequent analysis of ACT I and II trials has highlighted the importance of early mucosal healing: those patients with complete mucosal healing (Mayo Clinic endoscopy subscore of 0) at 8 weeks were four times as likely to be in remission at 30 weeks of inflix-imab treatment [82]. The presence of deep ulceration is a prequel to perforation and therefore associated with colec-tomy in order to prevent perforation occurring. In a group of 85 patients with acute severe colitis, 93 % of those with extensive deep colonic ulceration came to colectomy with ulceration reaching at least to the circular muscle layer in 42 of the 43 colectomy specimens [83]. One needs to be cautious of the circular argument as clinicians who are convinced of the prognostic importance of deep ulcers are more likely to perform colectomy in patients with deep ulceration.

## Impact of Different Activity Indices on Clinical Trial Outcomes

In clinical trials the endpoint of treatment is generally remis-sion, although the index selected and definition of remission are usually study specific. Differences in the threshold set-ting of remission have a substantial impact on the remission rates in the placebo arm of clinical trials, which range from 0 to 40 % in UC [84]. Placebo remission rates are influenced by factors including trial duration, number of study visits, design features used to enrol patients with more active dis-ease and intensity of endoscopic follow-up, but a stricter remission definition can be expected to drive down placebo rates [84]. The range of clinical trial endpoints (all described as "remission") is large and includes complete remission (DAI=0), a modified UCDAI $\leq 1$, UCDAI $\leq 2$, CAI $\leq 4$ and a Mayo Clinic score $\leq 2$ with no individual subscore >1 (ref below); [34, 40, 43, 44, 46] Inconsistency in the definition of remission results in clinically significant differences in out-comes for patients and clinicians. The lack of standardisation makes interpretation of trials difficult, because important symptoms such as bleeding or increased stool frequency can be hidden in low scores.

Differences in defining remission within a clinical trial can have a significant impact on the apparent efficacy of a drug [42, 85]. An example comes from two large prospective randomised double-blind controlled trials which included a total of 687 patients with mild to moderately active UC, treated with 2.4 g or 4.8 g mesalazine [37, 38]. In a retro-spective analysis using three different definitions of remis-sion for the results, the remission rate varied more than twofold [6, 42]. In a further example, the effect of epidermal growth factor (EGF) on UC was assessed by three different indices of disease activity: the Powell-Tuck, UCDAI and Simple Clinical Colitis Activity Index, where remission thresholds were set at score $\leq 4$, 0–1 and 0 respectively. Remission rates varied between 33 and 83 % depending on the index used [85].

The lack of a standardised definition of remission has considerable implications for patients. Specific aspects of the quality of life that are important to patients are not addressed by most indices. For instance, while the majority of compos-ite clinical indices contain some measure of patient well-being, only the Simple Clinical Colitis Activity Index (SCCAI) incorporates urgency and incontinence. In registra-tion trials where the main aim is to obtain a drug licence, urgency and incontinence are not assessed; hence the drug development process overlooks the control of key symptoms that are hugely important to patients.

## Conclusions

Metrics help with clinical decision-making in the manage-ment of UC. Comparison of different indices is challenging due to the lack of validation of most indices or their termi-nology. There are, however, well-validated indices for the four components for evaluating disease activity: quality of life (which matters most to patients), the clinical symptom score in children (PUCAI), endoscopic assessment of activ-ity (UCEIS) and histopathology (Geboes Index). What is now needed for clinical trials, let alone clinical practice, is not more indices but validation of current indices according to well-established statistical criteria, to determine their responsiveness and their role in predicting longer term out-come. There is a perceptible move to using separate vali-dated indices for the different components, because all convey different information of relevance. The difficulty for clinical trials is to select a single index as a primary outcome measure. It may be that a composite primary outcome that involves more than one of these validated indices is the way forward, but the risk (in economic and drug regulatory terms) of a therapeutic trial failing to reach its primary endpoint is such that sponsors are cautious. For the time being, there-fore, the dominance of the Mayo Clinic score (a composite, but unvalidated index) will remain. This will change when independently validated indices can be shown to predict long-term outcomes that matter to patients and payors.

## References

1. D'Haens G, Sandborn WJ, Feagan BG, et al. A review of activity indices and efficacy end points for clinical trials of medical therapy in adults with ulcerative colitis. Gastroenterology. 2007;132: 763–86.
2. Turner D, Otley AR, Mack D, et al. Development, validation, and evaluation of a pediatric ulcerative colitis activity index: a prospec-tive multicenter study. Gastroenterology. 2007;133:423–32.
3. Travis SPL, Schnell D, Krzeski P, et al. Development of an ulcerative colitis endoscopic index of severity (UCEIS). Gut. 2012; 61:535–42.

4. Geboes K, Riddell R, Öst A, Jensfelt B, Persson T, Löfberg R. A reproducible grading scale for histological assessment of inflammation in ulcerative colitis. Gut. 2000;47:404–9.

5. Irvine EJ, Feagan B, Rochon J, et al. Quality of life: a valid and reliable measure of therapeutic efficacy in the treatment of inflammatory bowel disease. Canadian Crohn's Relapse Prevention Trial Study Group. Gastroenterology. 1994;106:287–96.

6. Travis SPL, Higgins PDR, Orchard T, et al. Defining remission in ulcerative colitis. Aliment Pharmacol Ther. 2011;34:113–24.

7. Truelove SC, Richards WC. Biopsy studies in ulcerative colitis. Br Med J. 1956;1:1315–8.

8. Wright JG, Feinstein AR. A comparative contrast of clinimetric and psychometric methods for constructing indexes and rating scales. J Clin Epidemiol. 1992;45:1201–18.

9. Marx RG, Bombardier C, Hogg-Johnson S, Wright JG. Clinimetric and psychometric strategies for development of a health measurement scale. J Clin Epidemiol. 1999;52:105–11.

10. Noble A, Turner D. Clinical outcomes in pediatric inflammatory bowel disease. In: Mamula P, Markowitz J, Baldassano R, editors. Pediatric inflammatory bowel disease, vol. 1. Berlin: Springer; 2008. p. 744.

11. Lohr KN. Assessing health status and quality-of-life instruments: attributes and review criteria. Qual Life Res. 2002;11:193–205.

12. Yoshida EM. The Crohn's Disease Activity Index, its derivatives and the inflammatory bowel disease questionnaire: a review of instruments to assess Crohn's disease. Can J Gastroenterol. 1999;13:65–73.

13. Sandborn WJ, Sands BE, Wolf DC, et al. Repifermin (keratinocyte growth factor-2) for the treatment of active ulcerative colitis: a randomized, double-blind, placebo-controlled, dose-escalation trial. Aliment Pharmacol Ther. 2003;17:1355–64.

14. Walmsley RS, Ayres RCS, Pounder RE, Allan RN. A simple clinical colitis activity index. Gut. 1998;43:29–32.

15. Lichtiger S, Present D. Preliminary report: cyclosporin in treatment of severe active ulcerative colitis. Lancet. 1990;336:16–9.

16. Feagan BG, Greenberg GR, Wild G, et al. Treatment of ulcerative colitis with a humanized antibody to the α4β7 integrin. N Engl J Med. 2005;352:2499–507.

17. Beattie RM, Nicholls SW, Domizio P, Williams CB, Walker-Smith JA. Endoscopic assessment of the colonic response to corticosteroids in children with ulcerative colitis. J Pediatr Gastroenterol Nutr. 1996;22:373–9.

18. Schroeder KW, Tremaine WJ, Ilstrup DM. Coated oral 5-aminosalicylic acid therapy for mildly to moderately active ulcerative colitis. N Engl J Med. 1987;317:1625–9.

19. Sutherland LR, Martin F, Greer S, et al. 5-Aminosalicylic acid enema in the treatment of distal ulcerative colitis, proctosigmoiditis, and proctitis. Gastroenterology. 1987;92:1894–8.

20. Powell-Tuck J, Bown RL, Lennard-Jones JE. A comparison of oral prednisolone given as single or multiple daily doses for active proctocolitis. Scand J Gastroenterol. 1978;13:833–1.

21. Rachmilewitz D. Coated mesalazine (5-aminosalicylic acid) versus sulphasalazine in the treatment of active ulcerative colitis: a randomised trial. Br Med J. 1989;298:82–6.

22. Seo M, Okada M, Yao T, et al. An index of disease activity in patients with ulcerative colitis. Am J Gastroenterol. 1992;87:971–6.

23. Truelove S, Witts LJ. Cortisone in ulcerative colitis. Final report on a therapeutic trial. Br Med J. 1955;2:1041–8.

24. Silverberg MS, Satsangi J, Ahmad T, et al. Toward an integrated clinical, molecular and serological classification of inflammatory bowel disease: report of a working party of the 2005 Montreal World Congress of Gastroenterology. Can J Gastroenterol. 2005;19(Suppl A):5–36.

25. Baron JH, Connell AM, L-J JE. Variation between observers in describing mucosal appearances in proctocolitis. Br Med J. 1964;1:89–92.

26. Naganuma M, Ichikawa H, Inoue N, et al. Novel endoscopic activity index is useful for choosing treatment in severe active ulcerative colitis patients. Gastroenterology. 2010;45:936–43.

27. Riley SA, Mani V, Goodman MJ, Dutt S, Herd ME. Microscopic activity in ulcerative colitis: what does it mean? Gut. 1991;32:174–8.

28. Saverymuttu SH, Camilleri M, Rees H, Lavender JP, Hodgson HJF, Chadwick VS. Indium 111-granulocyte scanning in the assessment of disease extent and disease activity in inflammatory bowel disease: A comparison with colonoscopy, histology, and fecal indium 111-granulocyte excretion. Gastroenterology. 1986;90:1121–8.

29. Irvine EJ, Zhou Q, Thompson AK. The Short Inflammatory Bowel Disease Questionnaire: a quality of life instrument for community physicians managing inflammatory bowel disease. CCRPT Investigators. Canadian Crohn's Relapse Prevention Trial. Am J Gastroenterol. 1996;91:1571–8.

30. W-y C, Garratt AM, Russell IT, Williams JG. The UK IBDQ – a British version of the inflammatory bowel disease questionnaire: development and validation. J Clin Epidemiol. 2000;53:297–306.

31. Drossman D, Leserman J, Li Z, Mitchell C, Zagami E, Patrick D. The rating form of IBD patient concerns: a new measure of health status. Psychosom Med. 1991;53:701–12.

32. Travis S, Farrant JM, Ricketts C, et al. Predicting outcome in severe ulcerative colitis. Gut. 1996;38:905–10.

33. Turner D, Seow CH, Greenberg GR, Griffiths AM, Silverberg MS, Steinhart AH. A systematic prospective comparison of noninvasive disease activity indices in ulcerative colitis. Clin Gastroenterol Hepatol. 2009;7:1081–8.

34. Rutgeerts P, Sandborn WJ, Feagan BG, et al. Infliximab for induction and maintenance therapy for ulcerative colitis. N Engl J Med. 2005;353:2462–76.

35. Harvey RF, Bradshaw JM. A simple index of Crohn's disease activity. Lancet. 1980;315:514.

36. Plevy S, Salzberg B, Van Assche G, et al. A phase I study of visilizumab, a humanized anti-CD3 monoclonal antibody, in severe steroid-refractory ulcerative colitis. Gastroenterology. 2007;133:1414–22.

37. Sandborn WJ, Colombel JF, Frankel M, et al. Anti-CD3 antibody visilizumab is not effective in patients with intravenous corticosteroid-refractory ulcerative colitis. Gut. 2010;59:1485–92.

38. Travis S. Does it all ADA up? Adalimumab for ulcerative colitis. Gut. 2011;60:741–2.

39. Walsh AJ, Brain AOS, Keshav S, et al. How variable is the Mayo score between observers and might this affect trial recruitment or outcome? J Crohns Colitis. 2009;3:S71.

40. Hanauer SB, Sandborn WJ, Kornbluth A, et al. Delayed-release oral mesalamine at 4.8 g//day (800 mg tablet) for the treatment of moderately active ulcerative colitis: the ASCEND II trial. Am J Gastroenterol. 2005;100:2478–85.

41. Hanauer SB, Sandborn WJ, Dallaire C, et al. Delayed-release oral mesalamine 4.8 g/day (800 mg tablets) compared to 2.4 g/day (400 mg tablets) for the treatment of mildly to moderately active ulcerative colitis: the ASCEND I trial. Can J Gastroenterol. 2007;21:827–34.

42. Katz S, Higgins P, Eusebio R, Yacyshyn B. Different definitions of remission for ulcerative colitis result in large variations of clinical outcome scores. Gastroenterology. 2006;130 Suppl 2:A-482.

43. Marteau P, Probert CS, Lindgren S, et al. Combined oral and enema treatment with Pentasa (mesalazine) is superior to oral therapy alone in patients with extensive mild/moderate active ulcerative colitis: a randomised, double blind, placebo controlled study. Gut. 2005;54:960–5.

44. Kamm MA, Sandborn WJ, Gassull M, et al. Once-daily, high-concentration MMX mesalamine in active ulcerative colitis. Gastroenterology. 2007;132:66–75.

45. Higgins PD, Schwartz M, Mapili J, Krokos I, Leung J, Zimmermann EM. Patient defined dichotomous end points for remission and clinical improvement in ulcerative colitis. Gut. 2005;54:782–8.

46. Kruis W, Kiudelis G, Rácz I, et al. Once daily versus three times daily mesalazine granules in active ulcerative colitis: a double-blind, double-dummy, randomised, non-inferiority trial. Gut. 2009; 58:233–40.

47. Seo M, Okada M, Yao T, et al. Evaluation of disease activity in patients with moderately active ulcerative colitis: comparisons between a new activity index and Truelove and Witts' classification. Am J Gastroenterol. 1995;90:1759–63.

48. Järnerot G, Hertervig E, Friis-Liby I, et al. Infliximab as rescue therapy in severe to moderately severe ulcerative colitis: a randomized, placebo-controlled study. Gastroenterology. 2005;128: 1805–11.

49. Turner D, Walsh CM, Steinhart AH, Griffiths AM. Response to corticosteroids in severe ulcerative colitis: a systematic review of the literature and a meta-regression. Clin Gastroenterol Hepatol. 2007; 5:103–10.

50. Dinesen LC, Walsh AJ, Protic MN, et al. The pattern and outcome of acute severe colitis. J Crohns Colitis. 2010;4(4):431–7.

51. Brown SR, Haboubi N, Hampton J, George B, Travis SPL. The management of acute severe colitis: ACPGBI position statement. Colorectal Dis. 2008;10:8–29.

52. Kornbluth A, Sachar DB. Ulcerative colitis practice guidelines in adults: American College of Gastroenterology, Practice Parameters Committee. Am J Gastroenterol. 2010;105:501–23.

53. Van Assche G, Dignass A and Travis SPL (steering group) for the European Crohn's and Colitis Organisation (ECCO). The second European evidence-based Consensus on the diagnosis and management of ulcerative colitis. J Crohns Colitis. 2013;7(1):1–33.

54. Powell-Tuck J, Day DW, Buckell NA, Wadsworth J, Lennard-Jones JE. Correlations between defined sigmoidoscopic appearances and other measures of disease activity in ulcerative colitis. Dig Dis Sci. 1982;27:533–7.

55. Rutegard I, Ahsgren L, Stenling R, Nilsson T. A simple index for assessment of disease activity in patients with ulcerative colitis. Hepatogastroenterology. 1990;37 Suppl 2:110–2.

56. Colombel JF, Rutgeerts P, Reinisch W, et al. Early mucosal healing with infliximab is associated with improved long-term clinical outcomes in ulcerative colitis. Gastroenterology. 2011;141:1194–201.

57. Osada T, Ohkusa T, Yokoyama T, et al. Comparison of several activity indices for the evaluation of endoscopic activity in UC: inter- and intraobserver consistency. Inflamm Bowel Dis. 2010;16:192–7.

58. Flavell Matts SG. The value of rectal biopsies in the diagnosis of ulcerative colitis. QJM. 1961;30:393–407.

59. Blackstone MO. Inflammatory bowel disease. In: Blackstone MO, editor. Endoscopic interpretation. New York: Raven; 1984. p. 464–94.

60. Kamm MA, Lichtenstein GR, Sandborn WJ, et al. Randomised trial of once or twice daily MMX mesalazine for maintenance of remission in ulcerative colitis. Gut. 2008;57:893–902.

61. Travis SPL, Schnell D, Krzeski P, et al. Reliability and initial validation of the Ulcerative Colitis Endoscopic Index of Severity (UCEIS). Gastroenterology. 2013;145:987–95.

62. Thia KT, Loftus EV, Pardi DS, et al. Measurement of disease activity in ulcerative colitis: interobserver agreement and predictors of severity. Inflamm Bowel Dis. 2011;17:1257–64.

63. Wright R, Truelove S. Serial rectal biopsy in ulcerative colitis during the course of a controlled therapeutic trial of various diets. Dig Dis Sci. 1966;11:847–57.

64. Burger DC, Thomas SJ, Walsh AJ, et al. Depth of remission may not predict outcome of UC over 2 years. Gut. 2011;60 Suppl 1:A133.

65. Sandborn WJ, Moro L, Ballard ED, Travis SPL. Induction of remission of mild to moderately active ulcerative colitis with budesonide-MMX 9 mg: a multicentre, randomised, double-blind placebo-controlled trial in North America and India. Gut. 2011 (UEGW presentation).

66. Stange EF, Travis SPL, Vermeire S, et al. European evidence-based consensus on the diagnosis and management of ulcerative colitis: Definitions and diagnosis. J Crohns Colitis. 2008;2:1–23.

67. Hoivik ML, Bernklev T, Moum B. Need for standardization in population-based quality of life studies: a review of the current literature. Inflamm Bowel Dis. 2010;16:525–36.

68. Irvine EJ. Quality of life of patients with ulcerative colitis: past, present, and future. Inflamm Bowel Dis. 2008;14:554–65.

69. Ware JEJ, Sherbourne CD. The MOS 36-Item short-form health survey (SF-36): I conceptual framework and item selection. Medical Care. 1992;30:473–83.

70. The EQ-5D quality of life questionnaire. http://www.euroqol.org/eq-5d/what-is-eq-5d.html. Accessed 16 Jan 2012.

71. The CONSTRUCT Trial. http://www.construct.swansea.ac.uk. Accessed 16 Jan 2012.

72. Levenstein S, Li Z, Almer S, et al. Cross-cultural variation in disease-related concerns among patients with inflammatory bowel disease. Am J Gastroenterol. 2001;96:1822–30.

73. Travis S, Satsangi J, Lémann M. Predicting the need for colectomy in severe ulcerative colitis: a critical appraisal of clinical parameters and currently available biomarkers. Gut. 2011 2011;60:3-9.

74. Turner D, Griffiths AM, Mack D, et al. Assessing disease activity in ulcerative colitis: patients or their physicians? Inflamm Bowel Dis. 2010;16:651–6.

75. Waljee AK, Joyce JC, Wren PA, Khan TM, Higgins PD. Patient reported symptoms during an ulcerative colitis flare: a Qualitative Focus Group Study. Eur J Gastroenterol Hepatol. 2009;21:558–64.

76. Umanskiy K, Fichera A. Health related quality of life in inflammatory bowel disease: the impact of surgical therapy. World J Gastroenterol. 2010;16:5024–34.

77. Turner D, Mack D, Leleiko N, et al. Severe pediatric ulcerative colitis: a prospective multicenter study of outcomes and predictors of response. Gastroenterology. 2010;138:2282–91.

78. Lennard-Jones JE, Ritchie JK, Hilder W, Spicer CC. Assessment of severity in colitis: a preliminary study. Gut. 1975;16:579–84.

79. Turner D, Walsh CM, Benchimol EI, et al. Severe paediatric ulcerative colitis: incidence, outcomes and optimal timing for second-line therapy. Gut. 2008;57:331–8.

80. Ho GT, Mowat C, Goddard CJR, et al. Predicting the outcome of severe ulcerative colitis: development of a novel risk score to aid early selection of patients for second-line medical therapy or surgery. Aliment Pharmacol Ther. 2004;19:1079–87.

81. Benazzato L, D'Incà R, Grigoletto F, et al. Prognosis of severe attacks in ulcerative colitis: effect of intensive medical treatment. Dig Liver Dis. 2004;36:461–6.

82. Colombel JF, Rutgeerts P, Reinisch W, et al. Early mucosal healing With infliximab is associated with improved long-term clinical outcomes in ulcerative colitis. Gastroenterology. 2011;141:1194–201.

83. Carbonnel F, Lavergne A, Lémann M, et al. Colonoscopy of acute colitis. Dig Dis Sci. 1994;39:1550–7.

84. Su C, Lewis JD, Goldberg B, Brensinger C, Lichtenstein GR. A meta-analysis of the placebo rates of remission and response in clinical trials of active ulcerative colitis. Gastroenterology. 2007; 132:516–26.

85. Sinha A, Nightingale JMD, West KP, Berlanga-Acosta J, Playford RJ. Epidermal growth factor enemas with oral mesalamine for mild-to-moderate left-sided ulcerative colitis or proctitis. N Engl J Med. 2003;349:350–7.

# Medical Management of Toxic Megacolon

Subrata Ghosh and Marietta Iacucci

**Keywords**

Toxic megacolon • Ulcerative colitis • Dilatation • Colon • Intravenous corticosteroids • Colectomy • Megacolon

## Introduction

Toxic megacolon is a rare but extremely severe form of acute severe ulcerative colitis characterized by both toxicity and dilatation of the colon. The features of toxic megacolon include abdominal pain, tenderness and distension, reduced or absent bowel sounds, tachycardia, fever, hypotension in some patients, neutrophilia, and raised C-reactive protein and erythrocyte sedimentation rate [1]. A number of terms are used interchangeably with toxic megacolon such as fulminant colitis or acute severe colitis, but toxic megacolon should be used as a specific term indicating features of both megacolon and toxicity. Indicators of toxicity are shown in Table 33.1 [2]. As such it is an extreme presentation of acute severe colitis. Megacolon is defined as non-obstructive dilatation of the colon with a diameter of 5.5 cm or greater, segmental or total, demonstrated on a plain X-ray or on plain CT scan [3]. Some authorities consider the cutoff dimension of the colon as >6 cm, but it is important to recognize that it is the toxicity rather than the exact measurement of the colon that determines the clinical severity of toxic megacolon. Such an assessment of colonic dilatation may also be

S. Ghosh, M.D., F.R.C.P. (✉)
Department of Medicine, Foothills Medical Center,
University of Calgary, North Tower 9th floor Room 930,
1403 29th St NW, Calgary, AB, Canada T2N 2T9
e-mail: subrata.ghosh@albertahealthservices.ca

M. Iacucci, M.D., Ph.D.
Division of Gastroenterology, Department of Medicine,
University of Calgary, TRW Building, 3280 Hospital Drive NW,
Calgary, AB, Canada T2N 1N4
e-mail: miacucci@ucalgary.ca

misleading within 24 h of a colonoscopy or flexible sigmoidoscopy. It is important to note that the frequency of bowel movements with diarrhea or amount of rectal bleeding may no longer be reliable indicators of severity of ulcerative colitis once toxic megacolon sets in. Therefore, standard ulcerative colitis disease activity indices generally cannot be applied. Toxic megacolon complicating Crohn's colitis is unusual but may occur.

Toxic megacolon is a medical emergency, potentially fatal if not appropriately managed, and if the patient presents with features suggestive of toxic megacolon, it is mandatory for the patient to be admitted and managed jointly by the gastroenterology and surgical team. It is preferable for a colorectal surgeon experienced in management of inflammatory bowel disease to be directly involved. A patient with acute severe colitis may also develop toxic megacolon while an in-patient undergoing treatment, and immediate joint management by the surgical and gastroenterology team is necessary. The patient should be closely monitored in a high dependency unit. There is high risk of colonic perforation and peritonitis with associated mortality. The mortality of acute severe colitis is 1 %, and the mortality when toxic megacolon develops is much higher though population-based data is scant in this condition.

## Different Scenarios of Toxic Megacolon

Approximately 5 % of patients with acute severe colitis admitted to hospital will have toxic dilatation [3]. Toxic megacolon may present de novo in the emergency in a patient known to suffer from ulcerative colitis or rarely as the first presentation of ulcerative colitis. Toxic megacolon is unusual

**Table 33.1** Indicators of toxicity in acute severe ulcerative colitis [2]

| At least three of the following signs and laboratory findings: |
| --- |
| Heart rate > 120/min |
| Temperature > 38.6 °C |
| White cell count > $10.5 \times 10^3$/mm$^3$ |
| Anemia |
| AND, at least one of the following: |
| Dehydration |
| Altered mental status |
| Electrolyte disturbances |
| Hypotension |

**Table 33.2** Risk factors associated with development of toxic megacolon [3]

| Hypokalemia |
| --- |
| Hypomagnesemia |
| Narcotic analgesics |
| Antidiarrheals, including narcotic antidiarrheals |
| Infections, especially *Clostridium difficile* |
| Bowel preparation especially barium enema |

in patients with longstanding colitis with shortened, chronically inflamed colon. Careful assessment of the patient is necessary jointly by medical and surgical teams and options discussed. Significant abdominal pain is an indicator of impending perforation and such patients should undergo emergency colectomy. Otherwise the patients may be managed medically and the therapeutic options are delineated below. The therapeutic options depend on the presentation and previous treatment as well as the time course of the development of toxic megacolon and presence of reversible risk factors. A patient suffering from severe ulcerative colitis and already an in-patient on intravenous steroids may also deteriorate and develop toxic megacolon. The majority of such patients will undergo emergency colectomy, and only a few selected patients may be offered second-line salvage therapy with infliximab or ciclosporin if in the opinion of the colorectal surgeon such an option is safe and signs of impending perforation are absent. Careful monitoring is mandatory. In a patient already on salvage therapy such as infliximab or ciclosporin, development of toxic megacolon mandates emergency colectomy.

## Risk Factors for Toxic Megacolon

Risk factors predisposing to toxic megacolon include hypokalemia, hypomagnesemia, bowel preparation, and the use of antidiarrheal therapy as well as coinfections such as *Clostridium difficile* (Table 33.2). Small bowel distension may predict the onset of toxic megacolon. Early diagnosis of acute severe colitis using the Truelove and Witts or the American College of Gastroenterology criteria and in pediatric patients using the Pediatric UC Activity Index (PUCAI) may help the introduction of timely intensive medical management and if necessary timely colectomy before toxic megacolon may set in. Recognizing and dealing with the risk factors associated with toxic megacolon, advising the patients appropriately and prevention by early intensive management of acute severe ulcerative colitis are the best strategies to reduce incidence of toxic megacolon [4].

## Monitoring of a Patient with Toxic Megacolon

The patients need to have their vital signs monitored at least every 4 h and a CT scan of the abdomen and pelvis or an abdominal X-ray with the lower chest taken to exclude perforation and determine the severity of megacolon every day. In some instances of severe toxic megacolon, abdominal X-ray may be done twice daily [1]. Infections need to be excluded by stool culture, *Clostridium difficile* toxin assay or real-time PCR, CMV quantitative PCR in blood (as obtaining colonic histology in toxic megacolon may be difficult), and blood culture as patients are usually febrile. A complete blood count, C-reactive protein (or erythrocyte sedimentation rate), electrolytes and creatinine, and urea concentrations should be monitored every day, and plasma albumin concentrations and liver function tests should be monitored every 3–4 days. The patients need to be reviewed by the gastroenterologist and colorectal surgeon every day. In a patient with known ulcerative colitis, procedures such as flexible sigmoidoscopy or colonoscopy should be avoided, but a cautious diagnostic flexible sigmoidoscopy with minimal insufflation may be performed without bowel preparation or enema if the diagnosis is not known.

## General Management

It is important to optimize general supportive management of these very ill patients as this may make a significant difference to overall outcome.

## Prophylaxis of Thromboembolic Complications

Patients with toxic megacolon are very ill, often confined to bed, and dehydrated and have a hypercoagulable state. Active inflammation may play a direct role in producing a thrombophilic state [5] and all patients should receive prophylactic heparin. Administration of heparin is safe and does not increase the incidence of colonic bleeding [6].

Either unfractionated or low molecular weight heparin may be used for prevention of venous thrombosis, at least as long as the patient is on intravenous steroids or is confined to bed [7].

## Management of Nutritional Status

Oral feeding should be avoided when toxic megacolon is diagnosed [8]. Bowel rest via total parenteral nutrition has no therapeutic benefit in reducing the inflammation in toxic megacolon. However, a number of patients are admitted with very poor nutritional status and are too ill to have adequate oral nutritional intake. A dietician should always be involved in managing such patients, and parenteral nutrition should be considered on nutritional grounds if oral intake has been persistently inadequate, so that emergency surgery in a nutritionally debilitated patient can be avoided. As these patients are at high risk of colectomy and are kept nil by mouth, supported nutrition by parenteral route is even more important.

## Management of Fluid and Electrolyte Disturbances

Many of these patients are dehydrated and hypokalemic especially after high doses of steroids, and careful monitoring and replacement are necessary. In the presence of toxic megacolon, intravenous fluids will be required and tailored to vital signs and renal and electrolyte monitoring. In some cases hypokalemia may be a precipitating cause of megacolon and early restoration of electrolyte balance may help reversal of megacolon. In elderly patients, consideration has to be given to possible drug related electrolyte imbalance.

## Blood Transfusion

Anemia may be due to inflammation, blood loss, and inadequate nutrition [9]. Blood transfusion with packed red cells and parenteral iron replacement should be considered in patients in order to maintain a hemoglobin concentration above 10 g/dL. This is important in terms of keeping a patient in a fit state for surgery if medical management fails.

## Antibiotics

In the absence of infections, there is no evidence for empiric use of antibiotics. In hospitalized patients with developing toxic megacolon, oral vancomycin may be considered till the stools are negative for *Clostridium difficile*. Real-time PCR on feces might permit a rapid diagnosis of *Clostridium difficile* and early treatment with vancomycin. Broad-spectrum antibiotics are occasionally used in patients with significant abdominal tenderness [1]; however, there is no definite evidence for efficacy and there is the risk of *Clostridium difficile* infection. There is scant evidence for fecal microbial transplant in toxic megacolon associated with *Clostridium difficile* in the setting of severe ulcerative colitis.

## Abdominal Decompression

Naso-enteral decompression tubes do not help in reducing colonic dilatation but may be considered if there is accompanying significant small bowel ileus. Changing position to evacuate gas may only be considered after flexible sigmoidoscopy but is generally unnecessary. Patients are generally too ill to roll around in bed or lie in knee-elbow position every 30 min though it is recommended in some guidelines [8].

## Management of Abdominal Pain

Narcotic analgesics should be avoided as it may worsen colonic dilatation. Severe pain in the setting of toxic megacolon generally represents transmural inflammation and impending perforation, and hence, surgical review and emergency colectomy may be required rather than pain management. It is important that adequate vigilance is maintained to trigger surgical intervention as a matter of urgency in the event of severe abdominal pain.

## Principles of Specific Management

The initial medical management of toxic megacolon is similar to management of acute severe ulcerative colitis, and these patients require hospitalization and close monitoring, as the colectomy rates even if the patient initially responds to initial treatment is high. Therefore, it is important to monitor the patient in a gastroenterology (not a general) ward with an accurate record of stool frequency, blood in stool, temperature, pulse rate, and abdominal tenderness. Infection must be eliminated by stool culture and *Clostridium difficile* toxin assay, but commencement of treatment should not wait until the stool culture reports become available. The management of severe ulcerative colitis patients is a team effort between gastroenterologists, surgeons, inflammatory bowel disease nurses, dieticians, and clinical psychologists. In a patient admitted with acute severe ulcerative colitis and dilatation of the colon, joint assessment by a gastroenterologist and a

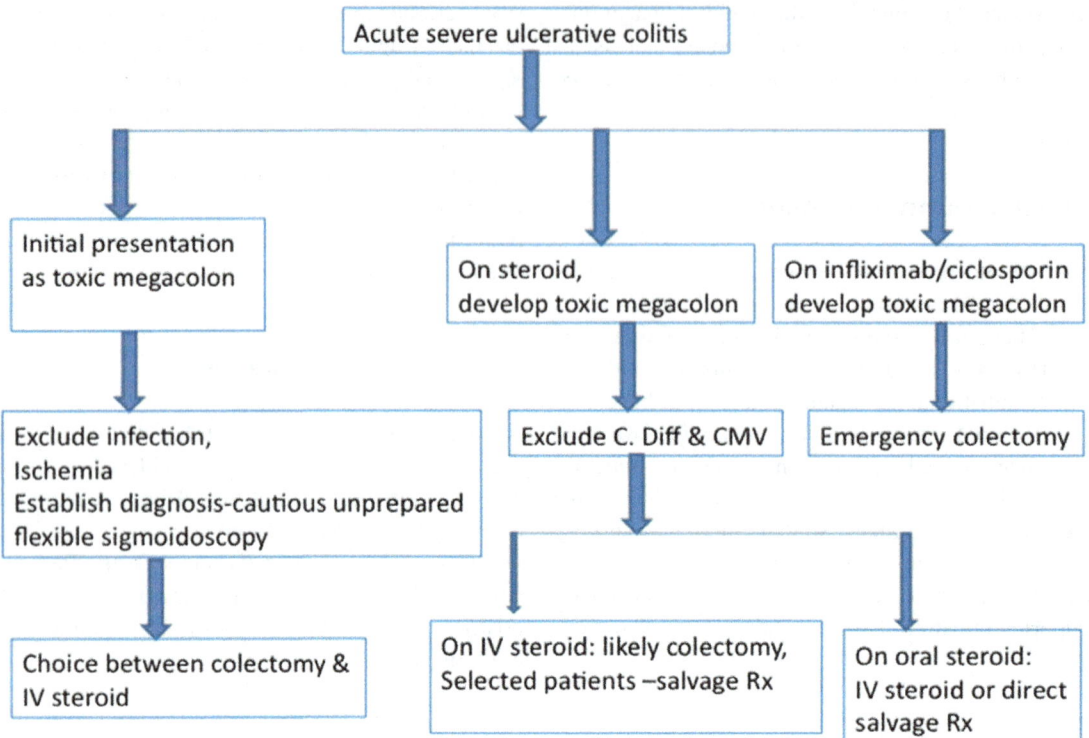

**Fig. 33.1** Different presentations of toxic megacolon and specific management choices. Colectomy is always an important management choice as delayed surgery may be life threatening, but medical management with close monitoring is a viable option with early surgery if there is inadequate response

colorectal surgeon is required urgently. In all other patients admitted with acute severe colitis, a colorectal surgical assessment will be required within 24 h, but vital signs should be monitored to trigger alarm at signs of impending toxic megacolon. The different scenarios in which toxic megacolon may develop will necessitate different strategies of management as illustrated in Fig. 33.1.

## Initial Therapy

The standard initial therapy of acute severe ulcerative colitis, including toxic megacolon where medical therapy is chosen, consists of intravenous corticosteroids [1, 4, 9, 10]. Intravenous corticosteroids generally chosen include hydrocortisone 100 mg four times a day or methylprednisolone 60 mg/daily by continuous infusion. Addition of rectal therapy has no clear advantages and is generally poorly tolerated by patients in the acute severe phase—rectal therapy is hazardous in toxic megacolon and should not be used. Overall, patients hospitalized for acute severe colitis and treated with intravenous steroids may have a colectomy rate between 29 and 46 % over the next 90 days [1, 8].

## Managing Intravenous Steroid Refractory Acute Severe Colitis with Toxic Megacolon

Close monitoring should lead to early recognition of those patients who fail to respond to intravenous steroids. Such recognition may be aided by formal rules, but clinical judgment is paramount based on the monitoring parameters noted in Table 33.1 and daily abdominal CT scan or abdominal plain X-rays. The two commonly used rules, which are very similar to each other, are the Travis index [11] and the fulminant colitis (Sweden) index [12]. However, these rules have not been validated in toxic megacolon and are unlikely to be very reliable as both rely heavily on stool frequency. Some patients respond initially to intravenous steroids but continue to have symptoms. These patients should be offered salvage therapy 5–7 days after initiation of intravenous corticosteroids as the colectomy rate is high in this group. This latter group may also benefit from a careful flexible sigmoidoscopy, as demonstration of severe inflammation with deep ulceration indicates a poor prognosis and consideration of salvage therapy or surgery (Fig. 33.2). Overall, a high proportion of patients failing intravenous steroids will undergo colectomy.

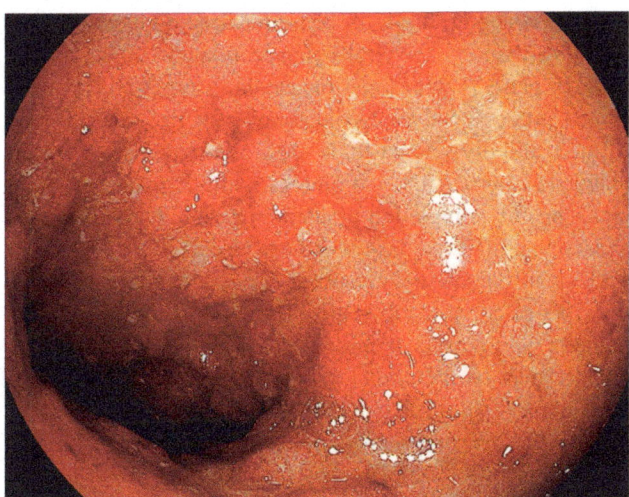

**Fig. 33.2** A patient with toxic megacolon after treatment with intravenous hydrocortisone for 7 days with improvement in toxicity features and colonic dilatation but significant inflammation and friability (Mayo endoscopic subscore 3) at careful flexible sigmoidoscopy with minimum insufflation and no bowel preparation. The patient was commenced on salvage therapy with infliximab but underwent colectomy after a further 2 weeks

Patients who develop toxic megacolon while on intravenous steroid therapy will require urgent and serious consideration of emergency colectomy. Two principal medical salvage therapies are currently available, ciclosporin and infliximab. The role of these salvage therapies in patients with toxic megacolon is limited and should be considered perhaps in patients who are admitted with toxic megacolon after failing ambulatory high-dose oral corticosteroids as an alternative to intravenous steroids or patients with contraindication to high-dose steroids or patients who are relatively stable after 72 h of intravenous steroids to permit consideration of additional salvage therapy.

## Infliximab

The chimeric anti-TNF antibody infliximab was used in intravenous steroid refractory ulcerative colitis in a pivotal Scandinavian study in which a single 5 mg/kg infusion of infliximab was used [12]. Patients unresponsive to IV corticosteroids at day 3 were randomized to additional single dose of 5 mg/kg of infliximab or placebo. Patients who were not considered unresponsive at day 3 but remained symptomatic at day 5–7 were also randomized to a single 5 mg/kg dose of infliximab or placebo. Overall, 29 % of patients underwent colectomy in the infliximab arm compared with 67 % in the placebo arm. In an Italian cohort study, patients who had received multiple doses of infliximab had better outcome than those receiving a single dose of infliximab in a group of intravenous steroid-resistant acute severe colitis

patients [13]. Keeping this in mind, it may be wise to administer infliximab at 0, 2, and 6 weeks and thereafter every 8 weeks till the patient is in remission. Therapeutic drug level monitoring of infliximab may be useful in optimizing infliximab therapy. Subsequently, in those patients who are azathioprine/6-mercaptopurine naïve, this drug may be used in combination only after the patient has responded, as such combination is superior to monotherapy with anti-TNF [14]. In patients who developed acute severe intravenous steroid-resistant colitis while on azathioprine or 6-mercaptopurine, infliximab should preferably be continued long term, rather than consider ciclosporin.

Though patients failing ciclosporin may respond to infliximab, repeated salvage therapy generally results in unacceptable delay to surgery and profound immunosuppression [15] with increased mortality. Therefore, only one form of salvage therapy should be decided upon after discussion with the patient, and failure of such therapy should lead to surgery. This is especially true in patients presenting with toxic megacolon.

## Ciclosporin

Ciclosporin, a cyclic peptide of 11 amino acids, acts by binding to cyclophilin and thereby inhibiting calcineurin. Inhibition of calcineurin prevents transcription of interleukin-2 (IL-2) and activation of T lymphocytes. With the demonstration that treatment with 2 mg/kg of ciclosporin is as effective as the conventional 4 mg/kg with fewer occurrences of some side effects such as hypertension [16], the lower dose is now accepted as standard therapy in most hospitals. Once the patient has responded and is feeling better, the intravenous preparation may be replaced by oral microemulsion ciclosporin 5 mg/kg. It is no longer necessary to exclude patients with low plasma cholesterol due to risk of seizures, as the intravenous preparation does not contain the incriminating chromophore. In a patient who responds to ciclosporin, the drug is continued as oral therapy for 3–4 months, while corticosteroids are tapered and discontinued, and azathioprine 2.5 mg/kg or 6-mercaptopurine 1.5 mg/kg is introduced at the time of discharge as long-term maintenance therapy. Such patients are quite severely immunosuppressed, and therefore, a high vigilance for opportunistic infections and prophylaxis for *Pneumocystis carinii* with co-trimoxazole is necessary. Ciclosporin is associated with a number of serious adverse events including an appreciable mortality.

## Infliximab or Ciclosporin

The question of whether to choose ciclosporin or infliximab as salvage medical therapy in toxic megacolon is important. In a parallel open-labeled randomized controlled trial, ciclosporin was not more effective than infliximab over a 14-week follow-up period in hospitalized acute severe ulcerative colitis patients refractory to intravenous corticosteroids [17]. Treatment failure defined by predetermined criteria occurred in 60 % of patients who received ciclosporin and in 54 % of patients who received infliximab over the 14-week period. The dosing regimen for ciclosporin was 2 mg/kg adjusted subsequently by drug trough levels—patients who responded at 7 days were switched to oral ciclosporin 4 mg/kg. The dosing regimen for infliximab was 5 mg/kg and patients who responded received further doses at weeks 2 and 6. Both groups received azathioprine started in responders at day 7. The initial clinical response at day 7 was 86 % in the ciclosporin group and 84 % in the infliximab group. The incidence of serious adverse events was 16 % in the ciclosporin group and 25 % in the infliximab group. The physician and Inflammatory Bowel Disease Center experience should guide the treatment choice but most centers are now more familiar with the use of anti-TNF therapy. In addition, ciclosporin therapy is associated with a 1–2 % mortality rate. In a cohort study in Australia, infliximab salvage therapy in acute severe steroid refractory colitis was associated with lower rates of severe adverse events and colectomy compared with ciclosporin salvage therapy [18].

## Surgery

A well-timed operation is an invaluable part of appropriate management of acute severe ulcerative colitis complicated by toxic megacolon and can be life saving. With toxic megacolon, close monitoring is necessary and if toxicity or megacolon does not improve within 72 h colectomy is generally recommended, and indeed any worsening of status after intensive medical management requires immediate surgery. With the availability of more salvage therapy choices, it is important that these are offered early to patients failing steroid therapy; therefore, in many instances, surgery will be offered after failure of second-line salvage therapy. An exception may be patients presenting with toxic megacolon who may be ill enough to undergo surgery if they do not rapidly improve after intravenous corticosteroids. Severe hemorrhage, perforation, and toxic megacolon developing on treatment are indications for emergency surgery. Mortality of patients undergoing emergency surgery may be as high as 5 % and even higher in the elderly patients with multiple comorbidities [19].

Surgery should be discussed with all patients admitted with acute severe ulcerative colitis with toxic megacolon. The colorectal surgeon, gastroenterologist, stoma therapist, and inflammatory bowel disease specialist nurse will all play a role in discussing surgery. In toxic megacolon appropriately timed surgery as a matter of urgency is life saving, and discussion about long-term consequences of colectomy and pouch formation is generally inappropriate in taking a decision. In patients with toxic megacolon, surgery has to be a staged process. Subtotal colectomy with ileostomy is performed initially, increasingly laparoscopy-assisted in specialized centers. After 3–6 months with the patient in much better health, completion proctectomy with ileal pouch anal anastomosis (IPAA) is performed. Use of salvage therapy such as infliximab or ciclosporin does not appear to increase the risks of complications after colectomy. In a minority of patients with poor anal sphincter function, a permanent ileostomy may be preferable to avoid disabling incontinence. Careful psychological support and counseling throughout the process are invaluable, especially in patients who lose their colon after only a short spell of illness and toxic megacolon.

## References

1. Pola S, Patel D, Ramamoorthy S, et al. Strategies for the care of adults hospitalized for active ulcerative colitis. Clin Gastroenterol Hepatol. 2012;10:1315–25.
2. Jalan KN, Sircus W, Card WI, et al. An experience of ulcerative colitis. I. Toxic dilation in 55 cases. Gastroenterology. 1969;57:68–82.
3. Gan SI, Beck PL. A new look at toxic megacolon: an update and review of incidence, etiology, pathogenesis, and management. Am J Gastroenterol. 2003;98:2363–71.
4. Dignass A, Lindsay JO, Sturm A, et al. Second European evidence-based consensus on the diagnosis and management of ulcerative colitis. Part 2: current management. J Crohn's Colitis. 2012;6:991–1030.
5. Danese S, Papa A, Saibeni S, Repici A, Malesci A, Vecchi M. Inflammation and coagulation in inflammatory bowel disease: the clot thickens. Am J Gastroenterol. 2007;102:174–86.
6. Shen J, Ran ZH, Tong JL, Xiao SD. Meta-analysis: the utility and safety of heparin in the treatment of active ulcerative colitis. Aliment Pharmacol Ther. 2007;26:653–63.
7. Nguyen GC, Bernstein CN, Bitton A, et al. Consensus statements on the risk, prevention, and treatment of venous thromboembolism in inflammatory bowel disease: Canadian Association of Gastroenterology. Gastroenterology. 2014;146:835–48.
8. Kornbluth A, Sachar DB. Ulcerative colitis practice guidelines in adults: American College of Gastroenterology, Practice Parameters Committee. Am J Gastroenterol. 2010;105:501–23.
9. Van Assche G, Dignass A, Bokemeyer B, et al. Second European evidence-based consensus on the diagnosis and management of ulcerative colitis. Part 3: special situations. J Crohn's Colitis. 2013;7:1–33.
10. Truelove SC, Jewell DP. Intensive intravenous regimen for severe attacks of ulcerative colitis. Lancet. 1974;1:1067–70.
11. Travis SPL, Farrant JM, Ricketts C. Predicting outcome in severe ulcerative colitis. Gut. 1996;38:905–10.
12. Jarnerot G, Hertervig E, Friis-Liby I, Blomquist L, Karlen P, Granno C, et al. Infliximab as rescue therapy in severe to moderately severe ulcerative colitis: a randomized, placebo-controlled study. Gastroenterology. 2005;128:1805–11.
13. Kohn A, Daperno M, Armuzzi A, Capello M, Biancone L, Orlando A. Infliximab in severe ulcerative colitis: short-term results of different infusion regimens and long-term follow-up. Aliment Pharmacol Ther. 2007;26:747–56.

14. Panaccione R, Ghosh S, Middleton S, et al. Combination therapy with infliximab and azathioprine is superior to monotherapy with either agent in ulcerative colitis. Gastroenterology. 2014;146: 392–400.

15. Chaparro M, Burqueno P, Iglesias E, et al. Infliximab salvage therapy after failure of ciclosporin in corticosteroid-refractory ulcerative colitis: a multicentre study. Aliment Pharmacol Ther. 2012;35:275–83.

16. Van Assche G, D'Haens G, Noman M. Randomised, double blind comparison of 4 mg/kg vs 2 mg/kg intra-venous cyclosporine in severe ulcerative colitis. Gastroenterology. 2003;125:1025–31.

17. Laharie D, Bourreille B, Branche J, et al. Ciclosporin versus infliximab in patients with severe ulcerative colitis refractory to intravenous steroids: a parallel, open label randomised controlled trial. Lancet. 2012;380:1909–15.

18. Croft A, Walsh A, Doecke J, et al. Outcomes of salvage therapy for steroid-refractory acute severe ulcerative colitis: ciclosporin versus infliximab. Aliment Pharmacol Ther. 2013;38:294–302.

19. Tottrup A, Erichsen R, Svaerke C, et al. Thirty-day mortality after elective and emergency total colectomy in Danish patients with inflammatory bowel disease: a population based nationwide cohort study. BMJ Open. 2012;2:e000823.

# Management of Acute and Chronic Pouchitis

Yue Li and Bo Shen

**Keywords**

Chronic pouchitis • Acute pouchitis • Familial adenomatous polyposis • Ileal pouch-anal anastomosis • Proctocolectomy • Permanent ileostomy • Inflammation • Diagnosis • Management • Etiology

## Introduction

A significant number of patients with ulcerative colitis (UC) and the majority of patients with familial adenomatous polyposis (FAP) will eventually need colectomy. Restorative proctocolectomy with ileal pouch-anal anastomosis (IPAA) is a preferred approach to proctocolectomy with permanent ileostomy, since the IPAA procedure preserves intestinal continuity and improves health-related quality of life. However, this bowel-anatomy-altering procedure is often associated with complications. The most frequently observed long-term complication of IPAA is acute and chronic idiopathic inflammation of the ileal reservoir, i.e., pouchitis. In this chapter, we provide up-to-date information on the etiology, diagnosis, and management of pouchitis.

## Incidence and Prevalence of Pouchitis

Pouchitis occurs almost exclusively in patients with underlying UC who undergo restorative proctocolectomy, rarely in FAP patients undergoing the same surgical procedure [1, 2].

Y. Li, M.D.
Department of Gastroenterology, Peking Union Medical College Hospital, and Digestive Disease Institute, Cleveland Clinic Foundation, Beijing, China
e-mail: liy8@ccf.org

B. Shen, M.D. (✉)
Department of Gastroenterology, Cleveland Clinic Foundation, 9500 Euclid Avenue, Cleveland 44195, OH, USA
e-mail: shenb@ccf.org

We speculate that etiopathogenesis of UC- and FAP-associated pouchitis may be different. It was estimated that initial episode of pouchitis happening within the first year after ileostomy closure occurs in 5 % of patients with FAP [3]. In contrast, reported cumulative frequencies of pouchitis 10–11 years after IPAA surgery for UC range from 23 to 46 % [4–7]. Approximately 50 % of patients who have undergone IPAA surgery for UC would develop at least one episode of pouchitis [8]. The risk for developing pouchitis may be higher in the first year following ileostomy closure [9, 10]. However, other studies reported that the risk continues to increase with longer follow-up [11]. While it has been difficult to estimate the true annual incidence of pouchitis, the reported incidence was 40 % in a randomized trial of a probiotic agent for the primary prophylaxis of pouchitis [9].

## Etiology and Pathogenesis of Pouchitis

The etiology and pathogenesis of pouchitis remain elusive. It is generally believed that pouchitis results from alternations in commensal luminal microflora (i.e., dysbiosis), leading to changes in mucosal immune response in genetically susceptible hosts [12]. Clinical evidence indicates that bacteria play a critical role in the initiation and disease progression in pouchitis, as conventional pouchitis hardly occurs in patients before stoma closure (except diversion pouchitis), and initial episodes of pouchitis in a majority of patients typically respond to antibiotic therapy. Investigators have also reported bacterial flora alterations, specifically a decrease in the number of lactobacilli and an increase in the number of anaerobes, *Clostridium perfringens*, and sulfate-reducing bacteria [13, 14].

With advances in molecular microbiology, investigators were able to depict a clearer picture of bacterial flora of the ileal pouch. Bacterial profiles of UC pouches and FAP pouches appear to be different [15, 16]. In addition to commensal bacteria, pathogenic microbes have been reported in pouchitis, including *Clostridium difficile* [17, 18], *Campylobacter* spp. [19], and *Cytomegalovirus* (CMV) [20–22].

Alterations in innate and adaptive mucosal immunity in the pouch and pouchitis have also been reported [23–28]. In addition, several genetic factors reported which may be associated with pouchitis are polymorphisms of interleukin-1 receptor antagonist [29, 30] and NOD2/CARD15 [31] and non-carrier status of tumor necrosis factor (TNF) allele 2 [30]. The presence of the NOD2 insC mutation was found to be associated with poor pouch outcome among patients with UC and IPAA [32]. The presence of NOD2/CARD15 mutations was also found to correlate with severe pouchitis after IPAA [33].

## Risk Factors

Factors associated with pouchitis have been extensively studied. The identification of risk factors may have a direct impact on the decision for the need and timing of IPAA and disease prevention of pouchitis. Patients' basic demographics (including age, race, and sex) and surgical techniques of IPAA (e.g., pouch anatomy, number of stages, laparoscopic vs. open) may have a limited impact on the risk for development of pouchitis [34–37]. Immunogenetic studies showed genetic polymorphisms such as those of IL-1 receptor antagonist [29], and NOD2 [30] may increase the risk for pouchitis. Other reported risk factors include the presence of extensive UC preoperatively [38, 39], the presence of backwash ileitis [10, 38], the presence of precolectomy thrombocytosis [40], the presence of concurrent primary sclerosing cholangitis (PSC) [10, 41, 42] or arthralgia or arthropathy [35], the presence of seropositivity to perinuclear antineutrophil cytoplasmic antibodies (p-ANCA) [5, 43, 44] or anti-CBir1 flagellin [5], being a non-smoker [5, 35, 39], the regular use of non-steroidal anti-inflammatory drugs (NSAIDs) [39, 42], and the presence of concurrent autoimmune disorders [45].

There were discrepancies in reported risk factors associated with subsequent development of pouchitis among different groups of investigators. These variations could largely be due to the difference in study design, sample size, diagnostic criteria used for pouchitis, referral pattern, and statistical methods. To complicate the matter, the diagnosis of acute and/or chronic pouchitis can be a moving target. For example, chronic pouchitis can evolve from acute pouchitis and other categories of pouch disorders such as pouch anatomic abnormalities.

## Diagnosis and Classification

Establishing the diagnosis of pouchitis is not always straightforward, since the patients typically present with nonspecific symptoms and signs. Patients with pouchitis have a wide range of clinical presentations, ranging from increased stool frequency, fecal urgency, fecal incontinence, and nighttime seepage to abdominal and/or pelvic discomfort. These symptoms, however, can be present in other inflammatory and noninflammatory disorders of the pouch, such as cuffitis, Crohn's disease (CD) of the pouch, and irritable pouch syndrome. In addition, the severity of symptoms does not necessarily correlate with the degree of endoscopic and/or histologic inflammation of the pouch [34, 46]. Patients with pouchitis due to enteric infections from pathogenic bacteria and viruses often present with constitutional symptoms, such as fever, general malaise, or weight loss. Therefore, a combined assessment of symptoms and endoscopic and histologic features is advocated for the diagnosis and differential diagnosis of pouchitis [34, 47]. Pouch endoscopy provides the most valuable information on severity and extent of mucosal inflammation, the presence of neo-ileitis, CD of the pouch or cuffitis, or other anatomic abnormalities, such as polyp, stricture, sinus, and fistula (Fig. 34.1).

Although histology has a limited role in grading the degree of pouch inflammation, it provides valuable information on some special features, such as granulomas, viral inclusion bodies (for CMV infection), pyloric gland metaplasia (a sign of chronic mucosal inflammation) [48], neoplasia [49], ischemia, or prolapse. A diagnostic and treatment algorithm is proposed (Figs. 34.2 and 34.3).

Laboratory testing is often necessary as a part of the evaluation of patients with pouch disorders, particularly in patients with chronic pouchitis. In patients with persistent symptoms, celiac sprue serology, salicylate screening, and microbiological assays for *Clostridium difficile* and CMV infections should be performed [50]. Fecal assays of lactoferrin and calprotectin have been evaluated for the diagnosis and differential diagnosis of pouchitis. However, the use of laboratory tests may not replace pouch endoscopy as the first-line evaluation for the diagnosis and differential diagnosis of pouchitis.

The natural history of pouchitis is poorly defined. Pouchitis likely represents a disease spectrum from acute, antibiotic-responsive, bacteria-associated entity to chronic, antibiotic-refractory, immune-mediated entity. Based on the etiology, disease duration and activity, and response to medical therapy, pouchitis can be categorized into: (1) idiopathic vs. secondary (with etiology such as NSAID use and *Clostridium difficile* or CMV infection), (2) acute vs. chronic (with a cutoff of 4 weeks of persistent symptoms being defined as chronic pouchitis), (3) infrequent episodes vs.

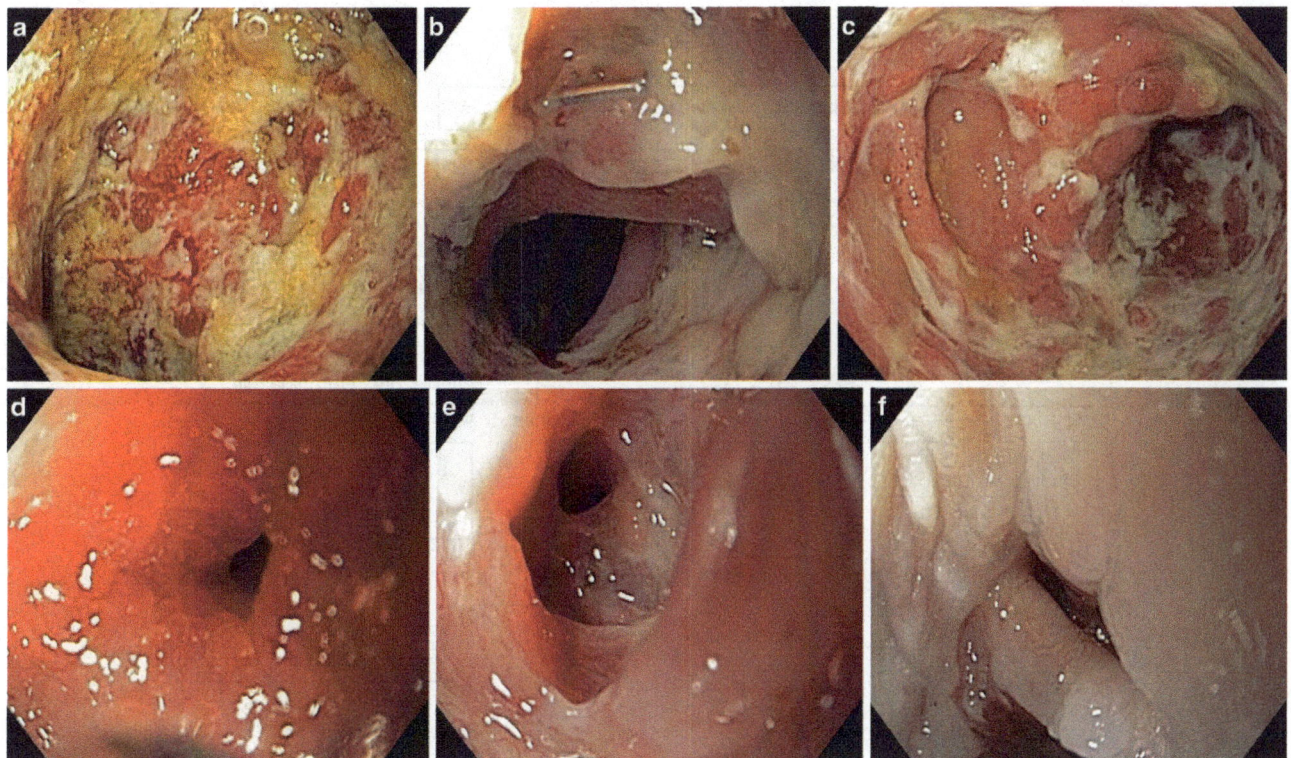

**Fig. 34.1** Endoscopy of inflammatory and noninflammatory disorders of the pouch. (**a**) severe diffuse pouchitis, (**b**) cuffitis, (**c**) Crohn's disease of the pouch—ulcers at the neo-terminal ileum, (**d**) pinhole pouch inlet stricture, (**e**) pouch anastomotic sinus, and (**f**) opening of cryptoglandular fistula at the dentate line

relapsing vs. continuous, and (4) responsive vs. refractory to antibiotic therapy [51]. Classification based on the response to antibiotic therapy is useful in clinical practice [52].

The various classification categories for pouchitis are noted in Table 34.1.

We recently proposed a new disease category of pouchitis, namely, "autoimmune pouchopathy" [45]. The patients often presented with symptoms similar to "bacteria-associated" pouchitis, such as increased stool frequency, cramps, and urgency. On endoscopic examination, there was mucosal inflammation of the pouch body, with or without a long segment of inflammation in the afferent limb. Although there are currently no established diagnostic criteria, the diagnosis of "autoimmune pouchopathy" may be suspected if a patient has antibiotic-refractory pouchitis, concurrent autoimmune disorders (such as rheumatoid arthritis and Hashimoto's thyroiditis), serum autoantibodies, and the presence of increased epithelial apoptosis (authors' unpublished data).

We recently also described IgG4-associated pouchitis. We found that a subgroup of symptomatic pouch patients with concurrent autoimmune disorders had an increased number of IgG4-expressing plasma cells in the lamina propria of the pouch and/or afferent limb biopsies [53, 54].

On the other hand, we also found that the degree of tissue IgG4-expressing plasma cells on pouch biopsy did not necessarily correlate with the serum level of IgG4, a marker for autoimmune pancreatitis. In a separate study we demonstrated that a high-level serum IgG4 was also associated with chronic antibiotic-refractory pouchitis [55]. The description of the new disease entity of the pouch suggests that abnormal mucosal B-cell immunity may play a role in the disease process of pouchitis and potentially provide a new therapeutic target.

PSC was reported to be associated with not only pouchitis but also long-segment backwash ileitis [54]. Typically, pouch patients with concurrent PSC often had a long segment of enteritis, with an endoscopic and histologic pattern similar to that of diffuse pouchitis. We speculate that pouchitis in those patients may represent a separate disease entity of the pouch, i.e., PSC-associated pouchitis/enteritis.

## Differential Diagnosis

There are overlaps in clinical presentations between a variety of inflammatory diseases of the pouch (such as pouchitis, cuffitis, and CD of the pouch) and some anatomic diseases

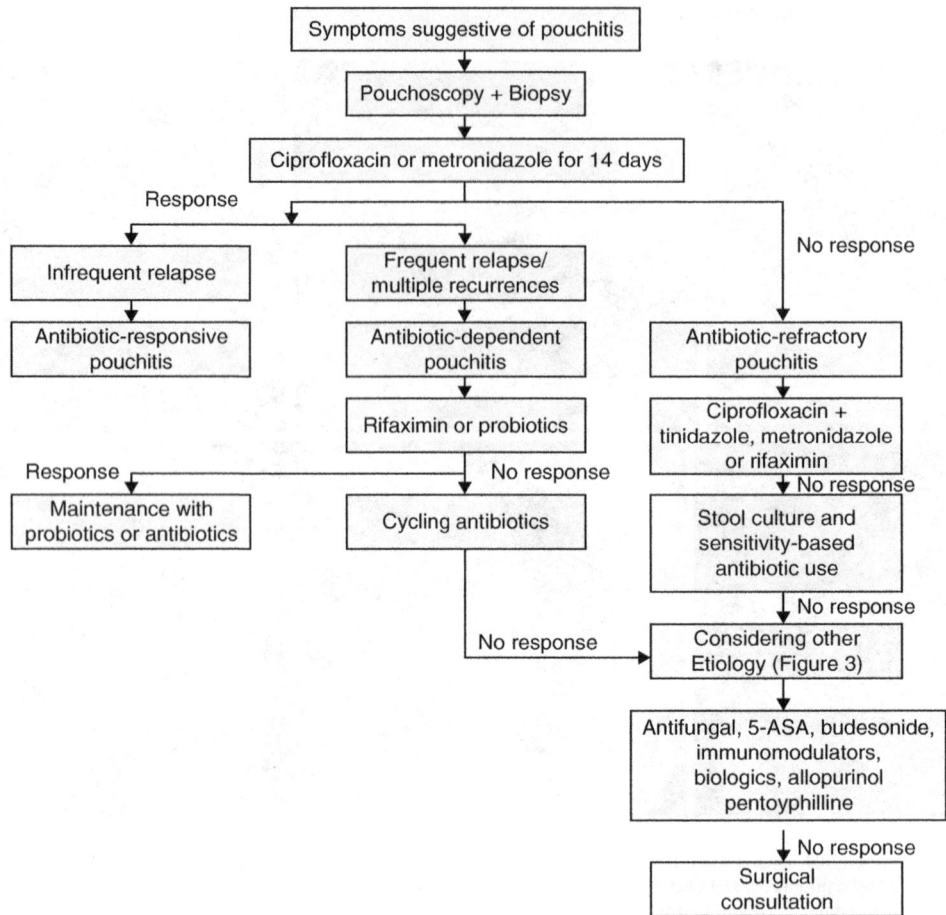

**Fig. 34.2** Diagnostic and treatment algorithm of pouchitis

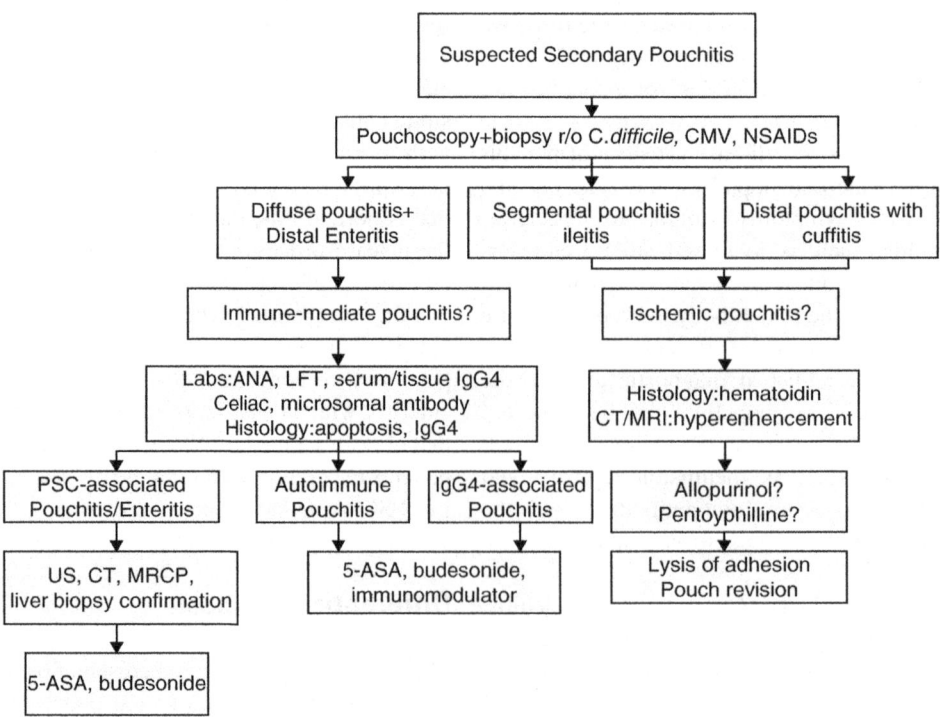

**Fig. 34.3** Diagnostic and treatment algorithm of secondary pouchitis

**Table 34.1** Classification of pouchitis

| Based on etiology | |
|---|---|
| Idiopathic | With unidentified pathogens or triggering factors |
| Secondary | • *Clostridium difficile*-associated<br>• *Cytomegalovirus*-associated<br>• Other pathogen-associated<br>• NSAID-induced<br>• Ischemic<br>• Autoimmune or IgG4-associated<br>• PSC-associated pouchitis/enteritis |
| **Based on duration of symptoms** | |
| Acute | Less than 4 weeks |
| Chronic | Greater than 4 weeks |
| **Based on symptom pattern** | |
| Infrequent | <3 episodes per year |
| Relapsing | ≥3 episodes per year or recurrence within 1 month of successful antibiotic therapy |
| **Based on response to antibiotic therapy** | |
| Antibiotic-responsive | Responds to a course of antibiotics |
| Antibiotic-dependent | Requires ongoing antibiotic therapy to maintain response |
| Antibiotic-refractory | Does not respond to a standard course of antibiotics |

(such as afferent limb or efferent limb obstruction, pouch sinus which is defined as a blind tract that may lead to an abscess cavity, and strictures).

Cuffitis occurs primarily in patients with a stapled pouch-anal anastomosis, in whom a segment of rectal mucosa is left in place and becomes inflamed [56, 57]. Cuffitis typically represents a recurrence of UC in the residual mucosa. However, other disease process may also contribute to the development of cuffitis, such as CD and ischemia [58]. Patients with cuffitis often present with bloody bowel movements, which seldom occur in conventional pouchitis.

One of the other common inflammatory disorders is CD of the pouch. CD of the pouch can occur after IPAA which is intentionally performed in a selected group of patients with CD with no small intestinal or perianal diseases [59]. CD is also inadvertently found in proctocolectomy specimens in patients with a preoperative diagnosis of UC or indeterminate colitis. However, a majority of patients with CD of the pouch were considered to develop the disease de novo. IPAA surgery with fecal stasis, sutures and anastomosis, ischemia, and re-routing of bowel may create a "CD-friendly" environment. Whether CD of the pouch or CD-like condition of the pouch is a true de novo, IBD is not known. Clinical phenotypes of CD of the pouch can be inflammatory, fibrostenotic, or fistulizing. The diagnosis of CD of the pouch often needs a combined assessment of symptoms, endoscopy, histology, radiography, and sometimes examination under anesthesia.

Patients with anatomic diseases (such as pouch leaks, sinus tracts, fistula, and abscesses) and pouch ischemia can present with symptoms resembling symptoms of patients with pouchitis. Again, pouch endoscopy is considered the first-line diagnostic modality. Additional evaluation with radiography or examination under general anesthesia may be helpful.

Irritable pouch syndrome is a functional disorder in patients with IPAA [60]. There are great overlaps in clinical presentation between irritable pouch syndrome and pouchitis. Currently, irritable pouch syndrome is a diagnosis of exclusion with symptoms but absence of endoscopic, radiographic, or histologic abnormalities. Pouch endoscopy is the diagnostic modality of choice for the distinction between pouchitis and irritable pouch syndrome.

## Management

While acute pouchitis is easy to treat, chronic pouchitis remains difficult to manage. The management strategies vary based on the etiology, triggering factors, and classification of pouchitis (Figs. 34.2 and 34.3) [61].

## Antibiotics

Since the majority of pouchitis is of bacterial etiology, antibiotic therapy is the mainstay of therapy. For antibiotic-responsive acute pouchitis, the first-line therapy includes a 14-day course of metronidazole (15–20 mg/kg/day) or ciprofloxacin (1,000 mg/day) [62, 63]. A randomized trial of ciprofloxacin (1,000 mg/day) and metronidazole (20 mg/kg/day) showed that patients treated with ciprofloxacin experienced a greater reduction in the disease activity scores and fewer adverse effects (0 % vs. 33 %) than those treated with metronidazole [63]. Most patients with acute pouchitis initially respond to ciprofloxacin at a dose of 500–1,000 mg/day or metronidazole at doses of 750–1,500 mg/day. Symptomatic improvement usually occurs within 1–2 days after initiation of therapy. Patients with relapsing or continuous pouchitis may require chronic maintenance ciprofloxacin therapy with doses ranging from 250 mg every third day up to 1,000 mg/day. Combination therapy with ciprofloxacin and metronidazole for 28 days was shown to be effective in treating backwash ileitis in a recent open-labeled trial [64]. Furthermore, diffuse pouchitis can be associated with backwash ileitis, particularly in patients with concurrent PSC. Those patients may be treated with antibiotics or oral budesonide (see below).

Rifaximin, a non-absorbed antibiotic frequently used in pouchitis, was not shown to be more effective than placebo in a small controlled trial [65]. However, rifaximin maintenance therapy appears to be effective in preventing relapse in a majority of patients with antibiotic-dependent pouchitis after induction of remission with a variety of antibiotics [66]. In this study, 51 patients began maintenance therapy with rifaximin (median dose 200 mg/day); 33 (65 %) maintained remission through 3 months. Of these 33 patients, 26 (79 %) successfully continued maintenance for 6 months after beginning maintenance, 19 (58 %) successfully continued for 12 months, and 2 (6 %) successfully continued for 24 months. Other oral antibiotics were also reported in open-labeled trials to be effective, including tetracycline, clarithromycin, amoxicillin/clavulanic acid, and doxycycline [67].

The management of chronic antibiotic-refractory pouchitis often poses a challenge. In fact, this phenotype of pouchitis is one of the most common causes for pouch failure requiring pouch excision or diversion. It is important to investigate contributing causes related to failure to antibiotic therapy. Fecal coliform sensitivity testing was shown to be helpful in guiding choice of appropriate antibiotics in patients with antibiotic-refractory pouchitis [68]. In this study, 80 % of patients achieved a clinical remission with individualized therapy based on sensitivity results.

For chronic antibiotic-refractory pouchitis, a combined use of antibiotic agents with a prolonged course may be attempted. In open-labeled trials, a combined therapy of ciprofloxacin (1,000 mg/day) with rifaximin (2,000 mg/day) [69, 70], metronidazole (1,000 mg/day) [71], or tinidazole (1,000–1,500 mg/day) for 4 weeks was reported to be effective [72]. However, maintenance of remission in this group of patients after a successful induction therapy with the dual antibiotic therapy remains to be challenging [73].

Chronic antibiotic-refractory pouchitis is often associated with secondary causes, such as NSAID use, concurrent *Clostridium difficile* [74], CMV [20, 21], or fungal infection [75], celiac disease, and other autoimmune disorders. Targeted therapy is a key.

## 5-ASA Agents

There are no randomized trials comparing oral or topical 5-aminosalicylate (5-ASA) therapy with placebo in management of pouchitis. Anecdotal reports suggest that topical (enema) or oral mesalamine may be of benefit [76, 77]. Topical mesalamine is also reported to be of benefit in management of cuffitis [56]. Recently, a pilot, open-labeled study showed that oral sulfasalazine (3,000 mg/day) leads to pouchitis in remission in 63 % of patients [78]. Sulfasalazine may be particularly indicated in patients with concurrent pouchitis and arthralgia or arthropathy, as NSAID is normally contraindicated in patients with IPAA.

## Corticosteroids

Oral prednisone is hardly used in the treatment of pouchitis due to its side effect profile and the lack of long-term efficacy. The only exception is pouchitis episode in pregnant women, in authors' experience. On the other hand, oral and topically active budesonide has been used in both acute and chronic pouchitis. A randomized controlled trial budesonide enema was conducted in comparison with oral metronidazole [79]. Improvement was similar in both groups, but budesonide enemas had a more favorable side effect profile. Budesonide suppositories for 4 weeks were showed to result in endoscopic improvement or remission in patients with acute pouchitis, but six of ten (60 %) patients relapsed 8 weeks later [80]. For patients who fail antibiotics, oral budesonide may be an option. In an open-labeled study of 20 patients with chronic antibiotic-refractory pouchitis, oral budesonide (9 mg/day orally for 8 weeks) induced remission in 15 (75 %) patients [81]. In a separate open-labeled series, budesonide induced a 60 % response rate in patients with antibiotic-refractory pouchitis [82].

With the description of autoimmune pouchitis, IgG4-associated pouchitis, and PSC-associated pouchitis/enteritis, oral budesonide has been routinely used in the authors' practice. Our anecdotal experience highlighted that some of the patients responded favorably to the therapy. We typically used oral budesonide 9 mg/day, with broken capsules, for treatment and 3–6 mg/day for maintenance therapy. As capsulated oral budesonide was designed for the pharmacologic action at the distal small bowel and autoimmune-associated pouchitis often involves whole small bowel and pouch, we expect that the administration of broken capsules may help drug delivery in a larger area of GI tract. Bone mineral density and blood glucose should be monitored in patients on long-term budesonide therapy.

## Immunomodulators

There are scant data on immunomodulator therapy for pouchitis. For patients with chronic pouchitis who are dependent on long-term maintenance therapy with antibiotics or topical and/or oral steroids, immunomodulators such as azathioprine and 6-mercaptopurine may be an alternative. Our anecdotal experience suggests that 6-mercaptopurine may be beneficial for patients with autoimmune pouchitis or IgG4-associated pouchitis. Anecdotal reports also suggested the efficacy of calcineurin inhibitors such as cyclosporine [83] and tacrolimus for therapy of chronic pouchitis.

## Biologics

Tumor necrosis factor alpha (TNF-α) expression has been shown significantly higher in mucosal pouch biopsies of patients with pouchitis than noninflamed pouches in UC patients [84]. Biological agents which have been routinely used in CD of the pouch have also been used in chronic refractory pouchitis [85]. Short-term treatment (10 weeks) with infliximab was reported to be effective in a small group (n=10) of patients with chronic antibiotic-refractory pouchitis complicated with ileitis [86]. Clinical remission was achieved in nine patients, and endoscopic remission with a complete healing of all lesions was observed in eight patients. Infliximab was also reported to be effective on a long-term basis in patients with refractory luminal inflammation and in some patients whose disease is complicated with pouch fistulas [87]. In this retrospective study, after a median follow-up of 20 months, 56 % showed sustained clinical response while three out of seven fistula patients showed sustained fistula response.

## Probiotics

It has been recommended by some individuals that patients with chronic pouchitis who achieve remission following antibiotic therapy but relapse more than three times per year should be treated with maintenance therapy [88]. Probiotics have been used as maintenance therapy for patients with antibiotic-dependent pouchitis or relapsing pouchitis (secondary prophylaxis), and also in prevention of pouchitis after IPAA surgery (primary prophylaxis). In addition, high-dose probiotics have been used for treating pouchitis. In a study of a probiotic agent, VSL#3®, 3,600 billion bacteria/day in treating mild pouchitis, 16 of 23 patients (69 %) were in remission after treatment [89]. A prospective, randomized, double-blind, placebo-controlled trial highlighted that treatment with VSL#3® at a dose of 900 billion bacteria/day was also effective in the prevention of the onset of acute pouchitis

and improved quality of life of patients with IPAA [90]. A randomized trial of VSL#3® at a dose of 6 g/day was conducted for the maintenance therapy to prevent relapse of pouchitis, after remission was induced by oral ciprofloxacin (1,000 mg/day) plus rifaximin (2,000 mg/day). During the 9-month trial of 40 patients with relapsing pouchitis, 15 % in the probiotic group relapsed vs. 100 % in the placebo group relapsed [91]. A separate randomized trial of VSL#3® in patients with antibiotic-dependent pouchitis showed that 17 of 20 patients (85 %) in the VSL#3® group maintained clinical remission, compared to remission in 1 of 16 patients (6 %) in the placebo group [92]. A meta-analysis of five randomized, placebo-controlled clinical trials was performed. Pooling of the results from these trials yielded an odds ratio of 0.04 in the treatment group in comparison with the placebo group. The benefit of probiotics in the management of pouchitis after IPAA operation was confirmed by the meta-analysis [93]. However, the routine use of probiotics for the induction and maintenance therapy of pouchitis has stirred some controversy. Some post-market open-labeled studies reported a much lower response rate of pouchitis that was originally reported. The above outstanding results have been challenged by two recent post-market open-labeled trials. In a study of 31 patients with antibiotic-dependent pouchitis treated with VSL#3® for maintenance therapy after 2 weeks of treatment with ciprofloxacin, 25 patients (81 %) had stopped the agent at 8 months, mainly because of the lack of efficacy or development of adverse effects [94]. Similar results were reported in a separate open-labeled trial [95].

## Other Agents

Other agents, including allopurinol [96, 97], bismuth carbomer enema [98, 99], short-chain fatty acid (SCFA) enemas, and glutamine enemas, have been reported to be of benefit from uncontrolled data. However, based on currently available controlled data, bismuth and allopurinol cannot be advocated as a therapy for pouchitis [100]. Considering the low overall response rates observed during open therapy with SCFA or glutamine, it appears not beneficial for pouchitis and cannot be advocated as standard therapy [100]. Recently, leukocytapheresis [101] and AST-120 (spherical carbon adsorbent) [102] showed benefit in patients with acute pouchitis. Randomized, placebo-controlled trials are warranted for assessing the long-term efficacy of these strategies.

## Endoscopic Polypectomy

Chronic pouchitis can be associated with single or multiple, small or large inflammatory polyps. Large (>1 cm) pouch polyps can occasionally cause bleeding and can be dysplastic. Endoscopic polypectomy is feasible, which may be helpful in controlling patients' symptoms, in conjunction with medical therapy [103].

## Summary and Conclusions

Pouchitis is the most common long-term complication of IPAA, which represents a spectrum of disease processes with different clinical phenotypes, risk factors, pathogenetic pathways, natural history, and prognosis. Pouch endoscopy is the most valuable tool for diagnosis and differential diagnosis. While the majority of patients with pouchitis respond favorably to antibiotic therapy, antibiotic-dependent or antibiotic-refractory diseases have posed a therapeutic challenge. Management of pouchitis, particularly chronic pouchitis, can be difficult. The search for a secondary etiology of pouchitis, such as *Clostridium difficile* infection, should be performed. Medical treatment of pouchitis is largely empiric, and only a few small randomized, placebo-controlled trials have been conducted. To date, there were no FDA-approved agents for pouchitis or other pouch disorders. A multidisciplinary approach involving gastroenterologists and colorectal surgeons, together with a team of GI pathologists and GI radiologists is advocated.

## References

1. Penna C, Tiret E, Kartheuser A, et al. Function of ileal J pouch-anal anastomosis in patients with familial adenomatous polyposis. Br J Surg. 1993;80:765–7.
2. Tjandra JJ, Fazio VW, Church JM, et al. Similar functional results after restorative proctocolectomy in patients with familial adenomatous polyposis and mucosal ulcerative colitis. Am J Surg. 1993;165:322–5.
3. Banasiewicz T, Marciniak R, Kaczmarek E, et al. The prognosis of clinical course and the analysis of the frequency of the inflammation and dysplasia in the intestinal J-pouch at the patients after restorative proctocolectomy due to FAP. Int J Colorectal Dis. 2011;26(9):1197–203.
4. Penna C, Dozois R, Tremaine W, et al. Pouchitis after ileal pouch-anal anastomosis for ulcerative colitis occurs with increased frequency in patients with associated primary sclerosing cholangitis. Gut. 1996;38:234–9.
5. Fazio VW, Ziv Y, Church JM, et al. Ileal pouch-anal anastomosis complications and function in 1005 patients. Ann Surg. 1995;222:120–7.
6. Ferrante M, Declerck S, De Hertogh G, et al. Outcome after proctocolectomy with ileal pouch-anal anastomosis for ulcerative colitis. Inflamm Bowel Dis. 2008;14:20–8.
7. Fleshner P, Ippoliti A, Dubinsky M, et al. Both preoperative perinuclear antineutrophil cytoplasmic antibody and anti-CBir1 expression in ulcerative colitis patients influence pouchitis development after ileal pouch-anal anastomosis. Clin Gastroenterol Hepatol. 2008;6:561–8.
8. Stocchi L, Pemberton JH. Pouch and pouchitis. Gastroenterol Clin North Am. 2001;30:223–41.
9. Gionchetti P, Rizzello F, Helwig U, et al. Prophylaxis of pouchitis onset with probiotic therapy: a double-blind placebo controlled trial. Gastroenterology. 2003;124:1202–9.
10. Abdelrazeq AS, Kandiyil N, Botterill ID, et al. Predictors for acute and chronic pouchitis following restorative proctocolectomy for ulcerative colitis. Colorectal Dis. 2008;10:805–13.
11. Meagher AP, Farouk R, Dozois RR, et al. J ileal pouch-anal anastomosis for chronic ulcerative colitis: complications and long-term outcome in 1310 patients. Br J Surg. 1998;85:800–3.
12. Wu H, Shen B. Pouchitis and pouch dysfunction. Gastroenterol Clin North Am. 2009;38:651–68.
13. Ohge H, Furne JK, Springfield J, et al. Association between fecal hydrogen sulfide production and pouchitis. Dis Colon Rectum. 2005;48:469–75.
14. Gosselink MP, Schouten WR, van Lieshout LM, et al. Eradication of pathogenic bacteria and restoration of normal pouch flora: comparison of metronidazole and ciprofloxacin in the treatment of pouchitis. Dis Colon Rectum. 2004;47:1519–25.
15. Komanduri S, Gillevet PM, Sikaroodi M, et al. Dysbiosis in pouchitis: evidence of unique microfloral patterns in pouch inflammation. Clin Gastroenterol Hepatol. 2007;5:352–60.
16. McLaughlin SD, Walker AW, Churcher C, et al. The bacteriology of pouchitis: a molecular phylogenetic analysis using 16S rRNA gene cloning and sequencing. Ann Surg. 2010;252:90–8.
17. Mann SD, Pitt J, Springall RG, et al. Clostridium difficile infection-an unusual cause of refractory pouchitis: report of a case. Dis Colon Rectum. 2003;46:267–70.
18. Shen B, Goldblum JR, Hull TL, et al. Clostridium difficile-associated pouchitis. Dig Dis Sci. 2006;51:2361–4.
19. Shen B. Campylobacter infection in patients with ileal pouches. Am J Gastroenterol. 2010;105:472–3.
20. Munoz-Juarez M, Pemberton JH, Sandborn WJ, et al. Misdiagnosis of specific cytomegalovirus infection of ileoanal pouch as a refractory idiopathic chronic pouchitis: report of two cases. Dis Colon Rectum. 1999;42:117–20.
21. Mooka D, Furth EE, MacDermott RP, et al. Pouchitis associated with primary cytomegalovirus infection. Am J Gastroenterol. 1998;93:264–6.
22. Casadesus D, Tani T, Wakai T, et al. Possible role of human cytomegalovirus in pouchitis after proctocolectomy with ileal pouch-anal anastomosis in patients with ulcerative colitis. World J Gastroenterol. 2007;13:1085–9.
23. Kroesen AJ, Leistenschneider P, Lehmann K, et al. Increased bacterial permeation in long-lasting ileoanal pouches. Inflamm Bowel Dis. 2006;12:736–44.
24. DeSilva HJ, Jones M, Prince C, et al. Lymphocyte and macrophage subpopulations in pelvic ileal reservoirs. Gut. 1991;32:1160–5.
25. Hirata I, Berrebi G, Austin LL, et al. Immunohistological characterization of intraepithelial and lamina propria lymphocytes in control ileum and colon and inflammatory bowel disease. Dig Dis Sci. 1986;31:593–603.
26. Stallmach A, Schafer F, Hoffman S, et al. Increased state of activation of CD4 positive T cells and elevated interferon gamma production in pouchitis. Gut. 1998;43:499–505.
27. Thomas PD, Forbes A, Nicholls RJ, et al. Altered expression of the lymphocyte activation markers CD30 and CD27 in patients with pouchitis. Scand J Gastroenterol. 2001;36:258–64.
28. Goldberg PA, Herbst F, Beckett CG, et al. Leukocyte typing, cytokine expression and epithelial turnover in the ileal pouch in patients with ulcerative colitis and familial adenomatous polyposis. Gut. 1996;38:549–53.
29. Carter K, Di Giovine FS, Cox A, et al. The interleukin 1 receptor antagonist gene allele 2 as a predictor of pouchitis following colectomy and IPAA in ulcerative colitis. Gastroenterology. 2001;121:805–11.

30. Aisenberg J, Legnani PE, Nilubol N, et al. Are pANCA, ASCA, or cytokine gene polymorphisms associated with pouchitis? Long-term follow-up in 102 ulcerative colitis. Am J Gastroenterol. 2004;99:432–41.

31. Meier C, Hegazi RA, Aisenberg J, et al. Innate immune receptor genetic polymorphisms in pouchitis: is NOD2/CARD15 a susceptibility factor? Inflamm Bowel Dis. 2005;11:965–71.

32. Tyler AD, Milgrom R, Xu W, et al. The NOD2 insC risk allele is associated with poor pouch outcome following IPAA in patients with ulcerative colitis. Gastroenterology. 2011;140:S-271.

33. Sehgal R, Berg A, Hegarty JP, et al. NOD2/CARD15 mutations correlate with severe pouchitis after ileal pouch-anal anastomosis. Dis Colon Rectum. 2010;53:1487–94.

34. Shen B, Achkar J-P, Lashner BA, et al. Endoscopic and histologic evaluations together with symptom assessment are required to diagnose pouchitis. Gastroenterology. 2001;121:261–7.

35. Shen B, Fazio VW, Remzi FH, et al. Risk factors for diseases of ileal pouch-anal anastomosis in patients with ulcerative colitis. Clin Gastroenterol Hepatol. 2006;4:81–9.

36. Heuschen UA, Hinz U, Allemeyer EH, et al. One- or two-stage procedure for restorative proctocolectomy: rationale for a surgical strategy in ulcerative colitis. Ann Surg. 2001;234:788–94.

37. Tiainen J, Matikainen M. Long-term clinical outcome and anemia after restorative proctocolectomy for ulcerative colitis. Scand J Gastroenterol. 2000;35:1170–3.

38. Schmidt CM, Lazenby AJ, Hendrickson RJ, et al. Pre-operative terminal ileal and colonic resection histopathology predicts risk of pouchitis in patients after ileoanal pull-through procedure. Ann Surg. 1998;227:654–62.

39. Achkar JP, Al-Haddad M, Lashner B, et al. Differentiating risk factors for acute and chronic pouchitis. Clin Gastroenterol Hepatol. 2005;3:60–6.

40. Okon A, Dubinsky M, Vasilauskas EA, et al. Elevated platelet count before ileal pouch–anal anastomosis for ulcerative colitis is associated with the development of chronic pouchitis. Am Surg. 2005;71:821–6.

41. Hata K, Watanabe T, Shinozaki M, et al. Patients with extraintestinal manifestations have a higher risk of developing pouchitis in ulcerative colitis—multivariate analysis. Scand J Gastroenterol. 2003;38:1055–8.

42. Lepistö A, Kärkkäinen P, Järvinen HJ. Prevalence of primary sclerosing cholangitis in ulcerative colitis patients undergoing proctocolectomy and ileal pouch-anal anastomosis. Inflamm Bowel Dis. 2008;14:775–9.

43. Fleshner PR, Vasiliauskas EA, Kam LY, et al. High level perinuclear antineutrophil cytoplasmic antibody (pANCA) in ulcerative colitis patients before colectomy predicts the development of chronic pouchitis after ileal pouch-anal anastomosis. Gut. 2001;49:671–7.

44. Kuisma J, Jarvinen H, Kahri A, et al. Factors associated with disease activity of pouchitis after surgery for ulcerative colitis. Scand J Gastroenterol. 2004;39:544–8.

45. Shen B, Remzi FH, Bennett AE, et al. Association between immune-associated disorders and adverse outcomes of ileal pouch-anal anastomosis. Am J Gastroenterol. 2009;104:655–64.

46. Moskowitz RL, Shepherd NA, Nicholls RJ. An assessment of inflammation in the reservoir after restorative proctocolectomy with ileoanal ileal reservoir. Int J Colorectal Dis. 1986;1:167–74.

47. Sandborn WJ, Tremaine WJ, Batts KP, et al. Pouchitis after ileal pouch-anal anastomosis: a pouchitis disease activity index. Mayo Clin Proc. 1994;69:409–15.

48. Kariv R, Plesec TP, Gaffney K, et al. Pyloric gland metaplasia and pouchitis in patients with ileal pouch-anal anastomoses. Aliment Pharmacol Ther. 2010;31:862–73.

49. Kariv R, Remzi FH, Lian L, et al. Preoperative colorectal neoplasia increases risk for pouch neoplasia in patients with restorative proctocolectomy. Gastroenterology. 2010;139:806–12.

50. Shen B, Fazio VW, Bennett AE, et al. Effect of withdrawal of non-steroidal anti-inflammatory drug use in patients with the ileal pouch. Dig Dis Sci. 2007;52:3321–8.

51. Sandborn WJ. Pouchitis: Risk factors, frequency, natural history, classification and public health prospective. In: McLeod RS, Martin F, Sutherland LR, Wallace JL, Williams CN, editors. Trends in Inflammatory Bowel Disease 1996. Lancaster, UK: Kluwer Academic Publishers; 1997. p. 51–63.

52. Shen B. Diagnosis and management of patients with pouchitis. Drugs. 2003;65:453–61.

53. Shen B, Bennett AE, Navaneethan U. IgG4-associated pouchitis. Inflamm Bowel Dis. 2011;17:1247–8.

54. Navaneethan U, Shen B. Hepatopancreatobiliary manifestations and complications associated with inflammatory bowel disease. Inflamm Bowel Dis. 2010;16:1598–619.

55. Navaneethan U, Venkatesh PG, Kapoor S, et al. Elevated serum IgG4 is associated with chronic antibiotic-refractory pouchitis. J Gastrointest Surg. 2011;15(9):1556–61.

56. Shen B, Lashner BA, Bennett AE, et al. Treatment of rectal cuff inflammation (cuffitis) in patients with ulcerative colitis following restorative proctocolectomy and ileal pouch-anal anastomosis. Am J Gastroenterol. 2004;99:1527–31.

57. Thompson-Fawcett MW, Mortensen NJ, Warren BF. "Cuffitis" and inflammatory changes in the columnar cuff, anal transitional zone, and ileal reservoir after stapled pouch-anal anastomosis. Dis Colon Rectum. 1999;42:348–55.

58. Shen B, Liu X. De novo collagenous cuffitis. Inflamm Bowel Dis. 2011;17:1249–950.

59. Panis Y, Poupard B, Nemeth J, et al. Ileal pouch-anal anastomosis for Crohn's disease. Lancet. 1996;347:854–7.

60. Shen B, Achkar J-P, Lashner BA, et al. Irritable pouch syndrome: a new category of diagnosis for symptomatic patients with ileal pouch-anal anastomosis. Am J Gastroenterol. 2002;97:972–7.

61. Nicholls RJ. Review article: Ulcerative colitis-surgical indications and treatment. Aliment Pharmacol Ther. 2002;16:25–8.

62. Madden MV, McIntyre AS, Nicholls RJ. Double-blinded crossover trial of metronidazole versus placebo in chronic unremitting pouchitis. Dig Dis Sci. 1994;39:1193–6.

63. Shen B, Achkar JP, Lashner BA, et al. A randomized trial of ciprofloxacin and metronidazole in treating acute pouchitis. Inflamm Bowel Dis. 2001;7:301–5.

64. McLaughlin SD, Clark SK, Bell AJ, et al. An open study of antibiotics for the treatment of pre-pouch ileitis following restorative proctocolectomy with ileal pouch-anal anastomosis. Aliment Pharmacol Ther. 2009;29:69–74.

65. Isaacs KL, Sandler RS, Abreu M, Crohn's and Colitis Foundation of America Clinical Alliance, et al. Rifaximin for the treatment of active pouchitis: a randomized, double-blind, placebo-controlled pilot study. Inflamm Bowel Dis. 2007;13:1250–5.

66. Shen B, Remzi FH, Lopez AR, et al. Rifaximin for maintenance therapy in antibiotic-dependent pouchitis. BMC Gastroenterol. 2008;8:26 [electronic journal].

67. Scott AD, Phillips RK. Ileitis and pouchitis after colectomy for ulcerative colitis. Br J Surg. 1989;76:668–9.

68. McLaughlin SD, Clark SK, Shafi S, et al. Fecal coliform testing to identify effective antibiotic therapies for patients with antibiotic-resistant pouchitis. Clin Gastroenterol Hepatol. 2009;7:545–8.

69. Gionchetti P, Rizzello F, Venturi A, et al. Antibiotic combination therapy in patients with chronic treatment-resistant pouchitis. Aliment Pharmacol Ther. 1999;13:713–8.

70. Abdelrazeq AS, Kelly SM, Lund JN, et al. Rifaximin-ciprofloxacin combination therapy is effective in chronic active refractory pouchitis. Colorectal Dis. 2005;7:182–6.

71. Mimura T, Rizzello R, Helwig U, et al. Four-week open-label trial of metronidazole and ciprofloxacin for the treatment of recurrent or refractory pouchitis. Aliment Pharmacol Ther. 2002;16:909–17.

72. Shen B, Fazio VW, Remzi FH, et al. Combined ciprofloxacin and tinidazole in the treatment of chronic refractory pouchitis. Dis Colon Rectum. 2007;50:498–508.

73. Viscido A, Kohn A, Papi C, et al. Management of refractory fistulizing pouchitis with infliximab. Eur Rev Med Pharmacol Sci. 2004;8:239–46.

74. Shen B, Jiang Z-D, Fazio VW, et al. Clostridium difficile infection in patients with ileal pouch-anal anastomosis. Clin Gastroenterol Hepatol. 2008;6:782–8.

75. Kühbacher T, Ott SJ, Helwig U, et al. Bacterial and fungal microbiota in relation to probiotic therapy (VSL#3) in pouchitis. Gut. 2006;55:833–41.

76. Miglioli M, Barbara L, Di Febo G, et al. Topical administration of 5-aminosalicylic acid: a therapeutic proposal for the treatment of pouchitis. N Engl J Med. 1989;320:257.

77. Pardi DS, D'Haens G, Shen B, et al. Clinical guidelines for the management of pouchitis. Inflamm Bowel Dis. 2009;15:1424–31.

78. Belluzzi A, Serrani M, Roda G, et al. Pilot study: the use of sulfasalazine for the treatment of acute pouchitis. Aliment Pharmacol Ther. 2010;31:228–32.

79. Sambuelli A, Boerr L, Negreira S, et al. Budesonide enema in pouchitis- a double-blind, double-dummy, controlled trial. Aliment Pharmacol Ther. 2002;16:27–34.

80. Belluzzi A, Campieri M, Miglioli M, et al. Evaluation of flogistic pattern in "pouchitis" before and after treatment with budesonide suppositories. Gastroenterology. 1992;102:A593.

81. Gionchetti P, Rizzello F, Poggioli G, et al. Oral budesonide in the treatment of chronic refractory pouchitis. Aliment Pharmacol Ther. 2007;25:1231–6.

82. Chopra A, Pardi DS, Loftus Jr EV, et al. Budesonide in the treatment of inflammatory bowel disease: the first year of experience in clinical practice. Inflamm Bowel Dis. 2006;12:29–32.

83. Hait EJ, Bousvaros A, Schuman M, et al. Pouch outcomes among children with ulcerative colitis treated with calcineurin inhibitors before ileal pouch anal anastomosis surgery. J Pediatr Surg. 2007;42:31–4.

84. Patel RT, Bain I, Youngs D, et al. Cytokine production in pouchitis is similar to that in ulcerative colitis. Dis Colon Rectum. 1995;38:831–7.

85. Viscido A, Habib FI, Kohn A, et al. Infliximab in refractory pouchitis complicated by fistulae following ileoanal pouch for ulcerative colitis. Aliment Pharmacol Ther. 2003;17:1263–71.

86. Calabrese C, Gionchetti P, Rizzello F, et al. Short-term treatment with infliximab in chronic refractory pouchitis and ileitis. Aliment Pharmacol Ther. 2008;27:759–64.

87. Ferrante M, D'Haens G, Dewit O, et al. Efficacy of infliximab in refractory pouchitis and Crohn's disease-related complications of the pouch: a Belgian case series. Inflamm Bowel Dis. 2010;16:243.

88. Pardi DS, Sandborn WJ. Systematic review: the management of pouchitis. Aliment Pharmacol Ther. 2006;23:1087–96.

89. Gionchetti P, Rizzello F, Morselli C, et al. High-dose probiotics for the treatment of active pouchitis. Dis Colon Rectum. 2007;50:2075–84.

90. Gionchetti P, Rizzello F, Helwig U, et al. Prophylaxis of pouchitis onset with probiotic therapy: a double-blind, placebo-controlled trial. Gastroenterology. 2003;124:1202–9.

91. Gionchetti P, Rizzello F, Venturi A, et al. Oral bacteriotherapy as maintenance treatment in patients with chronic pouchitis: a double-blind, placebo-controlled trial. Gastroenterology. 2000;119:305–9.

92. Mimura T, Rizzello F, Helwig U, et al. Once daily high dose probiotic therapy (VSL#3®) for maintaining remission in recurrent or refractory pouchitis. Gut. 2004;53:108–14.

93. Elahi B, Nikfar S, Derakhshani S, et al. On the benefit of probiotics in the management of pouchitis in patients underwent ileal pouch anal anastomosis: a meta-analysis of controlled clinical trials. Dig Dis Sci. 2008;53:1278–84.

94. Shen B, Brzezinski A, Fazio VW, et al. Maintenance therapy with a probiotic in antibiotic-dependent pouchitis—experience in clinical practice. Aliment Pharmacol Ther. 2005;22:721–8.

95. McLaughlin SD, Johnson MW, Clark SK, et al. VSL#3 for chronic pouchitis; experience in UK clinical practice. Gastroenterology. 2008;134 Suppl 1:A711.

96. Levin KE, Pemberton JH, Phillips SF, et al. Role of oxygen free radicals in the etiology of pouchitis. Dis Colon Rectum. 1992;35:452–6.

97. Joelsson M, Andersson M, Bark T, et al. Allopurinol as prophylaxis against pouchitis following ileal pouch-anal anastomosis for ulcerative colitis. A randomized placebo-controlled double-blind study. Scand J Gastroenterol. 2001;36:1179–84.

98. Giochetti P, Rizzello F, Venturi A, et al. Long-term efficacy of bismuth carbomer enemas in patients with treatment-resistant chronic pouchitis. Aliment Pharmacol Ther. 1997;11:673–8.

99. Tremaine WJ, Sandborn WJ, Wolff BG, et al. Bismuth carbomer foam enemas for active chronic pouchitis: a randomized, double-blind, placebo-controlled trial. Aliment Pharmacol Ther. 1997;11:1041–6.

100. Holubar SD, Cima RR, Sandborn WJ, et al. Treatment and prevention of pouchitis after ileal pouch-anal anastomosis for chronic ulcerative colitis (Review). Cochrane Database Syst Rev. 2010;16, CD001176.

101. Araki Y, Mitsuyama K, Nagae T, et al. Leukocytapheresis for the treatment of active pouchitis: a pilot study. J Gastroenterol. 2008;43:571–5.

102. Shen B, Pardi DS, Bennett AE, et al. The efficacy and tolerability of AST-120 (spherical carbon adsorbent) in active pouchitis. Am J Gastroenterol. 2009;104:1468–74.

103. Schaus BJ, Fazio VW, Remzi FH, et al. Large polyps in the ileal pouch in patients with underlying ulcerative colitis. Dis Colon Rectum. 2007;50:832–8.

# Medical Management of Extraintestinal Manifestations of Ulcerative Colitis

Randy S. Longman and Ellen J. Scherl

---

**Keywords**

Medical management • Extraintestinal manifestations • Ulcerative colitis • Pathogenesis • Epidemiology

---

## Introduction

Inflammatory bowel disease (IBD) is a group of disorders characterized by a dysregulated immune response to environmental antigens in genetically susceptible individuals. Typical clinical, endoscopic, and pathologic characteristics of intestinal disease divide IBD into ulcerative colitis (UC) and Crohn's disease (CD). While intestinal characteristics define the type of disease, the systemic nature of the underlying immune disorder is revealed clinically by extraintestinal manifestations (EIMs). Classical EIMs include joint, skin, ocular, and hepatobiliary manifestations; however, as our knowledge of the systemic effects of IBD expands, additional organ systems have been included under the umbrella of EIMs, including hematologic and pulmonary manifestations. Often these EIMs can cause significant morbidity and mortality and pose significant challenges for the managing physician.

In this chapter, we focused on the medical management of EIMs primarily associated with UC. There is considerable overlap with respect to particular EIMs associated with UC or CD, and the current evidence for management is frequently extrapolated from non-IBD cases. Notable cases are highlighted to provide the evidence for practical management. Diagnostic and epidemiologic data are discussed where applicable to enhance management algorithms or treatment strategies, but a comprehensive review of all EIMs in IBD is beyond the scope of this review.

While the characterization of EIMs is based on the clinical phenotype, the elucidation of the underlying pathogenic mechanisms offers the promise of improving diagnostic and therapeutic modalities. Genetic susceptibility and environmental triggers likely converge to produce clinical manifestations of disease. Genome-wide association studies have uncovered numerous disease susceptibility genes involved in T cell activation (e.g., *STAT3, IL23R*) and response to microbial stimuli (e.g., *NOD2, ATG16L*). With large networks of intestinal lymphoid tissue in close proximity to a high density of luminal bacteria, the gut is the likely portal of entry for the dysregulated immune response. Intestinal microbes can provide "danger" signals to break the immune system's tolerance to "self"-antigens. Alternatively, microbial-derived antigens may stimulate autoimmune responses by mimicking tissue antigens. Emerging data from both human and mouse models have begun to define how the microbiome (the collection of organisms residing in the intestine) shape the systemic immune response. Studies of the microbiome have revealed notable differences for patients with IBD compared to non-IBD controls [1–3], but a microbial cause of IBD remains elusive. Further studies defining the genetics and microbiology in IBD patients with EIMs will ultimately drive improved immunophenotyping and therapeutic strategies. As such, we have included the emerging clinical and research data on the etiopathogenesis of

R.S. Longman, M.D., Ph.D. (✉) • E.J. Scherl, M.D., A.G.A.F., F.A.C.G.
Division of Gastroenterology and Hepatology,
Department of Medicine, The Jill Roberts Center for IBD,
New York Presbyterian Hospital/Weill Cornell Medical Center,
Weill Cornell Medical College, 1315 York Avenue,
Mezzanine Level, New York, NY 10021, USA
e-mail: ral2006@med.cornell.edu; ejs2005@med.cornell.edu

G.R. Lichtenstein (ed.), *Medical Therapy of Ulcerative Colitis*,
DOI 10.1007/978-1-4939-1677-1_35, © Springer Science+Business Media New York 2014

EIMs to highlight the emerging role for a molecular taxonomy of disease subtypes with distinct prognostic and therapeutic significance [4].

## Classification

EIMs can be classified under three main groups: reactive manifestations in various organ systems, non-IBD-specific autoimmune manifestations (hemolytic anemia, thyroid disease, vitiligo, and insulin-dependent diabetes mellitus), and IBD-related complications (metabolic bone disease, nephrolithiasis, amyloidosis). Reactive manifestations can be associated with disease activity (type I peripheral arthritis, erythema nodosum, aphthous stomatitis) or independent (pyoderma gangrenosum, uveitis, ankylosing spondylitis, primary sclerosing cholangitis, type II arthritis). While the classification of these manifestations by intestinal activity has been incorporated into the canonical teaching of IBD, in practice these associations offer general guidelines rather than absolute characterizations [5]. Given the variable association of EIMs with intestinal disease and the desire to offer a clear approach according to manifestation, this chapter is organized by symptom/organ system.

## Epidemiology

Retrospective analysis of case records of 700 patients found EIMs in 36 % of the entire series, of which 202 carried a diagnosis of UC [6]. The majority of these EIMs (23 %) were associated with joint inflammation. The analysis of the National Cooperative Crohn's Disease Study reported a similar 24 % incidence in a cohort of 569 patients with Crohn's disease [7]. Prospective analysis of 792 patients (343 with UC) followed for up to 20 years revealed a 25.8 % occurrence of at least one EIM [8]. More recent prospective population-based analysis of 850 IBD patients from Switzerland supported these estimates, revealing 61 % of CD and 39 % of UC patients with at least one ongoing EIM. Similarly, peripheral arthritis (defined as "pain, swelling, and redness in one or several joints") in this cohort accounted for 33.3 and 21.3 % of EIM in CD and UC, respectively [9]. Population-based, longitudinal analysis of patients from the Manitoba IBD database revealed a 10-year prevalence of 5.5 and 7 % for CD and UC, respectively [10]. Notably, these data exclude arthritis/arthralgia which likely accounts for the drastic differences reported for EIM prevalence.

In this chapter, we have focused on the medical management of EIMs associated with UC. Although joint symptoms are reported more frequently in CD, they are also the most frequent EIM in UC (11–21.3 %) [8, 9] and will be discussed

below. Similarly, erythema nodosum and aphthous stomatitis are more common in CD [6, 9], but found in >3 % of UC patients and discussed below. Other skin manifestations such as pyoderma gangrenosum are less frequently reported overall (0.8–2.2 %), but are associated more commonly with ulcerative colitis. Primary sclerosing cholangitis (PSC) is similarly more frequently found in the setting of UC. Ocular manifestations and axial spondyloarthropathies are common in both UC and CD.

## Pathogenesis

### Adaptive Immunity

While the clinical association of IBD with EIMs was described almost a century ago, the mechanisms underlying the pathogenesis have not been well characterized. Genome-wide association studies revealed polymorphisms in genes involved in the maintenance of epithelial barrier integrity, innate pattern recognition, and T cell function [11], but the impact of these genetic susceptibility alleles on particular EIMs has not been reported. Familial studies of EIMs in IBD show high concordance rates between first-degree relatives [12, 13] suggesting a genetic predisposition. Although significant genetic heterogeneity exists within IBD, major histocompatibility alleles DRB1*103 (8.3 % vs. 3.2 % in controls) and DRB1*12 are implicated in inherited susceptibility to IBD [14], particularly in patients with EIMs including arthritis, aphthous stomatitis, and uveitis [13, 15]. These associations highlight the importance of dysregulated adaptive immunity in the pathogenesis of EIMs. Of note, aberrant expression of chemokine CCL25 by hepatic sinusoidal endothelium enables the recruitment of these inflammatory intestinal T cell to the liver in PSC [16]. Autoantibodies against various isoforms of tropomyosin have been reported in patients with UC, and the cross-reactivity against tropomyosin in extraintestinal organs may underlie the systemic immune response [17].

### Intestinal Microbes Drive Systemic Inflammation

Microbial antigen at the mucosal interface may likely trigger the dysregulated immune response. This hypothesis is supported by the clinical observation that EIMs are much more frequently associated with colonic or ileocolonic disease compared to isolated small bowel enteritis (42 % in colonic disease vs. 23 % in isolated small bowel) [6]. The colon (in particular, the cecum) contains a higher microbial burden than the small intestine, and the colonic intestinal microbiota may regulate lamina propria immune cell activation. In particular, the colon is an important site for microbial-dependent induction of regulatory CD4+ T cell function [18]. Regulatory T cells produce the cytokine interleukin (IL)-10 which regulates the production of inflammatory cytokines [19]. Clostridium clusters IV and XIVa induce regulatory T cells in the colon and protect mice from chemically induced colitis [18]. Lachnospiraceae, which include clostridium clusters IV and XIVa, are decreased in patients with IBD [3]. Moreover, reduction in *Faecalibacterium prausnitzii*, a member of cluster IV, correlates with higher incidence of postoperative recurrence of ileal Crohn's disease [20]. Enhancing regulatory T cell function can protect against colitis and systemic arthritis [21, 22]. In addition to regulatory T cells, the genetic importance of the IL-23 receptor in IBD highlighted the importance of IL-23 responsive T cells, which produce proinflammatory cytokines IL-17 (called "Th17" cells). Notably, Th17 cells play an important role in human [23] and mouse models of arthritis [24, 25]. The colonization of the terminal ileum by segmented filamentous bacteria is sufficient to induce intestinal Th17 [26] and systemic manifestations of autoimmunity [27].

Microbial regulation of innate immunity may also play an important role. Mouse models of UC revealed a crucial role for the transcription factor T-bet in colonic dendritic cells (DCs), which protect against intestinal disease [28]. Interestingly, T-bet functions in peripheral DCs to enhance immune inflammation in the joints [29] suggesting that the dysregulation of DC function may be central to the link between intestinal and systemic immune activation. T-bet-dependent UC is transmissible by intestinal microbiota, and sequencing of the bacteria revealed that *Klebsiella pneumoniae* and *Proteus mirabilis* (in the presence of maternally transmitted microbiota) can induce disease [30]. Although a microbial cause for EIMs remains to be identified, ongoing studies evaluating the pathogenesis in human may ultimately improve diagnostic immunophenotyping to allow for targeted therapy either by microbial manipulation (e.g., antibiotics/fecal bacteriotherapy) or medical regulation of signaling in immune cells.

## Joint Manifestations

Joint pain is the most common EIM occurring in 6–33 % of patients with IBD [9, 31]. Symptoms are reported more frequently in CD [32, 33], but population-based studies indicate rates of 15–21 % in patients with UC. IBD-associated joint pain is clustered with seronegative spondyloarthritis (SpA), which also includes reactive arthritis, psoriatic arthritis, ankylosing spondylitis, and undifferentiated SpA. IBD-associated SpA may either be peripheral or axial. IBD-associated peripheral arthritis (PeA) has been characterized clinically as either type I or type II [31]. Type I PeA is an acute, pauciarticular arthritis, affecting <5 joints, one of

which is a large, weight-bearing joint. Type I PeA is often associated with intestinal inflammation and occurs frequently in patients with other EIMs (particularly erythema nodosum and uveitis). Type II PeA is a persistent polyarticular arthropathy with a median duration of 3 years. Symptoms are generally independent of intestinal inflammation, but may be associated with uveitis. Large cross-sectional analysis of 976 UC patients reports rates of 3.6 % type I and 2.5 % type II. These low rates reflect strict exclusion of patients with arthralgias in comparison to population-based studies [9, 34]. Type I PeA is associated with HLA-B27 [31], validating its inclusion as a seronegative SpA, as well as a rare major histocompatibility II allele HLA-DRB1*0103. HLA-B44 is associated with type II arthritis (RR2.1) suggesting the possibility of different immune-mediated mechanism.

In addition to peripheral arthropathy, axial spondyloarthropathy including ankylosing spondylitis is frequent in IBD. Although back pain is present in 20–30 % of patients and radiographic imaging of sacroiliitis is present in 20–25 %, only 2–10 % of patients with IBD fulfill the criteria of ankylosing spondylitis [35]. The recent development of new criteria by the Assessment of SpondyloArthritis international Society (ASAS) has increased the sensitivity and specificity of diagnosis to 83 and 84 %, respectively, and may improve early detection of AS in IBD. These criteria include radiographic imaging (X-ray or MRI) of sacroiliitis plus one feature of SpA or the presence of HLA-B27 with two clinical features of SpA [36].

The differential diagnosis of joint pain in IBD includes delayed infusion reactions or drug-induced lupus, osteoarthritis, infection, tendonitis, and fracture. Red and warm joints signal inflammation compared to simple arthralgia. Multiple joints suggest systemic inflammation or medication reaction compared with isolated joints reflecting trauma or infection. Complaints of back or hip pain should precipitate evaluation for ankylosing spondylitis, psoas abscess with CD, or avascular necrosis in a patient with previous steroid exposure. Laboratory evaluation will often involve ESR and CRP as serologic markers of systemic inflammation and antibody titers of ANA and anti-dsDNA. Notably, infliximab and adalimumab can be associated with drug-induced ANA positivity or lupus-like arthralgias; transition to certolizumab (which lacks the Fc portion) resolves this immune-mediated phenotype [37]. HLA-B27 may be important to exclude ankylosing spondylitis and imaging may be important to help clarify the diagnosis. In general, IBD-associated SpA is nonerosive; evidence of erosive joint should prompt further evaluation and rheumatology consultation. CT or MRI may be necessary to evaluate for abscess or soft tissue infections.

The therapeutic management of IBD-associated SpA includes general measures, symptomatic measures, and management of underlying disease. Rest and analgesics are universally recommended. Nonsteroidal anti-inflammatories (NSAIDs) are very effective in treating joint swelling and are primary therapy in patients with AS; however, NSAIDs are largely avoided in patients with IBD given the concern for disease relapse. One notable retrospective case-control study using a large pharmacy database found an odds ratio of 1.77 and 1.93 for current and recent NSAIDs use, respectively, in patients evaluated in the emergency room for colitis exacerbation [38]. However, the majority of the data associating NSAIDs and IBD flares stems from retrospective studies [reviewed in [39]]. A major caveat to these associations is the fact that disease-associated symptoms precipitated the use of NSAIDs. One prospective trial of IBD patients without joint pains treated with either non-selective NSAIDs compared to COX-2 selective NSAIDs or acetaminophen revealed increased rates (17–28 %) of flares in patients given nonselective NSAIDs (naproxen or nabumetone) [40]. Although two retrospective studies of COX-2 selective NSAIDs (celecoxib or rofecoxib) revealed a higher incidence of discontinuation for GI disturbance [41, 42], the largest randomized controlled trial of patients with quiescent UC revealed no increase in disease exacerbation in patients treated with celecoxib compared to placebo for up to 2 weeks [43]. Thus, celecoxib may be safe for patients with well-controlled UC, particularly if they have taken that medication in the past and it will be used for short duration; however, given the concern for any NSAID to exacerbate intestinal disease, NSAIDs should be avoided if possible and attempts made to treat underlying disease while maximizing analgesia and rest.

Joint pain, particularly arthralgias and type I arthropathy, often accompanies disease activity and improves with management of intestinal disease. Sulfasalazine is effective for inducing remission of UC at 4–6 g/day. Although metanalysis revealed no benefit of sulfasalazine on functional outcomes for patients with AS, limited subgroup analysis suggested benefit in patients with the early disease, high ESR, or peripheral arthropathy [44]. Mesalamine showed some clinical and laboratory effect in two open-label studies suggesting that the 5-ASA (and not the sulfapyridine) may be the effective moiety in treatment of SpA [45, 46]. Steroids are effective in controlling EIMs when required to treat intestinal UC. High-dose steroids have been used anecdotally for refractory ankylosing spondylitis [47]. Although 6-mercaptopurine and azathioprine are important steroid-sparing agents in the management of UC, there is little data supporting their role in IBD-associated SpA or AS [48]. Furthermore, a metanalysis of three randomized controlled trials found no clear benefit of oral methotrexate [49].

The effectiveness of anti-TNFα biologics in the management of IBD-associated peripheral and axial spondyloarthritis can be extrapolated from CD-based trials. In patients with mild to moderate (defined by a Crohn's Disease Activity Index of 220–450) joint symptoms that are refractory to steroids, 6-MP, and methotrexate, 61 % reported improvement in joint symptoms at 12 weeks, and 46 % reported no persistent symptoms [50]. Notably, only 25 % of the patients had true arthritis with arthralgias, whereas 75 % had only arthralgias. Using a more strict definition of SpA, an open-label trial of 24 patients treated with infliximab showed a more rapid resolution of peripheral arthritis and enthesitis [51]. Similar results have been reported with the use of adalimumab in infliximab primary nonresponders [52]. Anti-TNFα biologics are indicated for the treatment of AS which cannot be controlled with either sulfasalazine or NSAIDs [53]. Despite the role for etanercept in the medical management of arthritis, retrospective analysis suggests a higher risk of IBD flares associated with etanercept [54] and is therefore avoided in the management of IBD.

Additional strategies for the management of IBD-associated SpA may be required in refractory cases. Interestingly, retrospective analysis of patients treated with ileocecectomy reveals less frequent arthritis complications, suggesting that the location and interaction with microbiota may alter disease pathogenesis [55]. Pilot studies suggest that probiotics may improve clinical outcomes [56], but randomized controlled trials are needed. Total proctocolectomy when required for active, refractory UC can improve joint pains; however, occasionally arthritis and spondylitis will persist [57, 58].

## Skin Manifestations

Major cutaneous manifestations occur in 2–34 % patients with IBD [5, 59]. These manifestations include erythema nodosum, pyoderma gangrenosum, and aphthous stomatitis, but other conditions including infection and skin cancer may be equally likely. A two- to threefold increased risk of psoriasis has been reported in both UC and CD [34, 60]. Frequently, a thorough history will help reveal the diagnosis, including association of symptoms with intestinal symptoms, recent travel, steroids, new medications, or recent infusion; however, dermatology consultation may be prudent if the diagnosis is uncertain or assistance with therapy is required. Exclusion of malignancy is important, particularly if there is a history of exposure to thiopurines. Large cohort studies including 26,974 patients with UC revealed an overall increased relative risk of 1.47 compared to case-matched controls [61]. Nested case-control analysis revealed an association of malignancy with thiopurine use. Although this finding was not corroborated by other retrospective studies [62], prospective analysis by the CESAME study group revealed significantly higher incidence rates for patients with ongoing (hazard ratio 5.90) or previous (HR 3.94) thiopurine exposure [63]. In addition several recent findings have confirmed these findings.

## Erythema Nodosum

The diagnosis of erythema nodosum (EN) can often be made clinically with classic raised, tender, red subcutaneous nodules usually present on the extensor surfaces of the lower extremities. Less frequently, nodules may occur on the calves, trunk, and face. The course of EN is usually self-limiting. Superficial discoloration may persist for weeks, but dermal ulceration or scarring does not occur. Histology reveals a focal panniculitis without vasculitis. Biopsy is rarely needed to make the diagnosis, but, if required, should be excisional to include the subcutaneous adipose tissue. The etiology appears to be mediated by immune complex deposition in the venules of subcutaneous connective tissue [64]. The majority of IBD-associated EN (~90 %) occurs in the setting of IBD relapse [65]. As such, EN in the absence of intestinal inflammation should prompt investigation for other causes. Underlying conditions commonly associated with EN include infections (poststreptococcal, primary tuberculosis), sarcoidosis, pregnancy, Behcet's disease, medications (OCP, penicillins, sulfonamides), and hematologic malignancy [64, 66, 67].

EN is more frequently associated with colonic CD (6–15 %) [6, 7, 10] compared to UC (2–9 %) [6, 10, 68] and two- to fivefold more common in women [10, 65]. Clinical findings of EN are increased in patients with type I peripheral arthritis. A polymorphism at the −1031C position in the *TNFA* promoter region associates with manifestations of EN and correlates with increase TNFa production, which may underlie the genetic susceptibility [65].

Treatment for EN is largely supportive given that the manifestations are generally self-limiting. In a cohort of 39 patients with EN, the maximum duration was 12 weeks; however, 1/5 had recurrence of symptoms [65]. The focus of treatment is on intestinal symptoms. In a prospective study of 792 IBD patients, 48 patients with EN responded to medical therapy of IBD [8]. Supportive management should also include leg elevation, support stockings, and rest. Acetylsalicylic acid (650 mg QID) and NSAIDs including naproxen [69] and indomethacin (25 mg QID) [70] have been used for controlling symptoms, but NSAIDs should be minimized given the risk of exacerbating underlying intestinal disease. Preferred analgesics include acetaminophen and low-dose opiates when needed. Potassium iodide has been used in small, uncontrolled cohorts of patients with EN at doses of 400 mg to 900 mg daily [71, 72]. These trials showed dramatic results within 2 weeks of initiating potassium iodide; however, larger controlled trials are lacking. A case report of a CD patient with recurrent EN despite steroids and immunomodulator therapy reports resolution to 1,500 mg daily of potassium iodide [73]. This report, however, was prior to the availability of anti-TNFα biologics, and the degree of intestinal remission was not assessed endoscopically. Of note, potassium iodide is contraindicated during pregnancy as excess iodine may cause goiter in the developing fetus [74]. Finally, successful case reports of the management of IBD-associated EN with 5 mg/kg of infliximab have been reported in the pediatric literature [75]. However, the improvement of EN may simply reflect the superiority of combined therapy in achieving mucosal healing and deep remission.

## Oral Lesions

Aphthous stomatitis or ulcers appear as shallow round ulcers with an erythematous halo base [64]. Aphthae may also be associated with several immune disorders including HIV/AIDS, Behcet's, Reiter's, and celiac disease. Infectious etiologies including HSV may need to be excluded. Aphthous stomatitis is common in both UC and CD (10 % CD, 4 % UC) [9]. Oral ulceration has also been described as a side effect of methotrexate used to treat IBD [76].

Similar to EN, aphthous stomatitis generally parallels intestinal disease activity. As such, therapy is directed at controlling underlying bowel inflammation and providing analgesia. Topical anesthetic including 2 % viscous lidocaine or benzocaine lozenge is routinely used [77]. Sucralfate suspension may be used to coat the lesion and provide topical analgesia [78]. Intralesional injection of triamcinolone (10 mg/mL given 0.1–0.5 mL per lesion) is recommended only for painful deep aphthae [77]. Recurrent aphthous stomatitis may require systemic immune modulating therapy. An open-label trial of colchicine at 1–2 mg/day showed a 63 % improvement at 3 months [79]. Similar success was seen with pentoxifylline, but placebo-controlled trials reported only a modest benefit in pain- and ulcer-free days [80]. Prednisone may be used (10–30 mg/day) during an attack and is safe during pregnancy. Azathioprine (1–2 mg/kg/day) and infliximab are effective in placebo-controlled trials [81]; but similar to the response of EN, this may reflect better control of intestinal disease. Thalidomide is useful in the management of aphthous stomatitis in HIV patients [82] and in our experience is similarly effective for patients with IBD.

## Pyoderma Gangrenosum

Pyoderma gangrenosum (PG) is a noninfectious, neutrophilic dermatosis occurring frequently on the legs, but may appear on the extremities, torso, or face. Numerous cases of perianal or peristomal PG have been described. Often patients will report a recent trauma or inciting injury at the site. The differential diagnosis is broad including infectious and noninfectious ulcerative lesions. There are no pathognomonic features of PG in laboratory evaluation, and biopsy is avoided to prevent further tissue damage when clinical exam is sufficient to make the diagnosis. When biopsy is performed, the characteristic histology of ulcerative PG reveals a neutrophilic infiltrate surrounding central ulceration with a lymphocytic infiltrate at the periphery [64]. PG may occur as ulcerative, pustular, bullous, or vegetative. Pustular and ulcerative PG are most common in IBD, whereas bullous PG is associated with myeloproliferative disorders [83]. Although cultures may be sent to exclude secondary infection, wound culture is generally of minimal benefit. Surgical debridement should be avoided to prevent extension and further tissue damage, although some centers with expertise have reported success with Epidex grafting [84].

The association between UC and PG was promoted by several case series. The initial description of ulcerative PG included four out of five patients with UC [85]. Although this association was emphasized early, subsequent reports estimate about 1/3 of patients with ulcerative PG have IBD [86]. While some reports revealed a higher incidence of PG in CD [10], PG is generally found to be more commonly associated with UC compared to CD at a frequency of about 3 % in recent population-based studies [9, 34]. PG occurs equally in men and women [34, 83].

Controversy exists as to whether PG parallels or is independent of intestinal disease activity. Traditionally, PG is felt to occur independently of bowel activity [87]. Supporting this assertion is the description of patients with PG following total proctocolectomy [88]; however, it is unclear from these studies if a cuff of colonic tissue remained postoperatively. More recent studies report active intestinal symptoms in 70–80 % of UC patients with PG [34, 68]. This discrepancy may be explained by the fact that PG may precede intestinal activity [89].

Therapy for PG includes local wound management and systemic immunomodulatory therapy. Supportive care including leg elevation and occlusive wound dressing is recommended to minimize secondary infections [90]. Analgesics are recommended for symptomatic relief. Although controlled trials are lacking given the low incidence of PG, steroids are generally considered the treatment of choice based on case series data. Prednisone (1–2 mg/kg/day) for several weeks and pulse therapy with methylprednisolone (1 g IV/day) for 3 days are reported to achieve good clinical response [91]. Retrospective analysis of 86 patients revealed that 80 % required systemic therapy with steroids [92]. The average time to skin resolution was 6 months with average 13 months until discontinuation of prednisone. 5.8 % of patients in this series had refractory disease.

Given the frequency of relapse and risk associated with prolonged steroid exposure, the role of anti-TNFα biologics in the management of PG is evolving particularly in IBD-associated PG. Open-label experience with infliximab for CD revealed that it allowed skin healing and steroid reduction [93]. The largest randomized placebo-controlled trial of 30 patients (19 with IBD) showed 69 % response and 21 % remission at 6 weeks [94]. Alternate steroid-sparing therapies may similarly be efficacious in steroid-refractory PG. A retrospective review of 11 IBD patients with steroid-refractory PG (5 of which had UC) treated with 4 mg/kg/day of IV cyclosporine for 7–22 days followed by oral cyclosporine 4–7 mg/kg/day (then transitioned to azathioprine or 6-MP) revealed the efficacy of cyclosporine [95]. Only one patient who could not tolerate 6-MP had a recurrence of PG. Other case reports have noted the efficacy of IV cyclosporine with methylprednisolone pulse therapy [96]. In addition to cyclosporine, there are case reports of thalidomide [97], methotrexate [98], tacrolimus [99, 100], dapsone [101], cyclophosphamide [102], and colchicine [103], but larger studies are required to determine the role of these medicines in routine therapy.

Topical therapy may be appropriate in situations of limited or mild disease that is not associated with bowel activity. Numerous case reports of topical therapy have been described: nitrogen mustard [104], aqueous benzoyl peroxide [105], sodium cromoglycate [106], and intralesional injection of triamcinolone [107]. Topical aminosalicylates may provide local improvement, but frequently systemic therapy is required to control deteriorating intestinal symptoms [108].

## Ocular Manifestations

Ocular manifestations are commonly associated with IBD and frequently occur with other EIMs. Larger retrospective and population-based studies have reported frequencies of 1–4 % [6, 9, 10, 34], but these numbers may significantly underestimate clinically silent ophthalmologic involvement [109]. Classic ophthalmologic EIMs include episcleritis, scleritis, and uveitis; however, case reports of optic neuritis [110] and retinal vasculitis [109] have been described. Steroid-induced cataract should also be considered in patients with a history of significant steroid use. The majority of the data for medical management is drawn from a limited set of case series, the majority of which are non-IBD associated [111].

Episcleritis is the most frequent ocular manifestation of IBD. It is often painful, but there is no associated vision loss, photophobia, or papillary abnormality. Ocular exam reveals focal or patchy redness with intervening white patches of sclera with dilated episcleral vessels, often in the interpalpebral zone [112]. Episcleritis is often associated with bowel inflammation, and treatment is focused on controlling intestinal flare. Cold compresses and steroid eyedrops (fluorometholone acetate 0.1 % or prednisolone acetate 1 %) are frequently used for symptom management [111].

In contrast to episcleritis, scleritis features edema and cellular infiltration of the entire thickness of the sclera. Disease severity ranges from self-limited episodes to necrotizing disease that may threaten vision. Visual disturbances should prompt urgent evaluation by an ophthalmologist. Scleritis is often accompanied by significant dull pain and tenderness to palpation. Ocular exam reveals patchy redness with a violaceous intervening [112]. Similar to episcleritis, scleritis generally parallels intestinal activity, and primary treatment should be geared towards controlling intestinal symptoms; however, in contrast to episcleritis, 60 % of patients with scleritis had complications including 16 % with permanent visual impairment. NSAIDs such as indomethacin are effective in uncomplicated scleritis (particularly anterior nodular scleritis), but should be avoided in patients with active IBD. Given the risk of permanent visual impairment with recurrent scleritis, the majority of patients will require systemic medication. Prednisone 1 mg/kg/day is recommended for refractory anterior scleritis, necrotizing scleritis, or posterior scleritis. The dose is generally tapered 1 month after symptom resolution. Immunomodulatory therapy including cyclosporine, methotrexate, or alkylating agents may be used in steroid-refractory or necrotizing scleritis [113, 114]. There is an emerging literature on the efficacy of biologic therapy, particularly infliximab, in the treatment of refractory scleritis particularly in patients with underlying IBD.

Uveitis is inflammation of the vascular lining of the eye. Anterior uveitis involves the iris and the ciliary body, while posterior uveitis involves the vitreous choroid and retina. Anterior uveitis (or iridocyclitis) is more frequently associated with CD, but occurs in 2–5 % of UC [9, 10, 34, 115]. Anterior uveitis in the context of IBD is frequently associated with arthritis or EN, while posterior inflammation is rarely associated with IBD. Uveitis presents clinically with pain, visual blurring, and photophobia. Ocular exam reveals a miotic pupil and a "ciliary flush" or intense erythema juxtaposed to the iris. Slit lamp exam reveals anterior chamber flare, corneal edema, and conjunctival injection. Visual loss may suggest posterior involvement or retinitis. The etiopathogenesis of uveitis is unclear, but genetic association with HLA-B27, B58, and HLA-DRB1*0103 [65] suggests an immune-mediated component which may be directed at overlapping antigens expressed in both colonic tissue and the eye [116].

In contrast to episcleritis and scleritis, uveitis does not generally parallel intestinal activity. Prompt treatment with topical and/or systemic therapy is required to prevent complications, such as glaucoma, cataract, and synechiae (adhesions of the iris to other ocular structures). Topical treatment with glucocorticoids (1 % prednisolone acetate) is primary therapy. Dilating agents such as scopolamine, cyclopentolate, or homatropine may be helpful to relieve pain due to spasm of the ciliary muscle and to prevent synechiae formation.

Systemic treatment may be necessary in cases of refractory disease, bilateral involvement, or patients unable to tolerate steroid eyedrops. Prednisone 40–60 mg daily tapering to lowest dose to sustain remission is considered first-line therapy. Only anecdotal reports support the use of steroid-sparing agents such as methotrexate, cyclosporine, and azathioprine in refractory cases [117].

Anti-TNFα biologics are emerging as second-line therapy for uveitis associated with IBD; however, the data supporting these recommendations are largely extrapolated from Behcet's patients with refractory uveitis. Conventional infliximab therapy resulted in better visual acuity, reducing the number and duration of relapses of uveitis [118]. Adalimumab is similarly effective in patients intolerant of infliximab [119]. Case reports describe the efficacy of infliximab for recurrent uveitis in patients with CD [120, 121], but further studies are needed to assess the efficacy of anti-TNFα in treatment of UC-associated uveitis.

## Hepatobiliary Manifestations

IBD is associated with numerous hepatobiliary manifestations that are either related to underlying inflammatory disease or medication induced. Primary sclerosing cholangitis (PSC) is frequently associated with underlying UC, but the etiopathogenesis remains unclear. Portal vein thrombosis can also be associated with inflammatory-mediated hypercoagulability. Cholelithiasis is frequent, particularly in ileal CD, given the interruption of bile salt absorption. Thiopurines, azathioprine, and less commonly mesalamine can cause medication-induced pancreatitis, while thiopurines, methotrexate, sulfasalazine, cyclosporine, and biologic agents can cause hepatotoxicity. Given the array of manifestations, abnormal liver function test or evidence of cholestasis should prompt evaluation in the patient with UC.

## Primary Sclerosing Cholangitis

PSC is a chronic cholestatic liver disease caused by periductal inflammation, fibrosis, and stricturing of medium and large intra- and extrahepatic bile ducts. Progression of disease can lead to malabsorption, cirrhosis, and portal hypertension. Definitive therapy is liver transplantation [122], but diagnosis is crucial for effective medical management of symptoms. The majority of PSC cases occur in the context of IBD [123, 124]; however, the chronic periductal inflammation does not generally parallel intestinal activity in IBD patients. Furthermore, total proctocolectomy does not affect the natural history of PSC [125].

On a population level, the prevalence of primary sclerosing cholangitis ranges from 2 to 7 % [9, 10, 126].

UC is more common than CD in patients with PSC, and PSC is rarely seen with isolated small bowel CD [6]. The majority of UC patients with PSC are men, while the non-IBD PSC individuals are predominantly women [10]. Although northern European-based cohorts report 62–83 % association with IBD [123], reports from southern Europe [127, 128] and Japan [129] suggest a lower incidence and association with IBD. Diagnosis of PSC in the context of UC defines a unique disease phenotype with high risk for colorectal cancer (OR 6.9 compared to well-controlled UC) [130]. As such, annual screening colonoscopy for UC patients with PSC is recommended starting at the time of diagnosis. Patients with PSC are similarly at increased risk for cholangiocarcinoma. Although no studies show outcomes benefit [131], 2010 guidelines from the AASLD recommend annual screening ultrasound [132].

The pathogenesis of PSC remains unknown. Pathologic evidence reveals that the inflammation associated with PSC liver disease is T cell mediated. T cell-mediated immune pathogenesis is supported by the strong HLA association. Major histocompatibility complex I HLA-B7 [133] and B8 [134, 135], as well as MHCII HLA-DR3 and DQ2, have been associated with PSC [136]. HLA-DR4 and DQ8 are associated with progression to cholangiocarcinoma. Molecular mimicry may drive T cell activation by shared epitopes on colonic and biliary epithelium [137], but antigenic peptides driving the T cell response in PSC need to be defined.

The clinical association with large bowel disease suggests the importance of dysregulated interaction of colonic bacteria with the intestine. Portal bacteremia in patients with UC may drive this systemic reaction [138]. Early investigation in rats revealed that bacterial overgrowth resulted in hepatic inflammation with histologic characteristics similar to PSC. Clinical use of metronidazole in patients with PSC (of which 80 % had UC) resulted in a reduction in alkaline phosphatase and PSC Mayo risk score, but histologic parameters were not statistically improved [139]. Data from the pediatric literature [140] shows that patients treated with oral vancomycin have improvement in liver chemistry, ESR, and clinical symptoms, particularly in patients without cirrhosis. Further work is required to identify a microbial causative agent, diagnostic criteria for microbial-driven PSC, and antimicrobial treatment regimens to alter the natural history of the disease.

Liver chemistry abnormalities or clinical symptoms should prompt evaluation in any patient with IBD. Serologic and virologic evaluation as well as ultrasound should be performed to rule out common causes of hepatocellular or infiltrative diseases. MRCP is the diagnostic test of choice with specificity of 94 % and sensitivity of 86 % [141]. Clinical or laboratory evidence of obstructive physiology should prompt ERCP for dilation and brushings of stricture. Liver biopsy may be performed if an ERCP is equivocal or to exclude overlap syndrome. ANA and p-ANCA are frequently seen in patients with PSC [142] and may be helpful in guiding diagnosis in cases of clinical suspicion. In addition, IgG4 levels should be checked to exclude IgG4-associated sclerosing cholangitis.

Although liver transplantation is the only curative therapy, medical management is important for preventing cholestatic complications and progression of underlying liver disease. Based on the efficacy of ursodeoxycholic acid (UDCA) in primary biliary cirrhosis [143], UDCA was evaluated in the treatment of PSC. Randomized controlled trials of patients with PSC treated with 13–15 mg/kg showed improvement in laboratory values, but no change in the primary endpoint defined as death, liver transplantation, histologic progression, or complications of portal hypertension (i.e., varices, ascites, encephalopathy) [144]. Initial studies with high-dose (20–30 mg/kg) UDCA suggested improved 4-year survival [145, 146], but subsequent larger randomized controlled trial of 28–30 mg/kg was halted prematurely because interim analysis suggested an increased likelihood to reach the primary endpoint of death, need for liver transplant, or development of varices [147]. As such, the 2010 AASLD guidelines recommend against the use of UDCA for the treatment of PSC [132].

Adding complexity to the management algorithm is the reported beneficial role for UDCA in preventing IBD-associated colorectal cancer (CRC). Initial data from a cross-sectional study of 59 patients found a lower frequency of colonic dysplasia in patients with UC and PSC taking ursodiol (mean 9 mg/kg, duration 3.5 years) [148]. Post hoc analysis of the PSC-UCDA study [144] supported these conclusions, revealing a relative risk of 0.26 of colonic dysplasia in patients taking ursodiol [149]. Furthermore, a historical cohort of 105 patients shows a trend in reduction of dysplasia and a statistically significant benefit in overall survival, about half of which was due to colonic malignancy [150]. More recent data, however, has called into question the efficacy of UDCA in CRC prevention. Post hoc analysis of high-dose UDCA (28–30 mg/kg) described above showed an increased risk of IBD-associated dysplasia [151]. Recent metanalysis of eight trials of UCDA in PSC has suggested [152] that no beneficial effect on mortality or liver complications could be shown, but none of the trials were of low risk of bias. As such, there is insufficient data to recommend the use of UDCA for either chemoprophylaxis or preventing cholestatic complications. Newer bile acids are currently under development. 24-*nor*-ursodeoxycholic acid (norUDCA) has a side-chain modification of UDCA that confers relative resistance to amidation. This pharmacologic property may account for increased cholehepatic shunting and bicarbonate-rich hypercholeresis that protects from cholestatic injury in mouse models of PSC [153].

While a variety of immunosuppressive and anti-inflammatory agents have been tried, none have shown a consistent benefit in overall or transplant-free survival to support medical therapy. Steroids have been largely avoided given multiple side effects particularly in the PSC population prone to metabolic bone disease. A small study of 21 patients with PSC found no effect of 9 mg/day of budesonide on histologic progression of liver disease, but a marked loss of bone density at the femoral neck and lumbar spine was seen [154]. Treatment with methotrexate and FK506 revealed an improvement in liver enzymes, but no survival effect was seen [155, 156]. Similarly, colchicine, penicillamine, and pirfenidone have shown little value [157–160]. Case reports of N-acetylcysteine as a mucolytic may improve liver chemistries, but further studies are required to determine the effect on outcomes [161]. Angiotensin II receptor blocker candesartan and propranolol have antifibrotic effects in animal models of cholestatic liver disease [162], but further studies are needed to evaluate the clinical efficacy of these therapeutic strategies for PSC.

Although PSC is generally asymptomatic, there are some important metabolic manifestations that require evaluation and medical management. A decreased secretion of conjugated bile acids may manifest as malabsorption of fat-soluble vitamins. Vitamin A deficiency is most common. PSC patients should be screened for fat-soluble vitamin deficiency and repleted as needed. In addition to vitamin D deficiency, metabolic bone disease, with a predisposition to osteoporosis, bone pain, and fractures, is increased in patients with PSC. A recent retrospective analysis of 237 patients with PSC found a prevalence of 15 % of osteoporosis at the time of diagnosis [163]. Thirty-nine percent of these patients were vitamin D deficient compared to 21 % of the non-osteoporotic patients. Multivariate analysis revealed age >54 (OR 7.8), BMI<=24 (OR 4.9), and duration of IBD>=19 years (OR 3.6) as independent predictors that can be used to identify patients at risk. As such, bone mineral density should be evaluated at the time of diagnosis. Based on AASLD guidelines, repeat evaluation every 2–3 years is appropriate for PSC patients; however, surveillance may need to be intensified in patients with increased clinical risk factors. Interestingly, cumulative corticosteroid dose does not predict risk for osteoporosis; however, given the risk for osteoporosis, steroids should be avoided in IBD patients with PSC. Controlled trials for medical osteoporosis therapy in PSC patients have not been reported, but bisphosphonates are well tolerated and effective in the setting of cholestatic liver disease [164] and should be considered for PSC with osteoporosis.

## Hematologic Manifestations

### Anemia

Anemia is common in IBD. Guidelines suggest monitoring hemoglobin every 6 months for patients in remission and every 3 months for patients with active disease [165].

Iron deficiency and anemia of chronic disease are the most common causes of anemia in patients with UC. In addition, vitamin B12 and folate deficiencies are not infrequent causes of anemia, and drug-induced myelosuppression should also be considered in patients taking sulfasalazine or thiopurines. Autoimmune hemolytic anemias and myelodysplastic syndromes are much less frequent. Laboratory evaluation of iron saturation and ferritin will help to distinguish iron deficiency from anemia of chronic disease. In the absence of sufficient iron stores, serum ferritin is generally <30 μg/L; however, active inflammation may raise the serum ferritin in iron-deficient patients. Thus, a serum ferritin <100 μg/L and an iron saturation <16 % in anemic patients support the diagnosis of iron deficiency [165].

Iron deficiency anemia in UC should be treated with iron repletion. Open-label randomized trial suggests iron sucrose (7 mg/kg followed by 200 mg at 1–2-week intervals) was associated with less GI intolerance and quicker recovery of iron stores [166]. Although the short-term efficacy and overall tolerability are likely the same, intravenous repletion is favored in patients with intolerance to oral iron, severe anemia (<10), or inappropriate response to oral iron repletion. Furthermore, there is a theoretical concern that the release of reactive oxygen species (via Fenton reaction) will aggravate intestinal inflammation. Although previous formulations of intravenous iron with dextran were associated with anaphylaxis, the risk with iron sucrose and iron gluconate is minimal. These formulations, however, deliver significantly less total iron per injection. Newer formulations such as ferric carboxymaltose may allow larger iron delivery in a single injection, thereby decreasing the number of injections needed and the overall cost [167]. In mild cases of anemia particularly in patients in remission who prefer the convenience of self-administering, oral repletion may be appropriate. The maximal intestinal absorption is 10–20 mg of elemental iron/day, which is provided by low-dose 100–200 mg iron sulfate, but the optimal oral dosing has not been defined. Response to treatment is assessed by hemoglobin and transferrin saturation; ferritin may less accurately reflect iron stores during repletion. The appropriate erythropoietic response to adequate iron repletion is an increase of 2 g/dL by 4 weeks.

In contrast to iron deficiency, the treatment of anemia of chronic disease is aimed at controlling the underlying disease. Cytokine activation or sequestration of iron in the reticuloendothelial system may contribute to the underlying pathogenic mechanisms. In patients with anemia <10 mg/dL and refractory to 4 weeks of iron repletion, erythropoietin may be considered to increase hemoglobin levels [168]. However, improved control of disease with anti-TNFα therapy will increase erythropoietin production and improve anemia [169].

Autoimmune hemolytic anemia (AIHA) occurs in 1–2 % of patients with IBD [170]. The underlying pathogenic mechanism is driven by red cell autoantibodies produced by colonic mononuclear cells [171]. In general, AIHA parallels intestinal disease activity, and treatment is aimed at controlling disease symptoms. Standard medical management is high-dose corticosteroids, with or without cyclophosphamide or azathioprine; if unsuccessful splenectomy is indicated [172]. Colectomy has been indicated as a treatment modality in refractory cases, but case report described UC-associated AIHA following colectomy [173]. Refractory cases of UC-associated AIHA have been managed with cyclosporine [174], infliximab [175], and autologous stem cell transplant [176].

## Thrombotic Complications

IBD is associated with a hypercoagulable state. Both acute and chronic inflammation can increase procoagulants (fibrinogen, factors V, VIII, IX) and decrease anticoagulants (proteins C, S, antithrombin III). Decreased fibrinolysis and enhanced platelet aggregation may also contribute. In addition to inflammatory-mediated hypercoagulability, IBD patients are often postsurgical and immobile and have increased risk for malignancy. These factors lead to a threefold increased risk in venous thromboembolism (VTE) in population studies of patients with IBD [177]. Thrombotic complications most frequently include DVT and PE, but cerebral sinovenous, portal, and mesenteric thrombosis have been described. A large cohort-controlled trial revealed an even higher, 8.4-fold increase of VTE risk in IBD patients within 120 days of a recent flare of intestinal symptoms requiring steroids [178]. While colonic involvement is associated with VTE, retrospective analysis revealed that 25 % occurred after colectomy, and moreover, colectomy did not prevent VTE recurrence [179].

The management of VTE complications in IBD is similar to the management of complications in non-IBD patients. Heparin is more effective and practical in the short term or during active disease, but transition to warfarin may be appropriate in stable disease. Of note, thiopurine-based therapy may mediate warfarin resistance [180]. Anticoagulation should be continued for 3–6 months followed by complete evaluation for underlying thrombophilia. IVC filter should be considered for patients with contraindications to anticoagulation. In the case of life-threatening thromboembolic complications, catheter-directed thrombolysis may be appropriate in patients with lower bleeding risk [181].

Isolated VTE in the setting of trauma or surgery does not generally require long-term anticoagulation, but the risk of recurrent VTE in IBD patients is not known. A recent retrospective analysis revealed almost 30 % recurrence at 5 years for IBD with unprovoked VTE [182]. Further prospective studies, as well as an assessment of long-term anticoagula-

tion bleeding risks, will be required to determine appropriate long-term secondary prophylaxis. Primary prevention studies of high-risk patients, including some patients with IBD, have shown a nearly 50 % reduction in the risk of VTE [183]. Moreover, given the 8.4-fold increased risk of VTE in hospitalized patients with IBD flare, primary prophylaxis with LMWH or compression stockings should be considered in hospitalized IBD patients.

Arterial thrombotic complications have also been associated with IBD. Two population studies have revealed increased incidence in ischemic heart disease [184, 185]. Interestingly, traditional risk factors for coronary artery disease, including BMI, chronic kidney disease, dyslipidemia, smoking, gender, and family history, did not explain increased risk suggesting that alternative surrogates are required for inflammatory-mediated CAD. In patients with traditional risk factors and stable disease, primary prophylaxis with aspirin may be indicated, but further studies are needed to identify those at risk and assess the benefit of primary prophylaxis.

## Pulmonary Manifestations

Although clinically severe pulmonary manifestations are rare, bronchopulmonary symptoms with no other etiology have been attributed to extraintestinal manifestations of IBD [186]. Pulmonary manifestations include airway disease, interstitial lung disease, and neutrophilic necrotic nodules mimicking Wegener's granulomatosis [187]. Although the incidence of clinically significant pulmonary disease is unclear, emerging data suggest that almost half of UC patients have abnormal PFTs (most commonly a decreased FEV1 and abnormal DLCO) [188, 189]. Impairment in DLCO correlates with histopathologic grade of intestinal activity [190] suggesting a shared inflammatory mechanism between embryologically related colonic and respiratory epithelia. Further supporting this inflammatory link, alveolar lymphocytosis correlates with disease activity and impairment in PFTs [191], but the cellular mechanism and underlying genetic susceptibility remain obscure.

Although 25–48 % of patients present with symptoms of pulmonary manifestations including pleuritic chest pain, cough, and dyspnea [115, 192], further clinical and laboratory evaluation can clarify the diagnosis. Current or previous exposure to anti-TNFα biologics should precipitate evaluation for tuberculosis. Both sulfasalazine [193] and mesalamine [194] can rarely induce interstitial lung disease that resolves with discontinuation of the medication. Laboratory evaluation for c-ANCA and ACE level may be helpful to evaluate for concurrent Wegener's granulomatosis or sarcoidosis, respectively; however, c-ANCA + IBD-associated pulmonary manifestations have been described [195].

High-resolution CT scan can be effectively used to identify peribronchial thickening associated with airway disease underlying abnormal PFTs [196]. There are no prospective trials to provide guidance for managing UC-associated pulmonary manifestations. However, since disease may progress independently of intestinal activity, early diagnosis and management are prudent. IBD-associated large airway disease can be managed with inhaled steroids (high-dose beclomethasone and budesonide). In contrast, small airway disease is generally less responsive to inhaled steroids and variably responsive to oral steroids. Interstitial lung disease responds favorably to oral steroids. There are no data to suggest that colectomy or control of intestinal symptoms with biologics improves pulmonary disease.

## Conclusions

Extraintestinal manifestations provide clinical reminders of the systemic nature of immune dysregulation in association with IBD. Medical management of these manifestations plays a crucial role in the overall care of patients with IBD. The etiology of the immune dysregulation stems from both genetic and environmental/microbial exposure. A more complete understanding of the immune pathogenesis offers the promise of molecular-based diagnoses and targeted therapeutic strategies to improve the clinical management of IBD.

## References

1. Willing BP, et al. A pyrosequencing study in twins shows that gastrointestinal microbial profiles vary with inflammatory bowel disease phenotypes. Gastroenterology. 2010;139(6):1844–54 e1.
2. Qin J, et al. A human gut microbial gene catalogue established by metagenomic sequencing. Nature. 2010;464(7285):59–65.
3. Frank DN, et al. Molecular-phylogenetic characterization of microbial community imbalances in human inflammatory bowel diseases. Proc Natl Acad Sci U S A. 2007;104(34):13780–5.
4. McInnes IB, Schett G. The pathogenesis of rheumatoid arthritis. N Engl J Med. 2011;365(23):2205–19.
5. Levine JS, Burakoff R. Extraintestinal manifestations of inflammatory bowel disease. Gastroenterol Hepatol. 2011;7(4):235–41.
6. Greenstein AJ, Janowitz HD, Sachar DB. The extra-intestinal complications of Crohn's disease and ulcerative colitis: a study of 700 patients. Medicine (Baltimore). 1976;55(5):401–12.
7. Rankin GB, et al. National Cooperative Crohn's Disease Study: extraintestinal manifestations and perianal complications. Gastroenterology. 1979;77(4 Pt 2):914–20.
8. Veloso FT, Carvalho J, Magro F. Immune-related systemic manifestations of inflammatory bowel disease. A prospective study of 792 patients. J Clin Gastroenterol. 1996;23(1):29–34.
9. Vavricka SR, et al. Frequency and risk factors for extraintestinal manifestations in the Swiss inflammatory bowel disease cohort. Am J Gastroenterol. 2011;106(1):110–9.
10. Bernstein CN, et al. The prevalence of extraintestinal diseases in inflammatory bowel disease: a population-based study. Am J Gastroenterol. 2001;96(4):1116–22.
11. Van Limbergen J, Wilson DC, Satsangi J. The genetics of Crohn's disease. Annu Rev Genomics Hum Genet. 2009;10:89–116.
12. Satsangi J, et al. Clinical patterns of familial inflammatory bowel disease. Gut. 1996;38(5):738–41.
13. Roussomoustakaki M, et al. Genetic markers may predict disease behavior in patients with ulcerative colitis. Gastroenterology. 1997;112(6):1845–53.
14. Satsangi J, et al. Contribution of genes of the major histocompatibility complex to susceptibility and disease phenotype in inflammatory bowel disease. Lancet. 1996;347(9010):1212–7.
15. van Sommeren S, Janse M, Karjalainen J, Fehrmann R, Franke L, Fu J, Weersma RK. Extraintestinal manifestations and complications in inflammatory bowel disease: from shared genetics to shared biological pathways. Inflamm Bowel Dis. 2014;20(6):987–94.
16. Eksteen B, et al. Hepatic endothelial CCL25 mediates the recruitment of CCR9+ gut-homing lymphocytes to the liver in primary sclerosing cholangitis. J Exp Med. 2004;200(11):1511–7.
17. Mirza ZK, et al. Autoimmunity against human tropomyosin isoforms in ulcerative colitis: localization of specific human tropomyosin isoforms in the intestine and extraintestinal organs. Inflamm Bowel Dis. 2006;12(11):1036–43.
18. Atarashi K, et al. Induction of colonic regulatory T cells by indigenous Clostridium species. Science. 2011;331(6015):337–41.
19. Uhlig HH, et al. Characterization of Foxp3+CD4+CD25+ and IL-10-secreting CD4+CD25+ T cells during cure of colitis. J Immunol. 2006;177(9):5852–60.
20. Sokol H, et al. Faecalibacterium prausnitzii is an anti-inflammatory commensal bacterium identified by gut microbiota analysis of Crohn disease patients. Proc Natl Acad Sci U S A. 2008;105(43):16731–6.
21. Zanin-Zhorov A, et al. Protein kinase C-theta mediates negative feedback on regulatory T cell function. Science. 2010;328(5976):372–6.
22. Zaiss MM, et al. Regulatory T cells protect from local and systemic bone destruction in arthritis. J Immunol. 2010;184(12):7238–46.
23. Hot A, Miossec P. Effects of interleukin (IL)-17A and IL-17F in human rheumatoid arthritis synoviocytes. Ann Rheum Dis. 2011;70(5):727–32.
24. Hirota K, et al. Preferential recruitment of CCR6-expressing Th17 cells to inflamed joints via CCL20 in rheumatoid arthritis and its animal model. J Exp Med. 2007;204(12):2803–12.
25. Sakaguchi N, et al. Altered thymic T-cell selection due to a mutation of the ZAP-70 gene causes autoimmune arthritis in mice. Nature. 2003;426(6965):454–60.
26. Ivanov II, et al. Induction of intestinal Th17 cells by segmented filamentous bacteria. Cell. 2009;139(3):485–98.
27. Wu HJ, et al. Gut-residing segmented filamentous bacteria drive autoimmune arthritis via T helper 17 cells. Immunity. 2010;32(6):815–27.
28. Garrett WS, et al. Communicable ulcerative colitis induced by T-bet deficiency in the innate immune system. Cell. 2007;131(1):33–45.
29. Wang J, et al. Transcription factor T-bet regulates inflammatory arthritis through its function in dendritic cells. J Clin Invest. 2006;116(2):414–21.
30. Garrett WS, et al. Enterobacteriaceae act in concert with the gut microbiota to induce spontaneous and maternally transmitted colitis. Cell Host Microbe. 2010;8(3):292–300.
31. Orchard TR, et al. Clinical phenotype is related to HLA genotype in the peripheral arthropathies of inflammatory bowel disease. Gastroenterology. 2000;118(2):274–8.
32. Gravallese EM, Kantrowitz FG. Arthritic manifestations of inflammatory bowel disease. Am J Gastroenterol. 1988;83(7):703–9.

33. Orchard TR, Wordsworth BP, Jewell DP. Peripheral arthropathies in inflammatory bowel disease: their articular distribution and natural history. Gut. 1998;42(3):387–91.

34. Yuksel I, et al. Mucocutaneous manifestations in inflammatory bowel disease. Inflamm Bowel Dis. 2009;15(4):546–50.

35. Turkcapar N, et al. The prevalence of extraintestinal manifestations and HLA association in patients with inflammatory bowel disease. Rheumatol Int. 2006;26(7):663–8.

36. Rudwaleit M, et al. The development of Assessment of SpondyloArthritis international Society classification criteria for axial spondyloarthritis (part I): classification of paper patients by expert opinion including uncertainty appraisal. Ann Rheum Dis. 2009;68(6):770–6.

37. Verma HD, et al. Anti-nuclear antibody positivity and the use of certolizumab in inflammatory bowel disease patients who have had arthralgias or lupus-like reactions from infliximab or adalimumab. J Dig Dis. 2011;12(5):379–83.

38. Evans JM, et al. Non-steroidal anti-inflammatory drugs are associated with emergency admission to hospital for colitis due to inflammatory bowel disease. Gut. 1997;40(5):619–22.

39. Feagins LA, Cryer BL. Do non-steroidal anti-inflammatory drugs cause exacerbations of inflammatory bowel disease? Dig Dis Sci. 2010;55(2):226–32.

40. Takeuchi K, et al. Prevalence and mechanism of nonsteroidal anti-inflammatory drug-induced clinical relapse in patients with inflammatory bowel disease. Clin Gastroenterol Hepatol. 2006; 4(2):196–202.

41. Matuk R, et al. The spectrum of gastrointestinal toxicity and effect on disease activity of selective cyclooxygenase-2 inhibitors in patients with inflammatory bowel disease. Inflamm Bowel Dis. 2004;10(4):352–6.

42. Mahadevan U, et al. Safety of selective cyclooxygenase-2 inhibitors in inflammatory bowel disease. Am J Gastroenterol. 2002; 97(4):910–4.

43. Sandborn WJ, et al. Safety of celecoxib in patients with ulcerative colitis in remission: a randomized, placebo-controlled, pilot study. Clin Gastroenterol Hepatol. 2006;4(2):203–11.

44. Chen J, Liu C. Sulfasalazine for ankylosing spondylitis. Cochrane Database Syst Rev. 2005;2, CD004800.

45. Thomson GT, et al. Clinical efficacy of mesalamine in the treatment of the spondyloarthropathies. J Rheumatol. 2000;27(3): 714–8.

46. Dekker-Saeys BJ, Dijkmans BA, Tytgat GN. Treatment of spondyloarthropathy with 5-aminosalicylic acid (mesalazine): an open trial. J Rheumatol. 2000;27(3):723–6.

47. Peters ND, Ejstrup L. Intravenous methylprednisolone pulse therapy in ankylosing spondylitis. Scand J Rheumatol. 1992;21(3): 134–8.

48. Dougados M, et al. Conventional treatments for ankylosing spondylitis. Ann Rheum Dis. 2002;61 Suppl 3:iii4–50.

49. Chen J, Liu C, Lin J. Methotrexate for ankylosing spondylitis. Cochrane Database Syst Rev. 2006;4, CD004524.

50. Herfarth H, et al. Improvement of arthritis and arthralgia after treatment with infliximab (Remicade) in a German prospective, open-label, multicenter trial in refractory Crohn's disease. Am J Gastroenterol. 2002;97(10):2688–90.

51. Generini S, et al. Infliximab in spondyloarthropathy associated with Crohn's disease: an open study on the efficacy of inducing and maintaining remission of musculoskeletal and gut manifestations. Ann Rheum Dis. 2004;63(12):1664–9.

52. Lofberg R, et al. Adalimumab produces clinical remission and reduces extraintestinal manifestations in Crohn's disease: results from CARE. Inflamm Bowel Dis. 2012;18(1):1–9.

53. Braun J, et al. First update of the international ASAS consensus statement for the use of anti-TNF agents in patients with ankylosing spondylitis. Ann Rheum Dis. 2006;65(3):316–20.

54. Braun J, et al. Differences in the incidence of flares or new onset of inflammatory bowel diseases in patients with ankylosing spondylitis exposed to therapy with anti-tumor necrosis factor alpha agents. Arthritis Rheum. 2007;57(4):639–47.

55. Orchard TR, Jewell DP. The importance of ileocaecal integrity in the arthritic complications of Crohn's disease. Inflamm Bowel Dis. 1999;5(2):92–7.

56. Karimi O, Pena AS, van Bodegraven AA. Probiotics (VSL#3) in arthralgia in patients with ulcerative colitis and Crohn's disease: a pilot study. Drugs Today (Barc). 2005;41(7):453–9.

57. Isdale A, Wright V. Seronegative arthritis and the bowel. Baillieres Clin Rheumatol. 1989;3(2):285–301.

58. Wright V, Watkinson G. The arthritis of ulcerative colitis. Br Med J. 1965;2(5463):670–5.

59. Tavarela Veloso F. Review article: skin complications associated with inflammatory bowel disease. Aliment Pharmacol Ther. 2004;20 Suppl 4:50–3.

60. Lee FI, Bellary SV, Francis C. Increased occurrence of psoriasis in patients with Crohn's disease and their relatives. Am J Gastroenterol. 1990;85(8):962–3.

61. Long MD, et al. Increased risk for non-melanoma skin cancer in patients with inflammatory bowel disease. Clin Gastroenterol Hepatol. 2010;8(3):268–74.

62. van Schaik FD, et al. Risk of nonmelanoma skin cancer in patients with inflammatory bowel disease who use thiopurines is not increased. Clin Gastroenterol Hepatol. 2011;9(5):449–50 e1. author reply 450–1.

63. Peyrin-Biroulet L, et al. Increased risk for nonmelanoma skin cancers in patients who receive thiopurines for inflammatory bowel disease. Gastroenterology. 2011;141(5):1621–28 e1–5.

64. Trost LB, McDonnell JK. Important cutaneous manifestations of inflammatory bowel disease. Postgrad Med J. 2005;81(959):580–5.

65. Orchard TR, et al. Uveitis and erythema nodosum in inflammatory bowel disease: clinical features and the role of HLA genes. Gastroenterology. 2002;123(3):714–8.

66. Mert A, et al. Erythema nodosum: an experience of 10 years. Scand J Infect Dis. 2004;36(6–7):424–7.

67. Anan T, et al. Erythema nodosum and granulomatous lesions preceding acute myelomonocytic leukemia. J Dermatol. 2004; 31(9):741–7.

68. Mir-Madjlessi SH, Taylor JS, Farmer RG. Clinical course and evolution of erythema nodosum and pyoderma gangrenosum in chronic ulcerative colitis: a study of 42 patients. Am J Gastroenterol. 1985;80(8):615–20.

69. Lehman CW. Control of chronic erythema nodosum with naproxen. Cutis. 1980;26(1):66–7.

70. Elizaga FV. Erythema nodosum and indomethacin. Ann Intern Med. 1982;96(3):383.

71. Schulz EJ, Whiting DA. Treatment of erythema nodosum and nodular vasculitis with potassium iodide. Br J Dermatol. 1976; 94(1):75–8.

72. Horio T, et al. Potassium iodide in the treatment of erythema nodosum and nodular vasculitis. Arch Dermatol. 1981;117(1):29–31.

73. Marshall JK, Irvine EJ. Successful therapy of refractory erythema nodosum associated with Crohn's disease using potassium iodide. Can J Gastroenterol. 1997;11(6):501–2.

74. Requena L, Requena C. Erythema nodosum. Dermatol Online J. 2002;8(1):4.

75. Kugathasan S, et al. Dermatologic manifestations of Crohn disease in children: response to infliximab. J Pediatr Gastroenterol Nutr. 2003;37(2):150–4.

76. Bauer J, et al. Ulcerative stomatitis as clinical clue to inadvertent methotrexate overdose. Hautarzt. 1999;50(9):670–3.

77. Altenburg A, et al. Practical aspects of management of recurrent aphthous stomatitis. J Eur Acad Dermatol Venereol. 2007;21(8): 1019–26.

78. Rattan J, et al. Sucralfate suspension as a treatment of recurrent aphthous stomatitis. J Intern Med. 1994;236(3):341–3.

79. Fontes V, et al. Recurrent aphthous stomatitis: treatment with colchicine. An open trial of 54 cases. Ann Dermatol Venereol. 2002;129(12):1365–9.

80. Thornhill MH, et al. A randomized, double-blind, placebo-controlled trial of pentoxifylline for the treatment of recurrent aphthous stomatitis. Arch Dermatol. 2007;143(4):463–70.

81. Haugeberg G, Velken M, Johnsen V. Successful treatment of genital ulcers with infliximab in Behcet's disease. Ann Rheum Dis. 2004;63(6):744–5.

82. Jacobson JM, et al. Thalidomide for the treatment of oral aphthous ulcers in patients with human immunodeficiency virus infection. National Institute of Allergy and Infectious Diseases AIDS Clinical Trials Group. N Engl J Med. 1997;336(21):1487–93.

83. Powell FC, Su WP, Perry HO. Pyoderma gangrenosum: classification and management. J Am Acad Dermatol. 1996;34(3):395–409. quiz 410–2.

84. Hafner J, Kuhne A, Trueb RM. Successful grafting with EpiDex in pyoderma gangrenosum. Dermatology. 2006;212(3):258–9.

85. Brunsting HA. Pyoderma gangrenosum in association with chronic ulcerative colitis. Ohio Med. 1954;50(12):1150–1.

86. Powell FC, et al. Pyoderma gangrenosum: a review of 86 patients. Q J Med. 1985;55(217):173–86.

87. Johnson ML, Wilson HT. Skin lesions in ulcerative colitis. Gut. 1969;10(4):255–63.

88. Cox NH, Peebles-Brown DA, MacKie RM. Pyoderma gangrenosum occurring 10 years after proctocolectomy for ulcerative colitis. Br J Hosp Med. 1986;36(5):363.

89. Thornton JR, et al. Pyoderma gangrenosum and ulcerative colitis. Gut. 1980;21(3):247–8.

90. Miller J, et al. Pyoderma gangrenosum: a review and update on new therapies. J Am Acad Dermatol. 2010;62(4):646–54.

91. Johnson RB, Lazarus GS. Pulse therapy. Therapeutic efficacy in the treatment of pyoderma gangrenosum. Arch Dermatol. 1982;118(2):76–84.

92. Bennett ML, et al. Pyoderma gangrenosum. A comparison of typical and atypical forms with an emphasis on time to remission. Case review of 86 patients from 2 institutions. Medicine (Baltimore). 2000;79(1):37–46.

93. Regueiro M, et al. Infliximab for treatment of pyoderma gangrenosum associated with inflammatory bowel disease. Am J Gastroenterol. 2003;98(8):1821–6.

94. Brooklyn TN, et al. Infliximab for the treatment of pyoderma gangrenosum: a randomised, double blind, placebo controlled trial. Gut. 2006;55(4):505–9.

95. Friedman S, et al. Intravenous cyclosporine in refractory pyoderma gangrenosum complicating inflammatory bowel disease. Inflamm Bowel Dis. 2001;7(1):1–7.

96. Futami H, et al. Pyoderma gangrenosum complicating ulcerative colitis: Successful treatment with methylprednisolone pulse therapy and cyclosporine. J Gastroenterol. 1998;33(3):408–11.

97. Rustin MH, Gilkes JJ, Robinson TW. Pyoderma gangrenosum associated with Behcet's disease: treatment with thalidomide. J Am Acad Dermatol. 1990;23(5 Pt 1):941–4.

98. Teitel AD. Treatment of pyoderma gangrenosum with methotrexate. Cutis. 1996;57(5):326–8.

99. Lyon CC, Kirby B, Griffiths CE. Recalcitrant pyoderma gangrenosum treated with systemic tacrolimus. Br J Dermatol. 1999;140(3):562–4.

100. Jolles S, Niclasse S, Benson E. Combination oral and topical tacrolimus in therapy-resistant pyoderma gangrenosum. Br J Dermatol. 1999;140(3):564–5.

101. Galun E, Flugelman MY, Rachmilewitz D. Pyoderma gangrenosum complicating ulcerative colitis: successful treatment with methylprednisolone pulse therapy and dapsone. Am J Gastroenterol. 1986;81(10):988–9.

102. Kaminska R, Ikaheimo R, Hollmen A. Plasmapheresis and cyclophosphamide as successful treatments for pyoderma gangrenosum. Clin Exp Dermatol. 1999;24(2):81–5.

103. Kontochristopoulos GJ, et al. Treatment of Pyoderma gangrenosum with low-dose colchicine. Dermatology. 2004;209(3):233–6.

104. Tsele E, Yu RC, Chu AC. Pyoderma gangrenosum-response to topical nitrogen mustard. Clin Exp Dermatol. 1992;17(6): 437–40.

105. Nguyen LQ, Weiner J. Treatment of pyoderma gangrenosum with benzoyl peroxide. Cutis. 1977;19(6):842–4.

106. Cave DR, Burakoff R. Pyoderma gangrenosum associated with ulcerative colitis: treatment with disodium cromoglycate. Am J Gastroenterol. 1987;82(8):802–4.

107. Goldstein F, Krain R, Thornton JJ. Intralesional steroid therapy of pyoderma gangrenosum. J Clin Gastroenterol. 1985;7(6):499–501.

108. Sanders CJ, Hulsmans RF. Successful treatment of pyoderma gangrenosum with topical 5-aminosalicylic acid. Cutis. 1993;51(4): 262–4.

109. Felekis T, et al. Spectrum and frequency of ophthalmologic manifestations in patients with inflammatory bowel disease: a prospective single-center study. Inflamm Bowel Dis. 2009;15(1):29–34.

110. Barabino AV, et al. Sudden blindness in a child with Crohn's disease. World J Gastroenterol. 2011;17(38):4344–6.

111. McGavin DD, et al. Episcleritis and scleritis. A study of their clinical manifestations and association with rheumatoid arthritis. Br J Ophthalmol. 1976;60(3):192–226.

112. Mintz R, et al. Ocular manifestations of inflammatory bowel disease. Inflamm Bowel Dis. 2004;10(2):135–9.

113. Hakin KN, Ham J, Lightman SL. Use of cyclosporin in the management of steroid dependent non-necrotising scleritis. Br J Ophthalmol. 1991;75(6):340–1.

114. Sainz de la Maza M. Scleritis therapy. Ophthalmology. 2012; 119(1):51–8.

115. Yilmaz S, et al. The prevalence of ocular involvement in patients with inflammatory bowel disease. Int J Colorectal Dis. 2007; 22(9):1027–30.

116. Bhagat S, Das KM. A shared and unique peptide in the human colon, eye, and joint detected by a monoclonal antibody. Gastroenterology. 1994;107(1):103–8.

117. Dick AD, Azim M, Forrester JV. Immunosuppressive therapy for chronic uveitis: optimising therapy with steroids and cyclosporin A. Br J Ophthalmol. 1997;81(12):1107–12.

118. Tugal-Tutkun I, et al. Efficacy of infliximab in the treatment of uveitis that is resistant to treatment with the combination of azathioprine, cyclosporine, and corticosteroids in Behcet's disease: an open-label trial. Arthritis Rheum. 2005;52(8):2478–84.

119. Takase K, et al. Successful switching to adalimumab in an infliximab-allergic patient with severe Behcet disease-related uveitis. Rheumatol Int. 2011;31(2):243–5.

120. Fries W, et al. Treatment of acute uveitis associated with Crohn's disease and sacroileitis with infliximab. Am J Gastroenterol. 2002;97(2):499–500.

121. Ally MR, Veerappan GR, Koff JM. Treatment of recurrent Crohn's uveitis with infliximab. Am J Gastroenterol. 2008;103(8):2150–1.

122. Murray KF, Carithers Jr RL. AASLD practice guidelines: evaluation of the patient for liver transplantation. Hepatology. 2005; 41(6):1407–32.

123. Kingham JG, Kochar N, Gravenor MB. Incidence, clinical patterns, and outcomes of primary sclerosing cholangitis in South Wales, United Kingdom. Gastroenterology. 2004;126(7): 1929–30.

124. Karlsen TH, Schrumpf E, Boberg KM. Update on primary sclerosing cholangitis. Dig Liver Dis. 2010;42(6):390–400.

125. Goudet P, et al. Characteristics and evolution of extraintestinal manifestations associated with ulcerative colitis after proctocolectomy. Dig Surg. 2001;18(1):51–5.

126. Raj V, Lichtenstein DR. Hepatobiliary manifestations of inflammatory bowel disease. Gastroenterol Clin North Am. 1999; 28(2):491–513.

127. Escorsell A, et al. Epidemiology of primary sclerosing cholangitis in Spain, Spanish Association for the Study of the Liver. J Hepatol. 1994;21(5):787–91.

128. Okolicsanyi L, et al. Primary sclerosing cholangitis: clinical presentation, natural history and prognostic variables: an Italian multicentre study. The Italian PSC Study Group. Eur J Gastroenterol Hepatol. 1996;8(7):685–91.

129. Takikawa H, et al. Analysis of 388 cases of primary sclerosing cholangitis in Japan; Presence of a subgroup without pancreatic involvement in older patients. Hepatol Res. 2004;29(3):153–9.

130. Jess T, et al. Risk factors for colorectal neoplasia in inflammatory bowel disease: a nested case-control study from Copenhagen county, Denmark and Olmsted county, Minnesota. Am J Gastroenterol. 2007;102(4):829–36.

131. Bergquist A, et al. Hepatic and extrahepatic malignancies in primary sclerosing cholangitis. J Hepatol. 2002;36(3):321–7.

132. Chapman R, et al. Diagnosis and management of primary sclerosing cholangitis. Hepatology. 2010;51(2):660–78.

133. Donaldson PT, et al. Dual association of HLA DR2 and DR3 with primary sclerosing cholangitis. Hepatology. 1991;13(1):129–33.

134. Schrumpf E, et al. HLA antigens and immunoregulatory T cells in ulcerative colitis associated with hepatobiliary disease. Scand J Gastroenterol. 1982;17(2):187–91.

135. Chapman RW, et al. Association of primary sclerosing cholangitis with HLA-B8. Gut. 1983;24(1):38–41.

136. Boberg KM, et al. The HLA-DR3, DQ2 heterozygous genotype is associated with an accelerated progression of primary sclerosing cholangitis. Scand J Gastroenterol. 2001;36(8):886–90.

137. Das KM, Vecchi M, Sakamaki S. A shared and unique epitope(s) on human colon, skin, and biliary epithelium detected by a monoclonal antibody. Gastroenterology. 1990;98(2):464–9.

138. Eade MN, Brooke BN. Portal bacteraemia in cases of ulcerative colitis submitted to colectomy. Lancet. 1969;1(7603):1008–9.

139. Farkkila M, et al. Metronidazole and ursodeoxycholic acid for primary sclerosing cholangitis: a randomized placebo-controlled trial. Hepatology. 2004;40(6):1379–86.

140. Davies YK, et al. Long-term treatment of primary sclerosing cholangitis in children with oral vancomycin: an immunomodulating antibiotic. J Pediatr Gastroenterol Nutr. 2008;47(1):61–7.

141. Dave M, et al. Primary sclerosing cholangitis: meta-analysis of diagnostic performance of MR cholangiopancreatography. Radiology. 2010;256(2):387–96.

142. Duerr RH, et al. Neutrophil cytoplasmic antibodies: a link between primary sclerosing cholangitis and ulcerative colitis. Gastroenterology. 1991;100(5 Pt 1):1385–91.

143. Lindor KD. Effects of ursodeoxycholic acid on survival in patients with primary biliary cirrhosis. Gastroenterology. 1996; 110(5):1515–8.

144. Lindor KD. Ursodiol for primary sclerosing cholangitis. Mayo Primary Sclerosing Cholangitis-Ursodeoxycholic Acid Study Group. N Engl J Med. 1997;336(10):691–5.

145. Harnois DM, et al. High-dose ursodeoxycholic acid as a therapy for patients with primary sclerosing cholangitis. Am J Gastroenterol. 2001;96(5):1558–62.

146. Mitchell SA, et al. A preliminary trial of high-dose ursodeoxycholic acid in primary sclerosing cholangitis. Gastroenterology. 2001;121(4):900–7.

147. Lindor KD, et al. High-dose ursodeoxycholic acid for the treatment of primary sclerosing cholangitis. Hepatology. 2009; 50(3):808–14.

148. Tung BY, et al. Ursodiol use is associated with lower prevalence of colonic neoplasia in patients with ulcerative colitis and primary sclerosing cholangitis. Ann Intern Med. 2001;134(2):89–95.

149. Pardi DS, et al. Ursodeoxycholic acid as a chemopreventive agent in patients with ulcerative colitis and primary sclerosing cholangitis. Gastroenterology. 2003;124(4):889–93.

150. Wolf JM, Rybicki LA, Lashner BA. The impact of ursodeoxycholic acid on cancer, dysplasia and mortality in ulcerative colitis patients with primary sclerosing cholangitis. Aliment Pharmacol Ther. 2005;22(9):783–8.

151. Eaton JE, et al. High-dose ursodeoxycholic acid is associated with the development of colorectal neoplasia in patients with ulcerative colitis and primary sclerosing cholangitis. Am J Gastroenterol. 2011;106(9):1638–45.

152. Poropat G, et al. Bile acids for primary sclerosing cholangitis. Cochrane Database Syst Rev. 2011;1, CD003626.

153. Halilbasic E, et al. Side chain structure determines unique physiologic and therapeutic properties of norursodeoxycholic acid in Mdr2−/− mice. Hepatology. 2009;49(6):1972–81.

154. Angulo P, et al. Oral budesonide in the treatment of primary sclerosing cholangitis. Am J Gastroenterol. 2000;95(9):2333–7.

155. Knox TA, Kaplan MM. A double-blind controlled trial of oral-pulse methotrexate therapy in the treatment of primary sclerosing cholangitis. Gastroenterology. 1994;106(2):494–9.

156. Van Thiel DH, et al. Tacrolimus (FK 506), a treatment for primary sclerosing cholangitis: results of an open-label preliminary trial. Am J Gastroenterol. 1995;90(3):455–9.

157. Olsson R, et al. Colchicine treatment of primary sclerosing cholangitis. Gastroenterology. 1995;108(4):1199–203.

158. Lindor KD, et al. The combination of prednisone and colchicine in patients with primary sclerosing cholangitis. Am J Gastroenterol. 1991;86(1):57–61.

159. LaRusso NF, et al. Prospective trial of penicillamine in primary sclerosing cholangitis. Gastroenterology. 1988;95(4):1036–42.

160. Angulo P, et al. Pirfenidone in the treatment of primary sclerosing cholangitis. Dig Dis Sci. 2002;47(1):157–61.

161. Ozdil B, et al. New therapeutic option with N-acetylcysteine for primary sclerosing cholangitis: two case reports. Am J Ther. 2011;18(3):e71–4.

162. Strack I, et al. beta-Adrenoceptor blockade in sclerosing cholangitis of Mdr2 knockout mice: antifibrotic effects in a model of non-sinusoidal fibrosis. Lab Invest. 2011;91(2):252–61.

163. Angulo P, et al. Bone disease in patients with primary sclerosing cholangitis. Gastroenterology. 2011;140(1):180–8.

164. Zein CO, et al. Alendronate improves bone mineral density in primary biliary cirrhosis: a randomized placebo-controlled trial. Hepatology. 2005;42(4):762–71.

165. Gasche C, et al. Guidelines on the diagnosis and management of iron deficiency and anemia in inflammatory bowel diseases. Inflamm Bowel Dis. 2007;13(12):1545–53.

166. Schroder O, et al. Intravenous iron sucrose versus oral iron supplementation for the treatment of iron deficiency anemia in patients with inflammatory bowel disease – a randomized, controlled, open-label, multicenter study. Am J Gastroenterol. 2005;100(11):2503–9.

167. Evstatiev R, et al. FERGIcor, a randomized controlled trial on ferric carboxymaltose for iron deficiency anemia in inflammatory bowel disease. Gastroenterology. 2011;141(3):846–53 e1–2.

168. Schreiber S, et al. Recombinant erythropoietin for the treatment of anemia in inflammatory bowel disease. N Engl J Med. 1996; 334(10):619–23.

169. Bergamaschi G, et al. Prevalence and pathogenesis of anemia in inflammatory bowel disease. Influence of anti-tumor necrosis factor-alpha treatment. Haematologica. 2010;95(2):199–205.

170. Giannadaki E, et al. Autoimmune hemolytic anemia and positive Coombs test associated with ulcerative colitis. Am J Gastroenterol. 1997;92(10):1872–4.

171. Yates P, et al. Red cell autoantibody production by colonic mononuclear cells from a patient with ulcerative colitis and autoimmune haemolytic anaemia. Br J Haematol. 1992;82(4):753–6.

172. Altman AR, Maltz C, Janowitz HD. Autoimmune hemolytic anemia in ulcerative colitis: report of three cases, review of the literature, and evaluation of modes of therapy. Dig Dis Sci. 1979;24(4):282–5.

173. Alonso MJ, et al. Autoimmune hemolytic anemia associated with ulcerative colitis arising after colectomy. Rev Esp Enferm Dig. 1994;85(4):277–80.

174. Molnar T, et al. Successful treatment of steroid resistant ulcerative colitis associated with severe autoimmune hemolytic anemia with oral microemulsion cyclosporin – a brief case report. Am J Gastroenterol. 2003;98(5):1207–8.

175. Leo Carnerero E, et al. Autoimmune hemolytic anemia associated with ulcerative colitis: response to infliximab. Am J Gastroenterol. 2009;104(9):2370–1.

176. Yu LZ, et al. A case of ulcerative colitis associated with autoimmune hemolytic anemia successfully treated by autologous hematopoietic stem cell transplantation. Am J Gastroenterol. 2010;105(10):2302–4.

177. Bernstein CN, et al. The incidence of deep venous thrombosis and pulmonary embolism among patients with inflammatory bowel disease: a population-based cohort study. Thromb Haemost. 2001;85(3):430–4.

178. Grainge MJ, West J, Card TR. Venous thromboembolism during active disease and remission in inflammatory bowel disease: a cohort study. Lancet. 2010;375(9715):657–63.

179. Solem CA, et al. Venous thromboembolism in inflammatory bowel disease. Am J Gastroenterol. 2004;99(1):97–101.

180. Vazquez SR, Rondina MT, Pendleton RC. Azathioprine-induced warfarin resistance. Ann Pharmacother. 2008;42(7):1118–23.

181. Tabibian JH, Streiff MB. Inflammatory bowel disease-associated thromboembolism: a systematic review of outcomes with anticoagulation versus catheter-directed thrombolysis. Inflamm Bowel Dis. 2012;18(1):161–71.

182. Novacek G1, et al. Inflammatory bowel disease is a risk factor for recurrent venous thromboembolism. Gastroenterology. 2010;139(3):779-87. doi: 10.1053/j.gastro.2010.05.026. Epub 2010 Jun 12.

183. Samama MM, et al. A comparison of enoxaparin with placebo for the prevention of venous thromboembolism in acutely ill medical patients. Prophylaxis in Medical Patients with Enoxaparin Study Group. N Engl J Med. 1999;341(11):793–800.

184. Bernstein CN, Wajda A, Blanchard JF. The incidence of arterial thromboembolic diseases in inflammatory bowel disease: a population-based study. Clin Gastroenterol Hepatol. 2008;6(1): 41–5.

185. Yarur AJ, et al. Inflammatory bowel disease is associated with an increased incidence of cardiovascular events. Am J Gastroenterol. 2011;106(4):741–7.

186. Kraft SC, et al. Unexplained bronchopulmonary disease with inflammatory bowel disease. Arch Intern Med. 1976;136(4): 454–9.

187. Camus P, et al. The lung in inflammatory bowel disease. Medicine (Baltimore). 1993;72(3):151–83.

188. Herrlinger KR, et al. Alterations in pulmonary function in inflammatory bowel disease are frequent and persist during remission. Am J Gastroenterol. 2002;97(2):377–81.

189. Godet PG, et al. Pulmonary function abnormalities in patients with ulcerative colitis. Am J Gastroenterol. 1997;92(7):1154–6.

190. Marvisi M, et al. DLCO correlates with intestinal inflammation in ulcerative colitis, but albuminuria does not. Minerva Gastroenterol Dietol. 2007;53(4):321–7.

191. Mohamed-Hussein AA, Mohamed NA, Ibrahim ME. Changes in pulmonary function in patients with ulcerative colitis. Respir Med. 2007;101(5):977–82.

192. Douglas JG, et al. Respiratory impairment in inflammatory bowel disease: does it vary with disease activity? Respir Med. 1989;83(5): 389–94.

193. Peters FP, Engels LG, Moers AM. Pneumonitis induced by sulphasalazine. Postgrad Med J. 1997;73(856):99–100.

194. Lazaro MT, Garcia-Tejero MT, Diaz-Lobato S. Mesalamine-induced lung disease. Arch Intern Med. 1997;157(4):462.

195. Kasuga A, et al. Pulmonary complications resembling Wegener's granulomatosis in ulcerative colitis with elevated proteinase-3 anti-neutrophil cytoplasmic antibody. Intern Med. 2008;47(13):1211–4.

196. Mahadeva R, et al. Clinical and radiological characteristics of lung disease in inflammatory bowel disease. Eur Respir J. 2000; 15(1):41–8.

# Mimics of Ulcerative Colitis

## 36

Xinjun Cindy Zhu and Richard P. MacDermott

### Keywords

Ulcerative colitis • Mimics • Infectious colitis • Pathogens • Crohn's • Ischemic colitis • Radiation colitis • Eosinophilic colitis • Colorectal cancer • Irritable bowel syndrome • Allergic reaction to medications

## Introduction

The management of ulcerative colitis (UC) begins with accurately establishing the patient's diagnosis. In patients with established UC, relapses of symptoms can be due to the development of an additional gastrointestinal illness that mimics UC. Many other disease processes can mimic UC. Infectious colitides such as *Clostridia difficile*, hemorrhagic *E. coli, Campylobacter, Aeromonas, and Salmonellosis* can often present as severe ulcerative colitis. Other infectious pathogens which also need to be included in the differential diagnoses include *Amebiasis, Shigellosis, Cytomegalovirus, and Rotavirus*. Inflammatory diseases of the colon which can present as UC include Crohn's disease, ischemic colitis, radiation colitis, eosinophilic colitis, colorectal cancer, irritable bowel syndrome, and allergic reactions to medications such as mesalamine products, NSAIDS, and antibiotics. After the differential diagnosis of UC has been evaluated and other etiologies have been excluded, appropriate therapy can be started.

X.C. Zhu, M.D., M.S. (✉)
Division of Gastroenterology, Department of Medicine,
Albany Medical Center, 47 New Scotland Ave.,
Alba, NY 12208, USA
e-mail: zhux@mail.amc.edu

R.P. MacDermott, M.D., M.A.C.G., A.G.A.F.
Department of Gastroenterology, Albany Medical Center,
47 New Scotland Ave., Alba, NY 12208, USA
e-mail: macderr@mail.amc.edu

## Infectious Colitides in Patients with Ulcerative Colitis

The clinical presentations of acute infectious colitis and UC are indistinguishable and can pose a significant diagnostic challenge to the clinician. Most bacterial infections of the gastrointestinal tract result in acute self-limited diarrhea, but others can cause persistent infections, resulting in mucosal invasion with inflammation and/or ulceration and typically causing bloody diarrhea. The most common invasive bacterial pathogens in the developed world are *Campylobacter, Shigella, Salmonella, and Shiga* toxin-producing *E. coli (STEC)*, including *E. coli* 0157:H7. Invasive organisms such as *Campylobacter jejuni and Shigella* penetrate the mucosa, spread within the epithelial cells, and cause erosions and mucosal abscesses similar to those seen with UC. Symptoms from both UC and infectious colitides include severe diarrhea with abdominal cramping and systemic symptoms of fever, chills, malaise, and myalgias. Patients with established UC often display a relapsing, progressive, and remitting course [1]. Those patients who persistently exhibit UC symptoms despite appropriate therapy and also those patients whose symptoms recur after a good response to treatment must be carefully evaluated for other causes of their symptoms. Having UC does not protect a patient from contracting an infectious diarrheal illness, particularly when so many of our UC patients travel or are intermittently treated with antibiotics. This is particularly important in light of the marked overlap in symptoms between UC and infectious intestinal pathologies. Furthermore, UC complicated with unrecognized coexisting infection can lead to significant pathological consequences such as toxic megacolon [2]. The differential diagnosis should include, but may not be limited to, the following infectious agents: *Clostridium difficile, Campylobacter, E. coli 015:H7, Salmonella, Shigella*, Amebiasis, and CMV.

## *Clostridium difficile* Colitis

Superinfection of the colon with *C. difficile* is often associated with the use of antibiotics resulting in the suppression of normal microflora with the concomitant explosive overgrowth of *C. difficile*. Pseudomembranous colitis, a life-threatening complication of *C. difficile*, is a significant risk with immunocompromised patients in health-care settings. The incidence, severity, mortality, and recurrence of *C. difficile* are increasing, especially in patients [3, 4]. Increased risk factors for the development of *C. difficile* in IBD patients are age greater than 65 years, extended use of broad-spectrum antibiotics, longer periods of hospitalization, systemic usage of steroids and/or immunosuppressants, use of gastric acid-suppressing agents, and use of enemas [5–7].

Over the last decade, the emergence of a quinolone-resistant highly virulent strain of *C. difficile*, referred to as NAP1/BI/027, has accounted for the increased rates of *C. difficile* treatment failures with metronidazole. This strain, with high prevalence in North America and Northern Europe [8], carries a truncating mutation in the *tcdC* gene, a putative repressor of toxins A and B production, thus allowing the production of high levels of toxins A and B [9, 10].

Recent epidemiological data indicate more cases of *C. difficile* in IBD patients than controls. Similarly, effective therapeutic resolution of *C. difficile* is reduced in patients who also have IBD [11, 12]. *C. difficile* symptoms can mimic those of a flare-up of UC, with watery or bloody diarrhea with or without fever, leukocytosis, and hypoalbuminemia. Patients with *C. difficile* can present with a wide spectrum of symptoms ranging from those of mild, self-limiting illness to those of severe pseudomembranous colitis with toxic megacolon. Mild to moderate *C. difficile* is defined as leukocytosis with WBCs <15,000/μl and a serum creatinine <1.5 times the baseline level. Severe *C. difficile* is defined as leukocytosis with WBCs >25,000/μl and a serum creatinine level 1.5 times greater than baseline. Complicated severe *C. difficile* is defined as the coexistence of hypotension, shock, ileus, or toxic megacolon.

Risk factors for increased rates of emergency colectomy, morbidity, and mortality in severe presentations of *C. difficile* in IBD are advanced age and moderate to severe left-sided UC or Crohn's disease. With severe complicated *C. difficile*, the clinician must consider emergency surgical intervention with a subtotal colectomy, particularly with patients who develop septic shock, toxic megacolon, and colonic perforation.

A definitive diagnosis of *C. difficile* is made when stool samples are positive for *C. difficile* toxins A and B by glutamate dehydrogenase (GDH) EIA or PCR, the latter considered the most sensitive method of toxin detection. Likewise, a diagnosis of *C. difficile* can be made following colonoscopy revealing pseudomembranous colitis. However, it is critical to note that in IBD patients with *C. difficile*, pseudomembranes are absent in half of the patients on colonoscopy. Histological findings may also establish the existence of a coexisting infection, such as CMV and HSV.

The initial therapy for *C. difficile* in patients with IBD is to discontinue, when possible, the use of broad-spectrum antibiotics and to treat with vancomycin. Metronidazole (Flagyl) should not be used in IBD patients with *C. difficile*, due to the high resistant and recurrence rates. Oral vancomycin is currently the primary antibiotic recommended in IBD patients with severe initial or recurrent *C. difficile* or with posttreatment recurrent infections. Up to 30 % of IBD patients will develop recurrent *C. difficile* and will require repeated treatment. Patients with relapsing *C. difficile* may require tapered or pulse-chased oral vancomycin therapy [13].

A recent phase III comparative trial, in normal patients without IBD or other underlying illnesses, by Louie [14] demonstrated that fidaxomicin (200 mg p.o. twice a day), a poorly absorbed, macrocyclic antibiotic, having a narrow antimicrobial spectrum, had similar effectiveness as vancomycin against *C. difficile* (125 mg p.o. four times daily) yet achieved a 45 % reduction in recurrent *C. difficile*. However, fidaxomicin has not yet been evaluated in IBD patients with *C. difficile* in a controlled fashion.

In addition to the use of antibiotics to treat patients with refractory or recurrent *C. difficile*, the recent introduction of fecal microbial transplantation (FMT) has come to clinical practice as a treatment for the *C. difficile* [15, 16]. In patients without IBD, the overall success rate of FMT in recurrent infections is estimated to be 90 %. Preliminary results presented from the only placebo controlled trial to date to treat patients with active ulcerative colitis did not demonstrate benefit for FMT as primary treatment in patients with active ulcerative colitis (who did not have *C. difficile* infection) [17].

## Invasive *Escherichia coli*

Two *E. coli* strains characterized as enteroinvasive (EIEC) and enterohemorrhagic (EHEC) are significant causes of inflammation, invasion, and hemorrhagic enterocolitis. Infection with these organisms presents clinically as fever with watery and/or bloody diarrhea. Of the two strains, EHEC causes the more significant pathology and will be the focus of the remainder of this section.

EHEC disease is caused by the production of enterotoxins variously referred to as verotoxins or *Shiga* toxins. Indeed, the immunobiological activity of these toxins is identical to those produced by strains of *Shigella dysenteriae*. Infections with *E. coli* serotype *O157:H7*, a hypertoxigenic strain, typically begin as watery diarrhea that rapidly becomes bloody. The systemic response to *Shiga* toxin can lead to the development of hemolytic uremic syndrome (HUS) and thrombotic thrombocytopenic purpura (TTP) as *Shiga* toxin can circulate in the blood and bind to the renal tissue, causing glomerular swelling and deposition of fibrin and platelets in blood vessels. This typically occurs within 2 weeks after onset of diarrhea and is especially significant in children under 5 and in adults older than 65 years of age. Toxic megacolon is a significant complication of HUS caused by *E. coli O157:H7*. A growing number of foods, both raw and prepared, are associated with infections with *E. coli O157:H7*. These include undercooked ground beef, unpasteurized fruit juices, and raw fruits and vegetables. EHEC should be considered with symptomatic younger children presenting with ischemic changes in the right colon, often with severe mural edema, hemorrhage, and mucosal erosions.

EHEC is diagnosed by stool cultures with serotypic confirmation of the presence of appropriate somatic (O) and flagellar (H) antigens. Isolation and identification of *E. coli O157:H7* is facilitated by the use of MacConkey agar containing sorbitol as the majority of EHEC strains do not ferment this carbohydrate. Diagnostic samples for stool culture should be taken as early as possible in the course of infection. Colon biopsy samples may be processed with immunohistochemical staining using anti-O and anti-H antisera.

When diarrhea is severe, supportive treatment is indicated with intravenous replacement of fluids and electrolytes early in the disease; however, antibiotics and antidiarrheals are contraindicated as they increase risks of developing severe complications such as *Henoch-Schonlein purpura, hemolytic uremic syndrome,* and thrombocytopenic purpura. In particular, patients who had higher leukocyte count and used antibiotics in the first week of *E. coli O157:H7* infections are at risk to develop oligoanuric hemolytic uremic syndrome [18]. The use of plasma therapy during the acute phase has been found to be associated with poor long-term outcome, and a long-term follow-up for at least 5 years is recommended to detect late sequel, such as hypertension, neurological symptoms, impaired glomerular filtration rate, and proteinuria [19].

## Salmonella

*Salmonella* are a genus of Gram-negative enteric bacteria that are not normal inhabitants of the human gut. Although there are more than 2,000 recognized serotypes of *Salmonella*, all are now recognized to belong to a single species—*Salmonella enterica*. For example, the old names of *S. typhi* and *S. paratyphi* are currently rendered *S. enterica*, serotype *Typhi,*

and *S. enterica*, serotype *Paratyphi*. However, due to historical usage, medical personnel often continue to use the traditional species names. For clarity and historical reasons, names will be shown in parenthesis.

Nontyphoidal gastroenteritis develops in approximately 75 % of patients infected with *S. enterica, serotype Typhimurium* (*S. typhimurium*), and *S. enterica, serotype Enteritidis* (*S. enteritidis)* infections. Most human infections are from the consumption of contaminated food or water. The normal course of infection is lengthy, up to 4 week in duration, with fever, cramping abdominal pain, and diarrhea from acute ileitis and ileocolitis. Infection with *S. enterica, serotype Typhi* (*S. typhi*), leads to the development of typhoid fever in about 10 % of cases with typical symptoms of prolonged fever >103 F, decreased pulse, rash, abdominal pain, diarrhea or constipation, and intestinal bleeding or perforation [20]. *Salmonella* outbreaks in the past few years have been associated with the consumption of contaminated spinach, peanut butter, eggs, and vegetable snacks. Patients with hypochlorhydria or treated with immunosuppressive drugs are more susceptible to infection.

Patients with IBD should be advised to avoid contact with reptiles such as pet lizards, turtles, and aquatic frogs, as these are natural carriers of *Salmonellae*. Our UC patients commonly travel, and *Salmonella* is a common cause for infectious colitis to develop. Vaccination, either oral administration or injection, is recommended to those who travel to endemic areas. However, oral vaccination with live, attenuated Ty21a-based vaccines is contraindicated for IBD patients who are under immunosuppressive treatment or with any patient with impaired immunity.

Antibiotic treatment is necessary in patients who have severe disease, are younger than 1 or older than 50, immunosuppressed, and with underlying diseases including hemoglobinopathies, vascular grafts, and artificial joints. IBD patients who are infected with *Salmonella* also require treatment. Ciprofloxacin is the drug of choice for nonpregnant patients although increasing quinolone-resistant strains have been reported. Ceftriaxone is an alternative treatment choice for pregnant patients or children. If relapses occur, patients are retreated with antibiotics. Prolonged treatment is needed in carrier states, which occur in 3–5 % of those infected. Removal of the gallbladder is often required with chronic *Salmonella* carriers.

## Shigella

*Shigellae* represent four species, *Shigella dysenteriae, Shigella flexneri, Shigella boydii, and Shigella sonnei, and* are Gram-negative members of the *Enterobacteriaceae*. While all four species are globally distributed, *S. dysenteriae* and *S flexneri* have caused endemic and pandemic disease in developing countries, while *S. sonnei* is associated with outbreaks of shigellosis in the United States and Western Europe. Shigellosis is spread via the fecal-oral route of inoculation and is highly contagious, requiring <100 organisms to establish infection. *Shigella* invades the intestinal epithelium and causes the death of epithelial cells resulting in an acute proctocolitis with occasional involvement of the ileum as well.

Clinical symptoms usually start with fever, malaise, and watery diarrhea that rapidly progresses to grossly bloody diarrhea. Infections with *Shiga* toxin-producing strains of *S. dysenteriae* can cause life-threatening fulminant colitis with toxic megacolon and intestinal perforation [21]. *Shigella sonnei,* rarely a cause of severe infections, has been reported with infection requiring a subtotal colectomy [22]. Histological features of *Shigella* infection vary from early changes of acute infectious colitis with superficial neutrophilic infiltrates, edema, cryptitis, crypt abscesses, ulceration and exudates, and pseudomembranes to later changes that mimic UC, with increased mucosal destruction, mixed inflammatory infiltration of the lamina propria with architectural distortion, and glandular destruction.

It should be noted that because UC patients commonly travel to other countries, *Shigella* infection is common for them to expose to. Diagnosis is made by multiple cultures from freshly collected stool. Treatment of choice is with quinolones and sulfamethoxazole/trimethoprim. Relapse may occur in patients with immunodeficiency and may require prolonged antibiotic treatment [23].

## Amebiasis

*Entamoeba histolytica* is an amoeboid protozoan parasite with global distribution. Ingestion of cysts, the infective form of the parasite, typically occurs with contaminated food and water. The trophozoite, the actively motile stage of the parasite, causes various gastrointestinal manifestations, which include diarrhea, abdominal pain, cramps, and tenesmus. Diarrhea, while usually present, may be intermittent in some cases and can be accompanied by periods of constipation that can last for months to years. Complications of fulminating infections may include liver abscess, hemorrhagic colitis, perforation of the bowel, and toxic megacolon.

Endoscopic findings with acute amebic colitis reveal a wide range of erosions, flask-shaped ulcers, exudates, and bumps caused by edematous mucosa due to acute inflammation which is indistinguishable from that caused by UC, as well as by other agents of infectious colitis. The cecum is most often affected, but frequently the rest of the colon is involved as well. The most predictive endoscopic signs of amebic colitis are the presence of a multiplicity of typical exudative cecal lesions [24]. Diagnosis can made by stool microscopy for parasite, coproantigen ELISA with fecal samples, and hematoxylin and eosin staining of the tissue showing amebae with foamy cytoplasm and nuclei with smooth, evenly distributed peripheral chromatin with a small, central endosome. Ameboid trophozoites with typical morphology and containing ingested erythrocytes are pathognomonic for amebic dysentery. PCR is recommended for confirmation of the diagnosis of *Entamoeba* spp. [25].

For asymptomatic carriers, chemotherapeutic agents active against cysts, such as paromomycin or iodoquinol, are usually sufficient. A tissue amebicide, such as metronidazole or tinidazole, combined with paromomycin, should be used for treating symptomatic (active) infections [23].

## Campylobacter

*Campylobacter* is the most commonly identified bacterial pathogen of the gut in the developed world. Infections with *Campylobacter jejuni* are characterized by acute enteritis of 1–7 days duration. Symptoms vary from nausea and vomiting and mild watery diarrhea to grossly bloody stool. Although usually self-limited, *C;ampylobacter* infections rarely progress to severe life-threatening disease or produce complications such as toxic megacolon. The majority of patients develop ileitis and some degree of segmental colitis. A case of pancolitis mimicking UC has been reported [26]. Of note, *Campylobacter* infections are a leading cause of *Guillain-Barre syndrome.* As *Campylobacter* naturally colonizes poultry and a variety other domestic animals, it is frequently associated with zoonotic transmission of disease in humans via contaminated foods [27]. Diagnosis is made by stool culture and microscopic examination for curved Gram-negative *bacilli*. A higher yield from colonic tissue culture can be achieved for *C. jejuni*. Successful treatment can be achieved with quinolones, erythromycin, and tetracycline [23].

Ternhag et al. found an elevated risk for UC and reactive arthritis as well among *Campylobacter* infections [28]. Superinfection of *Campylobacter jejuni* was more commonly found in 17.6 % IBD patients with flares, being probably related to the consumption of chicken meal or drinking from contaminated water sources [29]. Although *Campylobacter jejuni* continues to be one of the most common causes of infectious diarrhea in the United States, a growing number of other clinically significant *Campylobacter species* have been identified. *Campylobacter concisus, C. upsaliensis, and C. ureolyticus* have been recognized as emerging human and animal pathogens and have been associated with gastrointestinal diseases, particularly in patients with underlying IBD and in children with newly diagnosed Crohn's disease [30].

## *Yersinia enterocolitica*

*Yersinia enterocolitica* is a Gram-negative bacterium belonging to the *Enterobacteriaceae* family of enteric organisms. Infections with *Y. enterocolitica* are associated with consumption of contaminated foods, often pork and unpasteurized milk. The natural reservoirs of the organism are various animals, particularly pigs, livestock, rodents, and rabbits. The most common forms of disease are hemorrhagic enterocolitis, terminal ileitis, and mesenteric lymphadenitis, often mimicking appendicitis and Crohn's disease [21, 31].

Dysentery is due to the penetration of the submucosa of the terminal ileum, the cecum, and the proximal ascending colon, with acute abdominal pain, often in the lower right quadrant. *Yersinia* granulomatous appendicitis may be seen with small bowel obstruction at the terminal ileum due to granulomatous inflammation, mural fibrosis, aphthous ulcers, and transmural lymphoid hyperplasia. Mesenteric adenopathy is frequently seen on CT scans.

*Yersinia* infection may be associated with migratory polyarthritis, Reiter's syndrome, and erythema nodosum which is indistinguishable to extraintestinal manifestations of IBD. *Yersinia* infection can also be a trigger of chronic IBD as evident by the fact that in some cases new onset of UC was demonstrated at diagnosis of *Y. enterocolitica* infection [32]. Most of time conventional cultures failed to detect obligate pathogenic bacteria; however, *Yersinia* species were detected by PCR in surgically resected intestinal specimens from patients with Crohn's disease and ulcerative colitis [33].

Colonoscopy typically reveals a thickened wall with inflammatory masses; round or oval elevations with or without ulcers in the ileum, right colon, and appendix; and histological features indistinguishable from Crohn's disease. Some cases show focal ulceration from the rectum to the cecum [34]. Diagnosis can be made from stool cultures using cold enrichment techniques with cefsulodin-irgasan-novobiocin agar, a medium specifically designed for the isolation of *Yersinia* spp. Serological techniques are of limited value in diagnosis as they are unable to determine the serotype of the infecting organism. In addition, there are cross-reacting antigens with the *Yersiniae*, *Brucellae*, and other bacteria that complicate diagnosis by serological means alone. Hemagglutination titers of ≥1:128 with consistent signs and symptoms may suggests *Yersinia* infection. Treatment is required for patients with severe disease. Ciprofloxacin, tetracycline, or trimethoprim/sulfamethoxazole is effective in the treatment of yersiniosis [23].

## Cytomegalovirus (CMV)

CMV-induced colitis remains the most common form of disease due to CMV, although CMV can affect the entire GI tract in immunosuppressed patients. Superimposed CMV infections are common in UC patients with severe disease and have been identified in up to 36 % of UC patients with a history of treatment failure. The use of steroids and other immunomodulating drug is also associated with high CMV loads [35]. Interestingly, CMV colitis has also been linked with coinfections with *C. difficile,* both of which are significant causes of toxic megacolon.

Segmental and/or linear ulcerative lesions can often be seen on colonoscopy, due to CMV colitis, with the presence of single, multiple, superficial or deep, or well-circumscribed "punched out"-appearing lesions in the bowel epithelium. Diagnosis of CMV infection can be made by viral culture as well as by histopathology of tissue specimens from the ulcer base. Histopathology provided the highest diagnostic yield with the presence of characteristic "giant" cells containing eosinophilic intranuclear inclusions and basophilic intracytoplasmic inclusions. Detection of viral antigens by immunohistochemistry and/or in situ DNA hybridization in biopsy specimens increases the yield of detection. Noninvasive molecular diagnostic techniques such as quantitative nucleic acid analysis using PCR and the CMV pp65 antigenemia assay are available.

Treatment is usually effective with intravenous ganciclovir, oral valganciclovir, or foscarnet. If gastrointestinal infections are complicated with CMV viremia, antiviral therapy should be continued until the viremia is cleared, determined by at least two consecutive negative CMV PCR tests. In patients with UC who have superimposed CMV, clearance of the CMV infection can be very difficult, and recurrent, refractory, and combined UC and CMV is common. Patients with both UC and CMV will often eventually need a colectomy.

## Rotavirus

Rotavirus is the most important etiologic agent of severe, acute gastroenteritis in infants and young children in the developed world. Adults with close contact to sick children can also become infected. In addition to watery diarrhea, patients with Rotavirus infections have a high incidence of vomiting, lethargy, and dehydration. In rare cases, Rotavirus gastroenteritis may be accompanied with convulsions, myositis, encephalitis, encephalopathy, and Reye's syndrome.

Elevated levels of alanine aminotransferase and aspartate aminotransferase have been reported, which appear linked with high levels of interleukin 6 [36]. Diagnosis of infection by Rotavirus can be made by detection of the virus in stool by PCR, ELISA, and direct viral culture. Treatment is mainly supportive with replacement of fluids and electrolytes and antiemetic therapy. Zinc supplements have been shown to have some effect in decreasing both the frequency and severity of diarrhea. However, antidiarrheal medicines and antibiotics should be avoided. Safe and effective vaccines against Rotavirus infection have been included in national immunization programs.

## Aspergillosis

Systemic infections with *Aspergillus* spp. frequently have gastrointestinal presentations; however, this infection is rarely seen with immunocompromised patients. Risk factors for invasive aspergillosis are prolonged severe neutropenia and the use of steroids and other immunosuppressors [37]. IBD patients who receive cyclosporine, steroids, and other 6-MP immunosuppressants have increased incidence of gastrointestinal aspergillosis as well as *Aspergillus fumigatus* pneumonia [38]. Clinical manifestations of infection include fever, abdominal pain, GI bleeding, abdominal tenderness, ileus, and toxic megacolon due to ischemia and infarction. In such cases, urgent surgical resection of the bowel may be indicated. *Aspergillus*-associated necrotizing enterocolitis has been reported [39]. Macroscopically lesions comprised ulcers of variable configurations, mucosal flecks, sloughed mucous membranes, polypoid masses, segmental lesions, and transmural invasion [40].

The diagnosis of aspergillosis requires either the culture of the organism from the tissues or the histopathological demonstration of typical broad, septate, branching hyphae morphologically consistent with that of *Aspergillus*. Aspergillosis in the presence of reduced lymphocytes in mesenteric nodes is suggestive of immunosuppression. The treatment of choice for invasive aspergillosis is voriconazole. Patients who cannot be treated with voriconazole are treated with amphotericin B.

## *Cryptosporidium parvum*

*C. parvum* is an intracellular protozoan parasite of intestinal epithelial cells and causes a secretory type of diarrheal disease. Severe and/or prolonged cryptosporidiosis is increased in patients with both cellular and humoral immune deficiencies. Risk factors include HIV infection, transplant-associated immunosuppression, IgA deficiency, and hypogammaglobulinemia [41]. IBD patients with cryptosporidiosis may present with symptoms of an acute UC or CD,

which include fever, malaise, abdominal cramps, rectal bleeding, and profound dehydrating diarrhea [42]. The diagnosis is primarily based on microscopic examination of stool which reveals *Cryptosporidium* trophozoites that line the surface of intestinal crypts, reactive atypia of epithelial cells, and increased numbers of inflammatory cells in the lamina propria. A modified acid-fast stain is used to show the presence of oocysts. Immunofluorescent-labeled monoclonal antibodies against components of the oocyte cell wall are used with stool or tissue samples. Treatment of immunocompetent individuals is supportive, as infections are usually self-limiting. Nitazoxanide is the drug of choice for use with immunocompromised patients.

## Microscopic Colitis

Microscopic colitis is defined histologically as either lymphocytic colitis (LC) or collagenous colitis (CC). Macroscopically in both cases, the colonic mucosa appears normal or near normal. LC is characterized by the infiltration of intraepithelial lymphocytes, whereas CC has an additional distinct subepithelial deposition appearing as a thickened band-like collagen structure. About 10 % of the patients, especially those older than 50 years of age with idiopathic watery diarrhea, have subsequently been found to have either LC or CC. The etiology of microscopic colitis is still unclear but is associated with immunological diseases, such as autoimmune thyroiditis, celiac disease, and IBD. A number of medications have been linked to the development of LC and CC, among which are NSAIDs and proton pump inhibitors [43]. Diagnosis of microscopic colitis is made based on characteristic histological features. Multiple tissue samples from both the left and right colon increase diagnostic yields as LC and CC can be manifest as focal or segmental colitis. Patients with microscopic colitis should be tested for celiac disease with appropriate serology and endoscopy and placed on a gluten-free diet if the diagnosis is established. NSAIDs and other potential contributing medications should be discontinued before therapy is initiated. Budesonide is the drug of choice for persistently symptomatic patients with LC or CC, as randomized controlled trials have shown its effectiveness in treating patients with either LC or CC. Patients usually respond to treatment within 2 weeks; however, relapse is common when budesonide is stopped. Treatment failures with budesonide may require use of other effective regimens, which include aminosalicylate, cholestyramine, and steroids [44].

## Crohn's Disease, IBD Unclassified, and Indeterminate Colitis

About 20 % of patients with Crohn's disease (CD) have involvement of only the colon, which complicates its differentiation from UC, especially in patients with moderate to severe disease. About 13 % of patients with presumed UC that undergo ileal pouch-anal anastomosis (IPAA) eventually develop de novo CD. Therefore, an accurate diagnosis of UC is important prior to performing an IPAA, as misdiagnosed UC patients with actual CD have increased postoperative complications such as pouchitis, perianal fistulizing disease, strictures, loss of pouch, and permanent ileostomy and are at increased risk for short bowel syndrome [45]. When chronic inflammatory disease has equivocal features for both UC and CD from biopsy specimens or from surgically resected colon specimens, it is referred to as IBD unclassified (IBDU) or indeterminate colitis (IC), respectively. Murrell ZA et al. reported that patients with IBDU or IC can undergo IPAA and expect a long-term outcome equivalent to patients with UC. However, about 12 % of these patients developed de novo CD [46]. Serologic markers such as anti-Saccharomyces cerevisiae antibodies (ASCA) and perinuclear antineutrophil cytoplasmic antibodies (pANCA) have been used to predict the development of CD or UC in patients with IC. A positive ASCA but negative pANCA predicts CD in 80 % of patients with IC, and a negative ASCA but positive pANCA predicts UC in 64 % of patients with IC [47]. Furthermore, a family history of CD was identified as a risk factor for CD after IPAA in patients originally presenting with IC.

## Irritable Bowel Syndrome (IBS)

It is sometime difficult to differentiate symptoms of IBS from those of IBD as both diseases share similar symptoms of diarrhea, abdominal pain, and sometimes weight loss. IBS symptoms are common among IBD patients. The prevalence of IBS in first-degree relatives of patients with IBD is elevated [48]. Coexistent IBS in the IBD patient can cause significant impairment in quality of life, increased anxiety and depression, and increased medical visits. A comprehensive history is critical to differentiate IBS from IBD. Patients with IBS present with watery diarrhea, bloating, and cramping abdominal pain, which is relieved after defecation. Certain foods, fruits, or drinks can aggravate IBS symptoms [49]. Normal ESR, CRP, and CBC favor the diagnosis of IBS. However, abnormal calprotectin levels have been reported with IBS-like symptoms in IBD patients in remission, suggesting a role of yet to be identified inflammatory factors causing IBS in those patients [50]. Patients with an IBD flare will present with diarrhea mixed with blood, constant abdominal pain without relief after defecation, and weight loss, accompanied with elevated ESR, CRP, and WBC and presence of anemia. Treatment of IBS in patients with IBD is similar to that of patients with IBS alone. It is critical to establish good patient-doctor relationship and provide ongoing patient education on the nature of the disease. It is also important to identify and avoid particular foods and beverages that induce IBS symptoms [49]. Antidiarrheals such as diphenoxylate, loperamide, and low-dose tricyclic antidepressants have been used for patients with IBS with diarrhea predominance. Rifaximin has also been shown to provide symptomatic improvement especially in diarrhea and bloating. The use of antispasmodic, anticholinergic medications such as dicyclomine and hyoscyamine can also be helpful in pain management with IBS patients.

## Eosinophilic Colitis

Eosinophilic colitis (EC), also known as allergic colitis, often occurs in infants and is an immune response to dietary or other antigens, resulting in extensive eosinophilic infiltration of the colonic mucosa and presenting as rectal bleeding, bloody diarrhea, and/or loose stool with mucus. In adults, involvement of both the ileum and colon, yet sparing the rectum, is a feature of EC that mimics those of Crohn's disease with focal erythema and friable-appearing mucosa, increased nodularity, and, in severe case, erosions and ulcers. In active IBD, eosinophils are also found to accumulate and become activated resulting in releasing cytotoxic proteins, such as eosinophil cationic protein (ECP) and eosinophil protein X (EPX), and infiltrating into the colonic mucosa [51]. Colonic biopsies are necessary to make the diagnosis of EC which is based on characteristic histological findings that demonstrate the presence of eosinophils $\geq 60/10HPF$ in lamina propria near the lymphoid aggregates, eosinophilic crypt abscess, and focal eosinophils in the intestinal epithelium and crypts. In active UC, eosinophils are also evident in colonic mucosa but with fewer number than that in EC. Tissue samples from each section of the colon must be placed into different containers, as each section of the colon has different numbers of eosinophils. Though serological ECP and EPX did not correlate with eosinophilic infiltration in colonic mucosa in patients with IBD in remission or with mild disease, the levels of ECP and EPX from stool samples have increased from the patients with active UC and CD [52]. Successful treatment of EC is based on the identification and removal of the causative antigen from the diet and is usually made by the use of dermal antigen sensitivity tests. An elemental diet may also be helpful. The better therapeutic approaches toward EC are yet to be established.

## Ischemic Colitis

Ischemic colitis is the most common sequelae of a compromised blood supply to the mesenteric vessels. It develops in older patients upon arterial or venous occlusion, low-flow states, or intestinal obstruction. Ischemic colitis often presents with acute abdominal pain, hematochezia, bloody diarrhea, and fever. It may be seen in younger patients with a history of use of oral contraceptives, cocaine, NSAIDs, phenylephrine, amphetamines, triptans, or underlying thrombophilia. Ischemic colitis has been reported in marathon runners as well as patients infected with *E. coli O157:H7* or CMV. Characteristic endoscopic features include a dusky or hemorrhagic appearance of the mucosa, marked edema and erythema, ulceration, and pseudomembrane with geographic distributions, of which the descending to the sigmoid colon are most affected, and the distal rectum is often spared. Brandt et al. reported that in patients with late-onset symptoms of IBD (>50 years of age), only 26 % of patients were found to have either UC (14 %), CD (5 %), or undetermined (7 %). The rest of patients were found to have either defined ischemic colitis (64 %) or possible ischemic colitis 10 % [53]. Colonoscopy with biopsy can confirm the diagnosis and assess severity and distribution. Isolated right-sided ischemic colitis requires more attention as it could be an early sign of impending small bowel infarct if left untreated. It is very important to early and liberally perform vascular imaging (CTA: Computed Tomography (CT) Angiography, MRA: Magnetic Resonance Angiogram, or MRV: Magnetic Resonance Venogram) and to use intra-arterial papaverine to decrease vascular spasms in order to make the diagnosis before intestinal infarct occurs, which has mortality rates of 70–90 %. Treatment includes supportive measures, discontinuance of offending agents, resection of involved segments, embolectomy, and/or arterial reconstruction. Broad-spectrum antibiotics should be immediately begun with the appearance of acute mesenteric ischemia. Appropriate anticoagulation for recurrent thrombosis should be started within 48 h after embolectomy or arterial reconstruction.

## Radiation-Induced Colitis

Radiation-induced colitis is caused by the therapeutic use of ionizing radiation which damages the colonic mucosa, blood vessels, and colonic wall. It commonly presents with diarrhea, bleeding, and pain due to colonic obstruction. Acute changes are normally self-limited and only require supportive care. However, chronic changes can be difficult to treat and may have lifelong consequences. With most cases, the diagnosis can be confirmed by colonoscopy or sigmoidoscopy, observing pallor of the mucosa with friability and multiple telangiectasias [54]. Characteristic histological features are eosinophilic cryptitis with eosinophilic infiltrations in the mucosa and lamina propria and subtlely withered-appearing crypts, which can be reversed. Chronic radiation colitis shows telangiectatic blood vessels with atypical endothelial cells, surrounded by hyalinized lamina

propria and marked crypt distortion where arterial damage leads to ischemic mucosa. A colonoscopy is indicated with patients who have received radiation treatment for prostate cancer or for gynecological cancers. Treatment of radiation-induced colitis includes supportive care in the acute phase, endoscopic thermotherapy such as argon plasma coagulation to cauterize bleeding and dilation of strictures using balloon or Savary dilators, as well as surgical resection of the bleeding or obstructed segmental colon. Therapy may also include the use of hyperbaric oxygen for nonhealing anorectal wounds and antibiotics for possible bacterial overgrowth. The use of topical corticosteroids or sucralfate may also be recommended.

## Segmental Colitis Associated with Diverticulosis (SCAD)

SCAD is defined as chronic segmental mucosal inflammation in the distribution of diverticula; however, SCAD is not related to diverticulitis. It is seen predominantly in the descending and sigmoid colon [55]. The incidence of SCAD is 0.2–1.4 cases per 100 colonoscopies and is markedly associated with the elderly with the median age of onset ≥64 years old. Clinical presentations include hematochezia, abdominal pain, diarrhea, obstruction, and possible fistula formation between the colon and the adjacent internal organs, such as the vagina and bladder [56]. Endoscopy reveals erythema of the mucosa surrounding the diverticula, with annular changes and microscopic features of chronic colitis with dense lymphoplasmacytic inflammation of the lamina propria, crypt distortion, and crypt abscesses. However, the mucosa both proximal and distal to the segment of diverticula is normal. CT scans show thickening of the colonic wall in the diverticular segments without signs of diverticulitis. Treatment includes control of constipation, segmental resection, antibiotics, and 5-ASA products [57].

## Colitis Due to Chronic, High-Dose NSAIDs

Up to 10 % of newly diagnosed colitis is associated with long-term use of high doses of NSAIDs. Patients typically present with anemia, bloody diarrhea, and abdominal pain. Colonoscopy reveals patchy erythema, localized erosion, and discrete ulcers in the colon, most commonly in the ileocecal region. Histological examination reveals patchy inflammation with focal areas of active colitis and various crypt distortions without increased intraepithelial lymphocytes. Treatment options include the discontinuation of NSAIDs and suppression of inflammation with sulfasalazine and metronidazole [58].

## Adverse Reactions to IBD Drugs

Intolerance to 5-ASA products as well as a variety of genetically engineered therapeutic proteins called "biologics" that are designed to inhibit inflammation can mimic symptoms associated with the recurrence of colitis. Bousseaden A. et al. observed the worsening of colitis symptoms after the oral or rectal administration of mesalamine [59], suggesting that sensitivity to mesalamine should be considered in the differential diagnosis of recrudescent ulcerative colitis. Clinically, patients intolerant to 5-ASA experienced abdominal pain and diarrhea within a few days of exposure to the drug. Endoscopy reveals active colitis mimicking ulcerative colitis. Histological characteristics feature eosinophilic infiltration to the mucosa and formation of eosinophilic crypt abscesses. Successful treatment usually involves discontinuation of mesalamine and administration of a short course of steroids.

## Ulcerative Colitis-Associated Colon Cancer

Patients with ulcerative colitis are at increased risk for developing colorectal cancer [60]. Risk factors for colorectal cancer for UC patients are advanced age of onset, longer duration of disease, more extensive disease, and coexisting primary sclerosing cholangitis. These observations provide supporting evidence for the etiological role of chronic inflammation in colon carcinogenesis. Additionally, patients with certain genetic markers are at risk for the development of colon cancer. Garrity-Park et al. reported that specific HLA-DR and HLA-DQ alleles within the class II region of the major histocompatibility complex (MHC) on chromosome 6p are highly associated with colon cancers [61]. Symptoms of colon cancer are change in bowel habits, blood in the stool, narrow caliber of the stool, abdominal cramping, chronic fatigue, and weight loss. Unfortunately, these symptoms also largely overlap those due to a flare-up of IBD, necessitating an accurate diagnosis for proper management. Colonoscopy with biopsy is the definitive means to differentiate between colon cancer and a flare-up of IBD. Annual or biennial colonoscopy is recommended for patients with ulcerative colitis 8–10 years after initial diagnosis. Total colectomy is warranted for colitis-associated dysplasia and colorectal cancer. Vigilant surveillance with shortened periods between examinations is advised with at-risk patients reluctant to elect surgery.

## Chemotherapy-Related Colitis

About 5–15 % patients who receive chemotherapy develop gastrointestinal mucositis, caused by highly reactive oxidative molecules that directly damage the intestinal epithelial cells. Fluoropyrimidine compounds such as 5-FU are commonly associated with chemotherapy-induced diarrhea. Clinical presentations typically include nausea, vomiting, diarrhea, and GI bleeding. The small intestine is the most common site for chemotherapy-related enteritis, whereas the colon is the least affected. Endoscopic findings include ulcers and erosions with histological evidence of epithelial apoptosis and cell death, with rare inflammation and dilated crypts [62]. The successful treatment of mucositis remained to be problematic. Palifermin, a recombinant human keratinocyte growth factor and a potent epithelial growth factor, which appears both to protect the mucosal epithelium from damage and to stimulate repair after chemotherapy or radiotherapy, is currently used in hematological malignancies [63].

## Vasculitis

A variety of vasculitides can affect the entire GI tract and include Behcet disease [64], Henoch-Schonlein purpura [65], enterocolic lymphocytic phlebitis [66], polyarteritis nodosa [67], Wegener granulomatosis [68], microscopic polyangiitis [69], Churg-Strauss syndrome [70], giant cell arteritis [47], rheumatoid arthritis, and systemic lupus erythematosus [71]. The small bowel and colon are the most affected sites with presentations of abdominal pain, GI bleeding, and diarrhea. Endoscopic findings often include edematous mucosa with ulcers, erosions, or changes that mimic ischemia. Histological features include inflammation in and around the vessel walls, fibrinoid necrosis of the vessel walls, and presence of thrombi. Treatment options are directed against the underlying disease.

In summary, patients with ulcerative colitis develop classic symptoms of colitis with diarrhea, blood in the stool, abdominal pain, and fever or chills. Most frequently, the differential diagnosis will lead to either acute self-limited colitis or new-onset UC. Established UC patients who experience symptoms of colitis that is unresponsive to treatment must be further evaluated to determine the most appropriate therapeutic regimen.

## References

1. Langholz E, Munkholm P, Davidsen M, Binder V. Course of ulcerative colitis: analysis of changes in disease activity over years. Gastroenterology. 1994;107:3–11.
2. Autenrieth DM1, Baumgart DC. Toxic megacolon. Inflamm Bowel Dis. 2012 Mar;18(3):584–91.
3. Ananthakrishnan AN, McGinley EL, Binion DG. Excess hospitalisation burden associated with Clostridium difficile in patients with inflammatory bowel disease. Gut. 2008;57:205–10.
4. Issa M, Vijayapal A, Graham MB, Beaulieu DB, Otterson MF, Lundeen S, Skaros S, Weber LR, Komorowski RA, Knox JF, Emmons J, Bajaj JS, Binion DG. Impact of Clostridium difficile on inflammatory bowel disease. Clin Gastroenterol Hepatol. 2007;5: 345–51.

5. Loo VG, Bourgault AM, Poirier L, Lamothe F, Michaud S, Turgeon N, Toye B, Beaudoin A, Frost EH, Gilca R, Brassard P, Dendukuri N, Beliveau C, Oughton M, Brukner I, Dascal A. Host and pathogen factors for Clostridium difficile infection and colonization. N Engl J Med. 2011;365:1693–703.

6. Howell MD, Novack V, Grgurich P, Soulliard D, Novack L, Pencina M, Talmor D. Iatrogenic gastric acid suppression and the risk of nosocomial Clostridium difficile infection. Arch Intern Med. 2010;170:784–90.

7. Sinh P, Barrett TA, Yun L. Clostridium difficile infection and inflammatory bowel disease: a review. Gastroenterol Res Pract. 2011;2011:136064.

8. Kuijper EJ, van Dissel JT, Wilcox MH. Clostridium difficile: changing epidemiology and new treatment options. Curr Opin Infect Dis. 2007;20:376–83.

9. Loo VG, Poirier L, Miller MA, Oughton M, Libman MD, Michaud S, Bourgault AM, Nguyen T, Frenette C, Kelly M, Vibien A, Brassard P, Fenn S, Dewar K, Hudson TJ, Horn R, Rene P, Monczak Y, Dascal A. A predominantly clonal multi-institutional outbreak of Clostridium difficile-associated diarrhea with high morbidity and mortality. N Engl J Med. 2005;353:2442–9.

10. Dupuy B, Govind R, Antunes A, Matamouros S. Clostridium difficile toxin synthesis is negatively regulated by TcdC. J Med Microbiol. 2008;57:685–9.

11. Ananthakrishnan AN, Issa M, Binion DG. Clostridium difficile and inflammatory bowel disease. Gastroenterol Clin North Am. 2009; 38:711–28.

12. Musa S, Thomson S, Cowan M, Rahman T. Clostridium difficile infection and inflammatory bowel disease. Scand J Gastroenterol. 2010;45:261–72.

13. Johnson S. Recurrent Clostridium difficile infection: causality and therapeutic approaches. Int J Antimicrob Agents. 2009;33 Suppl 1:S33–6.

14. Louie TJ, Miller MA, Mullane KM, Weiss K, Lentnek A, Golan Y, Gorbach S, Sears P, Shue YK. Group OPTCS: fidaxomicin versus vancomycin for Clostridium difficile infection. N Engl J Med. 2011;364:422–31.

15. Kao D, Hotte N, Gillevet P, Madsen K. Fecal microbiota transplantation inducing remission in Crohn's colitis and the associated changes in fecal microbial profile. J Clin Gastroenterol. 2014;48:625.

16. Smits LP, Bouter KE, de Vos WM, Borody TJ, Nieuwdorp M. Therapeutic potential of fecal microbiota transplantation. Gastroenterology. 2013;145(5):946–53.

17. Kassam Z, Lee CH, Yuan Y, Hunt RH. Fecal microbiota transplantation for Clostridium difficile infection: systematic review and meta-analysis. Am J Gastroenterol. 2013;108(4):500–8.

18. Wong CS, Mooney JC, Brandt JR, Staples AO, Jelacic S, Boster DR, Watkins SL, Tarr PI. Risk factors for the hemolytic uremic syndrome in children infected with Escherichia coli O157:H7: a multivariable analysis. Clin Infect Dis. 2012;55:33.

19. Rosales A, Hofer J, Zimmerhackl LB, Jungraithmayr TC, Riedl M, Giner T, Strasak A, Orth-Holler D, Wurzner R, Karch H, for the German-Austrian HUSSG. Need for long-term follow-up in enterohemorrhagic Escherichia coli-associated hemolytic uremic syndrome due to late-emerging sequelae. Clin Infect Dis. 2012;54:1413.

20. Matheson N, Kingsley RA, Sturgess K, Aliyu SH, Wain J, Dougan G, Cooke FJ. Ten years experience of Salmonella infections in Cambridge, UK. J Infect. 2010;60:21–5.

21. Ina K, Kusugami K, Ohta M. Bacterial hemorrhagic enterocolitis. J Gastroenterol. 2003;38:111–20.

22. Brodrick R, Sagar J. Toxic megacolon from sexually transmitted Shigella sonnei infection. Int J Colorectal Dis. 2012;27:415.

23. Pfeiffer ML, Dupont HL, Ochoa TJ. The patient presenting with acute dysentery - a systematic review. J Infect. 2012;64:374–86.

24. Nagata N, Shimbo T, Akiyama J, Nakashima R, Niikura R, Nishimura S, Yada T, Watanabe K, Oka S, Uemura N. Predictive value of endoscopic findings in the diagnosis of active intestinal amebiasis. Endoscopy. 2012;44:425–8.

25. Moon JH, Cho SH, Yu JR, Lee WJ, Cheun HI. PCR diagnosis of Entamoeba histolytica cysts in stool samples. Korean J Parasitol. 2011;49:281–4.

26. Siegal D, Syed F, Hamid N, Cunha BA. Campylobacter jejuni pancolitis mimicking idiopathic ulcerative colitis. Heart Lung. 2005; 34:288–90.

27. Man SM. The clinical importance of emerging Campylobacter species. Nat Rev Gastroenterol Hepatol. 2011;8:669–85.

28. Ternhag A, Torner A, Svensson A, Ekdahl K, Giesecke J. Short- and long-term effects of bacterial gastrointestinal infections. Emerg Infect Dis. 2008;14:143–8.

29. Dasti JI, Tareen AM, Lugert R, Zautner AE, Gross U. Campylobacter jejuni: a brief overview on pathogenicity-associated factors and disease-mediating mechanisms. Int J Med Microbiol. 2010;300: 205–11.

30. Man SM, Zhang L, Day AS, Leach ST, Lemberg DA, Mitchell H. Campylobacter concisus and other Campylobacter species in children with newly diagnosed Crohn's disease. Inflamm Bowel Dis. 2010;16:1008–16.

31. Kato Y, Chihara K, Daigo S, Iwasaki Y, Abe H. Regulation of growth hormone secretion. Horumon Rinsho Clin Endocrinol. 1977;25:131–41.

32. Saebo A, Vik E, Lange OJ, Matuszkiewicz L. Inflammatory bowel disease associated with Yersinia enterocolitica O:3 infection. Eur J Intern Med. 2005;16:176–82.

33. Kallinowski F, Wassmer A, Hofmann MA, Harmsen D, Heesemann J, Karch H, Herfarth C, Buhr HJ. Prevalence of enteropathogenic bacteria in surgically treated chronic inflammatory bowel disease. Hepatogastroenterology. 1998;45:1552–8.

34. Tuohy AM, O'Gorman M, Byington C, Reid B, Jackson WD. Yersinia enterocolitis mimicking Crohn's disease in a toddler. Pediatrics. 1999;104:e36.

35. Roblin X, Pillet S, Oussalah A, Berthelot P, Del Tedesco E, Phelip JM, Chambonniere ML, Garraud O, Peyrin-Biroulet L, Pozzetto B. Cytomegalovirus load in inflamed intestinal tissue is predictive of resistance to immunosuppressive therapy in ulcerative colitis. Am J Gastroenterol. 2011;106:2001–8.

36. Kawashima H, Ishii C, Ioi H, Nishimata S, Kashiwagi Y, Takekuma K. Transaminase in rotavirus gastroenteritis. Pediatr Int. 2012;54:86–8.

37. Martino R, Subira M, Rovira M, Solano C, Vazquez L, Sanz GF, Urbano-Ispizua A, Brunet S, De la Camara R, allo PIN-iCSotGEdTH. Invasive fungal infections after allogeneic peripheral blood stem cell transplantation: incidence and risk factors in 395 patients. Br J Haematol. 2002;116:475–82.

38. Caroli A, Fregonese D, Di Falco G, D'Inca R. Aspergillus fumigatus pneumonia during cyclosporine treatment for ulcerative colitis. Am J Gastroenterol. 2000;95:3016–7.

39. Andres LA, Ford RD, Wilcox RM. Necrotizing colitis caused by systemic aspergillosis in a burn patient. J Burn Care Res. 2007;28: 918–21.

40. Prescott RJ, Harris M, Banerjee SS. Fungal infections of the small and large intestine. J Clin Pathol. 1992;45:806–11.

41. Fayer R, Ungar BL. Cryptosporidium spp. and cryptosporidiosis. Microbiol Rev. 1986;50:458–83.

42. Banerjee D, Deb R, Dar L, Mirdha BR, Pati SK, Thareja S, Falodia S, Ahuja V. High frequency of parasitic and viral stool pathogens in patients with active ulcerative colitis: report from a tropical country. Scand J Gastroenterol. 2009;44:325–31.

43. Chetty R, Govender D. Lymphocytic and collagenous colitis: an overview of so-called microscopic colitis. Nat Rev Gastroenterol Hepatol. 2012;9:209–18.

44. Mahajan D, Goldblum JR, Xiao SY, Shen B, Liu X. Lymphocytic colitis and collagenous colitis: a review of clinicopathologic

features and immunologic abnormalities. Adv Anat Pathol. 2012; 19:28–38.

45. Martland GT, Shepherd NA. Indeterminate colitis: definition, diagnosis, implications and a plea for nosological sanity. Histopathology. 2007;50:83–96.

46. Murrell ZA, Melmed GY, Ippoliti A, Vasiliauskas EA, Dubinsky M, Targan SR, Fleshner PR. A prospective evaluation of the long-term outcome of ileal pouch-anal anastomosis in patients with inflammatory bowel disease-unclassified and indeterminate colitis. Dis Colon Rectum. 2009;52:872–8.

47. Trimble MA, Weisz MA. Infarction of the sigmoid colon secondary to giant cell arteritis. Rheumatology. 2002;41:108–10.

48. Aguas M, Garrigues V, Bastida G, Nos P, Ortiz V, Fernandez A, Ponce J. Prevalence of irritable bowel syndrome (IBS) in first-degree relatives of patients with inflammatory bowel disease (IBD). J Crohns Colitis. 2011;5:227–33.

49. MacDermott RP. Treatment of irritable bowel syndrome in outpatients with inflammatory bowel disease using a food and beverage intolerance, food and beverage avoidance diet. Inflamm Bowel Dis. 2007;13:91–6.

50. Keohane J, O'Mahony C, O'Mahony L, O'Mahony S, Quigley EM, Shanahan F. Irritable bowel syndrome-type symptoms in patients with inflammatory bowel disease: a real association or reflection of occult inflammation? Am J Gastroenterol. 2010;105:1788. 1789–1794; quiz 1795.

51. Hogan SP. Functional role of eosinophils in gastrointestinal inflammation. Immunol Allergy Clin North Am. 2009;29:129–40. xi.

52. Saitoh O, Kojima K, Sugi K, Matsuse R, Uchida K, Tabata K, Nakagawa K, Kayazawa M, Hirata I, Katsu K. Fecal eosinophil granule-derived proteins reflect disease activity in inflammatory bowel disease. Am J Gastroenterol. 1999;94:3513–20.

53. Brandt L, Boley S, Goldberg L, Mitsudo S, Berman A. Colitis in the elderly. A reappraisal. Am J Gastroenterol. 1981;76:239–45.

54. O'Brien PC, Hamilton CS, Denham JW, Gourlay R, Franklin CI. Spontaneous improvement in late rectal mucosal changes after radiotherapy for prostate cancer. Int J Radiat Oncol Biol Phys. 2004;58:75–80.

55. Lamps LW, Knapple WL. Diverticular disease-associated segmental colitis. Clin Gastroenterol Hepatol. 2007;5:27–31.

56. Sultan K, Fields S, Panagopoulos G, Korelitz BI. The nature of inflammatory bowel disease in patients with coexistent colonic diverticulosis. J Clin Gastroenterol. 2006;40:317–21.

57. Peppercorn MA. Drug-responsive chronic segmental colitis associated with diverticula: a clinical syndrome in the elderly. Am J Gastroenterol. 1992;87:609–12.

58. Ananthakrishnan AN, Higuchi LM, Huang ES, Khalili H, Richter JM, Fuchs CS, Chan AT. Aspirin, nonsteroidal anti-inflammatory drug use, and risk for Crohn disease and ulcerative colitis: a cohort study. Ann Intern Med. 2012;156:350–9.

59. Bousseaden A, Ajana FZ, Essamri W, Benelbarhdadi I, Afifi R, Benazzouz M, Essaid A. Mesalamine enema-induced exacerbation of ulcerative colitis. Int J Colorectal Dis. 2009;24:1359–60.

60. Ekbom A, Helmick C, Zack M, Adami HO. Ulcerative colitis and colorectal cancer. A population-based study. N Engl J Med. 1990;323:1228–33.

61. Garrity-Park MM, Loftus Jr EV, Sandborn WJ, Bryant SC, Smyrk TC. MHC Class II alleles in ulcerative colitis-associated colorectal cancer. Gut. 2009;58:1226–33.

62. Keefe DM. Intestinal mucositis: mechanisms and management. Curr Opin Oncol. 2007;19:323–7.

63. Blijlevens N, Sonis S. Palifermin (recombinant keratinocyte growth factor-1): a pleiotropic growth factor with multiple biological activities in preventing chemotherapy- and radiotherapy-induced mucositis. Ann Oncol. 2007;18:817–26.

64. Ebert EC. Gastrointestinal manifestations of Behcet's disease. Dig Dis Sci. 2009;54:201–7.

65. Tobino K, Shimizu Y, Miura S, Sugawara K, Takeda K, Tomino Y. Severe erosive lesions in the digestive tract of patients with Henoch-Schonlein Purpura (HSP) and its impact on prognosis - presentation of two cases and statistical review of adult-onset Japanese HSP. Clin Nephrol. 2011;75 Suppl 1:47–55.

66. Tuppy H, Haidenthaler A, Schandalik R, Oberhuber G. Idiopathic enterocolic lymphocytic phlebitis: a rare cause of ischemic colitis. Mod Pathol. 2000;13:897–9.

67. Vavricka SR, Dirnhofer S, Degen L. Polyarteritis nodosa mimicking inflammatory bowel disease. Clin Gastroenterol Hepatol. 2007; 5:A22.

68. Storesund B, Gran JT, Koldingsnes W. Severe intestinal involvement in Wegener's granulomatosis: report of two cases and review of the literature. Br J Rheumatol. 1998;37:387–90.

69. Villiger PM, Guillevin L. Microscopic polyangiitis: clinical presentation. Autoimmun Rev. 2010;9:812–9.

70. Kurita M, Niwa Y, Hamada E, Hata Y, Oshima M, Mutoh H, Shiina S, Nakata R, Ota S, Terano A, et al. Churg-Strauss syndrome (allergic granulomatous angiitis) with multiple perforating ulcers of the small intestine, multiple ulcers of the colon, and mononeuritis multiplex. J Gastroenterol. 1994;29:208–13.

71. Marcolongo R, Bayeli PF, Montagnani M. Gastrointestinal involvement in rheumatoid arthritis: a biopsy study. J Rheumatol. 1979; 6:163–73.

# The Role of Diet and Nutrition in Ulcerative Colitis

Anna M. Buchner and Gary R. Lichtenstein

---

**Keywords**

Inflammatory bowel disease • Ulcerative colitis • Crohn's disease • Diet • Nutrition

---

## Introduction

Inflammatory bowel disease (IBD) specifically both ulcerative colitis (UC) and Crohn's disease (CD) represent global diseases characterized by relapsing chronic inflammatory intestinal changes effecting dietary intake, digestion, and nutrient utilization and are associated with impairment of nutritional status. The etiology of these disorders remains unknown and various bacterial, genetic, and environmental factors have been proposed to be contributory. While diet and nutrition impact on health, their potential roles in inflammatory bowel disease have been explored. Over the last decades, various aspects of diet and nutrition have been investigated, including their role in the etiology of IBD as well as their role in the management of these disorders. This chapter will discuss the current evidence of diet as a risk factor for the development of IBD and as well as the role of various dietary and nutritional approaches in the management of the inflammatory bowel disease.

## The Role of Diet in the Etiology of IBD

Over the last decade, the incidences of inflammatory bowel have been increasing not only in industrialized western countries but also in many other countries initially thought to have lower incidences of this disease [1–3]. The changes in dietary consumption pattern related to the popular western diet, high in protein and fat and lower in vegetables and fruits, are thought to be the key environmental factors contributing to the rising incidence of IBD and also playing a potential role in the pathogenesis of inflammatory bowel disease. In general, literature investigating these associations has been limited by their design characteristics retrospective, observational studies with small sample size, and conflicting results.

A recent systemic review of the literature by Hou et al. [4] analyzed 19 studies with over 2,600 IBD patients and reported that high dietary intakes of total fats, n-6 polyunsaturated fatty acids (PUFAs), omega-6 fatty acids, and meats were associated with an increased risk of CD and UC. On the other hand, high fiber and fruit intakes were associated with a decreased Crohn's disease risk, while high vegetable intake was associated with a decreased UC risk. There was no consistent association between total carbohydrate intake and IBD risk [4].

A subsequent prospective cohort study by Ananthakarishnan et al. [5] concluded that long-term intake of dietary fiber, particularly from fruits, is associated with lower risk of CD but not UC. The same group demonstrated also that a high intake of dietary long-chain n-3 polyunsaturated fatty acids may be associated with a reduced risk of UC, while high intake of *trans*-unsaturated fats may be associated with an increased risk of UC [6]. The association

A.M. Buchner, M.D., Ph.D. (✉)
Department of Gastroenterology, University of Pennsylvania Hospital, 1 Convention Avenue/Penn Tower 9th Floor, Philadelphia, PA 19104, USA
e-mail: anna.buchner@uphs.upenn.edu

G.R. Lichtenstein, M.D., F.A.C.P., F.A.C.G., A.G.A.F.
Gastroenterology Division, Hospital of the University of Pennsylvania, University of Pennsylvania School of Medicine, Philadelphia, PA, USA
e-mail: gary.lichtenstein@uphs.upenn.edu

G.R. Lichtenstein (ed.), *Medical Therapy of Ulcerative Colitis*,
DOI 10.1007/978-1-4939-1677-1_37, © Springer Science+Business Media New York 2014

between *trans*-unsaturated fat and various systemic inflammatory changes has been recognized before, playing a role in conditions such as coronary artery disease and diabetes mellitus.

A recent study by Tjonneland et al. [7] demonstrated the presence of a potential association between higher intake of linoleic acid, a dietary n-6 polyunsaturated fatty acid, and increased risk of ulcerative colitis. The subsequent French prospective cohort study of female patients, aged 40–65 living in France, also noted increased risk of IBD with higher intake of animal protein in this group [8].

A few observational studies assessed the association diet with the natural history of IBD and reported that patients with higher consumptions of eggs, animal protein, sulfate, and alcohol intake have more frequent relapse [9–11]. Finally, the most recent study by Spooren et al. [12] provided a complete overview of 41 studies associating habitual diet with the onset of IBD and its association with relapses of IBD. The study pointed out that the current evidence is not sufficient yet to draw firm conclusions on the role of specific food components or nutrients in the etiology of IBD and large prospective controlled trials are needed.

The certain dietary patterns may result in increased amount of intestinal sulfate leading to increased inflammation and resulting to clinical and endoscopic disease flare-ups [9, 13]. The specific long-term diet may also lead to intestinal inflammation through its effects of the gut microbiota, antigen presentation, and enhanced prostaglandin production though no clear association path has been established yet [14, 15].

The potential link between the diet and the gut microbiome has been also recently explored. It is supported by the studies in postoperative CD demonstrating the recurrence of intestinal inflammation in the neoterminal ileum with the exposure to luminal content shortly after the surgery [16, 17].

It is known that gut microbes have been in a symbiotic relation with their human host by the participation in various physiological functions including the fermentation of the indigestible carbohydrates, transformation of conjugated bile acids, synthesis of vitamins, etc. The alteration of the gut microbiota dysbiosis has been seen in IBD, and it may play a role in the pathogenesis of IBD through the depletion of protective bacterial species and increase of more harmful species [18, 19]. Thus various dietary patterns may change the gut microbiota dysbiosis and lead to the development of the disease. Recent studies have evaluated this association between dietary patterns and the gut microbiota [20–22]. They revealed that the adaption of the microbiota to diet is similar across different mammalian lineages [20]. Various long-term dietary interventions were shown to be associated with specific enterotypes such as *Bacteroides* with particularly protein and animal fat and *Prevotella* with carbohydrates [21].

*Prevotella* and related bacteria are efficient at fermenting dietary fiber, leading to higher concentrations of short-chain fatty acids, which may be a protective factor against inflammation [11, 23]. On the other hand, high-fat diets, through dietary intake, induced changes in the gut microbiota, may increase bowel permeability, and thus contribute to pathogenesis of IBD, particularly CD [24].

The animal models help us to understand the possible dietary mechanisms leading to worsening inflammatory changes [25–27]. For instance, it is known that high-fat diets exacerbate dextran sodium sulfate-induced colitis in mice potentially by increasing colonic natural T killer cell [25]. The study by Devkota and colleagues [26] demonstrated also that intake of saturated milk fat lead to more aggressive colitis in Il-1-deficient mice, by expanding rare bacterial population that induces pathogenic T-helper 1 immune responses [26]. Furthermore, the production of hydrogen sulfide through bacterial fermentation of sulfur amino acids from high-protein-containing food may contribute to bowel inflammation by direct toxic effects and abnormal use of short-chain fatty acids [28, 29]. The recent study by Martinez-Medizna et al. [27] assessed further the effects of a high-fat and sugar western diet on gut microbiota composition, barrier integrity, and susceptibility in transgenic mice model. It demonstrated an increased intestinal permeability, decreased mucous layer thickness, increased TNF alpha secretion, and higher adherent-invasive *Escherichia coli* (AIEC) colonization with the western diet in genetically susceptible mice.

In summary, the influence of diet on the gut microbiota is the important environmental factor playing a role in the pathogenesis of IBD in susceptible hosts, and further investigations are warranted.

## The Role of Nutrition in the Management of IBD

Various dietary interventions and nutritional approaches have been studied in the management of inflammatory bowel disease with the goal of altering the course of the disease while attempting to induce and maintain remission, also in patient in the postoperative period of the disease. Several additional and well-recognized goals are to prevent and treat the disease complications such as malnutrition and to promote growth and proper development in the pediatric population of patients with IBD. These additional goals are achieved by careful assessment of the nutritional status in all IBD patients and identifying disease-related malnutrition (inadequate nutrition), weight loss, and suboptimal nutritional status presenting at any stage of IBD including patients who are in clinical remission [30, 31]. The causes of malnutrition are complex and include poor dietary intake, impaired nutrient digestion, and absorption as well as generally increase nutrient requirement.

Nutrition-related complications in IBD such as weight loss; hypoalbuminemia anemia related to iron, B12, and folic acid deficiencies; as well as bone-related complications due to calcium, vitamin D, magnesium, and vitamin K deficiency have been well recognized and their management endorsed in guidelines for IBD management [32, 33].

## Enteral Nutrition in Crohn's Disease for Induction or Remission and Maintenance of Remission

Exclusive enteral nutrition (EEN) therapy with elemental, semi elemental, and define formulas has been extensively studied, especially in pediatric population, and it has been frequently used for the induction and remission of the disease in specific regions including Europe [34]. It has been demonstrated that EEN acts to induce mucosal healing and prolongs clinical remission of the disease [35]. EEN is maintained with up to 8 weeks of liquid feedings with either elemental or polymeric formulas, while patients are not allowed to have any other dietary items except water and some beverage drinks [21]. At the end of a 6–8-week period, a low-residue diet is slowly introduced.

A Cochrane meta-analysis comparing elemental formulas based on fat content did not show a significant difference of term of efficacy of enteral nutrition and a nonsignificant trend toward low-fat and low-triglyceride diet was noted [36]. It assessed enteral formulas vs. corticosteroids in acute therapy and pointed out the potential benefits of steroids [36]. However, after inclusion of only high-quality studies, this benefit was not present anymore.

This EEN approach has been primarily applied in the pediatric population for patients with Crohn's disease, but in general it has not been widely utilized and accepted. It is not recommended as treatment for active or quiescent ulcerative colitis.

The guidelines of the European Society for Clinical Nutrition and Metabolism specifically reviewed the role of enteral nutrition in the management of IBD based on the available scientific data [37]. In active CD, EEN can be the first-line therapy in children and should be used as sole therapy in adults mainly when treatment with corticosteroids is not feasible. Among children with CD, the response rates to EEN exceed 80 %, while for the maintenance of remission resulted in 50 % [36]. In long-standing clinical remission and in the absence of nutritional deficits, a benefit of enteral nutrition or supplement has not been demonstrated [38].

Subsequent studies analyzes also the enteral nutrition vs. placebo for maintenance therapy with 50 % calories as enteral feeding vs. normal food as well as elemental feeding at night and low-fat diet during the day vs. normal food [39, 40].

There are a few studies investigating the efficiency of EEN based on the CD location suggesting poorer response in patients with colonic CD, while other studies suggest remission with EEN to be not related to disease location [41, 42]. In addition, a meta-analysis of pediatric studies comparing the efficacy of steroids to EEN in inducing remission demonstrated that corticosteroids and EEN are equally efficacious in inducing remission in pediatric population with CD [43, 44]. Furthermore, a Cochrane meta-analysis summarizing the role for EEN for the maintenance of remission also showed that EEN may be effective for the maintenance of remission for CD either alone or with combination with other therapies [45]. While larger studies are needed to confirm these findings, enteral nutrition supplementation could be considered as an alternative or as an adjunct to maintenance drug therapy in Crohn's disease.

It has been demonstrated that EEN acts primarily by inducing mucosal healing and thus may prolong clinical remission of the disease [28, 46, 47]. In open-label study by Borelli comparing polymeric formulas to corticosteroids, there were significantly more patients who achieved mucosal healing as compared to steroids (75 % vs. 33 %) [35]. It has been also suggested that EEN may have an anti-inflammatory action by modifying the gut microbiota based on the studies evaluating the effect of EEN on microflora in active CD [30, 48]. In the study by Tjellstrom et al., 79 % of the children with small bowel/colonic CD responded clinically positively to EEN treatment showing decreased levels of proinflammatory acetic acid as well as increased concentrations of anti-inflammatory butyric acids and also of valeric acids, similar to the levels in healthy age-matched children [49]. Table 37.1 summarizes various nutritional interventions including enteral feedings.

In spite of the evidence of the utility of EEN in induction and remission of CD, this therapy has been overall poorly accepted, and there is a wide variability in its use with only 4 % of North American gastroenterologists utilizing the nutritional therapy frequently versus 62 % of their Western European colleagues ($p < 0.0001$) [3] practicing the treatment of active CD in pediatric population [50].

## Various Nutritional and Dietary Approaches in the Management of IBD

There is evidence that restrictive diets may improve disease activity and prolonged time relapse [51, 52]. Rajendran et al. used food-specific IgG4 levels to exclude selective foods based on high levels of IgG4 including eggs and beef with the utilization of such a restrictive diet demonstrating significant symptomatic improvement and reduction in the erythrocyte sedimentation rate compared to the pretreatment period [52]. In addition a few defined diets have been

**Table 37.1** Summary of recent studies of nutritional interventions in IBD

| Type of nutritional interventions | Type of study | Number of study patients | Primary outcome | Results | Conclusion (p values) | Reference |
|---|---|---|---|---|---|---|
| Maintenance therapy in CD: enteral nutrition (EN) vs. control (CO) | | | | | | |
| A: 50 % calories as enteral feed vs. normal food | A: randomized controlled | 51 adults | Relapse | A: EN: 9/25 CO: 16/25 | A: EN beneficial (p=0.05) | A: 39 |
| B: Elemental feeding (EL) at night and low fat diet during day vs. normal diet | B: non-randomized controlled | 40 adults | Relapse | B: EL: 5/20 CO: 13/20 | B: EL beneficial (p=0.03) | B: 40 |
| Elemental vs. polymeric enteral nutrition for acute therapy in CD | Cochrane meta-analysis of 10 studies (2007) | 334 adults | Remission | Odds ratio: 1.10 (0.69–1.75) | Elemental is equal to polymeric diet (p=NS) | [36] |
| Low fat vs. high fat enteral nutrition as acute therapy in CD | Cochrane meta-analysis (2007) | 209 adults | Remission | OR 1.13 | NS | [36] |
| Enteral nutrition vs. corticosteroids for acute therapy in CD | Cochrane meta-analysis (2007) of 7 studies | 352 (37 children) | Remission | OR 0.33 (0.21,0.53) advantage of steroid treatment OR 1.18 with only high quality studies OR 1.18 | Advantage of steroids noted (p=<0.00001) | [36] |
| Enteral nutrition vs. corticosteroids for acute therapy in pediatric CD | Meta-analysis of 5 studies | 147 children | Remission | Equally efficious | <0.03 | [43] |
| Intravenous nutrition (TPN) vs. normal diet as control- (CON) as adjunct to corticosteroid therapy in IBD (UC and CD | Randomized controlled | 36: 27 UC and 9 CD pts | Colectomy | UC: TPN: 9/19 CON: 6/17 | NS | [65] |
| Intravenous nutrition (TPN) vs. normal diet as control- (CON) as adjunct to corticosteroid therapy in IBD | Randomized controlled | 43 pts (27 UC/16 CD) | Colectomy and fatal outcome | UC: TPN: 10/15 (1 death) CON: 6/12 (1 death) CD: none | NS | [66] |

*No difference when only high quality studies re-analyzed

considered as having a potential beneficial impact in patients with IBD [11]. These diets include the specific carbohydrate diet (SCD), the low FODMAP diet, the Paleolithic diet, and the semi-vegetarian diet. Both the SCD and the low FODMAP diets restrict the intake of cereal grains and meat with the FODMAP diet restricting certain fruits and vegetables, while the LSD diet allows their intake [11]. The data supporting the use of these restrictive diets is overall limited, and it mainly focuses on the FODMAP diet in IBD patients [53, 54].

Geary et al. evaluated the effect of low FODMAP diet in 72 patients with IBD (52 CD and 20 UC) and demonstrated overall symptomatic improvement with reduction of bloating, diarrhea, and abdominal pain in both CD and UC patients [54]. Specifically for Crohn's disease, efficacy was associated with dietary adherence and inefficacy with nonadherence [54]. There is also some evidence that the semi-vegetarian diet may be beneficial in IBD patients.

Chiba et al. showed an advantage of the semi-vegetarian diet as compared to an omnivorous diet in maintaining clinical remission (93 % vs. 33 %) [55]. Table 37.2 summarizes these various dietary interventions. The link between these diets and the presence of certain bacteria has been evaluated. These specific diets can lead to bacterial overgrowth. The presence of bacterial overgrowth may result in increased intestinal permeability as well as fermentation of carbohydrates leading to increased intestinal production of short-chain organic acids with direct toxic effects on the intestinal mucosa. This again brings us to the theory that food and enteric bacteria interact with each other and thus together play a role in the development and establishing the clinical course of the disease [15, 21].

The examples of other studied dietary interventions include the effects of omega-3 fatty acid supplements, glutamine, and TPN [56, 57]. Omega-3 fatty acid supplements have been found to be not effective on preventing relapses of CD based on the large study by Feagan et al. [56]. The Cochrane meta-analysis by Turner et al. evaluated the efficacy of omega-3 fatty acids vs. placebo for maintenance based on 1,039 studies and reported potential benefit of fish oils [58]. However, the results need to be interpreted with caution given significant heterogeneity noted between studies. Glutamine supplementation, known to ameliorate the inflammatory response in intensive care, has been also con-

**Table 37.2** Summary of the recent studies of various dietary interventions in IBD

| Type of dietary intervention | Type of study | Number of study patients | Primary outcome | Results | Conclusion $p$ values | Reference |
|---|---|---|---|---|---|---|
| Omega 3 fatty acids (fish oil) vs. placebo for maintenance in UC | Cochrane-meta-analysis of 6 studies | 1,039 with 38 children | Remission at 1 year | RR 0.77 (0.61, 0.98) | Potential benefit of fish oil though significant heterogeneity of the studies noted $p=0.03$ | [58] |
| Low FODMAP diet | Retrospective | 72 patients (20 UC patients) | Functional symptomatic improvement | Reduction of bloating, diarrhea abdominal pain in both CD and UC patients | Potential benefit of low FODMAP diet $p<0.02$ for all | [54] |
| Semi-vegetarian diet (SVD) vs. omnivorous diet (OVD) | Perspective, non-randomized | 22 | Maintaining clinical remission | SVD: 15/16 (94 %) OVD: 2/6 (33 %) | SVD effective in preventing relapse $p=0.0003$ | [55] |
| Curcumin supplement | Cochrane meta-analysis | 89 | Relapse | 4 % Relapse at 6 months in curcumin group vs. 18 % in placebo RR 0.24 (0.05–1.09) | 0.06 | [61] |

sidered, but there is no sufficient evidence supporting benefits of its use [59, 60]. Kumar et al. evaluated also the role of curcumin supplementation in maintenance therapy in patients with UC and reported some benefits in the use of this supplement [61]. While initial studies suggested the benefit of parenteral nutrition (TPN) in the improvement of CD symptoms during bowel rest, subsequent studies including meta-analysis demonstrated no advantages in inducing a maintained remission but considered adjunctive therapy for IBD patients requiring bowel rest and nutritional repletion [62–66].

## Summary

In summary, there is scientific evidence that diet may play a role in the pathogenesis of IBD and lead to an increased disease incidence. The diets high in total fat, polyunsaturated fatty acids (PUFAs), omega-6 fatty acids, and meat have been found to be associated with increased risk of IBD. A higher intake of fiber and fruits was noted to correlate with a decreased CD risk, while higher intake of vegetables with a decreased risk of UC [4, 67].

The recent studies including animal models have speculated the influence of diet on the gut microbiome and demonstrated interactions between specific diets, various bacteria, genetic susceptibility, and immune responses in IBD, allowing guidance in future human trials.

Various studies looking at the dietary and nutritional approaches in the management of IBD did not reveal any striking benefits; therefore, there are no enforced recommendations regarding the adherence to any specific dietary and nutritional interventions in the management of IBD. This is

likely caused by a lack of large prospective control trials investigating the benefits. However, available studies of various exclusive nutritional and dietary approaches including EEN, low FODMAP diet, and semi-vegetarian diet suggest a potential benefit for patients with IBD [68]. This may be achieved by minimal exposure of the intestinal lumen to the selected food and nutrients, thus reducing intestinal mucosal inflammation and leading to longer remission in IBD patients [11]. This has been particularly demonstrated through EEN interventions found to be used for induction and remission of CD in pediatric population [69, 70].

Future well-designed studies are mandated to investigate both rationale for the specific diet utilization and its efficacy. As for now, our general dietary and nutritional recommendations should be individualized and based on patient's ability to identify the diets and specific nutrients that can worsen their symptoms but also should take into account the current knowledge based on the available studies which in time will be strengthened by better designed and larger studies.

## References

1. Prideaux L, Kamm MA, De Cruz PP, Chan FK, Ng SC. Inflammatory bowel disease in Asia: a systematic review. J Gastroenterol Hepatol. 2012;27:1266–80.
2. Hou JK, El-Serag H, Thirumurthi S. Distribution and manifestations of inflammatory bowel disease in Asians, Hispanics, and African Americans: a systematic review. Am J Gastroenterol. 2009; 104:2100–9.
3. Molodecky NA, Soon IS, Rabi DM, et al. Increasing incidence and prevalence of the inflammatory bowel diseases with time, based on systematic review. Gastroenterology. 2012;142:46–54. e42. quiz e30.

4. Hou JK, Abraham B, El-Serag H. Dietary intake and risk of developing inflammatory bowel disease: a systematic review of the literature. Am J Gastroenterol. 2011;106:563–73.

5. Ananthakrishnan AN, Khalili H, Konijeti GG, et al. A prospective study of long-term intake of dietary fiber and risk of Crohn's disease and ulcerative colitis. Gastroenterology. 2013;145:970–7.

6. Ananthakrishnan AN, Khalili H, Konijeti GG, et al. Long-term intake of dietary fat and risk of ulcerative colitis and Crohn's disease. Gut. 2014;63:776–84.

7. Tjonneland A, Overvad K, Bergmann MM, et al. Linoleic acid, a dietary n-6 polyunsaturated fatty acid, and the aetiology of ulcerative colitis: a nested case-control study within a European prospective cohort study. Gut. 2009;58:1606–11.

8. Jantchou P, Morois S, Clavel-Chapelon F, Boutron-Ruault MC, Carbonnel F. Animal protein intake and risk of inflammatory bowel disease: the E3N prospective study. Am J Gastroenterol. 2010;105:2195–201.

9. Jowett SL, Seal CJ, Pearce MS, et al. Influence of dietary factors on the clinical course of ulcerative colitis: a prospective cohort study. Gut. 2004;53:1479–84.

10. Magee EA, Edmond LM, Tasker SM, Kong SC, Curno R, Cummings JH. Associations between diet and disease activity in ulcerative colitis patients using a novel method of data analysis. Nutr J. 2005;4:7.

11. Hou JK, Lee D, Lewis J. Diet and inflammatory bowel disease: review of patient-targeted recommendations. Clin Gastroenterol Hepatol 2013;pii: S1542–3565(13):01512-7.

12. Spooren CE, Pierik MJ, Zeegers MP, Feskens EJ, Masclee AA, Jonkers DM. Review article: the association of diet with onset and relapse in patients with inflammatory bowel disease. Aliment Pharmacol Ther. 2013;38:1172–87.

13. Magee EA, Curno R, Edmond LM, Cummings JH. Contribution of dietary protein and inorganic sulfur to urinary sulfate: toward a biomarker of inorganic sulfur intake. Am J Clin Nutr. 2004;80:137–42.

14. Sharon P, Ligumsky M, Rachmilewitz D, Zor U. Role of prostaglandins in ulcerative colitis. Enhanced production during active disease and inhibition by sulfasalazine. Gastroenterology. 1978;75:638–40.

15. Albenberg LG, Lewis JD, Wu GD. Food and the gut microbiota in inflammatory bowel diseases: a critical connection. Curr Opin Gastroenterol. 2012;28:314–20.

16. D'Haens GR, Geboes K, Peeters M, Baert F, Penninckx F, Rutgeerts P. Early lesions of recurrent Crohn's disease caused by infusion of intestinal contents in excluded ileum. Gastroenterology. 1998;114:262–7.

17. Rutgeerts P, Goboes K, Peeters M, et al. Effect of faecal stream diversion on recurrence of Crohn's disease in the neoterminal ileum. Lancet. 1991;338:771–4.

18. Sartor RB. Therapeutic correction of bacterial dysbiosis discovered by molecular techniques. Proc Natl Acad Sci U S A. 2008;105:16413–4.

19. Wu GD, Bushmanc FD, Lewis JD. Diet, the human gut microbiota, and IBD. Anaerobe. 2013;24:117–20.

20. Muegge BD, Kuczynski J, Knights D, et al. Diet drives convergence in gut microbiome functions across mammalian phylogeny and within humans. Science. 2011;332:970–4.

21. Wu GD, Chen J, Hoffmann C, et al. Linking long-term dietary patterns with gut microbial enterotypes. Science. 2011;334:105–8.

22. De Filippo C, Cavalieri D, Di Paola M, et al. Impact of diet in shaping gut microbiota revealed by a comparative study in children from Europe and rural Africa. Proc Natl Acad Sci U S A. 2010;107:14691–6.

23. Scheppach W, Weiler F. The butyrate story: old wine in new bottles? Curr Opin Clin Nutr Metab Care. 2004;7:563–7.

24. Cani PD, Bibiloni R, Knauf C, et al. Changes in gut microbiota control metabolic endotoxemia-induced inflammation in high-fat diet-induced obesity and diabetes in mice. Diabetes. 2008;57:1470–81.

25. Ma X, Torbenson M, Hamad AR, Soloski MJ, Li Z. High-fat diet modulates non-CD1d-restricted natural killer T cells and regulatory T cells in mouse colon and exacerbates experimental colitis. Clin Exp Immunol. 2008;151:130–8.

26. Devkota S, Wang Y, Musch MW, et al. Dietary-fat-induced taurocholic acid promotes pathobiont expansion and colitis in Il10–/– mice. Nature. 2012;487:104–8.

27. Martinez-Medina M, Denizot J, Dreux N, et al. Western diet induces dysbiosis with increased E coli in CEABAC10 mice, alters host barrier function favouring AIEC colonisation. Gut. 2014;63:116–24.

28. Pitcher MC, Cummings JH. Hydrogen sulphide: a bacterial toxin in ulcerative colitis? Gut. 1996;39:1–4.

29. Magee EA, Richardson CJ, Hughes R, Cummings JH. Contribution of dietary protein to sulfide production in the large intestine: an in vitro and a controlled feeding study in humans. Am J Clin Nutr. 2000;72:1488–94.

30. Pirlich M, Schutz T, Kemps M, et al. Prevalence of malnutrition in hospitalized medical patients: impact of underlying disease. Dig Dis. 2003;21:245–51.

31. O'Sullivan M, O'Morain C. Nutrition in inflammatory bowel disease. Best Pract Res Clin Gastroenterol. 2006;20:561–73.

32. Lomer MC. Dietary and nutritional considerations for inflammatory bowel disease. Proc Nutr Soc. 2011;70:329–35.

33. Carter MJ, Lobo AJ, Travis SP. Guidelines for the management of inflammatory bowel disease in adults. Gut. 2004;53 Suppl 5:V1–16.

34. Kansal S, Wagner J, Kirkwood CD, Catto-Smith AG. Enteral nutrition in Crohn's disease: an underused therapy. Gastroenterol Res Pract. 2013;2013:482108.

35. Borrelli O, Cordischi L, Cirulli M, et al. Polymeric diet alone versus corticosteroids in the treatment of active pediatric Crohn's disease: a randomized controlled open-label trial. Clin Gastroenterol Hepatol. 2006;4:744–53.

36. Zachos M, Tondeur M, Griffiths AM. Enteral nutritional therapy for induction of remission in Crohn's disease. Cochrane Database Syst Rev. 2007:CD000542.

37. Lochs H, Pichard C, Allison SP. Evidence supports nutritional support. Clin Nutr. 2006;25:177–9.

38. Volkert D, Berner YN, Berry E, et al. ESPEN guidelines on enteral nutrition: geriatrics. Clin Nutr. 2006;25:330–60.

39. Takagi S, Utsunomiya K, Kuriyama S, et al. Effectiveness of an 'half elemental diet' as maintenance therapy for Crohn's disease: a randomized-controlled trial. Aliment Pharmacol Ther. 2006;24:1333–40.

40. Yamamoto T, Nakahigashi M, Saniabadi AR, et al. Impacts of long-term enteral nutrition on clinical and endoscopic disease activities and mucosal cytokines during remission in patients with Crohn's disease: a prospective study. Inflamm Bowel Dis. 2007;13:1493–501.

41. Afzal NA, Davies S, Paintin M, et al. Colonic Crohn's disease in children does not respond well to treatment with enteral nutrition if the ileum is not involved. Dig Dis Sci. 2005;50:1471–5.

42. Buchanan E, Gaunt WW, Cardigan T, Garrick V, McGrogan P, Russell RK. The use of exclusive enteral nutrition for induction of remission in children with Crohn's disease demonstrates that disease phenotype does not influence clinical remission. Aliment Pharmacol Ther. 2009;30:501–7.

43. Heuschkel RB. Enteral nutrition in children with Crohn's disease. J Pediatr Gastroenterol Nutr. 2000;31:575.

44. Dziechciarz P, Horvath A, Shamir R, Szajewska H. Meta-analysis: enteral nutrition in active Crohn's disease in children. Aliment Pharmacol Ther. 2007;26:795–806.

45. Akobeng AK, Thomas AG. Enteral nutrition for maintenance of remission in Crohn's disease. Cochrane Database Syst Rev. 2007: CD005984.

46. Fell JM, Paintin M, Arnaud-Battandier F, et al. Mucosal healing and a fall in mucosal pro-inflammatory cytokine mRNA induced by a specific oral polymeric diet in paediatric Crohn's disease. Aliment Pharmacol Ther. 2000;14:281–9.

47. Yamamoto T, Nakahigashi M, Umegae S, Kitagawa T, Matsumoto K. Impact of elemental diet on mucosal inflammation in patients with active Crohn's disease: cytokine production and endoscopic and histological findings. Inflamm Bowel Dis. 2005;11:580–8.

48. Leach ST, Mitchell HM, Eng WR, Zhang L, Day AS. Sustained modulation of intestinal bacteria by exclusive enteral nutrition used to treat children with Crohn's disease. Aliment Pharmacol Ther. 2008;28:724–33.

49. Tjellstrom B, Hogberg L, Stenhammar L, et al. Effect of exclusive enteral nutrition on gut microflora function in children with Crohn's disease. Scand J Gastroenterol. 2012;47:1454–9.

50. Levine A, Milo T, Buller H, Markowitz J. Consensus and controversy in the management of pediatric Crohn disease: an international survey. J Pediatr Gastroenterol Nutr. 2003;36:464–9.

51. Riordan AM, Hunter JO, Cowan RE, et al. Treatment of active Crohn's disease by exclusion diet: East Anglian multicentre controlled trial. Lancet. 1993;342:1131–4.

52. Rajendran N, Kumar D. Food-specific IgG4-guided exclusion diets improve symptoms in Crohn's disease: a pilot study. Colorectal Dis. 2011;13:1009–13.

53. Croagh C, Shepherd SJ, Berryman M, Muir JG, Gibson PR. Pilot study on the effect of reducing dietary FODMAP intake on bowel function in patients without a colon. Inflamm Bowel Dis. 2007;13:1522–8.

54. Gearry RB, Irving PM, Barrett JS, Nathan DM, Shepherd SJ, Gibson PR. Reduction of dietary poorly absorbed short-chain carbohydrates (FODMAPs) improves abdominal symptoms in patients with inflammatory bowel disease-a pilot study. J Crohns Colitis. 2009;3:8–14.

55. Chiba M, Abe T, Tsuda H, et al. Lifestyle-related disease in Crohn's disease: relapse prevention by a semi-vegetarian diet. World J Gastroenterol. 2010;16:2484–95.

56. Feagan BG, Sandborn WJ, Mittmann U, et al. Omega-3 free fatty acids for the maintenance of remission in Crohn disease: the EPIC randomized controlled trials. JAMA. 2008;299:1690–7.

57. Lorenz-Meyer H, Bauer P, Nicolay C, et al. Omega-3 fatty acids and low carbohydrate diet for maintenance of remission in Crohn's disease. A randomized controlled multicenter trial. Study Group Members (German Crohn's Disease Study Group). Scand J Gastroenterol. 1996;31:778–85.

58. Turner D, Shah PS, Steinhart AH, Zlotkin S, Griffiths AM. Maintenance of remission in inflammatory bowel disease using omega-3 fatty acids (fish oil): a systematic review and meta-analyses. Inflamm Bowel Dis 2011;17:336–45.

59. Akobeng AK, Miller V, Stanton J, Elbadri AM, Thomas AG. Double-blind randomized controlled trial of glutamine-enriched polymeric diet in the treatment of active Crohn's disease. J Pediatr Gastroenterol Nutr. 2000;30:78–84.

60. Den Hond E, Hiele M, Peeters M, Ghoos Y, Rutgeerts P. Effect of long-term oral glutamine supplements on small intestinal permeability in patients with Crohn's disease. JPEN J Parenter Enteral Nutr. 1999;23:7–11.

61. Kumar S, Ahuja V, Sankar MJ, Kumar A, Moss AC. Curcumin for maintenance of remission in ulcerative colitis. Cochrane Database Syst Rev. 2012;10, CD008424.

62. Fischer JE, Foster GS, Abel RM, Abbott WM, Ryan JA. Hyperalimentation as primary therapy for inflammatory bowel disease. Am J Surg. 1973;125:165–75.

63. Issa M, Binion DG. Bowel rest and nutrition therapy in the management of active Crohn's disease. Nutr Clin Pract. 2008;23:299–308.

64. Mullen JL, Hargrove WC, Dudrick SJ, Fitts Jr WT, Rosato EF. Ten years experience with intravenous hyperalimentation and inflammatory bowel disease. Ann Surg. 1978;187:523–9.

65. Dickinson RJ, Ashton MG, Axon AT, Smith RC, Yeung CK, Hill GL. Controlled trial of intravenous hyperalimentation and total bowel rest as an adjunct to the routine therapy of acute colitis. Gastroenterology. 1980;79:1199–204.

66. McIntyre PB, Powell-Tuck J, Wood SR, et al. Controlled trial of bowel rest in the treatment of severe acute colitis. Gut. 1986;27:481–5.

67. Chapman-Kiddell CA, Davies PS, Gillen L, Radford-Smith GL. Role of diet in the development of inflammatory bowel disease. Inflamm Bowel Dis. 2010;16:137–51.

68. Yamamoto T. Nutrition and diet in inflammatory bowel disease. Curr Opin Gastroenterol. 2013;29:216–21.

69. Sandhu BK, Fell JM, Beattie RM, Mitton SG, Wilson DC, Jenkins H. Guidelines for the management of inflammatory bowel disease in children in the United Kingdom. J Pediatr Gastroenterol Nutr. 2010;50 Suppl 1:S1–13.

70. Cohen AB, Lee D, Long MD, et al. Dietary patterns and self-reported associations of diet with symptoms of inflammatory bowel disease. Dig Dis Sci. 2013;58:1322–8.

# Parenteral Nutrition Use in Ulcerative Colitis

# 38

Alan L. Buchman

**Keywords**

Parenteral nutrition • Ulcerative colitis • Total parenteral nutrition • Primary therapy • Adjunctive therapy

## Introduction

Total parenteral nutrition (TPN) is the provision of all known essential dietary substances. This includes macronutrients (carbohydrate, in the form of dextrose monohydrate; protein, in the form of free amino acids; and fat, in the form of a long-chain triglyceride-based lipid emulsion), fluid, electrolytes (sodium, potassium, bicarbonate in the form of acetate, chloride, and magnesium), minerals (phosphorous, in the form of a phosphate, and calcium), trace elements (zinc, copper, and selenium, and possibly chromium), and vitamins (A, thiamine, niacin, pyridoxine, riboflavin, B12, C, D, E, K, biotin, and pantothenic acid). Typically, this is administered as a 1–3-l solution via a large central vein. A more dilute solution can be administered via a peripheral vein. Parenteral nutrition (PN) is indicated when a patient is unable to consume sufficient nutrients and fluid necessary to maintain normal nutritional and hydration status or correct undernutrition *and* the gastrointestinal tract is either nonfunctional or not sufficiently functional as to allow sufficient oral consumption of nutrients and fluid or the administration of sufficient quantities of nutrient and fluid via a feeding tube. For patients with ulcerative colitis, this is a very unusual situation that manifests only when the patient has severe or fulminant colitis and/or develops abdominal pain or cramping that limits the amount of luminal nutrient that can be provided or in the postoperative patient (e.g., following colectomy) where there is a prolonged ileus (e.g., greater than 5–7 days). Under these circumstances, PN is used as an adjunctive therapy, but not as a primary therapy. Patients with toxic megacolon should be made nil per os and PN initiated, although it should be weaned off prior to surgery. Home PN is not indicated for a patient with ulcerative colitis with the exception of the extremely unusual patient who manifests moderately severe or severe malnutrition, cannot tolerate sufficient enterally provided nutrients, and requires colectomy once they have been repleted nutritionally. In general, aside from this degree of undernutrition, colectomy should not be postponed in an attempt to improve nutritional status. It must be recognized that in this situation, serum visceral protein concentrations are likely to be low on the basis of the acute phase response and protein-losing enteropathy/colopathy rather than because of undernutrition.

For the rare patient with ulcerative colitis that requires PN, a goal should be set with a time table delineated. A complete history and physical examination is the best tool for the gross assessment of the nutritional status of an individual patient. It must be recognized that individuals who have experienced significant weight loss (e.g., >10 % over a 6-month period) are at increased risk for development of both macro- and micronutrient deficiencies. A history should be geared toward assessment of the clinical symptoms of specific nutritional deficiencies, while attention during the physical examination should be provided to the detection of loss of subcutaneous fat, muscle wasting, dependent edema (of in the presacral region of a bed-ridden patient), ascites, and cutaneous rashes associated with specific nutritional deficiencies.

In general, the following guidelines may be used to determine the PN formula: 25–30 kcal/kg/day for nutritional

A.L. Buchman, M.D., M.S.P.H. (✉)
Division of Gastroenterology, Feinberg School of Medicine, Northwestern University, Chicago, IL, USA

959 Oak Drive, Glencoe, IL, USA
e-mail: a.buchman@hotmail.com

maintenance and 35 kcal/kg/day (or more if required) for weight gain and 1–1.5 g/kg/day of amino acids. Maintenance fluid is generally required at a dose of 1 ml per kcal, although patients with severe diarrhea may require additional fluid. Additional potassium, magnesium, and acetate may need to be provided to replace fecal losses and maintain normal acid/base status. Because of the substantial risk for contamination of the central venous catheter, appropriate catheter care technique should be utilized, and the catheter reserved for use of PN. This includes the complete avoidance of the catheter for sedation in the endoscopy suite! There is also a risk for development of central venous thrombosis, both within and surrounding the catheter, which may be increased during the heightened inflammatory state of severe colitis. These risks are no different with the use of a peripherally inserted central venous catheters (PICCs).

## Parenteral Nutrition in Patients with Ulcerative Colitis

There is very little data concerning the use of parenteral nutrition (PN) either as primary therapy or even as adjunctive therapy in patients with ulcerative colitis (UC). Most reports consist of open-labeled case series during which patients received concomitant corticosteroids. Often, patients with Crohn's colitis were grouped together with those having UC. Reported follow-up was often brief and generally included only the immediate hospitalization; little objective data was presented. Patients were categorized as being in "remission" or having a "response," although this was often described subjectively in the absence of objective criteria. This chapter will focus on the use of parenteral nutrition in patients with ulcerative colitis.

In 1970, Gimpel and Schilling from the University of Oklahoma reported that 72 days of postoperative total parenteral nutrition (TPN) improved the nutritional status of a malnourished patient with severe UC who required colectomy but who had been unable to eat sufficiently due to multiple postoperative complications [1]. This was the first time TPN had been used in a patient with UC, although it was used primarily for nutritional support rather than to induce remission of the underlying disease. In 1973, Fischer et al. described the use of TPN in four patients with UC who were prescribed complete bowel rest; concomitant medical therapy was not described [2]. Only one of the four patients avoided colectomy during that admission. In 1974, Truelove and Jewell described their experience with 49 patients with "severe" UC in whom a 5-day regimen of PN had been prescribed [3]. Thirty-six of the 49 patients had achieved "remission" by the end of the 5-day course of PN, and in addition, some patients were described as having a "partial response." All patients received concomitant corticosteroids.

Approximately 2/3 of the patients that achieved remission remained symptom-free for a mean of 3 years following PN. Subsequently, Truelove's experience in 100 patients was reported in which 60 % achieved remission [4]. In 1976, Dean et al. described five patients with UC that were provided with PN but in whom colectomy was still required in four of the five during the hospitalization [5]. Reilly et al. reported a series of 11 patients (including the four patients described by Fischer et al. [2]), all of which with the exception of one required colectomy during their hospital admission despite the use of PN. Postoperative complications were more frequent in a historic control group that had not received PN [6]. Most patients were treated with corticosteroids in addition to PN. Fazio reported 1/4 of patients that received PN achieved remission during their hospitalization and did not require colectomy [7]. Elson described the University of Chicago experience of ten patients, "refractory" to corticosteroids, in whom three had "significant" improvement after a mean of 21 days of PN [8]. These patients were able to avoid colectomy for 5–43 months.

Dickinson et al. reported the results of one of only two prospective, randomized, controlled trials of PN in UC [9]. The study was small and underpowered, although similar outcomes were described in patients that received PN (6 of 13 achieved remission) without oral food intake and the control group (8 of 16 achieved remission); there were some long-term remissions in both groups. All patients received corticosteroids. Sitzman et al. reported the results of a series of patients that failed oral prednisone (83 %) as outpatients and were admitted to hospital for TPN and intravenous corticosteroids (91 %) [10]. Five of 22 patients were discharged without requirement for colectomy, although only 4 of those achieved long-term remission that ranged between 15 and 56 months. McIntyre et al. reported the results of the other randomized, controlled trials. Similar to the results reported by Dickinson et al., 6 of 15 patients with "severe" UC who were nil per os (NPO) and received PN achieved remission, compared with 7 of 12 that achieved remission while on an oral diet; all patients received concomitant corticosteroid therapy [11]. Gonzalez-Huix et al. randomized patients with severe UC (using the Truelove-Witt criteria) to receive PN or total enteral nutrition, the latter of which utilized nasoenteric feeding with a polymeric formula [12]. Ten of 20 patients that received TPN achieved remission compared with 12 of 22 enterally fed patients.

The use of TPN does not appear to have clinical benefit as a primary means for induction of remission in patients with UC (Table 38.1). However, it may be a useful adjunctive therapy when patients have toxic megacolon or who are otherwise unable to eat because of severe abdominal cramping. There appears to be no additional benefit from PN itself in patients with UC who are otherwise able to eat or to receive enteral nutritional support. The use of PN in patients with

**Table 38.1** The use of parenteral nutrition in patients with ulcerative colitis

| Study | Remission rate | Follow-up |
|---|---|---|
| Gimpel/Schilling [1] | ? | 72 days |
| Truelove/Jewell [3] | 60/100 (60 %) | Up to 3 years |
| Dean et al. [5] | 1/5 (20 %) | Same admission |
| Reilly et al. [6] | 1/10 (10 %) | Same admission |
| Fazio et al. [7] | ¼ (25 %) | Same admission |
| Elson et al. [8] | 3/21 (15 %) | 5–43 months |
| Dickinson et al. [9] | 6/13 (46 %) | Same admission |
| Sitzman et al. [10] | 5/22 (23 %) | Same admission (15–56 months) |
| McIntyre et al. [11] | 6/15 (40 %) | Same admission |
| Gonzalez-Huix et al. [12] | 10/20 (50 %) | Same admission |

UC has been associated with increased mortality after adjustment for age, sex, comorbidity, health insurance, and geographic location and whether the hospital where they were hospitalized was urban/rural and teaching/nonteaching or whether the facility was small or large [13]. However, the severity of the underlying UC was a likely factor in that "sicker" patients who are more likely to be malnourished and less likely to have sufficient spontaneous oral intake (or in whom enteral nutritional support is not tolerated) are more likely to require or receive PN. In fact, an initial requirement for PN is a predictor for corticosteroid refractoriness [14] as well as increased hospital length of stay and in-hospital mortality [15]. Therefore, the European Society for Enteral and Parenteral Nutrition (ESPEN) concluded in their 2009 guidelines that "Except in complicated UC or in the peri-operative period, PN is not indicated to treat undernutrition in UC..." although "PN is indicated as an adjuvant to other forms of medical treatment—but not as primary treatment—and is used in severe attacks of UC only when enteral nutrition is not tolerated or there are contraindications for its use (e.g. impending or established toxic megacolon, colonic perforation, or massive colonic bleeding [16]). It was further concluded that "in contrast" to Crohn's disease, artificial nutrition—both enteral and PN—does not have a primary therapeutic effect in UC.

# References

1. Gimpel A, Schilling JA. Long-term hyperalimentation in ulcerative colitis. Oklahoma State Med Assoc J. 1970;68:371–5.
2. Fischer JE, Foster GS, Abel RM, et al. Hyperalimentation as primary therapy for inflammatory bowel disease. Am J Surg. 1973;125:165–75.
3. Truelove SC, Jewell DP. Intensive intravenous regimen for severe attacks of ulcerative colitis. Lancet. 1974;1:1067–70.
4. Truelove SC, Willoughby CP, Lee EG, Kettlewell MG. Further experience in the treatment of severe attacks of ulcerative colitis. Lancet. 1978;2:1086–8.
5. Dean RE, Campos MM, Barrett B. Hyperalimentation in the management of chronic inflammatory intestinal disease. Dis Col Rect. 1976;19:601–4.
6. Reilly J, Ryan JA, Strole W, Fischer JE. Hyperalimentation in inflammatory bowel disease. Am J Surg. 1976;131:192–200.
7. Fazio VW, Kodner I, Jagelman DG, et al. Parenteral nutrition as primary of adjunctive treatment. Dis Col Rect. 1976;19:574–8.
8. Elson CO, Layden TJ, Nemchausky BA, et al. An evaluation of total parenteral nutrition in the management of inflammatory bowel disease. Dig Dis Sci. 1980;25:42–8.
9. Dickinson RJ, Ashton MG, Axon ATR, et al. Controlled trial of intravenous hyperalimentation and total bowel rest as an adjunct to the routine therapy of acute colitis. Gastroenterology. 1980;79:1199–204.
10. Sitzman JV, Converse Jr RL, Bayless TM. Favorable response to parenteral nutrition and medical therapy in Crohn's colitis. Gastroenterology. 1990;99:1647–52.
11. McIntyre PB, Powell-Tuck J, Wood SR, et al. Controlled trial of bowel rest in the treatment of severe ulcerative colitis. Gut. 1986;27:481–5.
12. Gonzalez-Huix F, Fernandez-Banares F, Esteve-Comas M, et al. Enteral versus parenteral nutrition as adjunct therapy in acute ulcerative colitis. Am J Gastroenterol. 1993;88:227–32.
13. Nguyen GC, Munsell M, Harris ML. Nationwide prevalence and prognostic significance of clinically diagnosable protein-calorie malnutrition in hospitalized inflammatory bowel disease patients. Aliment Pharmacol Ther. 2008;14:1105–11.
14. Chow DKL, Sung JJY, Tsoi KKF, et al. Predictors of corticosteroid-dependent and corticosteroid-refractory inflammatory bowel disease: analysis of a Chinese cohort study. Aliment Pharmacol Ther. 2009;29:843–54.
15. Nguyen GC, Laveist TA, Brant SR. The utilization of parenteral nutrition during the in-patient management of inflammatory bowel disease in the United States: a national survey. Aliment Pharmacol Ther. 2007;26:1499–507.
16. Van Gossum A, Cabre E, Hebuterne X, et al. ESPEN guidelines on parenteral nutrition: gastroenterology. Clin Nutr. 2009;28:415–27.

Gerassimos J. Mantzaris

**Keywords**

Ulcerative colitis • Remission • Maintenance therapy

## Introduction

The natural history of ulcerative colitis (UC) is characterised by a relapsing-remitting course and less often by a continuous active course. More than half of patients will inevitably relapse within a calendar year following a flare of disease. In controlled clinical trials in quiescent UC, the annual relapse rate of placebo-treated patients ranges from 38 to 76 % [1, 2]. Repetitive flares and chronic active disease may lead on to complications and hospitalisations and increase the risk of colectomy and colorectal cancer. Therefore, it is recommended that all patients receive maintenance therapy [3]. An exception is probably a small proportion of patients with a very mild course of disease for which intermittent therapy may be an option [3, 4].

## Defining Remission in Ulcerative Colitis

Ulcerative colitis cannot be cured by medical therapy. The goal of maintenance therapy is to prolong periods of remission without steroids, improve the quality of life and social function and reduce the risk for colorectal cancer [3]. However, defining "remission" in real life and in the world of the clinical trials varies considerably [5, 6]. Patient's and physician's perception of "remission" is the absence of clinical symptoms of active disease and discontinuation of steroids, if these were used to control the most recent flare. In clinical trials, "remission" is usually defined by clinical (e.g. "absence of a flare" or

"time to a flare") and/or endoscopic (mucosal healing) but rarely histologic criteria. The stringency of these criteria varies remarkably. For instance, "flares" may be defined as the "appearance of bloody diarrhoea" or "the need for steroids," whereas mucosal healing may be graded by a different score of the same grading system, for instance, as score 0 or 1 in the Mayo grading system. In many recent trials, the true impact of maintenance therapy on remission cannot be ascertained because patients with active UC achieving remission on a therapeutic regimen continue on the same regimen in the maintenance phase without re-randomisation to active therapy or placebo [7–10]. These methodological limitations render clinical trials difficult to compare and may be accounted for some of the discrepancies in efficacy outcomes. Interestingly, many studies and even society guidelines [3, 4] have not incorporated histologic criteria in the definition of remission. The latter may underestimate the impact of sustained clinical (steroid-free remission), endoscopic (complete mucosal healing) and histologic remission (absence of persisting active mucosal inflammation and/or basal plasmacytosis) on the long-term outcome of disease [11–16]. A critical evaluation of clinical trials in UC reveals that tight control of endoscopic and histologic inflammation is associated with longer periods of remission, fewer complications, hospitalisations and colectomies, maintenance of social function and a decreased risk for colorectal cancer [4, 11].

## Selecting the Appropriate Maintenance Therapy

The medical armamentarium to prevent relapses of UC includes sulfasalazine and its 5-ASA derivatives, thiopurines and biological agents. Maintenance therapy should be cost

G.J. Mantzaris, M.D., Ph.D., A.G.A.F. (✉)
Department of Gastroenterology, Evangelismos Hospital,
45-47 Ypsilantou St., Athens, Attica 10676, Greece
e-mail: gman195@yahoo.gr; gjmantzaris@gmail.com

G.R. Lichtenstein (ed.), *Medical Therapy of Ulcerative Colitis*,
DOI 10.1007/978-1-4939-1677-1_39, © Springer Science+Business Media New York 2014

**Table 39.1** Factors determining the choice of maintenance therapy in ulcerative colitis

1. Disease-related
   (a) Extent of disease
   (b) Activity and severity of disease
      • Frequency of flares
      • Failure of prior maintenance therapy
      • Severity of the most recent flare
      • Mode of treatment of the most recent flare
2. Patient-related
   (a) Patient preferences
   (b) Adherence
3. Medication-related
   (a) Effectiveness
   (b) Appropriateness
   (c) Safety
   (d) Cost
   (e) Availability

Adapted from [3, 4]

**Table 39.2** Risk factors for relapse in ulcerative colitis

1. Adherence to treatment
2. Young, single status
3. Low-fibre diet
4. Intestinal infections
5. Medications
   (a) Nonsteroidal anti-inflammatory drugs (NSAIDs)
   (b) Antibiotics
6. Seasonal factors
7. Stressful events of life
8. Clinical factors
   (a) Disease activity and severity
      • Shorter interval between relapses
      • Severity of the most recent relapse
      • Need for steroids
      • Slow response to steroids
   (b) Active extra-intestinal manifestations
9. Persistent elevation of serum C-reacting protein
10. Endoscopic and histologic factors
   (a) Lack of mucosal healing
   (b) Persistent basal plasmacytosis and active inflammatory infiltrate at colonic histology

Adapted from [3, 4, 15, 16, 18]

**Table 39.3** Demographic, environmental, clinical, serological, endoscopic and histologic risk factors for relapse of ulcerative colitis

1. Demographic
   (a) Young age
   (b) Being single
2. Environmental
   (a) Perceived and/or actual "stressful" events of life
   (b) Low-fibre diet
   (c) Infections
   (d) Nonsteroidal anti-inflammatory drugs
   (e) Antibiotics
3. Clinical
   (a) Shorter interval between relapses
   (b) Severity of the most recent relapse
      • Need for steroids
      • Slow response to steroids
   (c) Presence of active extra-intestinal manifestations
4. Serological
   (a) Persistent elevation of serum C-reacting protein
5. Endoscopic
   (a) Lack of mucosal healing
6. Histology at colonic (rectal) biopsies
   (a) Persistent basal plasmacytosis
   (b) Active inflammatory infiltrate despite clinical remission

may lead onto proximal extension of ulcerative proctitis (UP) or left-sided colitis (L-UC) in up to 50 % of patients and usually marks a more refractory course of disease [17, 18]. Maintenance therapy should adapt to the clinical pattern and course of disease. A severe flare or frequent relapses indicate failure of prior maintenance therapy and mandate intensification of treatment to recapture steroid-free remission.

Adherence is the most important factor that determines relapse. Non-adherence to mesalamine increases the likelihood of relapse at least five times [19, 20].

Finally, close monitoring is vital to maintain sustained remission even in asymptomatic patients in order to prevent the long-term sequelae of disease.

## Effectiveness of Medications for Maintenance of Remission

### Aminosalicylates

#### Sulfasalazine and Oral Aminosalicylates
Several meta-analyses have assessed the efficacy and safety profile of sulfasalazine and the newer aminosalicylates for remission maintenance of quiescent UC [21–25]. Sulfasalazine in daily doses of 1–4 g has demonstrated a dose–response effect and can maintain remission in 71–89 % of patients [26, 27]. In the 2006 Cochrane systematic review, oral 5-ASA preparations at doses ranging from 0.8 to 4 g per day were superior to placebo in maintaining clinical and/or

effective, appropriate and safe. The choice should depend largely on careful evaluation of various individual risk factors for relapse, disease extent, activity and severity, patient preferences and ability to adhere to a lifelong therapy (see Tables 39.1, 39.2 and 39.3).

Extent of disease is important. Patients with extensive colitis (E-UC) are at higher risk for complications and colectomy and usually need more intensive therapy than patients with shorter extent of disease. In contrast, patients with distal disease are in higher needs of topical therapy. Suboptimal treatment endoscopic remission with a pooled odds ratio of 0.47 [95 % confidence interval (CI), 0.36–0.62 and a number needed to treat (NNT) of 6] [20]. This meta-analysis demonstrated that sulfasalazine was more effective [OR 1.29 (95 % CI, 1.05–1.57)] and had a similar adverse event profile to mesalamine [OR 1.16 and 1.31, respectively] but has been criticised for including only patients who tolerated sulfasalazine. These results have been challenged by the recent large meta-analysis of Ford et al. [22] that confirmed that sulfasalazine, mesalamine, balsalazide and olsalazine were effective at preventing clinical relapse [11 trials of 6–12 months duration, 849 5-ASA treated vs. 653 placebo-treated patients, RR of 0.65, p=0.02, NNT of 4], endoscopic relapse (3 trials, RR of 0.56, p=0.01, NNT of 4) or both (6 trials, RR of 0.59, NNT of 4) without any significant differences between 5-ASA formulations. Nonetheless, subgroup analysis showed superiority over placebo of sulfasalazine (RR of 0.45, NNT of 3) and mesalamine (RR of 0.65, NNT of 4) but not olsalazine (RR of 0.72). In another two meta-analyses, sulfasalazine and mesalamine were equally effective to balsalazide for remission maintenance, but balsalazide was superior to sulfasalazine for withdrawals due to adverse events (RR of 0.17, p=0.001) [23, 24]. Regarding comparisons between mesalamine formulations, Ito et al. [25] performed a 12-month non-inferiority trial and found no significant differences in the proportion of patients without bloody stools between a 2.4 g/day pH-dependent release and a 2.25 g/day time-dependent mesalamine formulation. 5-ASA formulations were shown to maintain remission irrespective of the extent of disease [26, 27].

Based on these results, sulfasalazine should be recommended as the first-choice maintenance treatment in UC due to its efficacy and lower cost, whereas mesalamine, olsalazine and balsalazide should be reserved for patients intolerant of sulfasalazine [4]. However, as the optimal maintenance dose of sulfasalazine (4 g/day) cannot be tolerated by a significant proportion of patients, most gastroenterologists incline to use the newer 5-ASA preparations because they are better tolerated at greater than equivalent doses of sulfasalazine [3, 28, 29].

The optimal maintenance mesalamine dose is unknown. An Italian study documented that 1.2 g/day oral mesalamine was equally effective to 2.4 g/day for remission maintenance [12]. In another study, the minimum effective dose of oral mesalamine was 0.8 g/day, but an incremental benefit for patients receiving 1.6 g/day was shown [30]. However, although a clear dose–response at doses over 0.8 g 5-ASA has never been convincingly demonstrated, dose-ranging studies in patients who required doses of mesalamine up to 4.8 g/day to achieve remission have not been performed [31]. In fact, there is some evidence that higher doses may be more effective. Thus, in a 1-year prospective controlled trial, per protocol analysis of data

demonstrated that 3.0 g of oral mesalamine (Salofalk®) once daily was superior to 1.5 g once daily or 0.5 g three times weekly (86 %, 67 % and 78 %, respectively, p=0.024) [32]. In a meta-analysis of seven randomised clinical trials, 5-ASA doses greater than 2.0 g/day were more likely to reduce the risk for relapse for 6–12 months compared to doses lower than 2.0 g/day, but the quality of the trials that were subjected to analysis was not optimal [22]. Indirect evidence comes also from a post hoc analysis of two clinical trials with Multi-Matrix (MMX) mesalamine in mild-to-moderate UC [10] where 196 of 218 (89.9 %) patients who achieved remission and were maintained on the induction dose of mesalamine were still relapse free after 1 year, indicating that the higher doses that induced remission are expected to maintain also high rates of remission.

Once-daily dose of mesalamine is equally effective and safe, better tolerated and preferred by patients over divided daily doses [12, 13, 33–35]. This effect appears to be similar across all studies irrespective of the mesalamine formulation. A single tablet of 1.2 g MMX mesalamine was as effective as twice-daily dosing (2.4 g) in maintaining clinical remission (88.9 % vs. 93.2 %) and combined clinical and endoscopic remission (64.4 % vs. 68.5 %) for 12 months; both dosing regimens demonstrated a similar adverse event profile and very high adherence rates [13]. In another single-blinded study, 2 g delayed-release 5-ASA granules (Pentasa®) once daily were superior to 1 g twice daily in maintaining remission of quiescent UC for 1 year (70.9 % vs. 58.9 %, respectively, p=0.024) [33]. In a very large study, 1.6–2.4 g mesalamine (Asacol®) once daily was not inferior to twice-daily dosing in maintaining remission of quiescent UC for 1 year (85.4 % vs. 85.4 %, respectively) [34]. Additionally, mesalamine granules once daily at a dose of 1.5 g daily was more effective than placebo to maintain remission over a 6-month period. Finally, 2.4 g MMX mesalamine once daily was equally effective to 2.4 g/day pH-modified release mesalamine (Asacol®) in divided doses at preventing clinical and/or endoscopic relapse of quiescent UC [35].

## Topical 5-ASA

The efficacy and safety of various formulations (suppositories, foam and liquid or gel enemas) and dosing regimens of rectally administered mesalamine have been assessed in controlled clinical trials and case series for maintenance of remission of UP, "distal" colitis ("proctosigmoiditis") and L-UC [36–41]. 5-ASA is delivered to the upper rectum by suppositories and to the rectosigmoid area by foam enemas. Liquid enemas may deliver the active compound up to the splenic flexure, but the actual area of distribution varies between individuals, depending on the length of the sigmoid colon, the volume and the viscosity of the enema.

The advantage of the topical (rectal) therapy is that delivering the active compound directly to the affected area in less frequent dosing schedules increases its effectiveness and reduces systemic availability and adverse effects. In controlled clinical trials, the overall efficacy of topical mesalamine to prevent clinical and/or endoscopic relapse of UP and L-UC for 1 year ranges between 52 and 80 % [4]. Corresponding figures for placebo-treated patients range between 11 % and 53 % and are statistically lower than active treatment in almost all clinical trials. Topical mesalamine administered intermittently three times or even twice weekly is at least equally effective to oral sulfasalazine and mesalamine [18, 38, 42, 43]. However, unlike older mesalamine formulations, oral MMX mesalamine which aims at delivering 5-ASA more evenly throughout the colon has not been tested against topical therapy in quiescent UC. The frequency of topical administration depends largely on patient tolerance, frequency of prior flares and treatment regimen used to induce remission of the most recent flare and may range from 1 g per day to 1–4 g every third day [18, 44]. Topical steroids including the newer formulations with low systemic bioavailability have not shown maintenance efficacy [3, 4, 18, 45].

## Combination of Oral and Topical 5-ASA

The combination of oral and topical 5-ASA is superior to oral or topical therapy alone at preventing relapse of quiescent UC [46, 47]. There are no additional safety signals compared to oral or topical therapy, but the long-term tolerance of treatment is debatable. Topical therapy is usually administered intermittently. Combined treatment should be considered as an escalation of therapy for patients who have relapsed despite optimal oral or topical 5-ASA monotherapy [3, 4, 18, 44].

## Thiopurines

The quality of evidence for the efficacy of thiopurines, azathioprine (AZA) and 6-mercaptopurine (6-MP) in maintaining remission of UC is rather poor. It comes from retrospective uncontrolled observational cohorts from tertiary centres, uncontrolled case series and small prospective controlled trials [48–63]. These studies being few, heterogeneous, of limited size, diverse methodology and varied outcome measures have yielded conflicting results. Consequently, meta-analyses and systematic reviews of the literature cannot offer a precise estimate of the efficacy of thiopurines as maintenance agents in UC. Thus, although in the 2007 Cochrane meta-analysis [64] based on four randomised controlled trials of 12-month duration AZA was superior to placebo at preventing relapse with an odds ratio of 0.41 (95 % CI 0.24–0.70), Leung et al. [65] in their recent review suggested that AZA is only modestly effective in inducing and maintaining remission in UC. In another meta-analysis of six trials that included 124

**Table 39.4** Indications for thiopurines as maintenance agents in ulcerative colitis

1. Intolerance of 5-ASA
2. Frequent relapses despite maximum dose of oral and topical 5-ASA
3. Intolerance of steroids
4. Mild-to-moderate steroid-dependent disease
5. Relapse soon after discontinuation of oral steroids
6. Oral steroid-refractory disease in combination with infliximab
7. Clinical response/remission[a] achieved on
   (a) IV steroids
   (b) IV cyclosporine or IV tacrolimus, infliximab, adalimumab, golimumab or vedolizumab

[a]Thiopurine-naïve patients

patients treated with AZA or 6-MP, the mean maintenance efficacy of thiopurines was 60 % versus only 37 % in controls (OR 2.56, 95 % CI 1.51–4.34) [66]. The pooled OR was 2.59 (95 % CI 1.26–5.3) with an absolute risk reduction of 23 % and a NNT of 5 when only studies of thiopurines versus placebo were analysed. However, these results have been criticised for methodological flaws of the studies that were included in the meta-analysis. Khan et al. [67] analysed recently only three randomized controlled trials, all with "unclear risk of bias", that included 127 patients with quiescent UC followed for 9–12 months and found that AZA was superior to placebo at preventing relapse (RR=0.60; 95 % CI=0.37–0.95; $p=0.03$, NNT=4). Additionally another meta-analysis found similar findings.

Despite published evidence, thiopurines have been recommended by experts and societies' practice guidelines [3, 4, 18] for nearly 40 years as steroid-sparing and remission maintenance agents (see Table 39.4). Thiopurines are especially indicated for patients who cannot tolerate, respond, be waned from or relapse early after discontinuation of oral steroids, for thiopurine-naïve patients who have achieved long-term sustained remission on infliximab (IFX) monotherapy or combined with AZA and are considered for discontinuation of IFX and, finally, for hospitalised thiopurine-naïve patients responding to intravenous steroids or to second-line therapy with a fast-acting agent, such as intravenous cyclosporine or tacrolimus who need to be bridged to a steroid-sparing agent [3, 68, 69]. For these indications, thiopurines are likely to maintain clinical remission in approximately 40–70 % of patients' mucosal healing [4] and steroid sparing [70], resulting in a significant reduction in hospitalisations and colectomies [58].

The daily dose of AZA is 2.5 mg/kg and of 6-MP is 1–1.5 mg/kg. Treatment may be started at low doses (50 mg AZA or 25 mg 6-MP) and increased gradually if tolerated by 50 mg for AZA or 25 mg for 6-MP in order to achieve the target dose over a period of 2 months. A dosing strategy based on TPMT testing is discussed in Chaps. 13 and 14. Frequent white blood cell (WBC) and platelet count should be performed to avoid early leucopenia. Since late leucopenia and liver toxicity may develop at any time, patients should be monitored at regular intervals with WBC and platelet counts and liver function tests. If the WBC and/or the platelet count drops below 3.000/ml and 80.000/ml, respectively, thiopurines should be tapered or stopped temporarily. Adherence can be monitored by frequent consultations, checking the mean volume of red blood cells (MCV) or by measuring 6-MP metabolites. There is insufficient evidence to recommend monitoring the response to thiopurines by sequential measurements of 6-MP metabolites over the traditional approach of frequent clinical consultations and laboratory tests [4].

Relative leucopenia, a higher MCV and being older may predict response to AZA [54]. Efficacy appears to be higher in patients with shorter disease duration [70, 71]. There are no studies comparing the efficacy of AZA to 6-MP for remission maintenance. The doses of 6-MP in observational cohorts are probably lower to AZA doses, but the overall efficacy appears to be similar [4, 49–54].

Co-administration of thiopurines and 5-ASA increases 6-TGN metabolites in a dose-dependent manner. This interaction may result in myelotoxicity in a small proportion of patients but may theoretically be beneficial for patients who are refractory to thiopurines [72]. Whether these are clinically meaningful is questionable. Two small studies and a Cochrane meta-analysis have suggested that 5-ASA offers no advantage to AZA for the maintenance of remission [63, 73, 74]. However, many gastroenterologists incline to continue 5-ASA as a colorectal cancer preventive agent.

Although there is limited evidence to recommend certain duration of treatment [3], treatment should probably be indefinite [75]. AZA-withdrawal studies have demonstrated consistently that UC will inevitably relapse shortly after abrupt cessation of treatment [63, 72]. In an Oxford cohort, the proportion of IBD patients in remission after withdrawal of AZA was 0.63 at 1 year and 0.35 at 5 years [54]. It is also unclear whether disease extent, duration of treatment and concomitant use of 5-ASA influence relapse [54, 72–74]. Prolonged use of thiopurines may increase the risk of lymphoma, but the magnitude of this risk has not been completely defined [3, 4, 76, 77]. A recent meta-analysis suggests that a minimum of 1 year is needed for the risk of lymphoma and also that this occurs more commonly in men than women. Men have a greater risk than women (RR = 2.05; $p < 0.05$); both sexes were at increased risk for lymphoma (SIR for men = 3.60; 95 % CI, 2.68–4.83 and SIR for women = 1.76, 95 % CI, 1.08–2.87). Patients younger than 30 years had the highest RR (SIR = 6.99; CI, 2.99–16.4); younger men had the highest risk. The absolute risk was highest in patients older than 50 years (1:377 cases per patient year). In any case the risk of prolonged treatment needs to be balanced against colectomy at an individual level.

It is also questionable whether the full dose of thiopurines is needed to maintain long-term remission. However, under-dosing may lead onto relapse of disease without preventing drug toxicity.

## Anti-TNFα Agents

### Infliximab

Two large studies, ACT 1 and ACT 2, have assessed the efficacy of IFX in patients with moderate-to-severe UC refractory to steroids, immunomodulators (ACT 1 and 2) and/or 5-ASA (ACT 2) [7]. Remission rates at week 30 (ACT 1 and 2) and at week 54 (ACT 1) were assessed only in patients who had achieved clinical response or remission at week 8 after induction with IFX (5 or 10 mg/kg at weeks 0, 2 and 6) or placebo and continued IFX schedule therapy (5 or 10 mg/kg) or placebo every 8 weeks. Remission rates were significantly higher for IFX groups in ACT 2 at week 30 (26 % vs. 36 % vs. 11 % for 5 mg/kg and 10 mg/kg IFX or placebo, respectively) and in ACT 1 at week 54 (34 % for combined IFX groups vs. 17 % for placebo). In ACT 1, complete mucosal healing defined as a Mayo score 0 or 1 at week 54 was superior for IFX than placebo-treated patients (55 %, 57 % and 22 %, for 5 mg/kg, 10 mg/kg IFX and placebo, respectively). Although the gain in steroid-free remission at week 54 (ACT-1) was only 14 % for the 5 mg/kg arm and 9 % for the 10 mg/kg IFX over placebo (10 %), IFX resulted in a significant reduction in hospitalisations and colectomies [78]. The degree of mucosal healing at week 8 did not predict subsequent outcome of UC but was associated with a significant reduction in the likelihood for colectomy at 1 year [79]. Extended treatment with IFX for up to three additional years was effective in maintaining remission and well tolerated without any additional safety signals [80].

Numerous uncontrolled case series have been reported on patients with UC of varied degrees of severity and refractoriness to prior therapies who were treated with IFX alone or combined with AZA for variable periods of time. Although these data are difficult to subject to group analysis, a nonsystematic review [81] and a systematic review [82] of the literature have confirmed the efficacy and safety of IFX to induce and maintain clinical response, remission, mucosal healing and wane steroids in a considerable proportion of patients with active moderate-to-severe UC.

Colectomy-free survival after IFX therapy was investigated in four studies. Gustavsson et al. [83] reported on a 3-year follow-up of patients who received a single infusion of 4–5 mg/kg IFX as salvage therapy for severe intravenous steroid-refractory UC. Overall, 12/24 (50 %) of IFX-treated patients versus 16/21 (76 %) of placebo-treated patients underwent colectomy ($p = 0.012$). Lack of mucosal healing at 3 months after the single infusion of IFX predicted subsequent colectomy. In a cohort of 121 patients from Leuven [84] and in a French cohort of 119 patients [85], who were treated with IFX for a median of 33 (IQR 17.0–49.8) months and 18 (IQR 8–32) months, respectively, predictors for colectomy were the lack of short-term response to IFX, baseline levels of CRP ≥5 mg/l [84] or ≥10 mg/l [85], prior treatment with intravenous steroids [84] and/or ciclosporin [84, 85] and an indication of IFX for severe UC [85]. In a Canadian cohort, 46/115 (40 %) of UC patients treated with IFX and/or immunomodulators came to colectomy after a median of 5.3 months. Patients with a detectable serum IFX trough level but not antibodies to IFX had higher rates of remission (69 % vs. 15 %; $p<0.001$) and endoscopic improvement (76 % vs. 28 %, $p<0.001$). In contrast, an undetectable serum IFX was highly predictive of increased risk for colectomy (55 % vs. 7 %, OR 9.3; 95 % CI 2.9–29.9; $p<0.001$). Concomitant use of immunomodulators did not influence the clinical outcomes [86].

In a recent trial involving patients with steroid-refractory UC who were naïve to immunomodulators and anti-TNF therapy, patients were assigned randomly to receive intravenous infusions of infliximab (5 mg/kg at weeks 0, 2, 6 and 14) plus daily oral placebo capsules, oral azathioprine 2.5 mg/kg daily plus placebo infusions on the infliximab schedule or combination therapy with the two drugs. Corticosteroid-free clinical remission was evaluated at week 16 as a primary end point. Corticosteroid-free remission at week 16 was achieved by 39.7 % (31 of 78) of patients receiving infliximab/azathioprine, compared with 22.1 % (17 of 77) receiving infliximab alone ($p=0.017$) and 23.7 % (18 of 76) receiving azathioprine alone ($p=0.032$). Mucosal healing at week 16 occurred in 62.8 % (49 of 78) of patients receiving infliximab/azathioprine, compared with 54.6 % (42 of 77) receiving infliximab ($p=0.295$) and 36.8 % (28 of 76) receiving azathioprine ($p=0.001$). Thus, in antitumour necrosis factor-alpha-naive patients with moderate-to-severe UC treated with infliximab plus azathioprine were more likely to achieve corticosteroid-free remission at 16 weeks than those receiving either monotherapy. Combination therapy treatment was associated with better mucosal healing than azathioprine monotherapy.

Whether UC patients in remission on combined AZA and IFX should discontinue AZA is currently unknown. In Crohn's disease, long-term combination therapy is associated with a higher IFX trough level [87] and lower rate of loss of response to IFX [88] than IFX monotherapy [88]. Whether the full dose of AZA is required to achieve these goals awaits clarification by future trials. However, the benefits of any long-term combination therapy should be balanced against the increased risk for infections and/or malignancies especially in young male patients [84, 88–91]. On the other hand, bridging with IFX to AZA monotherapy in AZA-naïve patients may be easier to achieve in UC than

in Crohn's disease. In any case, the decision to stop IFX and continue on AZA should be discussed only for patients in long-standing sustained steroid-free clinical, serologic (normal CRP), endoscopic (mucosal healing) and/or histologic remission who have a detectable IFX trough level. Again, safety issues, patient preferences, adherence, cost and also the risk of no response or allergic reaction upon re-treatment with IFX should be considered in decision-making.

## Adalimumab

Adalimumab (ADA) has been approved for the treatment of UC. Initially, preliminary evidence from small trials and retrospective case series suggests that ADA may be effective and safe in achieving and maintaining long-term clinical response or remission, mucosal healing, steroid sparing, improving quality of life and reducing colectomies in patients who have failed almost all prior therapies [92–97]. Concomitant use of AZA was the only independent factor predicting response to ADA in one trial [95]. Recently, a large controlled trial was reported in 494 patients with moderate-to-severe UC who had failed treatment with steroids, immunomodulators and/or IFX (40.3 % of the ITT population). Patients were randomised 1:1 to placebo or ADA ($n=248$, 160/80 mg sc at week 0 and 2 and then 40 mg every other week). Dose escalation of ADA was allowed. At weeks 8, 52 and both 8 and 52, significantly more patients on ADA achieved clinical remission and response. Significantly more patients with prior IFX failure achieved clinical remission or response on ADA than placebo at week 52 and sustained clinical response at both weeks 8 and 52. The therapeutic gain in steroid-free remission rate at week 52 was only 7.6 % in favour of ADA but was still significantly statistically superior to placebo (5.7 %, $p=0.035$). Adverse events were not significantly different between ADA and placebo [98].

## Golimumab

Golimumab is a subcutaneously administered fully human anti-TNF antibody, previously approved for the treatment of rheumatoid arthritis, ankylosing spondylitis and psoriatic arthritis. The treatment of ulcerative colitis recently gained regulatory approval for induction and maintenance of remission in patients who have moderate-to-severe ulcerative colitis based on the data in two registration trials. There has been one randomised placebo-controlled trial [Program of Ulcerative Colitis Research Studies Utilizing an Investigational Treatment-Subcutaneous (PURSUIT-SC)] that assessed induction therapy with subcutaneous golimumab in anti-TNF-α-naive patients with moderate-to-severe ulcerative colitis (Mayo score 6–12 points with an endoscopic subscore >2 points) not responding to conventional therapy with oral mesalamine, oral corticosteroids, and AZA/6-mercaptopurine or unable to taper corticosteroids without recurrence of ulcerative colitis activity. The subsequent PURSUIT-M randomised placebo-controlled trial assessed the efficacy and safety of golimumab in maintaining clinical response in patients who responded to induction treatment with golimumab in the preceding PURSUIT-SC trial. Golimumab was shown to be more efficacious than placebo in inducing clinical response, remission and mucosal healing and improving quality of life.

Based upon the date from these two clinical trials, Golimumab is initially administered subcutaneously at the dose of 200 mg at week 0 followed by 100 mg at week 2 and after that every 4 weeks.

## Vedolizumab

Vedolizumab is the most recent agent for treatment of ulcerative colitis (and Crohn's disease) to gain regulatory approval. The efficacy of treatment with vedolizumab in ulcerative colitis was assessed. 374 patients were randomised to either drug or placebo as part of induction. The response for week 6 was measured by the Mayo score and documented mucosal healing.

During induction, 47.1 % of the patients on vedolizumab versus 25.5 % of the patients on placebo achieved remission ($p < 0.001$). A second cohort of patients received open-label vedolizumab, and responders from both cohorts were included in the maintenance trial that evaluated clinical remission at week 52. Patients were randomised to receive the drug every 4 or 8 weeks or a placebo. A total of 41.8 % of patients maintained remission when receiving medication every 8 weeks compared to 44.8 % who received the drug every 4 weeks; patients who received placebo had maintenance of remission at a rate of 15.9 %. There was a statistically significant difference in maintenance of remission between patients who received the drug every 8 weeks versus placebo ($p < 0.001$) and those receiving the drug every 4 weeks versus placebo ($p < 0.001$). Based on this data, the drug was approved for use in adults with moderate-to-severe ulcerative colitis when one or more standard therapies (corticosteroids, immunomodulators or tumour necrosis factor blocker medications) have not resulted in an adequate response.

## Additional Therapies

### Methotrexate

Several small retrospective case series mostly in patients intolerant or unresponsive to thiopurines have claimed satisfactory results of methotrexate (MTX) for maintenance of remission in UC [55, 99–101]. However, a small subtherapeutic trial did not show maintenance efficacy of oral 12.5 mg MTX once weekly since 64 % of the 14 patients

receiving MTX compared to 44 % of 18 placebo-treated patients relapsed within 9 months of follow-up ($p = 0.25$) [102], and a Cochrane systematic review confirmed these negative results [103]. Based on these data, MTX is not currently recommended for maintenance therapy for UC [3]. At present, there is a multicentre trial (ClinicalTrials.gov Identifier: NCT01393405) evaluating the efficacy of methotrexate 25 mg subcutaneously once weekly as a maintenance therapy for patients with ulcerative colitis in remission.

## Omega-3 Fatty Acids (Fish Oil)

Several studies have evaluated the role of diverse formulations and dosing regimens of omega-3 fatty acids in the maintenance of remission of UC, yielding conflicting results [104–107]. A 2007 Cochrane meta-analysis did not show any maintenance benefit of omega-3 fatty acids over placebo [108]. A more recent meta-analysis included only two randomised controlled trials and concluded that enteric-coated preparations of fish oil are safe and probably effective at preventing relapses of UC [109]. However, data are still insufficient to recommend fish oil as a treatment modality for preventing relapses in quiescent colitis [3].

## Antibiotics and Probiotics

Small trials with the antibiotics ciprofloxacin and metronidazole offer insufficient evidence to recommend their use as maintenance treatment for UC [110–112].

The Nissle 1917 strain of E. coli is the most extensively studied probiotic for the maintenance of remission in UC. Evidence comes for three randomised controlled trials and one prospective open-label trial. All these studies have reported exceptionally high relapse rates. In the first study, 11 % of patients treated with 1.5 g/day 5-ASA relapsed after 3 months compared to 16 % of patients treated with E. coli Nissle 1917 [113]. The second was a randomised induction and maintenance of remission study where patients with active colitis who had achieved remission on 2.4 g/day 5-ASA or 200 mg/day E. coli strain Nissle 1917, in association with oral gentamicin, and variable doses of oral and/or rectal steroids were randomised to probiotic monotherapy ($n = 79$) or 1.2 g/day 5-ASA ($n = 87$). After 12 months, 67 % of patients on the probiotic versus 73 % on 5-ASA had relapsed [114]. The last study was a 12-month non-inferiority study conducted in 327 patents with long-standing quiescent UC. Relapse rates on 1.5 g/day 5-ASA were not significantly different from an equivalent dose of E. coli Nissle 1917 (36 % vs. 45 %, respectively) [115]. Similar results were obtained in a small prospective open-label 12-month trial in young patients with quiescent UC [116].

Based on these results, it can be assumed that *E. coli* strain Nissle 1917 may be an effective alternative for the maintenance of remission in patients who cannot tolerate or develop adverse events to 5-ASA.

Studies with other probiotics have usually serious methodological limitations to offer convincing evidence for effectiveness as maintenance agents for UC in adults. However, a large trial of Zocco et al. demonstrated that patients treated for 1 year with Lactobacillus GG ($18 \times 10^9$ viable bacteria/day), 5-ASA 2.4 g/day or the combination had similar clinical and endoscopic remission rates at 6 and 12 months [117].

## Appendectomy

Appendectomy performed for true acute appendicitis at a young age reduces significantly the risk for subsequent development of UC [118, 119]. Prior appendectomy may also influence the course of colitis, decreasing the needs for immunosuppressive treatment and colectomy [120]. Nonetheless, it is unclear whether appendectomy performed after the diagnosis of UC exerts a beneficial effect on the

subsequent course of colitis [121]. Consequently, there is insufficient evidence to recommend appendectomy as a potential disease modifier.

## Recommendations for Maintenance of Remission According to Location and Activity of Disease

### Extensive Colitis

In clinical practice, oral 5-ASA at doses >2 g/day (or equivalent) is used for induction of remission [3]. It is recommended that patients should continue on the same dose to prevent relapse (see Fig. 39.1) [10]. Although the optimal maintenance dose of mesalamine has not been documented, doses greater than the minimum effective dose (1.2 g/day) [12] may be necessary for patients who require higher doses to achieve remission [10]. Since analysis of efficacy data offers no direct evidence of superiority of any 5-ASA preparation, the choice of the oral 5-ASA agent for maintenance therapy should be based on local availability, cost, patient's

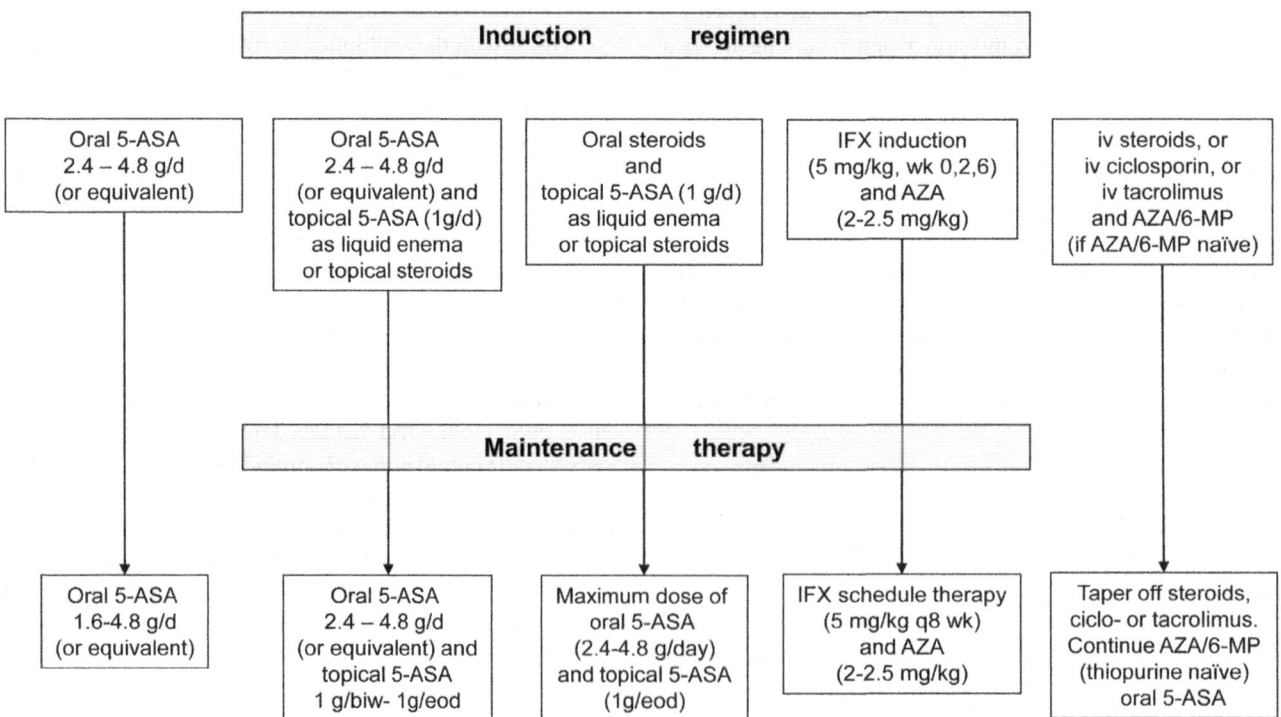

**Fig. 39.1** Management algorithm for patients with extensive ulcerative colitis according to the therapeutic regimen that was used to induce clinical remission of disease. *5-ASA* 5-aminosalicylic acid, *AZA* aza-thioprine, *6-MP* 6-mercaptopurine, *IFX* infliximab, *biw* twice weekly, *eod* every other day

preferences and potential to increase adherence and avoid side effects [3, 122]. Once-daily dosing increases adherence without compromising efficacy and safety. Renal function should be monitored at regular intervals.

Patients who relapse on oral 5-ASA will benefit from addition of topical 5-ASA. If remission is achieved, it should be maintained on combined oral and topical therapy [3, 4, 18]. The minimum effective dose of topical 5-ASA for E-UC is 1 g as liquid or gel enema three times a week. However, dosing schedules ranging from 1 g/day to 1 g once weekly may be required depending on disease behaviour. Patients achieving remission on oral steroids and/or 5-ASA or steroid enemas should receive the maximum dose of oral and topical 5-ASA for maintenance (see Fig. 39.1) [18].

Patients truly refractory to and/or intolerant of 5-ASA should receive thiopurines as maintenance therapy. A short course of steroids may bridge to the effect of thiopurines. Patients intolerant of 5-ASA may benefit from treatment with *E. coli* Nissle 1917 at a dose of 200 mg/day (corresponding to $50 \times 10^9$ viable *E. coli* bacteria), but there are currently insufficient data regarding its long-term efficacy; availability and reimbursement may constitute additional barriers for widespread use.

Patients with steroid dependency or intolerance should also be treated with thiopurines. 6-MP can substitute for AZA in patients who develop gastrointestinal intolerance to AZA. Concomitant use of 5-ASA may benefit patients who are refractory to thiopurine monotherapy but may increase the risk for leucopenia in some patients [72]. Patients who relapse on AZA/6-MP should be evaluated for adherence and treatment should be optimised before switching to another drug category.

IFX in combination with AZA should be the maintenance treatment of choice for ambulatory, thiopurine-naive patients with oral steroid-refractory UC who have responded to induction therapy with this regimen. The duration of combined treatment and the criteria for stopping IFX or AZA have already been discussed. The same strategy is advocated for hospitalised patients with intravenous steroid-refractory disease who have responded to second-line therapy with intravenous cyclosporine or tacrolimus, or IFX. However, IFX alone is probably the only option for patients with prior AZA/6-MP failure because it offers an effective exit strategy to long-term maintenance therapy. ADA and GOL are other options to consider for patients with moderate-to-severe ulcerative colitis. These agents can be used initially or can be used as treatment for patients who are intolerant or have lost response to IFX. Additionally, the use of vedolizumab is another option for patients who have had inadequate response to mesalamine, steroids, immunomodulators or even anti-TNF therapy.

## Left-Sided Colitis

For practical reasons, therapeutic trials with mesalamine or steroid enemas in L-UC included often patients with distal colitis or colitis extending to the splenic flexure but also patients with UP. In all these trials and in a meta-analysis of two randomised controlled trials, continuous or intermittent administration of rectal mesalamine appears to be at least equally effective to oral sulfasalazine, mesalamine and olsalazine but superior to placebo in maintaining clinical and endoscopic remission of UP and distal colitis for at least 1 year [38–44]. For patients with disease extending to the splenic flexure, mesalamine liquid or gel enemas were equally effective to oral sulfasalazine or 5-ASA preparations and are recommended as first-line maintenance therapy or as alternative to oral 5-ASA (Fig. 39.2) [3, 4, 18, 38–44].

An algorithm for treating L-UC is given in Fig. 39.3. Patients achieving remission on topical mesalamine should continue the same regimen for maintenance. If topical therapy cannot be tolerated, oral 5-ASA is an effective alternative. Oral 5-ASA should be added if topical therapy is insufficient. Patients achieving remission on combined oral and topical 5-ASA should continue on this regimen for maintenance of remission.

Recommendations for patients with quiescent L-UC intolerant or refractory to 5-ASA, steroids and/or thiopurines are similar to E-UC [3, 4, 18].

## Ulcerative Proctitis

Suppositories are the preferred mesalamine formulation for maintenance therapy in UP. 5-ASA foam enemas (not available in the United States) are an alternative if suppositories cannot be tolerated [123, 124]. The usual maintenance dose of mesalamine suppositories ranges from 0.5–1.0 g twice weekly to 1.0 g/day, depending on the course of UP (see Fig. 39.3). Intermittent administration improves adherence greatly. Some patients may not need maintenance treatment, but this carries a risk for proximal extension of disease. Patients intolerant of topical therapy should receive oral mesalamine at a daily dose of 1.6–2.4 g (or an equivalent dose of sulfasalazine or other 5-ASA preparations).

In patients who relapse despite adherence to topical therapy, dose escalation to 1.0 g/day 5-ASA at bedtime with adjunctive oral mesalamine at a dose of 1.6–2.4 g/day is usually sufficient to recapture and maintain remission. The addition of oral 5-ASA provides even greater efficacy than oral or rectal mesalamine monotherapy and may prevent proximal extension of disease [3, 4, 17]. Daily doses of topical mesalamine above 1.0 g do not increase the efficacy of maintenance therapy [3, 4].

## Left-sided UC: Maintenance of Remission According to Induction Regimen

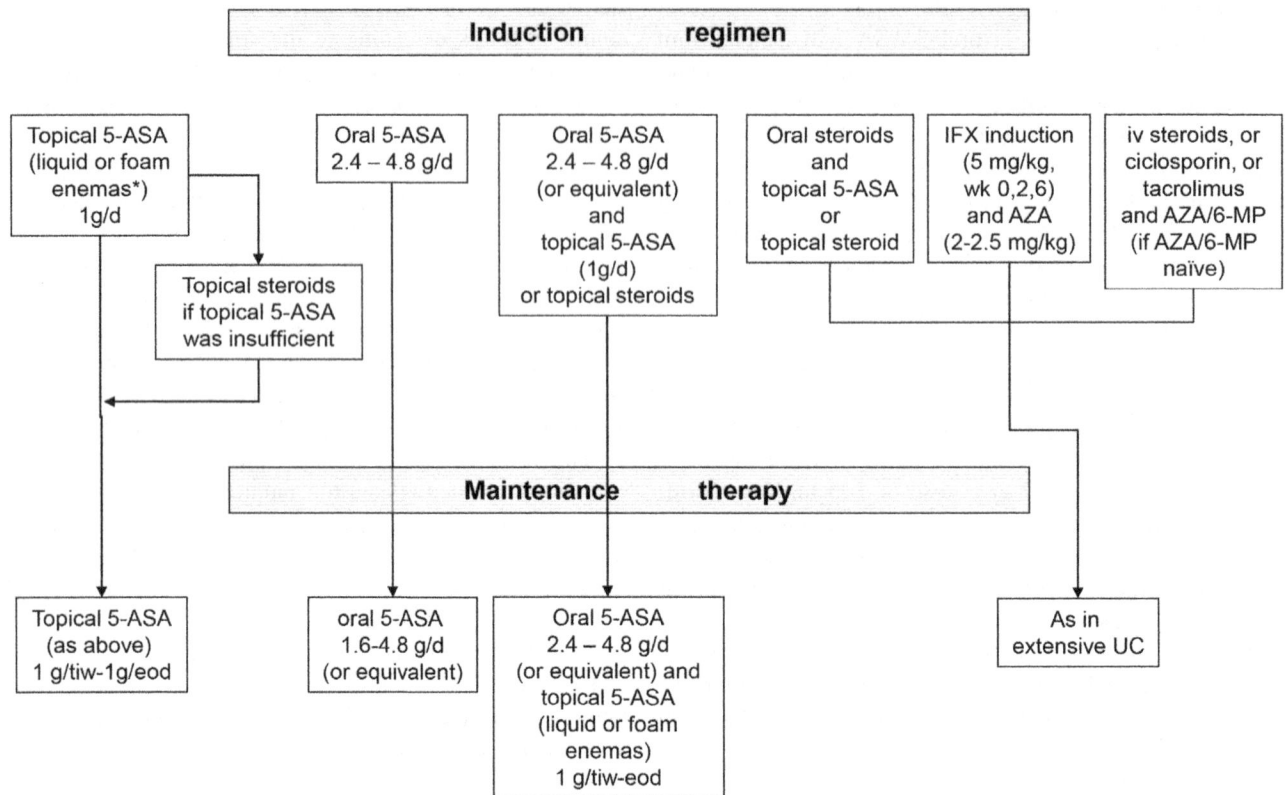

**Fig. 39.2** Management algorithm for patients with left-sided ulcerative colitis according to the therapeutic regimen that was used to induce clinical remission of disease. *5-ASA* 5-aminosalicylic acid, *AZA* azathioprine, *6-MP* 6-mercaptopurine, *IFX* infliximab, *tiw* three times weekly, *eod* every other day. *For topical therapy, liquid (or gel) enemas are recommended for disease extending to the splenic flexure and foam enemas for proctosigmoiditis [18]

Patients achieving remission on rectal steroids and oral mesalamine (2.4–4.8 g/day, or equivalent) or oral steroids and rectal 5-ASA or rectal steroids should be maintained on the maximum combined oral and topical mesalamine. Divided doses may be more efficacious in frequently relapsing proctitis because 5-ASA is applied more evenly to the affected mucosa for 24 h, but in active UP, 1 g mesalamine suppositories once daily were not inferior to 1 g in divided daily doses [125, 126].

Topical steroids are not recommended for maintenance treatment. Intermittent administration of topical steroids with low systemic availability has not been assessed in clinical trials for maintenance of remission in UP. Patients with steroid-dependent UP and those who cannot maintain remission on adequate doses of oral and rectal mesalamine should be treated with thiopurines as patients with E-UC.

The choice of maintenance therapy for refractory UP depends upon the therapeutic regimen that induced steroid-free remission and prior treatment with AZA/6-MP as discussed previously for E-UC. AZA/6-MP should be used if patients are naïve to thiopurines. Oral or rectal cyclosporine, oral or rectal tacrolimus and/or IFX schedule therapy have all been used as maintenance therapy in prior thiopurine failure. Additionally, adalimumab, golimumab and vedolizumab should be considered in this patient population. However, if disease cannot be controlled and clinical judgement ascertains that persisting symptoms truly impact negatively on patient's quality of life, social function and professional activities, surgical options should be discussed. This is because the outcome of elective restorative colectomy with pouch formation is excellent in patients with proctitis and distal colitis and provides a much better quality of life [127].

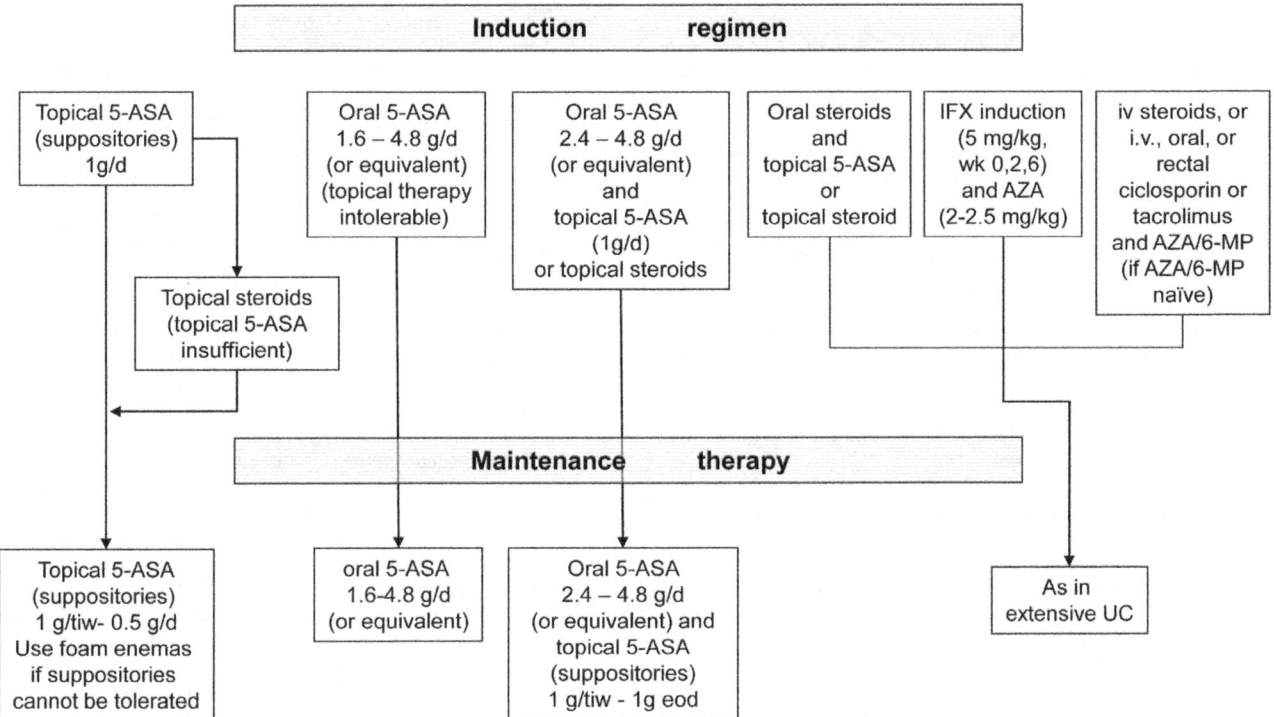

**Fig. 39.3** Management algorithm for patients with ulcerative proctitis according to the therapeutic regimen that was used to induce clinical remission of disease. *5-ASA* 5-aminosalicylic acid, *AZA* azathioprine, *6-MP* 6-mercaptopurine, *IFX* infliximab, *tiw* three times weekly, *eod* every other day

## References

1. Su C, Lewis JD, Goldberg B, Brensinger C, Lichtenstein GR. A meta-analysis of the placebo rates of remission and response in clinical trials of active ulcerative colitis. Gastroenterology. 2007;132:516–26.
2. Meyers S, Janowitz HD. The "natural history" of ulcerative colitis: an analysis of the placebo response. J Clin Gastroenterol. 1989;11:33–7.
3. Travis SP, Stange EF, Lemann M, et al. European evidence based consensus on the diagnosis and management of Crohn's disease: current management. Gut. 2006;55 Suppl 1:i16–35.
4. Kornbluth A, Sacher DA, the Practice Parameters Committee of the American College of Gastroenterology. Ulcerative colitis practice guidelines in adults: American College of Gastroenterology. Practice Parameters Committee. Am J Gastroenterol. 2010;105:501–23.
5. D'Haens G, Sandborn WJ, Feagan BG, et al. Clinical trials of medical therapy in adults with ulcerative colitis. Gastroenterology. 2007;132:763–86.
6. Travis SP, Higgins PDR, Orchard T, et al. Review article: defining remission in ulcerative colitis. Aliment Pharmacol Ther. 2011;34: 113–24.
7. Rutgeerts P, Sandborn WJ, Feagan BG, et al. Infliximab for induction and maintenance therapy for ulcerative colitis. N Engl J Med. 2005;353:2462–76.
8. Kamm MA, Sandborn WJ, Gassull M, et al. Once-daily, high-concentration MMX mesalamine in active ulcerative colitis. Gasroenterology. 2007;132:66–75.
9. Lichtenstein GR, Kamm MA, Boddu P, et al. Effect of once- or twice-daily MMX mesalamine (SPD476) for induction of remission in mild to moderately active ulcerative colitis. Clin Gastroenterol Hepatol. 2007;5:95–102.
10. Hanauer SB, Present DH, Rubin DT. Emerging issues in ulcerative colitis and ulcerative proctitis: individualizing treatment to maximize outcomes. Gastroenterol Hepatol (NY). 2009;5 Suppl 6:4–16.
11. Burger D, Thomas SJ, Walsh AJ, et al. Depth of remission may not predict outcome of ulcerative colitis over 2 years. J Crohn's Colitis. 2011;5:S4–5.
12. Paoluzi OA, Iacopini F, Pica R, et al. Comparison of two different daily dosages (2.4 vs. 1.2 g) of oral mesalazine in maintenance of remission in ulcerative colitis patients: 1-year follow-up study. Aliment Pharmacol Ther. 2005;21:1111–9.
13. Kamm MA, Lichtenstein GR, Sandborn WJ, et al. Randomised trial of once- or twice-daily MMX mesalazine for maintenance of remission in ulcerative colitis. Gut. 2008;57:893–902.
14. Dignass AU, Bokemeyer B, Adamek H, et al. Mesalamine once daily is more effective than twice daily in patients with quiescent ulcerative colitis. Clin Gastroenterol Hepatol. 2009;7:762–9.
15. Riley SA, Mani V, Goodman MJ, Dutt S, Herd ME. Microscopic activity in ulcerative colitis: what does it mean? Gut. 1991;32: 174–8.

16. Bitton A, Peppercorn MA, Antonioli DA, et al. Clinical, biological, and histologic parameters as predictors of relapse in ulcerative colitis. Gastroenterology. 2001;120:13–20.

17. Pica R, Paoluzi OA, Iacopini F, et al. Oral mesalazine (5-ASA) treatment may protect against proximal extension of mucosal inflammation in ulcerative proctitis. Inflamm Bowel Dis. 2004;10: 731–6.

18. Regueiro M, Loftus EV, Steinhart AH, Cohen RD. Clinical guidelines for the medical management of left-sided ulcerative colitis and ulcerative proctitis: summary statement. Inflamm Bowel Dis. 2006;12:972–8.

19. Kane S, Huo D, Aikens J, Hanauer S. Medication nonadherence and the outcomes of patients with quiescent ulcerative colitis. Am J Med. 2003;114:39–43.

20. Higgins PD, Rubin DT, Kaulback K, Schoenfield PS, Kane SV. Systematic review: impact of non-adherence to 5-aminosalicylic acid products on the frequency and cost of ulcerative colitis flares. Aliment Pharmacol Ther. 2009;29:247–57.

21. Sutherland L, Macdonald JK. Oral 5-aminosalicylic acid for maintenance of remission in ulcerative colitis. Cochrane Database Syst Rev. 2006; (19):CD000544.

22. Ford AC, Achkar JP, Khan KJ, et al. Efficacy of 5-aminosalicylates in ulcerative colitis: systematic review and meta-analysis. Am J Gastroenterol. 2011;106:601–16.

23. Nikfar S, Rahimi R, Rezaie A, Abdollahi M. A meta-analysis of the efficacy of sulfasalazine in comparison with 5-aminosalicylates in the induction of improvement and maintenance of remission in patients with ulcerative colitis. Dig Dis Sci. 2009;54:1157–70.

24. Rahimi R, Nikfar S, Rezaie A, Abdollahi M. Comparison of mesalazine and balsalazide in induction and maintenance of remission in patients with ulcerative colitis: a meta-analysis. Dig Dis Sci. 2009;54:712–21.

25. Ito H, Iida M, Matsumoto T, et al. Direct comparison of two mesalamine formulations for the induction of remission in patients with ulcerative colitis: a double-blind, randomized study. Inflamm Bowel Dis. 2010;16:1567–74.

26. Kruis W, Schreiber S, Theuer D, et al. Low dose balsalazide (1.5 g twice daily) and mesalazine (0.5 g three times daily) maintained remission of ulcerative colitis but high dose balsalazide (3.0 g twice daily) was superior in preventing relapses. Gut. 2001;49:783–9.

27. Green JR, Gibson JA, Kerr GD, et al. Maintenance of remission of ulcerative colitis: a comparison between balsalazide 3 g daily and mesalazine 1.2 g daily over 12 months. ABACUS Investigator Group. Aliment Pharmacol Ther. 1998;12:1207–16.

28. Dissanayake AS, Truelove SC. A controlled therapeutic trial of long-term maintenance treatment of ulcerative colitis with sulphazalazine (Salazopyrin). Gut. 1973;14:923–6.

29. Azad-Khan AK, Howes DT, Piris J, et al. Optimum dose for sulphasalazine for maintenance treatment in ulcerative colitis. Gut. 1980;21:232–40.

30. Hanauer S, Sninsky CA, Robinson M, et al. An oral preparation of mesalamine as long-term maintenance therapy for ulcerative colitis. Ann Intern Med. 1996;124:204–11.

31. Kamm MA, Lichtenstein GR, Sandborn WJ, et al. Effect of extended MMX mesalamine therapy for acute, mild-to-moderate ulcerative colitis. Inflamm Bowel Dis. 2009;15:1–8.

32. Kruis W, Jonaitis L, Pokrotnieks J, et al. Randomized clinical trial: a comparative dose-finding study of three arms of dual release mesalazine for maintaining remission in ulcerative colitis. Aliment Pharmacol Ther. 2010;32:990–9.

33. Diagnass A, Bokemeyer B, Adamek H, et al. Mesalamine once daily is more effective than twice daily in patients with quiescent colitis. Clin Gastroenterol Hepatol. 2009;7:762–9.

34. Sandborn WJ, Korzenik J, Lashner B, et al. Once-daily dosing of delayed-release oral mesalazine (400-mg tablet) is as effective as

twice-daily dosing for maintenance of remission of ulcerative colitis. Gastroenterology. 2010;138:1286–96.

35. Prantera C, Kohn A, Campieri M, et al. Clinical trial: ulcerative colitis maintenance treatment with 5-ASA: a 1-year randomized multicentre study comparing MMX with Asacol. Aliment Pharmacol Ther. 2009;30:908–18.

36. Biddle WL, Greenberger NJ, Swan JT, McPhee MS, Miner Jr PB. 5-Aminosalicylic acid enemas: effective agent in maintaining remission in left-sided ulcerative colitis. Gastroenterology. 1988;94:1075–9.

37. D'Arienzo A, Panarese A, D'Armiento FP, et al. 5-Aminosalicylic acid suppositories in the maintenance of remission in idiopathic proctitis or proctosigmoiditis: a double-blind placebo-controlled clinical trial. Am J Gastroenterol. 1990;85:1079–82.

38. Mantzaris GJ, Hatzis A, Petraki K, Spiliadi C, Triantaphyllou G. Intermittent therapy with high-dose 5-aminosalicylic acid enemas maintains remission in ulcerative proctitis and proctosigmoiditis. Dis Colon Rectum. 1994;37:58–62.

39. D'Albasio G, Paoluzi P, Campieri M, et al. Maintenance treatment of ulcerative proctitis with mesalazine suppositories: a double-blind placebo-controlled trial. The Italian IBD Study Group. Am J Gastroenterol. 1998;93:799–803.

40. Marteau P, Crand J, Foucault M, Rambaud JC. Use of mesalazine slow release suppositories 1 g three times per week to maintain remission of ulcerative proctitis: a randomised double blind placebo controlled multicentre study. Gut. 1998;42:195–9.

41. Hanauer S, Good LI, Goodman MW, et al. Long-term use of mesalamine (Rowasa) suppositories in remission maintenance of ulcerative proctitis. Am J Gastroenterol. 2000;95:1749–54.

42. Andreoli A, Spinella S, Levenstein S, Prantera C. 5-ASA enema versus oral sulphasalazine in maintaining remission in ulcerative colitis. Ital J Gastroenterol. 1994;26:121–5.

43. d'Albasio G, Trallori G, Ghetti A, et al. Intermittent therapy with high-dose 5-aminosalicylic acid enemas for maintaining remission in ulcerative proctosigmoiditis. Dis Colon Rectum. 1990;33: 394–7.

44. Cohen RD, Woseth DM, Thisted RA, et al. A meta-analysis and overview of the literature on treatment options for left-sided ulcerative colitis and ulcerative proctitis. Am J Gastroenterol. 2000;95:1263–76.

45. Lindgren S, Lofberg R, Bergholm L, et al. Effect of budesonide enema on remission and relapse rate in distal ulcerative colitis and proctitis. Scand J Gastroeterol. 2002;37:705–10.

46. d'Albasio G, Pacini F, Camarri E, et al. Combined therapy with 5-aminosalicylic acid tablets and enemas for maintaining remission in ulcerative colitis: a randomized double-blind study. Am J Gastroenterol. 1997;92:1143–7.

47. Yokoyama H, Takagi S, Kuriyama S, et al. Effect of weekend 5-aminosalicylic acid (mesalazine) enema as maintenance therapy for ulcerative colitis: results from a randomized controlled study. Inflamm Bowel Dis. 2007;13:1115–20.

48. Jewell DP, Truelove SC. Azathioprine in ulcerative colitis: final report on controlled therapeutic trial. Br Med J. 1974;4:627–30.

49. Adler DJ, Korelitz BI. The therapeutic efficacy of 6-mercaptopurine in refractory ulcerative colitis. Am J Gastroenterol. 1990;85: 717–22.

50. Steinhart AH, Baker JP, Brzezinski A, Prokipchuk EJ. Azathioprine therapy in chronic ulcerative colitis. J Clin Gastroenterol. 1990;12: 271–5.

51. Lobo AJ, Foster PN, Burke DA, Johnston D, Axon AT. The role of azathioprine in the management of ulcerative colitis. Dis Colon Rectum. 1990;33:374–7.

52. George J, Present DH, Pou R, Bodian C, Rubin PH. The long-term outcome of ulcerative colitis treated with 6-mercaptopurine. Am J Gastroenterol. 1996;91:1711–4.

53. Khan ZH, Mayberry JF, Spiers N, Wicks AC. Retrospective case series analysis of patients with inflammatory bowel disease on azathioprine. A district general hospital experience. Digestion. 2000;62:249–54.

54. Fraser AG, Orchard TR, Jewell DP. The efficacy of azathioprine for the treatment of inflammatory bowel disease: a 30 year review. Gut. 2002;50:485–9.

55. Mate-Jimenez J, Hermida C, Cantero-Perona J, Moreno-Otero R. 6-mercaptopurine or methotrexate added to prednisone induces and maintains remission in steroid-dependent inflammatory bowel disease. Eur J Gastroenterol Hepatol. 2000;12:1227–33.

56. Actis GC, Fadda M, Pellicano R, David E, Rizzetto M, Sapino A. The 17-year single-center experience with the use of azathioprine to maintain remission in ulcerative colitis. Biomed Pharmacother. 2009;63:362–5.

57. Jharap B, Seinen ML, de Boer NK, et al. Thiopurine therapy in inflammatory bowel disease patients: analyses of two 8-year intercept cohorts. Inflamm Bowel Dis. 2010;16:1541–9.

58. Gisbert JP, Nino P, Cara C, et al. Comparative effectiveness of azathioprine in Crohn's disease and ulcerative colitis: prospective, long-term, follow-up study of 394 patients. Aliment Pharmacol Ther. 2008;28:228–38.

59. Sood A, Midha V, Sood N, Kaushal V. Role of azathioprine in severe ulcerative colitis: one-year, placebo-controlled, randomized trial. Indian J Gastroenterol. 2000;19:14–6.

60. Sood A, Kaushal V, Midha V, Bhatia KL, Sood N, Malhotra V. The beneficial effect of azathioprine on maintenance of remission in severe ulcerative colitis. J Gastroenterol. 2002;37:270–4.

61. Sood A, Midha V, Sood N, Avasthi G. Azathioprine versus sulfasalazine in maintenance of remission in severe ulcerative colitis. Indian J Gastroenterol. 2003;22:79–81.

62. Ardizzone S, Maconi G, Russo A, Imbesi V, Colombo E, Bianchi PG. Randomised controlled trial of azathioprine and 5-aminosalicylic acid for treatment of steroid dependent ulcerative colitis. Gut. 2006;55:47–53.

63. Hawthorne AB, Logan RF, Hawkey CJ, et al. Randomised controlled trial of azathioprine withdrawal in ulcerative colitis. BMJ. 1992;305:20–2.

64. Timmer A, McDonald JW, Macdonald JK. Azathioprine and 6-mercaptopurine for maintenance of remission in ulcerative colitis. Cochrane Database Syst Rev. 2007; (1):CD000478.

65. Gisbert JP, Linares PM, McNicholl AG, Maté J, Gomollón F. Meta-analysis: the efficacy of azathioprine and mercaptopurine in ulcerative colitis. Aliment Pharmacol Ther. 2009;30:126–37.

66. Leung Y, Panaccione R, Hemmelgarn B, Jones J. Exposing the weaknesses: a systematic review of azathioprine efficacy in ulcerative colitis. Dig Dis Sci. 2008;53:1455–61.

67. Khan KJ, Dubinsky MC, Ford AC, Ullman TA, Talley NJ, Moayyedi P. Efficacy of immunosuppressive therapy for inflammatory bowel disease: a systematic review and meta-analysis. Am J Gastroenterol. 2011;106:630–42.

68. Actis GC, Bresso F, Astegiano M, et al. Safety and efficacy of azathioprine in the maintenance of ciclosporin-induced remission of ulcerative colitis. Aliment Pharmacol Ther. 2001;15:1307–11.

69. Domènech E, Garcia-Planella E, Bernal I, et al. Azathioprine without oral ciclosporin in the long-term maintenance of remission induced by intravenous ciclosporin in severe, steroid-refractory ulcerative colitis. Aliment Pharmacol Ther. 2002;16:2061–5.

70. Chebli LA, Chaves LD, Pimentel FF, et al. Azathioprine maintains long-term steroid-free remission through 3 years in patients with steroid-dependent ulcerative colitis. Inflamm Bowel Dis. 2010;16:613–9.

71. Cassinotti A, Actis GC, Duca P, et al. Maintenance treatment with azathioprine in ulcerative colitis: outcome and predictive factors after drug withdrawal. Am J Gastroenterol. 2009;104:2760–7.

72. de Boer NK, Wong DR, Jharap B, et al. Dose-dependent influence of 5-aminosalicylates on thiopurine metabolism. Am J Gastroenterol. 2007;102:2747–53.

73. Mantzaris GJ, Sfakianakis M, Archavlis E, et al. A prospective randomized observer-blind 2-year trial of azathioprine monotherapy versus azathioprine and olsalazine for the maintenance of remission of steroid-dependent ulcerative colitis. Am J Gastroenterol. 2004;99:1122–8.

74. Campbell S, Ghosh S. Effective maintenance of inflammatory bowel disease remission by azathioprine does not require concurrent 5-aminosalicylate therapy. Eur J Gastroenterol Hepatol. 2001;13:1297–301.

75. Holtmann MH, Krummenauer F, Claas C, et al. Long-term effectiveness of azathioprine in IBD beyond 4 years: a European multicenter study in 1176 patients. Dig Dis Sci. 2006;51:1516–24.

76. Su CG, Stein RB, Lewis JD, Lichtenstein GR. Azathioprine or 6-mercaptopurine for inflammatory bowel disease: do risks outweigh benefits? Dig Liver Dis. 2000;32:518–31.

77. Lewis JD, Gelfand JM, Troxel AB, et al. Immunosuppressant medications and mortality in inflammatory bowel disease. Am J Gastroenterol. 2008;103:1428–35.

78. Sandborn WJ, Rutgeerts P, Feagan BG, et al. Colectomy rate comparison after treating ulcerative colitis with placebo or infliximab. Gastroenterology. 2009;137:1250–60. quiz 1520.

79. Colombel JF, Rutgeerts P, Reinisch W, et al. Early mucosal healing with infliximab is associated with improved long-term clinical outcomes in ulcerative colitis. Gastroenterology. 2011;141:1194.

80. Reinisch W, Sandborn WJ, Rutgeerts P, et al. Long-term infliximab maintenance therapy for ulcerative colitis: the ACT-1 and ACT-2 extension studies. Inflamm Bowel Dis. 2012;18:201.

81. Van Assche G, Vermeire S, Rutgeerts P. Infliximab: the evidence for its place in therapy in ulcerative colitis. Core Evid. 2008;2:151–61.

82. Gisbert JP, Gonzalvez-Lama Y, Mate J. Systematic review: infliximab therapy in ulcerative colitis. Aliment Pharmacol Ther. 2007; 25:19–37.

83. Gustavsson A, Järnerot G, Hertervig E, et al. Clinical trial: colectomy after rescue therapy in ulcerative colitis - 3-year follow-up of the Swedish-Danish controlled infliximab study. Aliment Pharmacol Ther. 2010;32:984–9.

84. Ferrante M, Vermeire S, Fidder H, et al. Long-term outcome after infliximab for refractory ulcerative colitis. J Crohns Colitis. 2008;2:219–25.

85. Oussalah A, Evesque L, Laharie D, et al. Multicenter experience with infliximab for ulcerative colitis: outcomes and predictors of response, optimization, colectomy, and hospitalization. Am J Gastroenterol. 2010;105:2617–25.

86. Seow CH, Newman A, Irwin SP, Steinhart AH, Silverberg MS, Greenberg GR. Trough serum infliximab: a predictive factor of clinical outcome for infliximab treatment in acute ulcerative colitis. Gut. 2010;59:49–54.

87. Oussalah A, Chevaux JB, Fay R, Sandborn WJ, Bigard MA, Peyrin-Biroulet L. Predictors of infliximab failure after azathioprine withdrawal in Crohn's disease treated with combination therapy. Am J Gastroenterol. 2010;105:1142–9.

88. Van Assche G, Magdelaine-Beuzelin C, D'Haens G, et al. Withdrawal of immunosuppression in Crohn's disease treated with scheduled infliximab maintenance: a randomized trial. Gastroenterology. 2008;134:1861–8.

89. Cotlyar DS, Osterman MT, Diamond RH, et al. A systematic review of factors that contribute to hepatosplenic T-cell lymphoma in patients with inflammatory bowel disease. Clin Gastroenterol Hepatol. 2011;9:36–41.

90. Rahier JF, Ben-Horin S, Chowers Y, et al. European evidence-based Consensus on the prevention, diagnosis and management of opportunistic infections in inflammatory bowel disease. J Crohns Colitis. 2009;3:47–91.

91. Rahier JF, Yazdanpanah Y, Colombel JF, Travis S. The European (ECCO) Consensus on infection in IBD: what does it change for the clinician? Gut. 2009;58:1313–5.

92. Afif W, Leighton JA, Hanauer SB, et al. Open-label study of adalimumab in patients with ulcerative colitis including those with

prior loss of response or intolerance to infliximab. Inflamm Bowel Dis. 2009;15:1302–7.

93. Oussalah A, Laclotte C, Chevaux JB, et al. Long-term outcome of adalimumab therapy for ulcerative colitis with intolerance or lost response to infliximab: a single-centre experience. Aliment Pharmacol Ther. 2008;28:966–72.

94. Gies N, Kroeker KI, Wong K, Fedorak RN. Treatment of ulcerative colitis with adalimumab or infliximab: long-term follow-up of a single-centre cohort. Aliment Pharmacol Ther. 2010;32: 522–8.

95. Taxonera C, Estelles J, Blanco I, et al. Adalimumab for ulcerative colitis patients previously treated with infliximab: outcomes at short and long term and predictors of response. Aliment Pharmacol Ther. 2011;33:340–8.

96. Hudis N, Rajca B, Polyak S, et al. The outcome of active ulcerative colitis treated with adalimumab. Gastroenterology. 2009;136:A661.

97. Fiorino G, Peyrin-Biroulet L, Repici A, Malesci A, Danese S. Adalimumab in ulcerative colitis: hypes and hopes. Expert Opin Biol Ther. 2011;11:109–16.

98. Sandborn WJ, Van Assche G, Reinisch W, et al. Induction and maintenance of clinical remission by adalimumab in patients with moderate-to-severe ulcerative colitis. J Crohn's Colitis. 2011;5: S1–192.

99. Nathan DM, Iser JH, Gibson PR. A single center experience with methotrexate in the treatment of Crohn's disease and ulcerative colitis: a case for subcutaneous administration. J Gastronterol Hepatol. 2008;23:954–8.

100. Wahed M, Louis-Auguste JR, Baxter LM, et al. Efficacy of methotrexate in Crohn's disease and ulcerative colitis patients unresponsive or intolerant to azathioprine/mercaptopurine. Aliment Pharmacol Ther. 2009;30:614–20.

101. Cummings JR, Herrlinger KR, Travis SP, Gorard DA, McIntyre AS, Jewell DP. Oral methotrexate in ulcerative colitis. Aliment Pharmacol Ther. 2005;21:385–9.

102. Oren R, Aber N, Odes S, et al. Methotrexate in chronic active ulcerative colitis: a double-blind, randomized, Israeli multicenter trial. Gastroenterology. 1996;110:1416–21.

103. El Matary W, Vandermeer B, Griffiths AM. Methotrexate for maintenance of remission in ulcerative colitis. Cochrane database Syst rev. 2009; (3):CD007560.

104. Aslan A, Triadafilopoulos G. Fish oil fatty acid supplementation in active ulcerative colitis: a double-blind, placebo-controlled, crossover study. Am J Gastroenterol. 1992;87:432–7.

105. Hawthorne AB, Daneshmend TK, Hawkey CJ, et al. Treatment of ulcerative colitis with fish oil supplementation: a prospective 12 month randomised controlled trial. Gut. 1992;33:922–8.

106. Greenfield SM, Green AT, Teare JP, et al. A randomized controlled study of evening primrose oil and fish oil in ulcerative colitis. Aliment Pharmacol Ther. 1993;7:159–66.

107. Mantzaris GJ, Archavlis E, Zografos C, et al. A prospective, randomized, placebo-controlled study of fish oil in ulcerative colitis. Hellenic J Gastroenterol. 1996;9:138–41.

108. Turner D, Steinhart AH, Griffiths AM. Omega 3 fatty acids (fish oil) for maintenance of remission in ulcerative colitis. Cochrane Database Syst Rev. 2007; (3):CD006443.

109. Rahimi R, Nifkar S, Rezaei A, Abdollahi M. A meta-analysis of the benefit of probiotics in maintaining remission of human ulcerative colitis: evidence for prevention of disease relapse and maintenance of remission. Arch Med Sci. 2008;4:185–90.

110. Gilat T, Leichtman G, Delpre G, Eshchar J, Bar MS, Fireman Z. A comparison of metronidazole and sulfasalazine in the maintenance of remission in patients with ulcerative colitis. J Clin Gastroenterol. 1989;11:392–5.

111. Turunen UM, Farkkila MA, Hakala K, et al. Long-term treatment of ulcerative colitis with ciprofloxacin: a prospective, double-blind, placebo-controlled study. Gastroenterology. 1998;115:1072–8.

112. Present DH. Ciprofloxacin as a treatment for ulcerative colitis-not yet. Gastroenterology. 1998;115:1289–91.

113. Kruis W, Schutz E, Fric P, Fixa B, Judmaier G, Stolte M. Double-blind comparison of an oral Escherichia coli preparation and mesalazine in maintaining remission of ulcerative colitis. Aliment Pharmacol Ther. 1997;11:853–8.

114. Rembacken BJ, Snelling AM, Hawkey PM, Chalmers DM, Axon AT. Non-pathogenic Escherichia coli versus mesalazine for the treatment of ulcerative colitis: a randomised trial. Lancet. 1999; 354:635–9.

115. Kruis W, Fric P, Poktrotnieks J, et al. Maintaining remission of ulcerative colitis with the probiotic Escherichia coli Nissle 1917 is as effective as with standard mesalazine. Gut. 2004;53:1617–23.

116. Henker J, Müller S, Laass MW, Schreiner A, Schulze J. Probiotic Escherichia coli Nissle 1917 (EcN) for successful remission maintenance of ulcerative colitis in children and adolescents: an open-label pilot study. Gastroenterology. 2008;46:874–5.

117. Zocco MA, dal Verme LZ, Cremonini F, et al. Efficacy of Lactobacillus GG in maintaining remission of ulcerative colitis. Aliment Pharmacol Ther. 2006;23:1567–74.

118. Koutroubakis IE, Vlachonikolis IG. Appendectomy and the development of ulcerative colitis: results of a metaanalysis of published case-control studies. Am J Gastroenterol. 2000;95:171–6.

119. Andersson RE, Olaison G, Tysk C, Ekbom A. Appendectomy and protection against ulcerative colitis. N Engl J Med. 2001;344: 808–14.

120. Cosnes J, Carbonnel F, Beaugerie L, Blain A, Reijasse D, Gendre JP. Effects of appendicectomy on the course of ulcerative colitis. Gut. 2002;51:803–7.

121. Bolin TD, Wong S, Crouch R, Engelman JL, Riordan SM. Appendicectomy as a therapy for ulcerative proctitis. Am J Gastroenterol. 2009;104:2476–82.

122. Sandborn WJ. Rational selection of oral 5-aminosalicylic acid formulations and prodrugs for the treatment of ulcerative colitis. Am J Gastroenterol. 2002;27:2939–41.

123. Moody GA, Eaden JA, Helyes Z, Mayberry JF. Oral or rectal administration of drugs in IBD? Aliment Pharmacol Ther. 1997;11:999–1000.

124. Casellas F, Vaquero E, Armengol JR, Malagelada JR. Practicality of 5-aminosalicylic acid suppositories for long-term treatment of inactive distal ulcerative colitis. Hepatogastroenterology. 1999;46: 2343–6.

125. Andus T, Kocjan A, Müser M, et al. International Salofalk Suppository OD Study Group. Clinical trial: a novel high-dose 1 g mesalamine suppository (Salofalk) once daily is as efficacious as a 500-mg suppository thrice daily in active ulcerative proctitis. Inflamm Bowel Dis. 2010;16:1947–56.

126. Lamet M. A Multicenter, Randomized study to evaluate the efficacy and safety of mesalamine suppositories 1 g at bedtime and 500 mg twice daily in patients with active mild-to-moderate ulcerative proctitis. Dig Dis Sci. 2011;56:513–22.

127. Brunel M, Penne C, Tiret E, Balladur P, Parc R. Restorative proctocolectomy for distal ulcerative colitis. Gut. 1999;45:542–5.

# Management of Irritable Bowel Syndrome in the Patient with Ulcerative Colitis

40

Philip M. Ginsburg and Theodore M. Bayless

**Keywords**

Irritable bowel syndrome • Ulcerative colitis • Diarrhea • IPAA • Proctosigmoiditis • Prevalence • Inflammation

Irritable bowel syndrome (IBS) is one of the most common disorders in gastroenterology, affecting 10–15 % of the US population [1] and accounting for one-quarter to one-half of all visits to digestive health specialists. With such a high prevalence, it may be inferred that a significant number of patients with ulcerative colitis (UC) also suffer from coexisting IBS. Indeed, it is widely believed that the prevalence of IBS is greater in patients with inflammatory bowel disease (IBD), affecting an estimated one-third of UC patients in remission [2–5]. Recent research demonstrating a possible association between low-grade inflammation and IBS highlights the interconnecting relationship between inflammatory and functional disorders.

Many patients with UC are initially misdiagnosed with IBS, leading to delays in initiating effective medical therapies and increasing the risk of disease-related complications. Conversely, long after the diagnosis of IBD is made, patients and/or their caregivers may either forget a preexisting IBS diagnosis or assume that preexisting IBS symptoms were actually the unappreciated (and undiagnosed) onset of IBD. This becomes an issue when physicians are confronted with cases of "refractory UC." Differentiating between inflammatory and functional symptoms is crucial to avoiding inappropriate escalation of misdirected treatments that are often ineffective, increase the risk of side effects and drug-induced toxicities, and negatively impact on the patient-physician relationship.

These difficult issues raise several important questions: (1) How does one make the diagnosis of IBS in a patient with established UC? (2) Does "stress" trigger UC flares? (3) Can UC or its treatment aggravate IBS? (4) Can IBS be the cause for refractory symptoms in a UC patient? (5) How do we treat IBS in our UC patients?

## Prevalence

In the USA, two-thirds of patients who seek medical attention for IBS are women. A survey of healthy college students at the University of North Carolina found that 15 % of respondents report symptoms attributable to IBS [1]. Thompson and Heaton reported a 14 % prevalence of functional complaints among a healthy English population, most of whom had not consulted a doctor [6]. Among patients with IBD, the problem is at least equivalent in scope. In a population-based prospective cohort study from Manitoba, 14 % of newly diagnosed IBD patients with symptoms for >3 years were considered to also have likely or possible IBS [7].

The prevalence of IBS may be higher among patients with IBD, probably more so in Crohn's disease (CD) but clinically relevant in UC nonetheless. Isgar et al. found that 33 % of patients with quiescent UC described symptoms that met criteria for IBS compared with 7 % of healthy controls [2]. In a Swedish survey, 33 % of UC and 57 % of CD patients who had been in remission for at least 1 year reported IBS-like symptoms [3]. Another study reported 32 % of UC and

P.M. Ginsburg, M.D., F.A.C.G. (✉)
Gastroenterology Center of Connecticut, Yale-New Haven Hospital, 2200 Whitney Avenue, Suite 360, Hamden, CT 06518, USA
e-mail: pginsburg@gastrocenter.org

T.M. Bayless, M.D.
Division of Gastroenterology, Johns Hopkins Medical Institutions, 600 N. Wolfe St., Baltimore, MD 21287, USA
e-mail: tbayless@jhmi.edu

G.R. Lichtenstein (ed.), *Medical Therapy of Ulcerative Colitis*,
DOI 10.1007/978-1-4939-1677-1_40, © Springer Science+Business Media New York 2014

431

42 % of CD patients in remission met Rome II criteria for IBS versus 8 % of controls [4]. Keohane et al. found that 39 % of UC and 60 % of CD patients fulfilled Rome II criteria for IBS despite being considered to be in clinical remission by predefined criteria, although fecal calprotectin levels were higher in these groups compared with those without IBS-type symptoms [5]. The prevalence of IBS-like symptoms in a group of Iranian patients with UC in remission was 46 % based on Rome II criteria versus 13 % of controls [8].

These reports highlight the challenges in performing epidemiological studies because the Rome criteria are not applicable to patients with IBD and no objective bioassay reliably distinguishes between IBD activity and functional symptoms. Regardless, the magnitude of the problem among IBD patients is at least comparable with the general population, probably higher.

## Diagnosis

How does one make the diagnosis of IBS in a patient with UC? This is a common clinical dilemma. IBS remains a clinical diagnosis which relies on a careful history. One common refrain among patients is "I've always had a nervous stomach." A history of typical functional symptoms going back to childhood is an important clue. IBS usually begins in the teenage years or in the early 20s, and one-third of patients can recall symptoms going back to adolescence. Since one of the hallmarks of colitis is rectal bleeding, it is often much simpler to date the initial onset of UC as compared with Crohn's. Patients with coexisting IBS may report functional symptoms such as alternating bowel habits, postprandial urgency, pain and/or bloating relieved by defecation, or stress-related diarrhea, especially in the morning or worse with certain foods. When such symptoms predate the initial onset of rectal bleeding, one may infer that there is a noninflammatory component. This can be especially challenging when UC began in childhood.

Certainly these symptoms can also occur when UC is active, but this is where a sigmoidoscopy can help because symptoms that are disproportionate to objective findings strongly suggest the presence of coexisting IBS. The typical patient with predominantly functional symptoms may complain of marked urgency and diarrhea, yet have only minimal or quiescent endoscopic disease activity. Other objective tests such as fecal calprotectin have also proven useful [9]. It is very important to differentiate between inflammatory and noninflammatory causes of symptoms. Although IBS patients often have a perception that their symptoms are due to active UC, caregivers must avoid reinforcing such misperceptions.

Inappropriately starting or escalating IBD therapies in such patients may have several deleterious consequences, including: (1) potential toxicities of misdirected treatments, (2) side effects of some IBD medications can actually worsen IBS, (3) failure to respond leading to being mislabeled as "refractory UC," (4) somatic symptoms may be reinforced and perpetuate a negative cycle that occasionally leads to narcotic dependence and/or depression, and (5) the physician-patient relationship may suffer. The importance of establishing a functional cause for patient symptoms cannot be overstated.

There is much interest in developing reliable biomarkers and genetic techniques for both IBS and ulcerative colitis. In the future, objective and noninvasive tests may help distinguish between IBS and IBD. However, a careful history and selective use of endoscopy and adjunctive laboratory tests are usually adequate to make both diagnoses.

## Inflammation and IBS

Does IBD predispose to IBS? It is well known that inflammation is associated with intestinal irritability, motility disturbances, and visceral hypersensitivity [10–12]. Animal models of experimental and infectious colitis reveal that motility changes persist after resolution of acute inflammation [13, 14]. Interestingly, colonic irritability can be demonstrated even when a preceding infection was limited to the proximal small bowel. In humans, we have indirect evidence showing differences in colonic motility and visceral hypersensitivity in patients with quiescent versus active ulcerative colitis [15, 16]. Small bowel and gastric dysmotility have been demonstrated in patients with ulcerative colitis [17], suggesting that active UC may lead to more generalized gut-motor dysfunction even in areas distant from the inflammation.

Immunology has traditionally been the realm of IBD, but recent interest has focused on the presence of immune activation in IBS. This pertains to both innate and adaptive immune responses as evidenced by numerous studies which have demonstrated increased activation of proinflammatory cytokines, mast cells, and monocytes in the peripheral blood and mucosa of subpopulations of patients with IBS [18]. There is experimental evidence in IBS that increased epithelial barrier permeability, and gut bacteria may drive a host immune response characterized by T-cell activation and chronic low-grade inflammation [18]. Sounds familiar? While a complete review of the immunopathogenesis of IBS is beyond the scope of this chapter, it is interesting to speculate: Are shared pathways of immune activation in IBD and IBS responsible for the significant overlap between these two syndromes frequently encountered in the clinic?

It is unknown whether ulcerative colitis causes IBS because its very presence affects measurable parameters such as motility and permeability. However, there is a condition which may provide insight: postinfectious IBS.

## Postinfectious IBS

First described in 1962 [19], postinfectious IBS (PI-IBS) is a condition wherein sensory-motor dysfunction persists long after resolution of an acute enteric infection. PI-IBS has been reported to occur in up to 30 % of individuals following acute bacterial gastroenteritis. Predictors include severity of the infection, psychological distress, and persistent low-grade inflammation. Indeed, it has been hypothesized that psychological stress during an acute infection may result in permanent alterations in central and enteric nervous system pathways which lead to visceral hypersensitivity and motility disturbances [20]. Drossman has also proposed that psychological distress may lead to a perpetuation of gut inflammation through psychoimmunologic mechanisms. Even in endoscopically normal appearing mucosa, studies in humans with PI-IBS have suggested a continuing presence of chronic low-grade inflammation with increased gut permeability following resolution of acute bacterial gastroenteritis.

Several valuable lessons may be drawn from the PI-IBS model. The first is that acute inflammation is an important determinant of subsequent irritability. The second is that inflammation and factors important in IBS (motor disorder, visceral hypersensitivity) may be linked. Thirdly, the combination of acute inflammation and psychological distress increases the likelihood of developing irritable bowel syndrome. Lastly, it is possible that psychological distress or even IBS itself may cause or potentiate chronic low-grade inflammation. In other words, can IBS cause or worsen IBD? Additional studies are needed to address this intriguing question.

## Management of IBS in UC Patient

How do we treat IBS when it occurs in patients with UC? A constructive physician-patient relationship is important. So is a careful history. First, the patient and physician must each recognize when symptoms are due to IBS and avoid misattributing them to UC. Indeed, we believe that insight and acceptance as to the functional nature of some symptoms are fundamental to effective care of the IBS/IBD patient. In this respect, the first (and perhaps most important) step in management is education and gentle redirection in the form of a thoughtful conversation.

## Diet

Medical management starts with conservative dietary and lifestyle modifications. Many patients report a perception that certain foods aggravate their colitis. When ulcerative colitis is active, especially when there is severe inflammation, it is true that certain foods, especially high residue or fatty foods, may be difficult for an inflamed colon to handle, and this can result in worsened symptoms of pain, bloating, and diarrhea. However, it is important to note that no single dietary factor has been consistently shown to affect disease activity in UC. Patients should be educated that certain foods may exacerbate symptoms, but what they eat will not worsen their disease because UC is an immune system disorder. When UC is active, the primary focus should be to first treat the inflammation with appropriate medical therapies and then address any residual irritability afterward.

Once UC is in remission, dietary management of lingering symptoms is similar to standard recommendations for IBS with some important distinctions. A thorough dietary history is important, and some patients are helped by keeping a food and symptom diary and then modifying their diets accordingly. A useful list for gassy and diarrhea patients is included in Table 40.1. Attempts should be made to lessen steatorrhea, gas production, and stool volume by avoiding caffeine, lactose, fructose, sorbitol, and "gassy" foods and adhering to a low-fat diet. Given the high prevalence of lactose intolerance, selected patients should be encouraged to adhere to a lactose-free diet. If lactose intolerance is questionable, patients may test themselves with two glasses of skim milk on an empty stomach and check for symptoms over the next 2–4 h. Lactose-hydrolyzed milk and lactase enzymes are widely available. Soy derivatives are also a useful alternative. Fructose, found in many fruits and fruit juices, is an often underappreciated cause of symptoms. Sorbitol is a laxative that is also used as a sugar substitute in sugarless gums and many dietetic candies. Patients should be told to read labels carefully and avoid sorbitol-containing foods. Large, high-fat, greasy meals may increase intestinal motility and can be particularly troublesome to patients with a spastic bowel, hence, the importance of a low-fat diet. Carbonated beverages and gassy foods such as certain raw or uncooked vegetables should be avoided because colonic fermentation of undigested carbohydrates can produce large amounts of gas, which distends the spastic colon. In IBS patients with longstanding UC, the colon may be foreshortened, tubular, or poorly compliant as a result of prior inflammation. The result can be significant pain, bloating, and diarrhea. Close coordination with a dietician can be helpful for those with persistent symptoms.

Caffeine is a potent secretagogue, which deserves special mention. Even modest amounts (75–300 mg) cause transient net small bowel secretion. Dietary methylxanthines inhibit phosphodiesterases in small bowel mucosa causing chloride and fluid secretion into the lumen via increased intracellular cAMP. Normal people do not have diarrhea because the colon can reabsorb this increased fluid load.

**Table 40.1** Gassy foods

| Gassy foods | |
| --- | --- |
| Vegetables (raffinose, soluble fiber) | Artichokes |
| | Asparagus |
| | Beans |
| | Broccoli |
| | Brussels sprouts |
| | Cabbage |
| | Carrots |
| | Cauliflower |
| | Celery |
| | Cucumbers |
| | Green peppers |
| | Lentils |
| | Onions |
| | Peas |
| | Potatoes |
| | Radishes |
| | Shallots |
| | Scallions |
| Fruits (fructose or sorbitol) | Apples |
| | Apricots |
| | Bananas |
| | Oranges |
| | Peaches |
| | Pears |
| | Prunes |
| | Raisins |
| Dairy (lactose) | Cheese |
| | Ice cream |
| | Milk |
| | Processed foods containing milk products |
| | Frozen Yogurt |
| Whole grains (certain types of fiber) | Barley |
| | Flax seed |
| | Oat bran |
| | Wheat |
| Beverages (fructose, sorbitol, carbonation) | Beer |
| | Diet sodas |
| | Fruit juices |
| | Soft drinks |
| | Wine |

However, in patients with both IBS and UC, excessive caffeine intake (such as 1,000 mg per day) can cause severe diarrhea. A typical 12 oz cup of coffee has roughly 200 mg of caffeine, though this varies widely (a "grande" brewed coffee from a specialty coffee shop may have more than 400 mg). We have found that patients often do not appreciate the amount of caffeine they consume in various forms. However, it is important to remember that the average consumption of caffeinated beverages has risen significantly in recent years, and patients frequently fail to report even large quantities of regular intake either because they don't realize it or due to a misperception that their intake is not excessive. Once identified, this problem is easily corrected with a simple dietary adjustment.

## Adjunctive Therapies

There has been much interest in the use of antibiotics in IBS. There is circumstantial evidence that gut flora may play a role in the pathophysiology of IBS. Indeed, a 2-week course of rifaximin, a minimally absorbed antibiotic, at 550 mg three times a day was found to significantly improve symptoms of bloating, abdominal pain, and loose or watery stools among patients who had IBS without constipation [21]. This therapeutic approach for IBS was not given FDA approval. On the other hand, it may be premature to conclude that small intestinal bacterial overgrowth (SIBO) causes IBS [22]. To our knowledge there are no data in patients with coexisting IBS/IBD. However, SIBO can complicate IBD and this is more of a problem in Crohn's than in UC. Although commonly used in clinical practice, commercially available breath tests have been criticized for being inaccurate at diagnosing SIBO [22]. Instead, they do accurately measure the speed of small bowel transit, which is often increased in IBS patients. We will occasionally give a short course of rifaximin for patients with IBS/UC with bloating, cramps, and diarrhea or if SIBO is suspected on clinical grounds. It is important to avoid repeated courses of certain antibiotics due to the high risk of *C. difficile* in UC patients. The role of the fecal microbiome in patients with UC and in patients with IBS is evolving. Perhaps a better understanding of the differences will lead to better disease-specific treatments [23].

Antispasmodics can be used as an adjunct for crampy abdominal pain or urgency, especially when symptoms occur immediately after eating. We have also found them to be useful for patients who have difficulty holding mesalamine enemas (instruct patient to take a dicyclomine or hyoscyamine tablet and a warm bath before administering the enema to help relax the spastic response to rectal and sigmoid distension). Antidiarrheals are helpful for controlling symptoms of diarrhea, although patients should be warned to take only as directed. Fiber supplements are also very good adjuncts. For diarrhea, fiber provides bulk to the stool and takes in water. For constipation or those with pellet-like or ribbonlike stools, fiber supplements taken with plenty of water help to regularize and give form to movements. For alternators who bounce between the two extremes, we have found that fiber drives patients' bowel habits toward the middle. Care should be taken to avoid certain types of dietary or over-the-counter fiber formulations such as psyllium that worsen gassiness (Table 40.1). Our experience with using tricyclic antidepressants to treat functional gastrointestinal disorders suggests that they may provide important benefit in selected circumstances. We have also referred some patients for psychotherapy, which may help with coping.

## Complementary Therapies

Alternative therapies such as hypnosis, acupuncture, yoga, and other complementary approaches are often employed by our patients and should be encouraged when appropriate. However, patients should be cautioned to avoid herbal remedies, which may contain laxatives, nonsteroidal antiinflammatory drugs (NSAIDS), or psychotropic ingredients. Many such agents also have potent active pharmaceutical ingredients that may have toxic effects. Since most herbal remedies are not regulated and have not been rigorously evaluated in large-scale multicenter randomized placebo-controlled studies, the risks versus benefits of individual products are unknown, and there is at least theoretical potential that certain ingredients may worsen IBD.

Probiotics are generally considered to be complementary therapies. Although various probiotic formulations have been used for both IBS and IBD, evidence-based data in patients with IBS is lacking and there is no current consensus regarding efficacy. In IBD, there are some reasonable data in antibiotic-responsive pouchitis patients and in maintenance of moderate UC in remission. It is recognized that (a) patients often make use of probiotic supplements, (b) probiotics are not subject to FDA regulation, (c) most formulations appear to be safe, (d) many are costly and not covered by prescription benefit plans, and (e) further research is needed. This is an area of interest in both the IBS and IBD communities.

## Special Populations

The following examples describe commonly encountered clinical situations and highlight how a thorough understanding of underlying pathophysiological mechanisms may aid in constructing a comprehensive treatment plan for patients with IBS/IBD.

## Postcholecystectomy Syndrome

Postcholecystectomy syndrome is a particular problem in patients with coexisting IBS and UC. The colon in patients with IBS is hypersensitive to distension. This can be modeled experimentally with balloon studies, which induce painful spastic contractions in patients with IBS. The clinical correlate occurs when increased volume of gas, fluid, and stool enters the left colon after a fatty meal. The increased volume in the colon can cause spasm and pain in

a patient with IBS and UC. Surgical removal of the gallbladder in patients who already have this physiology can result in a "perfect storm" because bile salt wasting and maldigestion of dietary fats magnify the problem. The combination of IBS, UC, and cholecystectomy can result in severe pain, gassiness, and diarrhea. This syndrome can be effectively treated with a low-fat diet, bile salt sequestrants such as cholestyramine, and/or antidiarrheals. Narcotics are to be carefully avoided. If narcotics are prescribed for left sigmoid colon pain, a vicious cycle of chronic pain may ensue because narcotic medications enhance the spastic response to distension.

## Active Proctosigmoiditis

We are all familiar with the splenic flexure syndrome in which there is a postprandial contraction of the sigmoid colon, followed by often painful distension of the proximal colon, especially in the area of the more cephalad bowel. Since the colons of some patients with IBS are more sensitive to this distension, the pain produced in the left upper quadrant can be quite severe. Constipation even in healthy subjects can cause one or more symptoms of IBS.

Active colitis produces colonic motor changes that are magnified in patients with coexisting IBS. An inflamed left colon worsens the spastic response to distension and also results in increased speed of transit, which may exacerbate motility disturbances in patients with coexisting IBS. On the other hand, in patients with active proctitis or proctosigmoiditis, there can be severe spasm in the sigmoid, which may result in seemingly paradoxical complaints of pellet- or ribbonlike stools, incomplete evacuation, bloating, and left upper quadrant pain similar to splenic flexure syndrome.

The clinical correlate is left lower quadrant pain and diarrhea in a patient with IBS and proctosigmoiditis. Patients with IBS have exaggerated sigmoid contractions after eating, due to an enhanced gastrocolic reflex. This is especially true after large fatty meals, which may worsen the pain even further. Active proctosigmoiditis compounds the problem because the inflamed rectum and/or sigmoid is even more sensitive to distension, and alterations in neurovisceral responses produce hyperalgesia. However, symptoms can occur even in the absence of significant inflammation. In this case, one must be careful to avoid misdirected and potentially harmful escalation of IBD therapies. Also, in patients with proctitis, one may be led to the mistaken impression that inflammation has extended up the left side of the colon, as occurs in half of such patients.

Another example is paradoxical constipation and left-sided abdominal pain in a patient with active proctitis or proctosigmoiditis. Splenic flexure syndrome occurs when postprandial sigmoid contractions are followed by painful distension of the hypersensitive proximal colon. In patients with IBD, this can occur with or without constipation. It is important to recognize this problem. We have seen patients with significant active IBD being treated with laxatives on the erroneous assumption that the constipation was functional. Indeed, a significant amount of stool may become retained in the noninflamed proximal colon. This can be seen on imaging, which often shows a dilated stool-filled colon leading down to an inflamed sigmoid and rectum. Sigmoidoscopy confirms the presence of active proctosigmoiditis. Here, the treatment is to escalate IBD therapies, which is in contrast to the first example. Again, a thorough understanding of the underlying pathophysiology will help the astute clinician to distinguish between these situations.

Alerting patients to the coexistence of two syndromes—IBS and IBD—helps them to understand the need to treat both disorders simultaneously. In both examples, we treat the proctosigmoiditis by stepping up IBD therapies and we treat the IBS component with a multifaceted approach. As before, conservative dietary approaches include instructing patients to avoid large high-fat meals, lactose-containing products, and gassy foods (Table 40.1) and to lessen their intake of carbonation, to utilize dietary bulk such as polycarbophil, and to avoid secretagogues such as caffeine. In the first example, antidiarrheals and antispasmodics may be employed as adjuncts, together if needed. In the case of paradoxical constipation, the gentle use of a laxative such as polyethylene glycol-soluble powder should be considered in combination with aggressive therapy of the IBD, including the use of topicals such as mesalamine enemas. Individuals with severe proctosigmoiditis may find it very difficult to tolerate enemas. The problem can be overcome by advising people to take an oral or sublingual antispasmodic immediately prior to introduction of the enema. Warm baths are also helpful in lessening the discomfort from spasm. Narcotic medications should be carefully avoided in both instances, because they themselves cause a hyperactive sigmoid response, creating a vicious cycle of colonic pain and spasm. Emotional stress is known to produce severe colonic spasms in susceptible individuals. To that extent, psychosocial interventions and/or antidepressant medications are occasionally beneficial.

It is important to avoid misattributing functional symptoms as "unresponsive colitis." This may lead to unnecessary and potentially detrimental administration of corticosteroids, immunomodulators, biologics, and even surgery. Also, the potential negative impact on the physician-patient relationship cannot be underestimated.

## Diarrhea After Colectomy with IPAA

A loop of grossly normal small intestine is used to create an ileal pouch for an ileoanal anastomosis (IPAA). These pouches are expected to store about 300 mL of ileal effluent prior to evacuation. Although the normal ileum gradually adapts to this new role, patients' pouches have differing capacities and there is variation in the numbers of bowel movements that may be expected in a 24-hs period. It is important to remember that in patients with IBS the small bowel is as irritable as the colon once was. After IPAA, the pouch is hyperreactive to distension, resulting in diminished pouch capacity, excessive movements, and painful spasms [24]. Such patients might have relatively more bowel movements or marked urgency or even painful spasm after meals or when the pouch is distended. They can only expel half the contents of the already small pouch. Irritable pouch syndrome (IPS) is characterized by decreased pouch compliance, visceral hypersensitivity to balloon distension, and lower-volume thresholds for stool sensation in the absence of pouchitis [25]. Its prevalence at a tertiary referral center with a special pouch disorder clinic was 43 % of 61 consecutive symptomatic IPAA patients [26].

The typical patient has functional pain and/or diarrhea prior to surgery. This may include a lifelong history of IBS symptoms predating the diagnosis of IBD or pain/diarrhea which is disproportionate to objective findings preoperatively. After surgery, patients with severe IPS may suffer greatly, with significant pain and diarrhea as well as seepage, nighttime symptoms, marked urgency, and fecal incontinence. Some patients are willing to accept significant symptoms (and may not even report them to their doctor) because of a fear of needing a permanent ileostomy. On the other hand, it is important to elicit the diagnosis because IPS has been associated with significant morbidity and poor quality of life. Other disorders such as pouchitis, Crohn's, and cuffitis can be excluded with a pouchoscopy. In the appropriate clinical context with absence of related pouch complications, the diagnosis of IPS is made.

Clinical experience has suggested that this special population of patients with IPS have poor outcomes. As before, reassurance and patient education as to the underlying problem forms the cornerstone of conservative therapy and also helps solidify the doctor-patient relationship. Because IPS is a relatively recently described entity, there is a dearth of literature regarding medical treatments. Experience suggests that patients with IPS can be treated with dietary modifications (low-fat diet), adjunctive agents (anticholinergics, antidiarrheals, antispasmodics, bile acid sequestrants), tricyclics, and/or an empiric trial of antibiotics for bacterial overgrowth. Studies in this disorder of biofeedback, cognitive psychotherapy, and naturopathic or complementary therapies are needed. We have found that refractory cases occasionally require pouch excision. Along these lines, careful consideration should be given to avoiding IPAA surgery in patients with severe IBS. One of our patients with IPS reportedly committed suicide.

## Physician-Patient Relationship

We have found it very helpful to explain to the patient with irritable bowel syndrome and inflammatory bowel disease that he or she has two disorders and that each may cause its own symptoms. Explaining the pathophysiology helps the patient understand the nature of their condition. Oftentimes patients respond to gentle redirection and reassurance. Insight into the role that anxiety plays may go a long way to alleviating stress-related symptoms. It is important that patients receive positive reinforcement and feel that their complaints are being listened to, because adherence with medical recommendations is enhanced by a constructive doctor-patient relationship. This is increasingly important in the current medical climate.

## References

1. Sandler RS, Drossman DA, Nathan HP, et al. Symptom complaints and health care seeking behavior in subjects with bowel dysfunction. Gastroenterology. 1984;87:314–8.
2. Isgar B, Harman M, Kaye M, et al. Symptoms of irritable bowel syndrome in ulcerative colitis in remission. Gut. 1983;24:190–2.
3. Simrén M, Axelsson J, Gillberg R, Abrahamsson H, Svedlund J, Björnsson ES. Quality of life in inflammatory bowel disease in remission: the impact of IBS-like symptoms and associated psychological factors. Am J Gastroenterol. 2002;97(2):389–96.
4. Minderhoud IM, Oldenburg B, Wismeijer JA, van Berge Henegouwen GP, Smout AJ. IBS-like symptoms in patients with inflammatory bowel disease in remission; relationships with quality of life and coping behavior. Dig Dis Sci. 2004;49(3):469–74.
5. Keohane J, O'Mahony C, O'Mahony L, O'Mahony S, Quigley EM, Shanahan F. Irritable bowel syndrome-type symptoms in patients with inflammatory bowel disease: a real association or reflection of occult inflammation? Am J Gastroenterol. 2010;105(8):1788. 1789-94; quiz 1795. doi: 10.1038/ajg.2010.156. Epub 2010 Apr 13.
6. Thompson WG, Heaton KW. Functional bowel disorders in apparently healthy people. Gastroenterology. 1980;79:283–8.
7. Burgmann T, Clara I, Graff L, et al. The Manitoba Inflammatory Bowel Disease Cohort Study: prolonged symptoms after diagnosis—how much is irritable bowel syndrome? Clin Gastroenterol Hepatol. 2006;4:614–20.
8. Ansari R, Attari F, Razjouyan H, et al. Ulcerative colitis and irritable bowel syndrome: relationships with quality of life. Eur J Gastroenterol Hepatol. 2008;20:46–50.
9. Chang MH, Chou JW, Chen SM, Tsai MC, Sun YS, Lin CC, Lin CP. Faecal calprotectin as a novel biomarker for differentiating between inflammatory bowel disease and irritable bowel syndrome. Mol Med Rep. 2014;10(1):522–6.
10. Geboes K, Collins S. Structural abnormalities of the nervous system in Crohn's disease and ulcerative colitis. Neurogastroenterol Motil. 1998;10:189–202.
11. Shanahan F. Enteric neuropathology and inflammatory bowel disease. Neurogastroenterol Motil. 1998;10:185–7.
12. Collins SM. The immunomodulation of enteric neuromuscular function: implications for motility and inflammatory disorders. Gastroenterology. 1996;111:1683–99.
13. MacPherson BR, Shearon NL, Pfeiffer CJ. Experimental diffuse colitis in cats: observations on motor changes. J Surg Res. 1978;25:42–9.
14. Barbara G, Vallance BA, Collins SM. Persistent intestinal neuromuscular dysfunction after acute nematode infection in mice. Gastroenterology. 1997;113:1224–32.
15. Rao SS, Read NW. Gastrointestinal motility in patients with ulcerative colitis. Scand J Gastroenterol Suppl. 1990;172:22–8.
16. Farthing MJ, Lennard-Jones JE. Sensibility of the rectum to distension and the anorectal distension reflex in ulcerative colitis. Gut. 1978;19:64–9.
17. Manousos ON, Salem SN. Abnormal motility of the small intestine in ulcerative colitis. Gastroenterologia. 1965;104:249–57.
18. Ohman L, Simren M. Pathogenesis of IBS: role of inflammation, immunity, and neuroimmune interactions. Nat Rev Gastroenterol Hepatol. 2010;7:163–73.
19. Chaudhary NA, Truelove SC. The irritable colon syndrome. A study of the clinical features, predisposing causes, and prognosis in 130 cases. Q J Med. 1962;31:307–22.
20. Drossman DA. Mind over matter in the postinfective irritable bowel. Gut. 1999;44:306–7.
21. Pimentel M, Lembo A, Chey WD, et al. Rifaximin therapy for patients with irritable bowel syndrome without constipation. N Engl J Med. 2011;364:22–32.
22. Spiegel B. Questioning the bacterial overgrowth hypothesis in irritable bowel syndrome: an epidemiologic and evolutionary perspective. Clin Gastroenterol Hepatol. 2011;9:461–9.
23. Shanahan F, Quigley EM. Manipulation of the microbiota for treatment of IBS and IBD-challenges and controversies. Gastroenterology. 2014;146(6):1554–63.
24. Schmidt CM, Horton KM, Sitzmann JV, et al. Simple radiographic evaluation of ileoanal pouch volume. Dis Colon Rectum. 1996;39:66–73.
25. Bernstein CN, Rollandelli R, Niazi N, et al. Characterization of afferent mechanisms in ileoanal pouches. Am J Gastroenterol. 1997;92:103–8.
26. Shen B, Achkar JP, Lashner BA, et al. Irritable pouch syndrome: a new category of diagnosis for symptomatic patients with ileal pouch-anal anastomosis. Am J Gastroenterol. 2002;97:972–7.

# 41

# Medical Therapy of Hepatobiliary Diseases Associated with Ulcerative Colitis

Chalermrat Bunchorntavakul and K. Rajender Reddy

## Keywords

Hepatobiliary disease • Ulcerative colitis • Medical therapy • Liver function tests • Pancolitis • Liver abnormality • Remission • Pathogenesis • Primary sclerosing cholangitis • Epidemiology • Genetics • Biliary epithelial cells • Hepatobiliary transporters • Microorganisms • Ursodeoxycholic acid (UDCA) • Cholangiocarcinoma • Hepatitis B • Hepatitis C

## Introduction

Ulcerative colitis (UC) is associated with a variety of extraintestinal manifestations, and these include a spectrum of hepatobiliary diseases. Abnormal liver function tests (LFTs) are not infrequently observed in patients with UC. Transient alanine aminotransferase (ALT) elevation has been reported in up to one-third of patients during active UC, particularly in those with pancolitis [1, 2]. This type of liver abnormality does not need specific treatment apart from management of UC itself and generally resolves within a few weeks to months after remission of UC [1, 2].

Hepatobiliary diseases associated with UC can manifest at any time during the course, or even precede the diagnosis, of UC. They may present either with symptoms (i.e., pruritus, jaundice) and abnormal LFTs or they may have an incidental abnormal finding on imaging studies done for a variety of nonspecific reasons. Persistently elevated levels of ALT and/or alkaline phosphatase (ALP) have been reported in 6–17 % of patients with UC [2–4], regardless of disease activity. A number of hepatobiliary diseases have been linked to UC and can have protean manifestations which can be classified into 3 groups: (1) hepatobiliary diseases with association to UC or possibly shared pathogenesis with UC, (2) hepatobiliary disease with association to UC therapy, and (3) hepatobiliary diseases encountered in UC, which may relate to physiological changes from UC (Table 40.1). Among these abnormalities, the most common conditions include primary sclerosing cholangitis (PSC), liver steatosis, gallstones, and drug-induced liver injury (DILI) [2–6]. Unlike several extraintestinal manifestations of IBD, such as the skin, eyes, and joints, in which their activity often parallels the course of UC, hepatobiliary diseases typically do not follow the disease severity course of UC [5]. In addition, immunosuppressive agents (ISAs) used for UC can be associated with various forms of drug-induced liver injury (DILI), as well as with potential reactivation of chronic hepatitis B.

C. Bunchorntavakul, M.D.
Division of Gastroenterology and Hepatology,
Department of Medicine, Hospital of the
University of Pennsylvania, 3400 Spruce Street,
Phialdephia, PA 19104, USA

Division of Gastroenterology and Hepatology,
Department of Medicine, Rajavithi Hospital, 2 Phaya-Thai road,
Ratchathewi, Bangkok 10400, Thailand
e-mail: dr.chalermrat@gmail.com

K.R. Reddy, M.D. (✉)
Division of Gastroenterology and Hepatology,
Department of Medicine, Hospital of the
University of Pennsylvania, 3400 Spruce Street,
Phialdephia, PA 19104, USA
e-mail: rajender.reddy@uphs.upenn.edu

G.R. Lichtenstein (ed.), *Medical Therapy of Ulcerative Colitis*,
DOI 10.1007/978-1-4939-1677-1_41, © Springer Science+Business Media New York 2014

## Hepatobiliary Diseases with Association to UC or Possibly Shared Pathogenesis with UC

### Primary Sclerosing Cholangitis (PSC)

PSC is a chronic cholestatic liver disease characterized by chronic inflammation and progressive obliterating fibrosis of the intrahepatic and extrahepatic bile ducts. It eventually leads to portal hypertension, biliary cirrhosis, and liver failure requiring consideration of liver transplantation. Further, patients with PSC are at risk for the development of cholangiocarcinoma (CHCA), as well as extrahepatic malignancy [7–9]. There is a strong but incompletely understood relationship between PSC and inflammatory bowel disease (IBD), particularly UC. The pathogenesis of PSC has not been clearly elucidated; however, it appears to be multifactorial and is closely linked to IBD.

### Epidemiology

PSC is an uncommon disease in the general population. Three large population-based cohort epidemiological studies from the United Kingdom, the United States, and Canada have reported an incidence of PSC to be 0.41, 0.90, and 0.92 cases per 100,000 person-years, respectively [10–12]. Geographic variation in the prevalence of PSC exists; the prevalence of PSC, as well as IBD, is lower in the Middle East and Asia [13, 14]. PSC generally affects young and middle-aged individuals with male preponderance with a male to female ratio of approximately 2:1 [5, 10–12]. Interestingly, a recent cohort from the United Kingdom found that approximately 50 % of PSC patients presented after the age of 55 years and also demonstrated a nonstatistically significant trend toward increasing incidence of PSC, over time, during the 10-year study period [11]. PSC has been shown to be strongly associated with IBD and is now considered the most common hepatobiliary manifestation of IBD [6]. Majority of patients with PSC have associated IBD that may be diagnosed at any time during the course of PSC and vice versa. Notably, the diagnosis of UC precedes PSC in most cases. Most series from Northern America and Northern Europe have reported the prevalence of IBD in patients with PSC to range between 70 and 81 % [9, 10, 12, 15, 16]. In patients with IBD and PSC, approximately 50–90 % have UC, whereas the remaining have Crohn's disease (CD) [5, 8, 12]. Importantly, CD in patients with PSC usually involves the entire colon (Crohn's colitis or ileocolitis) [17]. Though the prevalence ratio between UC and CD among IBD patients is not exactly known, most data have suggested that UC is more prevalent than CD. The prevalence of CD in PSC is relatively lower in patients with IBD and PSC than in those with IBD alone. The reasons for these differences in prevalence between the two IBD conditions are unclear.

Conversely, the prevalence of PSC in those with IBD is much lower and ranges from 2.4 to 7.5 % in patients with UC [5, 18] and 1.4 to 3.4 % in patients with CD [5, 17]. Among UC patients, the prevalence of PSC is higher in patients with substantial colitis (5.5 %) as opposed to limited and distal colitis (0.5 %) [18]. Most of these epidemiological data have been derived from IBD-specialized centers in Northern America and Northern Europe. However, the data from other regions of the world appear to be different and vary substantially. Although not as high as in certain regions in the Northern Hemisphere, the prevalence of IBD in patients with PSC has been reported to be 21–32 % in Japan [19, 20], 44 % in Spain [21], 50 % in India [22], and 62 % in the United Kingdom [23]. The reason for this variation is unclear, but possibly is due to multifactorial factors such as differences in genetic predilection and in the rates of performing colonoscopy with multiple biopsies in PSC patients across different centers, which may then possibly translate into the under- and overestimation of colitis [24]. In addition, in some regions with a high prevalence of IgG4-associated disease such as in Japan, the reported cases of PSC- and IgG4-associated cholangitis (IAC) may somewhat overlap, and the former may be classified as the latter condition, thus an underreporting of PSC.

### Pathogenesis

The pathogenesis of PSC has been extensively investigated, but not completely elucidated. A variety of concepts have been implicated (i.e., autoimmunity, host genetic susceptibility, immunobiology model); however, a single hypothesis has not explained all the pathological and clinical features of this disease [7, 25–27]. As in IBD, the interaction between microorganisms and host immune response related either directly or indirectly to the biliary system, particularly in the background of genetic susceptibility, seems to be the most convincing concept.

### Autoimmunity

Evidence of immune dysregulation in patients with PSC is suggested indirectly by the presence of a variety of autoantibodies, which are often detected in the serum of patients with PSC. The prevalence of autoantibodies in patients with PSC has been reported at a rate of 50–88 % for antinuclear cytoplasmic antibody (ANCA), 7–77 % for antinuclear antibody, 13–20 % for anti-smooth muscle antibody, 35 % for anti-endothelium antibody, 4–66 % for anticardiolipin antibody, 4 % for thyroglobulin antibodies, and 15 % for rheumatoid factor [8, 28]. Antinuclear-specific antibodies are detected in up to 88 % of patients with PSC. The immunofluorescence microscopy patterns of these antibodies are distinct from that produced by c-ANCA or classic p-ANCA in vasculitic diseases [28]. Atypical p-ANCAs (so-called antineutrophil nuclear antibody or ANNA) are nonspecific and can be detected in patients with UC (40–87 %) and autoimmune hepatitis type 1 (50–96 %) [28]. Recently, Terjung et al. suggested that a target autoantigen for atypical p-ANCAs is a neutrophil envelop protein called beta-tubulin isotype 5 (TTB-5) [29].

Autoimmune disorders, such as type I diabetes mellitus (DM) and Grave's disease, are common in PSC-IBD patients which may further suggest the role of autoimmunity in PSC. Saarinen et al. reported that 25 % of patients with PSC had concurrent autoimmune disease(s), compared to 9 % of patients with IBD alone [30]. In addition, PSC patients have an increased frequency of the HLA B8, DR3, and DC2 haplotypes, which are also common to several autoimmune diseases, such as type 1 DM, myasthenia gravis, and thyrotoxicosis [26]. However, PSC is more common in men, in contrast to female predominance in the majority of other autoimmune diseases, and also does not respond to an immunosuppressive therapy such as corticosteroids. Further, specific autoantibodies against biliary system have not been identified in PSC. The autoantibodies generally are present at low levels and are not useful for the diagnosis or determining the prognosis of PSC [8, 26]. Therefore, PSC is not a classic autoimmune disease, but layers of evidences do suggest a pivotal role for immune-mediating processes in the pathogenesis of PSC.

## Role of Genetics

The prevalence of PSC in first-degree relatives and siblings is 0.7 % and 1.5 %, respectively [31]. This represents a nearly 100-fold increased risk for PSC compared with general populations, which in turn suggest genetic predisposition for the development of PSC [31]. In genetic terms, PSC is considered a complex trait whereby polymorphisms in several genes together with environmental factors are required for disease development [27]. The major histocompatibility complex (MHC) on the short arm of chromosome 6 encodes the HLA molecules that have a critical role in T-cell response, and along with MHC class I chain-like (MIC) α-molecules, which are involved in the innate immune function, especially as ligands for natural killer cells, may play a role in the pathogenesis [7]. An association between the haplotypes HLA A1-B8-DR3 (particularly with the presence of MICA5.1 and MICB24), DR6, and DR2 and susceptibility to PSC is well documented, whereas HLA DR4, DR11, and MICA*002 may be protective [25–27].

A number of non-MHC genes have been evaluated in association to PSC, including those related to cytotoxic lymphocyte antigen-4 (CTLA-4), chemokine receptor-5 (CCR-5), intracellular adhesion molecule-1 (ICAM-1), and matrix metalloproteinases (MMPs) [7, 26, 27]. The role of these immunoregulatory genes in PSC remains unsettled since the studies have revealed conflicting results.

Whether or not PSC and IBD share similar genetic susceptibility remains inconclusive. A large Scandinavian cohort found that IBD-associated polymorphisms in the CARD15, TLR-4, CARD4, SLC22, DLG5, and MDR1 genes failed to demonstrate their role in patients with PSC [32]. HLA associations found in PSC have been mostly distinct from those seen in UC, and no significant differences were noted between PSC patients with or without concurrent UC [33]. However, recent 3 genome-wide association studies (GWASs) identified 9 PSC risk loci outside the HLA complex including 2q13, 2q16, 2q35, 3p21, 4q27, 6p21, 9q34, 10p15, and 13q3 [34–36]. Several of these loci are also reported to be associated with UC and harbor the putative candidate genes REL, IL2, and CARD9 and bile acid receptor TGR-5 [36, 37].

## Biliary Epithelial Cells and Hepatobiliary Transporters

The biliary epithelial cell (BEC) is the primary target of immune injury in PSC. Normal BECs express only HLA class I, but HLA class II antigens (HLA-DR, DQ, and DP) do express in BECs of patients with PSC, and these antigens have a potential to initiate immune response triggered by either autoantigens or exogenous antigens [26]. Unlike in controls and patients with other liver diseases, autoantibodies against a cross-reactive peptide shared by colon and BECs were identified in up to two-thirds of cases of PSC [38]. Thus, anti-BEC antibodies can stimulate the production of inflammatory cytokines and the expression of CD44 from BECs through TLR-4, TLR-9, and extracellular signal-related kinase (ERK) and transcription factor [39, 40]. An increased nitric oxide production from stimulated BECs has been shown to cause ductular cholestasis by inhibition of bile secretion [41].

Genetic polymorphisms in hepatocellular transport system may play a role in PSC. The steroid and xenobiotic receptor (SXR) is a ligand-dependent transcription factor involved in bile acid homeostasis. Genetic polymorphisms in SXR genes appear to adversely modify the disease course of PSC [42]. Knockout of multidrug resistance (MDR2) gene, which encodes for canalicular transport of phospholipids in mice, results in biliary changes resembling human PSC [43]. However, a study in humans did not find an association between PSC and genetic variations of canalicular membrane transporters bile salt export pump (BSEP) and multidrug resistance protein type 3 (MDR3) [44].

## Role of Microorganisms

A role for bacterial or viral antigens in the development of PSC has been proposed. Chronic inflammation of the bowel promotes translocation of bacteria and their products, through a leaky gut wall into portal circulation, and activates Kupffer cells, resulting in peribiliary cytokine/chemokine

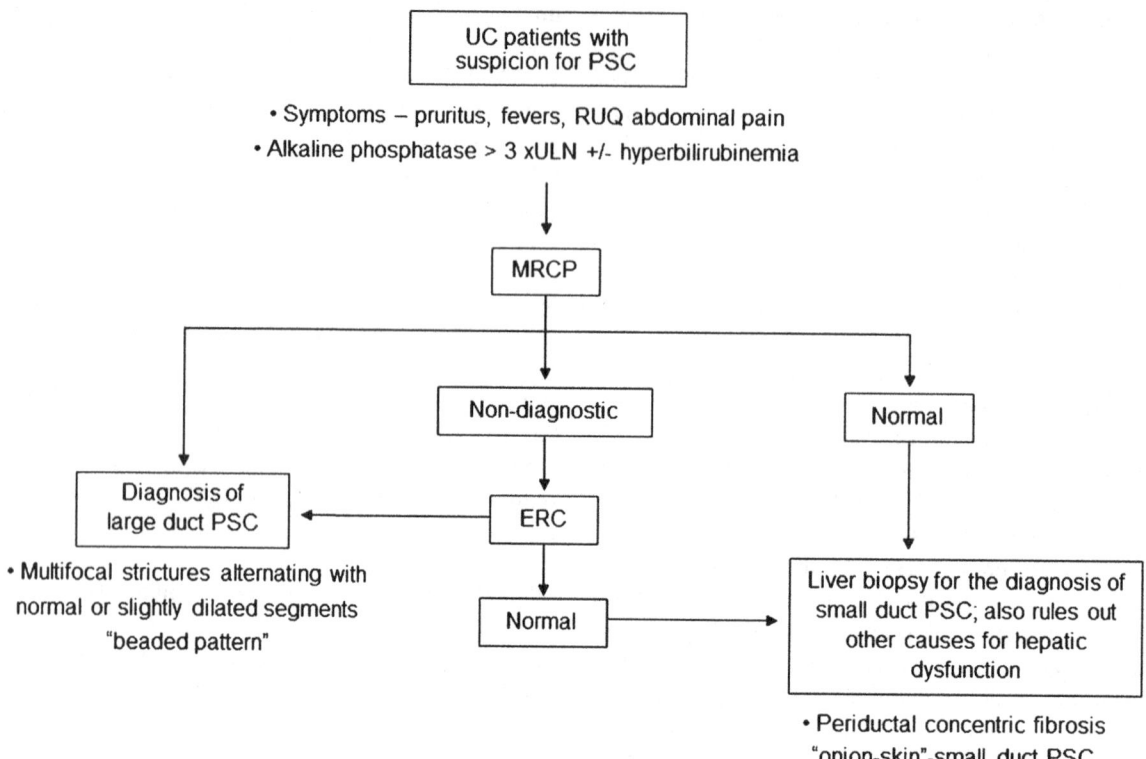

**Fig. 41.1** Algorithm for the diagnosis of primary sclerosing cholangitis in patients with ulcerative colitis

release, which in turn likely activates inflammation, ischemia, and fibrosis of the biliary system [26]. More recent concepts suggest a role for microorganisms as a molecular mimic, triggering immune responses directed against biliary epithelium, particularly in the immunogenetically susceptible host [7, 25, 26]. A potential bacterial antigen that may mimic autoantigen is the bacterial cell wall division protein FtsZ [29]. This bacterial protein shares high degree of structural homology with human TBB-5 and conserves across broad range of bacterial species in gut [29, 45]. The role of certain other microorganisms that included *Helicobacter pylori*, cytomegalovirus, and *Candida spp.* in the pathogenesis of PSC remains controversial [7].

Though there is data to support the model of immunobiology in PSC, significant peripheral and portal bacteremia has not been frequently noted in patients with severe UC who have undergone colectomy [46]. Small bowel bacterial overgrowth leads to strictures in a rat model, but it, as well as an increased intestinal permeability, does not seem to play an important role in patients with PSC [7, 47].

## Diagnosis and Clinical Features

The clinical presentation of PSC is variable. Majority of patients are asymptomatic at presentation and develop symptoms over time [5]. Symptomatic patients commonly

present with right upper quadrant abdominal discomfort (30–40 %), pruritus (20–40 %), fever (11–35 %), jaundice (27–30 %), and weight loss (10–15 %) [7, 15, 16, 48]. Jaundice typically occurs in the setting of disease complications, i.e., dominant strictures, cholangitis, or in those who develop advanced cirrhosis. Fatigue is nonspecific and does not correlate with liver disease severity. Though fatigue is common in PSC patients, its prevalence seems to be similar to those with IBD alone [49]. Physical examination is often unremarkable, though hepatomegaly (44–55 %) and splenomegaly (~30 %) may be detected by abdominal ultrasound (US) [7, 48]. Liver function tests typically show persistent elevation of ALP (~3–10 times of the upper limit of normal), and majority of patients have mildly elevated serum ALT and IgG, with normal bilirubin levels at the time of diagnosis [8]. However, normal LFTs do not exclude the diagnosis of PSC [8]. Serum autoantibodies have neither acceptable sensitivity nor specificity for the diagnosis of PSC [7, 8].

A diagnosis of PSC is based on a constellation of an appropriate clinical and biochemical profile and characteristic cholangiographic features (Fig. 41.1) [8]. Typical cholangiographic changes include multifocal, short, annular strictures with intervening segments of normal or dilated ducts, the so-called beaded-like pattern, and which involve the intra- and/or extrahepatic biliary system. Traditionally, endoscopic retro-

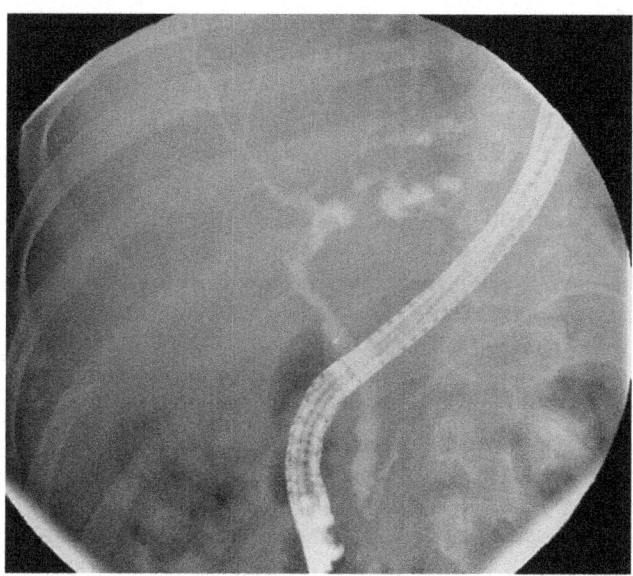

**Fig. 41.2** Typical endoscopic retrograde cholangiographic findings in primary sclerosing cholangitis

grade cholangiography (ERC) has been regarded as the gold standard for the diagnosis of PSC. However, ERC is invasive and is associated with risk of complications requiring hospitalization (i.e., cholangitis, pancreatitis) in over 10 % of PSC patients despite the use of antibiotic prophylaxis [50]. Given its noninvasive nature, magnetic resonance cholangiography (MRC) has become a diagnostic procedure of choice for PSC (Fig. 41.2), and ERC should be reserved for those patients who need endoscopic therapeutic intervention [8]. MRC has a demonstrated sensitivity of 80–91 %, a specificity of 85–99 %, and a diagnostic accuracy of 83–93 %, which is comparable or slightly inferior to ERC, for the diagnosis of PSC [5]. Nevertheless, early changes in PSC may be missed by MRC, and ERC is still helpful when MRC views are not optimal [8].

Both intra- and extrahepatic ducts are often involved (60–70 %), whereas localized intrahepatic duct (~25 %) or extrahepatic duct disease alone (<5 %) is less common [8, 48]. The cystic duct, pancreatic duct (PD), and gallbladder may be also involved. Severity of cholangiographic changes, scored by Amsterdam classification, has been noted to inversely correlate with transplant-free survival [51].

It should be noted that several conditions (i.e., ischemia, malignancy, chronic infection, and inflammation) can cause sclerosing and multifocal stricturing process of the biliary tract by nonimmune-mediated mechanism, and these may have cholangiographic features similar to those of PSC, the so-called secondary sclerosing cholangitis [8].

The findings on computer tomography (CT) and US are nonspecific. Thickening and/or saccular dilatations of the bile ducts and evidence of portal hypertension (i.e., varices, splenomegaly, and ascites) may be present. Contract

enhancement of thickened bile duct wall is suggestive of an inflammatory process. Interestingly, abdominal lymphadenopathy, particularly in perihepatic and celiac axis groups, is often detected in PSC (66–100 %) and does not imply malignancy and should not exclude a patient from undergoing liver transplantation (LT) [52, 53].

In the presence of an abnormal cholangiogram, a liver biopsy is not required for the diagnosis of large-duct PSC. Periductal concentric (onionskin) fibrosis is a characteristic histopathologic feature. However, it is uncommonly encountered in a percutaneous biopsy specimen and may also be observed in secondary sclerosing cholangitis [8]. Importantly, liver biopsy may be essential to establish the diagnosis of small-duct PSC and PSC/autoimmune hepatitis (AIH) overlap as well as to exclude other causes of liver disease.

## Natural History of PSC With and Without UC and Vice Versa

The clinical course of PSC is variable. The median time from diagnosis of PSC to death or LT has ranged from 9.6 to 21 years [1, 7, 26], and the overall survival is significantly decreased (approximately threefold) compared to the general population, even when asymptomatic at diagnosis [11, 16]. The clinical course is characterized by recurrent episodes of cholangitis, during which time the disease slowly progresses. Clinical features of pruritus and jaundice gradually develop overtime, and finally end-stage liver disease can appear [7]. Cholangiocarcinoma (CHCA) may complicate the course of PSC in 8–15 % of patients (annual incidence 0.6–1 %) [5, 7, 9]. Of interest is that the duration of PSC may not be a risk factor for CHCA, and, in fact, in approximately 50 % of patients with PSC plus CHCA, the malignancy is detected at the time of diagnosis or within the first year suggesting that superimposed CHCA may lead to the diagnosis of PSC [8, 54]. Compared to the general population, PSC patients are at higher risk for developing cancers (two- to tenfold for any cancers and 40–160-fold for colon cancer) [9, 11]. Patients with PSC are prone to develop complications of ESLD and portal hypertension (i.e., ascites, varices, encephalopathy). In some patients, esophageal varices may present early in the course of their liver disease, which is possibly explained by localized vascular damage in the portal triad from bile duct inflammation causing presinusoidal portal hypertension [5].

Serum bilirubin, albumin, and age at the diagnosis of PSC were independent prognostic factors in a time-dependent model [55]. Although the traditional Child-Pugh classification system is informative with regard to outcomes, the Mayo score model (includes age, bilirubin, AST, albumin, and history of variceal bleeding) may provide more reproducible and more accurate prognostic information without the need for liver biopsy, especially in patients with early disease [8, 56]. However, this model is not superior to the

Child-Pugh system in predicting survival and related economic outcomes after LT [57]. The addition of cholangiographic findings in the model may provide some additional prognostic value [8, 48, 51].

The association between coexisting PSC and the disease extension and activity of UC remains inconclusive. UC patients with coexisting PSC tend to have higher incidence of pancolitis, backwash ileitis, and rectal sparing than UC patients without PSC [5]. However, patients with PSC-UC may have lower grade of colonic inflammation and more often run a quiescent course of colitis than UC patients without PSC [5, 58]. Colectomy with ileal pouch-anal anastomosis (IPAA) does not appear to alter the disease course of PSC [5].

## Medical Therapy for PSC

A number of medical treatments that are targeted to alleviate inflammation and cholestasis have been investigated in PSC. However, unlike primary biliary cirrhosis (PBC), the efficacy of these therapies is somewhat limited. The uncertainty in the pathogenesis of PSC may present a barrier for the development of significant disease-modifying agents in PSC.

## Ursodeoxycholic Acid (UDCA)

Ursodeoxycholic acid (UDCA) is a hydrophilic, tertiary bile acid which has been used for the treatment of a variety of chronic cholestatic conditions [59]. It has been shown to be an effective therapy in PBC [60]. After oral administration, UDCA is absorbed mainly in the small intestine, and then it has an enterohepatic circulation. At a daily dose of 13–15 mg/kg body weight/day, UDCA constitutes 40–50 % of total bile acid pool and results in a decrease in relative contribution of the more hepatotoxic endogenous hydrophobic bile acids [59]. Several mechanisms have been proposed by which UDCA may protect against cholestatic liver injury, and these include the choleretic effect by increasing bile flow, protection of injured cholangiocytes from toxic bile acids, stimulation of detoxification of hydrophobic bile acids, inhibition of hepatocyte apoptosis, and direct cytoprotective and immunomodulatory effects [29, 59].

The majority of the early studies of UDCA in PSC were small and/or uncontrolled. Many of these studies demonstrated liver function test improvement by using doses of 10–15 mg/kg body weight/day [8, 26, 61]. Lindor et al. conducted a randomized controlled trial (RCT) of UDCA 13–15 mg/kg/day, for 2–5 years, in 105 PSC patients. The results demonstrated improvement in LFTs but not symptoms and the time to treatment failure (defined by histologic progression by two stages, development of cirrhosis or esophageal varices, liver decompensation, LT, or death) [62]. On the basis that higher doses of UDCA may be required to provide sufficient delivery of UDCA to the bile pool and also enhance immunomodulatory effects in the setting of cholestasis and

bile duct injury in PSC, several studies using higher dose of UDCA were conducted and published in the early 2000s. An RCT from Oxford using UDCA 20–25 mg/kg/day in 26 PSC patients found significant improvement in LFTs, histology, as well as cholangiographic features. However, no benefit in symptoms and survival was demonstrated [63]. Two studies comparing different doses of UDCA suggested that higher daily dose (25–30 mg/kg) was well tolerated and provided benefits, which included survival benefit in one study, compared to a lower dose (10–20 mg/kg) [64, 65].

Despite somewhat convincing data on benefits with higher doses, a large Scandinavian RCT evaluating UDCA at 17–23 mg/kg/day in 219 PSC patients for 5 years found no significant favorable effect on survival, symptoms, and prevention of CHCA although there was a nonsignificant trend toward improvement in LFTs and survival [66]. Recently, a multicenter RCT from the United States comparing high-dose UDCA (28–30 mg/kg/day) with placebo, in 150 PSC patients, was terminated prematurely at 6 years due to a higher incidence of adverse outcomes (i.e., death, LT, esophageal varices) in the UDCA group [67]. The likelihood of developing serious adverse outcomes was not predicted by biochemical response, but was predicted by advanced liver disease at presentation [67]. Therefore, currently there is no established role for UDCA in slowing the progression of PSC. Further, high-dose UDCA may be harmful in late-stage disease [8, 60].

## Immunosuppressive Therapy

Unlike most of other immune-mediated diseases, treatment with corticosteroids and other ISAs has not demonstrated consistent benefits in PSC, and most evidence is derived from pilot studies. Corticosteroids demonstrated no benefit in PSC and were associated with significant worsening of osteoporosis [68–70]. Corticosteroids may be considered only in patients with PSC/AIH overlap and IgG4-associated cholangitis [8]. No controlled trial of azathioprine (AZA) has been reported as monotherapy to date. A combination of AZA, prednisolone, and UDCA (500–750 mg/day) for PSC was reported in a case series of 15 PSC patients. All patients had ALP improvement (seven patients had been previously treated with UDCA, but ALP improved only after prednisolone and AZA were added), and 60 % had histological improvement after 41 months [71]. Methotrexate (MTX) may minimally improve ALP levels, but does not impact clinical outcomes of PSC [72]. Addition of MTX to UDCA was associated with toxicity and without further improvement in LFTs [73]. Mycophenolate mofetil (MMF) was poorly tolerated (56 %) and did not demonstrate clinical benefit in PSC [74]. Further, combination of MMF and UDCA did not provide additional benefits [73]. Tacrolimus [75] and cyclosporin [76] had no significant effects on PSC disease outcomes and were poorly tolerated although they provided benefits in UC [76]. A pilot RCT in 10 PSC patients failed to demonstrate clinical efficacy of infliximab (5 mg/kg) on the course of liver disease [77].

## Miscellaneous Treatment

Based on the observation that elevated hepatic copper levels are universally detected in patients with chronic cholestasis, D-penicillamine was evaluated in an RCT of 70 PSC patients. However, it was not associated with clinical benefit and has considerable toxicity, which led to treatment discontinuation in 21 % of patients [78]. Colchicine, an anti-fibrogenic agent, either alone or in combination with prednisone failed to show beneficial effects in two RCTs [70, 79]. Silymarin, a milk thistle extract, which potentially has several hepatoprotective properties, was evaluated in an open-label pilot study of 30 PSC patients for 1 year [80]. One-third of patients achieved substantial improvement in LFTs, but no significant change in Mayo risk score [80]. Several agents, such as nicotine, bezafibrate, pirfenidone, minocycline, and probiotics, have been preliminarily evaluated in PSC but without clear demonstrable benefits [8, 61, 81].

## Medical Management for Complications of PSC
### Cholangiocarcinoma (CHCA)

CHCA, a dreadful complication of PSC, develops in 8–15 % of patients [5, 7, 9]. Risk factors include the duration of UC, colonic dysplasia, variceal bleeding, proctocolectomy, alcohol consumption, and polymorphisms in the NKG2D gene [8, 82]. The diagnosis of CHCA in the setting of PSC is often challenging, particularly for the periductal infiltrative type. The presence of mass-like lesion or a long biliary stricture, particularly in the hilar area, on an imaging study strongly raises the possibility of CHCA. In PSC patients with clinical suspicion for CHCA, CA 19-9 at a cutoff of 129 U/mL has value in determining the likelihood for CHCA; positive predictive value was 57 % and negative predictive value 99 % [83]. However, caution must be exercised since CA 19-9 is undetectable in person with Lewis-negative blood type and can be elevated in other conditions (i.e., cholangitis, nonbiliary cancers) [84]. A combination of cross-sectional liver imaging studies, tumor biomarkers, and cholangiography with tissue sampling is often required, and is recommended, to make the accurate diagnosis of CHCA (Fig. 41.3) [8, 54, 84].

The prognosis of CHCA in PSC is dismal with a 3-year survival of less than 20 % even in surgically resected patients [8]. Recent data suggests that neoadjuvant therapy followed by LT in highly selected patients may result in a better outcome with a 5-year survival of ~70 % [85]. The benefit of other palliative modalities, such as external beam radiation, endoscopic ablative therapy, and systemic chemotherapy, has not been clearly demonstrated [8].

## Colorectal Neoplasia

PSC has been shown to be an independent risk factor for the development of colorectal neoplasia in patients with UC (OR 4.79, 95%CI; 3.58–6.41) [86]. Colorectal neoplasia associated with PSC can be diagnosed at any time during the course of PSC, and it appears to occur predominantly in the right colon [87]. This risk appears to persist even after LT [5, 24]. Therefore, colonoscopy surveillance for colonic neoplasia is recommended to begin at the time of the diagnosis of PSC [8]. There are controversial data suggesting a benefit of UDCA in preventing the development of colorectal neoplasia [8, 60]. The current US guideline recommends against the use of UDCA as chemoprevention in patients with PSC-UC [8], while the European guideline suggests the use of UDCA in high-risk patients, such as those with strong family history of colorectal cancer, previous history of colorectal neoplasia, or long-standing extensive colitis [60].

## Gallbladder Disease

Gallbladder abnormalities are commonly observed in patients with PSC, and these include gall stones (26 %), PSC involving the gallbladder (15 %), and gallbladder neoplasms (4–14 %) [8, 88]. Remarkably, 40–60 % of gallbladder polyps detected in patients with PSC are malignant [89, 90]. Therefore, surveillance by ultrasound should be done annually. In patients with a gallbladder mass lesion, cholecystectomy is recommended regardless of lesion size since the 1-cm rule may not reliably predict malignant potential of the gallbladder polyp in the setting of PSC [8, 91].

## Bacterial Cholangitis

Patients with PSC are susceptible to repeated episodes of bacterial cholangitis, especially after biliary tract manipulation [92]. If cholangitis occurs without biliary intervention, the presence of stones, dominant strictures, or CHCA should be considered. Most common causative organisms are gram-negative enteric bacteria and enterococci [92]. The majority of patients respond to broad-spectrum intravenous antibiotic plus biliary drainage. Patients with recurrent bacterial cholangitis may benefit from long-term antibiotic prophylaxis [8].

## Portal Hypertension and End-Stage Liver Disease (ELSD)

Management of portal hypertension and its complications in patients with PSC does not differ from other etiologies. The ultimate treatment for end-stage liver disease (ESLD) associated with PSC is LT with 5-year survival rates of approximately 85 % [8]. Resection of the extrahepatic biliary tree along with a Roux-en-Y choledochojejunostomy is widely accepted as a method of choice for biliary reconstruction in LT for PSC [60]. As in non-PSC, the Model for End-Stage Liver Disease (MELD) score is most widely utilized for organ allocation for PSC patients, although the presence of dominant strictures may affect MELD score by increasing bilirubin levels, and this may not necessarily mean advanced disease and liver failure. Other unique indications for LT in PSC patients include intractable pruritus, recurrent bacterial

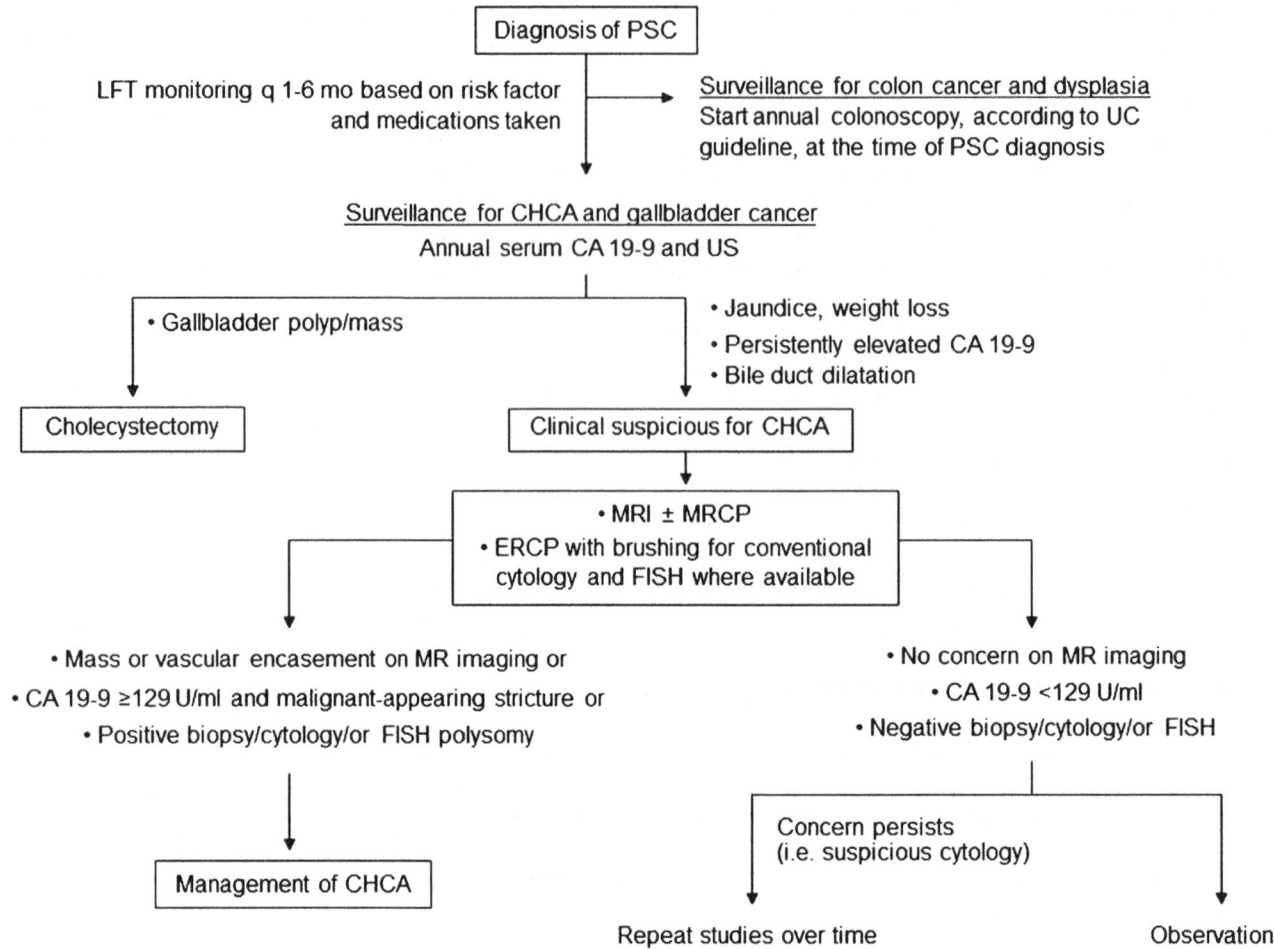

**Fig. 41.3** Algorithm for the surveillance and the diagnosis of malignancy in patients with ulcerative colitis and primary sclerosing cholangitis

cholangitis, and CHCA [8]. Recurrence of PSC occurs in 20–25 % of the liver grafts after 5–10 years following LT [8, 93], but this is sometimes difficult to assess due to the similarities in biliary changes seen with ischemic and preservative injury, infections, and chronic rejection.

The activity of UC following LT is heterogeneous. Contrary to general wisdom, while on liver transplant-related immunosuppression, the majority of PSC-IBD patients experience a deterioration of their IBD following LT [94]. Further, the increased risk of developing colorectal neoplasia persists after LT [95]. The guideline for the management of UC exacerbation after LT has not been established, and the long-term effect of anti-TNF agents on liver graft is unknown.

**Metabolic Bone Disease**
Patients with long-standing IBD, and particularly with the prolonged use of corticosteroid therapy, frequently have

decreased bone mass density (BMD) [96]. The presence of PSC, with or without cirrhosis, further negatively impacts BMD by several mechanisms, such as vitamin D malabsorption, altered bone turnover rate, and hypogonadism [97]. A recent study of 237 PSC patients with 10 years of follow-up reported that patients with PSC lost 1 % of their BMD per year. Osteoporosis was detected in 15 % of patients (24-fold higher rate than matched population) and risk factors included older age, low body mass index, and long duration of IBD [98]. The surveillance and management of osteoporosis in PSC does not substantially differ from other situations, and there is particular emphasis on calcium and vitamin D supplementation [8, 96]. Oral bisphosphonates may induce esophageal ulcerations which could precipitate variceal hemorrhage. Therefore, parenteral bisphosphonates may be a reasonable approach for patients with esophageal varices [8].

## PSC Variants

### Small-Duct PSC

Small-duct PSC, previously termed as pericholangitis, refers to a subgroup of patients who have biochemical and histological features compatible with PSC, but with normal cholangiography. Small-duct PSC represents approximately 6–11 % of patients with sclerosing cholangitis and often coexists with IBD (~80 %). It is a disease that is potentially progressive but is associated with a better long-term prognosis as compared with large-duct PSC (LT-free survival 13 years vs. 10 years, respectively; $p<0.0001$) [99]. Cholangiocarcinoma does not seem to occur in patients with small-duct PSC. Approximately one-fourth of patients eventually progressed to large-duct PSC over a median of 7.4 years, and some patients progressed to end-stage liver disease requiring LT without developing large-duct disease [99]. Given a relatively small number of patients with small-duct PSC, the management is not well defined, and there is no controlled prospective study reported to date. In a longitudinal cohort of 42 patients from Mayo Clinic followed up to 25 years, UDCA 13–15 mg/kg/day improved liver biochemistries, but did not significantly delay disease progression [100].

### PSC/Autoimmune Hepatitis (AIH) Overlap

PSC/AIH overlap is an ill-defined immune-mediated disorder, which is predominantly encountered in children and young adults [101]. A diagnosis of PSC/AIH overlap is made when both typical cholangiographic features of PSC and definitive diagnosis of AIH, based on modified AIH score, are present [101, 102]. The prevalence of PSC/AIH overlap in patients with PSC has varied from 7 to 14 % based on the revised AIH criteria, and majority of these patients (50–88 %) have underlying IBD [101]. The presentation of PSC/AIH overlap may be either simultaneous or sequential. Particularly in the setting of IBD, patients with PSC with an elevation of ALT should prompt a search for AIH. On the other hand, PSC should be considered in AIH patients with cholestasis, histological bile duct injury, and in those who show a poor response to therapy [101]. Patients with PSC/AIH overlap seem to benefit from UDCA and ISA, and survival is apparently better than in classical PSC, but with a poorer outcome than AIH [103, 105]. In a prospective Italian study (N=7 PSC/AIH, 34 PSC), a combination of UDCA (15–20 mg/kg/day), prednisolone (0.5 mg/kg/day, then tapered to 10–15 mg/day), and azathioprine (50–75 mg) reported a good biochemical response (ALT, but not ALP) in patients with PSC/AIH overlap [104].

### IgG4-Associated Cholangitis

IgG4-associated cholangitis (IAC) is a biliary tract disease of unclear pathogenesis and with cholangiographic features indistinguishable from PSC. It has been described in patients with autoimmune pancreatitis (AIP) as a part of a systemic autoimmune process associated with IgG4 [61, 105]. The clinical entity is characterized by pancreatic enlargement, elevated serum IgG4 levels, histologic evidence of lymphoplasmacytic infiltrate in the pancreas, and extrapancreatic manifestations, such as sclerosing cholangitis, sialadenitis, and retroperitoneal fibrosis [61, 105]. It is important to distinguish PSC from IAC, which is at times challenging due to the fact that pancreatic disease may not be evident (8 %) and IgG4-associated sclerosing colitis, mimicking IBD or UC itself, may be present [61, 105, 106]. IAC appears to be histologically distinct from PSC, and it usually has a dramatic response to corticosteroids in contrast to the refractory nature in PSC [5, 61]. All patients with possible PSC should be tested for serum IgG4 levels to exclude IAC [8]. Interestingly, up to one-quarter of patients with biopsy-proven PSC have an increased IgG4 periductal plasma cell infiltrate, and 9–22 % have elevated serum IgG4 levels [107, 108]. These findings raise the question of whether PSC and AIP/AIC represent different ends of the same disease spectrum or are distinct disease entities, although current evidence favors the latter [8]. Of note is that PSC patients with elevated IgG4 levels tend to have more severe disease severity and course [107, 108]. Thus, a trial of corticosteroids may be considered; however, proven benefit has yet to be demonstrated in RCT [61, 108].

## Hepatobiliary Diseases Encountered in UC

### Fatty Liver

Nonalcoholic fatty liver disease (NAFLD) is the most common hepatobiliary disease encountered in IBD, with reported prevalence range of 2–80 % (median 29.5 %) in published studies with over 100 subjects [109]. Thus, it may account for approximately 40 % of cases of LFT abnormalities in those with IBD [3]. As in the general population, the prevalence of NAFLD is likely increasing among IBD population as well [109]. Apart from obesity and metabolic syndrome, NAFLD can be caused by IBD-related factors, such as malnutrition, protein loss, and medications (i.e., corticosteroids, MTX, anti-TNFs) [109]. There is no specific guideline for the management of NAFLD in IBD patients; periodic monitoring and counseling to avoid excessive weight gain would be reasonable.

### Portal Vein Thrombosis

Portal vein thrombosis (PVT) is rarely observed in IBD patients in a nonsurgical setting, but it is not uncommon in those with recent abdominal surgery [5]. Several factors associated with IBD, such as increased platelet counts, factor V, VII, and fibrinogen levels, state of active bowel inflammation, and infections, may contribute to the thrombotic complications [5]. Portal vein thrombosis has been detected by CT imaging in 25–45 % of UC patients who have undergone IPAA surgery and was more likely to be segmental, multiple, and occlusive [110–112]. Presentation of PVT following IPAA surgery includes abdominal pain, nausea/vomiting, prolonged ileus, and leukocytosis. Septic complications (i.e., liver abscesses, pelvic sepsis) subsequently occur in 0–50 % of patients [111, 112]. Anticoagulation and antibiotic treatments are generally associated with a good clinical response and resolution of PVT. Interestingly, postoperative PVT has been linked to an increased risk of subsequent pouchitis (46 % in patients with PVT and 15 % in those without after 36 months follow-up) [111].

## Miscellaneous Conditions

Several other hepatobiliary diseases have been reported to be more prevalent in IBD patients than in the general population, and these include PBC, gallstones, hepatic amyloidosis, and granulomatous hepatitis [5] (Table 41.2). These conditions have been reported more often in CD than UC (with the exception of PBC), and the mechanisms are unclear. UC patients with PBC typically present with elevated ALP and positive AMA. Interestingly, unlike classical PBC, UC-associated PBC seems to occur at a younger age and more often in men [113]. Hepatic amyloidosis classically occurs in patients with long-standing active IBD and presents with elevated ALP and hepatomegaly (with hard consistency). Involvement of other organs, particularly gastrointestinal tract and kidneys, is commonly observed [114]. Granulomatous hepatitis can be linked to either IBD itself (CD) or IBD-related factors, such as medications, particularly sulfasalazine, and infections. It often presents with isolated elevation of ALP, although other features, such as fever and hepatomegaly, can also be encountered [5, 115]. The diagnosis of hepatic amyloidosis and granulomas generally requires a liver biopsy.

## Hepatobiliary Diseases with Association to IBD Therapy (Tables 41.1 and 41.2)

### Drug-Induced Liver Injury (DILI)

#### 5-Aminosalicylic Acid (ASA) Compounds

Sulfasalazine-induced DILI in IBD is relatively uncommon, with three severe cases per million prescriptions reported in the United Kingdom [116]. Acute hepatocellular damage may develop alone or, less commonly, as a part of generalized

**Table 41.1** Hepatobiliary diseases associated with inflammatory bowel disease

|  | UC | CD |
|---|---|---|
| Hepatobiliary disease with association to IBD or possibly shared pathogenesis with IBD | | |
| • Primary sclerosing cholangitis (PSC) | ++ | + |
| • Small-duct PSC | ++ | + |
| • PSC/AIH overlap syndrome | ++ | + |
| • IgG4-associated cholangitis | ++ | + |
| Hepatobiliary disease encountered in IBD | | |
| • Fatty liver disease | ++ | ++ |
| • Portal vein thrombosis (PVT) | + | ++ |
| • Presinusoidal portal hypertension | ++ | +/− |
| • Gall stones | +/− | ++ |
| • Hepatic amyloidosis | +/− | ++ |
| • Granulomatous hepatitis | +/− | ++ |
| • Primary biliary cirrhosis | ++ | + |
| Hepatobiliary disease with association to IBD therapy | | |
| • Drug-induced hepatotoxicity | ++ | ++ |
| • Reactivation of hepatitis B | ++ | ++ |
| • Hepatosplenic T-cell lymphoma | +/− | ++ |

*IBD* inflammatory bowel disease, *UC* ulcerative colitis, *CD* Crohn's disease, *PSC* primary sclerosing cholangitis, *AIH* autoimmune hepatitis, *Ig* immunoglobulin

Adapted from Navaneethan U and Shen B. Hepatopancreatobiliary manifestations and complications associated with inflammatory bowel disease. Inflamm Bowel Dis. 2010;16:1598–619. With permission from John Wiley and Sons [5]

**Table 41.2** Differential diagnosis of hepatobiliary abnormalities associated with medications used in ulcerative colitis

| Clinical features | Medications |
|---|---|
| Acute hepatocellular injury | Sulfasalazine, 5-ASA, thiopurines, methotrexate |
| Hypersensitivity reaction | Sulfasalazine, 5-ASA, thiopurines |
| Autoimmune hepatitis features | Anti-TNF agents |
| Cholestasis | Sulfasalazine, 5-ASA, thiopurines, cyclosporin |
| Cirrhosis | Methotrexate |
| Steatohepatitis | Methotrexate |
| Nodular regenerative hyperplasia (NRH) | Thiopurines |
| Non-cirrhotic portal hypertension | Thiopurines |
| Sinusoidal obstruction syndrome (SOS) | Thiopurines |
| Peliosis hepatis | Thiopurines |
| Pancreatitis | Thiopurines |
| Reactivation of hepatitis B | Anti-TNF agents, corticosteroids, thiopurines, methotrexate, cyclosporin |
| Hepatosplenic T-cell lymphoma | Anti-TNF agents (typically in combination with thiopurines) |

*ASA* aminosalicylic acid, *TNF* tumor necrotic factor

hypersensitivity reaction, which is characterized by fever, malaise, lymphadenopathy, and hepatomegaly. It has been suggested that DILI, particularly a hypersensitivity reaction, is related to the sulfapyridine moiety; however, recent data reported similar incidence of overall DILI with sulfasalazine (sulfapyridine and 5-ASA) and mesalamine (5-ASA alone), suggesting that DILI is more likely from 5-ASA rather than the sulfa moiety [116, 117]. Cross-hypersensitivity reaction with mesalamine after a prior hypersensitivity reaction to sulfasalazine has been reported [118]. Hepatotoxicity can occur from as early as 6 days to 1 year after initiation of therapy. Other forms of DILI include granulomatous hepatitis, acute liver failure, chronic hepatitis, and cholestasis [5, 115].

## Thiopurines

Treatment of IBD with azathioprine (AZA), 6-mercaptopurine (6-MP), or 6-thioguanine (6-TG) can be associated with various forms of DILI, mainly acute hepatocellular injury, idiosyncratic cholestatic reaction, and hepatic vascular endothelial injury [3, 115, 119]. Recent data reported a prevalence of thiopurine-induced acute DILI in IBD patients to be 3.4–7.1 %, with an annual incidence of 1.4–2.6 % [3, 119]. Liver function test abnormalities are usually reversible and often occur soon after the initiation of treatment [115, 119–121]. In addition, hypersensitivity reaction and cholestatic hepatitis have also been reported [115]. Hepatotoxicity from AZA/6-MP is related to its metabolite 6-methylmercaptopurine ribonucleotide (6-MMP); however, the sensitivity and specificity of 6-MMP levels for DILI were poor [122]. In an effort to avoid the potential adverse events from AZA/6-MP, assessment of thiopurine methyltransferase (TPMT) genotype or phenotype before initiation of treatment is suggested [120, 123]. Individuals with low TPMT activity are at risk for myelotoxicity via higher levels of 6-TG, whereas individuals with high TPMT activity have lower 6-TG levels and can result in a suboptimal treatment response, as well as hepatotoxicity from higher levels of 6-MMP [115, 120, 123]. With close monitoring, allopurinol co-therapy with low-dose AZA/6-MP may help to avoid poor response and decrease risk of hepatotoxicity, especially in patients with very high TPMT activity [124]. In addition, split-dosing regimen of thiopurines, by decreasing 6-MMP levels, has been proposed to reduce the risk of DILI [122].

Most cases of idiosyncratic cholestatic reaction associated with AZA/6-MP occur within 2–5 months of treatment and with a male preponderance. Jaundice may not immediately resolve despite drug withdrawal [119].

Apart from direct hepatic injury, thiopurines can be associated with hepatic vascular endothelial lesions and their consequence, and these included nodular regenerative hyperplasia (NRH) and non-cirrhotic portal hypertension, sinusoidal obstruction syndrome (SOS or formerly called venoocclusive disease), and peliosis hepatis [5, 115]. Nodular regenerative hyperplasia has been reported to occur from 1.3 to 18 % of IBD patients who receive 6-TG, and it may develop as soon as few months or many years after therapy [125, 126]. The development of NRH seems to be dose related, as it is rarely seen with low-dose 6-TG (<20 mg/day) [115]. Male gender and small bowel resection of >50 cm appear to be additional risk factors [125]. Majority of patients are asymptomatic with mild abnormality in LFTs. The definite diagnosis of NRH is based on a liver biopsy, while MRI has a sensitivity of 77 % and a specificity of 72 % [126]. The natural course of NRH-associated with thiopurines is usually indolent and potentially reversible. However, adverse outcomes, such as portal hypertension, varices, and hepatocellular carcinoma, have also been reported [115].

## Methotrexate

Long-term use of MTX has been associated with liver fibrosis and cirrhosis in patients with psoriasis and rheumatoid arthritis, and often LFTs are normal. Risk factors for DILI from MTX include high cumulative dose, older age, alcohol, obesity, diabetes, and preexisting liver disease [5]. Since there is poor correlation between ALT and histologic changes, surveillance with liver biopsy is recommended to monitor for MTX hepatotoxicity, traditionally after a cumulative total dose of 1.5 g. Despite limited data, the incidence of MTX hepatotoxicity in IBD patients appears to be lower than in those with psoriasis and rheumatoid arthritis. In a series of 20 IBD patients receiving a cumulative MTX dose of 1.5–5.4 g, only one patient developed hepatic fibrosis on biopsy [127]. Concordantly, in a recent series of 87 IBD patients, MTX was commonly associated with LFT abnormalities (24 %), but these frequently normalized while still on therapy, and in only 5 % was drug discontinuation necessary. Among patients with LFT abnormalities, 44 % had underlying risk factors for DILI, and liver biopsy rarely showed substantive abnormalities [128]. Therefore, liver biopsy may not routinely be necessary for IBD patients without risk factor(s). Close monitoring with LFTs every 1–3 months is recommended, and liver biopsy should be performed if the majority of ALT values over 1-year period are elevated or if serum albumin is decreased (Fig. 41.4) [5, 123, 129]. Supplementation with folic acid may help to reduce hepatic adverse effects associated with MTX [130].

## Anti-TNF Agents

It is difficult to estimate the incidence of DILI associated with anti-TNF agents, since anti-TNFs are generally used along with thiopurines or MTX. Few cases of DILI have been reported with infliximab. However, in clinical trials with infliximab for IBD, liver injury was not seen or was seen at a similar rate compared to the placebo arm [115, 131]. Clinical features of infliximab-associated DILI typically resemble autoimmune hepatitis and include a positive ANA and/or ASMA and with female predominance [132]. In addition, cholestatic liver injury associated with infliximab has also been reported [5].

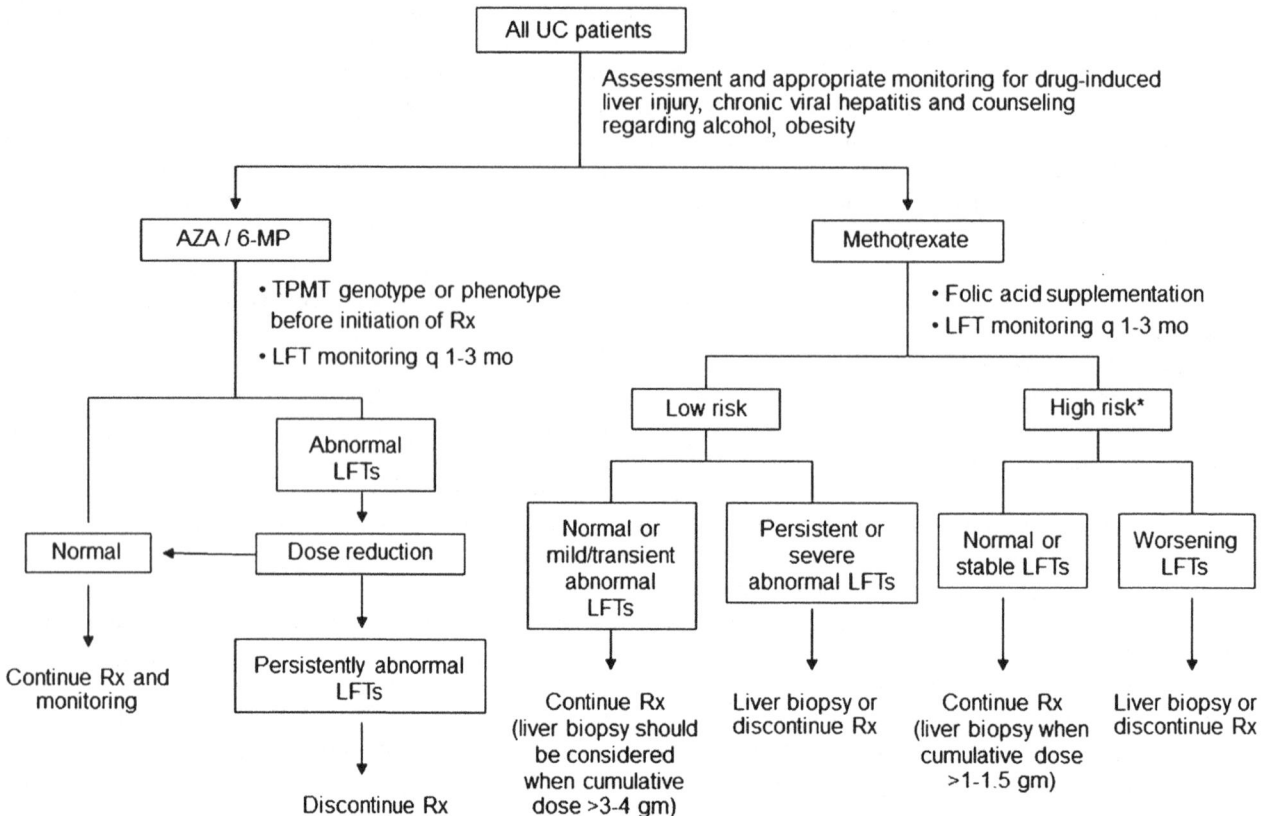

*Risk factors for MTX hepatotoxicity include older age, obesity, diabetes, long-term alcohol intake, pre-existing liver disease

**Fig. 41.4** Algorithm for the monitoring and the management of drug-induced liver injury in patients with ulcerative colitis

## Reactivation of Viral Hepatitis

Decades ago, patients with IBD were considered to be at risk for hepatitis B virus (HBV) and hepatitis C virus (HCV) infections, possibly related to frequent hospitalization, blood transfusion, and surgery. However, recent epidemiological studies have noted that the prevalence of HBV and HCV in IBD patients was similar to the general population, possibly as a result of improvement in IBD care, safety measures for blood transfusion, and universal HBV vaccination [121]. Treatment of UC may affect the clinical course of viral hepatitis, particularly HBV, and vice versa. Without antiviral prophylaxis, HBV reactivation following ISA can be associated with severe, or even fulminant, hepatitis.

## Hepatitis B
### Prevalence and Clinical Significance
Recent studies (after 2000) from North America and Europe have reported the prevalence of HBsAg-positive and anti-HBc-positive state in UC patients to be 0.6–2.3 % (weighted mean 0.8 %) and 1.6–17 % (weighted mean 8.1 %), respectively [121]. Reactivation of HBV replication has been reported in 20–50 % of HBV carriers undergoing ISA, and severity can range from self-limiting anicteric hepatitis to severe fulminant hepatitis [133]. Liver-related mortality in patients receiving cancer chemotherapy is reported to be 4–60 % [134]. A diagnosis of HBV reactivation is confirmed by an increase in serum HBV-DNA levels along with a positive HBsAg and can occur at any time during the treatment period, with the highest rates observed at either after initiation or withdrawal of ISA.

Incidence of HBV reactivation depends on the type and degree of immunosuppression and state of HBV infection when ISA is given. Cytotoxic chemotherapies, particularly in combination with corticosteroids and/or rituximab, carry the greatest risk (>60 %) of reactivation [135]. Reactivation of hepatitis B is uncommon, but has been reported, with long-term use of AZA, MTX, and low-dose corticosteroids [136]. Recently, HBV reactivation associated with anti-TNF

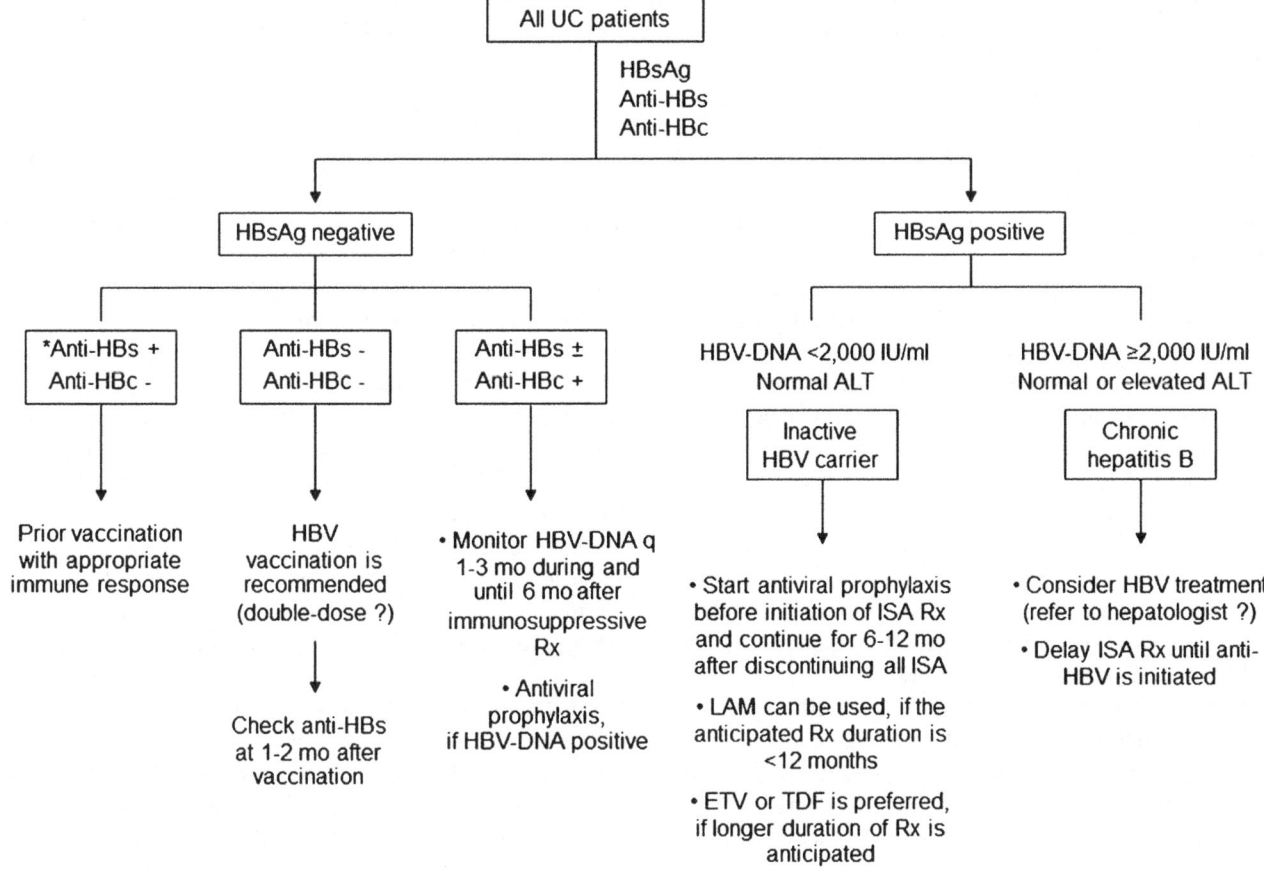

*Anti-HBs + is considered when titer ≥10 mlU/ml

**Fig. 41.5** Algorithm for the prophylaxis and the management of viral hepatitis B in patients with ulcerative colitis

has been increasingly reported in IBD patients, particularly in CD [121, 135]. All cases received infliximab, and nearly all cases received concomitant ISAs (AZA, corticosteroids). Duration of infliximab treatment ranged from 1 infusion to 2 years [121]. Several fatal cases and breakthrough reactivation despite lamivudine prophylaxis have also been reported [121]. Though there are no cases yet reported with the newer anti-TNF agents, such as adalimumab and certolizumab, one would need to use HBV prophylaxis in the appropriate patients at risk as these new agents also have the potential for promoting HBV reactivation.

A multicenter study from Spain assessed outcome of viral hepatitis in 129 IBD patients; 104 had positive anti-HBc, and 25 were HBsAg positive. Liver dysfunction was observed in 36 % (9/25) of HBsAg-positive patients and six of whom developed liver failure. Treatment with ≥2 ISAs was an independent predictor for reactivation, whereas HBV reactivation was infrequent with single ISA or in patients with positive anti-HBc alone [137].

## Screening and Management

All IBD patients should be screened for chronic HBV infection (Fig. 41.5). Screening should be performed at the diagnosis of IBD and the reasonable tests are HBsAg and anti-HBs. In patients without detectable HBsAg, HBV vaccination should be given in those who have negative or low levels of anti-HBs (<10 IU/L), before the initiation of ISA. Generally, three-dose regimen of a recombinant DNA vaccine at 0, 1, and 6 months is often effective [121, 135]. However, in a series of 129 IBD patients who received HBV vaccination, inadequate immune response was observed in more than half of patients, particularly in the elderly and in those previously or currently treated with ISA [138]. A recent study noted that a quick double-dose HBV vaccine regimen (0, 1, and 2 months) was associated with a higher response rate, and this strategy might be ideal in IBD patients [139]. Postvaccination anti-HBs levels should be obtained in all UC patients in order to confirm immune response. Data from non-IBD populations suggests that revaccination with either standard or double-dose regimens, using combined hepatitis A and B vaccine or intradermally administered vaccine, may be of benefit in suboptimal responders [140–142]. A high proportion of IBD patients with protective anti-HBs titers after vaccination lose them overtime particularly in those on anti-TNF therapy [143]. Therefore, periodic checking for anti-HBs levels is recommended, and booster dose should be considered in heavily immunosuppressed patients who are at risk for HBV infection.

The significance of isolated anti-HBc in this context remains controversial. Anti-HBc may be falsely positive in a low prevalence population. On the other hand, isolated positive anti-HBc can represent occult HBV infection (very low levels of HBsAg and HBV-DNA), particularly in high-risk or immunosuppressed patients [133, 135]. Several cases of HBV reactivation in patients with isolated positive anti-HBc have been reported in the setting of bone marrow transplantation or in patients who received rituximab; this is extremely rare in other settings. Therefore, antiviral prophylaxis is not recommended in isolated anti-HBc-positive patients [121, 133, 135]. Nevertheless, periodic monitoring of ALT and HBV-DNA should be considered.

Patients with chronic HBV infection (HBsAg-positive) warrant further evaluation, and antiviral treatment is considered in patients with active disease according to their HBV-DNA, HBeAg, and ALT status. In inactive HBV carriers, antiviral prophylaxis is recommended prior to undergoing treatment with any ISAs, including steroids, thiopurines, MTX, and biological agents. Prophylaxis should be continued until 6–12 months after discontinuation of all ISAs. Clinical studies, including 2 RCTs, demonstrated that prophylactic therapy with lamivudine can reduce the rate of HBV reactivation, severity of associated hepatitis flare, and mortality [133, 144]. Patients with UC often require long-term ISA, which overtime raises the concern of HBV resistance to lamivudine. Therefore, antivirals with high-genetic barrier for resistance, such as entecavir or tenofovir, should be considered, as opposed to lamivudine, in patients with HBV and the need for long-term ISAs for IBD [133, 135].

## Hepatitis C
### Prevalence and Clinical Significance
Recent studies (after 2000) from North America and Europe have reported the prevalence of anti-HCV positivity in UC patients to be 0.6–10.9 % (weighted mean 2.7 %) [121]. In post-LT setting, high-dose intravenous corticosteroids used in HCV-positive LT recipients are associated with a transient increase in HCV viremia, which may in turn promote HCV recurrence [145]. However, there are no convincing data that ISAs used in IBD patients, including corticosteroids, thiopurines, MTX, and anti-TNFs, have detrimental effect on the course of HCV [121, 135]. On the other hand, in vitro data

suggest that AZA, MMF, and anti-TNFs possess some anti-HCV activity [121, 145]. However, these findings have not yet been confirmed in the clinical arena.

### Screening and Management
It is reasonable to screen for anti-HCV in all IBD patients. Currently, there is no vaccine for HCV. There is little evidence to suggest that treatment of UC may negatively impact on the course of HCV. Antiviral prophylaxis is not recommended.

### Interferon Therapy and Its Impact on the Course of UC
Due to the immunomodulating properties of interferon-alfa used for the treatment of HBV and HCV, there is some concern that interferon may increase the risk of exacerbation of IBD. Theoretically, this is more likely to be in patients with CD which is predominantly characterized by Th1-type immune response [121]. In contrast to CD, earlier studies suggest a potential benefit of interferon-alfa in UC patients, but this finding was not confirmed by a Cochrane review in 2008 [146]. Though there were some case reports of new-onset UC or exacerbation of preexisting UC during interferon treatment [121], this is very unlikely to occur, particularly in those who are in clinical remission or have mildly active disease. A case-control study suggests that interferon-alfa can be safely administered to patients with HCV and IBD (10 CD and 11 UC patients), and virologic responses were similar to those observed in non-IBD HCV-matched controls [147].

## Hepatosplenic T-Cell Lymphoma (HSTCL)

HSTCL is a rare subtype of peripheral T-cell lymphoma and is associated with an aggressive course and dismal prognosis. Although uncommon, it has been increasingly reported in IBD patients, particularly CD [5, 148]. The development of HSTCL is possibly related to chromosomal abnormality induced by long-standing use of IBD medications [149]. HSTCL commonly presents with fever, fatigue, abnormal LFTs, pancytopenia, and hepatosplenomegaly. Most cases are young men (age <35 years) and have a history of receiving combination thiopurines and anti-TNF therapy [148].

## Summary

Hepatobiliary diseases are not uncommon in patients with UC. Among a variety of hepatobiliary diseases encountered in UC, PSC is the most common and likely to share pathogenesis with UC. A diagnosis of PSC is based on a constellation of clinical, biochemical, and typical cholangiographic features. The response to a variety of medical therapies for PSC has varied. The most common agent that has been widely utilized is UDCA, and there have been mixed results. Recent data found that high-dose UDCA may even be harmful. Cancer surveillance, management of portal hypertension and its complications, and treatment of manifestations of cholestasis in those with PSC are clinically relevant. To a lesser extent, PSC variants and overlap of PSC and AIH can also be encountered, in addition to other miscellaneous hepatobiliary conditions, such as fatty liver, PVT, PBC granulomatous hepatitis, and hepatic amyloidosis. ISAs used for UC can be associated with various patterns of DILI and can reactivate chronic hepatitis B. Anti-HBV prophylaxis is recommended in UC patients with chronic HBV prior to pursuing treatment with ISAs.

# References

1. Broome U, Glaumann H, Hellers G, Nilsson B, Sorstad J, Hultcrantz R. Liver disease in ulcerative colitis: an epidemiological and follow up study in the county of Stockholm. Gut. 1994;35(1):84–9.
2. Yamamoto-Furusho JK, Sanchez-Osorio M, Uribe M. Prevalence and factors associated with the presence of abnormal function liver tests in patients with ulcerative colitis. Ann Hepatol. 2010;9(4):397–401.
3. Gisbert JP, Luna M, Gonzalez-Lama Y, et al. Liver injury in inflammatory bowel disease: long-term follow-up study of 786 patients. Inflamm Bowel Dis. 2007;13(9):1106–14.
4. Riegler G, D'Inca R, Sturniolo GC, et al. Hepatobiliary alterations in patients with inflammatory bowel disease: a multicenter study. Caprilli & Gruppo Italiano Studio Colon-Retto. Scand J Gastroenterol. 1998;33(1):93–8.
5. Navaneethan U, Shen B. Hepatopancreatobiliary manifestations and complications associated with inflammatory bowel disease. Inflamm Bowel Dis. 2010;16(9):1598–619.
6. Bernstein CN, Blanchard JF, Rawsthorne P, Yu N. The prevalence of extraintestinal diseases in inflammatory bowel disease: a population-based study. Am J Gastroenterol. 2001;96(4):1116–22.
7. Weismuller TJ, Wedemeyer J, Kubicka S, Strassburg CP, Manns MP. The challenges in primary sclerosing cholangitis–aetiopathogenesis, autoimmunity, management and malignancy. J Hepatol. 2008;48 Suppl 1:S38–57.
8. Chapman R, Fevery J, Kalloo A, et al. Diagnosis and management of primary sclerosing cholangitis. Hepatology. 2010;51(2):660–78.
9. Bergquist A, Ekbom A, Olsson R, et al. Hepatic and extrahepatic malignancies in primary sclerosing cholangitis. J Hepatol Mar. 2002;36(3):321–7.
10. Bambha K, Kim WR, Talwalkar J, et al. Incidence, clinical spectrum, and outcomes of primary sclerosing cholangitis in a United States community. Gastroenterology. 2003;125(5):1364–9.
11. Card TR, Solaymani-Dodaran M, West J. Incidence and mortality of primary sclerosing cholangitis in the UK: a population-based cohort study. J Hepatol. 2008;48(6):939–44.
12. Kaplan GG, Laupland KB, Butzner D, Urbanski SJ, Lee SS. The burden of large and small duct primary sclerosing cholangitis in adults and children: a population-based analysis. Am J Gastroenterol. 2007;102(5):1042–9.
13. Shorbagi A, Bayraktar Y. Primary sclerosing cholangitis – what is the difference between east and west? World J Gastroenterol. 2008;14(25):3974–81.
14. Thia KT, Loftus Jr EV, Sandborn WJ, Yang SK. An update on the epidemiology of inflammatory bowel disease in Asia. Am J Gastroenterol. 2008;103(12):3167–82.
15. Broome U, Olsson R, Loof L, et al. Natural history and prognostic factors in 305 Swedish patients with primary sclerosing cholangitis. Gut. 1996;38(4):610–5.
16. Wiesner RH, Grambsch PM, Dickson ER, et al. Primary sclerosing cholangitis: natural history, prognostic factors and survival analysis. Hepatology. 1989;10(4):430–6.
17. Rasmussen HH, Fallingborg JF, Mortensen PB, Vyberg M, Tage-Jensen U, Rasmussen SN. Hepatobiliary dysfunction and primary sclerosing cholangitis in patients with Crohn's disease. Scand J Gastroenterol. 1997;32(6):604–10.
18. Olsson R, Danielsson A, Jarnerot G, et al. Prevalence of primary sclerosing cholangitis in patients with ulcerative colitis. Gastroenterology. 1991;100(5 Pt 1):1319–23.
19. Takikawa H, Manabe T. Primary sclerosing cholangitis in Japan – analysis of 192 cases. J Gastroenterol. 1997;32(1):134–7.
20. Tanaka A, Takamori Y, Toda G, Ohnishi S, Takikawa H. Outcome and prognostic factors of 391 Japanese patients with primary sclerosing cholangitis. Liver Int. 2008;28(7):983–9.
21. Escorsell A, Pares A, Rodes J, Solis-Herruzo JA, Miras M, de la Morena E. Epidemiology of primary sclerosing cholangitis in Spain. Spanish Association for the Study of the Liver. J Hepatol. 1994;21(5):787–91.
22. Kochhar R, Goenka MK, Das K, et al. Primary sclerosing cholangitis: an experience from India. J Gastroenterol Hepatol. 1996;11(5):429–33.
23. Kingham JG, Kochar N, Gravenor MB. Incidence, clinical patterns, and outcomes of primary sclerosing cholangitis in South Wales, United Kingdom. Gastroenterology. 2004;126(7):1929–30.
24. Broome U, Bergquist A. Primary sclerosing cholangitis, inflammatory bowel disease, and colon cancer. Semin Liver Dis. 2006;26(1):31–41.
25. Aoki CA, Bowlus CL, Gershwin ME. The immunobiology of primary sclerosing cholangitis. Autoimmun Rev. 2005;4(3):137–43.
26. Chandra NCS, Chapman RW. Primary sclerosing cholangitis. In: McDonald JWDBA, Feagan BG, Fennerty MB, editors. Evidence-based gastroenterology and hepatology. 3rd ed. Chichester, UK: Blackwell; 2010. p. 533–53.
27. Karlsen TH, Schrumpf E, Boberg KM. Genetic epidemiology of primary sclerosing cholangitis. World J Gastroenterol. 2007;13(41):5421–31.
28. Terjung B, Worman HJ. Anti-neutrophil antibodies in primary sclerosing cholangitis. Best Pract Res Clin Gastroenterol. 2001;15(4):629–42.
29. Terjung B, Sohne J, Lechtenberg B, et al. p-ANCAs in autoimmune liver disorders recognise human beta-tubulin isotype 5 and cross-react with microbial protein FtsZ. Gut. 2010;59(6):808–16.
30. Saarinen S, Olerup O, Broome U. Increased frequency of autoimmune diseases in patients with primary sclerosing cholangitis. Am J Gastroenterol. 2000;95(11):3195–9.
31. Bergquist A, Lindberg G, Saarinen S, Broome U. Increased prevalence of primary sclerosing cholangitis among first-degree relatives. J Hepatol. 2005;42(2):252–6.
32. Karlsen TH, Hampe J, Wiencke K, et al. Genetic polymorphisms associated with inflammatory bowel disease do not confer risk for primary sclerosing cholangitis. Am J Gastroenterol. 2007;102(1):115–21.
33. Karlsen TH, Boberg KM, Vatn M, et al. Different HLA class II associations in ulcerative colitis patients with and without primary sclerosing cholangitis. Genes Immun. 2007;8(3):275–8.
34. Karlsen TH, Franke A, Melum E, et al. Genome-wide association analysis in primary sclerosing cholangitis. Gastroenterology. 2010;138(3):1102–11.

35. Melum E, Franke A, Schramm C, et al. Genome-wide association analysis in primary sclerosing cholangitis identifies two non-HLA susceptibility loci. Nat Genet. 2011;43(1):17–9.

36. Janse M, Lamberts LE, Franke L, et al. Three ulcerative colitis susceptibility loci are associated with primary sclerosing cholangitis and indicate a role for IL2, REL, and CARD9. Hepatology. 2011;53(6):1977–85.

37. Hov JR, Keitel V, Laerdahl JK, et al. Mutational characterization of the bile acid receptor TGR5 in primary sclerosing cholangitis. PLoS One. 2010;5(8):e12403.

38. Mandal A, Dasgupta A, Jeffers L, et al. Autoantibodies in sclerosing cholangitis against a shared peptide in biliary and colon epithelium. Gastroenterology. 1994;106(1):185–92.

39. Karrar A, Broome U, Sodergren T, et al. Biliary epithelial cell antibodies link adaptive and innate immune responses in primary sclerosing cholangitis. Gastroenterology. 2007;132(4):1504–14.

40. Xu B, Broome U, Ericzon BG, Sumitran-Holgersson S. High frequency of autoantibodies in patients with primary sclerosing cholangitis that bind biliary epithelial cells and induce expression of CD44 and production of interleukin 6. Gut. 2002;51(1):120–7.

41. Spirli C, Fabris L, Duner E, et al. Cytokine-stimulated nitric oxide production inhibits adenylyl cyclase and cAMP-dependent secretion in cholangiocytes. Gastroenterology. 2003;124(3):737–53.

42. Karlsen TH, Lie BA, Frey Froslie K, et al. Polymorphisms in the steroid and xenobiotic receptor gene influence survival in primary sclerosing cholangitis. Gastroenterology. 2006;131(3):781–7.

43. Fickert P, Fuchsbichler A, Wagner M, et al. Regurgitation of bile acids from leaky bile ducts causes sclerosing cholangitis in Mdr2 (Abcb4) knockout mice. Gastroenterology. 2004;127(1):261–74.

44. Pauli-Magnus C, Kerb R, Fattinger K, et al. BSEP and MDR3 haplotype structure in healthy Caucasians, primary biliary cirrhosis and primary sclerosing cholangitis. Hepatology. 2004;39(3):779–91.

45. van den Ent F, Amos L, Lowe J. Bacterial ancestry of actin and tubulin. Curr Opin Microbiol. 2001;4(6):634–8.

46. Palmer KR, Duerden BI, Holdsworth CD. Bacteriological and endotoxin studies in cases of ulcerative colitis submitted to surgery. Gut. 1980;21(10):851–4.

47. Bjornsson E, Cederborg A, Akvist A, Simren M, Stotzer PO, Bjarnason I. Intestinal permeability and bacterial growth of the small bowel in patients with primary sclerosing cholangitis. Scand J Gastroenterol. 2005;40(9):1090–4.

48. Tischendorf JJ, Hecker H, Kruger M, Manns MP, Meier PN. Characterization, outcome, and prognosis in 273 patients with primary sclerosing cholangitis: a single center study. Am J Gastroenterol. 2007;102(1):107–14.

49. Bjornsson E, Simren M, Olsson R, Chapman RW. Fatigue in patients with primary sclerosing cholangitis. Scand J Gastroenterol. 2004;39(10):961–8.

50. Bangarulingam SY, Gossard AA, Petersen BT, Ott BJ, Lindor KD. Complications of endoscopic retrograde cholangiopancreatography in primary sclerosing cholangitis. Am J Gastroenterol. 2009;104(4):855–60.

51. Ponsioen CY, Reitsma JB, Boberg KM, Aabakken L, Rauws EA, Schrumpf E. Validation of a cholangiographic prognostic model in primary sclerosing cholangitis. Endoscopy. 2010;42(9):742–7.

52. Braden B, Faust D, Ignee A, Schreiber D, Hirche T, Dietrich CF. Clinical relevance of perihepatic lymphadenopathy in acute and chronic liver disease. J Clin Gastroenterol. 2008;42(8):931–6.

53. Johnson KJ, Olliff JF, Olliff SP. The presence and significance of lymphadenopathy detected by CT in primary sclerosing cholangitis. Br J Radiol. 1998;71(852):1279–82.

54. Fevery J, Verslype C, Lai G, Aerts R, Van Steenbergen W. Incidence, diagnosis, and therapy of cholangiocarcinoma in patients with primary sclerosing cholangitis. Dig Dis Sci. 2007;52(11):3123–35.

55. Boberg KM, Rocca G, Egeland T, et al. Time-dependent Cox regression model is superior in prediction of prognosis in primary sclerosing cholangitis. Hepatology. 2002;35(3):652–7.

56. Kim WR, Therneau TM, Wiesner RH, et al. A revised natural history model for primary sclerosing cholangitis. Mayo Clin Proc. 2000;75(7):688–94.

57. Talwalkar JA, Seaberg E, Kim WR, Wiesner RH. Predicting clinical and economic outcomes after liver transplantation using the Mayo primary sclerosing cholangitis model and Child-Pugh score. National Institutes of Diabetes and Digestive and Kidney Diseases Liver Transplantation Database Group. Liver Transpl. 2000;6(6):753–8.

58. Joo M, Abreu-e-Lima P, Farraye F, et al. Pathologic features of ulcerative colitis in patients with primary sclerosing cholangitis: a case-control study. Am J Surg Pathol. 2009;33(6):854–62.

59. Paumgartner G, Beuers U. Mechanisms of action and therapeutic efficacy of ursodeoxycholic acid in cholestatic liver disease. Clin Liver Dis. 2004;8(1):67–81. vi.

60. European Association for the Study of the Liver. Clinical practice guidelines: management of cholestatic liver diseases. J Hepatol. 2009;51(2):237–67.

61. Culver EL, Chapman RW. Systematic review: management options for primary sclerosing cholangitis and its variant forms – IgG4-associated cholangitis and overlap with autoimmune hepatitis. Aliment Pharmacol Ther. 2011;33(12):1273–91.

62. Lindor KD. Ursodiol for primary sclerosing cholangitis. Mayo Primary Sclerosing Cholangitis-Ursodeoxycholic Acid Study Group. N Engl J Med. 1997;336(10):691–5.

63. Mitchell SA, Bansi DS, Hunt N, Von Bergmann K, Fleming KA, Chapman RW. A preliminary trial of high-dose ursodeoxycholic acid in primary sclerosing cholangitis. Gastroenterology. 2001;121(4):900–7.

64. Harnois DM, Angulo P, Jorgensen RA, Larusso NF, Lindor KD. High-dose ursodeoxycholic acid as a therapy for patients with primary sclerosing cholangitis. Am J Gastroenterol. 2001;96(5):1558–62.

65. Cullen SN, Rust C, Fleming K, Edwards C, Beuers U, Chapman RW. High dose ursodeoxycholic acid for the treatment of primary sclerosing cholangitis is safe and effective. J Hepatol. 2008;48(5):792–800.

66. Olsson R, Boberg KM, de Muckadell OS, et al. High-dose ursodeoxycholic acid in primary sclerosing cholangitis: a 5-year multicenter, randomized, controlled study. Gastroenterology. 2005;129(5):1464–72.

67. Lindor KD, Kowdley KV, Luketic VA, et al. High-dose ursodeoxycholic acid for the treatment of primary sclerosing cholangitis. Hepatology. 2009;50(3):808–14.

68. Angulo P, Batts KP, Jorgensen RA, LaRusso NA, Lindor KD. Oral budesonide in the treatment of primary sclerosing cholangitis. Am J Gastroenterol. 2000;95(9):2333–7.

69. Giljaca V, Poropat G, Stimac D, Gluud C. Glucocorticosteroids for primary sclerosing cholangitis. Cochrane Database Syst Rev. 2010;1, CD004036.

70. Lindor KD, Wiesner RH, Colwell LJ, Steiner B, Beaver S, LaRusso NF. The combination of prednisone and colchicine in patients with primary sclerosing cholangitis. Am J Gastroenterol. 1991;86(1):57–61.

71. Schramm C, Schirmacher P, Helmreich-Becker I, Gerken G, zum Buschenfelde KH, Lohse AW. Combined therapy with azathioprine, prednisolone, and ursodiol in patients with primary sclerosing cholangitis. A case series. Ann Intern Med. 1999;131(12):943–6.

72. Knox TA, Kaplan MM. A double-blind controlled trial of oral-pulse methotrexate therapy in the treatment of primary sclerosing cholangitis. Gastroenterology. 1994;106(2):494–9.

73. Lindor KD, Jorgensen RA, Anderson ML, Gores GJ, Hofmann AF, LaRusso NF. Ursodeoxycholic acid and methotrexate for

primary sclerosing cholangitis: a pilot study. Am J Gastroenterol. 1996;91(3):511–5.

74. Talwalkar JA, Angulo P, Keach JC, Petz JL, Jorgensen RA, Lindor KD. Mycophenolate mofetil for the treatment of primary sclerosing cholangitis. Am J Gastroenterol. 2005;100(2):308–12.

75. Talwalkar JA, Gossard AA, Keach JC, Jorgensen RA, Petz JL, Lindor RN. Tacrolimus for the treatment of primary sclerosing cholangitis. Liver Int. 2007;27(4):451–3.

76. Sandborn WJ, Wiesner RH, Tremaine WJ, Larusso NF. Ulcerative colitis disease activity following treatment of associated primary sclerosing cholangitis with cyclosporin. Gut. 1993;34(2):242–6.

77. Hommes DW, Erkelens W, Ponsioen C, et al. A double-blind, placebo-controlled, randomized study of infliximab in primary sclerosing cholangitis. J Clin Gastroenterol. 2008;42(5):522–6.

78. LaRusso NF, Wiesner RH, Ludwig J, MacCarty RL, Beaver SJ, Zinsmeister AR. Prospective trial of penicillamine in primary sclerosing cholangitis. Gastroenterology. 1988;95(4):1036–42.

79. Olsson R, Broome U, Danielsson A, et al. Colchicine treatment of primary sclerosing cholangitis. Gastroenterology. 1995;108(4): 1199–203.

80. Angulo P, Jorgensen RA, Kowdley KV, Lindor KD. Silymarin in the treatment of patients with primary sclerosing cholangitis: an open-label pilot study. Dig Dis Sci. 2008;53(6):1716–20.

81. Silveira MG, Torok NJ, Gossard AA, et al. Minocycline in the treatment of patients with primary sclerosing cholangitis: results of a pilot study. Am J Gastroenterol. 2009;104(1):83–8.

82. Chalasani N, Baluyut A, Ismail A, et al. Cholangiocarcinoma in patients with primary sclerosing cholangitis: a multicenter case-control study. Hepatology. 2000;31(1):7–11.

83. Levy C, Lymp J, Angulo P, Gores GJ, Larusso N, Lindor KD. The value of serum CA 19-9 in predicting cholangiocarcinomas in patients with primary sclerosing cholangitis. Dig Dis Sci. 2005;50(9):1734–40.

84. Charatcharoenwitthaya P, Enders FB, Halling KC, Lindor KD. Utility of serum tumor markers, imaging, and biliary cytology for detecting cholangiocarcinoma in primary sclerosing cholangitis. Hepatology. 2008;48(4):1106–17.

85. Rea DJ, Rosen CB, Nagorney DM, Heimbach JK, Gores GJ. Transplantation for cholangiocarcinoma: when and for whom? Surg Oncol Clin N Am. 2009;18(2):325–37. ix.

86. Soetikno RM, Lin OS, Heidenreich PA, Young HS, Blackstone MO. Increased risk of colorectal neoplasia in patients with primary sclerosing cholangitis and ulcerative colitis: a meta-analysis. Gastrointest Endosc. 2002;56(1):48–54.

87. Shetty K, Rybicki L, Brzezinski A, Carey WD, Lashner BA. The risk for cancer or dysplasia in ulcerative colitis patients with primary sclerosing cholangitis. Am J Gastroenterol. 1999;94(6):1643–9.

88. Brandt DJ, MacCarty RL, Charboneau JW, LaRusso NF, Wiesner RH, Ludwig J. Gallbladder disease in patients with primary sclerosing cholangitis. Am J Roentgenol. 1988;150(3):571–4.

89. Lewis JT, Talwalkar JA, Rosen CB, Smyrk TC, Abraham SC. Prevalence and risk factors for gallbladder neoplasia in patients with primary sclerosing cholangitis: evidence for a metaplasia-dysplasia-carcinoma sequence. Am J Surg Pathol. 2007;31(6):907–13.

90. Buckles DC, Lindor KD, Larusso NF, Petrovic LM, Gores GJ. In primary sclerosing cholangitis, gallbladder polyps are frequently malignant. Am J Gastroenterol. 2002;97(5):1138–42.

91. Leung UC, Wong PY, Roberts RH, Koea JB. Gall bladder polyps in sclerosing cholangitis: does the 1-cm rule apply? ANZ J Surg. 2007;77(5):355–7.

92. Bonnel AR, Bunchorntavakul C, Reddy KR. Immune dysfunction and infections in patients with cirrhosis. Clin Gastroenterol Hepatol. 2011;9(9):727–38.

93. Alabraba E, Nightingale P, Gunson B, et al. A re-evaluation of the risk factors for the recurrence of primary sclerosing cholangitis in liver allografts. Liver Transpl. 2009;15(3):330–40.

94. Verdonk RC, Dijkstra G, Haagsma EB, et al. Inflammatory bowel disease after liver transplantation: risk factors for recurrence and de novo disease. Am J Transplant. 2006;6(6):1422–9.

95. Dvorchik I, Subotin M, Demetris AJ, et al. Effect of liver transplantation on inflammatory bowel disease in patients with primary sclerosing cholangitis. Hepatology. 2002;35(2):380–4.

96. Lichtenstein GR, Sands BE, Pazianas M. Prevention and treatment of osteoporosis in inflammatory bowel disease. Inflamm Bowel Dis. 2006;12(8):797–813.

97. Rouillard S, Lane NE. Hepatic osteodystrophy. Hepatology. 2001;33(1):301–7.

98. Angulo P, Grandison GA, Fong DG, et al. Bone disease in patients with primary sclerosing cholangitis. Gastroenterology. 2011; 140(1):180–8.

99. Bjornsson E, Olsson R, Bergquist A, et al. The natural history of small-duct primary sclerosing cholangitis. Gastroenterology. 2008;134(4):975–80.

100. Charatcharoenwitthaya P, Angulo P, Enders FB, Lindor KD. Impact of inflammatory bowel disease and ursodeoxycholic acid therapy on small-duct primary sclerosing cholangitis. Hepatology. 2008;47(1):133–42.

101. Boberg KM, Chapman RW, Hirschfield GM, Lohse AW, Manns MP, Schrumpf E. Overlap syndromes: the International Autoimmune Hepatitis Group (IAIHG) position statement on a controversial issue. J Hepatol. 2011;54(2):374–85.

102. Alvarez F, Berg PA, Bianchi FB, et al. International Autoimmune Hepatitis Group Report: review of criteria for diagnosis of autoimmune hepatitis. J Hepatol. 1999;31(5):929–38.

103. Al-Chalabi T, Portmann BC, Bernal W, McFarlane IG, Heneghan MA. Autoimmune hepatitis overlap syndromes: an evaluation of treatment response, long-term outcome and survival. Aliment Pharmacol Ther. 2008;28(2):209–20.

104. Floreani A, Rizzotto ER, Ferrara F, et al. Clinical course and outcome of autoimmune hepatitis/primary sclerosing cholangitis overlap syndrome. Am J Gastroenterol. 2005;100(7): 1516–22.

105. Ghazale A, Chari ST, Zhang L, et al. Immunoglobulin G4-associated cholangitis: clinical profile and response to therapy. Gastroenterology. 2008;134(3):706–15.

106. Narula N, Vasudev M, Marshall JK. IgG-related sclerosing disease: a novel mimic of inflammatory bowel disease. Dig Dis Sci. 2010;55(11):3047–51.

107. Zhang L, Lewis JT, Abraham SC, et al. IgG4+ plasma cell infiltrates in liver explants with primary sclerosing cholangitis. Am J Surg Pathol. 2010;34(1):88–94.

108. Mendes FD, Jorgensen R, Keach J, et al. Elevated serum IgG4 concentration in patients with primary sclerosing cholangitis. Am J Gastroenterol. 2006;101(9):2070–5.

109. McGowan CE, Jones P, Long MD, Barritt AS. Changing shape of disease: nonalcoholic fatty liver disease in Crohn's disease – a case series and review of the literature. Inflamm Bowel Dis. 2011;18(1):49–54.

110. Baker ME, Remzi F, Einstein D, et al. CT depiction of portal vein thrombi after creation of ileal pouch-anal anastomosis. Radiology. 2003;227(1):73–9.

111. Ball CG, MacLean AR, Buie WD, Smith DF, Raber EL. Portal vein thrombi after ileal pouch-anal anastomosis: its incidence and association with pouchitis. Surg Today. 2007;37(7):552–7.

112. Remzi FH, Fazio VW, Oncel M, et al. Portal vein thrombi after restorative proctocolectomy. Surgery. 2002;132(4):655–61. discussion 661–2.

113. Xiao WB, Liu YL. Primary biliary cirrhosis and ulcerative colitis: a case report and review of literature. World J Gastroenterol. 2003;9(4):878–80.

114. Wester AL, Vatn MH, Fausa O. Secondary amyloidosis in inflammatory bowel disease: a study of 18 patients admitted to

Rikshospitalet University Hospital, Oslo, from 1962 to 1998. Inflamm Bowel Dis. 2001;7(4):295–300.

115. Khokhar OS, Lewis JH. Hepatotoxicity of agents used in the management of inflammatory bowel disease. Dig Dis. 2010;28(3): 508–18.

116. Ransford RA, Langman MJ. Sulphasalazine and mesalazine: serious adverse reactions re-evaluated on the basis of suspected adverse reaction reports to the Committee on Safety of Medicines. Gut. 2002;51(4):536–9.

117. Rachmilewitz D. Coated mesalazine (5-aminosalicylic acid) versus sulphasalazine in the treatment of active ulcerative colitis: a randomised trial. BMJ. 1989;298(6666):82–6.

118. Hautekeete ML, Bourgeois N, Potvin P, et al. Hypersensitivity with hepatotoxicity to mesalazine after hypersensitivity to sulfasalazine. Gastroenterology. 1992;103(6):1925–7.

119. Gisbert JP, Gonzalez-Lama Y, Mate J. Thiopurine-induced liver injury in patients with inflammatory bowel disease: a systematic review. Am J Gastroenterol. 2007;102(7):1518–27.

120. Kornbluth A, Sachar DB. Ulcerative colitis practice guidelines in adults: American College of Gastroenterology, Practice Parameters Committee. Am J Gastroenterol. 2010;105(3):501–23. quiz 524.

121. Gisbert JP, Chaparro M, Esteve M. Review article: prevention and management of hepatitis B and C infection in patients with inflammatory bowel disease. Aliment Pharmacol Ther. 2011;33(6):619–33.

122. Shaye OA, Yadegari M, Abreu MT, et al. Hepatotoxicity of 6-mercaptopurine (6-MP) and Azathioprine (AZA) in adult IBD patients. Am J Gastroenterol. 2007;102(11):2488–94.

123. Lichtenstein GR, Abreu MT, Cohen R, Tremaine W. American Gastroenterological Association Institute technical review on corticosteroids, immunomodulators, and infliximab in inflammatory bowel disease. Gastroenterology. 2006;130(3):940–87.

124. Ansari A, Elliott T, Baburajan B, et al. Long term outcome of using allopurinol co-therapy as a strategy for overcoming thiopurine hepatotoxicity in treating inflammatory bowel disease. Aliment Pharmacol Ther. 2008;28(6):734–41.

125. Seksik P, Mary JY, Beaugerie L, et al. Incidence of nodular regenerative hyperplasia in inflammatory bowel disease patients treated with azathioprine. Inflamm Bowel Dis. 2011;17(2):565–72.

126. Seiderer J, Zech CJ, Reinisch W, et al. A multicenter assessment of liver toxicity by MRI and biopsy in IBD patients on 6-thioguanine. J Hepatol. 2005;43(2):303–9.

127. Te HS, Schiano TD, Kuan SF, Hanauer SB, Conjeevaram HS, Baker AL. Hepatic effects of long-term methotrexate use in the treatment of inflammatory bowel disease. Am J Gastroenterol. 2000;95(11):3150–6.

128. Fournier MR, Klein J, Minuk GY, Bernstein CN. Changes in liver biochemistry during methotrexate use for inflammatory bowel disease. Am J Gastroenterol. 2010;105(7):1620–6.

129. Kremer JM, Alarcon GS, Lightfoot Jr RW, et al. Methotrexate for rheumatoid arthritis. Suggested guidelines for monitoring liver toxicity. American College of Rheumatology. Arthritis Rheum. 1994;37(3):316–28.

130. Prey S, Paul C. Effect of folic or folinic acid supplementation on methotrexate-associated safety and efficacy in inflammatory disease: a systematic review. Br J Dermatol. 2009;160(3):622–8.

131. Rutgeerts P, Sandborn WJ, Feagan BG, et al. Infliximab for induction and maintenance therapy for ulcerative colitis. N Engl J Med. 2005;353(23):2462–76.

132. Mancini S, Amorotti E, Vecchio S, Ponz de Leon M, Roncucci L. Infliximab-related hepatitis: discussion of a case and review of the literature. Intern Emerg Med. 2010;5(3):193–200.

133. Lok AS, McMahon BJ. Chronic hepatitis B: update 2009. Hepatology. 2009;50(3):661–2.

134. Kohrt HE, Ouyang DL, Keeffe EB. Antiviral prophylaxis for chemotherapy-induced reactivation of chronic hepatitis B virus infection. Clin Liver Dis. 2007;11(4):965–91. x.

135. Hou JK, Velayos F, Terrault N, Mahadevan U. Viral hepatitis and inflammatory bowel disease. Inflamm Bowel Dis. 2010;16(6): 925–32.

136. Hoofnagle JH. Reactivation of hepatitis B. Hepatology. 2009;49 Suppl 5:S156–65.

137. Loras C, Gisbert JP, Minguez M, et al. Liver dysfunction related to hepatitis B and C in patients with inflammatory bowel disease treated with immunosuppressive therapy. Gut. 2010;59(10): 1340–6.

138. Vida Perez L, Gomez Camacho F, Garcia Sanchez V, et al. Adequate rate of response to hepatitis B virus vaccination in patients with inflammatory bowel disease. Med Clin (Barc). 2009;132(9):331–5.

139. Chaparro M, Nogueiras AR, Menchen LA, Marin-Jimenez I, Garcia-Sanchez V, Villagrasa JR, Gisbert JP. Comparative study to evaluate the effectiveness of two different vaccination protocols against hepatitis B virus in inflammatory bowel disease patients. Gastroenterology. 2011;140(5 (Suppl 1)):S587–8.

140. Barraclough KA, Wiggins KJ, Hawley CM, et al. Intradermal versus intramuscular hepatitis B vaccination in hemodialysis patients: a prospective open-label randomized controlled trial in nonresponders to primary vaccination. Am J Kidney Dis. 2009;54(1): 95–103.

141. Cardell K, Akerlind B, Sallberg M, Fryden A. Excellent response rate to a double dose of the combined hepatitis A and B vaccine in previous nonresponders to hepatitis B vaccine. J Infect Dis. 2008;198(3):299–304.

142. Goldwater PN. Randomized, comparative trial of 20 micrograms vs 40 micrograms Engerix B vaccine in hepatitis B vaccine nonresponders. Vaccine. 1997;15(4):353–6.

143. Chaparro M, Nogueiras AR, Villagrasa JR, Gisbert JP. Kinetics of the anti-HBs titers after vaccination against hepatitis B virus in patients with inflammatory bowel disease. Gastroenterology. 2011;140(5 (Suppl 1)):S589.

144. Katz LH, Fraser A, Gafter-Gvili A, Leibovici L, Tur-Kaspa R. Lamivudine prevents reactivation of hepatitis B and reduces mortality in immunosuppressed patients: systematic review and meta-analysis. J Viral Hepat. 2008;15(2):89–102.

145. Watt K, Veldt B, Charlton M. A practical guide to the management of HCV infection following liver transplantation. Am J Transplant. 2009;9(8):1707–13.

146. Seow CH, Benchimol EI, Griffiths AM, Steinhart AH. Type I interferons for induction of remission in ulcerative colitis. Cochrane Database Syst Rev. 2008;3, CD006790.

147. Bargiggia S, Thorburn D, Anderloni A, et al. Is interferon-alpha therapy safe and effective for patients with chronic hepatitis C and inflammatory bowel disease? A case-control study. Aliment Pharmacol Ther. 2005;22(3):209–15.

148. Kotlyar DS, Osterman MT, Diamond RH, et al. A systematic review of factors that contribute to hepatosplenic T-cell lymphoma in patients with inflammatory bowel disease. Clin Gastroenterol Hepatol. 2011;9(1):36–41 e31.

149. Kotlyar DS, Blonski W, Diamond RH, Wasik M, Lichtenstein GR. Hepatosplenic T-cell lymphoma in inflammatory bowel disease: a possible thiopurine-induced chromosomal abnormality. Am J Gastroenterol. 2010;105(10):2299–301.

Michelle Vu and Daniel W. Hommes

**Keywords**

Therapy • Ulcerative colitis • Step-up • Top-down

## Introduction

Ulcerative colitis (UC) is an inflammatory bowel disease (IBD) characterized by a heterogeneous disease course, unpredictable disease activity, and variable response to treatment [1]. Disease classification is based on clinical features such as number of stools with or without blood, abdominal pain, signs of systemic toxicity, and laboratory or imaging abnormalities [2]. UC usually develops in a younger population with few comorbidities [3] and carries significant potential to adversely affect a patient's welfare, thus presenting a protracted challenge for healthcare providers to stave off its debilitating consequences. Patients with UC more frequently reported lower health-related quality of life (HRQOL) [4], and selection of appropriate therapy is crucial.

The goal of medical management is to induce rapid remission, maintain long-term remission, improve quality of life, reduce the need for chronic steroids, minimize disease- or therapy-related complications, and avoid surgery. Mucosal healing has also been recently introduced as a more objective outcome measure [5, 6], and its lack has been associated with a more aggressive disease course and poorer patient outcomes [7, 8]. Over a 10-year period, approximately two-thirds of UC patients will suffer one or more relapses [9] which are associated with higher incidence of complications [10], increased healthcare spending [10–12], and decreased quality of life [4, 13].

Traditional therapy has included sulfasalazine, mesalamine, and corticosteroids, which are effective in a proportion of IBD patients with mild to moderate colitis. The development of immunomodulating and biologic agents has opened a new dialogue surrounding optimal setting for delivery of these medications. With the advent of innovative therapies, advances in surgical techniques, and improved understanding of pathophysiology, focus has shifted toward individualizing our management approach to IBD and optimizing utilization of current resources. Central to this discussion is whether the traditional "step-up" approach to therapy should be modified and if these more intensive therapies should be introduced earlier in the course of the disease.

Prior to the development of potential "top-down" treatment algorithms that begin with higher drug intensity selection, it is imperative to be able to justify exposure to potential drug toxicities by identifying those who will develop more complicated disease—a task that is currently impossible due to the unpredictable nature of UC. This chapter outlines the rationale for a *proactive* step-up approach to therapy in UC, identifies early indicators, which can help guide choice of therapy, and introduces treatment intensities for different severity scenarios.

M. Vu, M.D. (✉)
Division of Digestive Diseases, University of California,
Los Angeles, 10945 Le Conte Ave PVUB 2114 MC694907,
Los Angeles, CA, USA
e-mail: mvu@mednet.ucla.edu

D.W. Hommes, M.D., Ph.D.
Division of Digestive Diseases, UCLA Center for Inflammatory
Bowel Diseases, 10945 Le Conte Ave., Suite 2338E, Los Angeles,
CA 90095, USA
e-mail: dhommes@mednet.ucla.edu

## Disease Course

Established definitions classify disease activity and are widely applied in clinical trials and everyday practice [14], but they lack predictive power regarding overall disease course. UC follows a variable path, with more than 50 % of

**Fig. 42.1** Graphical presentation of the activity courses for 600 patients during 3–7 years after diagnosis. Adapted with permission from Elsevier [22]

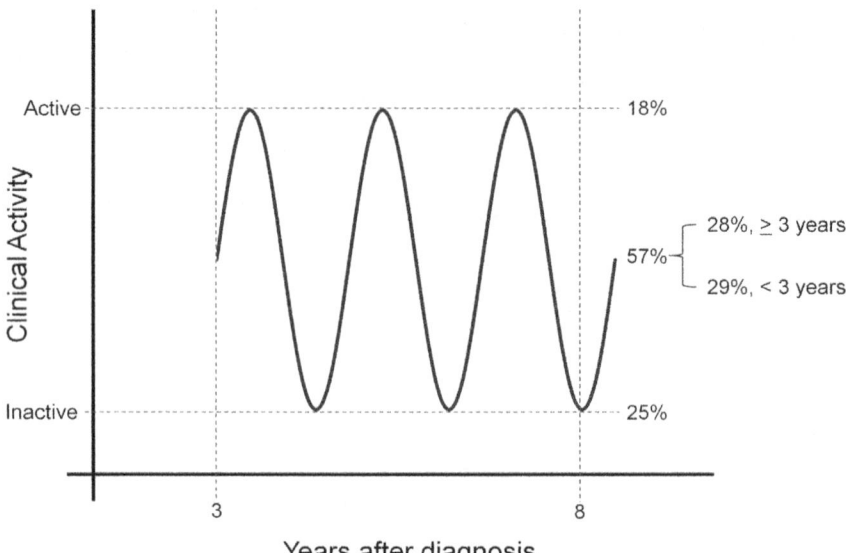

patients first manifesting with mild colitis and up to 19 % of patients initially presenting with severe colitis [15, 16]. Population-based studies of the natural history of UC found that the majority of patients experience indolent, intermittently relapsing disease pattern, with half of those cases being in remission at any point in time [17, 18]. A smaller fraction of patients have mostly quiescent disease, and the rest suffer from relentlessly active colitis [19, 20]. This distribution has held relatively constant despite advances in medical therapy. A longer length of period with flares or remission increases the likelihood of having a similar course in the following years, but by 25 years after diagnosis, it has been estimated that as many as 90 % of patients will continue to suffer from intermittent flares [21]. Figure 42.1, adapted from Langholz et al., demonstrates the varied and fluctuating nature of UC between years 3 and 7 after diagnosis, where 25 % of patients stayed in remission, 57 % had intermittent flares, and 18 % had active disease [22].

Investigations to uncover clinical predictors of long-term disease course have been unsuccessful. Ritchie et al. found that there was no relationship between future disease course and disease extent or severity at the first attack. However, there was an association between disease extent during an attack year and maximal disease severity that year [18], which was confirmed later by Langholz et al. [22]. These findings indicate that severity and disease extent during an exacerbation are prognostic of only the immediately subsequent clinical course, without providing information on long-term disease. Thus, while our arsenal has expanded, a semi-prophylactic approach utilizing higher-intensity therapeutics in low disease activity states does not make sense when accounting for the potential risks of these drugs.

Colectomy rates are higher in the first year after diagnosis as clinicians attempt to subdue disease activity [19], but an active therapeutic approach can bring overall rates as low as 9 % by 10 years after diagnosis [23]. However, moderate attacks of colitis carry a 20 % colectomy rate, and severe attacks have colectomy rates as high as 47 % despite IV corticosteroids [24]. Extent of disease is also a factor in stratifying disease severity, with as many as 60 % of patients with pancolitis requiring surgery at 3 months [25]. However, unlike with CD, there is no accurate model to predict whether an individual with UC will progress to easily controlled intermittent flares or acute spikes in activity requiring surgery.

## A Top-Down Strategy?

Certain differences must be underscored when explaining the divergence in approach to therapy for CD and UC. In CD, where clinical, serologic, genetic, and endoscopic data allow providers to forecast outcomes and surgical resection rates approach 80 % by 20 years after diagnosis, a top-down approach to inducing and maintaining remission has gained acceptance in clinical practice. The landmark ACCENT I study showed that CD patients who achieved mucosal healing with infliximab required fewer hospitalizations, surgeries, and ICU admissions [26]. This is logical given that unchecked inflammation will increase the complication rate and result in fistula or stricture formation [27]. To prevent these deleterious effects, a higher-intensity strategy aimed at suppressing inflammation has been successfully utilized in a subset of CD patients prone to a more severe disease outcome. However, this has not translated over to the treatment of UC, where disease course fluctuates as demonstrated in Fig. 42.1, and overall surgical rates are as low as 9 % at 10 years after diagnosis [23] and 20 % at 25 years of diagnosis [22]. With the established approach to therapy for UC, long-term survival rates equal those for age-matched controls, and there has been no difference from the general population in the capacity of UC patients to hold employment [19], with over 90 % of UC patients deemed fully capable of working after 10 years of diagnosis [22]. Since there is potential for a relatively benign disease course, adequate disease control is achievable with low-intensity therapy, and survival rates remain relatively high, our strategy in the treatment of UC continues to follow a step-up approach.

## A Proactive, Step-Up Approach

Given our inability to identify and initiate early treatment in patients who will suffer from severe disease, focus should be shifted toward swiftly instituting targeted therapy based on early markers for disease activity. Thus, clinicians need not take a passive approach to treating disease flares and wait for symptoms to erupt. Validated clinical scores gauging disease severity combined with objective markers indicating degree of brewing inflammation can enable providers to take a *proactive* step-up approach to decide appropriate treatment intensity. Formal research evaluating the validity of these early disease markers as diagnostic and prognostic tools in IBD should be an area of future investigation.

## How Is Disease Severity Best Measured?

Scoring scales have been validated to distinguish classes of disease severity. In 1955, Truelove and Witts published the first clinical criteria for classifying disease severity [28]. Mild disease was defined as fewer than four bowel movements per day with trace or no blood in the stool, without other signs of systemic toxicity, and a normal ESR. Severe disease was six or greater bloody stools daily, evidence of systemic toxicity (such as fever or tachycardia), anemia, and an elevated ESR. The American College of Gastroenterologists further clarified the definitions of moderate disease as cases with four stools daily with minimal signs of toxicity and fulminant disease for cases with more than ten bowel movements daily with continuous rectal bleeding, signs of systemic toxicity, abdominal tenderness or distension, anemia requiring transfusion, or colonic dilatation on imaging [2].

While symptom profile is the traditional measure to which therapy is titrated, mucosal healing has been implicated as a better gauge of long-term disease control and prognosis. Advances in endoscopy led to the inclusion of endoscopic

appearance in parallel with clinical features by scales such as the UC-DAI and the Mayo score [29, 30]. One early study revealed that 40 % of patients who also achieved endoscopic remission after acute treatment versus 18 % of patients who still had endoscopic disease remained asymptomatic during the following year [31]. Increased inflammation has been correlated with higher colectomy and hospitalization rates in UC patients [32], and mucosal healing may help prevent disease extension and development of dysplasia. During an active flare, mucosal inflammation is often seen, and therapy is subsequently "stepped-up." However, when evaluating the efficacy of maintenance therapy, we also propose that the presence of mucosal inflammation on endoscopy be a prompt for providers to consider "stepping-up" treatment intensity, especially in the presence of biomarker elevations which are outlined below.

## What Are Early Markers of Disease Activity?

Laboratory markers, such as serum C-reactive protein (CRP), fecal calprotectin, and fecal lactoferrin, have been studied with the goal of providing measurable objective markers of disease activity and to avoid costly, invasive procedures.

Serum C-reactive protein (CRP) has been a useful tool for gauging disease activity, as its production is not altered by immunosuppressive medications, and its levels correlate with clinical severity and endoscopic inflammation [33–35]. A CRP level >12 mg/L has been suggested to be a marker of severe and extensive disease [36], and sustained elevation despite medications is indicative of inadequacy of therapy [35]. High CRP levels may be predictive of need for colectomy, as shown by an early study correlating CRP >45 mg/L with colectomy by 4 months [37, 38] and a later population-based study which found that persistent CRP levels >10 mg/L after 1 year of treatment with surgery by 4 years [39]. Because CRP is not affected by immunosuppressive medication, a decrease in its level is considered an objective marker of the effect of medical therapy on intestinal inflammation, even if there is no change in symptomatology [35].

Fecal calprotectin and fecal lactoferrin, two proteins involved in regulating the inflammatory process, are noninvasive, objective biomarkers for grading mucosal disease activity in IBD. Their potential diagnostic and prognostic utility have been studied, but due to lack of coverage for these tests by insurance companies, they are not commonly used, even in academic centers.

Fecal calprotectin is an iron-binding protein found primarily in neutrophils, and stool concentrations are being used as a surrogate marker for gut inflammation given its correlation with neutrophil incursion into the gut lumen [39]. Stool concentrations are increased in active UC, with a level greater than 50 mcg/g having over 79 % specificity and 91 %

sensitivity for differentiating active versus inactive disease [39]. Stool calprotectin levels were found to correlate with degree of inflammation rather than disease extent [40], and concentrations in active UC patients were significantly higher than patients with inactive UC or control patients (402.16 mcg/g±48.0 vs. 35.93 mcg/g±3.39 vs. 11.5 mcg/g±3.42, $p < 0.01$) [39]. Additionally, a strong relationship between disease activity index (DAI) and fecal calprotectin was observed in the same cohort of patients ($r = 0.866$, $p < 0.001$), with calprotectin ranging from 100 to 500 mcg/g for DAI 6–9 and 500 to 1,000 mcg/g for DAI above 9 (more severe disease).

Fecal lactoferrin is another iron-binding protein secreted into the gut by activated neutrophils and is another surrogate for intestinal inflammation [41, 42]. It has been shown to be an accurate diagnostic tool for UC with a sensitivity of 92 % and specificity of 88 % [41] and can also be used to monitor disease activity. Lactoferrin concentrations are increased in active UC, with greater than 90 % correlation of levels to disease activity [42, 43]. Patients with active UC had significantly higher fecal lactoferrin levels than patients with inactive UC or control patients (median 51.1 mcg/mL, range 0–104 vs. 4.34 mcg/mL, 1–1,669 vs. 1.82 mcg/mL, 0–90) [44]. Patients with elevated fecal lactoferrin levels were also found to be prone to a disease flare when tapered off steroids [43]. These markers also have prognostic utility—with normalization of calprotectin predicting complete response to treatment and lactoferrin levels decreasing in correspondence to a decrease in Mayo score [45].

Findings of moderate-to-severe symptoms, endoscopic inflammation, or abnormal objective markers of inflammation, such as a persistently elevated fecal calprotectin >50 mg/kg, fecal lactoferrin, or serum CRP >12 mg/L despite 4 days of therapy, should prompt escalation to higher intensity of therapy.

## Matching Treatment Intensity to Severity Scenarios

A primary goal of therapy is to "do no harm"—therefore providers must select medications for which the risk benefit ratio is balanced. Figure 42.2 shows our step-up model and breakdown of classes of therapeutic intensity. Patients with controlled disease on no medications or 5-ASAs via the topical or systemic route only are receiving a low-intensity treatment. While moderately active UC had been recognized as a clinically and endoscopically distinct category, its therapeutic algorithm had often been borrowed from mild or severe disease. A moderate-intensity regimen is indicated in those not adequately controlled on systemic or topical 5-ASAs and includes topical or systemic 5-ASAs in conjunction with corticosteroids or the addition of immunomodulators for those intolerant of corticosteroids or requiring greater than two courses of corticosteroids within 1 year. A high-intensity strategy would be reserved for those with persistent symptoms on moderate-intensity medications and includes anti-TNF agents, cyclosporine, or experimental drugs not

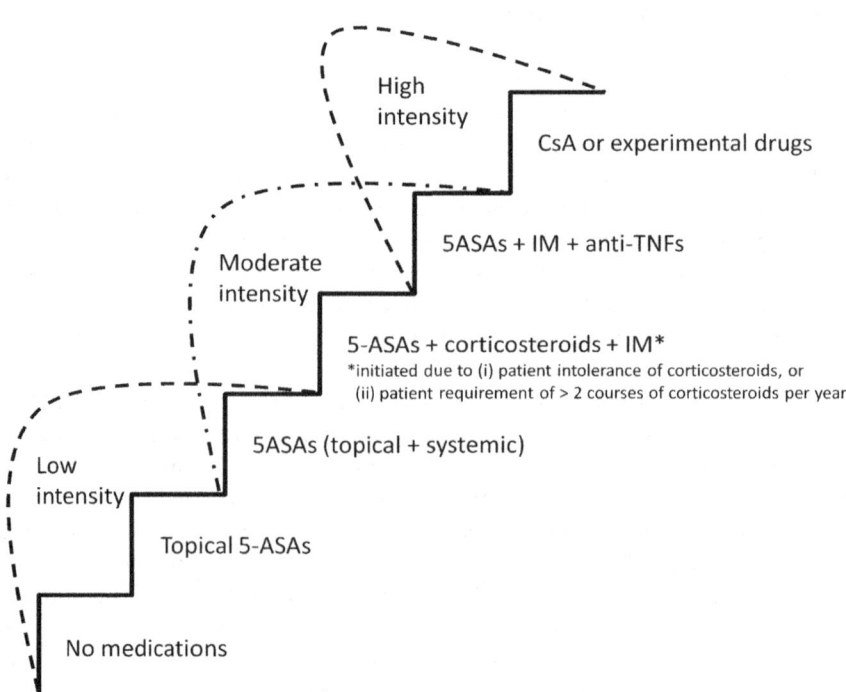

**Fig. 42.2** A step-up algorithm matching treatment intensity to disease severity. *5-ASAs* 5-aminosalicylates, *IM* immunomodulators, *anti-TNFs* anti-tumor necrosis factor agents, *CsA* cyclosporine

currently indicated for the treatment of UC. All these therapies are associated with potentially toxic effects, and these risks must be weighed against the need to attain disease control in every individual.

## Low-Intensity Therapy: Topical and Systemic 5-ASAs

### Systemic 5-ASAs

Aminosalicylates are the key to a low-intensity strategy to treatment of mildly active UC. Oral aminosalicylates are clearly effective at inducing therapeutic response in anywhere from 40 to 80 % of UC patients at 4 weeks, and their use as a first-line therapy in most UC patients has been widely accepted [2, 46, 47]. A recent 2012 Cochrane review investigated the ability of 5-ASAs versus placebo to induce remission in UC [48]. 5-ASA outperformed placebo for all endpoints—including adherence, adverse events, drug discontinuation, and clinical or endoscopic improvement—with 72 % of 5-ASA users versus 85 % of placebo patients failing to attain clinical remission (RR 0.86, 95 % confidence interval [CI] 0.81–0.91). There was also a trend toward 5-ASA superiority over sulfasalazine in inducing remission (RR 0.90, 95 % CI 0.77–1.04), and fewer 5-ASA patients had adverse events versus sulfasalazine users (15 % vs. 29 %, RR 0.48, 95 % CI 0.37–0.63).

After induction, mesalamine is used as maintenance therapy for UC [48–50]. A meta-analysis of mesalamine in the maintenance of remission in quiescent UC showed 5-ASA superiority over placebo, with 41 % of treatment versus 58 % of placebo patients suffering a relapse (RR 0.69, 95 % CI 0.62–0.77) [51]. The rate of adverse events between 5-ASA and placebo, different 5-ASA dosages, or various 5-ASA dosing strategies did not differ, and compliance rates were similar in all groups.

Although the above meta-analyses found no difference among various 5-ASAs, variations in dosing timing, delivery system, or volume reaching the colon are still believed to translate into some variation in clinical response [51]. Adherence to a regimen might be considered a more important factor than the 5-ASA formulation, as noncompliant patients are reported to have greater than a five times increased risk of recurrence (95 % CI 2.3–13, $p < 0.001$) [52, 53].

### Topical 5-ASAs

Rectal 5-ASAs achieve higher levels of 5-ASA in the distal colon, and findings of higher rectal 5-ASA concentrations in patients without bloody stools than those with bloody stools suggest that maintaining high mucosal concentrations may be the factor determining efficacy of 5-ASAs [54]. 5-ASA enemas can also be used in combination with oral 5-ASAs to control symptoms in patients with extensive disease [55, 56].

Safdi et al. showed that combining 2.4 g of oral mesalamine with mesalamine enemas resulted in more rapid and complete symptom control in left-sided colitis [56]. Limitations to this mode of delivery include patient preference, although there is strong evidence to support its use in the presence of distal colitis.

## Moderate-Intensity Therapy: 5 ASAs + Immunodilators, Steroids

### 5-ASAs

Higher doses lead to a higher mucosal concentration of 5-ASA, which is inversely related to endoscopic and histologic activity in UC ($r = 0.712, p < 0.001$) [57]. The ASCEND trials were randomized controlled phase 3 clinical trials that compared 4.8 g/day of mesalamine versus 2.4 g/day of mesalamine in achieving complete remission or response to therapy from baseline. Both ASCEND I and II demonstrated superiority of higher-dose mesalamine among patients with moderate UC, with a nonsignificant decrease in median time to achieving normal stool frequency and resolution of rectal bleeding [58, 59]. In ASCEND III, higher dose mesalamine was more effective in patients with difficult to treat disease who had previously required corticosteroids or multiple agents [60]. There was no difference in adverse events among the two dosing strategies [58–60].

The benefits of greater mesalamine doses in high-risk relapsers were further demonstrated by Frieri et al., where 18 patients had a decrease in recurrence episodes from 80 over 2 years to 8 over the following 2 years, after increasing the oral 5-ASA dose to 4.8 g daily and adding daily 5-ASA enemas [61]. There was a 100-fold increase in mucosal 5-ASA levels (median, 3–260 ng/mL) to which the authors attributed the striking clinical differences—over the first 2 years, there were 33 prescribed courses of corticosteroids, 93 hospital days, and 249 outpatient visits; this decreased to zero steroid courses or hospital days and 116 outpatient visits using higher-dose combination 5-ASA therapy. However, expecting patients to adhere to such a strict regimen is not realistic, and disease that is active despite systemic 5-ASAs often prompts consideration of higher-intensity strategies.

Initial treatment of active UC should be based on disease severity, with conventional 2.4 g/day dosing being effective in mild disease and higher doses providing incremental benefit for moderately active disease, especially those who have previously required corticosteroids or multiple agents to control symptoms.

### Thiopurines

Thiopurines have long been used in Crohn's disease [62], and this benefit has also been demonstrated in moderately active UC [63–65]. In 2008, a meta-analysis of thiopurines in

UC found that azathioprine was superior to placebo, with a failure to maintain remission of OR 0.41 (95 % CI 0.24–0.70) [66]. A 2011 meta-analysis confirmed that azathioprine was effective for preventing relapse in quiescent UC (RR 0.60, 95 % CI 0.37–0.95) and showed a trend toward benefit in active UC (RR 0.85, 95 % CI 0.71–1.01) [67]. This outcome has been attributed the ability of thiopurines in achieving long-term mucosal healing in UC [68].

Ardizzone et al. conducted an RCT of azathioprine versus 5-ASA for steroid-dependent UC and found that 50 % of patients using azathioprine versus 35 % of 5-ASA treated-patients achieved clinical and endoscopic remission to a degree that allowed for discontinuation of steroid therapy [69]. At 6 months, clinical remission rates were similar, but the azathioprine group had a significantly higher rate of endoscopic remission. Additionally, the 5-ASA group also required an additional course of steroids to achieve these effects, and the authors of this study hypothesized that aza-thioprine's ability to induce mucosal healing may be the reason for its efficacy.

Thiopurines are slow-acting drugs, and it can take up to 6 months to achieve a therapeutic response, thus limiting their utility in acute relapses. Use is further limited by the high rate of side effects, which typically manifest in the first month, and a significant toxicity profile [66]. Some dose-dependent toxicities include myelosuppression and hepato-toxicity; rarer dose-independent effects include pancreatitis, nausea, pneumonitis, and a slightly increased risk of lym-phoma [66, 70].

## Corticosteroids

Corticosteroids are successful at rapidly inducing remission for symptoms that persist or worsen despite medical therapy [28, 71], and their role has been firmly established for active UC. While immunologics and biologics expand our options against moderate-to-severe UC, steroids remain at the center of therapy given their established efficacy in inducing remission for moderate-to-severe disease. However, the metabolic, immunologic, and psychiatric side effects of cor-ticosteroids stemming from supraphysiologic doses, lengthy courses, and withdrawal have resulted in more judicious use in mild-to-moderate disease [72]. Additionally, around 60 % of patients have an incomplete response to steroids [25, 71, 73], and a considerable proportion become steroid-dependent or fail to respond over time [24, 71]. While newer therapies have yet to achieve perfect success controlling IBD, they expand our arsenal against moderate-to-severe cases of UC. Unlike corticosteroids, these agents may more reliably induce mucosal healing, which has been shown to alter disease course [74, 75]. Newer therapeutic algorithms incorporating these agents are being developed with the goals of maximizing remission, minimizing corticosteroid dependence, and staving off colectomy.

## High-Intensity Therapy: Anti-TNFs and Cyclosporine

### Infliximab

The success of anti-TNF agents for the treatment of CD prompted investigation in UC patients, with particular interest on those nonresponders to conventional therapy [76]. Infliximab has since been approved to treat symptoms of colitis, induce and maintain clinical remission, and act as a steroid-sparing agent in moderately to severely active UC patients [24, 77].

The ACT 1 and 2 trials were randomized, double-blind, placebo-controlled studies evaluating infliximab for induc-tion and maintenance of remission in UC patients who had failed immunosuppressives and/or corticosteroids [77]. The primary endpoint of both trials was a clinical response at 8 weeks, with secondary endpoints including clinical response at week 8 in steroid-refractory patients, discontinu-ation of steroids at week 30, and sustained clinical remission at week 30 in ACT-2 and week 54 in ACT-1. Almost one-third of the patients had steroid-refractory UC, defined as persistent symptoms despite an equivalent of ≥40 mg/day of prednisolone orally for two or more weeks or intravenously for one or more week. Clinical response was significantly greater with infliximab, and sub-analysis revealed preserva-tion of this effect in steroid-refractory patients. In both trials, infliximab-induced clinical remission was associated with the discontinuation of corticosteroid use at week 30.

An extension study of the ACT-1 and -2 cohorts evaluated those patients who achieved benefit from infliximab and fol-lowed them for three subsequent years of therapy. The initial improvement in PGA score or IBDQ scores continued for the duration of therapy, without an increase in adverse events [78]. Infliximab was associated with a 50 % decrease in the hospitalizations, which has been hypothesized to result in increased HRQOL [79, 80]. A post hoc analysis of the ACT-1 and ACT-2 data found that maintenance with infliximab resulted in an absolute risk reduction of 7 % in colectomy rates [81], confirming findings in earlier pilot studies [24, 82]; however, it should be noted that patients thought to require colectomy within 12 weeks of enrollment were excluded from the ACT trials. A 2008 retrospective review of acute severe UC found that although the risk of urgent colectomy was decreased with infliximab use in steroid-refractory patients, there was actually no difference in long-term elective colectomy rates [83].

Infliximab can have serious adverse effects, but mucosal healing with infliximab can potentially lead to improved out-comes [84, 85]. Toxicities include risk of infection, which is potentiated by concomitant steroid use, skin eruptions, and less commonly malignancy and neurologic diseases [86]. There is the additional risk of antibody formation to infliximab from infusion reactions, serum-like sickness, and attenuation of response [87]. Infliximab is contraindicated in certain settings—with active infection, multiple sclerosis, severe heart failure, or a history of optic neuritis or malignancy [87]. Clinicians must weigh the risks of infliximab toxicity against the potential benefits on long-term outcomes.

## Adalimumab

Given the success seen with infliximab in UC patients and adalimumab in CD patients, adalimumab was subsequently evaluated for the treatment of UC, with the rationale that anti-murine antibodies to infliximab would not influence the efficacy of a completely human anti-TNF monoclonal antibody. Anti-TNF-naïve and experienced UC patients were evaluated for short- and long-term response to adalimumab, with results indicating a role for adalimumab as a corticosteroid-sparing agent in UC [88] and long-term colectomy-free rates in these severely active UC patients reaching as high as to 59 % at 2 years [89].

The first randomized, double-blind placebo-controlled study evaluating adalimumab for induction and maintenance of remission in anti-TNF naïve patients with moderately to severely active UC who had failed immunosuppression found that adalimumab was safer and more effective than placebo in both induction of remission (19 % vs. 9 % at week 8) [90]. A second recently published trial, ULTRA 2, evaluated adalimumab in patients who had failed immunosuppressants or previous anti-TNF agents and showed that adalimumab was more effective in induction and maintaining remission, with response rates of 17 % vs. 9 % at weeks 8 and 52 [91]. Based on these results, adalimumab was recently approved for the treatment of moderately to severely active UC unresponsive to corticosteroids or thiopurines. Further studies evaluating its efficacy against currently used therapies have yet to be conducted.

## Golimumab

Golimumab is a fully humanized monoclonal immunoglobulin also directed against TNF-α. Genetically engineered mice were immunized with human anti-TNFα resulting in an antibody with a human-derived variable and regions that are constant. The variable region of golimumab binds to both the soluble and transmembrane bioactive forms of TNF-α and as a result inhibits the biological activity of TNF-α. Golimumab has been shown in vitro to modulate the biological effects mediated by TNF including the expression of adhesion proteins responsible for leukocyte infiltration (E-selectin, ICAM-1, and VCAM-1) and the secretion of proinflammatory cytokines (IL-6, IL-8, G-CSF, and GM-CSF).

Golimumab has been approved by the Food and Drug Administration in the United States to treat moderately to severely active rheumatoid arthritis (RA), active psoriatic arthritis, active ankylosing spondylitis (AS), and recently gained regulatory approval in 2013 for the treatment of moderate-to-severe UC patients who have had an inadequate response or intolerance to prior conventional treatments or who require continuous steroid therapy. Golimumab is given subcutaneously, and for UC, the dosage recommended is 200 mg initially at week 0 and then 100 mg at week 2 and then 100 mg every 4 weeks.

A combined double-blind placebo-controlled phase 2 dose-finding and phase 3 dose-confirmation trials demonstrated golimumab's efficacy for induction of a clinical response and remission in patients with moderate-to-severe ulcerative colitis (PURSUIT) [92, 93]. There were 1,064 adult patients with moderately to severely active UC (Mayo score: 6–12, endoscopy subscore $\geq 2$). Patients were randomly assigned to groups given golimumab doses of 100 mg and then 50 mg (phase 2 only), 200 mg and then 100 mg, or 400 mg and then 200 mg, 2 weeks apart. The phase 3 primary endpoint was a clinical response at week 6. The secondary endpoints included clinical remission, mucosal healing, and IBDQ score change at week 6. In phase 2, median changes from baseline in the Mayo score were −1.0, −3.0, −2.0, and −3.0 in placebo and 100 mg/50 mg, 200 mg/100 mg, and 400 mg/200 mg golimumab respectively. In phase 3, rates of clinical response at week 6 were 51.8 % and 55 % among patients given 200 mg/100 mg and 400 mg/200 mg golimumab respectively vs. 29.7 % in the placebo group ($p < 0.0001$). Rates of clinical remission and mucosal healing and mean changes in the IBDQ scores were significantly greater in both the golimumab and placebo groups ($p \leq 0.0005$).

In the phase 3, double-blind trial evaluating golimumab in the maintenance of a clinical response in patients with moderate-to-severe UC, patients who responded to the initial golimumab induction therapy were randomly assigned to groups given placebo or injections of 50 or 100 mg of golimumab every 4 weeks through week 52 [93]. Four hundred sixty-four patients were included in this study. Patients who responded to placebo in the induction study continued to receive placebo. Nonresponders in the induction study received 100 mg golimumab. The primary outcome was a clinical response maintained through week 54 and secondary outcomes included clinical remission and mucosal healing at week 30 and week 54. Clinical response was found to be maintained in 47.0 % receiving 50 mg golimumab, 49.7 % receiving 100 mg golimumab, and 31.2 % receiving placebo ($p = 0.010$ and $p < 0.001$ respectively). At weeks 30 and 54, 27.8 % patients who received 100 mg golimumab were in clinical remission and 42.4 % had mucosal healing compared to placebo (15.6 % and 26.6 %, $p = 0.004$ and $p = 0.002$, respectively) or 50 mg golimumab (23.2 % and 41.7 %).

## Vedolizumab

Natalizumab, a humanized IgG4 monoclonal antibody directed against the a4 integrin adhesion molecule involved in endothelial leukocyte migration, was approved by the Food and Drug Administration (FDA) for the treatment of Crohn's disease for both induction and maintenance of remission. Patient and physician concerns over its association with progressive multifocal leukoencephalopathy have led to a search for gut-specific anti-integrin action that would eliminate this risk. Drugs with selective effects in the alpha-4 beta-7 integrin and mucosal adhesion molecule (MadCAM-1) pathway were investigated. Vedolizumab, as a consequence of this pursuit, was born.

The results of the subsequent GEMINI studies investigating vedolizumab for both induction and maintenance in ulcerative colitis and Crohn's disease were published in 2013. In the Crohn's disease study, 368 patients were randomized to vedolizumab or placebo [94]. Disease activity was measured at week 6 by assessing the reduction of Crohn's disease activity index (CDAI).

Patients on vedolizumab had a statistically significant difference in clinical remission of 14.5 % versus 6.8 % in placebo ($p < 0.02$) but no difference in CDAI-100 response or reduction in mean C-reactive protein (CRP) levels. A second cohort was given open-label vedolizumab, and a total of 461 responders from both cohorts continued in the maintenance portion of the trial; patients were randomized to receive drug every 4 or 8 weeks or placebo for 52 weeks. There was statistical significance in clinical remission, CDAI-100 response, and glucocorticoid-free remission at week 52 in every 4- or 8-week group versus placebo ($p < 0.001$ and 0.004, respectively).

A similarly designed study was conducted for vedolizumab in ulcerative colitis; 374 patients were randomized to either drug or placebo as part of induction [95]. The response for week 6 was measured by the Mayo score and documented mucosal healing. During induction, 47.1 % of the patients on vedolizumab versus 25.5 % of the patients on placebo achieved remission ($p < 0.001$). A second cohort of patients received open-label vedolizumab, and responders from both cohorts were included in the maintenance trial that evaluated clinical remission at week 52. Patients were randomized to receive drug every 4 or 8 weeks or placebo. A total of 41.8 % maintained remission when receiving medication every 8 weeks compared with 44.8 % who received drug every 4 weeks; patients on placebo had maintenance of remission at a rate of 15.9 %. There was a statistically significant difference in maintenance of remission between patients who received drug every 8 weeks versus placebo ($p < 0.001$) and those receiving drug every 4 weeks versus placebo ($p < 0.001$). Based on these findings, the drug was approved for use in adults with moderate-to-severe ulcerative colitis and moderate-to-severe Crohn's disease when one or more standard therapies (corticosteroids, immunomodulators, or tumor necrosis factor blocker medications) have not resulted in an adequate response.

## Cyclosporine

Cyclosporine has long been used to rapidly induce remission in difficult cases but requires providers and patients to adhere to strict monitoring for toxicity. In an early study, intravenous cyclosporine was shown to be effective in severe UC refractory to IV glucocorticoids [96], where 9 out of 11 patients randomized to additional IV cyclosporine at 4 mg/kg had clinical improvement, and none of the 9 placebo patients improved despite continued IV corticosteroids. A later RCT of 20 steroid-refractory UC patients compared cyclosporine or continued steroids and was actually stopped early due to the benefits of cyclosporine [97]. Given the dose-dependent toxicity of IV cyclosporine, later studies investigated a lower dose of 2 mg/kg, which has been used in other immune-related diseases, and found it to be as efficacious as a 4 mg/kg dosing regimen [98, 99].

Laharie et al. published results from a head-to-head multicenter trial, which showed equivalency of infliximab and cyclosporine for induction of remission of severe, steroid-refractory UC patients [100, 101]. Patients were randomized to IV cyclosporine for 7 days followed by PO cyclosporine or IV infliximab at 0, 2, and 6 weeks. Responders were started on azathioprine at day 7, and steroids were tapered per protocol. There was no significant difference among treatment regimens, with a failure rate of 60 % with cyclosporine and 54 % with infliximab and day 7 response rates around 85 % in both groups [101].

Despite its established efficacy in induction of remission, use of cyclosporine is generally limited to experienced academic centers with the ability to monitor concentrations and toxicity according to institutional protocols. Cyclosporine toxicity is a real danger, with effects including nephrotoxicity, opportunistic infection, hypertrichosis, and a 1–2 % mortality rate [102]. Additionally, cyclosporine is not used as a maintenance drug and requires bridging to other medications also needing close surveillance, such as azathioprine or 6-mercaptopurine.

## Conclusions

The majority of UC patients have a low-to-moderate disease activity level which can be managed with a low-intensity strategy based on 5-ASAs. For more severe disease, rescue medications provide a palatable alternative to surgery. Investigations are currently aimed at individualizing therapy for those patients who will ultimately require more potent medical therapies. Top-down treatment strategies in certain patients could potentially help increase HRQOL and drive down indirect costs of therapy, thus offsetting the high up-front costs of anti-TNF or immunomodulating agents. Unfortunately, the side-effect profiles of these drugs and our current inability to identify those who will have more aggressive disease limit our use of moderate- or high-intensity medications to those experiencing moderately to severely active disease flares.

Future research will likely confirm that a *proactive* step-up approach to treatment, which incorporates traditional measures of disease severity and current diagnostic tools, can form a framework in which to stratify UC patients and match them to an appropriate therapeutic intensity regimen.

# References

1. Meyers S, Janowitz HD. The "natural history" of ulcerative colitis: an analysis of the placebo response. J Clin Gastroenterol. 1989;11:33–7.
2. Kornbluth A, Sachar DB, The Practice Parameters Committee of the American College of Gastroenterology. Ulcerative colitis practice guidelines in adults: American College of Gastroenterology. Practice Parameters Committee. Am J Gastroenterol. 2010;105:501–23.
3. Loftus Jr EV. Clinical epidemiology of inflammatory bowel disease: incidence, prevalence, and environmental influences. Gastroenterology. 2004;126:1504–17.
4. Robinson M, Hanauer S, Hoop R, et al. Mesalamine capsules enhance the quality of life for patients with ulcerative colitis. Aliment Pharmacol Ther. 1994;8:27–34.
5. Lichtenstein GR, Rutgeerts P. Importance of mucosal healing in ulcerative colitis. Inflamm Bowel Dis. 2010;16(2):338–46.
6. Travis SP, Higgins PD, Orchard T, et al. Review article: defining remission in ulcerative colitis. Aliment Pharmacol Ther. 2011;34(2):113–24.
7. Colombel JF, Rutgeerts P, Reinisch W, et al. Early mucosal healing with infliximab is associated with improved long-term clinical outcomes in ulcerative colitis. Gastroenterology. 2011;141(4):1194–201.
8. Ardizzone S, Cassinotti A, Duca P, et al. Mucosal healing predicts late outcomes after the first course of corticosteroids for newly diagnosed ulcerative colitis. Clin Gastroenterol Hepatol. 2011;9(6):483–9.
9. Hoie O, Wolters F, Riis L, et al. European Collaborative Study Group of Inflammatory Bowel Disease (EC-IBD). Ulcerative colitis: patient characteristics may predict 10-year disease recurrence in a European-wide population-based cohort. Am J Gastroenterol. 2007;102:1692–701.
10. Nguyen GC, Tuskey A, Dassopoulos T, et al. Rising hospitalization rates for inflammatory bowel disease in the United States between 1998 and 2004. Inflamm Bowel Dis. 2007;13:1529–35.
11. Kappelman MD, Rifas-Shiman SL, Porter C, et al. Direct health care costs of Crohn's disease and ulcerative colitis in US children and adults. Gastroenterology. 2008;135:1907–13.
12. Sonnenberg A, Chang J. Time trends of physician visits for Crohn's disease and ulcerative colitis in the United States, 1960–2006. Inflamm Bowel Dis. 2008;14:249–52.
13. Waljee AK, Joyce JC, Wren PA, et al. Patient reported symptoms during an ulcerative colitis flare: a Quality Focus Group Study. Eur J Gastroenterol Hepatol. 2009;21(5):558–64.
14. Turner D, Walsh C, Steinhart AH, Griffiths AM. Response to corticosteroids in severe ulcerative colitis: a systematic review of the literature and a meta-regression. Clin Gastroenterol Hepatol. 2007;5:103–10.
15. Sinclair TS, Brunt PW, Mowat NA. Nonspecific proctocolitis in northeastern Scotland: a community study. Gastroenterology. 1983;85:1–11.
16. Edwards FC, Truelove SC. The course and prognosis of ulcerative colitis. Gut. 1963;4:299–308.
17. Watts JMK, de Dombal FT, Watkinson G, et al. Long-term prognosis of ulcerative colitis. Br Med J. 1966;1:1447–553.
18. Ritchie JK, Powell-Tuck J, Lennard-Jones JE. Clinical outcome of the first ten years of ulcerative colitis and proctitis. Lancet. 1978;1:1140–3.
19. Hendriksen C, Kreiner S, Binder V. Long-term prognosis in ulcerative colitis – based on results from a regional patient group from the county of Copenhagen. Gut. 1985;26:158–63.
20. Stonnington CM, Phillips SF, Zinmeister AR, et al. Prognosis of chronic ulcerative colitis in a community. Gut. 1987;28:1261–6.
21. Bitton A, Sewitch MJ, Peppercorn MA, et al. Psychosocial determinants of relapse in ulcerative colitis: a longitudinal study. Am J Gastroenterol. 2003;98:2203–8.
22. Langholz E, Munkholm P, Davidsen M, et al. Course of ulcerative colitis: analysis of changes in disease activity over years. Gastroenterology. 1994;107:3–11.
23. Hoie L, Wolters FL, RIIS L, et al. Low colectomy rates in ulcerative colitis in an unselected European cohort followed for 10 years. Gastroenterology. 2007;132:507–15.
24. Jarnerot G, Hertervig E, Friss-Liby I, et al. Infliximab as rescue therapy in severe to moderately severe ulcerative colitis: a randomized, placebo-controlled study. Gastroenterology. 2005;128:1805–11.
25. Jarnerot G, Rolny P, Sandberg-Gertzen H. Intensive intravenous treatment of ulcerative colitis. Gastroenterology. 1985;89:1005–13.
26. Hanauer SB, Feagan BG, Lichtenstein GR, et al. Maintenance infliximab for Crohn's disease: the ACCENT I randomized trial. Lancet. 2002;359:1541–9.
27. Cosnes J, Cattan S, Blain A, et al. Long-term evolution of disease behavior of Crohn's disease. Inflamm Bowel Dis. 2002;8:244–50.
28. Truelove SC, Witts LJ. Cortisone in ulcerative colitis: final report on a therapeutic trial. Br Med J. 1955;2:1041–88.
29. Sutherland LR, Martin F, Greer S, et al. 5-Aminosalicylic acid enema in the treatment of distal ulcerative colitis, proctosigmoiditis, and proctitis. Gastroenterology. 1987;92:1894–8.
30. Schroeder KW, Tremaine WJ, Ilstrup DM. Coated oral 5-aminosalicylic acid therapy for mildly to moderately active ulcerative colitis. A randomized study. N Engl J Med. 1987;317:1625–9.
31. Wright R, Truelove SR. Serial rectal biopsy in ulcerative colitis during the course of a controlled therapeutic trial of various diets. Am J Dig Dis. 1966;11:847–57.
32. Rubin DT, Huo D, Hetzel JT, et al. Increased degree of histological inflammation predicts colectomy and hospitalization in patients with ulcerative colitis. Gastroenterology. 2007;132:A19. Abstract 103.
33. Prantera C, Davoli M, Lorenzetti R, et al. Clinical and laboratory indicators of extent of ulcerative colitis. Serum C-reactive protein helps the most. J Clin Gastroenterol. 1988;10:41–5.
34. Solem CA, Loftus EV, Tremaine WJ, et al. Correlation of C-reactive protein (CRP) with clinical, radiographic, and endoscopic activity in Inflammatory Bowel Disease (IBD). Gastroenterology. 2004;26(Suppl):A477.
35. Vermeire S, Van Assche G, Rutgeerts P. C-reactive protein as a marker for inflammatory bowel disease. Inflamm Bowel Dis. 2004;10:661–5.

36. Chouhan S, Gahlot S, Pokharna RK, Mathur KC, Saini K, Pal M. Severity and extent of ulcerative colitis: role of C-reactive protein. Indian J Gastroenterol. 2006;25:46–7.

37. Travis SP, Farrant JM, Ricketts C, et al. Predicting outcome in severe ulcerative colitis. Gut. 1996;38:905–10.

38. Henriksen M, Jahnsen J, Lygren I, et al. C-reactive protein: a predictive factor and marker of inflammation in inflammatory bowel disease. Results from a prospective population-based study. Gut. 2008;57:1518–23.

39. Xiang JY, Ouyang Q, Li GD, et al. Clinical value of fecal calprotectin in determining disease activity of ulcerative colitis. World J Gastroenterol. 2008;14:53–7.

40. Røseth AG, Aadland E, Jahnsen J, et al. Assessment of disease activity in ulcerative colitis by faecal calprotectin, a novel granulocyte marker protein. Digestion. 1997;58:176–80.

41. Dai J, Liu WZ, Zhao YP, et al. Relationship between fecal lactoferrin and inflammatory bowel disease. Scand J Gastroenterol. 2007;42:1440–4.

42. Kane SV, Sandborn WJ, Rufo PA, et al. Fecal lactoferrin is a sensitive and specific marker in identifying intestinal inflammation. Am J Gastroenterol. 2003;98:1309–14.

43. Walker TR, Land ML, Cook TM, et al. Serial fecal lactoferrin measurements are useful in the interval assessment of patients with active and inactive inflammatory bowel disease. Gastroenterology. 2004;126:A215.

44. Langhorst J, Elsenbruch S, Koelzer J, et al. Noninvasive markers in the assessment of intestinal inflammation in inflammatory bowel diseases: performance of fecal lactoferrin, calprotectin, and PMN-elastase, CRP, and clinical indices. Am J Gastroenterol. 2008;103:162–9.

45. Masoodi I, Kochhar R, Dutta U, et al. Fecal lactoferrin, myeloperoxidase and serum C-reactive are effective biomarkers in the assessment of disease activity and severity in patients with idiopathic ulcerative colitis. J Gastroenterol Hepatol. 2009;24:1768–74.

46. Lichtenstein GR, Kamm MA, Boddu P, et al. Effect of once- or twice-daily MMX mesalamine (SPD476) for the induction of remission of mild to moderately active ulcerative colitis. Clin Gastroenterol Hepatol. 2007;5:95–102.

47. Kamm MA, Sandborn WJ, Gassull M, et al. Once-daily high-concentration MMX mesalamine in active ulcerative colitis. Gastroenterology. 2007;132:66–75.

48. Feagan BG, Macdonald JK. Oral 5-aminosalicylic acid for induction of remission in ulcerative colitis. Cochrane Database Syst Rev. 2012; CD000543.

49. Hanauer SB, Sninsky CA, Robinson M, et al. An oral preparation of mesalamine as long-term maintenance therapy for ulcerative colitis: a randomized, placebo-controlled trial. Ann Intern Med. 1996;124(2):204–11.

50. Sutherland L, Macdonald JK. Oral 5-aminosalicylic acid for maintenance of remission in ulcerative colitis. Cochrane Database Syst Rev. 2006; CD000544.

51. Courtney MG, Nunes DP, Bergin CF, et al. Randomised comparison of olsalazine and mesalazine in prevention of relapses in ulcerative colitis. Lancet. 1992;339:1279–81.

52. Kane S, Huo D, Aikens J, et al. Medication nonadherence and the outcomes of patients with quiescent ulcerative colitis. Am J Med. 2003;114:39–43.

53. Kane S. Systematic review: adherence issues in the treatment of ulcerative colitis. Aliment Pharmacol Ther. 2006;23:577–85.

54. Naganuma M, Iwao Y, Ogata H, et al. Measurement of colonic mucosal concentrations of 5-aminosalicylic acid is useful for estimating its therapeutic efficacy in distal ulcerative colitis: comparison of orally administered mesalamine and sulfasalazine. Inflamm Bowel Dis. 2001;7(3):221–5.

55. Marteau P, Probert CS, Lindgren S, et al. Combined oral and enema treatment with Pentasa (mesalazine) is superior to oral therapy alone in patients with extensive mild/moderate active ulcerative colitis: a randomised, double blind, placebo controlled study. Gut. 2005;54:960–5.

56. Safdi M, DeMicco M, Sninsky C, et al. A double-blind comparison of oral versus rectal mesalamine versus combination therapy in the treatment of distal ulcerative colitis. Am J Gastroenterol. 1997;92:1867–71.

57. Frieri G, Gioacomelli M, Pimpo G, et al. Mucosal 5-aminiosalicylic acid concentration inversely correlates with severity of colonic inflammation in patients with ulcerative colitis. Gut. 2000;47:410–6.

58. Hanauer S, Sandborn W, Dallaire C, et al. Delayed-release oral mesalamine at 4.8 g/day (800 mg tablet) compared to 2.4 g/d (400 mg tablets) for the treatment of mildly to moderately active ulcerative colitis: the ASCEND I trial. Can J Gastroenterol. 2007;21:827–34.

59. Hanauer S, Sandborn W, Kornbluth A, et al. Delayed-release oral mesalamine at 4.8 g/day (800 mg tablet) for the treatment of moderately active ulcerative colitis: the ASCEND II trial. Am J Gastroenterol. 2005;100:2478–85.

60. Sandborn WJ, Requla J, Feagan BG, et al. Delayed-release oral mesalamine 4.8 g/day (800-mg tablet) is effective for patients with moderately active ulcerative colitis. Gastroenterology. 2009;137:1934–43.

61. Frieri G, Pimpo M, Galletti B, et al. Long-term oral plus topical mesalazine in frequently relapsing ulcerative colitis. Dig Liver Dis. 2005;37(2):92–6.

62. Fraser AG, Orchard TR, Jewell DP. The efficacy of azathioprine for the treatment of inflammatory bowel disease: a 30 year review. Gut. 2002;50:485–9.

63. Rosenberg JL, Wall AJ, Levin B, et al. A controlled trial of azathioprine in the management of chronic ulcerative colitis. Gastroenterology. 1975;69:96–9.

64. Hawthorne AB, Logan RF, Hawkey CJ, et al. Randomised controlled trial of azathioprine withdrawal in ulcerative colitis. Br Med J. 1992;305:20–2.

65. Kirk AP, Lennard-Jones JE. Controlled trial of azathioprine in chronic ulcerative colitis. Br Med J (Clin Res Ed). 1982;284:1291–2.

66. Timmer A, McDonald JW, Macdonald JK. Azathioprine and 6-mercaptopurine for maintenance of remission in ulcerative colitis. Cochrane Database Syst Rev. 2007; CD000478.

67. Khan KJ, Dubinsky MC, Ford AC, et al. Efficacy of immunosuppressive therapy for inflammatory bowel disease: a systematic review and meta-analysis. Am J Gastroenterol. 2011;106:630–42.

68. López-Palacios N, Mendoza JL, Taxonera C, et al. Mucosal healing for predicting clinical outcome in patients with ulcerative colitis using thiopurines in monotherapy. Eur J Intern Med. 2011;22(6):621–5.

69. Ardizzone S, Maconi G, Russo A, et al. Randomised controlled trial of azathioprine and 5-aminosalicylic acid for treatment of steroid dependent ulcerative colitis. Gut. 2006;55:47–53.

70. Kandiel A, Fraser AG, Korelitz BI, et al. Increased risk of lymphoma among inflammatory bowel disease patients treated with azathioprine and 6-mercaptopurine. Gut. 2005;54:1121–6.

71. Truelove SC, Jewell DP. Intensive intravenous regimen for severe attacks of ulcerative colitis. Lancet. 1974;303:1067–70.

72. Stein RB, Hanauer SB. Comparative tolerability of treatments for inflammatory bowel disease. Drug Saf. 2000;23:429–48.

73. Hawthorne AB, Travis SPL, the BSG IBD Clinical Trials Network. Outcome of inpatient management of severe ulcerative colitis: a BSG IBD Clinical Trials Network survey. Gut. 2002;50:A16.

74. Frøslie KF, Jahnsen J, Mourm BA, et al. Mucosal healing in inflammatory bowel disease: results from a Norwegian population-based cohort. Gastroenterology. 2007;133:412–22.

75. Solberg IC, Lygren I, Jøhnsen J, et al. Mucosal healing after initial treatment may be a prognostic marker for long-term outcome in inflammatory bowel disease. Gut. 2008;57 Suppl 2:A15.

76. Kornbluth A, Marion JF, Salomon P, Janowitz HD. How effective is current medical therapy for severe ulcerative and Crohn's colitis? An analytic review of selected trials. J Clin Gastroenterol. 1995;20:280–4.

77. Rutgeerts P, Sandborn WJ, Feagan BG, et al. Infliximab for induction and maintenance therapy for ulcerative colitis. N Engl J Med. 2005;353:2462–76.

78. Reinisch W, Sandborn WJ, Rutgeerts P. Long-term infliximab maintenance therapy for ulcerative colitis: the ACT-1 and -2 extension studies. Inflamm Bowel Dis. 2012;18:201–11.

79. Feagan BG, Reinisch W, Rutgeerts P, et al. The effects of infliximab therapy on health-related quality of life in ulcerative colitis patients. Am J Gastroenterol. 2007;102:794–802.

80. Cohen RD, Thomas T. Economics of the use of biologics in the treatment of inflammatory bowel disease. Gastroenterol Clin North Am. 2006;35:867–82.

81. Sandborn WJ, Rutgeerts P, Feagan BG, et al. Colectomy rate comparison after treatment of ulcerative colitis with placebo or infliximab. Gastroenterology. 2009;137:1250–60.

82. Sands BE, Tremaine WJ, Sandborn WJ, et al. Infliximab in the treatment of severe, steroid-refractory ulcerative colitis: a pilot study. Inflamm Bowel Dis. 2001;7:83–8.

83. Aratari A, Papi C, Clemente V, et al. Colectomy rate in acute severe ulcerative colitis in the infliximab era. Dig Liver Dis. 2008; 40:821–6.

84. Colombel J-F, Loftus EV, Tremaine WJ, et al. The safety profile of infliximab in patients with Crohn's disease: the Mayo Clinic experience in 500 patients. Gastroenterology. 2004;126:19–31.

85. Ljung T, Karlén P, Schmidt D, et al. Infliximab in inflammatory bowel disease: clinical outcome in a population based cohort from Stockholm County. Gut. 2004;53:849–53.

86. Lees CW, Ali AI, Thompson AI, et al. The safety profile of anti-tumour necrosis factor therapy in inflammatory bowel disease in clinical practice: analysis of 620 patient-years follow-up. Aliment Pharmacol Ther. 2009;29:286–97.

87. Rutgeerts P, Van Assche G, Vermeire S. Review article: infliximab therapy for inflammatory bowel disease – seven years on. Aliment Pharmacol Ther. 2006;23:451–63.

88. Taxonera C, Estellés J, Fernández-Blanco I, et al. Adalimumab induction and maintenance therapy for patients with ulcerative colitis previously treated with infliximab. Aliment Pharmacol Ther. 2011;33:340–8.

89. McDermott E, Murphy S, Keegan D, et al. Efficacy of adalimumab as a long term maintenance therapy in ulcerative colitis. J Crohns Colitis. 2013;7:150–3.

90. Reinisch W, Sandborn WJ, Hommes DW, et al. Adalimumab for induction of clinical remission in moderately to severely active ulcerative colitis: results of a randomized controlled trial. Gut. 2011;60:780–7.

91. Sandborn WJ, Colombel JF, D'Haens G, et al. One-year maintenance outcomes among patients with moderately-to-severely active ulcerative colitis who responded to induction therapy with adalimumab: subgroup analyses from ULTRA 2. Aliment Pharmacol Ther. 2013;37(2):204–13.

92. Sandborn WJ, et al. Subcutaneous golimumab maintains clinical response in patients with moderate-to severe ulcerative colitis. Gastroenterology. 2014;146(1):96–109.

93. Sandborn WJ, Feagan BG, Marano C, Zhang H, Strauss R, et al. Subcutaneous golimumab induces clinical response and remission in patients with moderate to severe ulcerative colitis. Gastroenterology. 2014;146:85–95.

94. Sandborn WJ, Feagan BG, Rutgeerts P, et al. Vedolizumab as induction and maintenance therapy for Crohn's disease. N Engl J Med. 2013;369:711–21.

95. Feagan BG, Rutgeerts P, Sands BE, et al. Vedolizumab as induction and maintenance therapy for ulcerative colitis. N Engl J Med. 2013;369:699–710.

96. Lichtiger S, Present DH. Preliminary report: cyclosporine in treatment of severe active ulcerative colitis. Lancet. 1990;336:16–9.

97. Lichtiger S, Present DH, Kornbluth A, et al. Cyclosporine in severe ulcerative colitis refractory to steroid therapy. N Engl J Med. 1994;330:1841–5.

98. Actis GC, Ottobrelli A, Pera A, et al. Continuously infused cyclosporine at low dose is sufficient to avoid emergency colectomy in acute attacks of ulcerative colitis without the need for high-dose steroids. J Clin Gastroenterol. 1993;17:10–3.

99. van Assche G, D'Haens G, Noman M, et al. Randomized, double-blind comparison of 4 mg/kg versus 2 mg/kg intravenous cyclosporine in severe ulcerative colitis. Gastroenterology. 2003;125: 1025–31.

100. Laharie D, Bourreille A, Branche J, et al. Cyclosporin versus infliximab in severe acute ulcerative colitis refractory to intravenous steroids: a randomized trial. Presented at Digestive Disease Week; May 7–10, 2011; Chicago, IL, Abstract 619.

101. Laharie D, Bourreille A, Branche J, et al. Cyclosporin versus infliximab in patients with severe ulcerative colitis refractory to intravenous steroids: a parallel, open-label randomized controlled. Lancet. 2012;380:1909–15.

102. Arts J, D'Haens G, Zeegers M, et al. Long-term outcome of treatment with intravenous cyclosporin in patients with severe ulcerative colitis. Inflamm Bowel Dis. 2004;10:73–8.

# Potential Conflict of Interest Declaration

| | |
|---|---|
| Abbott Corporation/Abbvie | Consultant |
| Actavis | Consultant |
| Alaven | Consultant |
| Clinical Advances in Gastroenterology | Editor (Honorarium) |
| Ferring | Consultant, Research |
| Gastroenterology and Hepatology | Editor (Honorarium) |
| Hospira | Consultant |
| Ironwood | Honorarium (CME Program) |
| Janssen Orthobiotech | Consultant, Research |
| Luitpold / American Regent | Consulting, Honorarium (CME Program) |
| Pfizer Pharmaceuticals | Consultant |
| Prometheus Laboratories, Inc. | Consultant, Research |
| Salix Pharmaceuticals | Consultant, Research |
| Santarus | Consultant, Research |
| Shire Pharmaceuticals | Consultant, Research |
| SLACK, Inc | Book Royalty |
| Takeda | Consultant |
| UCB | Consultant, Research |
| Warner Chilcotte | Consultant, Research, Grant |

G.R. Lichtenstein (ed.), *Medical Therapy of Ulcerative Colitis*,
DOI 10.1007/978-1-4939-1677-1, © Springer Science+Business Media New York 2014

# Index

## A

Abatacept, 201–202
Acetaminophen, 324
Active ulcerative colitis trials (ACT)
  clinical response, clinical remission, and mucosal healing, 177
  endoscopic response, 178–179
  hospitalization, colectomy, quality of life, and adverse events, 177–178
Activity Index (AI), 33
Acupuncture, 226–227
Acute kidney injury (AKI), 305
Acute pouchitis. *See* Pouchitis
Adalimumab (ADA), 50, 286
  efficacy, 185–186
  high-intensity therapy, 463
  *vs.* IFX and GLM, 187
  ULTRA1 trial, 186
  ULTRA2 trial, 186–187
Adherence medication, 329
AJM300, 199
Alicaforsen, 199–200
Alkaline phosphatase, 228–229
Allopurinol, 373
Aloe vera, 224
American College of Gastroenterology (ACG), 302
AMG 181, 198
Aminosalicylates, 49, 321–322
  infection, 297
  malignancy, 297–298
  remission
    oral aminosalicylates, 419, 420
    sulfasalazine, 418–419
    topical 5-ASA, 419–420
  renal injury, 298
5-Aminosalicylic acid (5-ASA), 35–36
  colorectal cancer, 292–293
  DILI, 448–449
  kidney injury, 298
  maintenance therapy, 263
  mimic, 401
  moderate intensity therapy, 461
  nonresponders, 260–261, 263–264
  oral therapy, 260
  pouchitis, 372
  rectal 5-ASA
    dosage, 259
    *vs.* oral 5-ASA, 258–259
    *vs.* placebo, 256
    *vs.* rectal corticosteroids, 257–258
    rectal formulations, 260
  systemic, 461
  topical therapy, 256, 461
  ulcerative proctitis, treatment of, 251–252
*Andrographis paniculata*, 204, 226
Anemia, 385–386
Antibiotics, 238
  pediatrics, 283
  role of, 209, 214
  ulcerative colitis, management of
    ciprofloxacin, 215, 216
    clinical trials, 216
    metronidazole, 214–215
    rifaximin, 215
Antidiarrheal therapy, 360
Antimetabolite therapy. *See* Methotrexate; Thiopurines
Antinuclear cytoplasmic antibody (ANCA), 440–441
Antispasmodics, 434
Anti-tumor necrosis factor (Anti-TNF), 323
  BPCI Act, 193
  chemoprevention, 294
  colorectal cancer, 294
  DILI, 449
  golimumab, 191–193
  remission
    adalimumab, 422
    golimumab, 422–423
    infliximab, 421–422
    vedolizumab, 423
Aphthous stomatitis, 381
Appendectomy, 245
Apriso®, 59, 61, 89
Arsenic (acetarsol), 230
Asacol®, 59, 61–63, 73, 81, 89
*Aspergillus fumigatus*, 305
Autoimmune hepatitis (AIH) overlap, 447
Autoimmune pouchopathy, 369
Azathioprine (AZA), 49, 252, 322–323. *See also* Thiopurines
  colorectal cancer, 293
  PSC, 444
  steroid-dependent ulcerative colitis, 313–314, 316

## B

Balsalazide, 57, 58, 63, 64, 81
Basiliximab, 195
Beclomethasone dipropionate (BDP)
  *vs.* 5-ASA, 126–127
  efficacy, 126
  enema, 126
Beclomethasone propionate enema, 105
Beta-tubulin isotype 5 (TTB-5), 441
Biliary epithelial cell (BEC), 441

Made in the USA
Monee, IL
25 August 2025

24181636R10273